Principles and Practice of Emergency Research Response

Editor-in-Chief Elizabeth S. Higgs
Managing Editor Robert A. Sorenson

Section Editors:
Mosoka P. Fallah
Nicole Lurie
Laura A. McNay
Peter G. Smith

Springer

Editor-in-Chief
Elizabeth S. Higgs
Division of Clinical Research
U.S. National Institute of Allergy and Infectious Diseases
National Institutes of Health
Rockville, MD, USA

Managing Editor
Robert A. Sorenson
Division of Clinical Research
U.S. National Institute of Allergy and Infectious Diseases
National Institutes of Health
Rockville, MD, USA

Section Editors
Mosoka P. Fallah
Directorate of Science and Innovation
Africa Centres for Disease Control and Prevention
Addis Ababa, Ethiopia

Nicole Lurie
Coalition for Epidemic Preparedness Innovations
Washington, DC, USA

Laura A. McNay
Operations and Management Branch
Division of Clinical Research
U.S. National Institute of Allergy and Infectious Diseases
National Institutes of Health
Rockville, MD, USA

Peter G. Smith
MRC International Statistics and Epidemiology Group
London School of Hygiene & Tropical Medicine
London, UK

This book is an open access publication.
ISBN 978-3-031-48407-0 ISBN 978-3-031-48408-7 (eBook)
https://doi.org/10.1007/978-3-031-48408-7

National Institute of Allergy and Infectious Diseases

Principles and Practice of Emergency Research Response has been funded in part with federal funds from the National Institutes of Health. The content of this publication does not necessarily reflect the views or policies of the NIH, the Department of Health and Human Services, or any other part of the U.S. Government, nor does mention of trade names, commercial products, or organizations imply endorsement by the U.S. Government.

This Springer imprint is published by the registered company Springer Nature Switzerland AG
The registered company address is: Gewerbestrasse 11, 6330 Cham, Switzerland

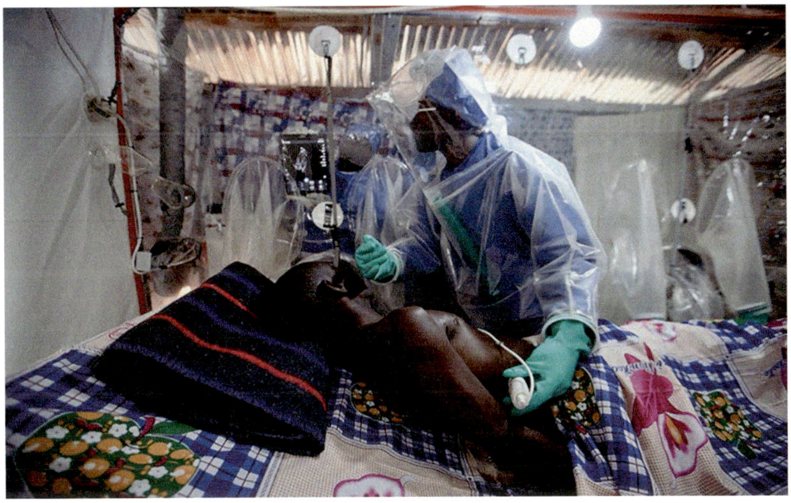

Dr. Richard Kojan, President of the Dakar-based Alliance for International Medical Action (ALIMA), performs a diagnostic ultrasound on an Ebola virus disease patient in the Democratic Republic of the Congo. This ALIMA Ebola Treatment Center (ETC) uses the CUBE modules ALIMA developed after the 2014–2016 Ebola outbreak in West Africa. The CUBE ensures infection control while allowing easier contact between patients and physicians, as well as the patients' families and friends. Previous ETC designs had cut patients off from the outside world and required medical care personnel to don hot, bulky personal protective equipment to provide close-in care. Clinical research and patient care complemented each other at the center shown and contributed to licensure of two Ebola therapeutic agents (see "In Practice," ▶ 17.1 and ▶ 40.1). (Photo: Ghinwa Daher/ALIMA)

Dedicated to all who have lost their lives to emerging and re-emerging infectious diseases.

Foreword

My interest in infectious diseases began one morning in 1997. I picked up a copy of the *New York Times*, and right there—on page A1—was an article that caught my attention. It was about diarrhea killing 3.1 million people every year, and almost all were young kids who lived in low-income countries in Africa and South Asia.

My eldest daughter, Jennifer, had recently been born. I couldn't believe that so many babies like her were dying of something treatable. I needed to know why, so I dove head-first into the subject of public health, reading dozens of textbooks like this one.

The more I read and spoke to experts, the more I understood why health outcomes differed so dramatically between high-income and low-income countries. In wealthy places, like where I lived in Seattle, diarrhea was mostly a minor inconvenience because we had access to basic treatments and vaccines. But those interventions weren't available in every country. In some places, everything was difficult to come by—not only vaccines for diarrhea-causing rotavirus, but also bed nets that prevent malaria and antiretrovirals for HIV/AIDS.

I wouldn't start studying pandemics in earnest for a few more years, but I suppose the writing was on the wall at that point: The world wasn't doing enough to fight the infectious diseases that had been around for centuries (or millennia)—*how could it be prepared for novel diseases that hadn't even appeared yet?*

After the Ebola outbreak of 2014, I outlined the gaps in the world's readiness for a pandemic, and eventually adapted that research into a TED talk. The title of the talk was "▶ The Next Epidemic? We're Not Ready." Unfortunately, most of the views on that video have been since the COVID-19 pandemic began—when it was already too late.

This is what happens in crises, whether they're longstanding ones like the rotavirus epidemic or more recent emergencies like COVID-19, people tend to react—if they react at all—only after the threat has materialized in wealthy countries. This approach is not sound at all, which is why I'm so enthusiastic that you've decided to study this book.

"Outbreaks are inevitable," the great epidemiologist Larry Brilliant once said, "but pandemics are optional." One day, another highly infectious, novel pathogen will emerge just as SARS-CoV-2 did in late 2019. That's inevitable, as Dr. Brilliant said, but the world can still stop a repeat of the COVID-19 pandemic so long as more people do exactly what you're doing right now—prepare. We need more people like you studying how to prevent pandemics before they happen.

Scientific research, the subject of this textbook, is especially crucial for pandemic preparedness.

SARS-CoV-2 has been an instructive adversary. It has thrown a spotlight on our R&D arsenal—informing us which innovations are highly effective at fighting pandemics, and which avenues of research need even more attention, like mRNA technology.

mRNA vaccines proved hugely effective against SARS-CoV-2, but they're temperature sensitive and need to be stored at around −70 °C following manufacture and can be at warmer temperatures for only a very short time before being administered. That cold chain is very difficult to maintain in rural and tropical areas and in places that lack the needed infrastructure. *Can researchers invent technologies that will help extend the cold chain to places where it didn't go before? Or can they develop mRNA vaccines that aren't so sensitive to temperature*? These are questions we need to answer.

We need to ask similar questions about immune protection. How do we give more people some level of immune protection more quickly? The COVID-19 vaccines were developed in record time. Yet it took a long time for manufacturing capacity to ramp up to provide enough doses for meaningful community protection.

I believe researchers must be on the frontlines of any outbreak. It is the only way we can effectively identify, track, and stop a novel disease when it enters the human population. One idea is a Global Health Emergency Corps that would act like an international firefighting battalion for infectious diseases, staffed by public health leaders and researchers like the ones you're training to become.

In fact, that may be the kind of career you're envisioning as you begin this textbook—hours spent in labs, studying viral genomes; designing vaccines and therapeutics to combat it; conducting clinical trials to ensure they are safe and effective; or on-the-ground in an outbreak hotspot, working with local partners to trace the spread of the pathogen and carry out clinical research before the outbreak turns into an pandemic. These are all important tasks, but I'd also argue that they aren't enough. If we are going to create a pandemic-free world, then researchers will have to do more. There are other equally important tasks that won't be in your formal job description.

COVID-19 taught us that stopping a pandemic requires more than just cutting-edge science. Leaders from different disciplines need to act in coordination—researchers and health workers, presidents and prime ministers, and the CEOs of pharmaceutical and logistics companies, among others. If one of the links in this network doesn't believe that pandemics are preventable (and it is worth spending the time and money to prevent them), then the whole enterprise fails.

As experts, you can be powerful advocates for public health and ambassadors for pandemic preparedness. You can credibly make the argument for why your work requires more funding and support. I often say that if we spend billions on work like yours, we can save trillions down the line. It is one of the wisest investments that we can make, but we need to remind people of that truth, over and over again.

I would also encourage you to always keep sight of the world's most vulnerable communities, who are often at the end of the line when it comes to receiving interventions that can help them fight epidemics. The next time a novel virus jumps into the human population, millions of lives may depend on that kind of advocacy. Not only that, but millions of lives can also be bettered when we apply the learnings gained from emergency responses to ongoing public health challenges—including the diarrheal diseases that brought me to this field so many years ago.

Thank you for your commitment to the field of pandemic preparedness and your willingness to learn even more through your coursework. Much of my life's work in technology and philanthropy has stemmed from a simple idea: Innovation can improve lives and solve important problems. The bedrock of innovation, and the foundation of a strong pandemic response, has always been scientific research.

With your passion and dedication to this work, I believe that COVID-19 can truly be humanity's last pandemic.

Bill Gates
Seattle, WA, USA
March 15, 2023

Preface

The need for principled, practical guidance on ethical, scientifically sound infectious disease research preparedness and research response is clearer than ever following the COVID-19 pandemic. Ironically, during the COVID-19 pandemic progress on this book on emergency infectious disease research, then based largely on the Ebola experience in West Africa, came to a halt. Nearly all the authors and editors, experts in various aspects of infectious disease research, devoted long hours to the pandemic emergency; many continue to work on COVID-19, mpox, or broader epidemic and pandemic issues. Although the magnitude of the COVID-19 research effort has been extraordinary, not all of it was optimally planned or executed, and much was unproductive. Better coordination of the research response is essential for future infectious disease outbreaks, epidemics, and/or the next Public Health Emergency of International Concern. *Principles and Practice of Emergency Response Research* elucidates standards, guidelines, and practical considerations to improve future research response. Much will depend on applying what we have learned from responses to past epidemics and pandemics, particularly over the last decade, to improve preparedness, including a willingness to leave unresolved issues between nations aside while humanity prepares to respond to future infectious disease threats. Collective political-scientific alliances committed to improved health security require focused improvements in global research systems, preparedness for response to known pathogens with pandemic potential, and rapid mobilization of resources to meet infectious disease emergencies as they arise. Nation states, international organizations, academia, NGOs, the private sector—all sectors of society—have lessons to learn and work to do. The principles and mechanisms for responding to potential pandemics, under negotiation in Geneva, New York, and national capitals as we go to press, need to be clarified to ensure a better response.

One premise of *Principles and Practice of Emergency Response Research*, based on recent ecological studies, is that outbreaks caused by pathogens new to humans are most likely to occur in countries where major changes in the wildlife-livestock-human interface occur near vulnerable human populations. As with SARS-CoV-2, the likelihood of new zoonotic infections first appearing in such a setting and the potential consequences remain high. The many response missteps seen in the most scientifically capable countries during the COVID-19 pandemic make a global effort to improve preparedness and response imperative. Hope of stopping such outbreaks early rests on there being sufficient local, national, and global capacity to rapidly mount a comprehensive response, including the development and deployment of safe, effective vaccines, therapeutics, and diagnostics (VTD). In the absence of already licensed or authorized VTDs, a prioritized research agenda for their development and evaluation must be integrated into disease outbreak response.

Many volumes analyzing the COVID-19 pandemic have already appeared or are in the pipeline. Building on the lessons learned from this and other major infectious disease outbreaks, we need to improve research response and preparedness now to have a better, more coordinated, and more rapid response to future infectious disease threats. This book, with many highly regarded, experienced research scientists and global health leaders among its authors, is one contribution to that effort. We hope to see it used in medical and public health schools to help train future generations of practitioners in the whys and wherefores of accelerated research response. We hope it buttresses the case that must be made in finance ministries for investment in health systems and research capacity. We hope to see it used in the field as a quick reference for implementing a research agenda. We believe the argument we had set out to make before the pandemic, that research can and must be part of infectious disease preparedness and response, hardly requires the evidence and argument we had originally planned, and we have therefore shifted our focus to how it must be done rather than why. Another major theme that runs through the book, often implicitly, is that meeting ethical and scientific standards is not only an imperative on its own terms, but a pragmatic necessity for successful emergency research response. Procedures may be accelerated and run in parallel rather than sequentially, but compliance with ethical and scientific standards is essential for research to produce reliable, actionable results.

Finally, while the COVID-19 pandemic has been devastating and we mourn its many victims, we must acknowledge that the lessons learned during the pandemic have made this volume better than it otherwise would have been. If our efforts are judged worthwhile and contribute to improving the response to the next pandemic, perhaps that can be counted among shreds of silver lining left behind by a pandemic that could be a harbinger of worse to come.

Elizabeth S. Higgs
Rockville, MD, USA

Robert A. Sorenson
Rockville, MD, USA

Mosoka P. Fallah
Addis Ababa, Ethiopia

Nicole Lurie
Washington, DC, USA

Laura A. McNay
Rockville, MD, USA

Peter G. Smith
London, UK
September 23, 2023

Learning Tracks: Fields of Study and Practice

Learning tracks are intended to help students, teachers, and practitioners find the material they need for formal and informal study using *Principles and Practice of Emergency Research Response* as best suits their interests, courses, and fields of practice. Reference information needs also benefit from electronic searches and, in both electronic and paper editions, the index and full tables of contents in each chapter. Note that there are also abundant cross-references from one chapter to another, hyperlinked in the electronic versions of the book, including the downloadable .pdf.

The learning tracks presented here may be used as suggestions for course syllabi or a program of self-study and are designed to allow the user to move easily from one portion of the book to others selected by the editors for their relevance to a field of study or practice.

Learning Tracks (Alphabetical Order)

1. Biostatistics
2. Clinical Research
3. Emergency Research Response, Research Operations
4. Global Health
5. Global Health Law
6. Health Policy, Multilateral Cooperation, International Governance
7. One Health
8. Preparedness
9. Public Health and Epidemiology
10. Research Ethics, Social Science Response Research
11. Social Science Research Response

Track	Academic courses or departments	Profession or practice	Suggested chapters	Selected sub-chapter headings (from chapters not listed at left)
Biostatistics	Biostatistics	Biostatisticians	► 4.1 In Practice: Vaccine Efficacy and Safety Testing—An Ethical Case for Individual Randomization	2.2 Evolution of Clinical Trial Methodology
			► 21.1 In Focus: The Impact and Mechanisms of Superspreading	
			► 22 Vaccine Trial Designs	
			► 22.1 In Focus: Ring Trial Design	
			► 23 Data and Safety Monitoring of Clinical Trials During Public Health Emergencies	
			► 23.1 In Practice: Monitoring the PALM Ebola Therapeutics Study in the Democratic Republic of the Congo	
			► 24 Mathematical Modeling for Emergency Response: Using Models to Inform and Direct Response Priorities and Shape the Research Agenda	
			► 25 Models in the COVID-19 Pandemic	
			► 25.1 Case Study: Modeling Fractional-Dose Emergency Vaccination Campaigns for Yellow Fever	

Clinical Research	Clinical research courses	Clinical research team practitioners at all levels	▶ 1 Introduction	
			▶ 2 Clinical Research on Infectious Diseases: An Overview	
			▶ 3 Guiding Principles for Emergency Research Response	
			▶ 4 Ethics of Pandemic Research	
			▶ 4.1 In Practice: Vaccine Efficacy and Safety Testing—An Ethical Case for Individual Randomization	
			▶ 5 Health Emergency Research amid Global Inequities: Some Considerations for Researchers	
			▶ 6 Meeting Regulatory Criteria and Seeking Licensure: Medicines Development Before and During Public Health Emergencies	
			▶ 7 Research, Sample, and Data Sharing During Outbreaks, Pandemics, and Beyond	
			▶ 9 Laboratory Needs for Research Response	
			▶ 12 Vaccine Candidates for Novel Pathogens	
			▶ 12.1 In Focus: Novel Manufacturing Platforms for Pandemic Preparedness and Emergency Response	

(continued)

Track	Academic courses or departments	Profession or practice	Suggested chapters	Selected sub-chapter headings (from chapters not listed at left)
			► 14 Accelerating Development of Therapeutics for Preparedness, Response, and a More Secure World	
			► 14.1 In Practice: RECOVERY Trial	
			► 15 ACTIV: A U.S. Public-Private Partnership Responds to COVID-19	
			► 15.1 In Practice: Leveraging an Integrated National Health System for Research Response—The UK National Institute for Health Research Respiratory Translational Research Collaboration	
			► 16 Challenges for Emergency Research Response and Preparedness in Fragile, Weak, and Failed Nation States	
			► 17 Integrating Clinical Research into Ebola Response: Liberia Case Study	
			► 17.1 In Practice: Integration of Clinical Research and Patient Care in the DRC PALM Ebola Therapeutics Trial	
			► 18 Good Participatory Practice: Social Mobilization, Communications, and Community Engagement	
			► 18.1 In Practice: Building Community Engagement for Clinical Research Response	
			► 18.2 In Practice: Adapting Social Analytics for Research Response	

			▶ 19 Understanding and Reporting the Natural History of an Infectious Disease	
			▶ 20 Turning Research Results into Clinical Practice Guidelines in Public Health Emergencies	
			▶ 22 Vaccine Trial Designs	
			▶ 22.1 In Focus: Ring Trial Design	
			▶ 23 Data and Safety Monitoring of Clinical Trials During Public Health Emergencies	
			▶ 24 Mathematical Modeling for Emergency Response: Using Models to Inform and Direct Response Priorities and Shape the Research Agenda	
			▶ 25 Models in the COVID-19 Pandemic	
			▶ 26 Social Science Evidence for Outbreak and Pandemic Response: Rapid Research and Analytics for Public Health Emergencies	
			▶ 30 Organizational Partnerships for Preparedness and Response to Emerging and Re-emerging Infectious Diseases	
			▶ 32 Launching a Clinical Research Operation	
			▶ 33 Ethical Review of Clinical Research During an Emergency Response	

(continued)

Track	Academic courses or departments	Profession or practice	Suggested chapters	Selected sub-chapter headings (from chapters not listed at left)
			► 35 Data Management in Emergency Response Research	
			► 36 Safety and Pharmacovigilance in Emergency Research Response	
			► 40 Selecting and Opening a Clinical Research Site in a Low-Resource Setting	
Emergency Research Response, Research Operations	MD, MPH, international development	Responsible officials and personnel—health ministries, development, defense, interior, government research institutes, NGOs	► 1 Introduction	2.3 Critical Ground Rules for Research Studies during Epidemics
			► 5 Health Emergency Research amid Global Inequities: Some Considerations for Researchers	8.3 Investing in Research Infrastructure before an Outbreak
			► 8 Building Biomedical Research Capacity in Low- and Middle-Income Countries: Why It Matters and Some of the Barriers to Success	
			► 9 Laboratory Needs for Research Response	
			► 13 Accelerating Vaccine Development: The 100 Days Mission	
			► 16 Challenges for Emergency Research Response and Preparedness in Fragile, Weak, and Failed Nation States	

			▶ 17 Integrating Clinical Research into Ebola Response: Liberia Case Study	
			▶ 18 Good Participatory Practice: Social Mobilization, Communications, and Community Engagement	
			▶ 18.1 In Practice: Building Community Engagement for Clinical Research Response	
			▶ 18.2 In Practice: Adapting Social Analytics for Research Response	
			Part VII Operations	
Global Health	MPH, MD, International Relations, Political Science, International Development	Government, NGOs, international and multilateral organizations	▶ 1 Introduction	2.3 Critical Ground Rules for Research Studies During Epidemics
			▶ 3 Guiding Principles for Emergency Research Response	2.4.8 Recommendations to Improve Clinical Research and Trials During Public Health Emergencies
			▶ 4 Ethics of Pandemic Research	
			▶ 5 Health Emergency Research amid Global Inequities: Some Considerations for Researchers	
			▶ 18 Good Participatory Practice: Social Mobilization, Communications, and Community Engagement	

(continued)

Track	Academic courses or departments	Profession or practice	Suggested chapters	Selected sub-chapter headings (from chapters not listed at left)
			► 22 Vaccine Trial Designs Part VI Governance	
Global Health Law	JD	Emergency response legal advisors, clinical research PIs, administrators, sponsors, funders	► 3 Guiding Principles for Emergency Research Response	2.3 Critical Ground Rules for Research Studies During Epidemics
			► 4 Ethics of Pandemic Research	4.6 Research Governance, Coordination, and Oversight During Pandemics
			► 5 Health Emergency Research amid Global Inequities: Some Considerations for Researchers	9.3.3 Laboratory Regulatory and Legal Concerns
			► 27 A Global Framework for Research Preparedness and Response	
			► 32 Launching a Clinical Research Operation	
			► 32.2 In Focus: Clinical Trial Insurance and Indemnification	
Health Policy, Multilateral Cooperation, International Governance	MPH, MD, international relations, political science, international development	Responsible government officials and personnel—ministries of health, foreign affairs, defense, development agencies	► 1 Introduction	4.6 Research Governance, Coordination, and Oversight During Pandemics
			► 3 Guiding Principles for Emergency Research Response	

			▶ 6 Meeting Regulatory Criteria and Seeking Licensure: Medicines Development Before and During Public Health Emergencies	
			▶ 7 Research, Sample, and Data Sharing During Outbreaks, Pandemics, and Beyond	
			▶ 8 Building Biomedical Research Capacity in Low- and Middle-Income Countries: Why It Matters and Some of the Barriers to Success	
			▶ 10 Understanding How and Where Pathogens Emerge: Preparedness and Response for Zoonotic Diseases	
			▶ 13 Accelerating Vaccine Development: The 100 Days Mission	
			▶ 16 Challenges for Emergency Research Response and Preparedness in Fragile, Weak, and Failed Nation States	
			Part VI Governance	
One Health	Human and veterinary infectious diseases, molecular biology, ecology, wildlife ecology and biology	Biosurveillance, wildlife biologists, veterinarians, laboratories, Ministries of Health, agriculture, development, environment, forestry, parks	▶ 7 Research, Sample, and Data Sharing During Outbreaks, Pandemics, and Beyond	

(continued)

Track	Academic courses or departments	Profession or practice	Suggested chapters	Selected sub-chapter headings (from chapters not listed at left)
			▶ 8 Building Biomedical Research Capacity in Low- and Middle-Income Countries: Why It Matters and Some of the Barriers to Success	
			▶ 9 Laboratory Needs for Research Response	
			▶ 10 Understanding How and Where Pathogens Emerge: Preparedness and Response for Zoonotic Diseases	
			▶ 21 Epidemiologic Research in the Setting of Outbreak Response	
			▶ 21.1 In Focus: The Impact and Mechanisms of Superspreading	
Preparedness	MPH, MD, international development	Responsible officials and personnel—ministries of health, development, disaster response agencies	▶ 1 Introduction	
			▶ 2 Clinical Research on Infectious Diseases: An Overview	
			▶ 8 Building Biomedical Research Capacity in Low- and Middle-Income Countries: Why It Matters and Some of the Barriers to Success	
			▶ 11 Accelerating Diagnostic Innovation for Pandemic Control	
			▶ 12 Vaccine Candidates for Novel Pathogens	

			► 12.1 In Focus: Novel Manufacturing Platforms for Pandemic Preparedness and Emergency Response	
			► 13 Accelerating Vaccine Development: The 100 Days Mission	
			► 14 Accelerating Development of Therapeutics for Preparedness, Response, and a More Secure World	
			► 16 Challenges for Emergency Research Response and Preparedness in Fragile, Weak, and Failed Nation States	
			► 18 Good Participatory Practice: Social Mobilization, Communications, and Community Engagement	
			► 18.1 In Practice: Building Community Engagement for Clinical Research Response	
			► 21 Epidemiologic Research in the Setting of Outbreak Response	
			► 21.1 In Focus: The Impact and Mechanisms of Superspreading	
			► 22 Vaccine Trial Designs	
			► 26 Social Science Evidence for Outbreak and Pandemic Response: Rapid Research and Analytics for Public Health Emergencies	

(continued)

Track	Academic courses or departments	Profession or practice	Suggested chapters	Selected sub-chapter headings (from chapters not listed at left)
			▶ 30 Organizational Partnerships for Preparedness and Response to Emerging and Re-emerging Infectious Diseases	
			▶ 30.1 In Focus: Research and Medical Humanitarian NGOs	
			▶ 32 Launching a Clinical Research Operation	
Public Health and Epidemiology	MPH, MD, anthropology, sociology	CDC, USPHS, NGOs	▶ 1 Introduction	
			▶ 2 Clinical Research on Infectious Diseases: An Overview	
			▶ 3 Guiding Principles for Emergency Research Response	
			▶ 4 Ethics of Pandemic Research	
			▶ 4.1 In Practice: Vaccine Efficacy and Safety Testing—An Ethical Case for Individual Randomization	
			▶ 5 Health Emergency Research amid Global Inequities: Some Considerations for Researchers	
			▶ 8 Building Biomedical Research Capacity in Low- and Middle-Income Countries: Why It Matters and Some of the Barriers to Success	
			▶ 10 Understanding How and Where Pathogens Emerge: Preparedness and Response for Zoonotic Diseases	

			▶ 18 Good Participatory Practice: Social Mobilization, Communications, and Community Engagement	
			▶ 18.1 In Practice: Building Community Engagement for Clinical Research Response	
			▶ 18.2 In Practice: Adapting Social Analytics for Research Response	
			▶ 21 Epidemiologic Research in the Setting of Outbreak Response	
			▶ 21.1 In Focus: The Impact and Mechanisms of Superspreading	
			▶ 22 Vaccine Trial Designs	
			▶ 23 Data and Safety Monitoring of Clinical Trials During Public Health Emergencies	
Research Ethics	MD, MPH, philosophy, anthropology, sociology	IRBs (RECs), clinical research practitioners, ethicists	▶ 1 Introduction	2.4 Lessons from Emergency Clinical Research
			▶ 3 Guiding Principles for Emergency Research Response	
			▶ 4 Ethics of Pandemic Research	
			▶ 4.1 In Practice: Vaccine Efficacy and Safety Testing—An Ethical Case for Individual Randomization	

(continued)

Track	Academic courses or departments	Profession or practice	Suggested chapters	Selected sub-chapter headings (from chapters not listed at left)
			▶ 4.2 In Practice: Research Ethics Committee Review in Public Health Emergencies	
			▶ 5 Health Emergency Research amid Global Inequities: Some Considerations for Researchers	
			▶ 18 Good Participatory Practice: Social Mobilization, Communications, and Community Engagement	
			▶ 18.1 In Practice: Building Community Engagement for Clinical Research Response	
			▶ 18.2 In Practice: Adapting Social Analytics for Research Response	
			▶ 17 Integrating Clinical Research into Ebola Response: Liberia Case Study	
			▶ 17.1 In Practice: Integration of Clinical Research and Patient Care in the DRC PALM Ebola Therapeutics Trial	
			▶ 26 Social Science Evidence for Outbreak and Pandemic Response: Rapid Research and Analytics for Public Health Emergencies	
			▶ 32 Launching a Clinical Research Operation	
			▶ 33 Ethical Review of Clinical Research During an Emergency Response	

			▶ 33.1 In Practice: Ethical Review During Emergencies: The Liberian Experience	
			▶ 33.2 In Practice: Independent Monitoring of Emergency Response Clinical Trials	
			▶ 33.3 In Practice: Capacity Building for Research Ethics Review in Low- and Middle-Income Countries	
			▶ 40 Selecting and Opening a Clinical Research Site in a Low-Resource Setting	
			▶ 40.1 In Practice: Improving Patient Care in the Field: The CUBE Isolation Unit	
Social Science Response Research	MD, MPH, anthropology, economics, sociology	Clinical research practitioners, social scientists	▶ 1 Introduction	2.4 Lessons from Emergency Clinical Research
			▶ 3 Guiding Principles for Emergency Research Response	
			▶ 5 Health Emergency Research amid Global Inequities: Some Considerations for Researchers	
			▶ 8 Building Biomedical Research Capacity in Low- and Middle-Income Countries: Why It Matters and Some of the Barriers to Success	
			▶ 16 Challenges for Emergency Research Response and Preparedness in Fragile, Weak, and Failed Nation States	

(continued)

Track	Academic courses or departments	Profession or practice	Suggested chapters	Selected sub-chapter headings (from chapters not listed at left)
			▶ 16.1 In Practice: Responding to an Infectious Disease Outbreak amid a Humanitarian Emergency	
			▶ 18 Good Participatory Practice: Social Mobilization, Communications, and Community Engagement	
			▶ 18.1 In Practice: Building Community Engagement for Clinical Research Response	
			▶ 18.2 In Practice: Adapting Social Analytics for Research Response	
			▶ 17 Integrating Clinical Research into Ebola Response: Liberia Case Study	
			▶ 17.1 In Practice: Integration of Clinical Research and Patient Care in the DRC PALM Ebola Therapeutics Trial	
			▶ 26 Social Science Evidence for Outbreak and Pandemic Response: Rapid Research and Analytics for Public Health Emergencies	
			▶ 33.3 In Practice: Capacity Building for Research Ethics Review in Low- and Middle-Income Countries	
			▶ 40 Selecting and Opening a Clinical Research Site in a Low-Resource Setting	
			▶ 40.1 In Practice: Improving Patient Care in the Field: The CUBE Isolation Unit	

Acknowledgments

There are many people whose help in preparing this volume for publication was invaluable, but whose names do not appear elsewhere in the book. The support of Cliff Lane, the Deputy Director for Clinical Research and Special Projects at the National Institute of Allergy and Infectious Diseases (NIAID), was essential throughout. Our editor at Springer, Alison Ball, stuck with us through the vagaries of the pandemic and many changes of plan. Linda Coe and Gelu Dobrescu were irreplaceable members of the editorial team preparing the book for publication. Bruce Agnew, Lori Dodd, Yolanda Jones, Gregg Larson, Yin Li, and Rob Taylor also contributed invaluable editorial work and advice during various phases of a long endeavor. Wade Green provided legal counsel, and Susan Yi, Tamara McDermott, and Sharon Gordon Smith helped get financing through federal procurement rules. Lizanne Selthoffer provided essential help and advice on personnel and financial matters.

NIAID employs many of the authors and provided funding to make the online version of this book open access.

Contents

III Preparedness for Emergency Research Response

IV Research Response

V Methodology for Research Response

VI Governance, Institutions, and Partnerships

VII Research Operations

Editors and Contributors

About the Editors

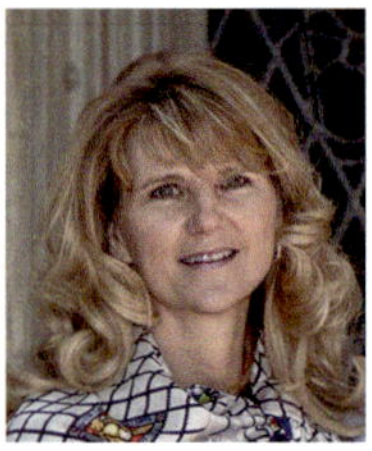

Elizabeth S. Higgs, MD, MIA, DTMH

is a clinical scientist, and pandemic preparedness research response policy expert working in the Division of Clinical Research at the U.S. National Institute of Allergy and Infectious Diseases (NIAID), National Institutes of Health (NIH). Throughout her career, Dr. Higgs has contributed to critical health emergencies, including H1N1, Ebola outbreaks in West Africa and the DRC, the 2018 Nipah outbreak in Kerala, India, mpox, and SARS-CoV-2, demonstrating that regulatory-level clinical trials during health emergencies are possible and contribute to medical countermeasures that accelerate the end of outbreaks.

Known for global health diplomacy while fostering interagency and multilateral collaborations, she actively engages in strategic global health security initiatives and policy groups, making impactful contributions to key policy documents such as the World Bank's *Money and Microbes*, the G7 Clinical Trials Charter, and the U.S. National Biosecurity Strategy and Global Health Security Strategy.

Her passions include nurturing sustainable clinical research capacity in low- and middle-income countries and promoting cooperative global clinical trial networks. With a foundation in internal medicine and infectious diseases, Dr. Higgs holds a doctorate in medicine, a master's degree in international affairs, an interdisciplinary bachelor's degree in bioethics, and a Diploma in Tropical Medicine and Hygiene. Through her commitment to response research, she is dedicated to safeguarding and enhancing the well-being of people worldwide in the face of health emergencies caused by emerging infectious disease.

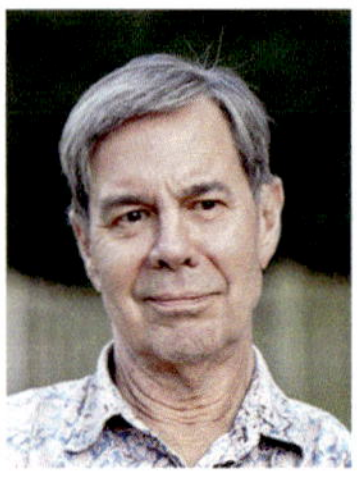

Robert A. Sorenson, MA

has worked with the NIAID Division of Clinical Research on infectious disease emergency response policy, especially urgent clinical research response to emerging pathogens, since 2016, after having worked on global health policy issues at the U.S. Department of State since 2009.

Mr. Sorenson was a Foreign Service and Civil Service Officer at State for 33 years. After 2001, when family circumstances curtailed his overseas career, he primarily served in the Bureau of Oceans, Environment, and Science, including terms as Deputy Director of the Offices of International Health and Biodefense, Environmental Policy, and Ecology and Terrestrial Conservation. His overseas experience, starting in 1986, included political, consular, environmental, and deputy chief of mission positions in Manila, Moscow, Osaka, Skopje, Tashkent, and Tirana, as well as several temporary duty assignments in crisis spots. He retired from State on New Year's Eve, 2017 and has since been a contractor with the NIAID Division of Clinical Research (DCR).

As managing editor of PPERR, Mr. Sorenson revived and updated his professional editorial experience, which dated to 1981–1986. He was a National Fellow at the Hoover Institution in 1999–2000 and has an MA in Russian literature from Cornell University and a BA from St. Olaf College.

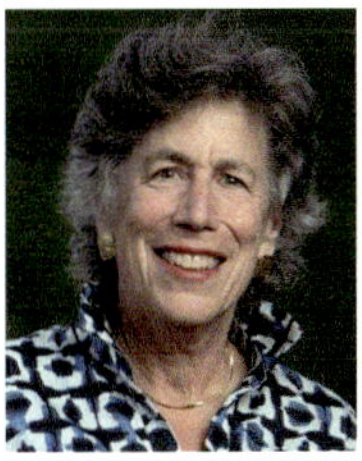

Nicole Lurie, MD, MSPH

is Executive Director for Preparedness and Response at the Coalition for Epidemic Preparedness Innovations (CEPI) and Director of CEPI-USA. She is also a Senior Lecturer at Harvard Medical School and Professor of Medicine at George Washington University School of Medicine.

She served an 8-year term as Assistant Secretary for Preparedness and Response at the U.S. Department of Health and Human Services (DHHS) from 2009 to 2017. In that role she led the HHS response to numerous public health emergencies, ranging from infectious disease to natural and man-made disasters, and is responsible for many innovations in emergency preparedness and response.

Prior to federal service, she was the Paul O'Neill Professor of Policy Analysis at RAND, and a Professor of Medicine and Public Health at the University of Minnesota. Her research has spanned access to and quality of care, health system redesign, health equity, mental health, public health, and preparedness. She is the recipient of numerous awards and is a member of the National Academy of Medicine. She continues to practice medicine in a community clinic in Washington DC.

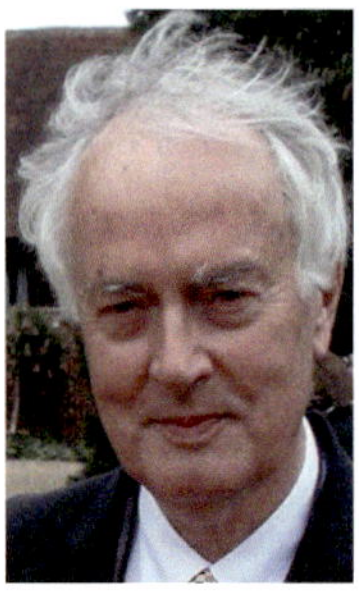

Peter G. Smith, CBE, DSc, FMedSci
is Professor of Tropical Epidemiology at the London School of Hygiene & Tropical Medicine (LSHTM).

He graduated in mathematics and statistics from City University, London, and in 1965 joined the Medical Research Council's Statistical Research Unit in London. Since then, he has worked on various aspects of epidemiological and statistical research based in Edinburgh, Kampala, Oxford, Boston, and Geneva. He joined LSHTM in 1979 to head the MRC International Statistics and Epidemiology Group. Research interests include large-scale intervention studies against tropical diseases, recently focusing on vaccines.

From 1999 to 2004 Dr. Smith chaired the UK Government Spongiform Encephalopathy Advisory Committee. He has chaired the WHO Global Advisory Committee on Vaccine Safety and the WHO Technical Expert Group on the RTS,S/AS01 malaria vaccine. He served as the Deputy Chair of the Nuffield Council on Bioethics and from 2004 to 2014 was a Governor of the Wellcome Trust. He has served on the Scientific Advisory Committees of the CEPI and the European and Developing Countries Clinical Trials Partnership (EDCTP). He chairs the WHO SAGE Working Group on malaria vaccines and serves on the WHO SAGE Working Group on SARS-CoV-2 vaccines.

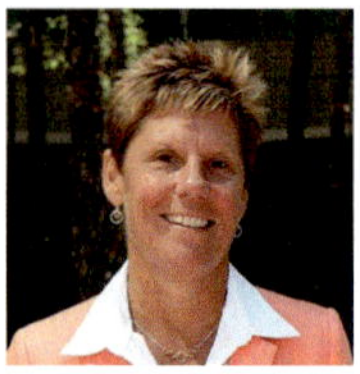

Laura A. McNay, MS
is the Deputy Director for Operations and Management in the Division of Clinical Research NIAID. She started her career at NIAID in 1991 and has served in many roles at NIAID over the past 32 years. During Ms. McNay's tenure with DCR, she has been responsible for the management and oversight of numerous small and large multinational clinical trials.

In addition to her role as DCR Deputy Director for Operations and Management, she serves as the DCR Project Lead for the Partnership for Research on Vaccines and Infectious Diseases in Liberia (PREVAIL). PREVAIL is a clinical research partnership between the U.S. Department of Health and Human Services and the Liberian Ministry of Health.

Ms. McNay attended the University of Maryland Baltimore County where she received her bachelor's degree in economics in 1987. In 2002, she received her Master of Science in Management and Healthcare Administration.

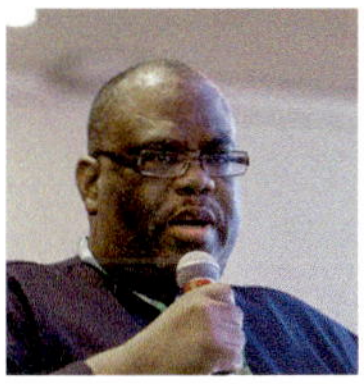

Mosoka P. Fallah, PhD, MPH, MA
is Acting Director of the Directorate of Science and Innovation, Africa Centres for Disease Control and Prevention and a visiting Lecturer in Global Health & Social Medicine, Harvard Medical School. Dr. Fallah completed his PhD in Immunology at the University of Kentucky and his MPH in Global Health/Infectious Disease Epidemiology at the Harvard T.H. Chan School of Public Health. For his work building community-level trust in the Ebola response, Dr. Fallah was named one of the Time Magazine Persons of the Year in 2014.

Dr. Fallah was also the co-founder and Director General of the National Public Health Institute of Liberia (NPHIL), which was founded in response to the devastation of the 2014–2016 Ebola outbreak in Liberia. He has also held positions as a health security technical consultant on pandemic diagnostics with the World Bank and senior consulting scientist at Medical Science & Computing, LLC. He continues to serve as President and CEO of Refuge Place International (RPI), a non-governmental organization dedicated to creating a replicable health care model for economically poor and disenfranchised people residing in the urban slums and poor rural communities of Liberia.

Contributors

Aishani Aatresh Harvard University, Cambridge, MA, USA

Jamila Aboulhab, MD Collaborative Clinical Research Branch, Division of Clinical Research, National Institute of Allergy and Infectious Diseases, Rockville, MD, USA

Sara Albert, MPH Clinical Monitoring Research Program Directorate, Frederick National Laboratory for Cancer Research, Frederick, MD, USA

Michele Andrasik, PhD, MSc, EdM, MA Social & Behavioral Sciences and Community Engagement, HIV Vaccine Trials Network, Vaccine and Infectious Disease Division, Fred Hutchinson Cancer Center, Seattle, WA, USA

Department of Global Health, University of Washington, Seattle, WA, USA

Julienne Ngoundoung Anoko, PhD RCCE/Social Sciences, EPR/EMP, WHO Regional Office for Africa, Brazzaville, Congo

Negin Atri, DrPH, MPH, BSc Division of Clinical Research, National Institute of Allergy and Infectious Diseases, Rockville, MD, USA

Moses Badio, MSc, BSc Partnership for Research on Ebola Virus in Liberia, Monrovia, Liberia

Kagisho Baepanye, MPH Hutchinson Centre Research Institute of South Africa, Johannesburg, South Africa

Marc Baguelin, PhD, MSc MRC Centre for Global Infectious Disease Analysis, Jameel Institute, School of Public Health, Imperial College London, London, UK

Sulzhan Bali, PhD, MSc Washington, DC, USA

Kenneth Ballie, BSc(Hons) MBChB PhD FRCA FRCP ISARIC (International Severe Acute Respiratory and Emerging Infection Consortium), University of Edinburgh, Edinburgh, UK

Emmanuel Baron, MD, MSc Epicentre, Paris, France

Kevin Barrett, RN, BScN International Clinical Research and Operations Branch, Division of Clinical Research, National Institute of Allergy and Infectious Diseases, Rockville, MD, USA

Beth Baseler, MSc, BSc Clinical Monitoring Research Program Directorate, Frederick National Laboratory for Cancer Research, Frederick, MD, USA

Nahid Bhadelia, MD, MALD Boston University Center on Emerging Infectious Diseases, Boston University, Boston, MA, USA

Section of Infectious Diseases, Boston University School of Medicine, Boston, MA, USA

Karin Bok, PhD, MSc Vaccine Research Center, National Institute of Allergy and Infectious Diseases, National Institutes of Health, Bethesda, MD, USA

Fatorma Bolay, PhD Liberian Institute of Biomedical Research, Monrovia, Liberia

Gail Broder, MSH Vaccine and Infectious Disease Division, Fred Hutchinson Cancer Center, Seattle, WA, USA

Kelly Cahill, RN, MSc, CCRC, RAC International Clinical Research and Operations Branch, Division of Clinical Research, National Institute of Allergy and Infectious Diseases, Rockville, MD, USA

Gail Carson, MD, MB ChB, MRCP International Severe Acute Respiratory and Emerging Infection Consortium (ISARIC), Global Outbreak Alert and Response Network (GOARN), Nuffield Department of Medicine, University of Oxford, Oxford, UK

Simone Carter, MSc Social Sciences Analytics Cell, UNICEF, Kinshasa, Congo

Marco Cavaleri, PhD European Medicines Agency, Amsterdam, The Netherlands

Patrick F. Chinnery, BMedSci, MBBS, PhD, MA, DSc MRC Mitochondrial Biology Unit, University of Cambridge, Cambridge, UK

Andrew Clements, PhD Office of Infectious Diseases, Emerging Threats Division, Bureau for Global Health, United States Agency for International Development, Washington, DC, USA

Francis S. Collins, MD, PhD National Institutes of Health, Bethesda, MD, USA

Ian Crozier, MD Clinical Monitoring Research Program Directorate, Frederick National Laboratory for Cancer Research, Frederick, MD, USA

David Cyprian, BA RootWise, LLC, Washington, DC, USA

Mimi Darko, BPharm, MBA Ghana Food and Drugs Authority, Accra, Ghana

Natalie E. Dean, PhD Department of Biostatistics & Bioinformatics, Rollins School of Public Health, Emory University, Atlanta, GA, USA

Jason T. DeBoer, BA Department of Pathology, Walter Reed National Military Medical Center, Bethesda, MD, USA

Yvette Delph, MBBS, DA Axle Informatics, Division of Clinical Research [C], National Institute of Allergy and Infectious Diseases, National Institutes of Health, Rockville, MD, USA

David L. DeMets, PhD Department of Biostatistics and Medical Informatics, School of Medicine and Public Health, University of Wisconsin Madison, Madison, WI, USA

Lennie Derde, MD, PhD, MSc European Clinical Research Alliance on Infectious Diseases, Randomised, Embedded, Multi-factorial, Adaptive Platform Trial for Community-Acquired Pneumonia (ReMAP-CAP), University Medical Center Utrecht, Utrecht, The Netherlands

Jestina Doe-Anderson, PhD Leidos Biomedical Research, Inc., The Clinical Monitoring Research Program Directorate, Frederick National Laboratory for Cancer Research, Frederick, MD, USA

Laurie K. Doepel, BA Division of Clinical Research, National Institute for Allergy and Infectious Diseases (ret.), Rockville, MD, USA

Nir Eyal, DPhil, MA Department of Philosophy, Center for Population-Level Bioethics, Rutgers University, New Brunswick, NJ, USA

Department of Health Behavior, Society & Policy, Rutgers School of Public Health, New Brunswick, NJ, USA

Mosoka P. Fallah, PhD, MPH, MA Directorate of Science and Innovation, Africa Centres for Disease Control and Prevention, Addis Ababa, Ethiopia

Global Health & Social Medicine, Harvard Medical School, Boston, MA, USA

Saving Lives and Livelihoods Initiative, Africa Centres for Disease Control and Prevention, Addis Ababa, Ethiopia

Refuge Place International, Monrovia, Liberia

Anthony S. Fauci, MD Georgetown University School of Medicine and the McCourt School of Public Policy, Georgetown University, Washington, DC, USA

National Institute of Allergy and Infectious Diseases, U.S. National Institutes of Health, Bethesda, MD, USA

Neil M. Ferguson, PhD, OBE FMedSci MRC Centre for Global Infectious Disease Analysis, Jameel Institute, School of Public Health, White City Campus, Imperial College London, London, UK

Mike Galcik, MSc Leidos Biomedical Research, Inc., Clinical Monitoring Research Program Directorate, Frederick National Laboratory for Cancer Research, Office of Clinical Research Policy and Regulatory Operations, National Institute of Allergy and Infectious Diseases, Frederick, MD, USA

Rogerio Gaspar, PhD, BPharm Department of Regulation and Prequalification, World Health Organization, Geneva, Switzerland

Nikki Gettinger, MPH, BSc Pamoja Tulinde Maisha (PALM), Leidos Biomedical Research, Inc., Frederick, MD, USA

Tedros Adhanom Ghebreyesus, PhD, MSc World Health Organization, Geneva, Switzerland

C. Taylor Gilliland, PhD National Institute of Biomedical Imaging and Bioengineering, National Institutes of Health, Bethesda, MD, USA

Nina Gobat, PhD Nuffield Department of Primary Care Health Sciences, University of Oxford, Oxford, UK

Rebecca F. Grais, PhD, MSc Epicentre, Paris, France

Dirceu Greco, MD, PhD Department of Internal Medicine and Infectious Diseases, School of Medicine, Federal University of Minas Gerais, Belo Horizonte, Brazil

Bradford Greening Jr, PhD Health Economics and Modeling Unit, Division of Preparedness and Emerging Infections, National Center for Emerging and Zoonotic Infectious Diseases, U.S. Centers for Disease Control and Prevention, Atlanta, GA, USA

Marion Gruber, PhD, MSc International AIDS Vaccine Initiative, New York, NY, USA

Louis Grue, RN, BSN Collaborative Clinical Research Branch, Division of Clinical Research, National Institute of Allergy and Infectious Diseases, Rockville, MD, USA

Birgit Grund, PhD School of Statistics, University of Minnesota, Minneapolis, MN, USA

Carol Han, MSc, BA Bureau for Humanitarian Assistance, U.S. Agency for International Development, Washington, DC, USA

Rachel Harrigan, MD Division of Clinical Research, National Institute of Allergy and Infectious Diseases, Rockville, MD, USA

Richard Hatchett, MD Coalition for Epidemic Preparedness Innovations, London, UK

William Heetderks, MD, PhD National Institute of Biomedical Imaging and Bioengineering, National Institutes of Health, Bethesda, MD, USA

Lisa E. Hensley, PhD, MSPH, MHS National Bio and Agro-Defense Facility, USDA Agricultural Research Service (ARS), Manhattan, KS, USA

Elizabeth S. Higgs, MD, MIA, DTMH Division of Clinical Research, U.S. National Institute of Allergy and Infectious Diseases, National Institutes of Health, Rockville, MD, USA

Peter Horby, PhD, MBBS Nuffield Department of Medicine, University of Oxford, Oxford, UK

Natsuko Imai, PhD, MSc MRC Centre for Global Infectious Disease Analysis, Jameel Institute, School of Public Health, White City Campus, Imperial College London, London, UK

Donna M. Jacobsen, BSc International Antiviral Society-USA, San Francisco, CA, USA

Melvin Johnson, RN, BScN, MSc Partnership for Research on Vaccines and Infectious Diseases in Liberia (PREVAIL), Monrovia, Liberia

Krishna Juluru, MD National Institute of Biomedical Imaging and Bioengineering, National Institutes of Health, Bethesda, MD, USA

Rebecca Kahn, PhD, MSc Center for Communicable Disease Dynamics, Department of Epidemiology, Harvard T.H. Chan School of Public Health, Boston, MA, USA

Luciana Kamel, MSc Vaccine and Infectious Disease Division, Fred Hutchinson Cancer Center, Seattle, WA, USA

Muhammad Karyana, MD, MPH Health Policy Agency, Ministry of Health of Indonesia, Jakarta, Indonesia

Rebecca Katz, PhD, MPH Center for Global Health Science and Security, Georgetown University Medical Center, School of Foreign Service, Georgetown University, Washington, DC, USA

Gerald T. Keusch, MD Boston University Schools of Medicine and Public Health, National Emerging Infectious Diseases Laboratory Institute, Boston University, Boston, MA, USA

Hassan Kiawu, MA Advanced Academic Programs, Johns Hopkins University, Baltimore, MD, USA

Matthew Carl Kirchoff, PharmD, MS, MBA U.S. Public Health Service, Rockville, MD, USA

Anthony Kirilusha, PhD, MSc National Institute of Arthritis and Musculoskeletal and Skin Diseases, National Institutes of Health, Bethesda, MD, USA

John D. Klena, PhD, BSc Viral Special Pathogens Branch, Centers for Disease Control and Prevention, Atlanta, GA, USA

Katie J. Knapek, DVM, MS, MLS(ASCP), DACLAM National Bio and Agro-Defense Facility, USDA Agricultural Research Service, Manhattan, KS, USA

Richard Kojan, MD The Alliance for International Medical Action, Dakar, Senegal

Ruth Kutalek, PhD, MA Center for Public Health, Department of Social and Preventive Medicine, Medical University of Vienna, Vienna, Austria

Martin Landray, MD, PhD, FRCP Nuffield Department of Population Health, University of Oxford, Oxford, UK

Gregg Larson, MA Leidos Biomedical Research, Inc., Minneapolis, MN, USA

University of Minnesota, Minneapolis, MN, USA

Tiffani B. Lash, PhD, BSc National Institute of Biomedical Imaging and Bioengineering, National Institutes of Health, Bethesda, MD, USA

Chuen-Yen Lau, MD, MS, MPH National Cancer Institute, National Institutes of Health, Rockville, MD, USA

Shelley Lees, PhD Anthropology of Public Health, London School of Hygiene and Tropical Medicine, London, UK

Nick R. Lemoine, MD, PhD, CBE, FRCPath, FMedSci CRUK Barts Centre, London, UK

NIHR Clinical Research Network, London, UK

Marc Lipsitch, PhD, MPH Center for Communicable Disease Dynamics, Harvard T.H. Chan School of Public Health, Cambridge, MA, USA

Department of Epidemiology, Harvard T.H. Chan School of Public Health, Cambridge, MA, USA

Department of Immunology and Infectious Diseases, Harvard T.H. Chan School of Public Health, Cambridge, MA, USA

Daniel J. Littlefield, MSc Modality Solutions LLC, Houston, TX, USA

Katherine Littler, BA(Hons), LLB, MA Health Ethics & Governance Unit on Ethics & COVID-19, World Health Organization, Geneva, Switzerland

Ira M. Longini Jr, PhD, MSc Department of Biostatistics, College of Public Health & Health Professions, College of Medicine, University of Florida, Gainesville, FL, USA

Nicole Lurie, MD, MSPH Coalition for Epidemic Preparedness Innovations, Washington, DC, USA

Claire Madelaine, PhD, MSc INSERM, ANRS Maladies Infectieuses Emergentes, Paris, France

Jonathan Marchand, MSc, BSc Leidos Biomedical Research, Inc., Frederick National Laboratory for Cancer Research, National Institutes of Health, Frederick, MD, USA

Henry Masur, MD, AB Critical Care Medicine Department, NIH Clinical Center, Bethesda, MD, USA

Placide Mbala Institut National de Recherche Biomédicale, Department of Epidemiology and Global Health, University of Kinshasa School of Medicine, Kinshasa, Democratic Republic of the Congo

Olivier Tshiani Mbaya, MD Institut National de la Recherche Biomédicale (DRC), Leidos Biomedical Research, Inc., Kinshasa, Democratic Republic of the Congo

Keith McAdam, MD, DL London School of Hygiene and Tropical Medicine, London, UK

Laura A. McNay, MSc Operations and Management Branch, Division of Clinical Research, National Institute of Allergy and Infectious Diseases, Rockville, MD, USA

Martin I. Meltzer, PhD, MSc Health Economics and Modeling Unit, Division of Preparedness and Emerging Infections, National Center for Emerging and Zoonotic Infectious Diseases, U.S. Centers for Disease Control and Prevention, Atlanta, GA, USA

Ian Mendenhall, PhD, BSc Office of Infectious Diseases, Emerging Threats Division, Bureau for Global Health, United States Agency for International Development, Washington, DC, USA

Todd Merchak, BSc National Institute of Biomedical Imaging and Bioengineering, National Institutes of Health, Bethesda, MD, USA

Nelson Michael, MD, PhD, MGH Center for Infectious Disease Research, Walter Reed Army Institute of Research, Bethesda, MD, USA

Alejandra Miranda, MSc, BA Leidos Biomedical Research, Inc., Collaborative Clinical Research Branch, Division of Clinical Research, National Institute of Allergy and Infectious Diseases, Frederick, MD, USA

Joel M. Montgomery, PhD Viral Special Pathogens Branch, Centers for Disease Control and Prevention, Atlanta, GA, USA

Vasee Moorthy, PhD, BMBCh, MA World Health Organization, Geneva, Switzerland

Lina Moses, PhD, MSPH Global Outbreak Alert and Response Network (GOARN), World Health Organization, Geneva, Switzerland

Melissa E. Moses Biosurveillance Division, MRIGlobal, Gaithersburg, MD, USA

Billy Sivahera Muyisa, PhD, MBA, DES Independent Consultant, Conakry, Guinea

Aaron Neal, PhD Collaborative Clinical Research Branch, Division of Clinical Research, National Institute of Allergy and Infectious Diseases, Rockville, MD, USA

Bjarke Frost Nielsen, PhD PandemiX Center, Department of Science and Environment, Roskilde University, Roskilde, Denmark

Niels Bohr Institute (NBI), University of Copenhagen, Copenhagen, Denmark

High Meadows Environmental Institute, Princeton University, Princeton, NJ, USA

Wissedi Njoh, MSc Nursing The Clinical Monitoring Research Program Directorate, Frederick National Laboratory for Cancer Research (FNLCR), Frederick, MD, USA

Alice Norton, PhD Scientific Secretariat, Global Research Collaboration for Infectious Disease Preparedness (GloPID-R), University of Oxford, Oxford, UK

Rhys O'Neill, BSc World Health Organization, Geneva, Switzerland

Gene G. Olinger, PhD, MBA MRIGlobal, Life Science and Global Health, Gaithersburg, MD, USA

Galveston National Laboratory, Microbiology & Immunology, University of Texas Medical Branch, Galveston, TX, USA

Linda Oseso, MPH Vaccine and Infectious Disease Division, Fred Hutchinson Cancer Center, Seattle, WA, USA

Francesco Paganini, MSc, MPH Bureau for Humanitarian Assistance, U.S. Agency for International Development, Washington, DC, USA

David Parrish, MSc Office of Planning and Operations Support, National Institute of Allergy and Infectious Diseases, Rockville, MD, USA

Muhammad Ali Pate, MD, MBA, MSc Gavi, The Vaccine Alliance, Geneva, Switzerland

Corey M. Peak, ScD, MSc Bill & Melinda Gates Foundation, Seattle, WA, USA

Leon Peto, DPhil, MRCP, FRCPath Nuffield Department of Population Health, University of Oxford, Oxford, UK

Alexandra L. Phelan, SJD, LLM, LLB Center for Health Security, Department of Environmental Health and Engineering, Johns Hopkins Bloomberg School of Public Health, Baltimore, MD, USA

Jerome F. Pierson, PhD, MS Office of Clinical Research Policy and Regulatory Operations, Division of Clinical Research, National Institute of Allergy and Infectious Diseases, Rockville, MD, USA

Calvin Proffitt, MA, BSc General Operations, Clinical Monitoring Research Program Directorate, Leidos Biomedical Research, Inc., Frederick National Laboratory, Frederick, MD, USA

Division of Clinical Research, National Institute of Allergy and Infectious Diseases, Frederick, MD, USA

Michael A. Proschan, PhD, MSc Biostatistics Research Branch, Division of Clinical Research, National Institute of Allergy and Infectious Diseases, Bethesda, MD, USA

Nicolas Pulik, MSc INSERM, ANRS Maladies Infectieuses Emergentes, Paris, France

Felicia Qashu, PhD, BSc Office of the Director, National Institutes of Health, Bethesda, MD, USA

V. Koneti Rao, MD, FRCPA Laboratory of Clinical Immunology and Microbiology, Division of Intramural Research, National Institute of Allergy and Infectious Diseases, Rockville, MD, USA

Sabina Faiz Rashid, PhD, MSc BRAC James P. Grant School of Public Health, BRAC University, Dhaka, Bangladesh

Emily Rasinski, MPA Bureau for Humanitarian Assistance, U.S. Agency for International Development, Washington, DC, USA

Arthur Reingold, MD, AB School of Public Health, University of California, Berkeley, Berkeley, CA, USA

Amanda Rojek, DPhil, MSc, MBBS Nuffield Department of Medicine, University of Oxford, Oxford, UK

Elizabeth Ross, BS, AA Bureau for Humanitarian Assistance, U.S. Agency for International Development, Washington, DC, USA

Michael S. Saag, MD Division of Infectious Diseases, Department of Medicine, Heersink School of Medicine, University of Alabama at Birmingham, Birmingham, AL, USA

Eric Barte de Sainte Fare Alliance for International Medical Action, Dakar, Senegal

Jen Sandrus, AA Leidos Biomedical Research, Inc., Frederick National Laboratory for Cancer Research, National Institutes of Health, Frederick, MD, USA

Daniel Schar, VMD, PhD Office of Infectious Diseases, Emerging Threats Division, Bureau for Global Health, United States Agency for International Development, Washington, DC, USA

Patricia Segura, RN, MPH Vaccine and Infectious Disease Division, Fred Hutchinson Cancer Center, Seattle, WA, USA

Cyrus Shahpar, MD, MBA Alameda, CA, USA

Douglas M. Sheeley, ScD, BSc Office of Strategic Coordination, Division of Program Coordination, Planning, and Strategic Initiatives, National Institutes of Health, Rockville, MD, USA

Office of the Director, National Institutes of Health, Rockville, MD, USA

Lone Simonsen, PhD, MA PandemiX Center, Department of Science and Environment, Roskilde University, Roskilde, Denmark

Barbara Sina, PhD Division of International Training and Research, Fogarty International Center, National Institutes of Health, Bethesda, MD, USA

Maxwell J. Smith, PhD, MSc Faculty of Health Sciences and Rotman Institute of Philosophy, Western University, London, ON, Canada

Mary Smolskis, BScN, MA Office of Planning and Operations Support, Division of Clinical Research, National Institute of Allergy and Infectious Diseases, Rockville, MD, USA

Kim Sneppen, PhD Niels Bohr Institute (NBI), University of Copenhagen, Copenhagen, Denmark

Mark Snyder, MD, BSc Deloitte Consulting LLP, McLean, VA, USA

Robert A. Sorenson, MA Division of Clinical Research, U.S. National Institute of Allergy and Infectious Diseases, National Institutes of Health, Rockville, MD, USA

Yves Souteyrand, PhD INSERM, ANRS Maladies Infectieuses Emergentes, Paris, France

Eric Stavale, MSc, BSc Leidos Biomedical Research, Inc., Frederick National Laboratory for Cancer Research, National Institutes of Health, Frederick, MD, USA

Paul Stoffels, MD Galapagos, Mechelen, Belgium

Johnson & Johnson, New Brunswick, NJ, USA

Soumya Swaminathan, MD, MBBS Science Division, World Health Organization, Geneva, Switzerland

Charlotte H. Taylor, MA Department of Health & Social Care, Antivirals Taskforce I, Therapeutics Taskforce, Global Health & Health Protection Group, London, UK

Marc Teitelbaum, MD, CPI Office of Clinical Research Policy and Regulatory Operations, Division of Clinical Research, National Institute of Allergy and Infectious Diseases, Frederick, MD, USA

Robert Fraser Terry, MPhil, BSc The Special Programme for Research and Training in Tropical Diseases, World Health Organization, Geneva, Switzerland

John Tierney, BSN, MPM Office of Clinical Research Policy and Regulatory Operations, Division of Clinical Research, National Institute of Allergy and Infectious Diseases, Rockville, MD, USA

Bruce Tromberg, PhD National Institute of Biomedical Imaging and Bioengineering, National Institutes of Health, Bethesda, MD, USA

Yven Van Herrewege, PhD, MSc Clinical Trial Unit, Institute of Tropical Medicine in Antwerp, Antwerp, Belgium

Harry van Loen, MSc Institute of Tropical Medicine in Antwerp, Antwerp, Belgium

Sofia S. Villar, PhD Clinical Trials Methodology Group, MRC Biostatistics Unit, School of Clinical Medicine, University of Cambridge, Cambridge, UK

Susan Vogel, RN, BSN Office of Clinical Research Policy and Regulatory Operations, Division of Clinical Research, National Institute of Allergy and Infectious Diseases, Rockville, MD, USA

Paul A. Volberding, MD Epidemiology & Biostatistics, School of Medicine, University of California San Francisco, San Francisco, CA, USA

Andrew Weitz, PhD, MSc, BSc National Institute of Biomedical Imaging and Bioengineering, National Institutes of Health, Bethesda, MD, USA

David Wholley, MPhil Foundation for the National Institutes of Health, Bethesda, MD, USA

Bartholomew Wilson, BSc Partnership for Research on Vaccines and Infectious Diseases in Liberia (PREVAIL), National Institutes of Health, Monrovia, Liberia

Michael Wolfson, PhD, MSc, BSc National Institute of Biomedical Imaging and Bioengineering, National Institutes of Health, Bethesda, MD, USA

Chris Worthington, MSc, BA Clinical Monitoring Research Program Directorate, Frederick National Laboratory for Cancer Research, Frederick, MD, USA

Joseph T. Wu, PhD Division of Epidemiology and Biostatistics, School of Public Health, University of Hong Kong, Hong Kong, China

Yazdan Yazdanpanah, MD, PhD, MSc ATIP-Avenir INSERM Team on Decision Analysis and Cost-Effectiveness in Infectious Diseases, Paris VII Medical School, Paris, France

Abbreviations

ACEGID	African Centre of Excellence for Genomics of Infectious Diseases
ACT-A	Access to COVID-19 Tools: Accelerating COVID-19 countermeasures
ACTIV	Accelerating COVID-19 Therapeutic Interventions and Vaccines
ADB	Asian Development Bank
AFC	African Risk Capacity Group
AfCDC	Africa Centres for Disease Control and Prevention
AfDB	African Development Bank
AFI	Acute febrile illness
AI	Artificial intelligence
AIDS	Acquired immunodeficiency syndrome
ALERRT	African Coalition for Epidemic Research, Response and Training
ALIMA	Alliance for International Medical Action
AMR	Anti-microbial resistance
AO	Area of operations
ARDS	Adult respiratory distress syndrome
ASEAN	Association of Southeast Asian Nations
ASHP	American Society of Health-System Pharmacists
ASPR	Assistant Secretary for Preparedness and Response (U.S. HHS)
AVAC	Global Advocacy for HIV Prevention
AVAREF	African Vaccine Regulatory Forum
BARDA	(U.S.) Biomedical Advanced Research and Development Authority
BHA	Bureau for Humanitarian Assistance (USAID)
BSL	Biosafety Level (scale is 1 [least secure] through 4 [most secure])
Cat-DDO	Catastrophic Demand Drawdown Option
CBD	Convention on Biological Diversity
CBPR	Community-based participatory research
CCP	Clinical characterization protocols
CDC	Centers for Disease Control and Prevention (USA)
CDISC	Clinical Data Interchange Standards Consortium
CDM	Clinical Data Management
CDMO	Contract Development and Manufacturing Organization
CDMS	Clinical Data Management Systems

CE	Community engagement
CEO	Chief executive officer
CEPI	Coalition for Epidemic Preparedness Innovations
CERC	Contingent Emergency Response Component
CFE	Contingency Fund for Emergencies
CFR	Case fatality rate
CFR	Code of Federal Regulations (USA)
CGD	Center for Global Development
CHIM	Controlled human infection model
CHMP	Committee for Medicinal Products for Human Use (EMA)
CIOMS	Council for International Organizations of Medical Sciences
CMC	Chemistry, manufacturing, and controls
CNS	Central nervous system
COHRED	Council on Health Research for Development
COVAX	COVID-19 Vaccines Global Access (Vaccine pillar of Access to COVID-19 Tools (ACT) Accelerator)
COVID-19	Coronavirus disease 2019
CoVPN	COVID-19 Prevention Network
CPG	Clinical practice guidelines
CRF	Case report form
CRF	Crisis Response Facility
CRO	Contract Research Organization
CRISPR	Clustered regularly interspaced short palindromic repeats
CRW	Crisis Response Window
CSMP	Clinical site monitoring plan
CUBE	Chambre d'urgence biosécurisée pour epidémies (individual, bio-secure, transportable treatment room)
DALY	Disability-adjusted life year
DART	Disaster Assistance Response Team (USAID)
DCR	Division of Clinical Research (NIAID)
DFID	Department for International Development (UK)
DHEW	Department of Health, Education, and Welfare (U.S. pre-1980, now HHS)
DM	Data management
DMID	Division of Microbiology and Infectious Diseases (U.S. NIH/NIAID)
DMP	Data management plan
DNA	Deoxyribonucleic acid
DRC	Democratic Republic of the Congo
DSMB	Data and Safety Monitoring Board

EAP	Expanded Access Program
EBOV	Ebola virus
EBRD	European Bank for Reconstruction and Development
EC	European Commission
ECOWAS	Economic Community of West African States
eCRF	Electronic case report form
ECRIN	European Clinical Research Infrastructure Network
EDC	Electronic data capture
EDCTP	European and Developing Countries Clinical Trials Partnership
EID	Emerging or re-emerging infectious disease
EMA	European Medicines Agency
eQMS	Electronic Quality Management System
ETC	Ebola treatment center
ETU	Ebola treatment unit
EU	European Union
EUA	Emergency Use Authorization
EUAL	Emergency Use Assessment and Listing
EUDRA	European Union Drug Regulatory Authorities (predecessor to EMA)
EUL	Emergency Use Listing
EVD	Ebola virus disease
FAIR	Findability, accessibility, interoperability, and reusability (of research data)
FAIRAT	Fairness, Autonomy, Integrity, Respect, Accountability, And Transparency
FDA	Food and Drug Administration (USA)
FDA(G)	Food and Drugs Authority (Ghana)
FETP	Field Epidemiology Training Program (U.S. CDC, others)
FIF	Financial Intermediary Fund
FIH	First-in-human studies
Gavi	Gavi, the Vaccine Alliance, formerly called the Global Alliance for Vaccines and Immunization (GAVI)
GCP	Good Clinical Practice
GDPR	General Data Protection Regulation (EU)
GLOPID-R	Global Research Collaboration for Infectious Disease Preparedness
GLP	Treatment guidelines panel
GMP	Good Manufacturing Practice
GOARN	Global Outbreak Alert and Response Network
GPG	Global public good

GPMB	Global Preparedness and Monitoring Board
GPP	Good Participatory Practice
GPP-EP	Good participatory practice guidelines for trials of emerging (and re-emerging) pathogens that are likely to cause severe outbreaks in the near future and for which few or no medical countermeasures exist
HCW	Health care worker
HEP	Health Emergencies Programme (WHO)
HEPR	Health Emergency Preparedness and Response
HHS	Department of Health and Human Services (USA)
HIPAA	Health Insurance Portability and Accountability Act
HIV-AIDS	Human immunodeficiency virus-Acquired immune deficiency syndrome
HPV	Human papillomavirus
HRH	Human resources for health
IAVI	International AIDS Vaccine Initiative
IBRD	International Bank for Reconstruction and Development
ICH	International Council for Harmonisation of Technical Requirements for Pharmaceuticals for Human Use
ICMRA	International Coalition of Medicines Regulatory Authorities
ICT	Information and communications technology
ID	Infectious disease
IDA	International Development Association
IDB	Inter-American Development Bank
IFI	International Financial Institution
IFPMA	International Federation of Pharmaceutical Manufacturers and Associations
IFR	Infection Fatality Rate
IHR (2005)	International Health Regulations (2005)
IMC	International Mercy Corps
IMF	International Monetary Fund
IMP	Investigational medicinal (or medical) product
IMS	Incident Management System

IMT	Incident management team
IND	Investigational new drug
INRB	Institut National de Recherche Biomédicale, National Biomedical Research Institute (DRC)
IOM	Institute of Medicine (USA, became National Academy of Medicine in 2015)
IP	Intellectual property
IPCC	Intergovernmental Panel on Climate Change
IPR	Intellectual property rights
IRB	Institutional review board (research ethics committee)
IT	Information technology
ITM	Institute of Tropical Medicine (Antwerp)
kb	Kilobase
LASV	Lassa (fever) virus
LDC	Least developed country
LGBTQ+	Lesbian, gay, bisexual, transgender, queer, etc.
LGBTQIA	Lesbian, gay, bisexual transgender, queer, intersex, asexual
LICs	Low-income countries
LMIC	Lower-middle-income country[1]
LMICs	Low- and middle-income countries
LSHTM	London School of Hygiene and Tropical Medicine
MAb	Monoclonal antibody
MCM	Medical countermeasure
MDGs	Millennium development goals
MDR-TB	Multi-drug resistant tuberculosis
MDTF	Multi-Donor Trust Fund
MedDRA	Medical Dictionary for Regulatory Activities (ICH)
MERS-CoV	Middle East respiratory syndrome coronavirus
MEURI	Monitored Emergency Use of Unregistered and Investigational Interventions (WHO)
MHRA	Medicines and Healthcare Products Regulatory Agency (UK)
ML	Machine learning
MoF	Ministry of Finance
MoH	Ministry of Health
MOP	Manual of Operations
MoU	Memorandum of Understanding

1 Usage of LMIC is inconsistent among various institutions and documents.

mRNA	Messenger ribonucleic acid
MSF	Médecins Sans Frontières (Doctors without Borders)
MTA	Material Transfer Agreement
NAM	National Academy of Medicine (USA)
NASEM	National Academies of Sciences, Engineering, and Medicine (USA)
NGO	Non-governmental organization
NHP	Non-human primate
NHRVR	National Healthy Volunteer Research Register
NHSRC	National Health Science and Research Ethics Committee (Liberia)
NIAID	National Institute for Allergy and Infectious Diseases (USA)
NIBIB	National Institute of Biomedical Imaging and Bioengineering (USA)
NIH	National Institutes of Health (USA)
NIHR	National Institute for Health Research (UK)
NLP	Natural language processing
NPHIL	National Public Health Institute of Liberia
NREB	National Research Ethics Board (Liberia)
NTD	Neglected tropical disease(s)
ODA	Official development assistance
OIE	International Organization for Animal Health (formerly the Office International des Epizooties)
OMB	Office of Management and Budget (USA)
OoC	Organs on a chip
OWS	Operation Warp Speed (U.S. Vaccine Development Program)
PAES	Post-authorization effectiveness study
PAHO	Pan-American Health Organization
PALM	Pamoja Tulinde Maisha (Swahili for "together save lives"): DRC Ebola therapeutics trial
PAS	Post-acute clinical sequelae
PASS	Post-authorization safety study
PCR	Polymerase chain reaction
PEF	Pandemic Emergency Financing Facility
PHE	Public health emergency

PHEIC	Public health emergency of international concern
PI	Principal investigator
POCTRN	Point of Care Technology Research Network
PPE	Personal protective equipment
PPP	Public-private partnership
PPPR	Pandemic prevention, preparedness, and response
PPR	Pandemic preparedness and response
PPR	Prevention, preparedness, and response
PREP	Pre-exposure prophylaxis
PREP Act	Public Readiness and Emergency Preparedness Act (USA)
PREVAIL	Partnership for Research on Ebola Vaccines in Liberia
PV	Pharmacovigilance
PVO	Private voluntary organization
QMS	Quality management system
R&D	Research and development
R&D&M	Research & Development & Manufacturing
RADx	Rapid Acceleration of Diagnostics
RCCE	Risk communication and community engagement
RCT	Randomized controlled trial
REC	Research ethics committee
RECOVERY	Randomised evaluation of COVID-19 therapy (trial)
REDISSE	Regional Disease Surveillance Systems Enhancement Program
RMT	Response Management Team (USAID)
RNA	Ribonucleic acid
RRNA	Rapid research needs appraisal
RSV	Respiratory syncytial virus
RT-PCR	Reverse transcription-polymerase chain reaction
rVSV-ZEBOV	Recombinant vesicular stomatitis virus–Zaire Ebola virus vaccine (Ervebo®)
RWE	Real world evidence
SAE	Serious adverse event
SAGE	Strategic Advisory Group of Experts
SARS	Severe acute respiratory syndrome

SARS-CoV	Severe acute respiratory syndrome coronavirus
SARS-Cov-2	Severe acute respiratory syndrome coronavirus 2 (virus causing COVID-19)
SATBHSS	Southern Africa Tuberculosis and Health Systems Support
SDGs	Sustainable development goals
SMC	Social mobilization, communications, and community engagement
SME	Subject matter expert
SMO	Site management organization
SMP	Safety management plan
SOC	Standard of care
SOPs	Standard Operating Procedures
SPRP	Strategic Preparedness and Response Program
SUSAR	Serious and unexpected suspected adverse reaction
TB	Tuberculosis
TORO	Transfer of Regulatory Obligations
TORs	Terms of reference
TRACE	Tracking Resistance and Coronavirus Evolution (U.S. NIH)
TTS	Thrombosis with thrombocytopenia syndrome
UHC	Universal health care
UHPR	Universal health and preparedness, review
UK	United Kingdom of Great Britain and Northern Ireland
UN	United Nations
UNAIDS	Joint United Nations Programme on HIV/AIDS
UNEP	UN Environmental Program
UNESCO	UN Educational, Scientific and Cultural Organization
UNICEF	United Nations Children's Fund
UNMEER	UN Mission for Ebola Emergency Response
UPS	Uninterruptible power supply
U.S./USA	The United States of America
USAID	U.S. Agency for International Development

USP	United States Pharmacopeia
VAC	Volts alternating current
VHF	Viral hemorrhagic fever
VSV	Vesicular stomatitis virus
VTD	Vaccines, therapeutics, and diagnostics
WAHO	West Africa Health Organization
WBG	World Bank Group
WHA	World Health Assembly (annual WHO governing body)
WHE	World Health Emergencies (Programme)
WHO	World Health Organization
WMA	World Medical Association
WOAH	World Organization for Animal Health (formerly the Office International des Epizooties (OIE))
YF	Yellow fever

Pandemic Preparedness and Research Response: A Necessary New Field

Elizabeth S. Higgs

Overview of Book Section I: introduces the new, multidisciplinary field of emergency research response and outlines why it is needed, the history and background behind it, and norms that are needed to govern the research conduct.

In his introduction, Anthony S. Fauci reminds the reader that infectious diseases have always been and will always be with us. Many emerging and re-emerging pathogens have threatened the world recently, including the first severe acute respiratory syndrome coronavirus (SARS-CoV-1) and a major outbreak, epidemic, and pandemics, respectively, of Ebola virus, Zika virus, SARS-CoV-2, and mpox. It is only recently that the scientific and medical communities have demonstrated the necessity— of integrating ethical, scientifically robust research into emergency response to infectious disease outbreaks. Standards for this research and how to conduct it are a lively subject of discussion, academically and within and among governments. Assimilating what we have learned through recent research responses to agree on scientific, ethical, and operational standards for accelerated emergency clinical research is an essential task.

In ► Chap. 2, Gerald T. Keusch and Keith McAdam provide a historical perspective on many of the subjects explored in this volume. Understanding something of the path from the earliest empirical medical studies to today's complex clinical trial landscape, as well as some of the crimes and blunders along the way, is useful for appreciating why things are the way they are as we seek to improve them.

Finally, Elizabeth S. Higgs (▶ Chap. 3) proposes six practical, normative guiding principles for using clinical research to mitigate, control, and help to end infectious disease outbreaks. These six principles are both ethically and practically necessary—bypassing basic moral and scientific norms in the name of urgency is not only wrong, but also ineffective. These principles, too, serve as background for the following chapters.

Contents

1 Introduction

Anthony S. Fauci and Tedros Adhanom Ghebreyesus

Learning Track Note: This chapter appears in Learning Tracks: Clinical Research; Emergency Research Response, Research Operations; Global Health; Health Policy, Multilateral Cooperation, International Governance; Preparedness; Public Health and Epidemiology; Research Ethics; Social Science Response Research

E. S. Higgs and R. A. Sorenson (eds.), *Principles and Practice of Emergency Research Response*,
https://doi.org/10.1007/978-3-031-48408-7_1

Emerging and re-emerging infectious diseases will always be with us. It seems that just as we control one disease, a new threat takes its place. For example, soon after the global community eradicated smallpox in the mid-1970s, Ebola was first detected in Central Africa in 1976. The human immunodeficiency virus was recognized a few years later, having spread undetected for decades. Since then, many other emerging and re-emerging pathogens have threatened the world, including the first severe acute respiratory syndrome coronavirus in 2002, major outbreaks of Ebola, Zika virus, and now of course the second severe acute respiratory syndrome coronavirus, SARS-CoV-2, the cause of coronavirus disease 2019 (COVID-19) (Fig. 1).

COVID-19 appeared suddenly at the end of 2019 and spread rapidly, causing both asymptomatic infections and severe clinical disease. Amid global societal and economic disruption and a rapidly mounting death toll, the research community had to quickly learn what public health measures would slow virus transmission, who was most affected, the clinical course of the disease, and how best to care for those sickened with COVID-19.

Researchers have chalked up remarkable achievements in response to COVID-19, notably in the development of safe and effective vaccines, diagnostics tests, and multiple therapeutics. Partly because of the SARS and Middle East respiratory syndrome (MERS) outbreaks earlier in the twenty-first century,

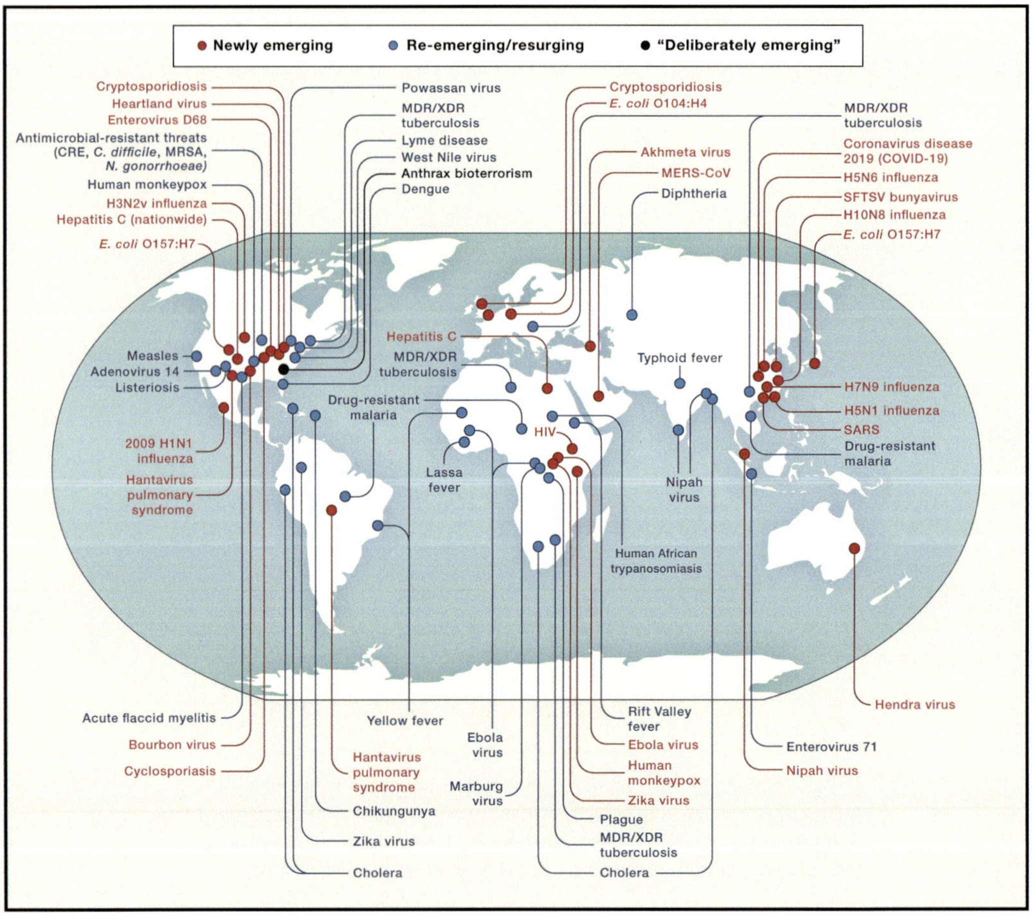

Fig. 1 Major emerging and re-emerging infectious diseases. (CC© from Morens and Fauci, ► https://doi.org/10.1016/j.cell.2020.08.021)

we were scientifically well prepared to respond to a new pandemic coronavirus.

There have also been notable shortcomings. Ineffective or even harmful treatments such as hydroxychloroquine were used at large scale despite lack of evidence. A large number of clinical trials were underpowered or poorly designed. Evidence for public health interventions sometimes came late, was at times inconsistent, and sometimes poorly implemented or not well communicated. An "infodemic," as the World Health Organization (WHO) calls it, has spread misinformation and undermined public trust in physicians, scientists, and public health officials. We must learn to communicate better with the public in a time of rapidly advancing scientific understanding amid growing distrust of scientific findings.

Both successes and failures in response to the COVID-19 pandemic remind us that preparedness and clinical research capacity are fundamental for responding to novel infectious diseases. Multiple research institutions around the world, including the U.S. National Institute of Allergy and Infectious Diseases (NIAID), are conducting and supporting research on multiple virus families known to infect humans so we can prepare to meet the challenge of a different novel pathogen when the time comes, hopefully before it can evolve into an epidemic or pandemic. With ethically sound scientific research, we can build our understanding of viruses and other pathogens and how they affect people. We devise and validate—or rule out—vaccines, therapeutics, and diagnostic tests to prevent, treat, and diagnose infection and disease (◘ Fig. 2).

In recent decades, the global public health community has greatly improved its ability to detect and respond to infectious disease threats. With many of the most dangerous diseases—yellow fever a century ago, Ebola and SARS-CoV-2 today—pivotal and relevant clinical research can best be done in the context of an outbreak. Such research has saved countless lives and will do so in the future, particularly when studies result in authorized or licensed vaccines and therapies. We must be prepared to conduct emergency response research far more rapidly than the "normal" pace of scientific research. We also need ongoing research to understand how changes in animal pathogens allow them to infect humans, how pathogens new to humans adapt to their new host, and how people's living conditions affect their vulnerability to disease. A number of research institutions, including NIAID, are pursuing the concept of developing new prototype vaccines and therapies against at least one virus from every virus family known to infect humans, something that should give us a head start if a new virus from any of those families causes an outbreak in humans. However, biomedical research alone is not sufficient to understand and address epidemics. Because human behavior is fundamental to how pathogens spread, a multisectoral approach that also involves social science, economics, and epidemiology is needed.

For decades, some worried that the conduct of research might impede the effectiveness of the public health response and that it should not be conducted during an outbreak. However, research that started during the 2014–2016 West Africa Ebola outbreak demonstrated that emergency clinical research can be vital to outbreak response. For example, the Partnership for Research on Ebola Vaccines in Liberia (PREVAIL) conducted rigorous, ethically sound research on Ebola vaccines and therapeutics, laying the groundwork for later studies including the *Ebola Ça Suffit* ring vaccination study coordinated by WHO in Guinea. This work enabled the emergency vaccination of more than 300,000 people during the 2018–2020 Ebola outbreak in the northeast Democratic Republic of the Congo (DRC), almost certainly helping bring the outbreak to an end.

The timely and broad sharing of research findings in emergencies is essential. During the 2014–2016 Ebola outbreak, WHO brought together international research stakeholders, including editors of the world's top medical journals, to agree that critical research gathered in emergencies should be made rapidly and publicly available, rather than being sealed during lengthy publishing embargoes. This major shift towards open access has

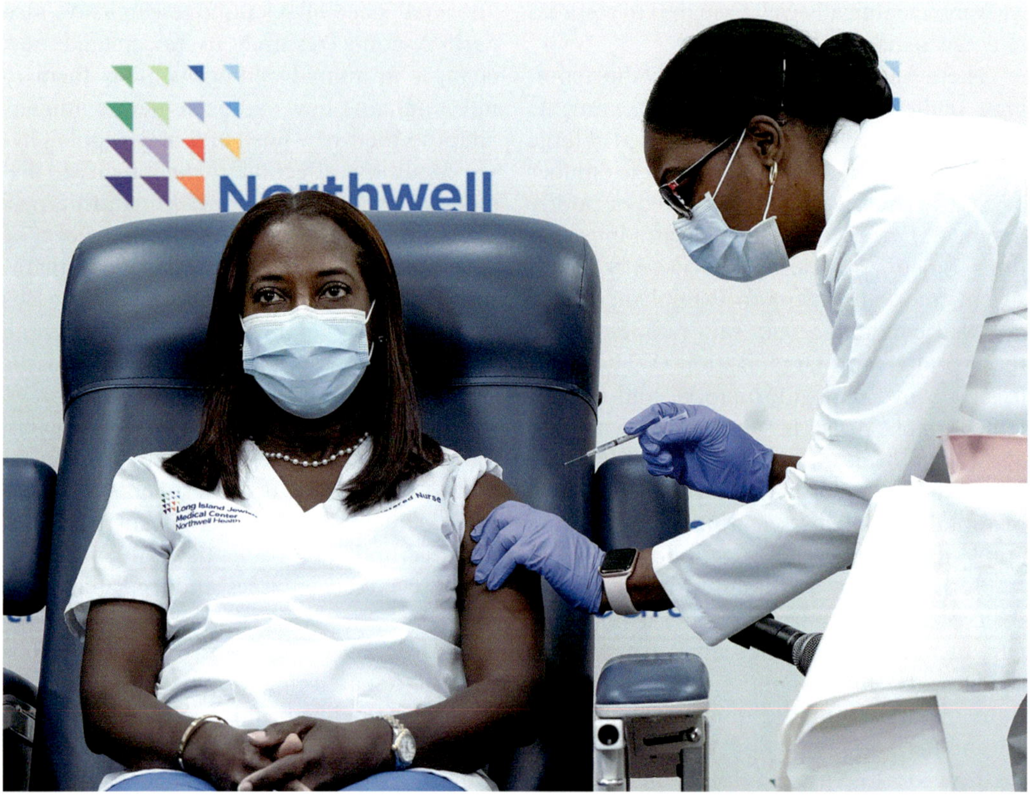

Fig. 2 Sandra Lindsay, an intensive care nurse at Long Island Jewish Medical Center, was the first person in the United States to receive the Pfizer/BioNTech COVID-19 vaccine, less than 12 months after the virus was identified and sequenced. (Courtesy Northwell Health)

shown significant benefits during the COVID-19 crisis, particularly with the use of pre-print dissemination before peer review (Fig. 3).

During the 2018–2020 DRC outbreak, the PALM trial (for *PAmoja TuLinde Maisha*, meaning "Together Save Lives" in Swahili) studied four therapeutic agents for Ebola virus disease and reached the clear conclusion that two of them were superior to the others. The emergency clinical research that began in 2014 resulted in two approved treatments and two approved vaccines for Ebola by early 2020, 44 years after the disease was first identified in the DRC. All those trials took place despite a near-total lack of pre-existing research infrastructure. The PALM trial achieved results despite harrowing circumstances, as research staff were threatened, attacked, and in a few cases killed amid civil conflict and a suspicious population.

SARS-CoV-2, of course, sparked an "all-hands-on-deck" global research response that has produced billions of courses of safe, effective vaccines in a remarkably short time. Efficacious monoclonal antibody treatments and antiviral therapeutics are also now available. The research response has taken advantage of many advances in biomedical research. We can share information on new pathogens electronically in the form of nucleic acid sequences. We have better diagnostic tools that allow us to identify diseases early. We have new ways of rapidly formulating and producing potential vaccines and therapeutics. There is a growing cadre of people with experience in rapidly implementing clinical studies to assess new vaccines and therapeutics.

Today, we can bring many scientific tools to emerging and re-emerging infectious disease outbreaks faster and more effectively

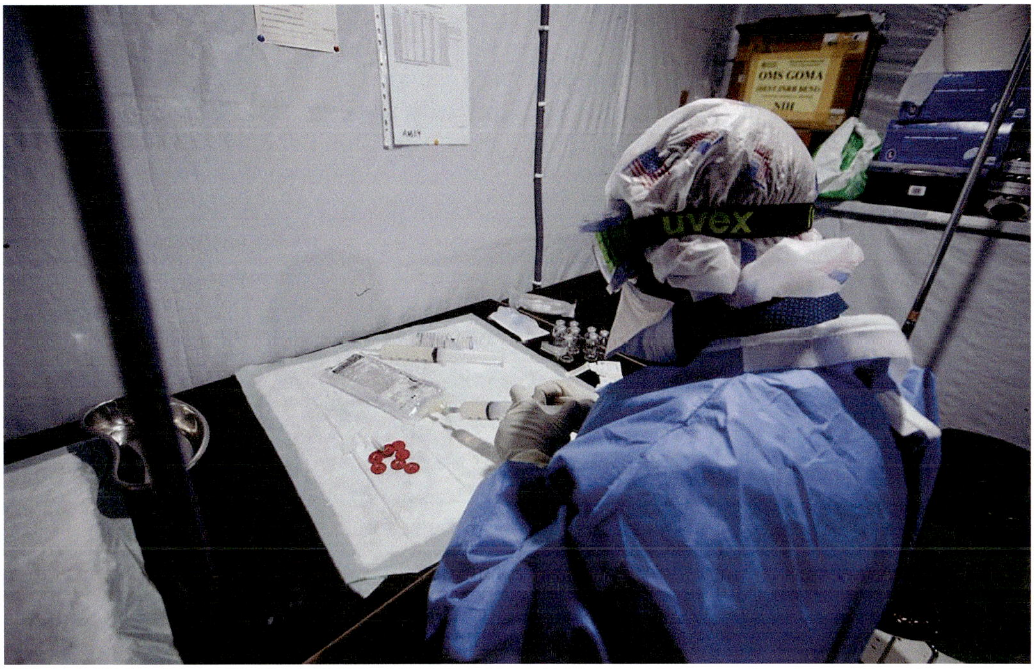

Fig. 3 A researcher in the PALM study prepares investigational therapies for administration to research participants. (Courtesy Alliance for International Medical Action (ALIMA))

than ever before. This means that research must be integrated into preparedness planning and emergency response. It is more essential than ever to bring in partners who will contribute to the success of the research, including humanitarian and multilateral organizations, non-governmental organizations (NGOs), government departments, international finance institutions, foundations, and others. To enhance readiness and response coordination, we must stimulate the field of research preparedness, so that procedures and capacities are response ready before outbreaks start. It is important also to address the current clutter of uncoordinated, small, and poorly designed research trials. Large, well-coordinated, high-quality international trials have proven much more beneficial for policy-making and product development.

While recognition of the need for response research has grown, so too has the understanding among governments that global health security is also national security. This perspective initially was spurred by concerns about bioterrorism, but it is now evident that naturally occurring emerging infectious diseases are the greater threat. Everyone working to diminish infectious disease threats understands that no one country, no single sector of society, can handle these threats alone. Governments, international organizations, and NGOs have begun to adapt accordingly.

Recent history has demonstrated that we can and must conduct integrated, ethically sound, scientifically robust research during infectious disease outbreaks. Yet, the concrete standards for this research are not entirely clear, nor are the best means by which to conduct high-quality studies on an emergency footing. Scientists, ministries of health, multilaterals, NGOs, non-health sectors, and others have questions about preparing for and executing response research, many of which have not been adequately addressed. The questions include:

- How does emergency response research differ from "regular" research?
- What are the best clinical study designs to produce statistically significant results quickly, while ensuring that participants are protected?

- How can you reconcile the research with the best possible patient care?
- What are the overriding ethical considerations? How do you build them into your research from beginning to end?
- What regulatory requirements need to be considered?
- How do you ensure that every country involved is a real partner?
- How can you ensure that the participants in the research will benefit?
- How do you engage communities during emergencies?
- How do you ensure that response research includes epidemiologic, clinical, social, and operational research?
- How do you ensure that participants, local partners, and their country will benefit most from the research?
- What are the best ways to communicate what you are doing, so that everyone from patients to country leaders understands?

Principles and Practices of Emergency Research Response gathers what we have learned over the last decade to accelerate research response to infectious disease outbreaks, and how to better prepare for the next outbreak. Where we have clear concepts of the scientific and ethical standards and how to meet them, we explain to the best of our ability. Where clear or accepted answers are lacking, we hope to convey an understanding of how we and others in the field are grappling with the issues, what principles govern research response during infectious disease emergencies, and the practical standards that apply. We expect to produce future editions reflecting progress as we continue to learn. Scientific research has ever-growing potential capacity to contribute to infectious disease outbreak response, so much so that it is now both a moral and practical imperative. Our goal is to make research response better for the benefit of all.

2 Clinical Research on Infectious Diseases: An Overview

Gerald T. Keusch and Keith McAdam

Contents

Learning Track Note: This chapter appears in Learning Tracks: Biostatistics (Sect. 2); Clinical Research; Emergency Research Response, Research Operations (▶ Sect. 3); Global Health (▶ Sects. 3 and 4.8); Global Health Law (▶ Sect. 3); Preparedness; Public Health and Epidemiology; Research Ethics (▶ Sect. 4); Social Science Response Research (▶ Sect. 4)

E. S. Higgs and R. A. Sorenson (eds.), *Principles and Practice of Emergency Research Response*, https://doi.org/10.1007/978-3-031-48408-7_2

Learning Objectives

This chapter will help readers understand and describe:

- Key milestones in the evolution of clinical research from precursors through the establishment of randomized controlled double-blind trials as standard practice.
- Reasons for use of control groups receiving placebo in clinical trials, even in a high-mortality disease outbreak where no established treatment exists.
- Important factors influencing decisions about whether to conduct controlled clinical trials during an infectious disease emergency.
- Why public communication is so important during a pandemic.
- Ways to mitigate fear and distrust in affected communities, including measures surrounding clinical trial implementation.
- Issues that arise from global efforts to mitigate the expanding number of microbial threats and implement effective interventions.
- How the evolution of bioethics has affected the conduct of clinical trials, and vice versa.
- Continuing topical issues in the application of bioethics to clinical trial design and implementation.

1 Introduction

Ever since humans gained the ability to communicate ideas with one another, we have made progress when we have been able to generate objective evidence to support our beliefs and guide our actions. An early example is the biblical story of Daniel and three other young Israelite nobles brought into service in the household of Babylonian King Nebuchadnezzar around 559 BC. The Book of Daniel, Chap. 1, says the four men refused to defile themselves by consuming their "daily portion of the king's food, and of the wine which he drank." Instead, Daniel proposed "Try thy servants, I beseech thee, ten days; and let them give us pulse to eat, and water to drink. Then let our countenances be looked upon before thee, and the countenance of the youths that eat of the king's food; and as thou seest, deal with thy servants" (Dan 1:12–13, JPS). The King's steward agreed to the proposal, and while this has been referred to as one of the earliest controlled clinical trials ever recorded in writing (Weingarten 2018), it contains a number of important study design shortfalls. For example, it lacks a detailed methods section, subjects were not randomly selected, and there is no accurate description of their clinical and demographic characteristics. The sample size of the "experimental diet" group is only four individuals, the outcome variables are vaguely defined, and the observation period is remarkably short, although it is possible this refers to some sort of "Biblical day." However, the result section, although circumscribed, is clear, "at the end of ten days their countenances appeared fairer, and they were fatter in flesh, than all the youths that did eat of the king's food. So, the steward took away their food, and the wine that they should drink, and gave them pulse," while the control group remained bound to the King's dietary preferences.

Fast forward 2200 years to 1747 when Dr. James Lind, Ship's Surgeon aboard *HMS Salisbury*, carried out a multi-arm therapeutic trial for scurvy, a well-known consequence of long sea voyages (Collier 2009). When the malady became evident, Lind selected a group of 12 affected seamen whom he described as clinically "similar as I could have them" and divided them into six groups of two men each. For six days, five groups were provided with different "experimental" diets, one of which included two oranges and one lemon per day, while standard ship's rations continued for the sixth group. The duration of the study was determined by the availability of oranges and lemons. Despite the limited observation period, Lind concluded that "the most sudden and visible good effects were perceived from the use of oranges and lemons." However, his interpretation of the findings in his 1753 report (◘ Fig. 1) remained that scurvy was the consequence of crowding and wet weather conditions on long voyages that affected the digestion and normal excretion of "putres-

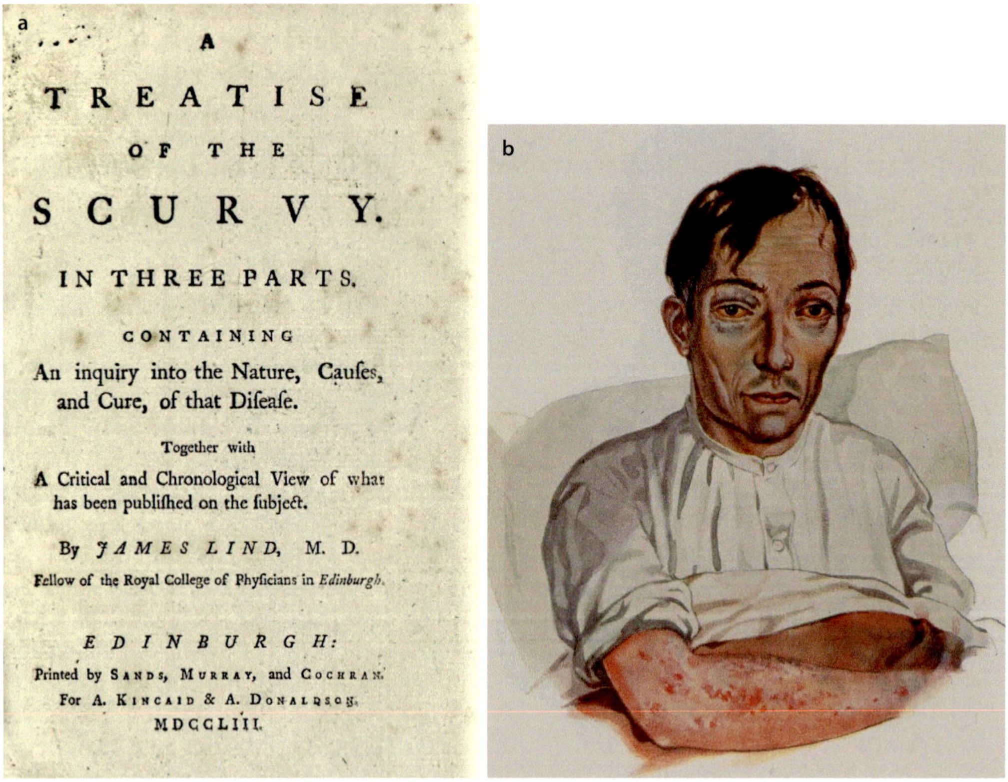

Fig. 1 **a** Title page, Lind's *Treatise of the Scurvy*, 1753 (Public Domain). **b** A 38-year-old man suffering from scurvy, from K.H. Baumgärtner, Kranken-Physiognomik, 1929. (Wellcome Images CC©)

cent … animal humours … insensibly perspired" across the skin (Lind 1753). Of course, he did not know about vitamins, that scurvy was the consequence of the dietary deficiency of vitamin C, or that provision of vitamin C-rich foods would prevent scurvy or result in rapid response for those afflicted, just as he observed in the sailors receiving citrus juice in their diet (Bartholomew 2002). During his long subsequent medical practice in the Royal Navy, he never imagined that there could be an effective dietary intervention or that the standard Ship's diet of unleavened bread and heavily salted meat was crucial in the pathogenesis of scurvy, and he never pushed the Royal Navy to include citrus juice in ship's provisions. It was left to others to make the case to finally establish new dietary standards for ships at sea, ironically around the time of Lind's death in 1794 (Bartholomew 2002).

The goal of this introductory chapter is to provide a broad historical perspective and background for the reader to better understand the progress and methodological advances in clinical research and trial design detailed in the chapters that follow and to serve as the backdrop to appreciate the necessary adaptations of study design to the challenge of implementing clinical research and trials during public health emergencies (Fleming and Ellenberg 2016; NASEM 2017). The focus throughout will be on severe emerging infectious diseases, using the 2014–2015 Ebola outbreak in West Africa and the coronavirus disease 2019 (COVID-19) pandemic of 2020–2023 as critical turning points to explore.

2 Evolution of Clinical Trial Methodology

Systematic study of investigational clinical interventions has undergone considerable change and development, particularly over the past century. Methodological rigor and both quantitative and qualitative approaches have evolved. Ethical principles as they apply to clinical trials have been elaborated and systematized to protect the interests, rights, and safety of trial subjects. Disagreements remain, however, as innovations open new avenues of clinical trial designs to evaluate therapeutics and vaccines during public health emergencies, such as infectious disease pandemics. At least four major issues must be considered, and the following discussion presents historical background for the current debate on best ethical and study design practices (▶ Chap. 22, In Practice 14.1, and In Focus 22.1).

2.1 The Inclusion of a Placebo Group in Clinical Trial Design

Clinical trials to evaluate the safety and efficacy of interventions to alter the natural history of diseases must have a comparison group which does not receive the intervention being studied. It has taken some time to agree that such a control group should consist of subjects with similar demographic characteristics and exposure to the condition under study, and it is essential that controls have similar clinical manifestations as the intervention group and differ only in the fact that they do not receive the treatment of interest. For the past 250 years, the control intervention has increasingly been a placebo, particularly something believed to be inert that is made to look like and be administered similarly to the actual intervention, e.g., a sugar pill or a safe medicinal product with no known or demonstrable physiological or clinical effect on the disease of interest. This practice traces back to at least the late eighteenth century, at first driven principally by pragmatic concerns to "satisfy the patient's demand [for treatment] and his expectations … for the satisfaction of the patient's mind, and not with the view of producing any direct remedial effect" (Jütte 2013). This was accomplished by providing "simple, feeble, or altogether powerless, non-perturbing medicines." The placebo's value in research was to create a comparison group managed as similarly as possible except for the therapeutic potential of the study intervention, but it took until the mid-twentieth century for the placebo-controlled, double-blinded trial to become the cornerstone of clinical research (Modell and Houde 1958; Shapiro and Shapiro 1997).

Over the past 75 years, as clinical trials have become indispensable in the development of therapeutic interventions, concerns about placebo control groups have emerged. For example, the ethical principle of beneficence, which mandates that physicians must act to minimize the risk of harm to their patients while maximizing potential benefits, raises the ethical dilemma of providing potential treatment to some and nothing but placebo to others in clinical trials. This seems especially egregious in the midst of an uncontrolled epidemic (Adebamowo et al. 2014). Uncertainties have also arisen about the potential impact of placebos on the evaluation of safety and efficacy in controlled clinical trials due to the clinical placebo effect. Indeed non-efficacious interventions will also have a placebo effect, so the placebo arm is needed for a proper comparison. The placebo effect is a phenomenon described as the "power of inert substances to provide striking relief for a wide variety of symptoms [as well as] the frequent occurrence of side-reactions following their use" (Lasagna et al. 1954). The effects have been attributed to the "eager confidence of the patient in the skill of his physician, and the firm expectation of relief by his means [and] sometimes a wonderful efficacy in restoring health" (Douglas 1754). Indeed, mounting interest in the therapeutic use of placebos has been the subject of a recent meta-analysis of 11 clinical trials for conditions as varied as back pain, cancer-related fatigue, attention deficit hyperactivity disorder, allergic rhinitis, major depression, irritable bowel syndrome, and menopausal symptoms, which concludes there is a statistically significant positive effect of placebo as treatment (von Wernsdorff et al. 2021). Currently, a number of ongoing open-label clinical trials are comparing control subjects, who may or may not be told they are receiving a placebo, with a so-called "nocebo" group who receive no placebo, with the intention of independently comparing each to the actual treatment intervention group.

2.2 Concurrent Versus Historical Control Groups

There are cogent arguments for the use of either concurrent or historical control groups in clinical trials, although the latter are based primarily on convenience, cost, and the argument by some that denying a possibly effective intervention for a severe potentially lethal disease is ethically unacceptable. The underlying concern for the latter, however, has recently been reframed by the "right to try" argument, particularly for individuals with fatal diseases who have nothing to lose by seeking direct access to a still unevaluated intervention, even if these may result in severe or lethal consequences (Frieden 2017b) above and beyond their potentially being ineffective, as, for example, the use of chloroquine or hydroxychloroquine to treat COVID-19 (Veatch 2020). The same argument can be used to challenge the use of placebo controls in clinical trials and is relevant as well to the choice between concurrent or historical control groups.

For the past 75 years, the "gold standard" trial design has been the randomized controlled trial (RCT) (Hariton and Locascio 2018). RCTs allow a reliable assessment of both the safety and efficacy of the intervention, removing time-dependent variables as sources of error. Statisticians and epidemiologists have tended to encourage large sample size trials, partly because multivariate analysis can allow for multiple comparisons between various intervention and control arms of a trial, making rigorous matching of the study groups less critical. There are other ways to minimize unintentional bias in the interpretation of trial results, for example, administering a placebo to the control group as noted above. In some circumstances, it is possible to randomize controls to receive a known safe medication or vaccine that is in clinical use for a different indication and is expected to have no effect on the condition being studied, other than a possible placebo effect. This can be particularly important when ongoing clinical experience with a disease leads to substantial improvements in standards of clinical care that, over time, radically alter the very outcomes that are the primary variables to assess in the clinical trial.

This was the case during the West Africa Ebola outbreak in 2014, when the mortality rate progressively diminished from the early days of the outbreak in May–June 2014 to the period from September to December 2014 because of improved clinical care (NASEM 2017). Although mortality among historical controls used for comparison in a study in Guinea of the antiviral drug favipiravir was considerably greater than the mortality rate during the subsequent single-arm clinical trial, the authors were unable to conclude whether the treatment was truly effective (Sissoko et al. 2016). Nonetheless, the treatment was adopted in the optimized standard care guidelines for Ebola in Guinea. The question of its efficacy remains uncertain, even after suggestive positive information emerged from later animal studies and extrapolation from mathematical modeling, because no human trial results are available to document this definitively (Madelain et al. 2020).

An often-cited argument for the use of historical controls is that of Stuart Pocock (1976), who emphasized their potential efficiency, especially the combination of historical and concurrent randomized controls in trials. Among the major considerations Pocock cited were the availability of historical control data before a new study began and the potential to minimize study risks, diminish the number of participants required, and thus reduce trial costs, shorten enrollment time, and lower potential bias due to dropouts. Pocock believed this procedure would also enhance participant accrual, attracting patients who would have been unwilling to be randomized to a control arm and accelerating trial completion and incorporation of new information into practice. These features would be of particular advantage for clinical trials in a pandemic emergency, when spiraling caseloads could cause clinical services to implode, require triage of patients to care or no care, and/or preclude admission to the hospital, let alone an intensive care unit, and interfere with provision of health services to patients with other health conditions. Such impacts were well-documented during the 2014–2016 West Africa Ebola epidemic (Brolin Ribacke et al. 2016) and the COVID-19 pandemic (Lau et al. 2022; Mak et al. 2022; SeyedAlinaghi et al. 2022).

There are major concerns beyond the fact that for a novel virus such as severe acute respiratory syndrome coronavirus 2 (SARS-CoV-2) there are no historical controls. For example, improved clinical diagnosis resulting in earlier identification of patients and initiation of supportive care early during a novel outbreak could by itself result in improved outcomes (Sissoko et al. 2016) independent of a therapeutic intervention. It may also be difficult to construct suitable comparative groups based on age, gender, racial, or other demographic characteristics (e.g., nutritional differences, co-morbidities, genetic susceptibility, or resistance to infection). You are stuck with the historical patients you have, and there is no opportunity to randomize patients and controls to the many variables of interest as the study is proceeding. Despite the potential benefit of smaller sample size, shorter duration, and reduced logistical complexity and costs, concurrent controls have generally been considered indispensable.

Yet historical controls, carefully identified and fully documented, may be of considerable value for certain clinical trials. For example, to identify treatments for rare diseases—their rarity, along with the possibility of a narrow time window when treatment has a positive impact, may limit the accumulation of matched control groups of sufficient size for analysis (Jansen-van der Weide et al. 2018). Whereas rare diseases may exhibit considerable phenotypic heterogeneity, they often can be identified over long periods of time, allowing for rare disease registries and identification of individuals who would be motivated to participate in clinical research. Jansen-van der Weide et al. (2018) have estimated there are over 700 active rare disease registries in Europe alone, with subject sizes sufficient to provide important insight into the natural history of the disease they track and the variability of the patient population to help in the design of single-arm clinical trials (Viele et al. 2014). Recent attention to methodological approaches to historical control groups for new clinical trials provides guidelines that can increase their statistical power and reduce type I errors or "false-positive" conclusions that the observed difference between an experimental and a control group is real instead of reflecting sampling or experimental errors (Schoenfeld et al. 2019; Viele et al. 2014). These insights can provide essential guidance in study design, including whether or not it would even be worthwhile to contemplate the use of historical controls in a particular study.

2.3 Randomization Versus Alternation in Enrollment

It had been common practice through the mid-1940s to alternate assignment of patients to an experimental intervention or a placebo control. This was the standard design in 1943 when a double-blind placebo-controlled trial was initiated to treat the common cold with Patulin, an extract of *Penicillium patulinum* (Patulin Clinical Trials Committee 1944). The statistician, Philip D'Arcy Hart, "decided on an alternation procedure for allocating subjects to study groups [and a] nurse made the allocations in strict rotation in a separate room." However, the trial showed no protective effect, "a disappointing outcome for a rigorously controlled clinical trial and perhaps the last of its kind" (D'Arcy Hart 1999). A few years later, a trial to study streptomycin for the treatment of pulmonary tuberculosis being designed by a committee including D'Arcy Hart and Austin Bradford Hill, an epidemiologist and expert statistician, accepted Bradford Hill's then-novel "allocation by random sampling numbers" approach (Marshall et al. 1948). The trial was a success, with a 6-month mortality rate of 7% (4/55) of patients treated with bedrest and 4 months of streptomycin versus 29% (15/52) of patients treated with bedrest alone ($p < 0.01$). According to D'Arcy Hart, "this was not a case of the doctrine of anecdotal experience knocking at the door and randomization emerging," because Bradford Hill had been advocating randomization for several years to "better conceal the allocation schedule" (D'Arcy Hart 1999). Some 75 years later, any trial that does not randomize allocation to the various study arms is considered less rigorous from the get-go, able at best to provide a hint of the true outcome that would still need to be confirmed in subsequent randomized double-blind prospective controlled trials.

Many different units or clusters of randomization can be applied, for example, communities or villages, or social groups such as families, households or religious congregations, schools, hospitals, or worksites, in which everyone in the unit is treated the same but the units are randomized to the different arms of the study (Moberg and Kramer 2015). When designing treatment trials for infectious diseases that spread within households, it might be tempting to randomize individuals within households to different arms of a clinical trial. However, this is seldom advisable because family members can be easily confused about which medicine they should be taking, often compare the type and schedule for the treatment they are receiving, and find it difficult to understand why family members are being treated differently. In some settings, this could lead to sharing of medication among the family members to be sure everyone accessed at least some of the active medication being studied. This has happened during HIV treatment trials with potential serious confounding of results during analysis (Moodley et al. 2016). Vaccine trial randomization within households, by contrast, makes sense since vaccine administration is discrete, supervised, and monitored.

In the Gambia Hepatitis B intervention study, immunization clinics were randomized following a stepped wedge design to receive supplies of the vaccine until all clinics in the country transitioned from control to intervention (Kirk et al. 2004). Every newborn infant in the country became part of the study when they presented at their local clinic for the standard Expanded Program of Immunization. Clinics that had also been supplied with the vaccine administered the HepB immunization as part of the National Childhood Vaccine rollout. The endpoint of the trial was the incidence of hepatoma (the most prevalent cancer in that part of the world) over the next 30 years. For the ultimate analysis of hepatoma prevention, several independent ways, including age, birthplace, and fingerprints, were available to trace whether a child had been immunized many years before. This very large longitudinal study demonstrated that Hep B vaccination was highly effective at preventing liver cancer and improved understanding of the pathogenesis of cirrhosis and cancer (Lin and Kao 2020).

In the successful international smallpox eradication program, a strategy of surveillance and containment around each case of smallpox led to a ring of immunization of all family and contacts (Fenner et al. 1988; Foege et al. 1975). Decades later, this basic design was implemented in a successful Ebola vaccine trial in which every case discovered led to a ring of immunization of all the patient's close contacts (Henao-Restrepo et al. 2017). The randomization occurred between groups immunized immediately or delayed for 21 days, and the end point was incident cases of Ebola virus disease. However, a heated academic debate emerged about the validity of this design and the statistical analysis of the results. While it was not a randomized controlled trial in the strict sense of the term, because all subjects received vaccine within a few weeks of one another, it provided data useful for subsequent trials and for international registration of the vaccine. Despite the difficulties of mounting well-controlled trials in the countries where Ebola outbreaks were occurring, "a worldwide partnership provided the foundation upon which a recombinant Vesicular Stomatitis Virus Zaire Ebola glycoprotein vaccine rVSV-ΔG-ZEBOV-GP [the Merck vaccine now approved and marketed as Ervebo]) could be successfully developed and licensed in approximately 5 years" (Wolf et al. 2021). This development required assembling a sufficiently sized database from multiple clinical trials in diverse populations and at the same time manufacturing vaccine for use in response to ongoing Ebola outbreaks.

Several new intervention protocols were suggested during recent Ebola epidemics, including adaptive designs in clinical trials. These adaptive designs were intended to make trials more flexible by utilizing results accumulating during the trial to modify the trial's course in accordance with prespecified rules. It has been claimed that "trials with an adaptive design are often more efficient, informative, and ethical than trials with a traditional fixed design," because they often make better use of resources, such as time and money, and might require fewer participants (Pallmann et al. 2018). Other experienced statisticians have questioned the validity of these assertions (Buyse 2012). This will be further discussed in ► Sect. 4.

2.4 Formal Ethical and Regulatory Frameworks

The dominant medical ethical framework before World War II was the Hippocratic oath commonly taken by physicians embarking on their studies and careers, pledging to adhere to the principle of *Primum non nocere*, "Above all, do no harm" (Smith 2005). The Nazi campaign beginning in 1933 to "cleanse German society of individuals viewed as biological threats to the nation's health" (U.S. Holocaust Memorial Museum 2022) and continuing through various medically supervised research experiments in the Nazi concentration camps from 1942 to 1945 demonstrated that the Hippocratic Oath alone cannot prevent atrocities from being conducted in the name of science (Roelcke 2004). The 1946–1947 Nuremberg medical trial documented many such experiments, though it underestimated the number of victims because it focused on the perpetrators who were arrested for conducting or abetting coerced research, most of them physicians and Nazi officials (Weindling et al. 2016). The Tribunal ultimately sentenced 12 defendants to death, three to life imprisonment, and four to long prison terms, while acquitting three.

The Nuremberg Code for the conduct of human research, still considered by some to be "the most important document in the history of the ethics of medical research" (Shuster 1997) and a transformative step forward, was a legacy of the trial. It included ten guidelines for research using human subjects (► Box 1), bookended by two critical principles: first that voluntary and informed consent of the subject was essential before a study began and last that the scientists in charge must terminate the experiment if there was probable cause to believe continuation would result in injury, disability, or death of the participant (Nuernberg Military Tribunals 1949).

Box 1: Nuremberg Code (Nuernberg Military Tribunals 1949)

1. The voluntary consent of the human subject is absolutely essential. The duty and responsibility for ascertaining the quality of the consent rests upon each individual who initiates, directs or engages in the experiment. It is a personal duty and responsibility which may not be delegated to another with impunity.
2. The experiment should be such as to yield fruitful results for the good of society, unprocurable by other methods or means of study, and not random and unnecessary in nature.
3. The experiment should be so designed and based on the results of animal experimentation and a knowledge of the natural history of the disease or other problem under study that the anticipated results will justify the performance of the experiment.
4. The experiment should be so conducted as to avoid all unnecessary physical and mental suffering and injury.
5. No experiment should be conducted where there is an a priori reason to believe that death or disabling injury will occur; except, perhaps, in those experiments where the experimental physicians also serve as subjects.

6. The degree of risk to be taken should never exceed that determined by the humanitarian importance of the problem to be solved by the experiment.
7. Proper preparations should be made and adequate facilities provided to protect the experimental subject against even remote possibilities of injury, disability, or death.
8. The experiment should be conducted only by scientifically qualified persons. The highest degree of skill and care should be required through all stages of the experiment of those who conduct or engage in the experiment.
9. During the course of the experiment, the human subject should be at liberty to bring the experiment to an end if he has reached the physical or mental state where continuation of the experiment seems to him to be impossible.
10. During the course of the experiment, the scientist in charge must be prepared to terminate the experiment at any stage, if he has probable cause to believe, in the exercise of the good faith, superior skill and careful judgment required of him that a continuation of the experiment is likely to result in injury, disability, or death to the experimental subject (◘ Fig. 2).

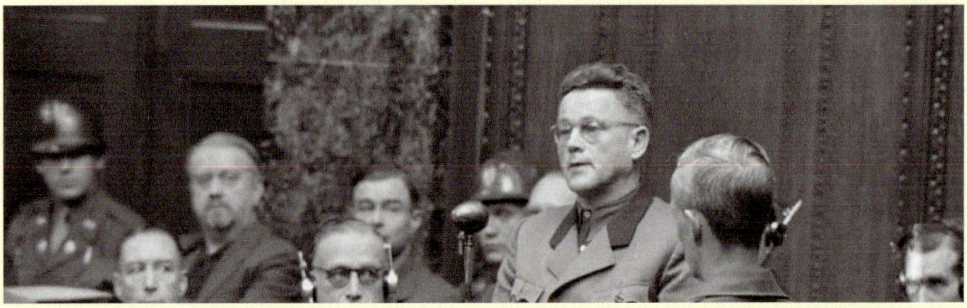

◘ **Fig. 2** Dr. Karl Gebhardt is shown as he pleads not guilty during the trial of the 23 German doctors who had conducted experiments on human "guinea pigs." Gebhardt was ultimately hanged for war crimes, including medical "experiments" at the Ravensbrück and Auschwitz camps. (Photograph by U.S. Army, T/4 Hewitt. Public domain)

But even in the United States, which prosecuted the Nuremberg medical trial, research that grossly violated the principles of the new Code would continue for another 25 years. The most infamous example is the Tuskegee syphilis study, which recruited 600 African-American males with diagnosed syphilis into a natural history experiment begun in 1932, when the only known treatments, arsenicals or mercury, were also known to be highly toxic (CDC 2021). But within a few years after a landmark 1944 set of articles on penicillin in the treatment of syphilis, widespread use of penicillin in all stages of syphilis (primary, secondary, tertiary, latent) resulted in dramatic decreases in the incidence of syphilis and associated mortality (Changing character of commercial penicillin, with suggestions as to the use of penicillin in syphilis 1946; Douglas Jr. 2009). Nonetheless, the Tuskegee study continued unchanged (◘ Fig. 3).

Fifteen years after the Nuremberg Trial, a 30-year review of the Tuskegee Study of Untreated Syphilis was published by CDC (Rockwell et al. 1964). The report documented increased mortality and morbidity in the infected cohort, nearly all of whom were positive by the fluorescent treponemal antibody absorption test, a marker of more advanced syphilis. In the interim, no systematic program to treat these individuals had been established, nor was there a plan to offer penicillin to any of the remaining survivors in 1963. Tuskegee remained an observational

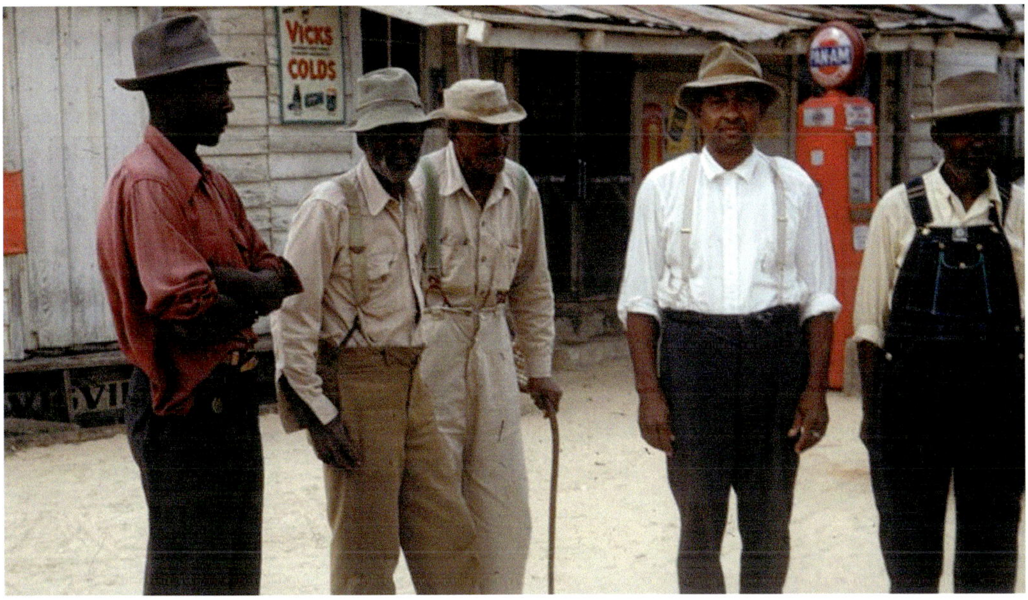

Fig. 3 Participants in the Tuskegee syphilis study. (Department of Health Education and Welfare via National Archives, USG Public Domain)

natural history study as far as the investigators and the CDC were concerned, and it continued unchanged.

In 1964, Henry Beecher and Jay Katz were each leading further transformations in thinking about the ethical conduct of human clinical research, focusing on informed consent and the responsibility of investigators to their subjects (Capron 2016). In the same year, the World Medical Association (WMA) issued its initial Declaration of Helsinki, affirming among other important precepts that the "nature, the purpose and the risk of clinical research must be explained to the subject by the doctor, … cannot be undertaken without his free consent after he has been informed, [and] the investigator or the investigating team should discontinue the research if in his or their judgement, it may, if continued, be harmful to the individual" (WMA 1964). The full impact of the changing standards for ethical conduct of clinical research and its codification for non-wartime practice by the WMA was not felt by those with ongoing responsibility for the Tuskegee study until Jean Heller of the Associated Press published an exposé on July 25, 1972, headlined "Syphilis Victims in U.S. Study Went Untreated for 40 Years," receiving immediate national attention (Heller 1972). The very first sentence was a blockbuster: "For 40 years the United States Public Health Service has conducted a study in which human beings with syphilis, who were induced to serve as guinea pigs, have gone without medical treatment for the disease and a few have died of its late effects, even though an effective therapy was eventually discovered."

The repercussions were swift. Public outcry led to the appointment of an Ad Hoc Advisory Panel by the Department of Health, Education and Welfare, to review the study's history. Its 1973 report concluded it was "ethically unjustified." Furthermore, although the report determined the subjects had agreed freely to be examined and treated there was no evidence the researchers had informed them of the real purpose of the study (HEW 1973). Far from being given all the facts required for informed consent, the participants had been misled. The report confirmed they were never offered penicillin after it became the drug of choice for syphilis, nor were they ever given the choice of quitting the study to receive penicillin when it became widely available in 1953. A class-action lawsuit was filed on behalf of the study participants and their families in

1973, leading to a US$10 million out-of-court settlement under which the U.S. government established the Tuskegee Health Benefits Program (THBP) to provide lifetime medical benefits and burial services to all living participants (Capron 2016). In 1975, THBP extended the benefits to wives, widows, and offspring of the participants. The last study participant died in January 2004, and the last widow receiving THBP benefits died in January 2009.

In the wake of the 1972 revelations, the U.S. government also established a National Commission for the Protection of Human Subjects of Biomedical and Behavioral Research under the National Research Act of 1974. Its mission was to identify "the basic ethical principles that should underlie the conduct of biomedical and behavioral research involving human subjects and [develop] guidelines to assure that such research is conducted in accordance with those principles" (National Commission for the Protection of Human Subjects of Biomedical and Behavioral Research 1979). The resulting Belmont Report[1] was published in 1979, and it continues to serve as a reference for clinical research ethics in the United States and elsewhere. It identified three basic ethical principles that must be operative in clinical research and trials involving human subjects: *respect for persons*, *beneficence* (including respecting their decisions, protecting them from harm, and making efforts to secure their well-being), and *justice* (in the sense of fairness in distribution). These principles were applied to informed consent, assessment of risk and benefit, and selection of subjects. Other efforts have provided additional guidance and perspective, including multiple revisions of the Helsinki Declaration, the latest in 2013 (WMA 2013), and several reports of the Council for International Organizations of Medical Sciences (CIOMS), often in collaboration with WHO. The latest, "International Ethical Guidelines for Health-Related Research Involving Humans," was published in 2016 (CIOMS). These substantial reports and the active dialog around the guidelines, recommendations, and rules have been usefully summarized by Christine Grady for the Hastings Center (Grady 2008) (▶ Box 2).

Box 2: Requirements of Ethical Clinical Research (Grady 2008)

Value: Ethical research should aim to answer a clinically, scientifically, or socially valuable question that will contribute to generalizable knowledge about health or be useful in improving health.

Validity: Ethical research should have an appropriate, rigorous, and feasible design, end points, methods, and implementation plans to ensure valid and interpretable data.

Fair subject selection: The process and outcomes of subject and site selection should be fair and based on scientific appropriateness, minimization of vulnerability and risk, and maximization of benefits.

Favorable risk-benefit: Research risks should be minimized and justified by potential benefits to participants and/or to society (the value of the knowledge).

Independent review: Independent review should evaluate adherence to ethical guidelines in the design, conduct, and analysis of research.

Informed consent: Research should include clear processes for providing adequate information to and promoting the voluntary enrollment of research participants.

Respect for enrolled: Both during and at the conclusion of research, actions should demonstrate respect for the rights and welfare of participants.

---

1 Named for the Belmont Conference Center of the Smithsonian Institution where the Commission met, not for a commissioner.

Ethical challenges are magnified when healthcare research is carried out in developing countries but funded by sponsors from higher-income countries; inequalities in resources and power pose a threat of exploitation. The Nuffield Council in the UK published a thorough review of ethical considerations for studies involving developing country populations in 2002 (Nuffield Council on Bioethics 2005). The ethical framework underpinning their approach was based on four principles or duties:

- Alleviate suffering
- Show respect for persons
- Be sensitive to cultural differences
- Not exploit the vulnerable

The last of these principles highlights the power of money and implicit expectations of the more affluent research partners to define the conditions of research, the scientific review process, and the nature of the ethics review process. The asymmetric power structure has been recognized, and an organizational learning tool to identify and address these issues has been developed by the Council on Health Research for Development (COHRED) and published as the Research Fairness Initiative or RFI (Research Fairness Initiative 2022).

In 2004, the Nuffield Council organized a joint workshop with the South African Medical Research Council, including many researchers and ethicists from low-income countries. The workshop report pointed out important challenges that were usually not considered in the application of imported ethical research standards to studies organized and funded by external entities and conducted in resource-limited settings (Nuffield Council on Bioethics 2005). Among them were inconsistencies in guidelines from different funders, varying requirements for informed consent, the standard of care offered to study participants including control groups, the use of placebos, and obligations to provide access to successful therapy to research participants when the studies end. Additional specific concerns were raised, including the challenges of obtaining consent in emergency settings, whether the proper standard of care for control groups in therapeutic or vaccine trials was to be the best available anywhere or the best available locally, and pragmatic barriers to faithful adherence to all provisions within these guidelines.

These discussions made it clear that before the research starts major negotiations among the partners are required around an internationally accepted agenda, oriented to creating a viable partnership between the local and international parties, including what happens after the research ends. Does the control arm in a randomized controlled trial gain access to a successful and helpful intervention? Does the country hosting the trial have broader access to the intervention and who pays for this, how much, and for how long? And, while there may be a scientific advantage to prolonging the study to document attributable longer-term adverse events, is there any financial commitment by the sponsor to care for those who suffer serious adverse events during a trial, including the potential for compensation and support well beyond the trial when these events are persistent or ultimately fatal? Are there any provisions for concomitant health care for other conditions among those enrolled in research studies?

Pretrial negotiations require competent negotiators on both sides to ensure that the vulnerable are not exploited. RFI provides a systematic approach and learning experience for all partners, for example, clarifying the standard of care to be afforded to control groups (Research Fairness Initiative 2022). Ideally, there should be a universal standard of care so that people in different countries receive the same basic level of care and treatment during research. In some circumstances, of course, it may not be possible to adopt such a universal standard of care, particularly when applicable technology is available in high-income countries but would not be feasible in low-income countries with limited technical capacity. In an ideal world, such variations in healthcare resources throughout the world would be eliminated, but this is not the direct responsibility of the clinical trial. However, when resources are limited and

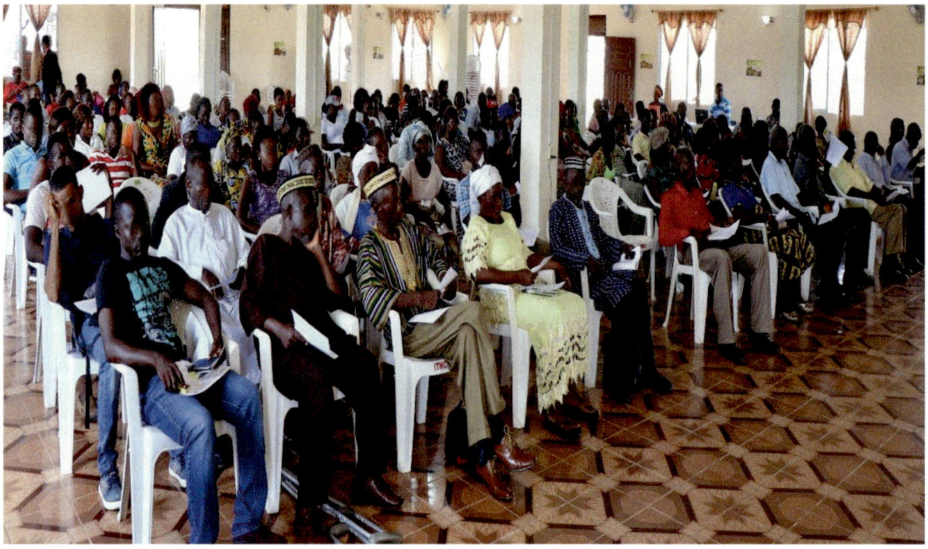

Fig. 4 Community meeting to discuss a clinical research project in West Africa. (Courtesy Laura McNay)

unequally distributed, it must at a minimum be assured that the best care available locally as part of the existing health system is provided to everybody. For a research program in practice, this means all subjects are enrolled in all arms of the research protocol (Fig. 4).

Several initiatives arising from these concerns have begun to diminish the gap in ethical standards for clinical trials among nations. First was the creation of ethics training programs based in resource-limited settings involving professionals from those countries and supported by outside research and training institutions (Millum et al. 2013). Second, the Global Forum on Bioethics in Research was established to provide a regular conference for research ethics practitioners from around the world to discuss, assess, and make recommendations to improve the ethical conduct of research (Hunt et al. 2019). Third, regional networks of bioethics experts were established to consult, learn, and collaborate with one another with the support of the World Health Organization (WHO) and the Pan American Health Organization. In January 2020, the Nuffield Council on Bioethics published a report on ethical considerations for research during health emergencies just as the COVID-19 pandemic began to spread within and outside of China (Nuffield Council on Bioethics 2020). This report will be discussed in ▶ Sect. 4, which addresses research during public health emergencies.

3 Critical Ground Rules for Research Studies During Epidemics

In addition to ensuring clinical trials are fair, ethical, and rigorous and produce evaluable results, the practice of clinical research during public health emergencies is complicated by the urgency stemming from the rapid spread of disease when effective tools and countermeasures may not exist or are in short supply. Capacity to identify and care for affected patients can be compromised by a grossly overloaded healthcare system, local authorities and health experts beset by a crisis for which they lack training and experience, and medical humanitarian organizations prioritizing immediate humanitarian response over research needs which they may view as unlikely to help mitigate or stop the outbreak. But in many cases such research can only be conducted while disease transmission continues and enough patients are available for enrollment in well-designed, approved clinical trials. To overcome such barriers, comprehensive, accepted ground rules are needed to guide the implementation and conduct of clinical research in general and trials in particular during epidemics.

3.1 Jurisdictional Levels and Collaborations

Pandemics by definition cross jurisdictions and require multidimensional collaborations that are challenging to manage. When an epidemic involves only one country, the national government and ministry of health are in control, even though the WHO country office is generally monitoring the situation. Under the International Health Regulations (IHR) of 2005, which came into force in 2007, countries experiencing outbreaks of infectious diseases, whether due to known agents or a new emerging pathogen, are responsible for surveillance to identify the event, report it to WHO, and take initial steps to control the outbreak (WHO 2016b). WHO applies a grading system of three levels of increasing concern to assess the urgency of a reported cluster of cases or a progressing outbreak within a country (▶ Box 3) (WHO 2017b).

Box 3: WHO Levels for Graded Emergencies

Ungraded: A public health event or emergency that is being monitored by WHO but that does not require a WHO operational response.

Grade 1: A single-country emergency requiring a limited response by WHO, but that still exceeds the usual country-level cooperation that the WHO Country Office (WCO) has with the member state. Most of the WHO response can be managed with in-country assets. Organizational and/or external support required by the WCO is limited. The provision of support to the WCO is coordinated by an emergency coordinator in the regional office.

Grade 2: A single-country or multicountry emergency, requiring a moderate response by WHO. The level of response required by WHO always exceeds the capacity of the WCO. Organizational and/or external support required by the WCO is moderate. The provision of support to the WCO is coordinated by an emergency coordinator in the regional office. An emergency officer is also appointed at headquarters to assist with the coordination of organization-wide support.

Grade 3: A single-country or multicountry emergency, requiring a major/maximal WHO response. Organizational and/or external support required by the WCO is major and requires the mobilization of organization-wide assets. The provision of support to WCO is coordinated by an emergency coordinator in the regional office(s). An emergency officer is also appointed at headquarters to assist with the coordination of organization-wide inputs. On occasion, the WHO executive director and regional director may agree to have the emergency coordinator based in headquarters. For events or emergencies involving multiple regions, an incident management support team at headquarters will coordinate the response across the regions (WHO 2017b).

The devil is in the details, and these include how minimal, moderate, or substantial public health consequences are defined and operationally addressed. The critical failures of the system during the initial months of the West Africa Ebola outbreak in 2014 resulted in a major revision of the structure for the entire WHO Health Emergencies Programme, with greater engagement and oversight at WHO Headquarters (Independent Panel for Pandemic Preparedness and Response 2021; WHO 2022b). Since 2016, the Executive Director of the WHO Health Emergencies Program in Geneva and WHO Regional Directors consult regularly when there are ongoing graded events and may jointly decide to move the emergency coordinator function to WHO Headquarters. When multiple regions are involved, an incident management support team is assembled at WHO Headquarters to coordinate the response.

If country-level measures fail to achieve control of a Grade 3 outbreak, further interventions come under the IHR (2005), which are legally binding for the 196 signatory nation states (WHO 2016b). When WHO identifies an uncontrolled outbreak and determines that it is potentially an international public health risk and may need a coordinated multiparty response, the Director General, with the advice of a standing emergency committee of experts, can declare a public health emergency of international concern (PHEIC) to mobilize and implement broad international responses. To the country or countries concerned, this action may appear to override national government authority and shift it to WHO and other outside organizations with more expertise, experience, and resources, including human capacity, materials, logistical support, and of course financing. Declaration of a PHEIC can be a difficult decision to make, and political interests and bureaucratic inertia can delay crisis response, especially when assessed in retrospect (Durrheim et al. 2020). A second major function of IHR (2005) is to set minimum requirements for the core capacities of nations to address outbreaks and to help resource-limited nations build the capability to rapidly detect an outbreak, report to WHO, and respond in an appropriate manner. WHO has lacked the human and financial resources for core capacity strengthening, and while there has been increased investment since the West Africa Ebola outbreak, for example, with financial and partnership inputs from the Global Health Security Agenda, the state of global preparedness overall can hardly be considered to meet required minimum standards (GHSA 2022; Kluge et al. 2018) (◘ Fig. 5).

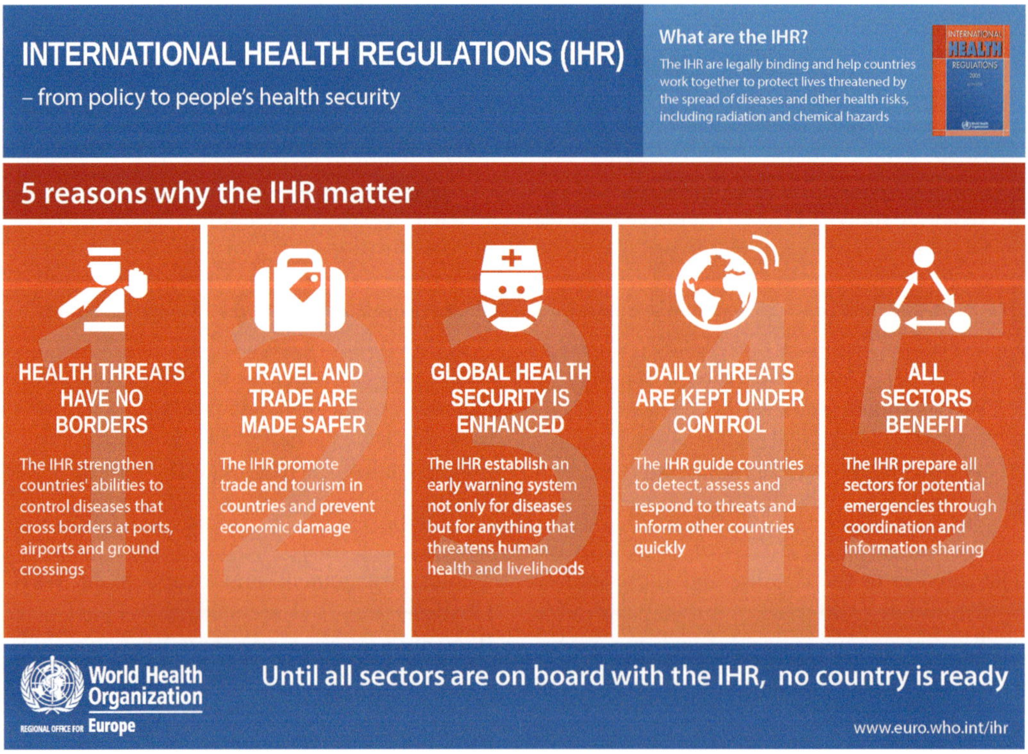

◘ **Fig. 5** Major goals of the International Health Regulations (2005) (► https://cdn.who.int/media/docs/default-source/documents/ihr-factsheet-euro.pdf?sfvrsn=2a5c364_6). (Courtesy WHO)

Seven PHEICs have been declared since the IHR went into effect in 2007 (► Box 4). The most recent two, for COVID-19 and mpox, were the most rapidly implemented, hopefully because recent experience has been translated into more efficient action. Affected countries may still resist declaration of a PHEIC, however, for fear of an economic hit and perceived loss of control over policy decisions to an international response. Implementation can be especially fraught in countries with limited facilities and insufficient human capacity to carry out the diverse response actions required. This is often complicated further by issues of mistrust between governments and affected communities, especially in countries with autocratic leadership and/or active conflict zones. Lessons from recent outbreaks make clear that WHO and its international partners must engage closely with national and local governments, their research and public health institutions, as well as local opinion leaders, religious leaders, traditional healers, media, and communications experts to establish informed support for appropriate interventions.

Box 4: PHEIC Declarations by WHO Under IHR (2005)

2009: Influenza A (H1N1): Declared in April 2009 because of rapid spread due to verified human-to-human transmission and sustained community-level outbreaks in multiple countries.

2014: Poliovirus: Declared in May 2014 because the international spread of polio was deemed a crisis for global polio eradication. This PHEIC continues because the risk of international spread of polio persists.

2014: Ebola Virus: Declared in August 2014 because of the uncontrolled Ebola outbreak in West Africa, and it was obvious the affected counties did not have the capacity to manage an outbreak of this size and complexity without organized international support.

2016: Zika Virus: Declared in February 2016 and driven primarily by a simultaneous epidemic of neurological anomalies, in particular congenital microcephaly, as cases spread primarily in South and Central America, and the Zika virus threatened to spread to other regions of the world.

2019: Ebola Virus: Declared in July 2019 following a year of uncontrolled spread in conflict areas of the Democratic Republic of Congo, with the threat of spread to contiguous countries and worldwide.

2020: SARS-CoV-2: Declared in late January 2020 because of spread to five WHO regions within the first month of the outbreak and documented human-to-human transmission.

2022: Monkeypox: Declared in July 2022 because of a rapidly escalating number of cases in countries where the virus had not previously been seen, especially in Europe.

3.2 Community Engagement

The West Africa Ebola outbreak of 2014–2016 demonstrated that close community engagement and communication to build consensus for effective health care and public health interventions were also critical to the success of a research program (Keusch and McAdam 2017; NASEM 2017). It was not until local community leaders were engaged and agreed to partner with national and international researchers to inform the population of the need for a research response and trust in the research team that essential clinical research, including clinical trials of therapeutics and vaccines, could move forward. Unfortunately, months were wasted due in part to the slow declaration of a PHEIC, logistical requirements in three least developed countries, and the time needed to establish effective communications between the research program and the local community. The delay effectively precluded the studies from reaching clear conclusions regarding efficacy and safety of the interventions they studied. By the time the studies began, public health measures had brought transmission down to the point that it was no longer possible to accrue enough events for reliable evaluation (NASEM 2017).

An avalanche of international advisors, high-level global health experts, nongovernmental organizations, leading research institutions, large funding agencies, even public figures from music, sports, and film, using different languages to convey different messages, is guaranteed to be confusing, if not intimidating. Leadership, coordination, and commitment to a shared agenda are critical. This may initially require a fine balance between representatives of the main actors, but establishing a broader coalition including local leaders quickly becomes essential. Interventions may range from altering traditional burial practices to the involvement of national and international military personnel with logistical support and, if necessary, security. These actions can ramp up the threat and fear felt by the community. Varying messaging, disinformation spread by local and social media, competition for priority and power among constituencies, mixed cues from heads of state and other leaders, and predictable misunderstandings are a good recipe for confusion and disorder. To cut through the chaos, specific methodologies for group engagement have been used successfully for engaging communities in research programs, including Appreciative Inquiry (Cooperrider and Fry 2020; Cooperrider and Whitney 2005), Community-Based Participatory Research (Appiah 2020; Salma and Giri 2021), and the WHO Community Engagement Framework (WHO 2017a) (▸ Chap. 18).

3.3 Identifying and Clarifying the Elements of Engagement

By including the multiple areas likely to engender distrust in the agenda of community outreach from the start, researchers can improve the likelihood of a successful outcome. We note seven critical steps:

1. Agreement on the processes of ethical assessment and approval
2. Detailed financial management and accountability plans
3. Provision of healthcare support and necessary laboratory capacity for those engaged in the care of research participants
4. Equitable ownership and sharing of data agreements
5. Capacity enhancement and training incorporated into every aspect of assistance
6. Addressing affordable access to therapeutics and vaccines to improve the standard of care after the trials are completed
7. Provisions to turn over new facilities and equipment enhancements to the national healthcare and health research systems in a long-term and sustainable manner

Many epidemics involve resource-limited countries where research facilities, experienced clinical investigators, trialists, and trained research personnel are in short supply. Support for these countries to develop and sustain the necessary capacities, usually through continuing collaborations, must be openly discussed, planned in detail, formally agreed upon, and budgeted collaboratively upfront.

Achieving high-quality "trusted institutions" (International Vaccines Task Force 2018) for clinical research in low- and even middle-income countries is a long-term goal, requiring national institutions with strong governance, dedicated clinical researchers, skilled staff trained in essential competencies and trusted to deliver high-level clinical services to the population, research expertise, and the capacity to manage large budgets and data sets accountably. This is a daunting challenge. Recent efforts have identified research and development partnerships with resources needed to prepare for and respond to a PHEIC of the future and the financial resources required (Lurie et al. 2021). Guidelines for developing and assessing trusted institutions, as well as evaluation frameworks for the fairness of research partnerships between national institutions and international partners, such as the COHRED Research Fairness Initiative, add credibility standards and meet the challenge of building networks of accredited clinical research institutions worldwide (Research Fairness Initiative 2022). Potter and Brough (2004) provide a practical framework for thinking through the capacity elements needed to build trusted institutions that are capable partners for emergency research response (▶ Chap. 8).

3.4 Broad-Based Scientific Participation

Clinical research and trials are not the sole domain of clinical investigators, clinical care staff, epidemiologists, biostatisticians, and other medical experts. Experience, particularly for pandemic-related research, has shown that the social and behavioral sciences are essential for managing the diverse societal challenges inherent in engaging the whole of society in a research response. Indeed, civil emergencies require transdisciplinary and cross-government responses based on understanding and consideration of deep-seated cultural mores and morals. One of the common denominators in epidemics is fear, from the uncertainty about a new, little-understood condition upending the stable orderliness of daily life to apprehension about one's own vulnerability at the individual, family, and community levels (Martin et al. 2020).

Fear is often easily initiated, sustained, and amplified, as observed early in the HIV pandemic where fears of exposure and infection were expressed by healthcare workers and the general population alike and were slow and difficult to overcome. Fear also fuels stigma and embarrassment, leading to rejection and sometimes violence in the community, with some people hiding signs of infection and delaying access to care and treatment. Others remain willing to acknowledge their diagnosis despite stigmatization and to participate in clinical trials in the hope of obtaining effective interventions. Physicians and other professionals with expertise in research skills are often poorly trained to engage with people caught up by such unknown, often overwhelming, social currents. It takes a village of skilled professionals, together with people from the community who look and think like the affected population, to turn fear into a commitment to common defense.

3.5 Communication and Messengers

The fears of infectious disease perceived by the public can be exacerbated by communication strategies intended to motivate action. For example, at the start of the HIV epidemic in the UK, a prominent media campaign showed toppling gravestones (AIDS: Monolith 1987). This memorable public health message was cancelled by the Chief Medical Officer, Donald Acheson, who preferred educating to frightening people. He replaced the campaign with a very different and more effective approach, HIV buddies, which many years later served as a model for community helpers during the COVID-19 pandemic (Berridge and Strong 1992; Omoto and Snyder 1995). Lessons learned from previous outbreaks have guided strategies to engage the public. For example, in February 2021, the U.S. National Academies of Science, Engineering, and Medicine published the results of a rapid expert consultation of the Academies' Societal Experts Action Network on risk communication, how perceptions and social norms shape action, and how to enhance vaccine uptake in the United States through public outreach (NASEM 2021). During the COVID-19 pandemic, changing sources of information, including the relatively new prominence of social media as a primary source of information and influence among the public, and their limited mechanisms to prevent or remove misinformation and deliberate deception, have been cause for concern and have required reexamination of the balance between free speech and accuracy of information (Cuan-Baltazar et al. 2020; Gabarron et al. 2021).

A recent representative survey experiment randomly assigned over 7000 respondents to read pro-vaccine communication materials emphasizing one of three messages: personal health risks, economic costs, or the collective public health consequences of not vaccinating. The message source was also randomly delivered by "ordinary people" or medical experts. The information was designed as "pre-bunking" communication to reduce the chances of recipients accepting misinformation about the rigorous standards of clinical trials (Motta et al. 2021). The findings demonstrated that "messages emphasizing the personal health risks and collective health consequences of not vaccinating significantly increase Americans' intentions to vaccinate." Much remains unknown, however, and there are many nuances and many more relevant research questions that need to be addressed within the context of public health interventions during epidemics.

Communications must be recognized as a vital part of epidemic response. In Liberia during the 2014–2015 Ebola epidemic, most mass communication was via local radio (NASEM 2017). There were upwards of 40 radio stations just around the capital, Monrovia, most in vernacular languages, along with social media, which led to widely different messaging and virtually no informed input to help accurately shape content. When the British Broadcasting Corporation was invited to help enhance local capacity for responsible journalism in Sierra Leone, the engagement itself, together with a useful monograph discussing the key principles of control, helped diminish differences and improve the validity of the communications among the many providers (Wilkinson 2016).

Language choice is also vitally important as people tend to prefer communication in their first language, which is often central to their cultural identity. It is remarkable, too, that whatever the age of the listener, popular music is most accurately recalled from their teenage "reminiscence bump" years (Munawar et al. 2018; Rao et al. 2021). Musical cues can be used most effectively when meaningful music styles from the adolescence of the listener are employed in the specific targeting of messages. In the Gambia, for example, health messages have been effectively passed on by Griots, local troubadours, and counterparts to medieval European minstrels (Rådelius 2016). They are a living archive of speech and song that maintains oral traditions. It is evident that the person communicating, intentionally or unintentionally, shapes messages according to gender, age, faith, dress, accent, humor, and personality. The message can easily have untoward effects if the messenger's demeanor appears self-aggrandizing or pompous to the audience (◘ Fig. 6).

The Ebola epidemic in West Africa also illustrated the importance of involving local decision-makers, including well-known community figures, faith leaders, traditional healers, traditional or tribal community leaders, and trusted elected government officials. In Guinea, an outside research team without "validation" by local decision-makers incited a local uprising that disrupted the progress of an important research program. "We don't want them in there at all," Marcel Dambadounou, a Guinea village chief told the *New York Times* in July, referring to doctors and aid workers battling Ebola. "We don't accept their presence at all. They are the transporters of the virus in these communities." He added, "we are absolutely afraid, and that's why we are avoiding contact with everybody—the whole world" (McCoy 2014). It required an intensive effort with local leaders to renegotiate the vaccine trial. When it became necessary to change deeply ingrained burial practices during the Ebola outbreak, anthropologists and local religious leaders helped to make alternative funeral arrangements more acceptable (Manguvo and Mafuvadze 2015).

This became even more problematic as patients entered Ebola treatment units (ETUs). Because of necessary isolation procedures, their family members were often unable to see or speak to them again before they died and were safely buried. The problems were often exacerbated by ignorance of local tradi-

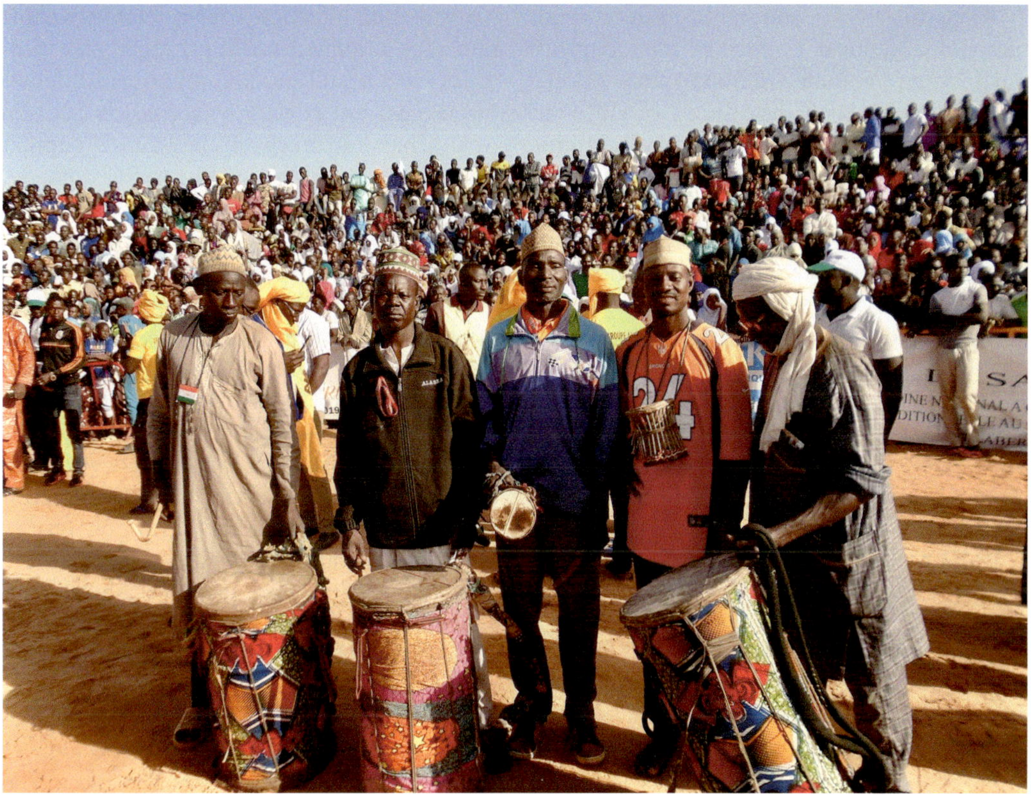

Fig. 6 Griots in Niger. (Credit: ▶ Amadouibrahim2 Wikimedia, CC© BY 4.0)

tions. For example, in Liberia, the dead were at first placed in black body bags because that was what the international teams brought with them. However, in this society, white is the color of mourning and of the traditional burial shroud (Ebola Communication Network 2015). In fact, a black shroud signaled disrespect. When the ETUs switched to white body bags, popular resistance dramatically decreased. While the outsider staff assumed it did not matter, it was important to the local community. As the Ebola Communication Network (2015) noted, "we don't know what we don't know, but anthropology can help us find out." Local religious leaders and faith groups were essential to translating messages from the response and research teams into terms compatible with cultural and religious tradition. Only when people in the community learned from trusted leaders why it was necessary to adapt established rites to the threat of Ebola were they able to overcome their reluctance to participate in Ebola response, clinical research, and trials.

The necessary transdisciplinarity of research during epidemics requires complicated international collaborations and respect for the different research approaches and methods. In addition to the essential research expertise, this process requires assistance from social scientists and ethnologists who understand and can effectively communicate with the local population. Collaboration among clinicians, public health practitioners, epidemiologists, statisticians, laboratory scientists, and humanitarian organizations—both local and international—likewise requires effort and is facilitated by the involvement of experienced social scientists, whose role may not have been recognized previously as essential to the research team.

Constructive communication with national and local politicians also requires outstanding communications and people skills. Working with individuals of different nationalities, languages, scientific disciplines, and prior experience in the stressful and urgent setting of an outbreak of severe disease in a limited resource setting is a test of leadership skills. It requires that participants have the necessary drive, spiced with humor and leavened with patience, along with outstanding communication and teamwork talents.

3.6 Special Considerations in Conflict Zones and Failed States

It is not surprising that emerging infectious disease outbreaks often occur in fragile, conflict, and violence zones as classified by the United Nations and the World Bank. The World Bank has taken note of the dramatic spike in violent conflict since 2010 on top of increasing sources of fragility, including climate change, rising inequality, demographic changes, poverty, illicit financial flows, and political and ideological factors (World Bank 2022a) (▶ Chap. 16). Even the provision of basic health care, including immunization of infants and children against childhood diseases, becomes more difficult under such circumstances. The literature is spotty, however, with most of it focused on a handful of countries in the Middle East and the impacts on healthcare workers rather than on the populations being served (Bou-Karroum et al. 2020). The Ebola outbreaks in West Africa in 2014–2016 and in the Democratic Republic of the Congo (DRC) in 2018–2020 have demonstrated how seriously conflict, fragility, and violence can degrade outbreak response. Such factors can delay recognition of an outbreak and identification of the pathogen involved, hinder swift action to contain and control it, and complicate critical clinical trials to develop and assess potential countermeasures. The COVID-19 pandemic, with multiple waves of infection over a relatively short time, has amplified existing stresses and inequities within and among countries; differential access to effective vaccines based on wealth has left much of the world's population waiting amid the health, social, political, economic, and moral crises the pandemic has created.

The exacerbation of infectious disease outbreaks in violent and conflict-ridden areas of the world includes the resurgence of polio in Syria; outbreaks of cholera in Yemen; Ebola in the northeast regions of the DRC; and at least 364 documented disease outbreaks in 108 refugee camps between 2009 and 2017 (Bousquet and Fernandez-Taranco 2020). Fragility and conflict invariably reverse development gains where they occur, particularly impact the poor, and especially disrupt educational opportunities for children and adolescents. Health systems are less able to respond to disease outbreaks as well as the usual healthcare needs. Interruptions in prenatal care and delivery services may lead to an increase in premature births and maternal and newborn mortality. The cessation of routine preventive services, such as infant and childhood immunization and malaria and tuberculosis programs, leads to an increased disease burden (Delamou et al. 2017; Masresha et al. 2020; Sun et al. 2017). Because the health services in such settings are commonly limited and difficult to access under "normal" circumstances, the additional burden of a major outbreak can be devastating, with long-term adverse implications for population health and for the healthcare system itself.

An emerging infectious disease emergency compounds the usual challenges of poverty, underdeveloped infrastructure, and the limited concern, attention, and local presence by the government in power to contain the outbreak. These factors may prevent timely clinical research when an outbreak produces enough cases for a statistically strong trial of interventions for a disease that normally occurs in small numbers in isolated populations. Institutional fragility, conflict, and violence besetting some populations are typically amplified by a concomitant lack of trust between community and government, both local and national, extending to hostility against healthcare workers and the healthcare system. They may all be labeled "outsiders," because they are not perceived by the local population as being in, from, and with the community, and can be suspected of operating with ulterior motives. The community response may be to ignore programmatic efforts at best, but at worst to actively resist. When the stakes are high, as in a PHEIC, and nonlocal and international health teams arrive in a convoy of sport utility vehicles (SUVs), they may at times be met with violence by the very community in need, as well as armed militias and other ideological groups (Wells et al. 2019a).

Over and above confronting an emerging infectious disease outbreak within a fragile, conflict-, or violence-affected country are the associated issue of refugees, potentially carrying disease agents with them, highly vulnerable to infection, and housed in makeshift, crowded camps with minimal access to health care, sanitation, and safe water and food. The World Bank has estimated that over 84 million people were forcibly displaced by mid-2021, with more than 68% from just five countries, over 85% staying in developing countries that are unable to adequately provide for their own populations, and about 75% displaced for 5 years or more (World Bank 2022b). In the context of trying to provide adequate health care for such populations, it may seem out of place to discuss the potential that research is urgently needed, how to assess the validity of informed consent, and how to preclude exploitation under such conditions. If a novel respiratory pathogen were to be found in such a population, that perspective might change quickly.

The scope and geographic spread of the COVID-19 pandemic have revealed how complex it is to intervene to reduce disease transmission, illness, and deaths, let alone to implement clinical trials (Blanc and Brown 2020) in fragile and violence-impacted countries. Both government (state actors) and autonomous individuals and groups (nonstate actors), often armed and violent, may use a crisis like COVID-19 to advance their ideology, political agendas, and power even though they are unable to favorably alter the pandemic and address its public health and economic consequences. The hope that warring factions would put their differences aside to jointly combat SARS-CoV-2 appears to have been naïve. Calls for a global or local ceasefire have been mostly ignored, as the opposing sides look for ways to exploit the calamity and consolidate their power or seize diplomatic advantage. Geopolitical strategy can lead to demonization of one foreign power or another, including alternative conspiracy stories like the alleged role of the United States or China in the origin, introduction, and spread of COVID-19 (Moritsugu 2021).

In some countries, the pandemic has provided opportunities for militias, parastatal groups, and other nonstate actors to increase their legitimacy by providing services. In many settings, government corruption, ineffective health and public health systems, minimal support of effective interventions, and inconsistent, sometimes false messaging to downplay the pandemic have added to the trust gap and increased tension between government authorities and citizens. This often leads to greater resistance and violent responses, including attacks on healthcare workers. While governments may try to conceal the facts of the outbreak, at some point it becomes obvious to the population that what is being said cannot be true.

Fragility, conflict, and violence reduce the ability to successfully implement clinical trials of promising medicines and vaccines. The core principles that allow clinical trials to provide reliable information on the risk-benefit assessment of drugs and vaccines are at the outset difficult for communities to understand and embrace. Why can't everybody get the intervention being tested? Or at least know whether they were given the test drug or vaccine or a placebo? Or clarify the difference between placebo and no treatment, and the relevance of providing an achievable standard of care to every participant? Will they really get access to proven interventions resulting from the trials? Conflict exacerbates the trust gap, which in turn will adversely affect decisions to participate in clinical trials. Ongoing conflicts can impede the simple practical ability of subjects to participate and study teams to collect data. Trials that are so interrupted that they cannot generate valid evidence in effect expose the participants to the potential risks of the intervention without the ability to assess their benefits.

Ongoing dangerous and uncertain societal conditions also limit the ability of trusted local leaders to help in the translation of information for the community when the focus turns from crisis to recovery and an opportunity to address the health sequelae and economic and social devastation of the pandemic and prepare for the future. Clinical researchers and trialists often underestimate the centrality of strategies to overcome distrust. This is a critical reason why diversely trained social scientists must be part of the research team from the very beginning (Ebola Communication Network 2015). Unless informed attention is focused on communicating with the local population and identifying trusted local leaders willing to learn why research is relevant and beneficial for their community and to deliver correct messages framed in the local language and consistent with prevailing belief systems, essential research stands little chance of being implemented timely enough to yield relevant results. Finally, when there is interpretable new information the findings and lessons learned that could benefit the community now or during the next outbreak need to be explained to the community leaders and members.

Attacks against healthcare workers and widely circulating mis- and disinformation are not restricted to conflict zones. A recent assessment of verbal and physical harassment and violence toward healthcare workers in the United States has revealed a rising level of incidents over the past decade, especially during the COVID-19 pandemic (Larkin 2021). This results from many factors, including isolation, stress, and loss of work and income, but also in part from consequences of misinformation that alleges, for example, that physicians are inflating the number of patients to increase their income. Such allegations have led to "alarming incidents of health workers being stigmatized, ostracized, harassed, or threatened for allegedly spreading the virus." Similar concerns have been identified in at least 40 other countries (Elsaid et al. 2022).

4 Lessons Learned from Emergency Clinical Research

Before 2014 there had been 24 recorded outbreaks of Ebola virus disease since the first cluster of cases was identified in 1976. All were similar: They occurred in relatively isolated rural areas in a number of endemic countries across central Africa, had high mortality rates, eventually "burned out" when the number of exposed individuals was reduced by identification and isolation of patients in ETUs, improved safety practices and availability of personal protective equipment (PPE) for health personnel caring for the patients, and introduced culturally sensitive safe burial practices. The 25th recorded outbreak was different. It rapidly spread from the rural epicenter of Guinea along the better roads to urban centers, to contiguous countries, and by air to five more distant countries, ultimately resulting in over 28,000 cases and more than 11,000 deaths (NASEM 2017). It exposed a number of problems in preparedness, response, cooperation, financing, and oversight that required attention and concerted corrective action to improve and coordinate health interventions and research (NASEM 2017).

4.1 The Genesis of the Ebola Epidemic in West Africa: The Consequences of Early Errors in Response

Reconstruction of the early events in Guinea identified an 18-month-old boy in the rural village of Meliandou, in Guéckédou, Guinea, as the first human link in a chain of rapidly fatal infections among family contacts and healthcare workers involved in their care from the end of December 2013 to the third week of January 2014 (Timothy et al. 2019). By this time, the head of the Meliandou health post had recognized an unusual cluster of five patients with severe and rapidly fatal diarrhea and had informed district health officials (Kaner and Schaack 2016). The report ultimately reached the Ministry of Health in the capital city, Conakry, and an MoH team was dispatched to investigate. The initial suspicion was cholera, known to be endemic in the area, and apparently confirmed when microorganisms resembling *Vibrio cholerae* were observed in patient stool samples (WHO 2015b). Unfortunately, despite the early recognition of the unusual cluster of cases, the lack of confirmatory evidence and prior experience with Ebola in the region resulted in the termination of the inquiry before other possibilities could be considered or investigated. Similar cases continued to occur and spread along travel routes to larger towns and regional hubs, reaching Conakry itself. Continuing spread and the death of a physician caring for these patients raised concerns again, and, in mid-March, the MoH considered the possibility it was a Lassa virus outbreak. With the help of a Médecins Sans Frontières (MSF) team, ironically working on cholera in the region, samples were sent to the Institut Pasteur in Lyon, France, where the diagnosis of Ebola was made and was reported by WHO on March 23, 2014 (WHO 2014). Unknowingly, Guinea had been almost three months into what would turn out to be the biggest Ebola outbreak ever, one that spread as people crossed borders into neighboring Sierra Leone and Liberia, and later by air to more distant destinations in Africa, Europe, and North America, thus becoming, in a sense, the first-ever global Ebola pandemic (WHO 2015b).

Although the early cluster of unusual, rapidly fatal illnesses was identified and reported quickly, the failure to correctly identify the etiology allowed precious time to be lost and delayed the chance to contain and control the outbreak and curtail its deadly consequences. The prolonged reliance of Guinea's MoH on prior experience alone turned out to be disastrous. This highlights the need to consider both likely and unlikely possibilities in differential diagnosis before reaching a conclusion. In the United States, this is often characterized by a well-known aphorism that a professional hearing hoofbeats outside should not only consider the most likely source, a horse, but also consider and discard unlikely possibilities by asking if this time could it be a zebra (Sotos 1989). In the West Africa Ebola outbreak, it turned out its course and consequences were a zebra.

But this was not the only failure to think out of the box during the outbreak and recognize and acknowledge that what was happening was different from the familiar patterns of the past. Although the local and regional WHO offices were immediately informed when the diagnosis of Ebola was confirmed in March 2014, the magnitude of the ongoing and expanding outbreak was consistently underestimated for several more months, because it was expected it too would burn out in a relatively short time as emergency teams isolated patients, initiated tracking and quarantine of contacts, took precautions in the care of patients, and implemented safe burial practices. However, the models of the past were from isolated rural areas, with limited means of travel from one community to the next, and few roads to the larger towns and cities. Responders were also misled by a decrease in WHO-reported cases in late April-early May 2014, suggesting the outbreak "might be nearing its end" (Kamradt-Scott 2016). The misimpression was reinforced at the 67th WHO World Health Assembly later that month by the Guinean Minister for Health who stated that the outbreak was essentially under control (WHO 2015a), even as Ebola was now being carried to larger and larger towns and cities via the better transportation routes in Guinea, Sierra Leone, and Liberia. The usual reluctance of WHO to escalate the classification of an outbreak to a PHEIC, because of its implications for transportation and trade in the affected member states, may have played a role (NASEM 2017). As a result, while MSF and other humanitarian organizations were struggling to provide services and crying out for help, no serious international assistance was provided at the required scale until after August 8, 2014, when WHO finally declared a PHEIC (Williams 2015). It then took weeks to mobilize resources and organize a response on the ground as the outbreak spread further.

4.2 Launching Clinical Trials of Therapeutics and Vaccines

Because of prior research on Ebola virus, particularly exploratory research to develop medical countermeasures supported by the Canadian Institutes of Health Research, a prototype Ebola vaccine (Canadian Institutes of Health Research 2015) and a potentially therapeutic mix of monoclonal antibodies (Branswell 2014) had been successfully tested in a small number of nonhuman primates and could be considered for initial human clinical trials under the emergency conditions of the escalating outbreak. It is important to understand that the unusual circumstance of such large numbers of naturally infected patients among large and accessible populations that could rapidly drive successful trials was a unique opportunity, compared to the usual limitations of small numbers of patients residing in isolated rural areas in resource-limited countries. The other option, human challenge studies, used to generate critical information for new or unproven vaccines for a few infectious diseases, such as cholera or typhoid fever (Darton et al. 2015), was deemed untenable because of the highly lethal nature of Ebola and the lack of a "rescue" intervention to terminate an experimental infection if necessary (WHO 2016a).

The desperate circumstances and logarithmic increase in cases in the three highly impacted countries in August and September 2014 were a clear signal to prioritize the launch of sufficiently powered clinical trials for the very first time in a hemorrhagic fever outbreak. Central to any subsequent trial design was the means to confirm the diagnosis, develop and adopt a uniform standard of care for all individuals enrolled in the proposed trials, provide effective PPE for the research and healthcare staff and training to upgrade their capacity to provide optimized care for patients in a containment setting within an ETU, identify additional cases through contact tracing, and ensure the safe burial of those who died. While clinical trials initiated as soon as possible could not have been more of a moral imperative, almost immediately these and other hurdles to that goal emerged.

4.3 Is it Ethical to Conduct Controlled Clinical Trials During a Public Health Emergency?

Some healthcare providers from the international humanitarian community, who had been in the trenches from the start caring for patients in the expanding West Africa Ebola outbreak, were concerned about the ethical basis for a randomized controlled trial design because it meant that only some patients enrolled in a study would be offered the intervention under investigation. As discussed earlier, the mandate in the Hippocratic Oath for physicians to "do no harm" (Smith 2005), and the similar Florence Nightingale Pledge for nurses (Gretter 2020), created an apparent ethical dilemma because individuals randomized to the control arm would be denied a potentially life-saving intervention. Instead, monoclonal antibodies against Ebola Zaire (ZMAPP), the first candidate therapy available, were distributed in a first come, first served manner until the supply was depleted. The National Academies of Sciences, Engineering, and Medicine (NASEM) report thoroughly explored the ethical dimensions of the use of placebo and randomization to experimental and control groups in the emergency setting of the outbreak and reached consensus on five critical principles (London et al. 2018; NASEM 2017) (▶ Chap. 3).

1. Research is essential, even in emergency settings
2. Study designs must generate reliable and evaluable safety and efficacy data

3. Clinical equipoise persists, even in the emergency setting
4. Informed consent from individuals and affected communities is required
5. Conducting trials that cannot be evaluated is itself unethical

This perspective is not universally accepted; for example, Adebamowo et al. (2014) argue that when the likelihood of survival without an intervention is very low and there are no alternatives to the proposed experimental product, it is immoral to give the experimental intervention to some and a placebo to others. The Nuffield Council on Bioethics (2020) report views "the successful establishment in the Democratic Republic of the Congo (DRC) in 2019 of a collaborative [adaptive] clinical trial, in which all participants with Ebola were randomized to one of four novel interventions (Mulangu et al. 2019) as a sensitive and appropriate way to address the concerns of populations facing devastating outbreaks, while still meeting the regulatory requirements necessary to license successful candidate interventions in the future." However, there were important nuances that may not be universally adaptable to future trials. In these DRC trials, a still experimental therapeutic consisting of a ZMapp cocktail had shown possible—but not statistically significant—efficacy in a controlled trial in West Africa initiated as that outbreak was waning (Prevail II Writing Group 2016). It was available and was chosen as one arm of the adaptive trial in the DRC, to be used as the comparator for the other interventions. In essence, then, ZMapp was selected by the study team to be a functional, possibly effective, control intervention for the other three products being studied, two of which proved to be statistically significantly more efficacious than ZMapp and the other test intervention. This sort of "solution" is not always available; adaptive study designs will be further discussed below.

A particularly cogent but undoubtedly still controversial concern was the fifth principle that a trial that cannot be evaluated—for example, a single-arm, nonrandomized trial—but exposes the subject to potential harm without benefit is itself unethical. A separate but related conflict was whether access to unproven experimental or repurposed interventions should be allowed for individual patients with limited options other than enrolling them in an RCT. Essentially, the question was whether clinical equipoise, that is, a genuine uncertainty within the scientific and medical community concerning the efficacy of a proposed intervention, remains under such conditions (Freedman 1987), or, in another formulation, whether the trial participant receiving the intervention has the right to choose to receive a potentially active product with no information on the possible adverse consequences of its use. However, many ethicists believe the argument that it is unethical to withhold a potentially beneficial intervention from patients in desperate need fails because it rests on an unwarranted assumption that early-stage interventions are more likely to be beneficial than to be ineffective or harmful. While this concern was not meant to "diminish the plight of the desperately ill or to denigrate the urgency of their needs ... the use of [unproven medical interventions] in an attempt to meet those needs implicates a broader set of interests, of a wider set of stakeholders, situated within a network of ethical concerns that extend far beyond the personal plight of the desperately ill" (London 2018).

4.4 Contentious Study Design Issues

The importance of using rigorous designs for clinical trials to assess interventions during an uncontrolled epidemic of a high consequence and often fatal infection was affirmed by *Integrating Clinical Research into Epidemic Response* (Ellenberg et al. 2018; NASEM 2017). One of the issues in need of resolution was the use of concurrent versus historic controls, already discussed in the context of changing mortality rates as medical staff becomes more experienced in the care of patients and the use of supportive treatment. This proved to be a concern even when the historical control information was obtained earlier in the same outbreak (Sissoko et al. 2016). An important additional consideration is that infected individuals do not necessarily have uniform or predictable outcomes, including diseases known to have a poor prognosis and despite patients appearing to be clinically similar when first seen. In other words, because it cannot be assumed there will be a consistent population outcome, randomly selected individual control subjects remain essential for valid analysis of the trial results.

The double-blinded administration of inactive or active placebos[2] (Jensen et al. 2017) ensures neither patients, their doctors, nor the researchers will be biased by their knowledge of who received the intervention being studied. The concern during an infectious outbreak that giving a placebo deprives the control group of a potentially efficacious, life-saving therapy has the potential to sow tensions among patients, their clinicians, and the clinical trialists. There are several ways to lower the temperature despite the heat of this situation. Most important is to ensure that the highest attainable standard of care in the setting of the outbreak is provided equally to all trial subjects, whether in the experimental or the control group. Even better is to admit all those ill to the treatment unit, whether or not they are enrolled in the trial, to provide the same optimized standard of care available to the trial subjects. This may also benefit the analysis of the trial because it provides a standard care control group to compare with the placebo control group and assess any placebo effects on the outcomes. Unfortunately, this is often impossible considering the number of patients, the size of the study unit and its staffing, and its available capacities and resources.

The most recent revision of the guidelines for clinical trials published by the Council for International Organizations of Medical Sciences (CIOMS) in 2016 adds support to the pushback against single-arm trials. CIOMS (2016) explicitly discourages the widespread use of unproven investigational treatments outside the context of a well-designed clinical trial. Objections to this view, referred to earlier as "right to try," have centered around the personal rights of desperately ill patients to access even unvalidated or potentially harmful medical interventions if they choose to, because they have reached the stage in their illness where they have nothing more to lose (Frieden 2017a; Veatch 2020). Proponents of right-to-try options argue that randomization to a control group implies an underlying coercion because it denies participants access to something to which they are otherwise entitled. The counter-argument, however, is strong "because self-allocation to receive an unvalidated experimental treatment does not advance the legitimate interests of any stakeholder—including the desperately ill—while preventing the generation of evidence necessary to help those stakeholders make informed better decisions" (London 2018).

4.5 The Relevance of Adaptive Clinical Trial Designs and Prepositioned Research and Patient Networks

The proponents of adaptive clinical trial designs also argue that a major reason they should be considered is because they "allow and even enforce continual modifications to key components of trial design while data are being collected" (Thorlund et al. 2018). Adaptive designs also present "the potential to reduce resource use, decrease time to trial completion, limit allocation of participants to inferior interventions, and improve the likelihood that trial results will be scientifically or clinically relevant." It is not surprising that adaptive clinical trial designs should be considered instead of standard randomized, double-blind, placebo-controlled trials for the

2 A product known to be safe but ineffective for the condition under study or a "safe but ineffective control intervention that mimics the side effects of the experimental interventions"(Jensen et al. 2017) may be used as an active placebo.

evaluation of experimental therapeutics or vaccines during outbreaks of infectious diseases with major consequences. Obtaining relevant information more quickly with sufficient reliability to determine whether or not emergency use authorization for the intervention is warranted during the outbreak itself would be of great added value. This contingency received serious consideration in the National Academies report on clinical research and trials during the West Africa Ebola outbreak of 2014–2015 (NASEM 2017). The report contextualized these opportunities and identified two principal issues relevant to both false-positive and false-negative outcomes (▶ Box 5).

Box 5: Adaptive Trial Design

The use of adaptive clinical trial design methodology, particularly adaptive randomization permitting changes in the randomization ratio, has been advocated to cut the time and cost of clinical trials in drug development. While some types of adaptive designs may provide greater flexibility and efficiency in some circumstances, there can be operational challenges with their implementation, including preplanning protocol deviations based on prior information and the need for extensive and continuous mathematical modeling (Gupta 2012; Mahajan and Gupta 2010). Further, adaptive designs can be less efficient than standard sequential designs that allow for early termination. Not surprisingly, considerable debate remains about the use of these models for clinical trials compared to more traditional RCT designs, especially during public health emergencies due to EIDs.

Two principal issues that must be addressed in adaptive trial design methods are:

1. "Whether the adaptation process has led to design, analysis, or conduct flaws that have introduced bias that increases the chance of a false conclusion that the treatment is effective (a Type I error)."
2. "Whether the adaptation process has led to positive study results that are difficult to interpret irrespective of having control of Type I error" (Chow and Chang 2012; FDA 2019).

The original ring vaccination strategy was used with great success in the smallpox eradication program, but it must be understood that it was not a clinical trial of smallpox vaccine, which was known to be effective and safe (Fenner et al. 1988; Foege 1998). The concept of a ring of intervention, however, served as the inspiration for an adaptive ring vaccination trial design to evaluate the experimental recombinant rVSV-ZEBOV Ebola (Zaire species) vaccine during the West Africa outbreak (Henao-Restrepo et al. 2015, 2017). The innovative and controversial aspect of this trial was the ethics of delaying administration of the vaccine by 21 days to some randomly selected rings (or clusters) of enrolled subjects, all of whom were exposed contacts or contacts of contacts of confirmed cases of the disease. The intent was to create a window of additional exposure from day of enrollment for this group to compare with the rings receiving the vaccine immediately to analyze outcomes during that interval. "While the ring vaccination study provided some evidence of efficacy, the trial was not designed to document long-term safety and vaccine efficacy because all participants were ultimately immunized within the space of 3 weeks, and the protocol only followed participants out to day 84" (NASEM 2017). The ring trial was followed by several standard RCTs in Sierra Leone and Liberia of the same and other vaccine candidates, but by the time they began it was already too late to accumulate enough patients for valid efficacy analysis. However, they provided enough follow-up information over a sufficiently long period to support the initial evidence that these vaccines were safe.

That information was critical background to further advance the rVSV-ZEBOV vaccine during the 2018–2020 Ebola outbreak in DRC. Within two weeks of the confirmation of the outbreak in rural Équateur Province in the DRC in April 2018, and its quick spread to a larger urban center, ring immunization with the rVSV-ZEBOV vaccine was implemented as a public health measure among front-line health professionals, contacts of confirmed cases, and contacts of these contacts. A total of 3330 subjects had been vaccinated by the time the outbreak was contained and declared over by WHO. During the two months of active transmission there were 55 cases, including 38 laboratory-confirmed, 15 probable, and two suspected infections, with 29 deaths (54.7%). Because there was no unvaccinated control group, vaccine efficacy could not be determined, although "DRC Minister of Health Oly Ilunga Kalenga [called] the vaccination program a 'game changer,' as it clearly boosted morale and encouraged other public health efforts… [and WHO noted that] none of the [initial] 53 cases occurred in a vaccinated person" (Cohen 2018). A subsequent adaptive innovative evaluation of the impact of this intervention involved the creation of "a framework that integrates a data-driven gravity model with population density, poverty, and geographic distance, calibrated to spatial Ebola incidence data during the outbreak but before initiation of the vaccination campaign" (Wells et al. 2019b). The model yielded estimates that the vaccination program contracted the geographical areas at risk for Ebola (Zaire species) by up to 70.4% and reduced the level of risk within the affected areas by up to 70.1%. "The early implementation of vaccination was critical. A delay of even 1 week would have reduced these effects to 33.3 and 44.8%, respectively."

On August 1, 2018, just a week after the outbreak in Équateur Province was declared over by WHO, another cluster of cases appeared on the other side of the country in North Kivu and Ituri provinces. Before it was over in 2019, 3444 cumulative cases (3310 confirmed and 134 probable) had been identified, with 2264 deaths (2130 confirmed and 134 probable) for a case fatality rate of 65.7%. But because appropriate regulatory approvals had already been obtained for the use of the rVSV-ZEBOV vaccine in the earlier DRC outbreak, ring vaccination could be initiated almost immediately to help contain the extent of the outbreak (Schindell et al. 2020). In April 2019, WHO released an interim data analysis of the vaccine's effectiveness, concluding that it demonstrated 97.5% protection among the more than 90,000 individuals who had been vaccinated. Of this group, 71 had developed Ebola virus disease, including 56 who became ill within 10 days of vaccination, before vaccinees developed full immunity. None of the cohort who became ill 10 or more days after vaccination died of the disease. The results were convincing enough for the vaccine to receive conditional marketing authorization from the European Commission on November 11, 2019, and approval from the U.S. Food and Drug Administration (FDA) on December 20, 2019. It is currently prequalified by WHO and licensed by 8 African countries (WHO 2021a). In February 2020, the CDC's Advisory Committee on Immunization Practices recommended the vaccine be approved for pre-exposure immunization of adults 18 years and older in the United States who are at the highest risk for occupational exposure to Ebola (Zaire species) virus. This included individuals who would respond to outbreaks of Ebola around the world, healthcare workers at the federally designated Ebola treatment centers in the Unites States, and staff working with Ebola virus at biosafety level 4 facilities in the United States (Choi et al. 2021).

Aside from the limited number of people at risk of occupational exposure to Ebola virus, there is no natural market for routine use of an Ebola vaccine because outbreaks are intermittent and unpredictable in a vast endemic region across Africa. The value of an Ebola vaccine (or for similar reasons other viral hemorrhagic fever vaccines) will be realized when it can be rapidly incorporated into an outbreak response. This possibility has been advanced by an agreement to create a vaccine stockpile involving Merck and the International Coordinating Group (ICG) on Vaccine Provision, consisting of WHO, United Nations Children's Fund (UNICEF), the International Federation of Red Cross and Red Crescent Societies, and MSF, with financial support from Gavi, the Vaccine Alliance (WHO 2021a). The stockpile, to be located in Switzerland, plans to maintain 500,000 doses of vaccine to allow countries to rapidly obtain the doses they need to contain a future Ebola epidemic with the support of humanitarian organizations.

Adaptive therapeutic trial designs using multiple simultaneous study arms have also proven to be useful, because they not only can achieve results more quickly, but can also use the same control group for all active arms of the study, and permit rapid removal of interventions that fail to meet pre-established outcome thresholds and substitute new experimental products already lined up for trial (Millen and Yap 2020). Such multi-arm, multistage clinical trials (known as MAMS trials) also allow the closure of an arm before recruitment is complete if the Data Safety Monitoring Board determines there is strong evidence of efficacy (this was the case in the PALM trial for Ebola therapeutics, when the DSMB dropped two of the four therapeutic arms because the scheduled interim analysis showed the impact of the other two on mortality was superior (Mulangu et al. 2019)) or to change target sample size or allocation ratios. Although there are variations in MAMS designs, the fundamental methods involve pairwise comparisons, stage by stage, between each treatment arm and a common control arm with the goal of identifying active treatments and dropping inactive ones as early as possible (Corey et al. 2011). Because of this and the use of a common control group for all the arms, such trials can be more efficient and provide information more rapidly to guide clinical choices. This would be especially advantageous during an emerging disease outbreak, and for these reasons, adaptive trials are considered by their proponents to be more ethical than traditional fixed designs where no interim adaptations are permitted. They may also be less expensive to run, particularly in contrast to the usual model in which a sequence of two-arm comparative trials is conducted to study multiple candidate interventions over time.

A particularly good example of the utility of a MAMS design is the Randomized Evaluation of COVID-19 Therapy (RECOVERY Trial) in the UK, which compared several clinical interventions for treatment of COVID-19 (RECOVERY trial 2022). The ability to rapidly implement these studies after the outbreak was identified was based on several factors. First, COVID-19 was rapidly spreading in high-income countries with significant research resources to apply, such as the UK. Second, and even more important, was the fact that the UK had already established a standing clinical research partnership across the country to insure more efficient planning and more rapid implementation of important research studies to guide clinical decision-making. Third, the initiative was embedded within the UK National Health Service, insuring there was a ready patient population to enroll in necessary studies and established mechanisms to follow individuals over time and collect data. COVID-19 challenged the system because the results were needed immediately, but the system performed extremely well (NIHR 2022; Pessoa-Amorim et al. 2021). Its success has led to suggestions that similar preexisting standing clinical research networks should be established across the world to address the needs of future pandemic infectious diseases (Lurie et al. 2021). Implementation of adaptive designs by the U.S. National Institutes of Health (NIH) (Accelerating COVID-19 Therapeutic Interventions and Vaccines or ACTIV partnership) (NCATS 2021; NIH 2021) and WHO (Access to COVID-19 Tools Accelerator, or ACT-Accelerator) (WHO 2021b) were slower to begin because the required infrastructure did not exist or was limited in low and middle-income countries. The latter trials did subsequently provide valuable clinical efficacy information (Goligher et al. 2021; Lawler et al. 2021; Ledford 2021; Lundgren et al. 2021; WHO Solidarity Trial Consortium 2021) (▶ Chap. 14, In Practice 14.1).

Designs to speed up vaccine trials can be even more controversial, especially when a first-studied vaccine has proven sufficiently safe and effective to use in an outbreak, such as the rVSV-ZEBOV vaccine in the 2018–2020 Ebola outbreak in the DRC (Schindell et al. 2020; WHO 2021a). WHO has published a guidance document for vaccine trials, which explores multiple issues, including comparator designs such as the delayed immunization of one group in order to create a window of exposure for evaluation, as employed in the Ebola ring vaccination study, or the use of an "active control" employing a known effective vaccine for a totally different disease for the control group (Dean et al. 2019). Additional considerations arise when a promising candidate or first approved vaccine for a high-consequence, potentially pandemic infection is known but other candidates are in development that may offer advantages, for example, simplified production, less stringent storage requirements, or ease of administration to individuals. While some have argued it would be unethical in these circumstances to initiate trials of novel vaccines when an effective vaccine already exists (Monrad 2020), or perhaps even worse an adaptive MAMS trial of multiple new experimental vaccines versus the proven effective vaccine as the comparator control group, this would have the practical effect of establishing the first to be licensed as the only option. It would preclude or delay improvements in efficacy, duration of protection, ease of manufacture, storage, administration, or improved safety profiles of second- and third-generation products to be identified and implemented.

Other adaptive features have been considered in the design of vaccine trials for HIV, which has proven to be notoriously recalcitrant to vaccine approaches. For example, "if multiple Phase II studies can be conducted in parallel, with the capability of examining efficacy endpoints and immune correlates in real time, the likelihood for advancing a successful vaccine to an efficacy trial in a more rapid time frame will increase greatly. Moreover, the ability to see common immunological findings either with different vaccine regimens or the same vaccine regimen in different populations (e.g., men versus women) provides more than circumstantial evidence that such responses have an underlying biological basis" (Corey et al. 2011). The ability to adapt the design after the trial begins and a study arm with efficacy is identified would permit a rapid switch to "vaccinating the placebo group for immune correlate analyses, adding a booster vaccination if vaccine efficacy appears to wane or expanding the trial design to include a higher risk population." Other adaptations such as sample size re-estimation would allow sample or event size to change during the trial as interim analysis provided more reliable estimates of vaccine efficacy and incidence rates or for "Bayesian historical borrowing to incorporate information from control arms of similar historical trials to augment data [or] to use the treatment information from a historical trial, which is commonly encountered in pediatric trials, e.g., extrapolation from the adult efficacy data to pediatric subjects" (Liu et al. 2021). The WHO global collaborative SOLIDARITY vaccine trial was designed to allow the investigators to "test several preventive candidate SARS-CoV-2 vaccines under development to enable the concurrent evaluation of the benefits and risks of each candidate" (WHO 2022c). In addition, the primary outcome variable was virologically confirmed COVID-19 disease independent of severity, and candidates could be added or dropped based on interim analysis compared to placebo or other vaccines. There has also been a push to use real-world data, meaning data "extracted from a broad range of sources such as patient registries, healthcare databases, claims databases, patient networks, social media, and patient-generated data from wearables" to improve the relevance of data from clinical trials (Baumfeld Andre et al. 2020). Tapping into "electronic health records (EHRs), vaccine registries, and patient-generated data using [a] mobile app can be beneficial for the clinical trial data collection, which does not require site visits for the subjects" and may provide additional analytical and efficiency benefits.

4.6 Achieving Trust and Support of the Affected Community

Research does not stand alone; it must be embedded in the healthcare system of the community. This integration is facilitated if community healthcare resources are effective, accessible to the population, affordable, and trusted in advance of an outbreak. If not, the ability to gain the confidence of people in the community and enroll them in research projects decreases dramatically, while active pushback is likely to increase—whether or not poverty, conflict, and violence are additional complicating concerns. The NASEM (2017) report emphasized that, in addition to strengthening capacity for clinical trials in countries, "sustained, coordinated international support for health systems in low- and middle-income countries is now of paramount importance. This includes investing in their medical infrastructure, enhancing their capacity to conduct public health surveillance and research and ensuring that collaborations provide lasting benefits to affected communities." Embedding research within a competent, patient-oriented healthcare system, as well as integrating research into the clinical, social, and humanitarian response to an outbreak, has been generally overlooked in the past but, following the West Africa Ebola outbreak, is now front and center in thinking and planning for the future. It remains an unfulfilled mandate, however, and solutions to the financial, management, and prioritization barriers to investing in healthcare system capacity are desperately needed. It should be noted that this is particularly difficult to implement in fragile and conflict-affected states (▶ Chap. 18).

When a previously unknown, consequential emerging infectious disease outbreak strikes an unprepared population, especially following the declaration of a PHEIC and an international intervention, the immediate reaction of the local community is concern and most likely fear. This is often rapidly translated into suspicions about "experts," particularly when they are unknown foreigners without a magical cure in hand, offering only a clinical trial the community is unprepared for and ill-equipped to understand. The trust gap is all too frequently amplified by long-standing distrust of national or local authorities from the political elite or the health ministry. While international global health professionals have been aware of such issues, even prior to the West Africa outbreak, experts in the conduct of clinical research—particularly from high-income countries with well-functioning, competent healthcare and research institutions—may have been much less aware and had limited if any prior collaboration on clinical research with social scientists who better understand the behavioral responses research projects can provoke (▶ Chap. 26).

In the 2014–2016 Ebola outbreak, early efforts to introduce clinical research protocols to the community were met with resistance until the research teams, with the help of anthropologists and others attuned to community engagement, figured out how to bridge the yawning credibility gap by connecting with respected local religious, civil, tribal, health, education, and other recognized community leaders to enlist their help as emissaries (NASEM 2017). The turn-around in attitudes and acceptance was often swift and impressive. Because of the compounded delays in getting clinical trial approvals and logistics arranged, however, direct clinical and public health interventions had already ramped up case identification and isolation, contact tracing, safe handling of infectious materials, and safe burial practices, and the trajectory of the outbreak was reversing when good community connections were in place (NASEM 2017). By the time proposed trials were fully approved and logistically ready to roll and enroll subjects, the number of eligible cases was fast diminishing. This is a major reason why so many trials in the West Africa Ebola outbreak failed to reach the required sample size and collect enough outcome events for a statistically valid analysis.

Similar issues of fear and distrust have played out in the COVID-19 pandemic, amplified in some countries, independent of their wealth and institutional resources, by the repeated denials of the serious nature of the disease and promotion of disinformation by political leaders at the national, state, or local level, celebrities, and even some research and healthcare professionals. These have been repeatedly echoed by some media sources and via social media, including directed attacks on the validity of evolving scientific information and denigration of the legitimacy of well-trained scientific experts. Increasing awareness and attempts to counteract the "infodemic" have not been enough to overcome its consequences, measurable in terms of morbidity, mortality, and stress on society, including healthcare systems. It has reinforced resistance among segments of the population in rich as well as poor countries, fueled by the din of inconsistent, sometimes deliberately false messages—manifested by refusals to self-quarantine if ill, or to wear face masks, maintain social distancing, and avoid large gatherings indoors or outside. This has remained so even though some of these crowded gatherings of mask-less unimmunized people have served as super-spreader events that have greatly expanded transmission in the community, ultimately leading to what has been characterized as a pandemic of the unimmunized (Angius et al. 2021).

The experience has made it clear there are fundamental principles and patterns of human behavior that apply across widely differing settings, from Ebola in isolated, resource-limited countries to COVID-19 in high-income, highly educated, and well-resourced nations. Widespread mistrust of government and authority figures has been a common theme, at times shamefully exploited for political gains; aided and abetted by dissemination of wishful thinking and deliberately false information in the context of poor scientific literacy, and amid sudden changes in social, cultural, and economic circumstances for almost everyone. This has played out as resistance to changes in personal behavior necessary to reduce transmission, increasing willingness to accept unproven and sometimes potentially or obviously dangerous remedies, along with hesitancy or outright refusal to accept well-documented safe and effective vaccines.

4.7 Speeding the Clinical Research Process and Regulatory Approval Without Compromising Safety

The COVID-19 pandemic has also demonstrated that it is possible to increase the speed and efficiency of vaccine development through well-conducted research and expedited evaluation and approval processes for medical countermeasures. The rapid development of candidate vaccines for SARS-CoV-2 and initiation of clinical trials were enabled by decades of investment in preparedness research and development (R&D). This investment led to a substantial background of prior basic knowledge, along with more recent investments in the creation of prototype vaccine approaches for the coronavirus family which includes SARS-CoV and MERS-CoV and SARS-CoV-2. Other virus families known to infect humans and potentially generate novel viruses with pandemic potential are also the subject of vaccine candidate development (Graham and Corbett 2020). As a direct consequence of these and other investments, concepts and prototypes were available as the outbreak began for researchers to apply immediately to SARS-CoV-2 in the first weeks of January 2020 (Lurie et al. 2020). The speed of development was increased further by:

- Encouraging parallel rather than sequential staging of R&D as in the past
- The evolution of more efficient adaptive clinical trial designs in therapeutics trials
- Better alignment of biomedical and social science perspectives in preparation for clinical trials
- Availability of public financial resources

- Willingness to invest in manufacture of promising candidates before evidence of their safety and effectiveness was available
- Expedited regulatory review with prioritized evaluation for emergency approval

For the FDA, this removed chokepoints from the system without compromising the agency's objective standards and rigor (Lurie et al. 2021). FDA provided emergency use authorization for three vaccines based on Phase III clinical trial data beginning less than a year after identification of the outbreak and began to approve and license them just 8 months later (▶ In Practice 4.2, Chaps. 6 and 12).

4.8 Recommendations to Improve Clinical Research and Trials During Public Health Emergencies

The NASEM (2017) report outlined seven recommendations to help meet the need for objective information obtained as rapidly as possible. They focus on identifying and providing safe and effective interventions while preventing the use of excessively risky or ineffective approaches that would expose recipients to increased risk without potential benefit (▶ Box 6). These opportunities to improve and speed the development of countermeasures against emerging infectious diseases also face major barriers of financing, engagement, collaboration across sectors, political will, and the need to invest at risk of failure before there is a reasonable indication of the potential success of the intervention. The private sector pharmaceutical industry's need to know that a product has a good chance to return profits on the investment has contributed to long delays in the traditional drug and vaccine development ecosystem. To the extent these recommendations are implemented, sustained, and aligned with an end-to-end R&D preparedness and response ecosystem, including R&D itself and the essential clinical research and clinical trials environment, improved efficiency of an independent regulatory process, and attention to manufacture

Box 6: Recommendations by the Committee on Clinical Trials During the 2014–2015 Ebola Outbreak

1. Support the development of sustainable health systems and research capacities in low-income countries.
2. Develop memoranda of understanding to facilitate data collection and sharing before an outbreak and provide resources to enable data collection and sharing at the start of an epidemic.
3. Facilitate capacity for rapid ethics reviews and legal agreements before an epidemic.
4. Ensure that capacity-strengthening efforts benefit the local population during an epidemic.
5. Enable the incorporation of research into national health systems before an epidemic.
6. Prioritize community engagement in research and response during an epidemic.
7. Fund training and research into community engagement and communication for research and response, coordinate international efforts in research and development for infectious disease pathogens, and establish and implement a cooperative international clinical research agenda at the outset of an epidemic (NASEM 2017).

and equitable distribution of the products wherever they are required, the time it will take from recognition of a disease to the availability of effective countermeasures will diminish. Success will be measured by the more rapid control of epidemic emerging infectious diseases, reduced consequences in individual morbidity and mortality, and less disruption to societal, cultural, economic, and political systems around the world.

4.9 The Emergence of SARS-CoV-2 and the COVID-19 Pandemic

At the end of 2019, the third human epidemic in under 20 years due to a betacoronavirus began. It is undisputedly the most serious and globally impactful public health disaster in the century since the 1918 influenza pandemic. At the same time, there were several positive innovations during the outbreak that must be sustained and further improved for the world to be better prepared to respond in the future.

First, COVID-19 was declared to be a PHEIC within a month of its recognition in Wuhan, China. WHO and its emergency mechanisms are now more prepared to recognize a public health emergency at earlier stages and to act in order to bring timely global attention and resources together in response. WHO will require additional support from its member states to staff and sustain an invigorated emergency management system for epidemic diseases and to improve the rollout of essential support.

Second, the recognition by clinicians of an unusual cluster of cases and their use of next-generation sequencing methods in Wuhan rapidly identified the cause as a novel betacoronavirus. This enabled the early development of molecular diagnostics, which in turn permitted surveillance of the population and diagnosis of affected individuals to proceed.

Third, nearly 20 years of research on betacoronaviruses, built on decades of basic research in virology, molecular pathogenesis, and vaccinology, was turned into vaccine candidates specific for the new pathogen, with the initiation of Phase I clinical trials within 10 weeks of the publication of the genetic sequence of the virus.

Fourth, innovative messenger RNA-based vaccines and adenovirus-based constructs completed Phase III trials, generating sufficient evidence to warrant authorization for emergency use by several regulatory agencies around the world and WHO, beginning 9 months from the start of Phase I trials. Additional vaccines were developed in China and Russia, initially for local use and then donated for vaccination campaigns in a number of low- and middle-income countries. They have not been evaluated or approved elsewhere, representing a failure of global coordination toward a common critical goal, control of the pandemic. Additional vaccines have been designed and produced in a number of middle-income countries, and some were rapidly approved for local use in those countries (Regulatory Affairs Professionals Society 2023). However, there is still no global mechanism for governance and oversight over the whole regulatory process.

Fifth, a new concept, "vaccine nationalism," has been applied to the policies of high-income countries to buy and co-opt most of the COVID vaccine supply available following emergency use authorization, using measures like pre-purchasing agreements and control over exportation of vaccines manufactured within those nations, not to mention higher bids for the products available on the open market (Bollyky and Brown 2020). The majority of the world's population remained vulnerable and without meaningful access to effective vaccines to control the ongoing pandemic far longer than those in the wealthiest countries (Our World in Data 2022). Failing to control transmission of the virus in so many countries has resulted in vast numbers of infected people, increasing the likelihood of selection of more readily transmitted and/or more virulent viral variants. In this way, inequitable distribution of vaccines in some parts of the world is having an adverse impact on control of the virus everywhere in the world (Wagner et al. 2021). Vaccine nationalism is not a rational global health management strategy.

Sixth, a pandemic of misinformation about the cause and evolution of the pandemic, and adoption of interventions, such as highly effective and safe vaccines, has further limited their uptake and impact on the pandemic, even where vaccine supplies are abundant, permitting further evolution of the virus into more transmissible or virulent variants. Vaccine hesitancy and refusal have been fueled by the ill-informed public statements of major political leaders and celebrities around the world and amplified by some media sources and many social media "influencers" preferentially over evidence-based information, sowing doubt about the views of accomplished scientific and public health leaders (van der Linden 2022).

Seventh, a global mechanism called COVAX was established by Gavi, the Coalition for Epidemic Preparedness Innovations (CEPI), and WHO to acquire and distribute vaccines to low- and middle-income countries in need. It is one pillar of the Access to COVID-19 Tools (ACT) Accelerator, along with equitable access to COVID-19 diagnostics and treatments. While the initiative had high hopes at the launch in April 2020, it was not able to obtain enough vaccine doses to perform as planned. Although distribution was much improved by mid-2022, slower-than-expected procurement and distribution of vaccine by COVAX lengthened the pandemic and permitted the emergence of additional variants of concern (WHO 2022a).

Eighth, geopolitics has slowed efforts to identify how SARS-CoV-2 emerged from an endemic virus of bats and was ultimately introduced into the human population. This has precluded a timely and thorough joint effort by international and Chinese experts to obtain essential evidence in the environment and laboratories in China and begin transparent, systematic explorations necessary to monitor virus spread and transmission and to implement measures to prevent or mitigate any similar emergence in the future.

Ninth, the cumulative global impact of a clinically serious, readily transmissible disease has first and foremost been the escalating morbidity and mortality around the world due to SARS-CoV-2. Healthcare facilities have been overwhelmed, not only in resource-limited developing countries but in the richest countries in the world as well, resulting in an inability to provide optimal care to all patients who need intensive care, mechanical ventilation, or skilled nursing. This has also delayed or preempted care for other serious diseases, with consequences for those affected that will likely never be fully known. The breakdown of preventive services, such as routine childhood immunizations and prenatal and delivery care in many countries around the world, will increase future disease burdens and require additional expenditures to remedy the shortfall to the extent possible. The long periods of social isolation and widespread quarantine have led to a widespread but underestimated and often poorly addressed mental health crisis. Childhood education, household income, and food security have been adversely affected. Poverty rates and homelessness have grown. On top of this, major global economic, social, cultural, and political consequences will continue to play out after the ongoing pandemic ends or, more likely, becomes a continuing endemic of lesser severity and extent and therefore of less concern as the vivid memories of its frightful early toll fade away.

Tenth, if we as a species have learned anything from the pandemic, we have done little to put the needed prevention and response measures in place. Financial mechanisms are needed to make the complex R&D ecosystem function more optimally and produce new drugs, vaccines, and diagnostics that are affordable, equitably distributed, and efficiently delivered to the point of greatest need. And better global health governance must begin to implement best practices for maximum global control over the pandemic for the most people, in the shortest time frame, and to ensure access to effective countermeasures (► Chap. 27).

5 Conclusions

The principles and practice of clinical research and clinical trials have evolved over time. Clinical research is now a specialty area of medicine of critical importance in the systematic and scientific development, evaluation, and implementation of treatment strategies and for the introduction of new or improved diagnostics, therapeutics, vaccines, and other essential products into medical practice. The advent of an increasing number of severe, often fatal, emerging infectious disease outbreaks, whether locally epidemic or globally pandemic, has added urgency to the need for action, without compromising safety for the approval and introduction of new products (Morens et al. 2004). Three overarching conclusions arise from the expanding number of microbial threats to human health and survival, in-depth analysis of how the R&D process has worked to make it more effective, efficient, and equitable, and assessment of how long it takes to obtain valid and objective conclusions and implement effective interventions.

First, the fundamental goals, context, and processes for clinical research and trials do not change when the topic is a mild or slowly advancing severe infectious disease or process or a rapidly progressive, severe, frequently fatal emerging infectious disease. It is the urgency of the need to begin studies that can produce solid results and the scope of consequences that differ with the nature of the disease. All the ethical, design, procedural, statistical, and regulatory standards remain as they are for any other clinical concern, although they may need different approaches to ensure they are fulfilled (▶ Chaps. 3 and 4).

Second, clinical research and clinical trials for emerging infectious diseases, especially those of high consequence in terms of direct and indirect threats to individuals and to human societies locally and internationally, must be embedded within the social, cultural, economic, and political systems of affected nations and effectively engage a broad range of trusted community leaders and the communities they serve. This is now a critical concern if people are to trust and participate in research studies and subsequently accept the information these generate on safety and efficacy of the resulting products. The community needs to appreciate that the rapid development of COVID-19 vaccines, while seemingly miraculous, was neither magical nor a conspiracy of the pharma and biotech industries to generate profits. The COVID-19 development was rather the result of prior investment in basic science and the exploration of platform technologies that could be adapted to an entirely new member of a pathogen family virtually overnight. To succeed, this effort requires a level of respect and trust between researchers and clinical trial participants and, more generally, between scientists and the public (▶ Chaps. 18 and 26).

Experience during COVID-19 has suggested that the biblical imagery of the Four Horsemen of the Apocalypse (usually portrayed as War, Famine, Pestilence and Death) is incomplete and should now be joined by a Fifth Horseman, Misinformation (◘ Fig. 7).

For these reasons, clinical research can no longer be seen as the domain of expert researchers and the statisticians who help design and analyze properly controlled and ethical clinical research and trials. Together, public health professionals, social scientists, and communication experts must engage the community in clinical trials to understand what information is essential to convey to people and how to convey it clearly and accurately, while sustaining dialog and communication between experts and the community as more information emerges and responses need to adapt accordingly.

Third, at the end of the R&D, clinical research and trials process, and required regulatory approval, the safe and effective products that emerge must be made rapidly available to all those who volunteered for clinical trials and those who did not initially receive them as soon as the products are available in sufficient quantities for everybody at risk around the world (Rogers et al. 2021). There should be no distinction in this respect between high-income countries and low- and middle-income countries (▶ Chap. 5). Sustainable, flexible global

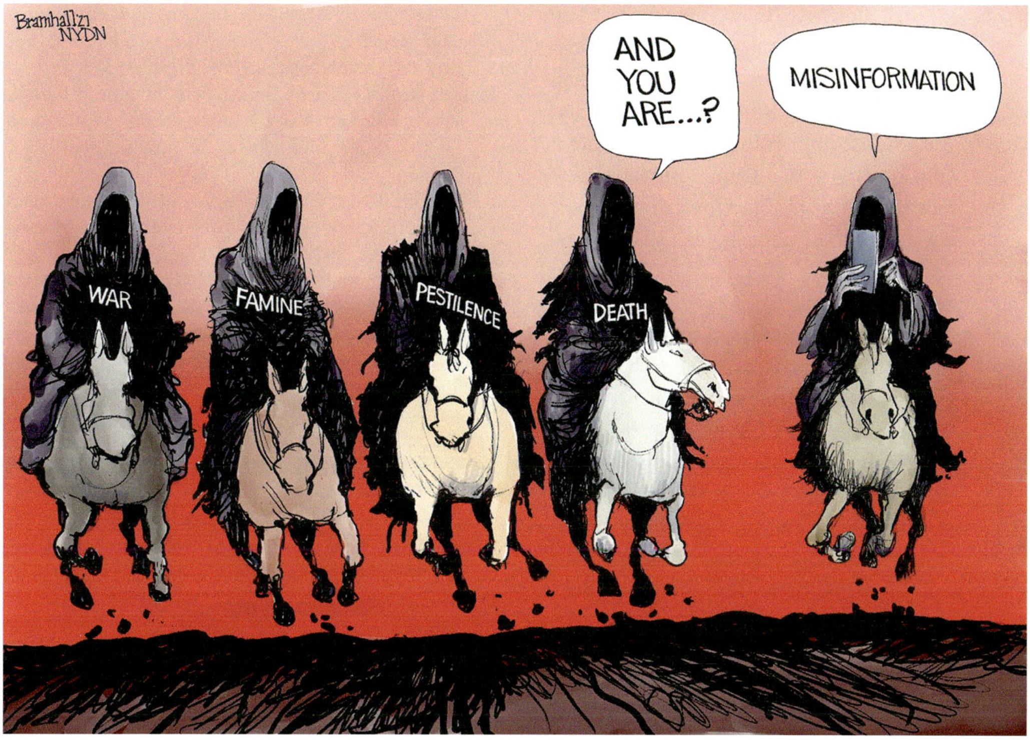

Fig. 7 Four Horsemen have a public relations manager! (Credit: Bill Bramhall/New York Daily News/TCA reprinted with permission)

mechanisms must be created to achieve these goals and ensure the necessary investments are made in research, development, evaluation, production, and global delivery of the products of the R&D process everywhere they are needed. The specter of "vaccine nationalism" must be replaced with the vision of "vaccine internationalism" for all products and tools emerging from the R&D system, clinical research, and the regulatory, manufacturing, and distribution systems essential for pandemic disease control.

Discussion Questions

1. Aldous Huxley once remarked, "The charm of history … [is that] nothing changes and yet everything is completely different." Discuss milestones in the long and fascinating journey of clinical research, culminating with the emergence of the randomly controlled, double-blind clinical trial. Also, briefly outline one or more developments in the evolution of medical ethics and remaining gaps and challenges.
2. Provide some cogent arguments for the use of placebo and of either concurrent or historical control groups in clinical trials. How do these arguments become more nuanced and difficult during pandemics or for people with high-mortality diseases who have nothing to lose?
3. What are the arguments for and against conducting controlled clinical trials during a public health emergency?
4. Fear and distrust often arise during pandemics (e.g., the Black Death, Ebola, and COVID-19) and seem to reflect universal patterns of human behavior. Propose some possible solutions, including methods of communication and community inclusion in clinical trials to mitigate these issues and rebuild trust and support in affected communities.

5. George Bernard Shaw remarked, "The single biggest problem in communication is the illusion that it has taken place." To avoid such illusion, discuss the critical importance of communication during a pandemic. Further, how can the fears of infectious disease perceived by the public be exacerbated by communication strategies intended to motivate action?
6. The fundamental ethical and scientific principles of clinical research have evolved since the Babylonian proto-trial of around 559 BCE. Contemporary principles of clinical research seem well established, but research study design, conduct, and location continue to stoke controversy. Discuss three overarching questions that arise from global efforts to mitigate the expanding number of microbial threats and implement effective interventions.

References

Adebamowo C, Bah-Sow O, Binka F, Bruzzone R, Caplan A, Delfraissy J-F, et al. Randomised controlled trials for Ebola: practical and ethical issues. Lancet. 2014;384(9952):1423–4. https://doi.org/10.1016/S0140-6736(14)61734-7.

AIDS: monolith. Richmond, UK: The National Archives; 1987.

Angius F, Pala G, Manzin A. SARS-CoV-2 and its variants: the pandemic of unvaccinated. Front Microbiol. 2021;12:749634. https://doi.org/10.3389/fmicb.2021.749634.

Appiah R. Community-based participatory research in rural African contexts: ethico-cultural considerations and lessons from Ghana. Public Health Rev. 2020;41(1):27. https://doi.org/10.1186/s40985-020-00145-2.

Bartholomew M. James Lind's treatise of the scurvy (1753). Postgrad Med J. 2002;78(925):695–6. https://doi.org/10.1136/pmj.78.925.695.

Baumfeld Andre E, Reynolds R, Caubel P, Azoulay L, Dreyer NA. Trial designs using real-world data: the changing landscape of the regulatory approval process. Pharmacoepidemiol Drug Saf. 2020;29(10):1201–12. https://doi.org/10.1002/pds.4932.

Berridge V, Strong P. AIDS policies in the United Kingdom: a preliminary analysis. In: Elizabeth Fee DMF, editor. AIDS: the making of a chronic disease. Berkeley: University of California Press; 1992. http://ark.cdlib.org/ark:/13030/ft9b69p35n/.

Blanc J, Brown FZ. Conflict zones in the time of coronavirus: war and war by other means. Washington, DC: Carnegie Endowment for International Peace; 2020.

Bollyky TJ, Brown CP. The tragedy of vaccine nationalism: only cooperation can end the pandemic. Foreign Aff. 2020;99(5):96.

Bou-Karroum L, El-Harakeh A, Kassamany I, Ismail H, El Arnaout N, Charide R, et al. Health care workers in conflict and post-conflict settings: systematic mapping of the evidence. PLoS One. 2020;15(5):e0233757. https://doi.org/10.1371/journal.pone.0233757.

Bousquet F, Fernandez-Taranco O. COVID-19 in fragile settings: ensuring a conflict-sensitive response. COVID-19 response. New York: United Nations; 2020.

Branswell H. How a Winnipeg lab became an Ebola research powerhouse. The Canadian Press; 2014.

Brolin Ribacke KJ, Saulnier DD, Eriksson A, von Schreeb J. Effects of the West Africa Ebola virus disease on health-care utilization—a systematic review. Front Public Health. 2016;4:222. https://doi.org/10.3389/fpubh.2016.00222.

Buyse M. Limitations of adaptive clinical trials. American Society of Clinical Oncology Educational Book, vol. 32. Alexandra, VA: American Society of Clinical Oncology; 2012. p. 133–7.

Canadian Institutes of Health Research. Showcasing a Canadian success story: the Ebola vaccine. Canadian Institutes of Health Research; 2015.

Capron AM. Henry Knowles Beecher, Jay Katz, and the transformation of research with human beings. Perspect Biol Med. 2016;59(1):55–77. https://doi.org/10.1353/pbm.2016.0025.

CDC. The Tuskegee timeline. Atlanta, GA: CDC; 2021. https://www.cdc.gov/tuskegee/timeline.htm. Accessed 17 May 2021.

Changing character of commercial penicillin, with suggestions as to the use of penicillin in syphilis. JAMA. 1946;131:271–5.

Choi MJ, Cossaboom CM, Whitesell AN, Dyal JW, Joyce A, Morgan RL, et al. Use of Ebola vaccine: recommendations of the Advisory Committee on Immunization Practices, United States, 2020. MMWR Recomm Rep. 2021;70(1):1–12. https://doi.org/10.15585/mmwr.rr7001a1.

Chow S-C, Chang M. Adaptive design methods in clinical trials. New York: Chapman and Hall; 2012.

CIOMS. International ethical guidelines for health-related research involving humans. Geneva: Council for International Organisations of Medical Sciences; 2016.

Cohen J. Congo's Ebola outbreak is all but over. Did an experimental vaccine help? Science. 2018; https://doi.org/10.1126/science.aau8236.

Collier R. Legumes, lemons and streptomycin: a short history of the clinical trial. CMAJ. 2009;180(1):23–4. https://doi.org/10.1503/cmaj.081879.
Cooperrider DL, Fry R. Appreciative inquiry in a pandemic: an improbable pairing. J Appl Behav Sci. 2020;56(3):266–71. https://doi.org/10.1177/0021886320936265.
Cooperrider DL, Whitney D. Appreciative inquiry: a positive revolution in change. San Francisco: Berrett-Koehler; 2005.
Corey L, Nabel GJ, Dieffenbach C, Gilbert P, Haynes BF, Johnston M, et al. HIV-1 vaccines and adaptive trial designs. Sci Transl Med. 2011;3(79):79ps13. https://doi.org/10.1126/scitranslmed.3001863.
Cuan-Baltazar JY, Muñoz-Perez MJ, Robledo-Vega C, Pérez-Zepeda MF, Soto-Vega E. Misinformation of COVID-19 on the internet: infodemiology study. JMIR Public Health Surveill. 2020;6(2):e18444. https://doi.org/10.2196/18444.
D'Arcy Hart P. A change in scientific approach: from alternation to randomised allocation in clinical trials in the 1940s. BMJ. 1999;319(7209):572–3. https://doi.org/10.1136/bmj.319.7209.572.
Darton TC, Blohmke CJ, Moorthy VS, Altmann DM, Hayden FG, Clutterbuck EA, et al. Design, recruitment, and microbiological considerations in human challenge studies. Lancet Infect Dis. 2015;15(7):840–51. https://doi.org/10.1016/s1473--3099(15)00068-7.
Dean NE, Gsell PS, Brookmeyer R, De Gruttola V, Donnelly CA, Halloran ME, et al. Design of vaccine efficacy trials during public health emergencies. Sci Transl Med. 2019;11(499). https://doi.org/10.1126/scitranslmed.aat0360.
Delamou A, Ayadi AME, Sidibe S, Delvaux T, Camara BS, Sandouno SD, et al. Effect of Ebola virus disease on maternal and child health services in Guinea: a retrospective observational cohort study. Lancet Glob Health. 2017;5(4):e448–e57. https://doi.org/10.1016/s2214-109x(17)30078-5.
Douglas J. The criterion: or, miracles examined with a view to expose the pretensions of pagans and papist. London: Millar; 1754.
Douglas JM Jr. Penicillin treatment of syphilis: clearing away the shadow on the land. JAMA. 2009;301(7):769–71. https://doi.org/10.1001/jama.2009.143.
Durrheim DN, Gostin LO, Moodley K. When does a major outbreak become a Public Health Emergency of International Concern? Lancet Infect Dis. 2020;20(8):887–9. https://doi.org/10.1016/s1473--3099(20)30401-1.
Ebola Communication Network. Anthropology and Ebola communication. Ebola Communication Network; 2015.
Ellenberg SS, Keusch GT, Babiker AG, Edwards KM, Lewis RJ, Lundgren JD, et al. Rigorous clinical trial design in public health emergencies is essential. Clin Infect Dis. 2018;66(9):1467–9. https://doi.org/10.1093/cid/cix1032.
Elsaid N, Ibrahim O, Abdel-Fatah ZF, Hassan HA, Hegazy MH, Anwar MM, et al. Violence against healthcare workers during coronavirus (COVID-19) pandemic in Egypt: a cross-sectional study. Egypt J Forensic Sci. 2022;12(1):45. https://doi.org/10.1186/s41935-022-00304-3.
FDA. Adaptive designs for clinical trials of drugs and biologics: guidance for industry. Silver Spring, MD: U.S. Food and Drug Administration; 2019.
Fenner F, Henderson D, Arita I, Ježek Z, Ladnyi I. Smallpox and its eradication. Geneva: World Health Organization; 1988.
Fleming TR, Ellenberg SS. Evaluating interventions for Ebola: the need for randomized trials. Clin Trials (London, England). 2016;13(1):6–9. https://doi.org/10.1177/1740774515616944.
Foege WH. Commentary: Smallpox eradication in West and Central Africa revisited. Bull World Health Organ. 1998;76(3):233–5.
Foege WH, Millar JD, Henderson DA. Smallpox eradication in West and Central Africa. Bull World Health Organ. 1975;52(2):209–22.
Freedman B. Equipoise and the ethics of clinical research. N Engl J Med. 1987;317(3):141–5.
Frieden T. Why the 'gold standard' of medical research is no longer enough. STAT; 2017a. https://www.statnews.com/2017/08/02/randomized-controlled-trials-medical-research/. Accessed 6 Sept 2021.
Frieden TR. Evidence for health decision making—beyond randomized, controlled trials. N Engl J Med. 2017b;377(5):465–75. https://doi.org/10.1056/NEJMra1614394.
Gabarron E, Oyeyemi SO, Wynn R. COVID-19-related misinformation on social media: a systematic review. Bull World Health Organ. 2021;99(6):455–63a. https://doi.org/10.2471/blt.20.276782.
GHSA. Global Health Security Agenda. 2022. https://ghsagenda.org/. Accessed 17 May 2022.
Goligher EC, Bradbury CA, McVerry BJ, Lawler PR, Berger JS, Gong MN, et al. Therapeutic anticoagulation with heparin in critically ill patients with Covid-19. N Engl J Med. 2021;385(9):777–89. https://doi.org/10.1056/NEJMoa2103417.
Grady C. Clinical trials. In: Crowley M, editor. Birth to death and bench to clinic: the Hastings Center bioethics briefing book for journalists, policymakers, and campaigns. Garrison, NY: The Hastings Center; 2008. p. 21–4.
Graham BS, Corbett KS. Prototype pathogen approach for pandemic preparedness: world on fire. J Clin Invest. 2020;130(7):3348–9. https://doi.org/10.1172/JCI139601.
Gretter L. The Nightingale pledge. The truth about nursing; 2020.
Gupta SK. Use of Bayesian statistics in drug development: advantages and challenges. Int J Appl Basic Med Res. 2012;2(1):3–6. https://doi.org/10.4103/2229-516x.96789.
Hariton E, Locascio JJ. Randomised controlled trials—the gold standard for effectiveness research: study

design: randomised controlled trials. BJOG. 2018;125(13):1716. https://doi.org/10.1111/1471-0528.15199.

Heller J. Syphilis victims in U.S. study went untreated for 40 years. New York Times. 1972.

Henao-Restrepo AM, Longini IM, Egger M, Dean NE, Edmunds WJ, Camacho A, et al. Efficacy and effectiveness of an rVSV-vectored vaccine expressing Ebola surface glycoprotein: interim results from the Guinea ring vaccination cluster-randomised trial. Lancet. 2015;386(9996):857–66. https://doi.org/10.1016/s0140-6736(15)61117-5.

Henao-Restrepo AM, Camacho A, Longini IM, Watson CH, Edmunds WJ, Egger M, et al. Efficacy and effectiveness of an rVSV-vectored vaccine in preventing Ebola virus disease: final results from the Guinea ring vaccination, open-label, cluster-randomised trial (Ebola Ca Suffit!). Lancet. 2017;389(10068):505–18. https://doi.org/10.1016/S0140-6736(16)32621-6.

HEW. Final report of the Tuskegee Syphilis Study Ad Hoc Advisory Panel. Washington, DC: U.S. Department of Health Education and Welfare; 1973.

Hunt A, Saenz C, Littler K. The Global Forum on Bioethics in Research meeting, "Ethics of alternative clinical trial designs and methods in low- and middle-income country research": emerging themes and outputs. Trials. 2019;20(Suppl 2):701. https://doi.org/10.1186/s13063-019-3840-3.

Independent Panel for Pandemic Preparedness & Response. The World Health Organization: an institutional review: background paper 15. Geneva: Independent Panel for Pandemic Preparedness & Response; 2021.

International Vaccines Task Force. Money and microbes: strengthening clinical research capacity to prevent epidemics. Washington, DC: World Bank; 2018.

Jansen-van der Weide MC, Gaasterland CMW, Roes KCB, Pontes C, Vives R, Sancho A, et al. Rare disease registries: potential applications towards impact on development of new drug treatments. Orphanet J Rare Dis. 2018;13(1):154. https://doi.org/10.1186/s13023-018-0836-0.

Jensen JS, Bielefeldt A, Hróbjartsson A. Active placebo control groups of pharmacological interventions were rarely used but merited serious consideration: a methodological overview. J Clin Epidemiol. 2017;87:35–46. https://doi.org/10.1016/j.jclinepi.2017.03.001.

Jütte R. The early history of the placebo. Complement Ther Med. 2013;21(2):94–7. https://doi.org/10.1016/j.ctim.2012.06.002.

Kamradt-Scott A. WHO's to blame? The World Health Organization and the 2014 Ebola outbreak in West Africa. Third World Q. 2016;37(3):401–18. https://doi.org/10.1080/01436597.2015.1112232.

Kaner J, Schaack S. Understanding Ebola: the 2014 epidemic. Global Health. 2016;12(1):53. https://doi.org/10.1186/s12992-016-0194-4.

Keusch GT, McAdam K. Clinical trials during epidemics. Lancet. 2017;389(10088):2455–7. https://doi.org/10.1016/s0140-6736(17)31602-1.

Kirk GD, Lesi OA, Mendy M, Akano AO, Sam O, Goedert JJ, et al. The Gambia Liver Cancer Study: infection with hepatitis B and C and the risk of hepatocellular carcinoma in West Africa. Hepatology. 2004;39(1):211–9. https://doi.org/10.1002/hep.20027.

Kluge H, Martín-Moreno JM, Emiroglu N, Rodier G, Kelley E, Vujnovic M, et al. Strengthening global health security by embedding the International Health Regulations requirements into national health systems. BMJ Glob Health. 2018;3(Suppl 1):e000656. https://doi.org/10.1136/bmjgh-2017-000656.

Larkin H. Navigating attacks against health care workers in the COVID-19 era. JAMA. 2021;325(18):1822–4. https://doi.org/10.1001/jama.2021.2701.

Lasagna L, Mosteller F, von Felsinger JM, Beecher HK. A study of the placebo response. Am J Med. 1954;16(6):770–9. https://doi.org/10.1016/0002--9343(54)90441-6.

Lau VI, Dhanoa S, Cheema H, Lewis K, Geeraert P, Lu D, et al. Non-COVID outcomes associated with the coronavirus disease-2019 (COVID-19) pandemic effects study (COPES): a systematic review and meta-analysis. PLoS One. 2022;17(6):e0269871. https://doi.org/10.1371/journal.pone.0269871.

Lawler PR, Goligher EC, Berger JS, Neal MD, McVerry BJ, Nicolau JC, et al. Therapeutic anticoagulation with heparin in noncritically ill patients with Covid-19. N Engl J Med. 2021;385(9):790–802. https://doi.org/10.1056/NEJMoa2105911.

Ledford H. International COVID-19 trial to restart with focus on immune responses. Nature. 2021; https://doi.org/10.1038/d41586-021-01090-z.

Lin CL, Kao JH. Hepatitis B: immunization and impact on natural history and cancer incidence. Gastroenterol Clin N Am. 2020;49(2):201–14. https://doi.org/10.1016/j.gtc.2020.01.010.

Lind J. A treatise on the scurvy. Printed by Sands, Murray and Cochran for A Kincaid and A Donaldson: Edinburgh; 1753.

Liu M, Li Q, Lin J, Lin Y, Hoffman E. Innovative trial designs and analyses for vaccine clinical development. Contemp Clin Trials. 2021;100:106225. https://doi.org/10.1016/j.cct.2020.106225.

London AJ. Social value, clinical equipoise, and research in a public health emergency. Bioethics. 2018;33(3):326–34. https://doi.org/10.1111/bioe.12467.

London AJ, Omotade OO, Mello MM, Keusch GT. Ethics of randomized trials in a public health emergency. PLOS Negl Trop Dis. 2018;12(5):e0006313. https://doi.org/10.1371/journal.pntd.0006313.

Lundgren JD, Grund B, Barkauskas CE, Holland TL, Gottlieb RL, Sandkovsky U, et al. A neutralizing monoclonal antibody for hospitalized patients with

Covid-19. N Engl J Med. 2021;384(10):905–14. https://doi.org/10.1056/NEJMoa2033130.

Lurie N, Saville M, Hatchett R, Halton J. Developing Covid-19 vaccines at pandemic speed. N Engl J Med. 2020;382(21):1969–73. https://doi.org/10.1056/NEJMp2005630.

Lurie N, Keusch GT, Dzau VJ. Urgent lessons from COVID 19: why the world needs a standing, coordinated system and sustainable financing for global research and development. Lancet. 2021;397(10280):1229–36. https://doi.org/10.1016/S0140-6736(21)00503-1.

Madelain V, Mentré F, Baize S, Anglaret X, Laouénan C, Oestereich L, et al. Modeling favipiravir antiviral efficacy against emerging viruses: from animal studies to clinical trials. CPT Pharmacometrics Syst Pharmacol. 2020;9(5):258–71. https://doi.org/10.1002/psp4.12510.

Mahajan R, Gupta K. Adaptive design clinical trials: methodology, challenges and prospect. Indian J Pharmacol. 2010;42(4):201–7. https://doi.org/10.4103/0253-7613.68417.

Mak IL, Wan EYF, Wong TKT, Lee WWJ, Chan EWY, Choi EPH, et al. The spill-over impact of the novel coronavirus-19 pandemic on medical care and disease outcomes in non-communicable diseases: a narrative review. Public Health Rev. 2022;43:1604121. https://doi.org/10.3389/phrs.2022.1604121.

Manguvo A, Mafuvadze B. The impact of traditional and religious practices on the spread of Ebola in West Africa: time for a strategic shift. Pan Afr Med J. 2015;22(Suppl 1):9. https://doi.org/10.11694/pamj.supp.2015.22.1.6190.

Marshall G, Blacklock J, Cameron C, Capon N, Cruickshank R. STREPTOMYCIN treatment of pulmonary tuberculosis. Br Med J. 1948;2(4582):769–82.

Martin GP, Hanna E, McCartney M, Dingwall R. Science, society, and policy in the face of uncertainty: reflections on the debate around face coverings for the public during COVID-19. Crit Public Health. 2020;30(5):501–8. https://doi.org/10.1080/09581596.2020.1797997.

Masresha BG, Luce R Jr, Weldegebriel G, Katsande R, Gasasira A, Mihigo R. The impact of a prolonged Ebola outbreak on measles elimination activities in Guinea, Liberia and Sierra Leone, 2014–2015. Pan Afr Med J. 2020;35(Suppl 1):8. https://doi.org/10.11604/pamj.supp.2020.35.1.19059.

McCoy T. Why the brutal murder of several Ebola workers may hint at more violence to come. Washington Post. 2014.

Millen GC, Yap C. Adaptive trial designs: what are multiarm, multistage trials? Arch Dis Child Educ Pract Ed. 2020;105(6):376–8. https://doi.org/10.1136/archdischild-2019-317826.

Millum J, Grady C, Keusch G, Sina B. Introduction: the Fogarty International Research Ethics Education and Curriculum Development Program in historical context. J Empir Res Hum Res Ethics. 2013;8(5):3–16. https://doi.org/10.1525/jer.2013.8.5.3.

Moberg J, Kramer M. A brief history of the cluster randomised trial design. J R Soc Med. 2015;108(5):192–8. https://doi.org/10.1177/0141076815582303.

Modell W, Houde RW. Factors influencing clinical evaluation of drugs; with special reference to the double-blind technique. JAMA J Am Med Assoc. 1958;167(18):2190–9. https://doi.org/10.1001/jama.1958.72990350005006.

Monrad JT. Ethical considerations for epidemic vaccine trials. J Med Ethics. 2020;46(7):465–9. https://doi.org/10.1136/medethics-2020-106235.

Moodley J, Naidoo S, Moodley J, Ramjee G. Sharing of investigational drug among participants in the Voice Trial. AIDS Behav. 2016;20(11):2709–14. https://doi.org/10.1007/s10461-016-1414-x.

Morens DM, Folkers GK, Fauci AS. The challenge of emerging and re-emerging infectious diseases. Nature. 2004;430(6996):242–9. https://doi.org/10.1038/nature02759.

Moritsugu K. China accuses US of politicizing COVID-19 origins research. Associated Press; 2021.

Motta M, Sylvester S, Callaghan T, Lunz-Trujillo K. Encouraging COVID-19 vaccine uptake through effective health communication. Front Polit Sci. 2021; https://doi.org/10.3389/fpos.2021.630133.

Mulangu S, Dodd LE, Davey RT Jr, Tshiani Mbaya O, Proschan M, Mukadi D, et al. A randomized, controlled trial of Ebola virus disease therapeutics. N Engl J Med. 2019;381(24):2293–303. https://doi.org/10.1056/NEJMoa1910993.

Munawar K, Kuhn SK, Haque S. Understanding the reminiscence bump: a systematic review. PLoS One. 2018;13(12):e0208595. https://doi.org/10.1371/journal.pone.0208595.

NASEM. Integrating clinical research into epidemic response: the Ebola experience. Washington, DC: National Academies of Sciences Engineering and Medicine Publications, National Academies Press; 2017.

NASEM. Strategies for building confidence in the COVID-19 vaccines. Washington, DC: National Academies of Sciences Engineering and Medicine Publications, National Academies Press; 2021.

National Commission for the Protection of Human Subjects of Biomedical and Behavioral Research. The Belmont report: ethical principles and guidelines for the protection of human subjects of research. Washington, DC: Department of Health, Education and Welfare; 1979. Contract No.: DHEW Publication No. (OS) 78-0012.

NCATS. A translational approach to addressing COVID-19. Bethesda, MD: National Center for Advancing Translational Sciences; 2021. https://ncats.nih.gov/covid19-translational-approach. Accessed 19 May 2022.

NIH. Accelerating COVID-19 therapeutic interventions and vaccines (ACTIV) governance. Bethesda, MD: National Institutes of Health; 2021. https://www.nih.gov/research-training/medical-research-initiatives/activ/governance. Accessed 26 Jul 2021.

NIHR. Clinical Research Network. 2022. https://www.nihr.ac.uk/explore-nihr/support/clinical-research-network.htm. Accessed 19 May 2022.

Nuernberg Military Tribunals. Trials of war criminals before the Nuernberg Military Tribunals under Control Law No. 10. Washington, DC: U.S. Government Printing Office; 1949.

Nuffield Council on Bioethics. The ethics of research related to healthcare in developing countries: a follow-up discussion paper based on the workshop held in Cape Town, South Africa 12–14th February 2004. London: Nuffield Council on Bioethics; 2005.

Nuffield Council on Bioethics. Research in global health emergencies: ethical issues. Oxford, UK: Nuffield Council on Bioethics; 2020.

Omoto AM, Snyder M. Sustained helping without obligation: motivation, longevity of service, and perceived attitude change among AIDS volunteers. J Pers Soc Psychol. 1995;68(4):671–86. https://doi.org/10.1037/0022-3514.68.4.671.

Our World in Data. Coronavirus (COVID-19) vaccinations. Oxford: Our World in Data; 2022. https://ourworldindata.org/covid-vaccinations. Accessed 20 May 2022.

Pallmann P, Bedding AW, Choodari-Oskooei B, Dimairo M, Flight L, Hampson LV, et al. Adaptive designs in clinical trials: why use them, and how to run and report them. BMC Med. 2018;16(1):29. https://doi.org/10.1186/s12916-018-1017-7.

Patulin Clinical Trials Committee. Clinical trial of patulin in the common cold: report of the Patulin Clinical Trials Committee, Medical Research Council. Lancet. 1944;244(6316):373–5. https://doi.org/10.1016/S0140-6736(00)45330-4.

Pessoa-Amorim G, Campbell M, Fletcher L, Horby P, Landray M, Mafham M, et al. Making trials part of good clinical care: lessons from the RECOVERY trial. Future Healthc J. 2021;8(2):e243–e50. https://doi.org/10.7861/fhj.2021-0083.

Pocock SJ. The combination of randomized and historical controls in clinical trials. J Chronic Dis. 1976;29(3):175–88. https://doi.org/10.1016/0021--9681(76)90044-8.

Potter C, Brough R. Systemic capacity building: a hierarchy of needs. Health Policy Plan. 2004;19(5):336–45. https://doi.org/10.1093/heapol/czh038.

Prevail II Writing Group. A randomized, controlled trial of ZMapp for Ebola virus infection. N Engl J Med. 2016;375(15):1448–56.

Rådelius E. "Shout to the people the reality, and they dance it!" A case study on the synergies and challenges between music, youth empowerment, sustainable development and social change in The Gambia. Bachelor thesis in Music and Education, Luleå University of Technology, Luleå, SE; 2016.

Rao CB, Peatfield JC, McAdam K, Nunn AJ, Georgieva DP. A focus on the reminiscence bump to personalize music playlists for dementia. J Multidiscip Healthc. 2021;14:2195–204. https://doi.org/10.2147/jmdh.S312725.

RECOVERY trial. University of Oxford, Oxford. 2022. https://www.recoverytrial.net/. Accessed 15 Apr 2022.

Regulatory Affairs Professionals Society. COVID-19 vaccine tracker. Rockville, MD: Regulatory Affairs Professionals Society; 2023. https://www.raps.org/news-and-articles/news-articles/2020/3/covid-19-vaccine-tracker. Accessed 13 Mar 2023.

Research Fairness Initiative. Council on Health Research for Development COHRED. 2022. https://rfi.cohred.org/. Accessed 15 May 2022.

Rockwell DH, Yobs AR, Moore MB Jr. The Tuskegee study of untreated syphilis; the 30th year of observation. Arch Intern Med. 1964;114:792–8. https://doi.org/10.1001/archinte.1964.03860120104011.

Roelcke V. Nazi medicine and research on human beings. Lancet. 2004;364:6–7. https://doi.org/10.1016/s0140-6736(04)17619-8.

Rogers AB, Barrie MB, Fallah MP, Kelly JD. Equitable and feasible distribution of SARS-CoV-2 vaccines for all in Africa. Am J Trop Med Hyg. 2021;105(2):278–80. https://doi.org/10.4269/ajtmh.21-0264.

Salma J, Giri D. Engaging immigrant and racialized communities in community-based participatory research during the COVID-19 pandemic: challenges and opportunities. Int J Qualitat Methods. 2021;20:16094069211036293. https://doi.org/10.1177/16094069211036293.

Schindell B, Kindrachuk J, Kuppalli K. What the 2018 DRC Ebola epidemic taught us about outbreak response and experimental countermeasures. Contagion. 2020;5(2).

Schoenfeld DA, Finkelstein DM, Macklin E, Zach N, Ennist DL, Taylor AA, et al. Design and analysis of a clinical trial using previous trials as historical control. Clin Trials (London, England). 2019;16(5):531–8. https://doi.org/10.1177/1740774519858914.

SeyedAlinaghi S, Karimi A, Barzegary A, Pashaei Z, Afsahi AM, Alilou S, et al. Mucormycosis infection in patients with COVID-19: a systematic review. Health Sci Rep. 2022;5(2):e529. https://doi.org/10.1002/hsr2.529.

Shapiro AK, Shapiro E. The powerful placebo, from ancient priest to modern physician. Baltimore, MD: Johns Hopkins University Press; 1997.

Shuster E. Fifty years later: the significance of the Nuremberg Code. N Engl J Med. 1997;337(20):1436–40. https://doi.org/10.1056/nejm199711133372006.

Sissoko D, Laouenan C, Folkesson E, M'Lebing AB, Beavogui AH, Baize S, et al. Experimental treatment with favipiravir for Ebola virus disease (the JIKI Trial): a historically controlled, single-arm proof-of-concept trial in Guinea. PLoS Med. 2016;13(3):e1001967. https://doi.org/10.1371/journal.pmed.1001967.

Smith CM. Origin and uses of primum non nocere—above all, do no harm! J Clin Pharmacol. 2005;45(4):371–7. https://doi.org/10.1177/0091270004273680.

Sotos JG. Zebra cards: an aid to obscure diagnosis. American College of Physicians; 1989.

Sun X, Samba TT, Yao J, Yin W, Xiao L, Liu F, et al. Impact of the Ebola outbreak on routine immunization in western area, Sierra Leone—a field survey from an Ebola epidemic area. BMC Public Health. 2017;17(1):363. https://doi.org/10.1186/s12889-017-4242-7.

Thorlund K, Haggstrom J, Park JJ, Mills EJ. Key design considerations for adaptive clinical trials: a primer for clinicians. BMJ. 2018;360:k698. https://doi.org/10.1136/bmj.k698.

Timothy JWS, Hall Y, Akoi-Boré J, Diallo B, Tipton TRW, Bower H, et al. Early transmission and case fatality of Ebola virus at the index site of the 2013–2016 west African Ebola outbreak: a cross-sectional seroprevalence survey. Lancet Infect Dis. 2019;19(4):429–38. https://doi.org/10.1016/s1473--3099(18)30791-6.

U.S. Holocaust Memorial Museum. Nazi racial science. Washington, DC: U.S. Holocaust Memorial Museum; 2022. https://www.ushmm.org/collections/bibliography/nazi-racial-science. Accessed 14 May 2022.

van der Linden S. Misinformation: susceptibility, spread, and interventions to immunize the public. Nat Med. 2022;28(3):460–7. https://doi.org/10.1038/s41591-022-01713-6.

Veatch RM. Clinical trials vs. right to try: ethical use of chloroquine for Covid-19, Clinical trials & research ethics. Covid-19 Ethics Resource Center, Hastings Bioethics Forum; 2020.

Viele K, Berry S, Neuenschwander B, Amzal B, Chen F, Enas N, et al. Use of historical control data for assessing treatment effects in clinical trials. Pharm Stat. 2014;13(1):41–54. https://doi.org/10.1002/pst.1589.

von Wernsdorff M, Loef M, Tuschen-Caffier B, Schmidt S. Effects of open-label placebos in clinical trials: a systematic review and meta-analysis. Sci Rep. 2021;11(1):3855. https://doi.org/10.1038/s41598--021-83148-6.

Wagner CE, Saad-Roy CM, Morris SE, Baker RE, Mina MJ, Farrar J, et al. Vaccine nationalism and the dynamics and control of SARS-CoV-2. Science. 2021;373(6562):eabj7364. https://doi.org/10.1126/science.abj7364.

Weindling P, von Villiez A, Loewenau A, Farron N. The victims of unethical human experiments and coerced research under National Socialism. Endeavour. 2016;40(1):1–6. https://doi.org/10.1016/j.endeavour.2015.10.005.

Weingarten S. Food in Daniel 1:5–16: the first report of a controlled experiment? JLL Bulletin: Commentaries on the history of treatment evaluation; 2018.

Wells CR, Pandey A, Ndeffo Mbah ML, Gauzere BA, Malvy D, Singer BH, et al. The exacerbation of Ebola outbreaks by conflict in the Democratic Republic of the Congo. Proc Natl Acad Sci U S A. 2019a;116(48):24366–72. https://doi.org/10.1073/pnas.1913980116.

Wells CR, Pandey A, Parpia AS, Fitzpatrick MC, Meyers LA, Singer BH, et al. Ebola vaccination in the Democratic Republic of the Congo. Proc Natl Acad Sci U S A. 2019b;116(20):10178–83. https://doi.org/10.1073/pnas.1817329116.

WHO. Ebola virus disease in Guinea. Geneva: World Health Organization; 2014.

WHO. Key events in the WHO response to the Ebola outbreak. Geneva: World Health Organization; 2015a.

WHO. One year into the Ebola epidemic: a deadly, tenacious and unforgiving virus. Geneva: World Health Organization; 2015b.

WHO. Human challenge trials for vaccine development: regulatory considerations. Geneva: WHO Expert Committee on Biological Standardization; 2016a. Contract No.: WHO Technical Report Series, No. 1004, 2017, Annex 10.

WHO. International Health Regulations (2005). 3rd ed. Geneva: World Health Organization; 2016b.

WHO. Community engagement framework for quality, people-centred and resilient health services. Geneva: WHO; 2017a.

WHO. Emergency response framework. 2nd ed. Geneva: World Health Organization; 2017b.

WHO. UNICEF, WHO, IFRC and MSF announce the establishment of a global Ebola vaccine stockpile. New York: World Health Organization; 2021a.

WHO. What is the Access to COVID-19 Tools (ACT) Accelerator, how is it structured and how does it work? Geneva: WHO; 2021b.

WHO. COVAX calls for urgent action to close vaccine equity gap. Geneva: World Health Organization; 2022a.

WHO. Emergencies. Geneva: World Health Organization; 2022b. https://www.who.int/emergencies/overview. Accessed 16 May 2022.

WHO. WHO COVID-19 solidarity trial vaccines. Geneva: World Health Organization; 2022c. https://www.who.int/emergencies/diseases/novel--coronavirus-2019/global-research-on-novel-coronavirus-2019-ncov/solidarity-trial-of-covid-19-vaccines. Accessed 7 Sept 2022.

WHO Solidarity Trial Consortium. Repurposed antiviral drugs for Covid-19—interim WHO Solidarity Trial results. N Engl J Med. 2021;384(6):497–511. https://doi.org/10.1056/NEJMoa2023184.

Wilkinson S. Using media and communication to respond to public health emergencies: lessons learned from Ebola. London: BBC Media Action; 2016.

Williams CL. Leading the charge: Médecins Sans Frontières receives the 2015 Lasker~Bloomberg Public Service Award. J Clin Invest. 2015;125(10):3737–41. https://doi.org/10.1172/jci84349.

WMA. Declaration of Helsinki: recommendations guiding doctors in clinical research. Helsinki: World Medical Association; 1964.

WMA. Declaration of Helsinki: ethical principles for medical research involving human subjects. Ferney-Voltaire, FR: World Medical Association; 2013.

Wolf J, Jannat R, Dubey S, Troth S, Onorato MT, Coller B-A, et al. Development of pandemic vaccines: ERVEBO case study. Vaccines (Basel). 2021;9(3):190. https://doi.org/10.3390/vaccines9030190.

World Bank. Fragility, conflict & violence. Washington, DC: World Bank; 2022a. https://www.worldbank.org/en/topic/fragilityconflictviolence. Accessed 31 Aug 2022.

World Bank. Fragility, conflict, and violence. Washington, DC: World Bank; 2022b. https://www.worldbank.org/en/topic/fragilityconflictviolence. Accessed 18 May 2022.

3 Guiding Principles for Emergency Research Response

Elizabeth S. Higgs

Contents

Learning Track Note: This chapter appears in Learning Tracks: Clinical Research; Global Health; Global Health Law; Health Policy, Multilateral Cooperation, International Governance; Public Health and Epidemiology; Research Ethics; Social Science Response Research

E. S. Higgs and R. A. Sorenson (eds.), *Principles and Practice of Emergency Research Response*, https://doi.org/10.1007/978-3-031-48408-7_3

Learning Objectives

This chapter will help readers understand and describe:

- The goals of an emergency research response to an emerging or re-emerging infectious disease outbreak.
- Six basic principles based on past infectious disease emergencies:
  - Principle 1: Research should be an integral part of preparedness and emergency response.
  - Principle 2: Research response must align with the three primary goals of an emergency response to: (a) save lives, (b) accelerate the end of the outbreak, and (c) develop measures to prevent and mitigate future outbreaks.
  - Principle 3: Response research should be implemented quickly and efficiently based on outbreak preparedness plans.
  - Principle 4: The scientific and ethical norms for human subject research do not change during health emergencies.
  - Principle 5: Research response should be led by the government of the country experiencing the health emergency.
  - Principle 6: Understanding cultures and communities through respectful dialogue ("Nothing about them without them") and including them as valued stakeholders in response efforts are critical to research in health emergencies.
- Some previous objections to inclusion of expedited research in emergency response
- More recent experience that has rendered the objections obsolete

1 Introduction

The debate is over. Following successive infectious disease outbreaks and pandemics resulting in millions of lives lost and dramatic economic disruptions, the world in 2024 accepts that immediate research response to infectious disease outbreaks is imperative for a secure world, and a key safeguard against loss of life, economic devastation, and social disruption (G7 2021; WHO 2022). The world is far from an ideal state of preparedness—one where all known pathogens have licensed, safe, and effective medical countermeasures approved, produced at scale, with widespread knowledge on optimal use among physicians, and a population ready to accept them. A prepared global clinical trial infrastructure conducting ongoing, rigorous clinical trials on endemic pathogens and pathogens of pandemic potential is essential to this preparedness state. Ideally, all nation-states will contribute to preparedness by developing a robust national clinical trial capacity.

There have been research response successes, yielding new vaccines, therapeutics, and diagnostics (VTDs) for pathogens with pandemic potential. For example, over the past decade, research responses have advanced medical countermeasures (MCMs) to contain and mitigate infectious diseases, such as Ebola virus disease (EVD) and coronavirus disease 2019 (COVID-19). Despite progress in these areas, additional severe acute respiratory syndrome coronavirus-2 (SARS-CoV-2) vaccine research is needed to elicit broader neutralization activity against continuously emerging sub-lineages and variants, and to achieve longer-lasting immunity after SARS-CoV-2 vaccination. Likewise, for Ebola virus the current 35% mortality in treated patients is unacceptably high; without a correlation of immunity, uncertainty remains on the need and intervals for vaccine boosting to ensure health care workers in increasingly endemic areas are protected.

The development of VTDs for existing and future emerging infectious disease pathogens requires clinical trials to generate reliable evidence for both safety and efficacy. Even when a vaccine or therapeutic is approved by the animal rule, as was the case for the 2022 mpox pandemic, research is needed to ensure that the products are safe and effective in the populations requiring their use. Though the need might seem obvious, the world has repeatedly demonstrated a short memory regarding the necessity of clinical research and the resources to ensure preparedness. Political and scientific leadership must work towards a standing global clinical research capacity that is continually ready to pivot towards strong clinical trials in the event of a health emergency. And though emergency research response must comply with international norms for the design, conduct, and human subject protections, it is not "business as usual" in terms of design, leadership, and speed.

Thus, a new field of research response and preparedness for health emergencies has emerged, requiring norms for the generation of timely, reliable actionable evidence. Research goals for any infectious disease health emergency include reducing mortality, accelerating the end of transmisison, and development of new tools to prevent and mitigate future outbreaks of the pathogen. By way of example, COVID-19 vaccines reduced mortality from the pandemic to a degree that is difficult to estimate; some inkling of the scale is suggested by a study estimating that COVID-19 vaccines averted about 300,000 deaths in Brazil alone in the first year of the vaccination program there (Santos et al. 2023). Over time, and with each research response, we are learning both what should be done and what should not be done to answer research questions effectively and efficiently. Having moved beyond the normative discussion about whether research should be part of emergency response, this chapter attempts to distill the wisdom collected over the past many health emergencies into six practical, normative principles for an effective research response. Experience and reflection have shown that compliance with these principles is both morally and pragmatically necessary for a successful research response.

Box 1: Six Principles to Guide Research Response

1. Research is an integral part of preparedness and emergency research response.
2. Research response must align with the three primary goals of an emergency response to: (a) save lives, (b) accelerate the end of the outbreak, and (c) develop measures to prevent and mitigate future outbreaks.
3. Research response should be implemented quickly and efficiently based on outbreak preparedness plans.
4. The scientific and ethical norms for human subject research do not change during a health emergency.
5. Research response should be led by the country experiencing the health emergency.
6. Good participatory practice (GPP) applies to research in health emergencies.

2 Principles

2.1 Principle 1: Research Should Be an Integral Part of Preparedness and Emergency Response

Integrating research into preparedness plans and early response efforts facilitates a successful research response and ensures that the research response is aligned with, and synergizes with, other response pillars. Clear early research leadership and response during a health emergency helps minimize proliferation of research that does not contribute to critical response efforts and can undermine it by using scarce resources and producing erroneous conclusions (Bugin and Woodcock 2021; Hanney et al. 2022).

There are many ways, at the country, regional, and global levels, that preparedness planning enables integration of early research response into overall response efforts. A primary means of ensuring preparedness is politically supported, continually operating clinical research infrastructure which pivots immediately to research response in a health emergency. Such capacity should be built on national clinical research capacity linked globally to tackle endemic diseases of concern to countries and regions and prepared to coordinate implementation of emergency response research when necessary. It is imper-

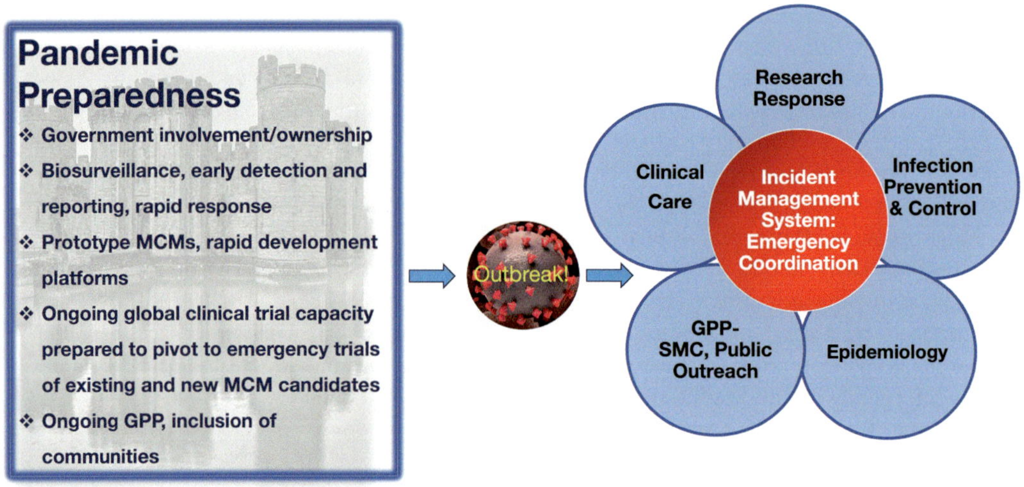

Fig. 1 Interacting elements of preparedness and response planning. *GPP-SMC* Good Participatory Practice-Social Mobilization, Communication, and Community Engagement, *MCMs* medical countermeasures. (Elizabeth Higgs and Robert Sorenson)

ative that research capacity is both supported by and responsive to governments to enable host country leadership of research response during emergencies. Countries can prepare for research response by adding a research pillar to their response structure and incident management systems, which ensures research interaction and integration with appropriate synergistic pillars, e.g., community engagement, case management, etc. The integration (Fig. 1) of the research pillar into the Incidence Management System was used successfully as early as 2014 by Liberia in West African Ebola outbreak (Brooks et al. 2016; Fallah et al. 2023).

Likewise, national research response leadership should be identified in advance. Doing so avoids delays, as identified leadership enables advance preparation of protocols for known pathogens. Clinical research capacity and the expertise necessary to implement rigorous, regulatory-level clinical trials must be in place and functioning. Ideally, an ongoing research capacity serving as a "warm base" for a quick transition to emergency research is already part of a global clinical research network. In non-emergency circumstances, the network can collaborate on pandemic preparedness research or on endemic diseases of local importance. In an emergency, a research site already working in the community can turn to emergency response more quickly and effectively than any outside effort. Its research can also be extended and integrated with other research response locations if the outbreak grows into an epidemic or pandemic.

Funders and governments should support global clinical research networks inclusive of geographic locations where there is a high likelihood of zoonotic infections in humans—not coincidentally, these are places likely to need better research capacity (Moorthy et al. 2024) (▶ Chap. 10). It is also necessary, both for ongoing and emergency research, that clinical research capacity include both inpatients and outpatients. A commitment to continuous clinical research facilitates advances in clinical care and population health and enables the development of equitable, global clinical trial capacity. Global "always on and always prepared" clinical trial capacity will ensure sufficient access to diverse populations enabling generalizable trial results. Interpandemic clinical research against endemic diseases, especially in the Global South will: benefit local populations by advancing MCMs and standards of care for endemic infectious diseases; attract support from governments, foundations, and international organizations; enrich popular understanding of research; and ensure preparedness to pivot to rapid research response in an emergency. Inclusion of response research in strategic planning for health emergencies helps ensure transparency, clear communication, advance engagement of communities with research plans, and integration of research into preparedness and response. Finally, advance planning can mitigate reactivity and research opportunism when an infectious disease emergency emerges.

2.2 Principle 2: Research Response Should Align with the Goals of the Health Emergency

The three primary goals of a response to an infectious disease emergency are to: (1) avert suffering and save lives, (2) accelerate the end of the emergency, and (3) identify tools to prevent and mitigate future outbreaks. Well-intentioned research that generates knowledge but does not align with the goals of the outbreak response during a health emergency can undermine the response in a myriad of ways, such as diverting resources needed for response, confusing communities, creating distrust, competing for research participants, etc. Research which undermines a response is arguably unethical. There are examples of well-intentioned research efforts with negative unintended consequences in almost every outbreak. The aim of aligning research with outbreak priorities is to leverage scientific innovation, capacity, and resources to address imperative outbreak goals.

A prioritized research agenda is an essential tool to outline the most pressing research questions posed by an outbreak and to choose the methodology for seeking answers that will most expeditiously contribute to outbreak goals. Every potential research endeavor during an outbreak should be evaluated for alignment with the three primary response goals. Those with the greatest potential benefit should be prioritized first; those unaligned with these goals or not meeting rigorous scientific and ethical standards should be dropped. A clear understanding of this principle by response and preparedness leaders will result in calm clarity of priorities once an emergency ensues, facilitating focus on the most critical elements of a research response. A well-planned research response will include coordination to allocate sufficient research resources to each prioritized goal and minimize duplicative research. All elements of the research system, including funders, oversight bodies such as data and safety monitoring boards (DSMBs), institutional review boards aka research ethics committees (IRBs or RECs), ministries of health and regulatory agencies, as well as preclinical and clinical investigators, have a responsibility to ensure that research conducted during an infectious disease emergency is scientifically and ethically rigorous and aligns with the emergency response goals.

2.3 Principle 3: Research Response Should Be Implemented Quickly and Efficiently Based on Outbreak Preparedness Plans

Time is of the essence in research response. Infectious disease health emergencies, simply by virtue of ongoing transmission of a pathogen with epidemic and/or pandemic potential, require immediate response. In the case of outbreaks, as opposed to larger or longer epidemics or pandemics, there may be only a limited window to launch and complete critical research. For a long list of known pathogens, outbreaks provide the only opportunity to acquire human safety and efficacy data for candidate therapeutics and clinical efficacy data for vaccines. Unfortunately, due to lack of preparedness, the brief opportunity to launch critical research has often been missed. This was a concern, for example, for the 2022 Sudan virus disease[1] outbreak in Uganda. Despite availability of candidate vaccines and therapeutics for Sudan virus, there were sev-

1 The common name Sudan virus is now used for *Sudan ebolavirus*, with the corresponding disease name Sudan virus disease (Kuhn 2017; Kuhn et al. 2019).

eral impediments to immediate clinical trial implementation, even though there was a great deal of clinical research capacity in neighboring Uganda. The primary problem, therefore, was not ability to rapidly conduct a research response, but research capacity that was not responsive to government priorities. Issues cited by others included absence of a protocol, inadequate supplies of investigational products to conduct the studies, and absence of clarity on research leadership prior to the emergency (Branswell 2022). To plan for success, we must prepare to quickly launch research programs to better understand the natural history and to evaluate the safety and efficacy of novel investigational products. Research priorities at the outset of an outbreak will depend largely on the etiologic pathogen and status of licensed and candidate VTDs. Nevertheless, there are anticipated evidence needs that apply to most outbreaks caused by a novel, re-emerging, or known pathogen, and, therefore, much research and epidemiologic investigation can be planned in advance.

A long list of evidence needs for novel emerging pathogens can be anticipated, including but not limited to:

- Pathogen identification and characterization
- Investigation of modes of transmission and pathogen viability on various surfaces
- Development of novel diagnostics
- Assessment of efficacy of non-pharmaceutical interventions to prevent spread
- Natural history studies to:
  - Elucidate pathogenesis
  - Characterize disease natural history and stages
  - Understand the role of existing comorbidities
- Demographics of high-risk groups
- Pathogen tropism, replication, persistence, and shedding
- Immunologic responses
- Correlates of protective immunity

Rigorous clinical trial protocols can be developed in advance, including platform randomized clinical trials with the necessary flexibility to further accelerate research response timelines. Early evidence can inform standards of care, health care equipment needs, and hospitalization projections. Early characterization of pathogens and pathogenesis elucidates potential mechanisms for putative therapeutics and enables screening of therapeutic candidates.

The prototype pathogen approach will advance preparedness for families of pathogens with pandemic potential, for example by developing VTD candidates for at least one additional virus in each of the virus families known to infect humans (Cassetti et al. 2022). Clinical research priorities for known pathogens can be identified in advance. Ideally therapeutic and vaccine candidates developed under the prototype pathogen approach will be in the pipeline, having completed Phase I, first-in-human studies, and with adequate investigational product supply ready for additional safety and efficacy studies when needed. Other innovations to speed the development of VTDs include well-tested "plug and play" vaccine platforms into which a gene sequence from a new pathogen can be inserted (▶ Chap. 12) and continual work to refine and accelerate computerized screening of small molecules for potential activity against novel pathogens (Bhati et al. 2021).

The entire research ecosystem must plan for speed in response to a pathogen with pandemic potential. Means to ensure this happens are discussed throughout this book. A few of them follow.

- Preapproved protocols which span outbreaks and countries
- Pre-identified research response leadership
- Rapid response teams
- Building local research capacity globally
- Emergency operating procedures for oversight bodies such as DSMBs, ethics review boards, and regulatory agencies
- Planning to accomplish needed actions concurrently rather than sequentially

Similarly, development plans for candidate VTDs need to ensure adequate supply of investigational products and prepositioned agreements for importation to countries where the pathogen has been found previously and, where possible, for advancing candidate VTD research through to Phase IIa. Once research is ongoing, study designs must be efficient, flexible, and adaptive to quickly incorporate findings (▶ Chaps. 22 and 23). We must plan to be successful.

There are known challenges to expedited research response at the global level which can be addressed in interpandemic periods. Many of these obstacles could be addressed through global cooperation, including differential requirements for individual country-level regulatory and ethical review, varying manufacturing practice, and complex labeling requirements. Advance protocol and ethical review, as well as import approvals for investigational products, should be possible for known pathogens, such as Ebola Zaïre in at-risk countries where the Ebola Zaïre virus has caused outbreaks in the past.[2]

2.4 Principle 4: The Scientific and Ethical Norms for Human Subject Research Do Not Change During a Health Emergency

The norms for scientific rigor and human subject protections do not change in an outbreak. Put another way, urgency is no excuse for either poor quality or unethical science (▶ Chap. 4 and In Practice 4.2) (NASEM 2017). To be ethical, clinical research must be both scientifically valid and adhere to international norms for human subject protections. Scientifically valid research by definition is designed to generate reliable, actionable evidence to support the outbreak goals (Principle 2). This does not preclude but rather requires innovation in trial design, implementation, consent processes, data capture, etc. The World Health Assembly recognized the need to strengthen global clinical trials to improve health security in 2022 by passing WHA Resolution 75.8, "Strengthening Clinical Trials to Provide High-Quality Evidence on Health Interventions and to Improve Research Quality and Coordination." During the COVID-19 pandemic poor quality clinical trial design and conduct resulted in significant research waste. Actionable, ethical, reliable clinical trials assessing the safety and efficacy of candidate vaccines and therapeutics must adhere to the accepted international norms as codified in CIOMS, the Declaration of Helsinki, and ICH guidance etc.

In resource-poor areas, the realities on the ground may need to be adapted to the needs of the research. This may mean substantial investments in host-country capacities, community outreach, and education in order to conduct the research, leveraging both partner and host country capabilities. The response to the 2014–2016 West Africa Ebola epidemic showed that this can be done in the midst of an emergency, even in a low-resource setting (NASEM 2017). With increasing recognition of the need to enhance global clinical research capacity to address inequity and share the benefits of the social value of research, especially in lower-income countries, preparedness activities should include a spectrum of initiatives to improve readiness in all countries (▶ Chap. 8) (WHO 2022).

2.5 Principle 5: Research Response Should Be Led by the Government of the Country Experiencing the Health Emergency

All United Nations member states have agreed to respect the sovereignty of country governments (with rare exceptions) (UN 1945). Though accepted and legally binding on states, this principle is repeatedly violated by well-meaning global actors, including other countries, non-governmental agencies (NGOs), academics, and external public

2 Ebola virus disease (EVD), the term formerly used for disease caused by any member of the genus *ebolavirus,* now officially denotes only disease caused by the species *Zaire ebolavirus.* The diseases caused by *Sudan ebolavirus* and *Bundibugyo ebolavirus* are now called Sudan virus disease (SVD) and Bundibugyo virus disease (BVD), respectively (Kuhn 2017; Kuhn et al. 2019).

health entities including international organizations. Preparedness plans are often misaligned with the clear need for the local government to lead response efforts, including research response.

The vulnerabilities of populations experiencing health emergencies are discussed elsewhere (▶ Chaps. 16 and 17), and the host government, with sovereign authority over its resources and territory, as well as leadership of the outbreak response, is best placed to ensure rapid implementation of research and application of research results. Host country leadership facilitates institutional and cultural understanding and the adaptations necessary to design and implement the research according to GPP, so that appropriate stakeholders are involved. Furthermore, in-country leaders may be best equipped to integrate research into overall response social mobilization, risk communication, and community engagement efforts. It may still be critical for the host country leadership, often the ministry of health, to shift operational authority to local and community leadership, which is often far more trusted by the population than central leadership. An early understanding of what information sources populations and social groups trust is needed for effective communication.

It should be noted that failed nation states offer special challenges. Not all governments have effective control or legitimacy over all their territory and people (▶ Chap. 16). In such cases, tragedy may ensue, as with cholera in Haiti or polio in Syria (Mbaeyi et al. 2021; Piarroux et al. 2022).

Lack of clear central national leadership during a health emergency can result in an uncoordinated, ineffective response (Muldoon et al. 2021). During interpandemic times, continuously operating research capacity must be developed and supported by governments so that capacity is responsive to government priorities. In low- and middle-income countries, governments may enter into partnerships with

Box 2: Why Government-Responsive Clinical Research Capacity Is Essential to Global Health Security

- Ensures ongoing support for needed clinical research capacities, ideally via a global clinical research infrastructure, continuously conducting needed clinical research on endemic diseases that burden populations where the research is conducted (national or regional). The clinical research capacity would be able to pivot quickly to emergency research response as determined by governments.
- Enables government to government partnerships for enhancing training, research capacity, and infrastructure development before an outbreak.
- Enables government to government regional clinical research coordination.
- Enables pre-positioned protocols through national regulatory bodies and RECs/IRBs for known re-emerging pathogens.
- Aligns research with country evidence needs with focus on population-level scale.
- Enables Good Participatory Practice.
- Ensures integration of research into response early in outbreak.
- Enables leveraging of country resources and talent during outbreak.
- Ensures coordination of research within country in alignment with country needs.
- Ensures consideration and preparation for scale of need for products after licensure (◘ Fig. 2).

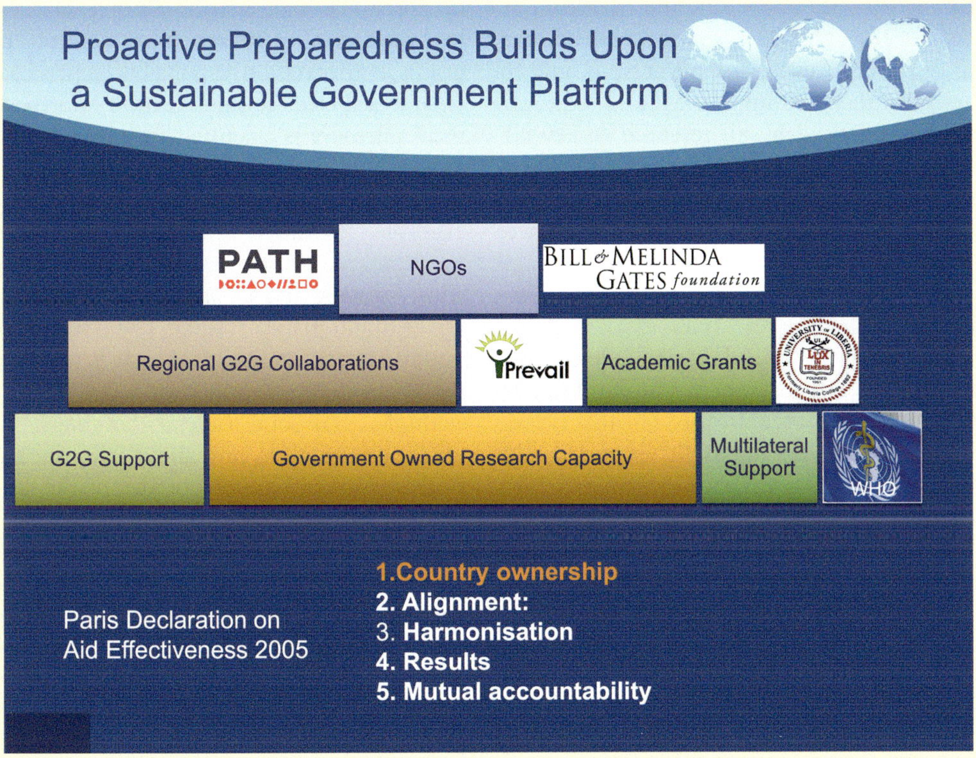

Fig. 2 The availability of government-owned clinical research capacity facilitates rapid research response. (Author)

other governments, foundations, international organizations, or the private sector to build capacity (▶ Chap. 8). A positive exemplar of government-responsive research capacity is integration of clinical research into the nationalized health system in the UK, which enabled the RECOVERY trial and other COVID-19 research (▶ In Practice 14.1). Fragmented research capacities unaligned with the government's prioritized research agenda during an emergency will likely result in wasted resources and ill-advised, if well-intentioned research detracting from more rigorous, coordinated research not only by diverting resources, but by generating flawed results (Bugin and Woodcock 2021).

A potential solution to the need to shift responsibility and authority to local governments for health emergencies is to develop research preparedness and response agreements under a political–scientific alliance.

2.6 Principle 6: Good Participatory Practice Applies to Research in Health Emergencies

"Nothing about them without them" is an axiomatic principle in development circles, acknowledging that well-intended efforts can be completely ineffectual or harmful unless they incorporate understanding of local culture, beliefs, rumors, community structures, and resources. Respect for all persons, and by extension their communities and cultures, must be practiced by all research stakeholders: research participants, community members, research staff, program and response managers, governments, funders, etc. There are many stakeholders—by definition, all those who are impacted by research or those who can impact the research.

The only way to understand cultures and communities is engagement via dialogue. In anthropological research this can take years, but basic understanding and trust can also be created in the face of emergencies, even though they may be fraught with dangers aside from infectious pathogens. Emergencies exacerbate existing mistrust in authorities and increase susceptibility to rumors, false information, and conspiracy theories. Emergencies are prime opportunities for paternalistic behavior by outsiders who make assumptions about what is and is not acceptable to participants, families, or communities with the excuse that the emergency does not allow time for nuances.

Good participatory practice (GPP) and its near equivalent in many African countries, social mobilization, communications, and community engagement (SMC), are not a nicety but a necessity in a health emergency. Following the West Africa 2014–2016 Ebola outbreak, in an effort to ensure that local participants, communities, and local health authorities were respected, heard, and treated respectfully, WHO adapted GPP, originally developed for HIV clinical trials, to pathogens with pandemic potential (WHO 2016). These were revised again in 2020, among other efforts to tailor community outreach to emergency situations (▶ Chap. 18) (Hankins et al. 2007; WHO 2020). Full community engagement is a necessary part of an effective response for pragmatic as well as ethical reasons. Though social science research can deepen GPP, in an emergency one can still understand and engage with relevant perspectives by involving communities and community leaders directly in the design and conduct of research—one reason among many for bringing local partners into research programs at all levels of responsibility. In a health emergency, clear communication informed by local partners is essential. In a given culture or community, even an English word can mean very different things. In Liberia for example, "research" in many communities was understood as something that is done with animals, and a "trial" was a process in the criminal justice system. The issue is compounded when multiple languages are in use: the Democratic Republic of the Congo, for example, has one official language, four national languages, and about 200 other languages spoken in the country (Translators without Borders 2022).

As seen in ◘ Fig. 3, stakeholders can be depicted by concentric circles, with the research participants at the center. The arguments about ethically acceptable study design during the 2014–2016 Ebola outbreak in West Africa too often took place at the periphery of these concentric circles, at the multinational level (WHO 2014). The target population to be enrolled from among those affected by a given heath emergency must be engaged early on in discussions of research. GPP opens an avenue of communications for explaining unanticipated events and coping with emergencies, whether directly related to the clinical trial or caused by external developments. Building trust in the research process is also essential for community confidence in research results and any VTDs validated in clinical trials. Much vaccine hesitancy during the COVID-19 pandemic, for example, stemmed from distrust of the accelerated research timeline. Media and government messages in the United States celebrating the wonders of the vaccine, without explaining the evidence of the many years of mRNA vaccine platform and coronavirus research that had preceded the COVID-19 vaccines, might have been better calibrated had there been better GPP (Tufekci 2021).

Written standards for community engagement are useful, but leaders and biomedical researchers must understand, practice, and

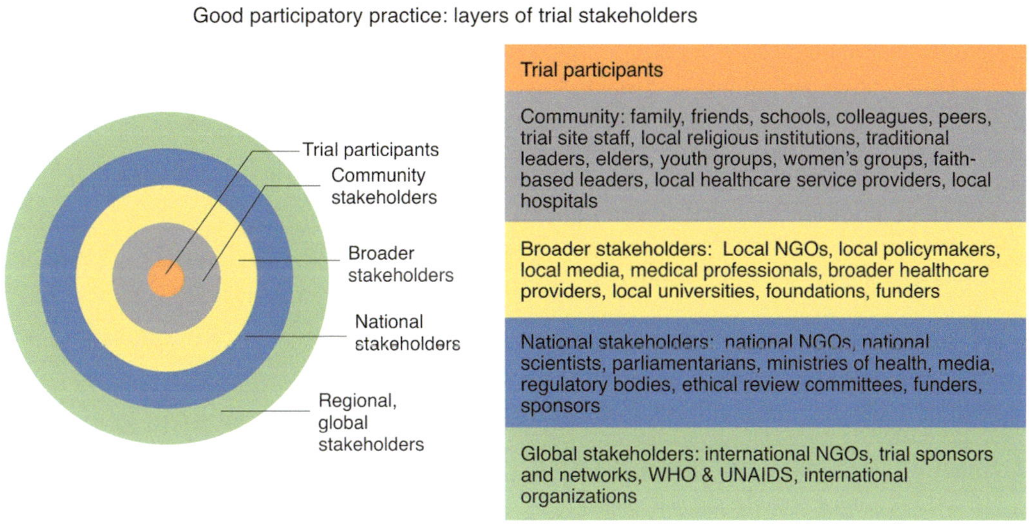

Fig. 3 GPP stakeholders (Wilson et al. 2021)

inculcate the principles and establish trust among research stakeholders through communications and collaboration, from study design and implementation through to publication and production of countermeasures. An attitude of superior wisdom should be discarded at the outset as wisdom and understanding are local. Assumptions about what the country, community, or individuals directly affected by the outbreak might want or believe is likely to be counterproductive. A core element of GPP is dialogue—meaning two-way communication, not merely telling people what to do.

3 Other Applicable Principles and Considerations

The six principles outlined here are applicable primarily to expedited clinical research in infectious disease emergencies. If there is a common thread, it is that such research needs to be integrated into both the continual practice of ongoing research and the practice of health emergency response. The principles governing these fields in "normal" circumstances fully apply to emergency research response.

Attempting to accelerate research response by loosening ethical standards or averting

Box 3: Differential Complexity and Actors in an Outbreak, Epidemic, and Pandemic

The subject of this book is response to an infectious disease outbreak, epidemic, or pandemic. What is the difference? It is the scale and speed of transmission that determines which term is most applicable. An outbreak refers to more cases of a disease than would commonly be expected among a given group of people or in a specific geographical area in a given period of time. An epidemic refers to a larger number of cases in a population or region in a short period of time. A pandemic is a global epidemic.

The phenomena they describe can vary vastly in scale, from, e.g., 23 Nipah virus cases in Kerala, India, in 2018 (Arunkumar et al. 2018) to the Black Death that reduced European populations by 30–50% from 1347 to 1351 (DeWitte 2014). The principles and practice of response to infectious disease emergencies are generally consistent at any one time, whatever the scale of the event.

The great hope of preparedness for research response is that an outbreak with pandemic potential can be contained while VTDs are developed, validated through clinical trials, and distributed to at-risk populations and areas. *All the measures needed for an outbreak will be needed in epidemics and pandemics as well*, which will require additional action to control and redress the consequences that arise with greater scale. Increasing scale naturally leads to greater complexity and politicization. There are many other possible differences between pandemics, e.g., the relatively gradual spread of HIV/AIDS vs. the rapid transmission of respiratory viruses like influenza and SARS-CoV-1&2. *Concerted interpandemic efforts to improve preparedness and response are essential.*

For an outbreak:

- Prompt global reporting and monitoring, data sharing, and consideration of response and research needs should begin at once for a novel pathogen, and potentially for a re-emerging one.
- Focus on modes of transmission immediately.
- Begin non-pharmaceutical interventions to help prevent pathogen spread; there should be a process in place to adjust NPIs based on accumulating research results.
- Conduct systematic natural history and laboratory studies urgently to
  - Characterize pathogenesis, stages and spectrum of disease, and pathogen replication and transmission
  - Improve clinical care
  - Discover pathogenic mechanisms for potential targeting with MCMs
- Conduct urgent VTD development and research, if possible while the outbreak remains contained.
- Preparedness for research implementation in low-resource environments could prevent an outbreak from growing into a pandemic.

In an epidemic, the measures above plus:

- Effective international engagement and leadership is likely to be necessary.
- International responders, like the World Health Organization (WHO), non-governmental organizations (NGOs), and research institutions bodies will need to begin active response or scale up existing efforts.

A global pandemic will require all measures listed above, but global partnership, coordination, and cooperation will become critical to marshal resources and use them wisely. Mitigating countries' predilection to prioritize the needs of their own populations over an effective global response will not be easy. Economic, social, and political consequences of the emergency will require national and global leadership. Funding may be abundant, but trained personnel, infrastructure, and supplies may be in short supply.

- Well-informed, credible leadership is essential to
  - Managing a coherent response
  - Maintaining popular confidence in countermeasures
  - Combating rumors and misinformation
- Funding is likely to be relatively abundant.
- Other resources, from health care systems to research assets, are likely to be overtaxed.
- Preparedness should focus on ensuring that efforts to counter the pandemic will be useful, e.g.,
  - To ensure clinical trials produce interpretable results
  - To minimize the popular appeal of ineffective clinical interventions

scientific rigor in clinical trial design or conduct can be a literally fatal mistake for trial participants and result in uninterpretable or unactionable clinical trial results. Rather, required procedural steps can be speeded up, for example by making ethical and scientific review immediate priorities for review bodies. Steps that are usually sequential can be taken in parallel, by, for example, beginning community outreach while funding is in process and protocols are being written, and by scaling up manufacturing with the proviso that the products might have to be discarded if clinical trials demonstrate that the investigational product has unexpected adverse effects or is not efficacious. Substantive requirements for human protections and scientific rigor have been developed over many decades to minimum risks to human subjects in developing novel vaccines, therapies, and diagnostics. These standards must not be relaxed because we are in a hurry.

Many of these additional principles are explained in detail in other chapters of this book. Let it be clear throughout that while emergency research response may be an urgent, life-and-death matter, the principles foundational to research and the practice of medicine are just as vital to successful response (◘ Fig. 4).

Objections to Integrating Research into Infectious Disease Emergency Response. Experiential Evidence to the Contrary.	
Objection	**Persuasive Refutation**
The process of developing medical countermeasures is too slow to produce results before an outbreak or pandemic wanes.	2014-2016 West African Ebola Outbreak Ebola vaccine research (Feldmann et al. 2018; Henao-Restrepo et al. 2017; Higgs et al. 2017; Kennedy et al. 2017)
An RCT interferes with medical response directed at saving patients' lives.	COVID-19 Pandemic RECOVERY, ACTT-1, Vaccine studies
Conducting an RCT with a placebo control arm in a high-mortality outbreak is unethical and even cruel, since it denies patients facing death their only hope of treatment.	ACTT-1, COVID-19 trials Pfizer & Moderna vaccines, Paxlovid (London 2018)
Proper clinical trials cannot be implemented in low-income countries with minimal health care systems.	Guinea Ring trial, PREVAIL 1, 2, 4 (Henao-Restrepo et al. 2017; Kennedy et al. 2017; Mulangu et al. 2019; Prevail II Writing Group 2016; PREVAIL III Study Group 2019)
Uneducated, often illiterate inhabitants of low-income areas cannot understand clinical trial participation and the stakes involved well enough to provide consent.	PALM 1, PREVAIL 1, PREVAC, (Mulangu et al. 2019)
Patients with novel emerging infectious diseases (EIDs) could not possibly provide genuine informed consent—can someone who is drowning consent to grasp at a straw?	DRC 2018-2020 Ebola outbreak PALM 1 Ebola treatment trial, demonstrated efficacy and products made available immediately after DSMB stopped study for efficacy (Mulangu et al. 2019).
Medical research primarily benefits those who can afford to pay high prices for pharmaceutical innovations – innovations that might eventually filter down to the research subjects and their communities once the patents expire.	Broad recognition that social value of research needs to accrue to those who will benefit most. This principle has been incorporated into several multilateral documents (G7 2021; WHO 2022a, c).

◘ **Fig. 4** Previous objections to inclusion of expedited research in emergency response. These considerations have been refuted or overcome with time. There is now a consensus that benefits from a well-designed research response outweigh the risks and difficulties. (Author)

Discussion Questions

1. Describe the results of an ideal research response to an outbreak with pathogen X.
2. Compliance with the six practical guiding principles collected over the past many health emergencies is both morally correct and practically necessary for development of improved VTDs and effective research response to existing and future novel pathogens.
   (a) Discuss implementation paths and benefits of Principle 1: research should be an integral part of preparedness and response. Also, what is the difference between an outbreak, epidemic, and pandemic and the actors involved in each?
   (b) For Principle 2, discuss how the research response should align with the three primary goals of an emergency response.
   (c) Time is of the essence in research response. Discuss why and how response research should be implemented quickly and efficiently based on preparedness plans (Principle 3).
   (d) Discuss the critical importance of Principle 4, which states that the norms of scientific rigor and ethical standards of protection for human research subjects do not change during health emergencies.
   (e) Discuss why research led by the host country government is essential to global health security (Principle 5).
   (f) Discuss Principle 6, which emphasizes that understanding cultures and communities through dialogue and respect ("Nothing about them without them") and involving them as trusted stakeholders in response efforts (GPP) are critical to research in health emergencies.
3. What are some previous objections to inclusion of expedited research in emergency response, which have been refuted or overcome with time?

References

Arunkumar G, Chandni R, Mourya DT, Singh SK, Sadanandan R, Sudan P, et al. Outbreak investigation of Nipah virus disease in Kerala, India, 2018. J Infect Dis. 2018;219(12):1867–78. https://doi.org/10.1093/infdis/jiy612.

Bhati AP, Wan S, Alfè D, Clyde AR, Bode M, Tan L, et al. Pandemic drugs at pandemic speed: infrastructure for accelerating COVID-19 drug discovery with hybrid machine learning- and physics-based simulations on high-performance computers. Interface Focus. 2021;11(6):20210018. https://doi.org/10.1098/rsfs.2021.0018.

Branswell H. An early lesson from the Uganda Ebola vaccine trial: shots must be ready to go before the next outbreak strikes. STAT; 2022.

Brooks JC, Pinto M, Gill A, Hills KE, Murthy S, Podgornik MN, et al. Incident management systems and building emergency management capacity during the 2014–2016 Ebola epidemic—Liberia, Sierra Leone, and Guinea. MMWR Suppl. 2016;65(3):28–34. https://doi.org/10.15585/mmwr.su6503a5.

Bugin K, Woodcock J. Trends in COVID-19 therapeutic clinical trials. Nat Rev Drug Discov. 2021;20:254. https://doi.org/10.1038/d41573-021-00037-3.

Cassetti MC, Pierson TC, Patterson LJ, Bok K, DeRocco AJ, Deschamps AM, et al. Prototype pathogen approach for vaccine and monoclonal antibody development: a critical component of the NIAID plan for pandemic preparedness. J Infect Dis. 2022;227:1433. https://doi.org/10.1093/infdis/jiac296.

DeWitte SN. Mortality risk and survival in the aftermath of the medieval Black Death. PLoS One. 2014;9(5):e96513. https://doi.org/10.1371/journal.pone.0096513.

Fallah MP, Lane HC, Higgs ES, Kennedy SB, Massaquoi MBF, Kieh MWS, et al. Clinical research as a critical component of epidemic response: the case of PREVAIL in Liberia. Lancet Glob Health. 2023;11(3):e321–3. https://doi.org/10.1016/s2214-109x(23)00040-2.

G7. G7 therapeutics and vaccines clinical trials charter. London: HMG Government (UK); 2021.

Hankins C, Warren M, Bass E, Sarche J, Wiysonge C, GPP Working Group. Communities matter! Guidelines for good participatory practice in HIV prevention trial (GPP). 2007.

Hanney SR, Straus SE, Holmes BJ. Saving millions of lives but some resources squandered: emerging lessons from health research system pandemic achievements and challenges. Health Res Policy Syst. 2022;20(1):99. https://doi.org/10.1186/s12961-022-00883-6.

Kuhn JH. Guide to the correct use of filoviral nomenclature. In: Mühlberger E, et al., editors. Marburg- and Ebolaviruses: from ecosystems to molecules, Current topics in microbiology and immunology. Cham: Springer Nature; 2017. p. 447–60.
Kuhn JH, Adachi T, Adhikari NKJ, Arribas JR, Bah IE, Bausch DG, et al. New filovirus disease classification and nomenclature. Nat Rev Microbiol. 2019;17(5):261–3. https://doi.org/10.1038/s41579-019-0187-4.
Mbaeyi C, Moran T, Wadood Z, Ather F, Sykes E, Nikulin J, et al. Stopping a polio outbreak in the midst of war: lessons from Syria. Vaccine. 2021;39(28):3717–23. https://doi.org/10.1016/j.vaccine.2021.05.045.
Moorthy V, Abubakar I, Qadri F, et al. The future of the global clinical trial ecosystem: a vision from the first WHO Global Clinical Trials Forum. The Lancet. 2024;403(10422):124–6.
Muldoon OT, Liu JH, McHugh C. The political psychology of COVID-19. Polit Psychol. 2021;42(5):715–28. https://doi.org/10.1111/pops.12775.
NASEM. Integrating clinical research into epidemic response: the Ebola experience. Washington, DC: National Academies of Sciences Engineering and Medicine Publications, The National Academies Press; 2017.
Piarroux R, Moore S, Rebaudet S. Cholera in Haiti. Presse Med. 2022;51(3):104136. https://doi.org/10.1016/j.lpm.2022.104136.
Santos CVB, Noronha TG, Werneck GL, Struchiner CJ, Villela DAM. Estimated COVID-19 severe cases and deaths averted in the first year of the vaccination campaign in Brazil: a retrospective observational study. Lancet Reg Health Am. 2023;17:100418. https://doi.org/10.1016/j.lana.2022.100418.
Translators without Borders. Language data for the Democratic Republic of Congo. Garden City, ID: Translators without Borders; 2022. https://translatorswithoutborders.org/language-data-for-the-democratic-republic-of-congo-drc. Accessed 17 Dec 2022.
Tufekci Z. 5 pandemic mistakes we keep repeating: we can learn from our failures. Atlantic. 2021.
UN, editor. Charter of the United Nations and statute of the International Court of Justice. San Francisco: United Nations Conference on International Organization; 1945.
WHO. Meeting summary of the WHO consultation on potential Ebola therapies and vaccines. Geneva: World Health Organization; 2014.
WHO. Good participatory practice guidelines for trials of emerging (and re-emerging) pathogens that are likely to cause severe outbreaks in the near future and for which few or no medical countermeasures exist (GPP-EP). Geneva: World Health Organization; 2016. p. 53.
WHO. Good Participatory Practice for COVID-19 clinical trials—a toolbox. Geneva: World Health Organization; 2020.
WHO. Strengthening clinical trials to provide high-quality evidence on health interventions and to improve research quality and coordination. WHA 75.8. Geneva: World Health Organization; 2022.
Wilson B, Wright K, Taylor R, Higgs E. Beyond recruitment: good participatory practice enhances the impact of research in a pandemic. Nat Med. 2021;27(3):369–71. https://doi.org/10.1038/s41591-021-01271-3.

Norms for Emergency Research Response

Robert A. Sorenson

Overview of Book Section II. Ethics is at the heart of the clinical research enterprise, in large part because the history of medical research contains questionable and even appalling episodes. Does the urgency of quelling a global disease outbreak justify bypassing accepted ethical standards? Perhaps pandemics *require* deviations from the usual ethical and scientific research standards? The editors and authors of this volume agree that the answer is "no." The urgency of understanding a novel or re-emerging disease and developing medical countermeasures, along with social and political pressure for fast results, do not justify relaxing fundamental standards that guard scientific integrity and human subject protections. But the urgency is real. How should research priorities be set during pandemics? Will research hinder efforts to care for affected patients in a high-mortality disease outbreak? From a broader perspective, what responsibilities do clinical research teams have to ameliorate current health inequities between rich and poor, inequities that make all of us more vulnerable to infectious disease?

Max Smith's introduction (► Chap. 4) to fundamental issues in pandemic research response sets the stage for considering the questions outlined here. Nir Eyal and Marc Lipsitch (► In Practice 4.1) argue cogently that randomly controlled clinical trials are usually the most ethical as well as the most efficient trial design, even when an untested intervention may be seen as the only hope for patients. V. Koneti Rao (► In Practice 4.2) outlines some of the ways research ethics committees can move quickly in an emergency. The inequity that makes health outcomes so uneven around the world, whether seen in unequal access to the products of research or to the basic health care that underlies their use, is the focus of a chapter by Dirceu Greco (► Chap. 5) that should make us all think again about global health justice.

Moving away from enduring moral questions, though certainly not leaving ethics behind, Marco Cavaleri and colleagues (► Chap. 6) outline how regulators adapt to emergency circumstances while ensuring the safety and efficacy of candidate medical countermeasures (MCMs). Robert Terry and Katherine Wright (► Chap. 7) review the state of biological sample and genetic data sharing—a necessity for accelerated emergency response research, but one that the world's countries continue to find difficult to negotiate given divergent North-South perspectives.

Contents

4 Ethics of Pandemic Research

Maxwell J. Smith

Contents

Learning Track Note: This chapter appears in Learning Tracks: Biostatistics; Clinical Research; Global Health; Global Health Law; Health Policy, Multilateral Cooperation, International Governance (► Sect. 6); Public Health and Epidemiology; Research Ethics

E. S. Higgs and R. A. Sorenson (eds.), *Principles and Practice of Emergency Research Response*, https://doi.org/10.1007/978-3-031-48408-7_4

Learning Objectives

This chapter will help readers understand and describe:

- Five foundational ethical questions and considerations facing researchers in pandemics:
- deviations from existing standards
- handling novel ethical issues
- prioritization
- research in relation to pandemic response
- governance and coordination
- Major stakeholders and how they collaborate

1 Introduction

It is critical to conduct research during pandemics and other infectious disease outbreaks. For starters, research conducted during pandemics can directly contribute to the emergency response and potentially mitigate morbidity and mortality and control the outbreak (e.g., by investigating novel medical countermeasures for pathogens that lack any effective vaccine or therapy). Second, some research questions can only be adequately investigated in the midst of a pandemic (e.g., investigating the effectiveness and impacts of public health countermeasures, or, if the disease rarely occurs in other circumstances, medical countermeasure [MCMs] as well). Finally, research conducted in this context can work to correct failures of the market to investigate and generate knowledge and products for neglected diseases that have epidemic or pandemic potential in a world where research and development (R&D) for neglected diseases has historically constituted less than 2% of all health R&D (WHO 2012). For these reasons, many argue there is an *ethical imperative* to conduct research during pandemics (Andersen et al. 2015; Bain et al. 2018; PAHO 2016; Schopper et al. 2017; Thompson 2016; WHO 2016a).

Yet, due to pressures of time, uncertainty, distress, the need for multi-country collaboration, and the potential for research to detract from pandemic response, the conduct of research during pandemics raises a number of profound ethical questions and concerns requiring scrutiny. This chapter examines five foundational ethical questions and considerations undergirding the nature and role of research in pandemic contexts, including:

1. Do pandemics necessitate or justify deviations from ethical and scientific standards for research?
2. Do pandemics raise novel ethical questions for research?
3. How should research priorities be set during pandemics?
4. How should research be conducted in the context of other response efforts?
5. How should pandemic research be governed and coordinated?

This chapter does not survey or focus on specific ethical issues likely to emerge in practice during the conduct of research in pandemics, such as informed consent and data sharing (▶ Chaps. 3, 7, 18, and 35 and In Practice 4.2), though it may touch on these in service of exploring other foundational questions. In other words, this chapter sets out to establish an understanding of the ethics *of* pandemic research, which may be contrasted with ethical issues *in* pandemic research.

Box 1: Correcting Market Failures via Research Conducted During Epidemics and Pandemics

The lack of an approved vaccine or effective therapy for Ebola virus disease (EVD) during the 2014–2016 epidemic in West Africa was in large part a result of limited investment in R&D activities in this area despite the identification of the virus several decades earlier in 1976 and the existence of two candidate vaccines. The threat posed by the epidemic created an opportunity for significant international research efforts, ultimately leading to the development and approval of more than one EVD vaccine within just 4 years. This illustrates an often-overlooked ethical reason to conduct research during epidemics and pandemics, i.e., to correct for market failures.

2 Do Pandemics Necessitate or Justify Deviations from Ethical and Scientific Standards for Research?

Pandemics require urgent research to understand the pathogen in question and to identify potential ways to diagnose, prevent, or mitigate its harmful effects. Pandemics may also require a degree of adaptability or flexibility in how research studies are designed and implemented, given practical or logistical limitations. Moreover, there is generally a short window of opportunity to conduct valuable research during pandemics, as it will often be difficult or impossible to answer some questions adequately outside the pandemic's acute phase. Consequently, some have asked whether the speed and adaptability required of research during pandemics might justify exceptions to ethical and scientific standards that otherwise govern research conduct. Put another way, some ask whether pandemics eliminate the "luxury" we otherwise have to demand such high standards for research, necessitating what might be called "pandemic research exceptionalism" (London and Kimmelman 2020). Indeed, there may be significant pressures, from the public or from decision makers, to cut corners in an effort to generate knowledge or provide countermeasures as quickly as possible (Bramstedt 2020). Such standards may include ethical standards, such as those that must otherwise be met during the ethics review process or during publication peer review, as well as scientific standards, such as those typically used to ensure rigor in study design, participant selection, blinding, masking, controls, sample size estimation, and so forth, which themselves have ethical dimensions and implications. Failing to get clarity and agreement on whether pandemics necessitate deviations from ethical and scientific standards for research runs the risk of fundamentally frustrating the prospect of effective collaboration between research stakeholders, establishing shared priorities for research, and so forth.

While it is attractive to think that research ought to be designed in whichever way is fastest and easiest to implement when faced with such a formidable threat, there are persuasive reasons to think that deviations from ethical and scientific standards of research due to a pandemic would not be ethically justified. As London and Kimmelman (2020) argue, "the moral mission of research remains the same: to reduce uncertainty and enable caregivers, health systems, and policymakers to better address individual and public health." The challenges that rigorous scientific methods are designed to address "do not disappear" in a pandemic, nor do researchers' obligations to protect the interests of research participants and align research conduct with the public interest, which are advanced by research ethics standards and regulations (London and Kimmelman 2020). Indeed, the ethical imperative to conduct research in a pandemic is not to conduct just *any* research; it is to generate the best possible data about questions of social value to inform decisions and provide better services (European Network of Research Integrity Offices 2020). And it remains unethical, even during a pandemic, to ask people to participate in research that is unlikely to produce meaningful results. Moreover, one ought not to discount the effects that lowering ethical or scientific standards could have on the public's trust in research studies, scientific institutions, and the products of research like therapeutics and vaccines (▶ Chap. 18). Erosion of trust can have deleterious effects on research participation, confidence in research findings, and uptake of the products of research that may be integral for mitigating or ending the pandemic. There is growing realization that social mobilization, community outreach, and well-designed communications with the community, also known as good participatory practice, are often essential, not only for recruiting trial participants but for public trust in research programs and in the results of the research, e.g., medical countermeasures against the disease under study (AVAC 2021; Hankins et al. 2007; Wilson et al. 2021).

Box 2: Research Ethics Standards

The U.S. Department of Health and Human Services (HHS) International Compilation of Human Research Standards has compiled over 1000 laws, regulations, and guidelines on human participants' protections in 131 countries and international organizations (OHRP 2020).

Due to the nature and complexity of pandemics, research conducted in this context may put research participants at heightened risk of harm and challenge existing mechanisms for ethical review and oversight (O'Mathúna 2010). Consequently, in contrast to lowering standards during pandemics, some argue that special scrutiny ought to exist in relation to research conducted in these contexts (Levine et al. 2004; Tansey et al. 2010).

Ultimately, pandemics do not obviate the need for rigorous scientific evaluation and adherence to universal ethical standards for social value, scientific validity, independent review, reasonable benefit–risk ratio, fair and voluntary participation, collaborative partnership, and equal moral respect for participants and affected communities (Emanuel et al. 2004; NASEM 2017; Smith et al. 2020a; WHO 2020b) (► Chap. 3). However, this is not to say that accepted ethical and scientific standards cannot be interpreted in light of, and adapted in response to, particular circumstances and contexts, or that different processes may not be used to advance those standards. For example, while ethical standards may remain the same, ethics review boards will likely need to modify their standard operating procedures to respond to time-sensitive protocols or put plans in place to facilitate expedited reviews in a manner that still accords with accepted standards (Schopper et al. 2017). Additionally, what might represent an ethical ideal may need to be revisited in contexts of time pressures and resource constraints; for instance, the imperative to achieve full partnership between medical and scientific colleagues in high-resource and low-resource countries may not be immediately achievable in an emergency (Canario Guzmán et al. 2017). In any case, adaptations must be explicitly ethically justified and reviewed through transparent and inclusive processes.

Discussion Question 1: Pressures to Revise Research Standards During Pandemics

A pandemic involving a novel pathogen has led to significant morbidity and mortality worldwide. There is no known effective therapy or prophylactic; however, a study of a novel therapy is about to be initiated. Given the immense burden of morbidity and mortality associated with the pandemic pathogen, the researchers leading the study are concerned that the use of placebo comparators in the trial would conflict with their duty of care and, more generally, with their compassion. They consider whether they ought to forgo randomization of some study participants to a placebo control arm given the dire prospects they otherwise face, despite the statistical control afforded by randomization. Others on the research team argue that it is uncertain whether the therapy is better than placebo in treating the disease or may actually cause harm—that is, clinical equipoise exists—and so no study participant will receive a standard of care inferior to any available alternative (► In Practice 4.1).

Discussion question: Do the dire circumstances faced by study participants created by a pandemic provide an ethical reason to adopt designs or methods that may be less capable of achieving statistical assurance of safety and efficacy?

3 Do Pandemics Raise Novel Ethical Issues for Research?

Arguably, pandemics can raise ethical issues for research that may not otherwise be encountered, either at all or with such intensity (Nuffield Council on Bioethics 2020). Pandemics may also create novel circumstances wherein familiar ethical issues in research must be uniquely navigated.

Consider the novel research ethics issues raised by the emergency use authorization of COVID-19 vaccines in the United States (and elsewhere), and specifically whether ongoing vaccine trials would be ethically justified in continuing to use placebo controls in this context. One might consult international research ethics standards on this question, including Article 33 of the Declaration of Helsinki, which states:

> » The benefits, risks, burdens and effectiveness of a new intervention must be tested against those of the best proven intervention(s), except in the following circumstances:
> - Where no proven intervention exists, the use of placebo, or no intervention, is acceptable; or
> - Where, for compelling and scientifically sound methodological reasons, the use of any intervention less effective than the best proven one, the use of placebo, or no intervention is necessary to determine the efficacy or safety of an intervention and the patients who receive any intervention less effective than the best proven one, placebo, or no intervention will not be subject to additional risks of serious or irreversible harm as a result of not receiving the best proven intervention. Extreme care must be taken to avoid abuse of this option (WMA 2013).

In other words, according to the Declaration of Helsinki, investigational COVID-19 vaccines should be tested against a placebo only in circumstances where no proven intervention exists. Yet, the emergency use authorization of COVID-19 vaccines raised the unique question of whether vaccines authorized by these means would meet the threshold of a "proven intervention" (WHO 2020a). If they do, then the continued use of placebo controls in those vaccine trials could be considered unethical. This situation led some to argue that participants of such vaccine trials should be offered the opportunity to be unblinded so they can make an informed decision about whether to withdraw from the trial and access the emergency authorized vaccine (Singh et al. 2021). By contrast, the continuation of trials with placebo controls even after emergency authorization is granted could be considered necessary in order to further characterize and understand the duration of protection provided by the vaccine, determine the effectiveness of the vaccine in populations not previously included in clinical trials, evaluate effectiveness for additional clinical endpoints not evaluated in previous clinical trials, and support the submission of applications for full market licensure. This debate arguably represents a novel ethical question and issue raised by the unique mechanisms that exist only in public health emergencies, like emergency use authorizations.

Other ethical issues that are salient in pandemics may not be novel but appear so due to their intensity, perceived relevance, or importance. For example, the COVID-19 pandemic prompted fierce debates regarding the ethical merits of human challenge studies, whereby healthy study participants are deliberately infected with a pathogen to rapidly test novel diagnostics, therapeutics, or vaccines (WHO 2020g). On the one hand, proponents argued that challenge studies could significantly accelerate the development of these crucial resources, which could in turn help to avert considerable morbidity and mortality. As Plotkin and Caplan (2020) put it, "extraordinary diseases require extraordinary solutions." On the other hand, opponents argued that challenge studies in this context represented an unfavorable risk–benefit ratio for study participants, particularly in the absence of a rescue therapy (Kahn et al. 2020) and uncertainty in longer term sequelae. Yet, these are not necessarily novel ethical issues or questions; human challenge studies have been conducted for hundreds of years and arguably raise similar ethical questions in non-pandemic contexts (Hope and McMillan 2004; Jamrozik and Selgelid 2021). But there is no doubt that pandemics can intensify the perceived need for challenge studies and consideration of their ethical merits and justification.

One could similarly argue that epidemics and pandemics, like the 2015–2016 Zika epidemic and COVID-19 pandemic, raise particularly urgent ethical questions regarding the inclusion of pregnant and breastfeeding people in related clinical research, such as trials for vaccines and therapeutics. Both Zika and COVID-19 illustrate how infectious diseases can uniquely affect the health interests of pregnant people and their offspring, highlighting the ethical importance of considering pregnant people and their offspring in vaccine trials and other pandemic research (Krubiner et al. 2019). However, the historical exclusion of such populations from research agendas and clinical trials has left an urgent need for additional data to ensure the safety of many medical countermeasures for pregnant and lactating individuals, so the ethical issue is hardly peculiar to pandemic research (Denne and Pediatric Policy Council 2019).

No matter whether pandemics raise novel ethical issues or simply create novel circumstances wherein familiar ethical issues in research must be navigated with greater urgency and intensity, the upshot is that researchers, regulators, and ethics review bodies require relevant guidance and mechanisms to effectively respond to them. This chapter returns to this point in its discussion of research governance, coordination, and oversight in ▶ Sect. 6.

4 Setting Research Priorities During a Pandemic

Research is not a value-neutral enterprise. What is studied tends to reflect the types of information, answers, and products considered to be of the highest priority or greatest value (Nuyens 2007). This is mediated through funding priorities, determinations of where and with whom research ought to be conducted, the nature of how research is conducted, where research is published, and so forth. It is therefore important to acknowledge that research priorities are necessarily set against a backdrop of inequity where the interests and values of some are seen to matter less. It is similarly important to acknowledge that research priority setting has the capacity to create or further exacerbate inequities insofar as it can dictate where scarce resources are prioritized as well as where research translation and research capacity strengthening occurs (Pratt and Loff 2014; Pratt et al. 2018). While much attention is paid to manifest injustices in allocation of the fruits of pandemic research (e.g., vaccines, therapeutics), injustices in research priority setting can also mean there simply are no vaccines or therapeutics for pathogens primarily affecting the least advantaged, notably the category of neglected tropical diseases (▶ Chap. 5).

? Discussion Question 2: Which Considerations Should Guide Research Priority Setting During Pandemics?

In their 2018 study, Pratt et al. (2018) report on an international workshop they convened to explore what might be ethically required for research priority setting at the national and global levels. Several substantive criteria that could be applied in global health research priority setting were suggested by workshop participants, including:

- Need
- Burden of disease
- Magnitude of benefits
- Equity
- The needs of vulnerable and disadvantaged groups
- Cost-effectiveness of research
- Cost-effectiveness of proposed interventions
- Likelihood of research success

Discussion questions: Which criterion, or combination of criteria, ought to guide pandemic research priority setting? Whose interests do different criteria serve or advance?

The research agenda in a pandemic is likely to be shaped by high-income countries, whose interests are overrepresented because of their financial and political power to exert influence or control over research priority setting processes and decisions, and because high-income countries are better resourced than low- and middle-income countries. Non-governmental funders are also usually influenced by high-income-country locations, staff, and funding as well. This may create or exacerbate inequities, as national governments of high-income countries who fund research will largely be expected to prioritize the health security of their own citizens when determining their funding objectives, which means that research with a greater likelihood of benefitting rich nations will be prioritized over research having a greater likelihood of benefitting poorer nations (Nuffield Council on Bioethics 2020). For example, greater priority may be given to high-tech innovations that rely on sophisticated infrastructure, with less priority given to low-tech local innovations that might be of greater value in low- and middle-income settings.

Correcting such inequities requires an understanding of who is affected by the pandemic and the research that may be conducted; fair and inclusive processes for including the interests, perspectives, and needs of all affected parties (and particularly those expected to be most disadvantaged by a given pandemic) when setting priorities; and in turn setting priorities themselves that aim to work to the benefit of the least advantaged. Some progress has been made to these ends in recent years, though considerable deficits remain (▶ Chap. 5). A few of the main organizations working to this end are

- The World Health Organization (WHO), through its R&D Blueprint, which aims to improve coordination between scientists and global health professionals, accelerate the research and development process, and develop new norms and standards to learn from and improve upon the global research response to infectious disease threats (WHO 2016b).
- The Global Research Collaboration for Infectious Disease Preparedness (GloPID-R), which brings funders together to facilitate a rapid and effective response to infectious disease outbreaks (GLOPID-R 2021).
- The Coalition for Epidemic Preparedness Innovations (CEPI), a global partnership between public, private, philanthropic, and civil society organizations to accelerate the development of vaccines against emerging infectious diseases (CEPI 2021).
- The Alliance for Accelerating Excellence in Science in Africa (AESA), a partnership aiming to shift the center of gravity for African science to Africa through agenda setting, mobilizing R&D funding, and managing continent-wide science, technology, and innovation programs (Alliance for Accelerating Excellence in Science in Africa 2021).
- The Access to COVID-19 Tools (ACT) Accelerator, a multilateral partnership dedicated to accelerating "development, production, and equitable access to COVID-19 tests, treatments, and vaccines," and its COVAX vaccine pillar, which in addition to the development and production of vaccines, seeks to "guarantee fair and equitable access for every country in the world" (WHO 2022a).

Box 3: Correcting Inequities in Research Priority Setting

In response to ethical concerns related to how decisions about research prioritization and funding are made during public health emergencies, the Nuffield Council on Bioethics has made the following recommendations to create a more collaborative approach between funders, ensure a wider range of voices is heard in determining the kind of research that should get funded, and shift the power balance in funding decisions towards lower-income countries:

- Collaboration between funders and relevant governments/national research institutions/UN bodies at the start of an emergency, to agree on research priorities
- A dedicated pooled funding resource for research in emergencies, with inclusive and diverse representation from research institutions around the world among its leadership and embedded in decision-making processes
- Innovative approaches among funders to find ways to support and incentivise researchers to include affected communities directly in plans for grant applications (Nuffield Council on Bioethics 2020).

But there are additional forces that may shape research priority setting which deserve ethical scrutiny. For example, pressures from the public or decision-makers may result in the prioritization of research dedicated to demonstrating the effectiveness of certain interventions, like occupancy limits or masking, where the merits of those interventions are called into question or resisted not for scientific reasons, but rather for political or ideological reasons. Conversely, research agendas may be shaped by public pressures to investigate interventions as a result of misinformation regarding the promise they show. These pressures, intense at times, have the capacity to influence the sorts of research conducted and the sorts of research seen as valuable. These influences are not necessarily unique to pandemics, but there is little doubt they are amplified in this context given the immense political and public pressures at play. Ethical scrutiny is therefore required so as not to divert scarce resources from other research priorities or unnecessarily expose research participants to harms.

It is also important to note that decisions about the kinds of research that ought to be conducted or prioritized during a pandemic are often informed by evidence generated from prior research. For example, some interventions, like therapeutics or vaccines, may be selected for testing based on evidence generated from previous trials. Due to the paucity of data and uncertainty that often characterizes pandemic contexts, evidence used to inform research priorities may be limited, sometimes stemming from only a handful of studies, or perhaps from mere signals emerging in unpublished studies or non-refereed publications (Smith et al. 2020b). What is published and, therefore, what makes up the limited evidence base upon which research priorities are based, has the potential for bias and may reflect important distortions, leading to distorted research priorities (Knox Clarke and Darcy 2014). This may in turn have consequences further down the line, for example, where a "positive results bias" (when statistically significant positive results from a study are more likely to be reported than negative results) leads to the use of certain measures in response to a pandemic when the effectiveness of those measures has been exaggerated or where an effect does not actually exist. Alternatively, research priorities during a pandemic may be particularly susceptible to "hot stuff bias," which occurs when a topic is popular within the scientific community, among public health authorities, popular media, politicians, or the public, such as hydroxychloroquine during the early days of the COVID-19 pandemic, leading to increased interest in research and publication on that topic, even if those results are preliminary or weak (Sacket 1979). Efforts to mitigate the ways in which biases in publication and in the evidence base are required for an effective, ethical pandemic response; these can include making data more accessible, introducing techniques for research registration and evidence synthesis, and examining the ways in which the interests of different stakeholders might contribute to bias or otherwise impact study effects (Smith 2015).

Finally, arriving at shared research priorities in a pandemic is threatened by the fact that the research enterprise comprises numerous organizations and stakeholders who may have conflicting priorities. Research governance and coordination are the subject of ▶ Sect. 6.

5 Research Versus Response or Research as Response?

Despite the ethical obligation to conduct research during pandemics, it is important to carefully balance the need to generate new knowledge in service of optimizing current and future pandemic response, including development of novel medical countermeasures, with efforts to directly respond to the current pandemic. There is good reason to believe that research should not impede response efforts or use resources that could be used for other response measures unless the research can itself contribute to the current response. In other words, if it can be expected that research might take away personnel, equipment, or other resources from those required for pandemic response (or from routine health care and public health services), then that research should not be conducted, at least not in ways that would run orthogonal to response efforts (WHO 2020b).

While the prospect of conducting rigorous clinical trials of medical countermeasures in a resource-limited environment once seemed so daunting as to require years of advance planning, the research experience that began in 2014 during the West Africa Ebola epidemic showed that it could be done and that it could contribute to eventual approval of vaccines and therapeutics (Bausch et al. 2008; FDA 2019, 2020; Mulangu et al. 2019; NASEM 2017), which accelerated the end of the Ebola outbreak. As demonstrated by the Ebola experience, and as broadly carried out during the COVID-19 pandemic, research response can be an integral and even a primary element of pandemic response, and in that case, it would arguably be misguided to say it takes resources away from response. The COVID-19 response is now the paradigm, for better or worse, of a relatively rapid research response to a major pandemic, and has set a new baseline for non-pharmaceutical interventions, evolving guidelines for treating patients, and the rapid development, clinical trials, and authorization or approval of medical countermeasures. Multifaceted research response will no longer be seen as an optional part of response to a novel pathogen, and the question in future outbreaks will be not whether but how to incorporate research into response while upholding ethical and scientific norms and standards.

Research response is no longer simply "nice to have." However, it remains critical to ensure research and other response elements operate in a manner that is complementary. That means doing a better job of ensuring resources go to well-planned, well-powered studies that can produce replicable, regulatory-level results (Bugin and Woodcock 2021). This is of particular ethical importance because of the interdependence of research and response, wherein the infrastructure necessary for research is also necessary for a well-functioning health system and pandemic response, and vice versa. Striking the right balance between research and response is also critical because research may not always be perceived as important (Nuffield Council on Bioethics 2020), especially where communities believe all available resources should be used to aid response efforts. Indeed, if the infrastructure undergirding research, particularly in low-resource settings, appears to be better supported than response efforts, including the provision of basic health services, then research may not be accepted (Parker 2019). While researchers, research funders, and research institutions may not always have control over response efforts and the provision of health services, they can partner with organizations who do in order to ensure research efforts complement response efforts (▶ In Practice 17.1). Respectful engagement and partnership with the communities where research is conducted and with research study participants themselves goes a long way to ameliorate community suspicions about the motives and professionalism of both research and humanitarian health care responders (▶ Chap. 18).

The line between research and other evidence-generating activities (e.g., surveillance as epidemiological research) that may be used in response is fuzzy and can easily become blurred in the context of a pandemic (Calain et al. 2009; Hunt et al. 2012; Sethi 2018; WHO 2010; Willison et al. 2014). This is also because research activities often comprise part of the response effort. Moreover, many activities straddle the categories of research even when they are not primarily seen as such. Disease surveillance, for example, may be seen primarily as a tool of epidemiological preparedness and response, but the data it generates can be used by researchers in various disciplines for research into, for example, social determinants of health or disease vector range mapping (Mitra and Sethi 2016). Precisely how research and response are distinguished has important implications in practice, since "research," "public health intervention," "clinical care," and so forth are governed by different regulations, laws, procedural guidance, codes of ethics, and ethical considerations. For example, research is generally required to undergo some form of independent ethics review (and is thus subjected to standard norms of research ethics), whereas interventions deemed not to be research generally are not. Consequently, the ethical stakes of getting this distinction right can be high. If scrutiny is not given to the nature and scope of different evidence-generating activities during a pandemic, some forms of evidence generation may end up proceeding with little or no consideration of their ethical implications, including harms that may arise for participants (Nuffield Council on Bioethics 2020). Conversely, requiring that routine public health surveillance or service evaluation adhere to research regulations would place unnecessary burdens on the public health sector, which may in turn impede response efforts.

Because it can be both conceptually and practically challenging to distinguish research practices from other activities conducted during a pandemic, the Nuffield Council on Bioethics has proposed that one first consider the nature of the ethical concerns raised by the particular activity and circumstance and then evaluate the most appropriate form of oversight to identify and respond to those concerns (Nuffield Council on Bioethics 2020). This approach is adopted by Public Health Ontario, which ensures ethical scrutiny and oversight is applied to all evidence-generating activities, but in a manner that is proportionate to the activity and attendant ethical concerns (Public Health Ontario 2012). As a result, the risk that activities will proceed without ethical scrutiny is attenuated, but without necessarily adding administrative or methodological burdens to activities where they are not required or would be disproportionate.

6 Research Governance, Coordination, and Oversight During Pandemics

During a pandemic, all of humanity has a shared interest in urgently developing safe and effective therapeutics, vaccines, and diagnostics to aid in pandemic response. There are also shared interests in better understanding the effectiveness and impacts of non-pharmaceutical countermeasures. Researchers (as well as research funders, publishers, etc.) the world over will therefore be motivated to pursue similar lines of research, which can result in a coordination challenge whereby duplication (of studies, of review of studies, etc.), competitive enrolment and underpowered studies, poor stewardship of scarce resources (e.g., investigational products, funding, research participants, etc.), and barriers to sharing information and learning from others are more likely to occur (Bugin and Woodcock 2021; Raynaud et al. 2021). Furthermore, research may continue to be funded and conducted on issues that have been thoroughly researched but for which results have simply not been published. Mechanisms to ethically govern and coordinate research efforts, including in setting research priorities, in a pandemic are therefore critical (G7 Therapeutics and vaccines clinical trials charter 2021).

Given the multiplicity of stakeholders involved in the conduct of pandemic research (e.g., research institutions, funders, regulatory authorities, humanitarian organizations, etc.), multi-center and multi-country collaboration is key. Such collaboration can be facilitated, in part, through creative trial platforms and so-called master protocols, such as the WHO Solidarity vaccine and therapeutics trials, which have adaptive designs that permit modifications to parameters of the trial (such as adding or dropping interventions as the trial progresses) while still proceeding under a common framework for research conducted across organizations and countries. The UK RECOVERY trial follows an analogous design using the infrastructure of the UK National Health Service (RECOVERY trial 2022; WHO 2021, 2022b). Many have argued that WHO possesses the legitimacy and convening power to take a leading role in coordinating research in this context (Nuffield Council on Bioethics 2020). Indeed, WHO's R&D Blueprint functions as an R&D model for global research coordination and product development efforts for epidemics and pandemics. Other existing collaborative networks, such as WHO's Thematic Platform for Health Emergency and Disaster Risk Management Research Network (TPRN), similarly represent progress in the effort to join up the global research community to improve the scientific evidence base in health emergency and disaster risk management (Kayano et al. 2019). Critically, a multiplicity of stakeholders is likely to also mean accountabilities to different, and often conflicting, interests, populations, regulations, and guidelines. Efforts to coordinate research efforts during pandemics must therefore be alive to, and in turn attempt to be transparent about, the responsibilities undertaken by different actors, like national governments, non-governmental organizations, funders, ethics review bodies, intergovernmental organizations, research institutions, and researchers (Moon et al. 2021).

Good governance and coordination of pandemic research is predicated, in part, on the capacities of researchers and their institutions and communities in different parts of the world to support, facilitate, and participate in such research. Yet, while pandemics are unique insofar as they can impact all countries, not all countries have similar capacities to conduct, facilitate, or review research. These capacities can be further limited where fragile health systems are already strained due to the pandemic. Good governance and coordination of research therefore demands that well-resourced countries and organizations support local researchers and ethics review boards in fragile or vulnerable settings to overcome these challenges, particularly to ensure research is conducted to high standards even in low-resource settings and that the benefits of research are shared equitably (Emanuel et al. 2004). In other words, existing global inequities, understood in terms of research capacity, health system capacity, and economic circumstances, have important consequences for the responsibilities countries and organizations have for research governance and coordination (Nuffield Council on Bioethics 2020).

Obligations of those with existing resources do not preclude local community leadership and agency in pandemic research. Local researchers and communities must still be meaningfully involved in the design, implementation, analysis, reporting, and publication of pandemic research as a matter of international equity in science and equal moral respect for affected communities, as well as to ensure studies respond to local realities and needs without jeopardizing pandemic response in those settings (Smith and Upshur 2018). Working with local partners to prepare for and respond to ethical issues in pandemics is therefore critical (Bain et al. 2018). This may require, among other things, building and strengthening capacity of ethics review bodies and their members in low- and middle-income countries, both in general and in relation to the ethical review of research conducted in emergency contexts (Bain et al. 2018; Gailits et al. 2019). Multiple tools could support capacity building to this end, including the development and sharing of model study protocols to be used by local research ethics committees (Macklin and Cowan 2009), template agreements for data and biospecimen ownership and governance (Alirol et al. 2017), case studies of common ethical issues expected to emerge in these contexts, model standard operating procedures for emergency ethics review (Saxena et al. 2019), and a repository of study protocols or protocol parts that articulate best practices in research design and implementation (WHO 2010). In all cases, capacity building efforts ought to be designed and positioned so as to encourage the bidirectionality of learning (Kohrt et al. 2019).

Ethical analysis, support, and oversight of research conducted during pandemics is of the utmost importance, particularly when such research is conducted in resource-poor settings or with already disadvantaged populations (O'Mathúna et al. 2013; Rid and Emanuel 2014; Schopper 2014; Sumathipala et al. 2010; Tansey et al. 2017). Among other reasons, this is because pandemics often necessitate a deviation from common research expectations (e.g., a faster roll-out of research or a shift from the relatively slow, traditional research ethics review processes to an expedited approach) (Bain et al. 2018; Calain 2018; Dahab 2017; Eckenwiler et al. 2015; Folayan et al. 2015; Mezinska et al. 2016; O'Mathúna 2010; Richardson et al. 2017; Thielman et al. 2016), research activities may impede response efforts or confuse potential research participants (O'Mathúna et al. 2013), potential participants who are already vulnerable may have increased vulnerability (Levine 2004), and because there may be a distortion of risk-benefit assessments, standards of care, and the quality of informed consent in these contexts (Adebamowo et al. 2014; Alirol et al. 2017; Andersen et al. 2015; Bain et al. 2018; Calain et al. 2009; Ellenberg et al. 2018; Joffe 2014; Kohrt et al. 2019; Leider et al. 2017; Millum et al. 2019; Sumathipala et al. 2010). These considerations or issues raise distinctive ethics and governance challenges (Mitra and Sethi 2016).

Existing regional, institutional, or national ethics review bodies provide ethics support, advice, review, and approval for research conducted both in general and during pandemics. Yet, not all countries or institutions have ethics review bodies, and some may not have the resources to function optimally, especially during pandemics (Schopper et al. 2009). Indeed, limited funding, limited training and expertise, and weak institutional support still plague many ethics review bodies in low- and middle-income countries (Bain et al. 2018; Eckenwiler et al. 2015). Even in well-resourced settings, many ethics review bodies or supports are largely designed to operate in non-emergency contexts and may lack relevant expertise related to pandemic research and its review, and therefore may not be capable of adequately adapting to the contexts of pandemics (Chan et al. 2019). Finally, significant collaboration and coordination deficiencies among ethics review bodies have been noted (both in general and in the context of public health emergencies), including the duplication of reviews, discordance between reviews and policies of different committees, and limited communication between committees (Ayukekbong 2016; Bain et al. 2018; Calain 2018; De Crop et al. 2016; Schopper et al. 2017). As a result, some have called for additional independent, international oversight of research (particularly clinical trials) to avoid inter-agency governance challenges (Thompson 2016). However, ethics review bodies must be adequately supported if they are to be expected address these deficits and successfully adapt to pandemic contexts, which was a shortcoming during the COVID-19 pandemic (Salamanca-Buentello et al. 2024).

It can also be said that there has been more attention to the ethics of emergency research (and to the ethics of research in low-income countries) in recent years, as the West Africa Ebola, Zika, and COVID-19 episodes have led to increasing reflection and writing more specifically related to this sort of research. The Nuffield Council on Bioethics (2020) published its report, "Research in global health emergencies: ethical issues" in January 2020 after several years of gestation, consultation, and writing. As 2020 rapidly became the year of the pandemic, WHO published several sets of ethical guidelines directly touching on research response (WHO 2020b, c, d, e, f, g). Whatever authority such guidelines may be lacking, they certainly provide food for reflection on the part of research ethics committees—if the latter can find time during the emergency to consult them—hence the need for both clinical investigators and review committees to get a thorough grounding in the ethics of emergency research before the emergency arrives.

Box 4: An Ethical Compass to Aid in the Navigation of Issues in Pandemic Research

The Nuffield Council on Bioethics (2020) has proposed an 'ethical compass' (Fig. 1) to inform policy approaches and help provide a common language and way of thinking through ethical dilemmas related to the conduct of research in emergencies, like pandemics. The ethical compass is comprised of three shared values:

- *Equal respect*: treating others as moral equals, including respecting their dignity, humanity and human rights.
- *Helping reduce suffering*: acting in accordance with fundamental duties, founded on solidarity, and humanity, to help those in need or suffering from disease.
- *Fairness*: including both duties of non-discrimination in the treatment of others, and of the equitable distribution of benefits and burdens.

The Council argues that, in many cases, these three values will suggest a clear course of ac-

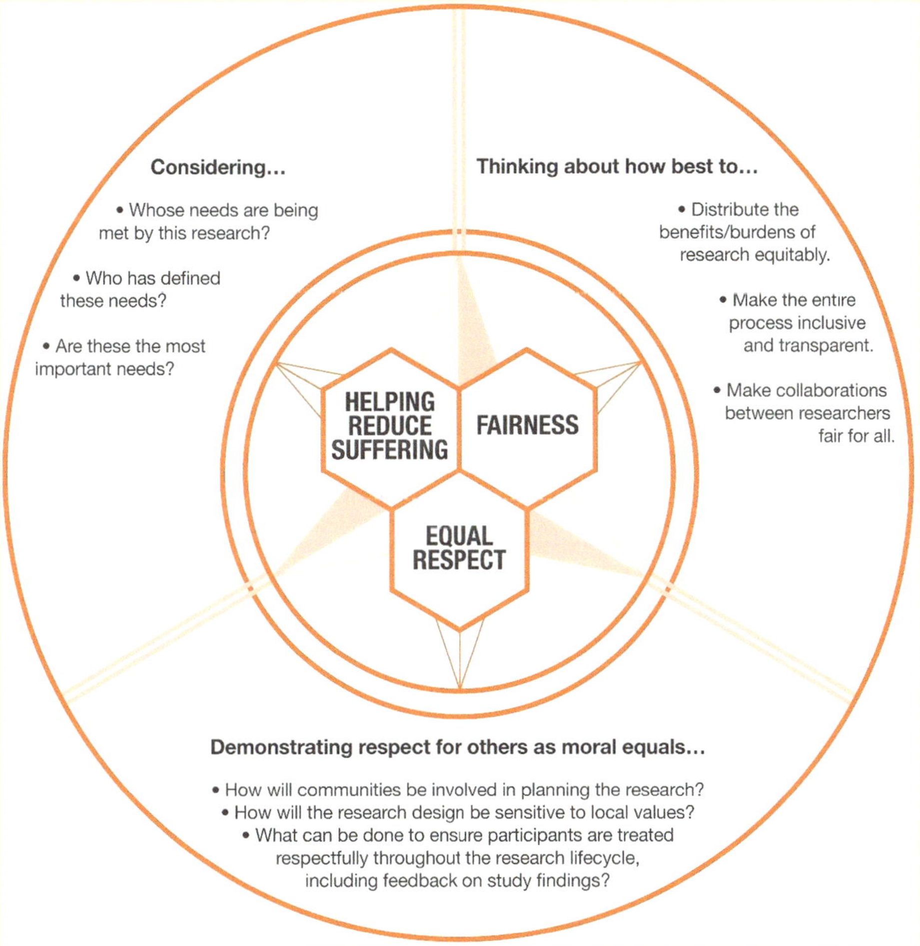

Fig. 1 The Nuffield ethical compass to aid in the navigation of issues in pandemic research, by Jade Rawling. (Nuffield Council on Bioethics 2020)

tion. In cases where this is not possible, these values act as an aid to thinking through whether ethical principles routinely applied to certain kinds of research might legitimately be adapted.

Perhaps the greatest challenge in navigating the application of these values occurs when the commitment to reduce suffering comes into conflict with the values of fairness. In other words, in a dire infectious disease outbreak like COVID-19, efforts to promote or achieve fairness in research may not always result in the greatest reduction in morbidity and mortality, and hence, reduction in suffering, which may cause some to ask whether commitments to fairness should be attenuated in service of minimizing the greatest amount of suffering as rapidly as possible.

Discussion questions: In what situations, if ever, should efforts to ensure fairness give way to the urgency to evaluate countermeasures in order to reduce suffering? Is there a way to reconcile commitments to reducing suffering and fairness?

7 Conclusion

Numerous ethical challenges can be expected to arise in research conducted during pandemics due to the urgent need to control morbidity and mortality and the challenging environments in which that research may have to take place. But fundamental ethical questions about the research enterprise itself and how it ought to operate in pandemics in many ways precede and ought to inform the ways in which we respond to those ethical challenges. The research enterprise is not a neutral endeavor. The justifications for what research is prioritized, how it is conducted, where it is conducted, and with whom it is conducted in light of a pandemic reflect judgments informed by values. This chapter has sought to examine prominent foundational ethical questions and considerations undergirding the research enterprise in pandemic contexts, including whether pandemics necessitate deviations from ethical and scientific standards for research, how research priorities are and ought to be set during pandemics, the ethics of conducting research alongside pandemic response efforts, and how pandemic research ought to be governed and coordinated. Preparing for the next pandemic will require a blueprint to accelerate the organization, coordination, and conduct of critical research and development. This requires innovative thinking about the tools, technologies, and mechanisms to support pandemic research. But such a blueprint will be distorted if it is not also explicitly grounded in ethical commitments, standards, and judgments capable of informing research priorities, collaboration and partnership, and equitable data and benefit sharing, and which exemplify an equal moral respect for all affected.

References

Adebamowo C, Bah-Sow O, Binka F, Bruzzone R, Caplan A, Delfraissy J-F, et al. Randomised controlled trials for Ebola: practical and ethical issues. Lancet. 2014;384(9952):1423–4.

Alirol E, Kuesel AC, Guraiib MM, de la Fuente-Núñez V, Saxena A, Gomes MF. Ethics review of studies during public health emergencies—the experience of the WHO ethics review committee during the Ebola virus disease epidemic. BMC Med Ethics. 2017;18(1):43. https://doi.org/10.1186/s12910-017-0201-1.

Alliance for Accelerating Excellence in Science in Africa. The Alliance for Accelerating Excellence in Science in Africa (AESA). 2021. https://www.aasciences.africa/aesa. Accessed 7 Dec 2021.

Andersen KG, Shapiro BJ, Matranga CB, Sealfon R, Lin AE, Moses LM, et al. Clinical sequencing uncovers origins and evolution of Lassa virus. Cell. 2015;162(4):738–50. https://doi.org/10.1016/j.cell.2015.07.020.

AVAC. Essential principles & practices for GPP compliance: engaging stakeholders in biomedical research during the era of COVID-19. New York: Global Advocacy for HIV Prevention (AVAC); 2021.

Ayukekbong JA. The 2014–2015 Ebola saga: lessons for the future. J Epidemiol Community Health. 2016;70(1):1–2.

Bain LE, Ebuenyi ID, Ekukwe NC, Awah PK. Rethinking research ethics committees in low- and medium-income countries. Res Ethics. 2018;14(1):1–7. https://doi.org/10.1177/1747016117692026.

Bausch DG, Sprecher AG, Jeffs B, Boumandouki P. Treatment of Marburg and Ebola hemorrhagic fevers: a strategy for testing new drugs and vaccines under outbreak conditions. Antivir Res. 2008;78(1):150–61. https://doi.org/10.1016/j.antiviral.2008.01.152.

Bramstedt KA. Luxembourg's approach to research integrity during the COVID-19 pandemic. Account Res. 2020;27(6):396–400. https://doi.org/10.1080/08989621.2020.1778473.

Bugin K, Woodcock J. Trends in COVID-19 therapeutic clinical trials. Nat Rev Drug Discov. 2021;20:254. https://doi.org/10.1038/d41573-021-00037-3.

Calain P. The Ebola clinical trials: a precedent for research ethics in disasters. J Med Ethics. 2018;44(1):3–8. https://doi.org/10.1136/medethics-2016-103474.

Calain P, Fiore N, Poncin M, Hurst SA. Research ethics and international epidemic response: the case of Ebola and Marburg hemorrhagic fevers. Public Health Ethics. 2009;2(1):7–29. https://doi.org/10.1093/phe/phn037.

Canario Guzmán JA, Espinal R, Báez J, Melgen RE, Rosario PAP, Mendoza ER. Ethical challenges for international collaborative research partnerships in the context of the Zika outbreak in the Dominican Republic: a qualitative case study. Health Res Policy Syst. 2017;15(1):82. https://doi.org/10.1186/s12961-017-0246-0.

CEPI. Who we are. Coalition for Epidemic Preparedness Innovations (CEPI), Oslo. 2021. https://cepi.net/about/whoweare/. Accessed 7 Dec 2021.

Chan EYY, Wright K, Parker M. Health-emergency disaster risk management and research ethics. Lancet. 2019;93(10167):112–3.

Dahab M. Operational challenges of implementing health research in humanitarian settings: lessons learned from R2HC funded studies. Cardiff: ELRHA; 2017.

De Crop M, Dela Mou A, Van Griensven J, Ravinetto R. Multiple ethical review in North-South collaborative research: the experience of the Ebola-Tx trial in Guinea. Indian J Med Ethics. 2016;1(2):76–82.

Denne SC, Pediatric Policy Council. Including pregnant women in clinical research: time to overcome the barriers. Pediatr Res. 2019;86:554–5. https://doi.org/10.1038/s41390-019-0553-y.

Eckenwiler L, Pringle J, Boulanger R, Hunt M. Real-time responsiveness for ethics oversight during disaster research. Bioethics. 2015;29(9):653–61.

Ellenberg SS, Keusch GT, Babiker AG, Edwards KM, Lewis RJ, Lundgren JD, et al. Rigorous clinical trial design in public health emergencies is essential. Clin Infect Dis. 2018;66(9):1467–9. https://doi.org/10.1093/cid/cix1032.

Emanuel EJ, Wendler D, Killen J, Grady C. What makes clinical research in developing countries ethical? The benchmarks of ethical research. J Infect Dis. 2004;189(5):930–7. https://doi.org/10.1086/381709.

European Network of Research Integrity Offices. Research integrity even more important for research during a pandemic. Helsinki: European Network of Research Integrity Offices; 2020.

FDA. ERVEBO. 2019. https://www.fda.gov/vaccines-blood-biologics/ervebo. Accessed 17 Oct 2021.

FDA. FDA approves treatment for Ebola virus. Washington, DC: U.S. Food and Drug Administration; 2020.

Folayan MO, Peterson K, Kombe F. Ethics, emergencies and Ebola clinical trials: the role of governments and communities in offshored research. Pan Afr Med J. 2015;22(Suppl 1):10. https://doi.org/10.11694/pamj.supp.2015.22.1.6216.

G7 Therapeutics and vaccines clinical trials charter. G7 Health Ministers' Meeting, June 2021, 4 Jun 2021, Oxford. London, UK Department of Health and Social Care; 2021. p. 2.

Gailits N, Nouvet E, Pringle J, Hunt M, Lu D, Bernard C, et al. Blurring lines: complexities of ethical challenges in the conduct of West African Ebola research. Hamilton, ON: Humanitarian Healthcare Ethics Research Group; 2019.

GLOPID-R. About us. 2021. https://www.glopid-r.org/about-us/. Accessed 7 Dec 2021.

Hankins C, Warren M, Bass E, Sarche J, Wiysonge C, GPP Working Group. Communities matter! Guidelines for good participatory practice in HIV prevention trial (GPP). IAS Conference on HIV Pathogenesis, Treatment and Prevention; 2007.

Hope T, McMillan J. Challenge studies of human volunteers: ethical issues. J Med Ethics. 2004;30(1):110–6. https://doi.org/10.1136/jme.2003.004440.

Hunt MR, Anderson JA, Boulanger RF. Ethical implications of diversity in disaster research. Am J Disaster Med. 2012;7:211–21. https://doi.org/10.5055/ajdm.2012.0096.

Jamrozik E, Selgelid MJ. Human challenge studies in endemic settings: ethical and regulatory issues, Springer briefs in ethics. Cham: Springer; 2021.

Joffe S. Evaluating novel therapies during the ebola epidemic. JAMA. 2014;312(13):1299–300.

Kahn JP, Meltzer Henry L, Matroianni AC, Chen WH, Macklin R. For now, it's unethical to use human challenge studies for SARS-CoV-2 vaccine development. Proc Natl Acad Sci USA. 2020;117(46):28538–42. https://doi.org/10.1073/pnas.2021189117.

Kayano R, Chan EY, Murray V, Abrahams J, Barber SL. WHO thematic platform for health emergency and disaster risk management research network (TPRN): report of the Kobe Expert Meeting. Int J Environ Res Public Health. 2019;16(7):1232. https://doi.org/10.3390/ijerph16071232.

Knox Clarke P, Darcy J. Insufficient evidence? The quality and use of evidence in humanitarian action. London: Active Learning Network for Accountability and Performance in Humanitarian Action; 2014. Report No.: ISBN: 978-0-9926446-4-2.

Kohrt BA, Mistry AS, Anand N, Beecroft B, Nuwayhid I. Health research in humanitarian crises: an urgent global imperative. BMJ Glob Health. 2019;4(6):e001870. https://doi.org/10.1136/bmjgh-2019-001870.

Krubiner C, Faden R, Karron R, Little M, Lyerly A, Abramson J, et al. Pregnant women & vaccines against emerging epidemic threats: ethics guidance for preparedness, research, and response. Vaccine. 2019;39:85. https://doi.org/10.1016/j.vaccine.2019.01.011.

Leider JP, DeBruin D, Reynolds N, Koch A, Seaberg J. Ethical guidance for disaster response, specifically around crisis standards of care: a systematic review. Am J Public Health. 2017;107(9):e1–9.

Levine C. The concept of vulnerability in disaster research. J Trauma Stress. 2004;17(5):395–402.

Levine C, Faden R, Grady C, Hammerschmidt D, Eckenwiler L, Sugarman J, et al. "Special scrutiny": a targeted form of research protocol review. Ann Intern Med. 2004;140(3):220–3. https://doi.org/10.7326/0003-4819-140-3-200402030-00013.

London AJ, Kimmelman J. Against pandemic research exceptionalism. Science. 2020;368(6490):476–7. https://doi.org/10.1126/science.abc1731.

Macklin R, Cowan E. Conducting research in disease outbreaks. PLoS Negl Trop Dis. 2009;3(4):e335. https://doi.org/10.1371/journal.pntd.0000335.

Mezinska S, Kakuk P, Mijaljica G, Waligóra M, O'Mathúna DP. Research in disaster settings: a systematic qualitative review of ethical guidelines. BMC Med Ethics. 2016;17(1):62. https://doi.org/10.1186/s12910-016-0148-7.

Millum J, Beecroft B, Hardcastle TC, Hirshon JM, Hyder AA, Newberry JA, et al. Emergency care research ethics in low-income and middle-income countries. BMJ Glob Health. 2019;4(Suppl

6):e001260. https://doi.org/10.1136/bmjgh-2018-001260.
Mitra AG, Sethi N. Conducting research in the context of global health emergencies: identifying key ethical and governance issues. Nuffield Council on Bioethics; 2016.
Moon S, Armstrong J, Hutler B, Upshur R, Katz R, Atuire C, et al. Governing the Access to COVID-19 Tools Accelerator: towards greater participation, transparency, and accountability. Lancet. 2021;399:487. https://doi.org/10.1016/s0140-6736(21)02344-8.
Mulangu S, Dodd LE, Davey RT Jr, Tshiani Mbaya O, Proschan M, Mukadi D, et al. A randomized, controlled trial of Ebola virus disease therapeutics. N Engl J Med. 2019;381(24):2293–303. https://doi.org/10.1056/NEJMoa1910993.
NASEM. Integrating clinical research into epidemic response: the Ebola experience. Washington, DC: National Academies of Sciences Engineering and Medicine Publications, The National Academies Press; 2017.
Nuffield Council on Bioethics. Research in global health emergencies: ethical issues. Oxford, UK: Nuffield Council on Bioethics; 2020.
Nuyens Y. Setting priorities for health research: lessons from low- and middle-income countries. Bull World Health Organ. 2007;85:319–20. https://doi.org/10.2471/blt.06.032375.
O'Mathúna D. Conducting research in the aftermath of disasters: ethical considerations. J Evid Based Med. 2010;3(2):65–75.
O'Mathúna D, Gordijn B, Clarke M. Disaster bioethics: normative issues when nothing is normal. Springer Science & Business Media; 2013.
OHRP. International compilation of human research standards. Wasington, DC: Office of Human Research Protection, U.S. Department of Health and Human Services; 2020.
PAHO. Zika ethics consultation: ethics guidance on key issues raised by the outbreak. Washington, DC: Pan American Health Organization; 2016.
Parker B. Aid community raises highest alert on Ebola. New Humanitarian. 2019.
Plotkin SA, Caplan A. Extraordinary diseases require extraordinary solutions. Vaccine. 2020;38(24):3987–8.
Pratt B, Loff B. A framework to link international clinical research to the promotion of justice in global health. Bioethics. 2014;28(8):387–96. https://doi.org/10.1111/bioe.12009.
Pratt B, Sheehan M, Barsdorf N, Hyder AA. Exploring the ethics of global health research priority-setting. BMC Med Ethics. 2018;19:94. https://doi.org/10.1186/s12910-018-0333-y.
Public Health Ontario. A framework for the ethical conduct of public health initiatives. Toronto: Queen's Printer for Ontario; 2012.
Raynaud M, Zhang H, Louis K, Goutaudier V, Wang J, Dubourg Q, et al. COVID-19-related medical research: a meta-research and critical appraisal. BMC Med Res Methodol. 2021;21(1):1. https://doi.org/10.1186/s12874-020-01190-w.
RECOVERY trial. University of Oxford, Oxford. 2022. https://www.recoverytrial.net/. Accessed 15 Apr 2022.
Richardson T, Johnston AM, Draper H. A systematic review of Ebola treatment trials to assess the extent to which they adhere to ethical guidelines. PLoS One. 2017;12(1):e0168975.
Rid A, Emanuel EJ. Ethical considerations of experimental interventions in the Ebola outbreak. Lancet. 2014;384(9957):1896–9. https://doi.org/10.1016/s0140-6736(14)61315-5.
Sacket D. Bias in analytic research. J Chronic Dis. 1979;32(1–2):51–63. https://doi.org/10.1016/0021-9681(79)90012-2.
Salamanca-Buentello F, Katz R, Silva D, Upshur REG, Smith MJ. Research ethics review during the covid-19 pandemic: an international study. PLOS One. 2024. https://doi.org/10.1371/journal.pone.0292512. https://journals.plos.org/plosone/article?id=10.1371/journal.pone.0292512.
Saxena A, Horby P, Amuasi J, Aagaard N, Kohler J, Gooshki ES, et al. Ethics preparedness: facilitating ethics review during outbreaks—recommendations from an expert panel. BMC Med Ethics. 2019;20(1):29. https://doi.org/10.1186/s12910-019-0366-x.
Schopper D. Research ethics governance in disaster situations. In: O'Mathúna D, Gordijn B, Clarke M, editors. Disaster bioethics: normative issues when nothing is normal. Springer Science & Business Media; 2014. p. 175–90.
Schopper D, Upshur R, Matthys F, Singh JA, Bandewar SS, Ahmad A, et al. Research ethics review in humanitarian contexts: the experience of the Independent Ethics Review Board of Médecins Sans Frontieres. PLoS Med. 2009;6(7):e1000115.
Schopper D, Ravinetto R, Schwartz L, Kamaara E, Sheel S, Selgelid MJ, et al. Research ethics governance in times of Ebola. Public Health Ethics. 2017;10(1):49–61. https://doi.org/10.1093/phe/phw039.
Sethi N. Research and global health emergencies: on the essential role of best practice. Public Health Ethics. 2018;11(3):237–50. https://doi.org/10.1093/phe/phy014.
Singh JA, Kochhar S, Wolff J, WHO ACT-Accelerator Ethics & Governance Working Group. Placebo use and unblinding in COVID-19 vaccine trials: recommendations of a WHO Expert Working Group. Nat Med. 2021;27:569–70. https://doi.org/10.1038/s41591-021-01299-5.
Smith M, Upshur R. Pandemic disease, public health, and ethics. In: Mastroianni AC, Kahn JP, Kass NE, editors. The Oxford handbook of public health ethics. New York: Oxford University Press; 2018.
Smith MJ. "Publication bias" and how it might affect the response to public health emergencies. In: WHO, editor. Ethics in epidemics, emergencies and disas-

ters: research, surveillance and patient care. Geneva: World Health Organization; 2015.
Smith MJ, Emanuel EJ, Thomé B, Upshur RE. Ethical conditions for accelerating COVID-19 vaccine research. Wellcome Open Res. 2020a;5:249. https://doi.org/10.12688/wellcomeopenres.16361.1.
Smith MJ, Upshur RE, Emanuel EJ. Publication ethics during public health emergencies such as the COVID-19 pandemic. Am J Public Health. 2020b;110(7):e1–2. https://doi.org/10.2105/AJPH.2020.305686.
Sumathipala A, Jafarey A, De Castro LD, Ahmad A, Marcer D, Srinivasan S, et al. Ethical issues in post-disaster clinical interventions and research: a developing world perspective. key findings from a drafting and consensus generation meeting of the Working Group on Disaster Research and Ethics (WGDRE) 2007. Asian Bioeth Rev. 2010;2(2):124–42.
Tansey CM, Herridge MS, Heslegrave RJ, Lavery JV. A framework for research ethics review during public emergencies. CMAJ. 2010;182(14):1533–7. https://doi.org/10.1503/cmaj.090976.
Tansey CM, Anderson J, Boulanger RF, Eckenwiler L, Pringle J, Schwartz L, et al. Familiar ethical issues amplified: how members of research ethics committees describe ethical distinctions between disaster and non-disaster research. BMC Med Ethics. 2017;18(1):44. https://doi.org/10.1186/s12910-017-0203-z.
Thielman NM, Cunningham CK, Woods C, Petzold E, Sprenz M, Russell J. Ebola clinical trials: five lessons learned and a way forward. Clin Trials (London, England). 2016;13(1):83–6. https://doi.org/10.1177/1740774515619897.
Thompson AK. Bioethics meets Ebola: exploring the moral landscape. Br Med Bull. 2016;117(1):5–13. https://doi.org/10.1093/bmb/ldv055.
WHO. Research ethics in international epidemic response: WHO technical consultation. Meeting report. Geneva: World Health Organization; 2010. Contract No.: WHO/HSE/GIP/ITP/10.1.
WHO. Research and development to meet health needs in developing countries: strengthening global financing and coordination. Geneva: World Health Organization; 2012. Report No.: ISBN: 978 92 4 150345 7.
WHO. Guidance for managing ethical issues in infectious disease outbreaks. Geneva: World Health Organization; 2016a.
WHO. An R&D blueprint for action to prevent epidemics: plan of action 2016. Geneva: World Health Organization; 2016b.
WHO. Emergency use designation of COVID-19 candidate vaccines: ethical considerations for current and future COVID-19 placebo-controlled vaccine trials and trial unblinding. Geneva: World Health Organization; 2020a. Contract No.: WHO/2019-nCoV/Policy_Brief/EUD_placebo-controlled_vaccine_trials/2020.1.
WHO. Ethical standards for research during public health emergencies: distilling existing guidance to support COVID-19 R&D. Geneva: World Health Organization; 2020b. COVID-19 WWGoE. Contract No.: WHO reference number: WHO/RFH/20.1.
WHO. Ethics review committee: review process. Geneva: Word Health Organization; 2020c. https://www.who.int/ethics/review-committee/review_process/en/. Accessed 20 Jan 2020.
WHO. Good Participatory Practice for COVID-19 clinical trials—a toolbox. Geneva: World Health Organization; 2020d.
WHO. Guidance for research ethics committees for rapid review of research during public health emergencies. Geneva: World Health Organization; 2020e.
WHO. Integrating ethics in infectious disease outbreaks. Geneva: World Health Organization; 2020f. https://extranet.who.int/ethics/home. Accessed 6 Oct 2020.
WHO. Key criteria for the ethical acceptability of COVID-19 human challenge studies. Geneva: World Health Organization; 2020g. Contract No.: WHO/2019-nCoV/Ethics_criteria/2020.1.
WHO. WHO COVID-19 solidarity therapeutics trial. Geneva: World Health Organization; 2021. https://www.who.int/emergencies/diseases/novel-coronavirus-2019/global-research-on-novel-coronavirus-2019-ncov/solidarity-clinical-trial-for-covid-19-treatments. Accessed 15 Oct 2021.
WHO. The Access to COVID-19 Tools (ACT) accelerator. Geneva: World Health Organization; 2022a. https://www.who.int/initiatives/act-accelerator. Accessed 2 Mar 2022.
WHO. WHO COVID-19 solidarity trial vaccines. Geneva: World Health Organization; 2022b. https://www.who.int/emergencies/diseases/novel-coronavirus-2019/global-research-on-novel-coronavirus-2019-ncov/solidarity-trial-of-covid-19-vaccines. Accessed 19 May 2022.
Willison DJ, Ondrusek N, Dawson A, Emerson C, Ferris LE, Saginur R, et al. What makes public health studies ethical? Dissolving the boundary between research and practice. BMC Med Ethics. 2014;15:61. https://doi.org/10.1186/1472-6939-15-61.
Wilson B, Wright K, Taylor R, Higgs E. Beyond recruitment: good participatory practice enhances the impact of research in a pandemic. Nat Med. 2021;27(3):369–71. https://doi.org/10.1038/s41591-021-01271-3.
WMA. Declaration of Helsinki: ethical principles for medical research involving human subjects. Ferney-Voltaire, France: World Medical Association; 2013.

4.1 In Practice: Vaccine Efficacy and Safety Testing—An Ethical Case for Individual Randomization

Nir Eyal and Marc Lipsitch

Contents

Learning Track Note: This chapter appears in Learning Tracks: Biostatistics; Clinical Research; Public Health and Epidemiology; Research Ethics

E. S. Higgs and R. A. Sorenson (eds.), *Principles and Practice of Emergency Research Response*,
https://doi.org/10.1007/978-3-031-48408-7_5

Learning Objectives

This chapter will help readers understand and describe:

- The ethical case for individually randomized, placebo-controlled clinical trials as the best trial designs in a high-mortality infectious disease emergency
- The ethical and practical dimensions of manufacturers providing vaccine, once it is authorized for use, to clinical trial participants who had received placebo during a Phase III trial
- Ethical advantages of individually randomized trials as compared to alternatives. The relevance of protections that benefit trial participants, including those receiving placebo

1 Introduction

What trial design is most ethical for assessing the efficacy of candidate vaccines against emerging infections? During the 2014–2016 Ebola outbreak, some suggested that, at least during highly lethal outbreaks against which there are no accepted vaccines or treatments, even when an individually randomized controlled trial would be most efficient, it is heartless to deny people the chance of receiving life-saving medical countermeasures (Cohen 2014; Cohen and Kupferschmidt 2014; Macklin 2014). The individuals randomized to not receive the candidate vaccine are effectively abandoned to a lethal disease. Indeed, some proffered alternative trial designs, which give all participants the candidate vaccine (as does a stepped-wedge design, which randomizes some groups of individuals to receive the experimental vaccine later, rather than denying it to them altogether); and still other trial designs contrasted with individual randomization (Caplan et al. 2015).

Strikingly, these claims were to our knowledge absent from the ethical debate about vaccine testing during COVID-19. But this may have reflected special characteristics of COVID-19, and it remains important for future outbreaks to see why these claims are misguided. As we shall explain, any individually randomized controlled trial tends to benefit all study participants or at least treat them fairly, especially in an outbreak of a lethal pathogen against which no approved vaccines or treatments exist. It can remain ethical in other respects as well.

2 Supporting Considerations

Forms of individually randomized trial will usually reach any level of statistical assurance of efficacy being sought faster, or with fewer participants, than any alternative to individual randomization. These alternatives include no study, an uncontrolled trial, a study design using historical controls, and a trial with cluster-randomized control (Dean et al. 2019; Kahn et al. 2018). It is true that, given feasibility constraints, some subtypes of the individually randomized trial are slower to reveal efficacy than some alternatives to such a trial (Lipsitch et al. 2015). Importantly, however, the fastest individually randomized trials—the only ones recommended for emergency circumstances—will reach any level of statistical confidence faster than alternatives (Lipsitch et al. 2015). We set aside the question whether other trial designs might better identify public health impact, partly because the latter is strongly sensitive to setting and hence less generalizable (Hitchings et al. 2018; Kahn et al. 2018) (◘ Fig. 1).

The expediency of the best individually randomized designs enhances their ethics. Especially when a vaccine candidate could reduce incidence of a highly lethal disease that puts many at risk and when no other protection exists, an expedient design is ethically urgent. Should the vaccine prove efficacious, a slower design will have delayed its approval and rollout to the broader population, including at-risk people. Study participants benefit from many protections that people at similar risk of infection do not receive, e.g., close monitoring, typically better clinician–patient ratios, and especially a

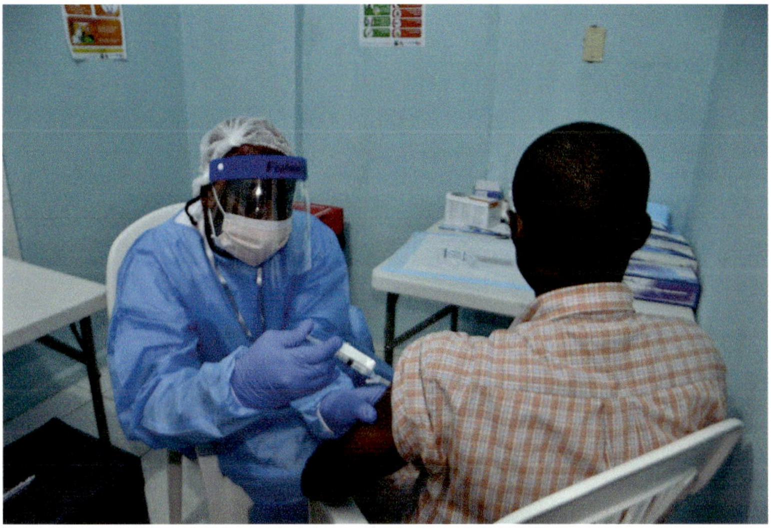

Fig. 1 A participant in a NIAID-supported vaccine study in West Africa receives an injection. Candidate vaccine or placebo? (Credit: PREVAIL)

chance to have been randomized to the preferred arm of the study (Bellan et al. 2014; Cox et al. 2014; Eyal and Lipsitch 2017). This typically better protection inside the trial rests not on trialists' having unjustly made the situation worse for anyone declining participation—trialists do nothing of the sort; it reflects the reality (emphasized by opponents of individual randomization) that no approved vaccines or treatments exist. The vaccine being tested remains experimental. It should not be widely available outside the trial; select "compassionate use" by non-participating communities can defeat the purpose; and often no doses exist for this use outside the trial (London 2018). While one can always further optimize the protection of participants at the expense of rapid protection of the broader population, that would arguably be unfair toward the latter. Numerous people at similar severe risk and with fewer protections depend on rapid results from the study.

It is true that a vaccine may be toxic or otherwise harmful to some or all trial participants, and that this harm may sometimes be discovered only in the process of efficacy testing (Lipsitch and Eyal 2017). But surely that cannot support complaints about individually randomized trials' failure to offer the untested vaccine to everyone.

Expediency can even be made to benefit study participants, including study controls, if all participants are promised access to the candidate vaccine as soon as data are analyzed (or, in some situations, collected) and the vaccine is shown to be effective. That means that when the candidate vaccine would improve recipients' prospects, all participants of fast individually randomized trials could access that benefit before some recipients of slower, non-individually randomized trials (Eyal and Lipsitch 2017; Lipsitch and Eyal 2017). But this arrangement complicates comparing the difference between study arms in longer-term outcomes.

Indeed, individual randomization can offer all participants a chance to get (the experimental) intervention even before data collection ends. The choice of individual randomization is compatible with delayed or active control, parallel or stepped rollout, various primary endpoints, and various choices of trial populations (Kahn et al. 2018), as well as either natural or deliberate (Eyal et al. 2020) viral exposure. Any ethical appeal based on giving everyone something during the trial is perfectly compatible with individually randomized design and its statistical advantages. These approaches can achieve the advantages of individual randomization while in some cases still providing the experimental intervention to all participants.

Thus, if the earliest possible vaccination of all trial participants were ethically necessary, a stepped-wedge design would remain unnecessary: in many if not all circumstances there would be scientifically preferable ways to vaccinate everyone earlier.

3 Conclusion

The strong default for testing candidate vaccine efficacy in most circumstances of an emerging infection should be an individually randomized design (Eyal and Lipsitch 2017; Lipsitch and Eyal 2017; London 2018; NASEM 2017). The case for individually randomized testing is strongest when the outbreak is of a highly lethal infection for which no drugs and vaccinations exist. Statistically weaker designs tend to be unnecessary and less ethical.

Discussion Questions

1. What are the arguments that individually randomized clinical trials are unethical in a high-mortality infectious disease emergency? What are their limitations?
2. What are some protections that benefit trial participants—even those who receive placebo—in individually randomized trials, benefits that people from the same population who are not enrolled in a trial might not receive?
3. Individually randomized trials will usually reach any given level of statistical evidence faster, or with fewer participants, than alternatives. What is the ethical import of this comparative advantage in reaching conclusions?
4. At the end of 2020, after receiving emergency use authorization for their vaccines, manufacturers provided vaccine to COVID-19 clinical trial participants who had received placebo during the trials. Was this justified? How? Did it have any disadvantages? What were they?

References

Bellan SE, Pulliam JRC, Dushoff J, Meyers LA. Ebola virus vaccine trials: the ethical mandate for a therapeutic safety net. BMJ (Clin Res Ed). 2014;349:g7518. https://doi.org/10.1136/bmj.g7518.

Caplan AL, Plunkett C, Levin B. Selecting the right tool for the job. Am J Bioeth. 2015;15(4):4–10. https://doi.org/10.1080/15265161.2015.1010993.

Cohen J. Issues continue to dog the testing of Ebola drugs and vaccines. Science. 2014.

Cohen J, Kupferschmidt K. Ebola vaccine trials raise ethical issues. Science. 2014;346(6207):289–90. https://doi.org/10.1126/science.346.6207.289.

Cox E, Borio L, Temple R. Evaluating Ebola therapies—the case for RCTs. N Engl J Med. 2014;371(25):2350–1. https://doi.org/10.1056/nejmp1414145.

Dean N, Gsell P-S, Brookmeyer R, De Gruttola V, Donnelly C, Halloran M, et al. Design of vaccine efficacy trials during public health emergencies. Sci Transl Med. 2019;11(499):eaat0360. https://doi.org/10.1126/scitranslmed.aat0360.

Eyal N, Lipsitch M. Vaccine testing for emerging infections: the case for individual randomisation. J Med Ethics. 2017;43(9):625–31. https://doi.org/10.1136/medethics-2015-103220.

Eyal N, Lipsitch M, Smith PG. Human challenge studies to accelerate coronavirus vaccine licensure. J Infect Dis. 2020; https://doi.org/10.1093/infdis/jiaa152.

Hitchings M, Lipsitch M, Wang R, Bellan S. Competing effects of indirect protection and clustering on the power of cluster-randomized controlled vaccine trials. Am J Epidemiol. 2018;187(8):1763–71. https://doi.org/10.1093/aje/kwy047.

Kahn R, Rid A, Smith P, Eyal N, Lipsitch M. Choices in vaccine trial design in epidemics of emerging infections. PLoS Med. 2018;15(8):e1002632. https://doi.org/10.1371/journal.pmed.1002632.

Lipsitch M, Eyal N. Improving vaccine trials in infectious disease emergencies. Science. 2017;357(6347):153–6. https://doi.org/10.1126/science.aam8334.

Lipsitch M, Eyal N, Halloran ME, Hernán MA, Longini IM, Perencevich EN, et al. Obtaining efficacy data in an environment of variable and uncertain incidence: Ebola and beyond. Science. 2015;348(6230):46–8. https://doi.org/10.1126/science.aaa3178.

London AJ. Social value, clinical equipoise, and research in a public health emergency. Bioethics. 2018;33(3):326–34. https://doi.org/10.1111/bioe.12467.

Macklin R. The ethics of the Ebola outbreak: who should receive experimental treatment? HuffPost; 2014.

NASEM. Integrating clinical research into epidemic response: the Ebola experience. Washington, DC: National Academies of Sciences Engineering and Medicine Publications, The National Academies Press; 2017.

4.2 In Practice: Research Ethics Committee Review in Public Health Emergencies

V. Koneti Rao

Contents

Learning Track Note: This chapter appears in Learning Tracks: Research Ethics

E. S. Higgs and R. A. Sorenson (eds.), *Principles and Practice of Emergency Research Response*,
https://doi.org/10.1007/978-3-031-48408-7_6

Learning Objectives

This chapter will help readers understand and describe:

- Advantages and disadvantages of a single research ethics board (REC) for clinical trial review and approval. What safeguards are needed in this case? What are the obstacles to a single ethical review board for a trial with international partners?
- Ethics of a small trial early in an outbreak on a medical countermeasure (MCM) that might work, based on biological mechanisms or on observed effects in patients, to get preliminary indications of safety and efficacy.
- Why the recommendation of a reputable clinician during a high-mortality outbreak is not sufficient for a regulatory authority to provide emergency use authorization.
- Minimum requirements for a REC decision on a request for regulatory concurrence on proof of principle to allow clinical research proposals that seek to provide actionable data to proceed.

1 Introduction

Consideration and debate among stakeholders, including funding agencies, government bodies, medical education and health care delivery systems, and the public continue in many venues on how to better prevent or prepare for the next global pandemic or other public health emergency (Nuffield Council on Bioethics 2020; WHO 2022). There are many ethical dimensions to the debate. The concept that a research program conceived in the initial phases of an outbreak can be implemented *during* the outbreak as a vital response element brings new considerations with it. The success of medical countermeasure (MCM) development during the coronavirus disease 2019 (COVID-19) pandemic has demonstrated that such research is an ethical necessity, not merely a potential additional response measure. To be of greatest benefit, such research must begin soon after a new pathogen appears to have the potential to spread widely. Yet, however urgent, emergency response research must go for review to a research ethics board (REC) or institutional review board (IRB)[1] to ensure compliance with ethical standards, including those governing interactions with individuals recruited as clinical trial participants (Packenham et al. 2021). Increasingly, these standards encompass not only individuals but their communities as well; emphasis on the plural since all of us belong to more than one community (MacQueen et al. 2001).

2 Historical Notes

The Nuremberg Code promulgated at the War Crimes Tribunal trial of 23 Nazi physicians and medical administrators in 1946–1949 has a fair claim as the watershed event in medical research ethics (Nuremberg Military Tribunals 1949). Perhaps the two most important points from the Nuremberg Code are the need for voluntary informed consent on the part of trial participants and a scientifically valid research design. However, widespread acceptance of the moral outrage and insight expressed by the justices in Nuremberg was a slow process in the United States and elsewhere. Indeed, much of the change in attitudes and establishment of guidelines came in response to abuses that demonstrated doctors could not be the sole judges of their own research (London 2022).

A few of the milestones on the way to wider acceptance of what are now globally accepted principles:

1. 1964: Declaration of Helsinki, World Medical Association (WMA 1964)
2. 1966: “Ethics and Clinical Research” article in the *New England Journal of Medicine* by H.K. Beecher (1966)

1 Editors’ note: Research ethics committee (REC) is the preferred term in this book because it is more descriptive than the rather opaque term usually used in the United States, institutional review board (IRB), as well as more familiar globally. Other equivalent terms include medical research ethics committee (MREC), *comité de protection des personnes* (CPP), research ethics board (REB), and human research ethics committee (HREC).

3. 1972: Associated Press story on Tuskegee study of untreated syphilis in Black men (Heller 1972)
4. 1977: The Belmont Report, National Commission for the Protection of Human Subjects of Biomedical and Behavioral Research (1979)

Pharmaceutical companies had research facilities for testing chemotherapeutics near prisons in the 1950s and 1960s (Ledford 2007). Even the U.S. National Institutes of Health (NIH) Clinical Center, when it opened in 1953, only required review of research involving healthy volunteers. The Belmont report established three principles that, in essence, continue to govern human-subjects research:

1. Respect for persons (dignity and autonomy requiring informed consent)
2. Beneficence (risks minimized and benefits maximized)
3. Justice (subject selection is equitable)

Routine ethical review of all research proposals began in earnest in the mid-1970s as well. In the United States today, all research sponsored or implemented by the Department of Health and Human Services (HHS) must be conducted under Federal Regulations embodying the Belmont report called, 45 CFR 46 or the Common Rule. This requires prospective review of any proposed research by an IRB. Most countries have analogous standards and regulations, though as noted earlier their capacity to conduct research and carry out ethical review varies greatly.

More recently, NIH and National Institute of Allergy and Infectious Diseases (NIAID) investigators have conducted expeditious scientific and ethical review of research studies to address public health emergencies including severe acute respiratory syndrome coronavirus (SARS-CoV-1), anthrax, various strains of influenza, Ebola, Zika, and Middle East respiratory syndrome coronavirus (MERS-CoV). Then, SARS-CoV-2 affected the entire planet starting in early 2020. In the wake of the 2009 H1N1 influenza pandemic, the Centers for Disease Control and Prevention (CDC) approached the NIH Office of Science Policy with concerns that ethical review of research protocols responding to emergent events could be too slow, delaying urgent research programs. The NIH Office of Science Policy (OSP) agreed to work with CDC and brought together a group including officials from the CDC, U.S. Food and Drug Administration (FDA), NIH (including the author), the Health and Human Services (HHS) Assistant Secretary for Preparedness and Response (ASPR), and the NIH Office of General Counsel to work out legal and ethical questions and logistics and explore the feasibility of establishing a REC/IRB with nationwide jurisdiction to review protocols in anticipation of, during, and after a public health emergency (Packenham et al. 2021). This process bore fruit with the publication of a new rule in 2016 mandating review by a single review board for research in the United States (Gordon et al. 2017).

3 Research Intervention in a Public Health Emergency

It is often thought that clinical investigators could have an inherent or perceived conflict of interest, as their medical training is oriented to promoting the welfare of individual patients, while their research program is aimed at developing medical countermeasures (MCMs) for society as a whole. For a century, "the axiom that the conscience of the investigator is an adequate judge of the ethics of an experiment" had been the basis of research ethics, but many of the abuses that led to the establishment of independent ethical review were committed by physicians making their own ethical decisions (Jonsen 1998). Seeking generalizable knowledge for the ultimate benefit of people other than participants in the research study requires another layer of peer review by a group of diverse, knowledgeable, and disinterested individuals to protect human subjects and ensure research standards are met. The ethical review process has become globally obligatory for virtually any research on humans that goes beyond pure observation.

A research ethics committee must review the risks and benefits to human participants in a proposed trial, considering their social circumstances and the applicable regulatory requirements. In an emergency, the ethics committee must act expeditiously, both because of the need to counter the outbreak if it continues, and because clinical trials are most productive when the risk of infection is high in the included population. If public health measures succeed in ending the outbreak, the opportunity to recruit enough participants to evaluate MCMs for future use may be lost (Higgs et al. 2017). The entire research operation needs to be adequately supported, funded, and implemented without burdensome delays. During an outbreak, the primary research goal is to mitigate morbidity and mortality and help end the emergency—not only to develop new medical countermeasures that might be available for future outbreaks. Vaccines against COVID-19 are now the paradigmatic example of what a rapid research response can accomplish during an emergency; they have saved millions of lives globally even though the pandemic continues. To be clear, it is not the role of a REC to develop protocols, but to review them before or during a public health emergency. To the extent anticipatory planning for emergency research response trials is not possible, there should at least be review of resources, available scientific knowledge, and potential methodologies that could form the basis of proposed studies. Finally, it is impossible to develop or complete all the scientific and ethical reviews to prepare for all exigencies in the absence of knowledge of the pathogen at issue.

Collecting epidemiological data to design public health and patient care interventions in the middle of an outbreak, and even more so conducting clinical trials on candidate medical countermeasures, present varied challenges, many of them the subject of other chapters in this book. Yet, the multiple scientific and organizational hurdles of clinical trials in an emergency may seem simple compared to the societal obstacles that we have seen with COVID-19. Social diversity, literacy levels, resistance to accepting both scientific uncertainty and scientific conclusions, and the prevalence of disinformation add a layer of intrigue beyond the remit of clinical sciences (▶ Chap. 18).

Preparations can be made for epidemiological research to begin immediately after an event (i.e., within a few days or a couple of weeks), along with biological sample and data collection, and non-pharmaceutical intervention studies that pose minimal risk. All of these can be based on previous experience with little initial knowledge about the pathogen at issue. Even for MCM trials, it is helpful to have generic, REC-approved protocol templates available in anticipation of some emergencies and to fill in the details later as and when a specific need arises. These could include several different trial designs to be adapted as needed (▶ Chap. 22). How to get research response started and then review an intervention depends in part on whether candidate interventions already exist or can be quickly identified, but also on geography, existing infrastructure, the experience and communication skills of the investigators, and the literacy levels and openness of the affected populations.

For an experimental study of vaccine or therapeutic candidates, the likely risks and/benefits, with or without a placebo arm, must be diligently assessed. An appropriate action sequence might be immediate utilization of an off-the-shelf protocol for data and sample collection, followed by consideration of appropriate intervention study protocols.

4 Seeking and Retaining Stakeholder Commitment

Generally speaking, a foreign-supported research study must be approved by RECs for both (or all) of the research organizations involved, including local ethics committees in developing countries that may have limited capacity to review a surge of research proposals during an infectious disease outbreak. That can lead to time-consuming delays which can be unacceptable in a public health emergency (PHE), although there are legitimate ways to expedite the process without weakening ethical review (▶ Chap. 33). Another possible solution would be single REC reviews of multicenter trials with adequate input to account for the specific laws, cultural concerns, languages, and literacy levels of the prospective research participants. The latest revision of the Declaration of Helsinki (completed in 2013 and currently being updated) requires that investigators must disclose funding, sponsors, and other potential conflicts of interest to both research ethics committees and study participants (Kimmelman et al. 2009; WMA 2013). Much study information is disclosed publicly, e.g., in clinical trial registries.

Research, notably research in developing countries, should benefit and be responsive to the health needs of the populations in which it is implemented (Emanuel et al. 2004). Suspicions about the motives of developed country researchers conducting research in lower income areas have sometimes been well founded, and the principle that clinical research should benefit the community in which it takes place is now widely accepted, even if the nature and extent of the benefit remains a topic of lively discussion (Pratt 2021). Among the reactions to previous research perceived as exploitative or unfair, there has been skepticism about whether placebo controls could ethically be used in clinical trials for MCMs in a high-mortality outbreak; insistence on more equal treatment for research partners in developing countries; and the need to publish results more fully, including complete data and negative findings (Adebamowo et al. 2014; ICMJE 2022).

During the 2014–2016 West Africa Ebola outbreak, collaborative efforts by all parties on ethical review (at NIH and in Liberia) for Ebola-related research including interventions and vaccinations led to development and use of a graphical interface-based consent process that augmented written and oral information sharing (Lavori et al. 1999). Social mobilization activities capitalized on the social mobilization pillar being established by the Liberian Ebola response framework. It engaged community leaders, including traditional and religious leaders, Liberian Cultural Ambassador Queen Julie Endi, and larger representation of the community in "town hall" meetings with local, tribal, and youth leaders (Kagan et al. 2021; NASEM 2017) (◘ Figs. 1–4 and 5).

It is generally accepted among investigators that a randomized, placebo-controlled trial is usually the most rapid route to identification of a safe and effective vaccine or novel therapeutic. There are other effective trial designs; ring trials, for example, can provide rigorous results and be more acceptable to the community than providing only a placebo to a patient at death's door (▶ In Focus 22.1). Multi-arm trials testing various interventions against each other can also find more favor among research participants (▶ Chap. 22). The importance of rigorous trial design was evident early in the COVID-19 pandemic, when numerous small, often non-randomized clinical trials led to widespread use of unproven or harmful medications like hydroxychloroquine and ivermectin in certain populations (Meyerowitz-Katz et al. 2022; Yogendrakumar et al. 2022). Well-planned, sufficiently powered, randomized controlled trials (RCTs) subsequently provided rigorous, expeditious assessment of safety and efficacy for both vaccines and therapies against SARS-CoV-2. It is an intellectually frustrating perplexity that therapies that showed little or no evidence of efficacy once they were assessed in well-designed trials remain more popular among certain population groups than rigorously tested vaccines and therapies (Schellack et al. 2022).

When reviewing protocols for trials of replicating viral vector vaccine candidates (modified adenovirus or vesicular stomatitis virus, for instance), we have considered it imperative to address potential risks to bystanders, i.e., individuals with whom the study participant may come in contact, in case the replicating virus can be transmitted to others. Similar risks could also occur with human challenge trials, in which participants are deliberately exposed to a pathogen against which they have been experimentally protected. In both cases this could be a household contact, intimate contact, or someone outside the protocol-defined group (infants, senior citizens, and pregnant or immunocompromised persons). Federal regulations mandate risk/benefit assessments for study participants conducted by the reviewing ethics committee and specify that it must consider "possible long-range effects" (CFR 2022). Potential risks to contacts of participants are thus included in the applicable protocols considered by the REC, along with consent documents and questionnaires to validate that study participants understand the risks adequately (Shah et al. 2018). We believe these measures make study participants aware of the risks while cautioning them to avoid exposing household and intimate contacts to potential infection. It should be noted that malaria challenge studies involve no bystander risk per se in United States, as *Anopheles* mosquitoes are no longer found there; research participants are still barred from donating blood for a year because of the potential risk to blood recipients.

Developing *reliance agreements* for multisite studies is critical to avoid wasting time and resources through duplication and mission creep (Resnik et al. 2018). However, other mechanisms are necessary to ensure buy-in from local communities. These fall under the rubric of good participatory practice (► Chap. 18) and must be included in the design, funding, and implementation of clinical research protocols. Funding agencies also need to decide who (experts with no conflict of interest) will

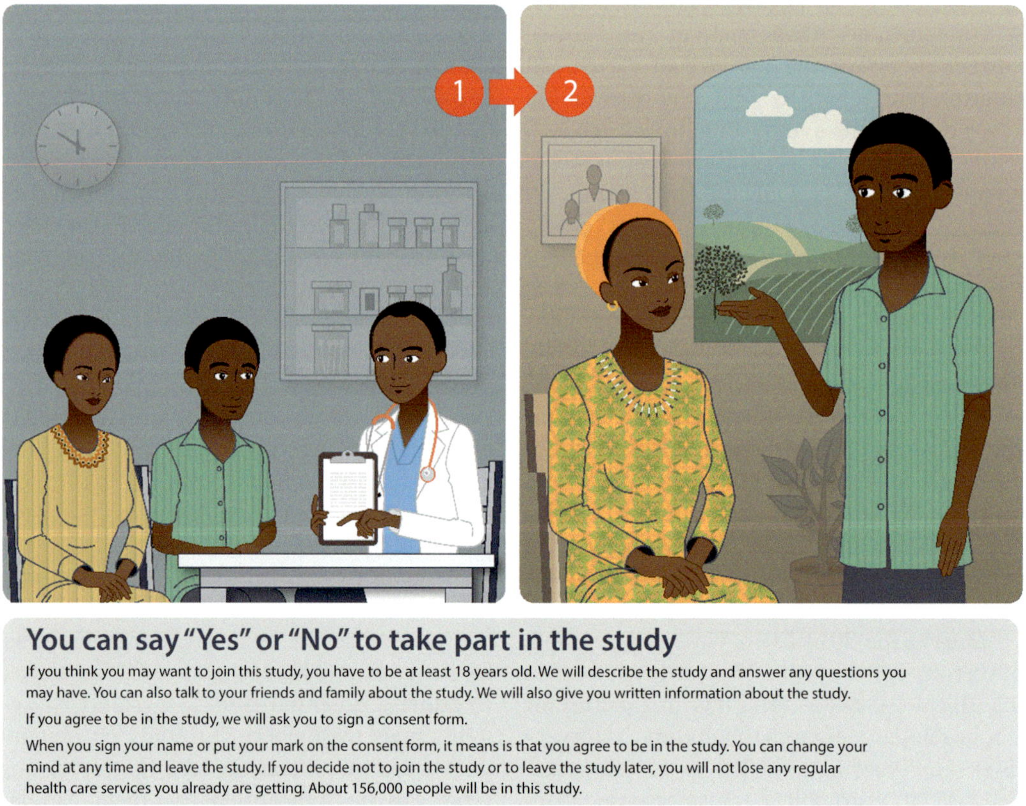

Figs. 1–4 Use of graphics to convey key clinical research concepts for informed consent. Pictures are a useful supplement to verbal explanation, especially when study participants may face linguistic, literacy, and cultural obstacles. At a bare minimum the participants must have a basic understanding of the trial they are enrolling in, be aware that they have the right to refuse participation and may get a placebo rather than an active investigational medical countermeasure, and be warned that there could be side effects and toxicities associated with the MCM. Research personnel must be satisfied that participation is not the result of coercion. (Figures courtesy Protocol Navigation/Protocol Development Program supporting NIAID and Scientific Publications, Graphics and Media, Frederick National Laboratory for Cancer Research. U.S. government work, public domain)

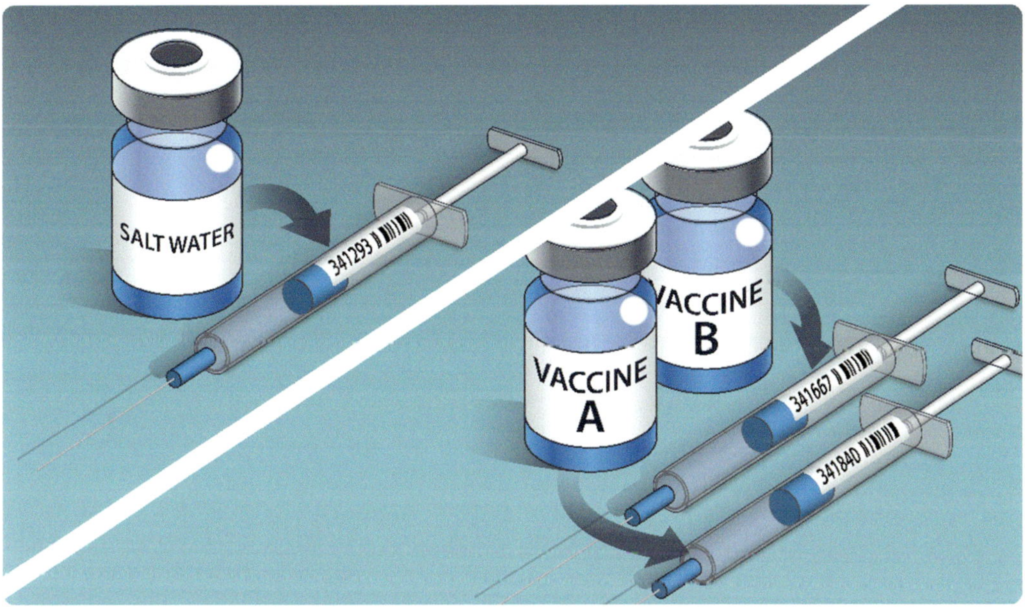

What is the salt water injection used for?

To find out if one of the vaccines works we need to compare it to getting something that does not have any effect on the body. This is called a placebo. The placebo is an injection of salt water. Using this is common in research studies.

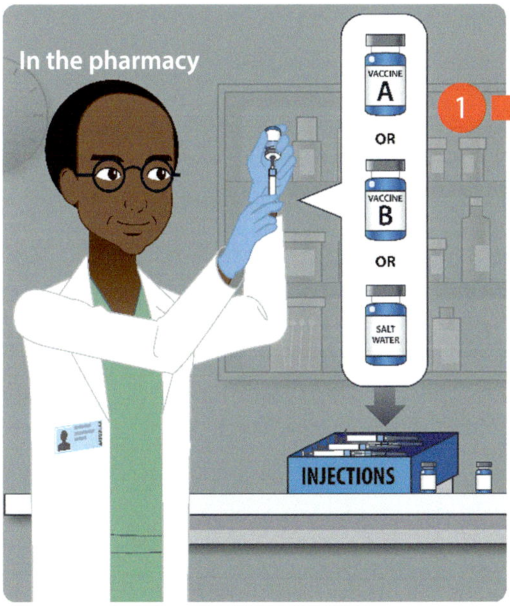

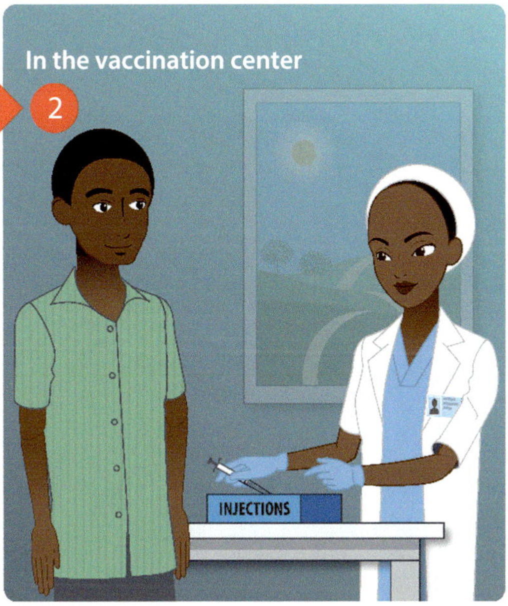

What will I get?

If you join the study, you will get an injection. The injection will be either Vaccine A, Vaccine B, or salt water.

What you get is decided by chance. Each person in the study will have a 2 out of 3 chance of getting Vaccine A or Vaccine B. If you do not get a vaccine, you will get the salt water.

The vaccines and the salt water injections all look the same. You and the study staff will not know what you are getting during the study. At the end of the study, we will attempt to contact you to let you know what you got. If we find out that a vaccines is safe and effective, we will offer it to you if you did not already get it during the study.

Figs. 1–4 (continued)

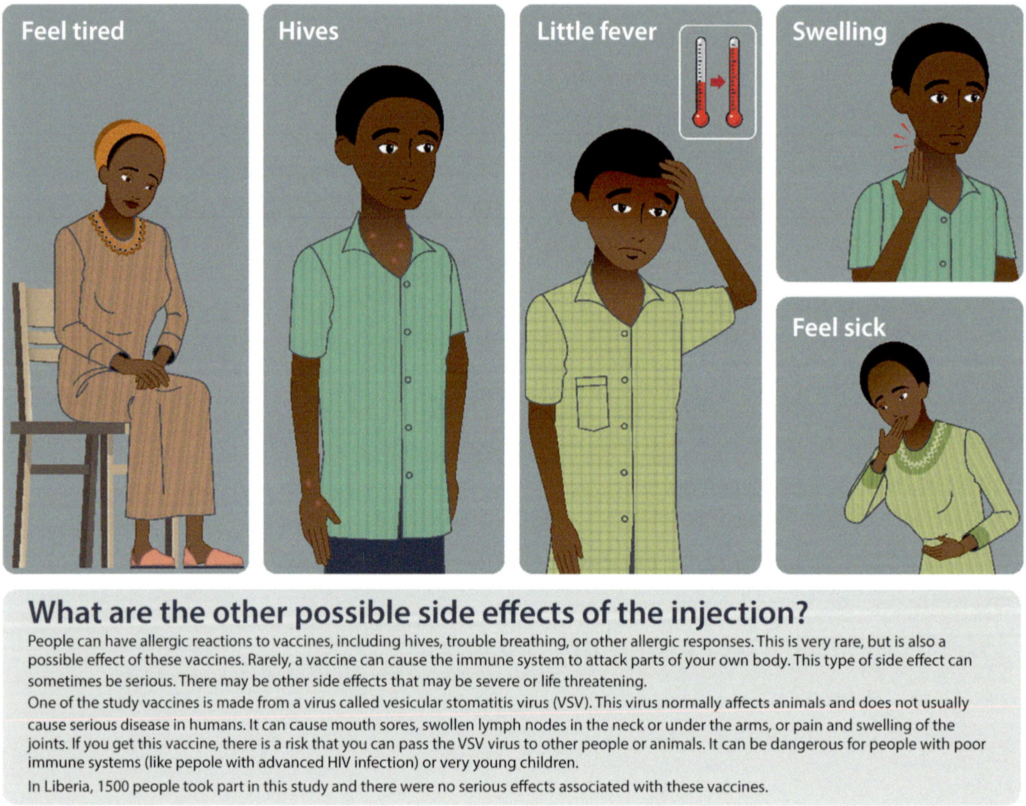

Figs. 1–4 (continued)

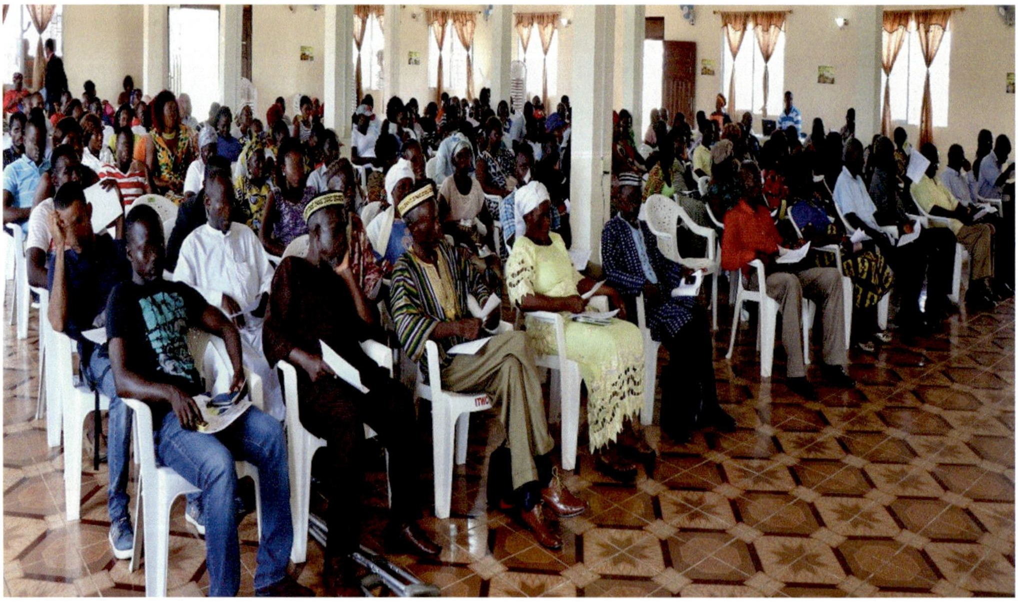

Fig. 5 Town meeting in Liberia: part of community engagement for controlled trials of Ebola MCMs (faces blurred). (Credit: Laura McNay)

undertake scientific review. It is axiomatic, or at least it should be, that research without a solid scientific grounding is by definition unethical—people must not be submitted to risk, however minimal, if there is no prospect of rigorous scientific results (CIOMS 2016).

Along the same lines, an assessment of capacity at the location where the research is being implemented is essential. There are complex, demanding logistical requirements for a large study, including personnel, supplies, facilities, patient care in the case of therapeutic interventions, and a huge, complex documentation flow in a large multi-site study. Ethics committees are one small element of a large undertaking, but as with many other small parts, the big machine will not work without it. Research committees must understand both study design and realistic implementation plans, whether for relatively straightforward observational studies, data or biological sample collection, or trials of innovative MCMs. International collaborations spanning academia and industry across geographic boundaries pose their additional coordination challenges, not least the frequent requirement for review by multiple ethics committees. Other considerations include wise stewardship of limited research resources—a failure seen early in the COVID-19 pandemic, for example (Bugin and Woodcock 2021; Resnik 2019). However, collaborations across international political and geographic boundaries should not entail duplication of unwarranted analysis and review efforts and squander precious time and resources needed for timely evaluations and interventions in public health emergency situations. A centralized single REC/IRB model has been conceptualized, mandated, and implemented in the context of NIH funded multi-site clinical research in the United States.

Trial designs providing for rigorous assessment of safety and efficacy should bolster confidence that the accumulated data will benefit humanity, whether in the course of an ongoing outbreak or pandemic or for future use if intervention strategies and pharmaceutical products can be used in wide-scale treatment, prophylaxis, or vaccination programs for the current pathogen, a related one, or a different emerging pathogen (such as a long-dormant pathogen released by permafrost melting in Arctic tundra) (Canavan 2019). Partnership with affected country investigators and officials on a concept that has scientific validity and a study design that ensures transparent and ethical partnership and avoids exploitation of vulnerable populations will be the most likely to yield salutary benefits for all affected in any given society.

5 Future Directions

Leveraging twenty-first century communications and molecular biology technologies for designing, implementing, assessing, and monitoring risks and benefits of clinical research interventions more reliably will be the next step. This requires adequate ethical safeguards and precautions in place for human subject safety, privacy, and confidentiality with no perception of bias or conflict of interest. Ensuring independent review and transparent scientific oversight, including independent data safety monitoring boards (▶ Chap. 23) free of conflicts of interest will allow successful conduct of clinical trials for emerging global challenges. All the stakeholders, including investigators in the field, research participants, and the broader populations at risk, need a basic understanding with a working knowledge of biomedical research and the uncertainty inherent in the endeavor. Objective and unbiased ethical and scientific research review, applying the best available resources and knowledge, is needed to assess the likely benefits of a research study proposal, not only for the human participants in the study and their communities, but for the wider at-risk population. Some have wisely posited that fostering a climate in which investigators perceive that they receive fair and unbiased treatment from ethics boards ensures likelihood of collegial compliance and confidentiality (Keith-Spiegel and Koocher 2005). Community acceptance of the review process that cleared the research to proceed is also an essential, though not sufficient, factor in ultimate public acceptance of MCMs that are implemented based on the findings of a research program (Wright et al. 2020). Review boards in each country involved should be highly qualified, with minimal conflicts of interest, and able to act on priority reviews quickly, while safeguarding the interests of participants and their communities. This process needs to minimize confirmation bias on the part of both the investigator proposing the research and the reviewing body, which can take the form of pride (Latin *superbia*) or hubris (Greek ὕβρις)—the original and most serious of the seven deadly sins. Many lessons have been learned from the recent global pandemic (Yogendrakumar et al. 2022). If we hope to meet the next outbreak of an infectious disease without engendering a crisis and manage it most effectively with transparency of purpose, we must not only absorb new technical knowledge; we must work to follow the most promising and transparent scientific leads, reducing the influence of selfish and parochial interests through broad inclusion of stakeholders and encouraging review boards to see themselves as guided by ethical and scientific principles, not by the institution where they happen to sit (Sisk et al. 2022; Solbakk 2011).

Discussion Questions

1. Should there be a single international REC so research projects would have to undergo only one in-depth ethics review? How could that be accomplished with adequate safeguards for local socioeconomic and cultural factors? What factors would make it difficult to realize in practice?
2. Is it ever ethical to conduct a small, nonrandomized trial on an MCM early in an outbreak caused by a novel pathogen, or should the study at least be randomized against a putative standard of care?
3. In a high-mortality outbreak, why should regulatory authorities hesitate to provide emergency use authorization (EUA) for any MCM that a reputable scientist recommends?
4. What are the minimum requirements for a REC decision on a request for regulatory concurrence on proof of principle, allowing clinical research proposals that seek to provide actionable data to proceed?

References

Adebamowo C, Bah-Sow O, Binka F, Bruzzone R, Caplan A, Delfraissy J-F, et al. Randomised controlled trials for Ebola: practical and ethical issues. Lancet. 2014;384(9952):1423–4. https://doi.org/10.1016/S0140-6736(14)61734-7.

Beecher HK. Ethics and clinical research. N Engl J Med. 1966;274(24):1354–60. https://doi.org/10.1056/nejm196606162742405.

Bugin K, Woodcock J. Trends in COVID-19 therapeutic clinical trials. Nat Rev Drug Discov. 2021; 20:254. https://doi.org/10.1038/d41573-021-00037-3.

Canavan BC. Opening Pandora's Box at the roof of the world: landscape, climate and avian influenza (H5N1). Acta Trop. 2019;196:93–101. https://doi.org/10.1016/j.actatropica.2019.04.021.

CIOMS. International ethical guidelines for health-related research involving humans. Geneva: Council for International Organisations of Medical Sciences; 2016.

Code of Federal Regulations. Title 45 Subtitle A Subchapter A Part 46 Subpart A § 46.111 Criteria for IRB approval of research. 2022.

Emanuel EJ, Wendler D, Killen J, Grady C. What makes clinical research in developing countries ethical? The benchmarks of ethical research. J Infect Dis. 2004;189(5):930–7. https://doi.org/10.1086/381709.

Gordon VM, Culp MA, Wolinetz CD. Final NIH policy on the use of a single institutional review board for multisite research. Clin Transl Sci. 2017;10(3):130–2. https://doi.org/10.1111/cts.12447.

Heller J. Syphilis victims in U.S. study went untreated for 40 years. New York Times. 1972.

Higgs ES, Dubey SA, Coller BAG, Simon JK, Bollinger L, Sorenson RA, et al. Accelerating vaccine development during the 2013–2016 West African Ebola virus disease outbreak. Curr Top Microbiol Immunol. 2017;411:229–61. https://doi.org/10.1007/82_2017_53.

ICMJE. Recommendations for the conduct, reporting, editing, and publication of scholarly work in medical journals. International Committee of Medical Journal Editors; 2022. p. 19.

Jonsen AR. The birth of bioethics. New York: Oxford University Press; 1998.

Kagan J, Lassa J, Zuckerman J, Cull E, Boan D, Lysander J, et al. Strategy management in collaborative clinical research partnerships. Contemp Clin Trials Commun. 2021;24:100833. https://doi.org/10.1016/j.conctc.2021.100833.

Keith-Spiegel P, Koocher GP. The IRB paradox: could the protectors also encourage deceit? Ethics Behav. 2005;15(4):339–49. https://doi.org/10.1207/s15327019eb1504_5.

Kimmelman J, Weijer C, Meslin EM. Helsinki discords: FDA, ethics, and international drug trials. Lancet. 2009;373(9657):13–4. https://doi.org/10.1016/s0140-6736(08)61936-4.

Lavori PW, Sugarman J, Hays MT, Feussner JR. Improving informed consent in clinical trials: a duty to experiment. Control Clin Trials. 1999;20(2):187–93. https://doi.org/10.1016/s0197-2456(98)00064-6.

Ledford H. Human-subjects research: trial and error. Nature. 2007;448(7153):530–2. https://doi.org/10.1038/448530a.

London AJ. For the common good: philosophical foundations of research ethics. New York: Oxford University Press; 2022.

MacQueen KM, McLellan E, Metzger DS, Kegeles S, Strauss RP, Scotti R, et al. What is community? An evidence-based definition for participatory public health. Am J Public Health. 2001;91(12):1929–38. https://doi.org/10.2105/ajph.91.12.1929.

Meyerowitz-Katz G, Wieten S, Medina Arellano MJ, Yamey G. Unethical studies of ivermectin for covid-19. BMJ. 2022;377:o917. https://doi.org/10.1136/bmj.o917.

NASEM. Engaging communities in research and response. In: Busta ER, Mancher M, Cuff PA, McAdam K, Keusch G, editors. Integrating clinical research into epidemic response: the Ebola experience. Washington, DC: National Academies of Sciences Engineering and Medicine Publications, National Academies Press; 2017. p. 199–222.

National Commission for the Protection of Human Subjects of Biomedical and Behavioral Research. The Belmont report: ethical principles and guidelines for the protection of human subjects of research. Washington, DC: Department of Health, Education and Welfare; 1979. Contract No.: DHEW Publication No. (OS) 78-0012.

Nuremberg Military Tribunals. Trials of war criminals before the Nuremberg Military Tribunals under Control Law No. 10. Washington, DC: U.S. Government Printing Office; 1949.

Nuffield Council on Bioethics. Research in global health emergencies: ethical issues. Oxford, UK: Nuffield Council on Bioethics; 2020.

Packenham JP, Rosselli R, Fothergill A, Slutsman J, Ramsey S, Hall JE, et al. Institutional Review Board preparedness for disaster research: a practical approach. Curr Environ Health Rep. 2021;8(2):127–37. https://doi.org/10.1007/s40572-021-00311-x.

Pratt B. Research for Health Justice: an ethical framework linking global health research to health equity. BMJ Glob Health. 2021;6(2):e002921. https://doi.org/10.1136/bmjgh-2020-002921.

Resnik DB. Stewardship of research resources. Account Res. 2019;26(3):246–51. https://doi.org/10.1080/08989621.2019.1585819.

Resnik DB, Taylor J, Morris K, Shi M. A study of reliance agreement templates used by U.S. research institutions. IRB. 2018;40(3):6–10. https://doi.org/10.1002/eahr.403002.

Schellack N, Strydom M, Pepper MS, Herd CL, Hendricks CL, Bronkhorst E, et al. Social media and COVID-19—perceptions and public deceptions of ivermectin, colchicine and hydroxychloroquine: lessons for future pandemics. Antibiotics (Basel). 2022;11(4):445. https://doi.org/10.3390/antibiotics11040445.

Shah SK, Kimmelman J, Lyerly AD, Lynch HF, Miller FG, Palacios R, et al. Bystander risk, social value, and ethics of human research. Science. 2018;360(6385):158–9. https://doi.org/10.1126/science.aaq0917.

Sisk BA, Baldwin K, Parsons M, DuBois JM. Ethical, regulatory, and practical barriers to COVID-19 research: a stakeholder-informed inventory of concerns. PLoS One. 2022;17(3):e0265252. https://doi.org/10.1371/journal.pone.0265252.

Solbakk JH. In the ruins of Babel: pitfalls on the way toward a universal language for research ethics and benefit sharing. Camb Q Healthc Ethics. 2011;20(3):341–55. https://doi.org/10.1017/S096318011100003X.

WHO. WHO Director-General's opening remarks at first meeting of the Intergovernmental Negotiating Body to draft and negotiate a WHO convention, agreement or other international instrument on pandemic prevention, preparedness and response. Geneva: World Health Organization; 2022.

WMA. Declaration of Helsinki: recommendations guiding doctors in clinical research. Helsinki: World Medical Association; 1964.

WMA. Declaration of Helsinki: ethical principles for medical research involving human subjects. Ferney-Voltaire, FR: World Medical Association; 2013.

Wright K, Parker M, Bhattacharya S, Blanchet K, Caney S, Ying Yang Chan E, et al. In emergencies, health research must go beyond public engagement toward a true partnership with those affected. Nat Med. 2020;26(3):308–9. https://doi.org/10.1038/s41591-020-0758-y.

Yogendrakumar V, Dewar B, McGuinty M, Dowlatshahi D, Dyason C, Kwok ES, et al. Many trials of hydroxychloroquine for SARS-CoV-2 were redundant and potentially unethical: an analysis of the NIH clinical trials registry. J Clin Epidemiol. 2022;143:73–80. https://doi.org/10.1016/j.jclinepi.2021.11.011.

5 Health Emergency Research amid Global Inequities: Some Considerations for Researchers

Dirceu Greco

Contents

Learning Track Note: This chapter appears in Learning Tracks: Clinical Research; Emergency Research Response, Research Operations; Global Health; Global Health Law; Public Health and Epidemiology; Research Ethics; Social Science Response Research

E. S. Higgs and R. A. Sorenson (eds.), *Principles and Practice of Emergency Research Response*,
https://doi.org/10.1007/978-3-031-48408-7_7

There have been as many plagues as wars in history; yet always plagues and wars take people equally by surprise.
Albert Camus, The Plague (1948)

Learning Objectives

This chapter will help readers understand and describe:

- The importance of urgent international medical research being ethically planned and conducted, particularly in low- and middle-income countries (LMICs)
- Familiarity with international research ethics codes, such as the Declaration of Helsinki, the UNESCO Universal Declaration on Bioethics and Human Rights, and the Council for International Organizations of Medical Sciences guidelines, as well as their shortcomings
- The basis for and extent of high-income countries' obligations to share research results with LMICs; the obligations of research programs to share results with stakeholders; and the role of an individual research program in ameliorating social and political injustices in countries where they are implemented
- Some ethical issues of conducting a research program sponsored by a high-income country in a low-income country in areas such as:
  - Partnerships with local scientists and institutions
  - Participation of civil society
  - Hiring local staff
  - Compensating research participants for their time and expenses
  - Health care for study participants who suffer from conditions other than the one being studied
  - Risks of exploitation
  - Post-trial access to products that have shown to be safe and effective in a given study

1 Introduction

Emergency research plans and their implementation must be ethically sound. Much of the professional and academic discussion of clinical research has focused on ensuring ethical interactions between a research program and research participants, in effect an extension of the discussion of how the research relationship differs from the default doctor–patient relationship, where the only goal is the well-being of the patient. But a full consideration of research ethics, especially for research in developing countries, requires taking into account the broader societal and global context of the research program, considering how the context falls short of established ethical and human rights principles, and determining how the research program must act in the face of deep-seated disparities. This complex task is all the more difficult in an emergency but must never be forgotten even amid the urgency of trying to control an infectious disease outbreak.

The United Nations (UN) Sustainable Development Goals (◘ Fig. 1) are a striking illustration of a still unequal world, where about 10% of the world's people still live on less than 2 dollars a day, and many more lack the basic elements of a dignified and secure livelihood (UN 2021). For all the remarkable achievements of the past two or three centuries, poverty, hunger, disease, and conflict remain the greatest burdens faced by humanity. In the past 2 years we have seen the rapid development and production of safe, effective vaccines against the severe acute respiratory syndrome coronavirus 2 (SARS-CoV-2) tarnished by the skewed distribution of vaccines to the wealthiest countries first, the less well-off later, and the least developed at the end of the line (Our World in Data 2022).

Every outbreak, epidemic, and pandemic occur in this global context, and every individual is embedded in multiple communities—geographical, ethnic, gender, religious, economic, linguistic, to name a few—and of course a nation-state. This chapter focuses on the social context of human-subject research through a wide-angle lens that takes in justice, fairness, and human-rights principles. Such principles are all the more applicable in an emergency when ordinary liberties may be curtailed, and research and medical resources are in high demand. We start from the research program's interactions with the local community (▶ Chap. 18), move outward to larger polities, and end with some reflections on the responsibilities of the "global community," to the extent that there is such a thing.

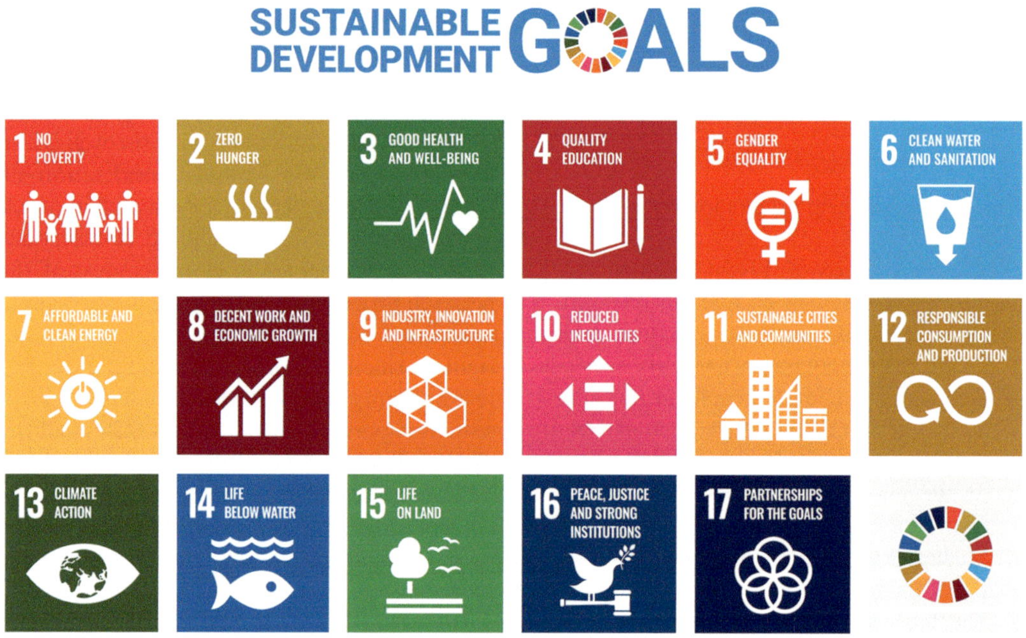

Fig. 1 The United Nations Sustainable Development Goals are a reminder of the many problems besetting humanity, as well as hopes for overcoming them. (Courtesy United Nations)

It is a commonplace now that COVID-19 has highlighted pre-pandemic inequities and injustices, both within societies and between nations and regions worldwide. Inequity and injustice have hardly been hidden from those paying attention, but perhaps the COVID-19 pandemic will help drive home the lesson that health care access for all is not only a moral imperative but also an effective measure of self-protection for everyone. It is obvious that economic losses alone during the pandemic dwarf the funding that would be required for the most ambitious plans for health-related assistance (CRS 2021; OECD 2022). Will enough leaders be able to see that our best chance of mitigating the human and economic damage of outbreaks and pandemics is to finance and implement adequate public health and health care systems everywhere, along with the strengthened scientific capacity to prevent or respond to emergent disease? Ultimately, scientific capacity must include the ability to develop and validate a broad range of medical countermeasures (MCMs), and health care systems must have the ability to deliver them to the populace.

Norman Daniels (2006) points out that disease outcomes are heavily determined by public and population health, which are highly dependent on social and economic status. But population-level issues have received much less attention from bioethicists than interpersonal relations between doctors or researchers and patients or research participants. COVID-19 may have brought discussion of inequities to the fore, but if the social determinants of health are not ameliorated, future epidemics or pandemics will continue to afflict the poor and vulnerable the most, be they the disadvantaged within societies or the populations of lower-income countries (Horton 2020; Singer et al. 2017). It is evident that we are entering an era of more frequent epidemics and pandemics. As the climate changes and population grows, emerging and re-emerging pathogens will have more opportunities to gain a foothold among the vulnerable and spread to the wider world (David et al. 2021; Folke et al. 2021). COVID-19 has most affected vulnerable groups within societies and is having a disproportionate impact on poorest countries (Bottan et al. 2020; Coalition 2021).

There is no question that novel pathogens causing severe disease outbreaks warrant immediate human research. We have seen again and again, most recently in the current

COVID-19 pandemic, the need for comprehensive efforts to keep research blueprints and road maps updated in preparation for emergencies, and how preparations always seem inadequate when the emergency comes. Every major infectious disease outbreak drives home the need for a robust, global discussion on how to ensure preparedness and rapidly deploy needed support during emergencies. There is no longer a debate about whether research should be part of preparedness; the question now is how to integrate it into preparedness and to do so ethically. The ethical dimension here also includes access to the fruits of successful research.

A great many preparedness issues have ethical and moral dimensions:

- Who has responsibility for intervening? How and when?
- Heightened risk to the most vulnerable communities and countries (due to poverty, health disparities, displacements, armed conflict, etc.).
- Insufficient local and international funding.
- Shortfalls of skilled local personnel and infrastructure in low- and middle-income countries (LMICs).
- Moral and practical necessity to understand and accommodate local health beliefs and cultural practices.
- Need for partnership with local stakeholders (individuals, communities, governments).
- Political, cultural, and religious obstacles that can impede dissemination of accurate information.
- The social and political motives for spreading misinformation and how to contest falsehoods.

Box 1: Ethics and Politics of Declaring a Public Health Emergency

Various interests may needlessly delay or accelerate declaration of a public health emergency. The declaration of an epidemic can be politically and economically sensitive, affecting international trade, travel and tourism, and in the case of COVID-19 all of these plus dramatic slowdowns in most of the world's major economies (Brodeur et al. 2021; Rull et al. 2015). The potential economic repercussions of declaring an emergency, loss of trust in the health institutions that failed to contain the outbreak, and the possibility of social unrest can delay a timely response. Measures to slow an outbreak and the research needed to help curb it and prevent future epidemics may get off to a slow start.

Regional and international dynamics play an important role; a glaring example—as most observers agreed—was the undue delay, until August 2014, before the World Health Organization (WHO) declared a Public Health Emergency of International Concern (PHEIC) in response to the 2014–2016 Ebola epidemic in West Africa. By March 2014, two countries—Guinea and Liberia—were reporting confirmed Ebola cases, and by May cases had been confirmed in Sierra Leone. One can argue that the internal politics and slow decision making at WHO played a significant role in the late declaration, but the International Health Regulations (IHR) provide override mechanisms, giving Director General Margaret Chan full powers to declare a PHEIC (Rull et al. 2015).

It is interesting to analyze the timing in light of events outside Africa: it was not until cases arrived in the United States and Europe that WHO declared Ebola a PHEIC, on 8 August 2014, some 8 months after the first cases were noted—though not at first identified as Ebola—in Guinea, and with confirmed, intense transmission ongoing in all three countries for months. Shortly thereafter, the UN Security Council declared the Ebola outbreak in West Africa a threat to international peace and security in the first Council meeting in its history to address a public health crisis (Rull et al. 2015). Many observers have concluded that the delay in international recognition of the epidemic allowed it to grow to the extent it did (Hoffman and Silverberg 2018).

Does the researcher have a role in ameliorating social and political conditions? How can a research program be ethical in an unjust or oppressive context? The 2014–2016 West Africa Ebola outbreak served as both a case study for and a harbinger of the enormous catastrophe of COVID-19. Ebola was a warning to prepare for similar emergencies, an alarm widely heard but little heeded after the Ebola outbreak ended. Both the Ebola outbreak and COVID-19 pandemic illuminate deep inequities within and among societies: the poor health conditions and medical care choices facing many populations, the social and economic conditions underlying their deprivation, and the need to redouble progress toward universal health care and re-examine global economic structures.

Adherence to accepted bioethical guidelines and codes of conduct is a sine qua non for research involving humans, during health emergencies as at all other times, and regardless of the country, ethnicity, race, gender, sexual orientation, education, and economic status of research participants. It is not only bioethical guidelines in question here, but broader norms of justice and human rights which researchers must consider. As the legal and political philosopher Norberto Bobbio told a conference on the foundations of human rights in 1964, "the fundamental problem concerning human rights today is not so much how to justify them, but how to protect them. This problem is political, not philosophical" (Bobbio 1996). Moreover, as Pratt and Loff (2014) observe, it is equally important that the responsibility for implementing broader norms of health justice be properly assigned to bodies that have the power to make needed changes and not stated as principle without a realistic means of implementation. An individual research program does not have the power to reform a national health system.

2 Research Participants and Communities

2.1 Research Participant Rights and Benefits

One major ethical concern about international clinical research is that researchers from developed countries may conduct research for the benefit of their own population back home, rather than for the benefit of the participants' communities. The very first criterion for justified research noted in the *Declaration of Helsinki* and the parallel ethical guidelines from the Council for International Organizations of Medical Sciences (CIOMS) is that "the research be responsive to the health needs and priorities of the host population or community" (CIOMS 2016; WMA 2013). Both these documents, and bioethicists more generally, also endorse the principle that "any interventions or products developed be made 'reasonably available' to the host community or population" (CIOMS 2016). Such precepts presuppose universally acceptable and adequate ethical principles, backed up by practical, culturally appropriate methodology for their implementation in research. In a practical sense, fulfilling such requirements seems to require a reasonably adequate health care system that can make medical interventions or medicinal products available to trial participants and their communities without the continued involvement of the research program. Licensure of a product, after all, may well come several years after the initial clinical research.

Guidelines, many of them developed over decades of practice and deliberation, are essential for ethical research and reproducible results. On the other hand, the sheer abundance of available guidance documents can become confusing, bringing the risk of guideline cherry-picking for the convenience of researchers. Perhaps more widespread is the formal adherence to ethical requirements without reflection on the principles the guidelines are meant to embody. Hence, the need for principal investigators, as well as other research personnel, to understand and incorporate not so much a checklist based on guidelines as the moral and ethical principles governing the conduct of their research. As we will see below, this can present special difficulties when researchers from wealthy nations come to work among the most impoverished citizens of lower-income countries. The current situation, where numerous guidance documents reflect varying perspectives, suggests the need for a comprehensive international convention on bioethics and patient/research participant rights approved by most countries. One possible model for a binding instrument is the Additional Protocol to the Convention on Human Rights and Biomedicine, concerning Biomedical Research, of the Council of Europe, which entered into force in 2009 (Council of Europe 2005). The global focus shifted in the wake of the COVID-19 pandemic to the negotiation of an international agreement on pandemic preparedness and response. WHO Director General Tedros Adhanom Ghebreyesus strongly emphasized equity in his remarks opening the negotiations. "Instead of solidarity," he said, "the [COVID-19] pandemic has been marred by inequity" (WHO 2022d).

In pandemics, global clinical trials must ensure sufficiently diverse enrollment for generalizability of results to a broad range of populations. Yet, health care systems differ significantly across the globe. In all research, including emergency response research, compliance with ethical standards and human subject protections is mandatory. Whatever the social context, human participants in clinical trials must be treated justly, and established ethical principles reinforce the norm that trial participants should receive benefits commensurate with the risks they undergo.

In developed countries, as Emanuel et al. (2004) point out, it is reasonable to presume that the benefits to society resulting from improved medical interventions developed in a clinical study will accrue to the members of the society, including clinical trial participants. In low-income developing countries, by contrast, one cannot assume that either trial participants or their communities have or will have access to health care that will provide them with the benefits of ongoing improvements in medical practice. Thus, the right of trial participants and their communities to access any successful products developed in a clinical trial has received widespread support, as explained in the 2021 UNAIDS/WHO *Guidance on Ethical Considerations in Biomedical HIV Prevention Trials* (Greco 2007; UNAIDS/WHO 2021).

The principle of justice as equality, meaning treating like cases alike, must be applied here, requiring that trial participants in high-, low-, and middle-income countries be treated equally with respect to post-trial access to study products. Ideally, this would apply to all and not just to trial participants, but full equality to this extent is far from realization. What researchers themselves may be able to achieve is limited, especially in an emergency. However, trial sponsors should ensure that baseline standards of care are similar across global trial sites. For example, the U.S. National Institutes of Health (NIH)-sponsored Accelerating COVID-19 Therapeutic Interventions and Vaccines trial of therapeutics in hospitalized patients (ACTIV-3) included intravenous (IV) remdesivir as part of the standard of care, based on data from the Adaptive COVID-19 Treatment Trial study demonstrating shorter hospital stays with remdesivir. ACTIV-3 was a global trial, so all study participants globally were provided with remdesivir in both investigational product and placebo arms (Lundgren et al. 2021). There has been much debate about how to balance the benefits of clinical research to broad populations when the inequality suffered by some communities of research participants cannot be quickly or easily overcome (Lie et al. 2004; Schuklenk 2004).

Fairness here is considered as the obligation of being just, ethical, and free from bias related to economic status, ethnicity, sexual orientation, gender, origin, and so on. This applies to all aspects of research planning, development, and implementation in urgent situations, just as it must be applied to research ethics in "normal" conditions. But to ensure fundamental fairness, measures to mitigate poverty, and especially inequality are urgent and imperative; this theme will be further elaborated.

2.2 Building Mutual Respect with Communities

2.2.1 Respect Community Beliefs and Cultural Practices; Include all Relevant Stakeholders

The UNAIDS *Good Participatory Practice Guidelines for Biomedical HIV Prevention Trials* (GPP), along with the companion *Ethical Considerations in Biomedical HIV Prevention Trials*, are seminal documents for establishing ethical relationships between investigators and research participants and for avoiding or counteracting insensitivity toward and exploitation of research participants (UNAIDS/AVAC 2011; UNAIDS/WHO 2021). Though these guidance documents were originally developed for HIV prevention trials, they have been widely used, serving as the starting point for, among others, *good participatory practice guidelines for trials of emerging (and re-emerging) pathogens* (GPP-EP) (WHO 2016a). This emphasizes emergency response research: "the foundational GPP-EP principles underpinning partnerships among trial stakeholders in situations of crisis are respect, fairness, integrity, transparency, accountability, and autonomy, while the benchmarks include mutual understanding, complementarity, and efficiency"; these have recently been adapted for COVID-19 trials (Greco 2008; WHO 2020b).

2.2.2 Avoid Exploitation and the Perception of Exploitation

Justice and beneficence require respecting the autonomy and equality of study participants and their communities. Beauchamp and Childress (2019) list autonomy as the first of their four foundational principles for medical ethics. Community involvement must also be part of EID outbreak response (▶ Chap. 18) for practical as well as ethical reasons. This includes participation of all stakeholders from the beginning of the project, with the assurance of transparency and clarity in all proposed interventions. Here it is worth mentioning the international intervention in the 2014–2016 Ebola outbreak. West African populations and communities were not familiar with the Ebola virus, which had previously infected humans primarily in Central Africa. International response teams, especially early in the response, lacked understanding of prevailing health practices, cultural norms, and customary behaviors that may have facilitated the spread of the disease. Messaging and response measure failures by both national governments and international responders may have contributed to conspiracy theories about the origin or even nonexistence of the virus, fueled in part by the arrival of foreign responders, and perhaps additionally by U.S. and British military engagement to help build field hospitals (Bayntun et al. 2014). There were violent clashes between police and citizens in Monrovia, the murder of a response team in Guinea by villagers who believed the team was bringing Ebola infection, and the passive reaction by some to dire warnings: "If Ebola was a death sentence, what was the point?" (BBC 2014; Stern 2014). Involvement of local communities, faith and traditional leaders, and anthropologists advising responders ultimately helped to convince most West Africans of the reality of Ebola and the effectiveness of means to prevent its transmission (Baggio et al. 2019; Kutalek et al. 2015; Wilkinson et al. 2017).

Guiding principles for community engagement that are common to GPP and GPP-EP include the points below, presented here in language taken from GPP-EP 4.4.C, "Good Participatory Practice for Protocol Development". See also ▶ Chap. 18.

- Trial sponsors provide opportunities and time for local research teams to engage actively in expedited trial protocol development. Local research teams provide opportunities and time for local stakeholders, in particular community stakeholders, to contribute to decisions about trial design issues and procedures, including the products to be tested, trial objectives, recruitment strategies, informed consent materials and procedures, reimbursement policies, counseling approaches, follow-up procedures, and post-trial access to trial products or procedures.

- Research teams maintain clear and transparent communication about the protocol development process with formal stakeholder advisory mechanisms and provide regular updates about protocol review and approval processes to relevant stakeholders.
- Researchers provide protocol summaries to relevant stakeholders and make technical information as accessible as possible by translating materials or facilitating workshops as necessary. They make full, final protocols of trials available and easily accessible to stakeholders.

2.3 Post-trial Access to Trial Products, Procedures, or Devices

One way to increase fairness in existing circumstances is by providing post-trial access to the products resulting from research for (a) individual participants in the research, (b) their communities, or (c) their countries. In Brazilian Research Ethics Guidelines regarding post-trial access, all participants are guaranteed "at the end of the study and for unlimited time, free access to the best prophylactic, diagnostic, and therapeutic methods that have proven their efficiency". There are also provisions to ensure particpants who have left the trial will continue to receive the same access as those still enrolled (National Council of Health (BR) 2012).

This has been a contentious issue in human research, but there are many reasons to make products or procedures shown to be efficacious in a trial available to research participants. The prevailing opinion is that participants must have access to drugs, vaccines, interventions, prevention strategies, and any other benefits resulting from the study (National Council of Health (BR) 2012; UNESCO 2005; WMA 2013). Post-trial access in "normal" research situations may be delayed by a host of factors (e.g., drug production delays, regulatory and licensing issues, and of course a finding that the investigational product was not efficacious). However, in emergency response, the balance between such hurdles and provision of efficacious trial products should mandate their earliest possible availability, while additional safety and efficacy information is collected through continued evaluation and follow-up. During design and implementation, community and other local stakeholders must have access to clear information on their rights, the access plan, and information on all anticipated factors that could hinder their access to the new product or procedure. The PREVAIL 1 study of Ebola vaccines is an example where post-trial access was provided many years after the study launch in February 2015. In 2021, once the Merck Ebola VSV vaccine had been licensed as Ervebo, the need for a booster dose was recognized, and the threat of an Ebola outbreak in Guinea near the border of Liberia loomed, the participants in PREVAIL 1 were vaccinated and/or revaccinated. WHO, via GAVI, the Vaccine Alliance, is making both the Merck and Johnson & Johnson Ebola vaccines available to countries when there is an Ebola-Zaire outbreak.

To mitigate hurdles related to post-trial access to research products, research teams and relevant stakeholders must clarify and resolve issues early in the process if possible. Trial funders, sponsors, and research teams conducting efficacy or effectiveness trials must negotiate and agree on responsibilities and funding with national governments concerning emergency use authorizations, licensure requirements, and access issues should the vaccine, therapeutic, or procedure under investigation during a pandemic or outbreak be shown to be safe and effective.

Certainly, during a PHEIC, trial teams and sponsors must work with LMIC research participants and participating countries to ensure appropriate post-research benefits, especially during the acute health emergency.

This has been done in the context of COVID-19 for vaccines and some therapeutics. Supply constraints can be expected during health emergencies, but all research stakeholders should work to ensure access to effective diagnostics, therapeutics, and vaccines during the health emergency. There is a very strong case for providing research participants and their communities with post-trial access to the products of emergency research, presumably medical countermeasures (MCMs) that will counter the pathogen in question. Ethical debate continues over the best ways to ensure that clinical research in developing countries contributes to global health justice or equity more generally. In regard to exploitation and injustice on research, Malmqvist (2017) has argued "that mutually beneficial and voluntary exploitation can be worse than neglect when—as is typically true of exploitative international research—it takes advantage of unjust background conditions" and that researchers may be "complicit in the injustice." In this respect, it is worth mentioning organizations and programs like GAVI, the Vaccine Alliance, the WHO-led Access to COVID-19 Tools Accelerator, or ACT-A, and especially COVID-19 Vaccines Global Access (COVAX), the effort to distribute vaccines against SARS-CoV-2 more universally and more equitably around the world (Gavi 2022; WHO 2022a).

3 Partnerships

3.1 Minimizing North-South Inequality in Research Partnerships

Collaboration among all relevant stakeholders, acting as equal partners, is indispensable to help overcome inequalities in research partnerships. International collaboration in AIDS research has demonstrated the need to re-examine legal and especially ethical aspects of research in general (Greco 2008). The practical difficulties faced by collaborative efforts in AIDS research and the issues and problems experienced in that epidemic can and should guide the response to other emerging or re-emerging illnesses. Indeed, one of the most ethically controversial international research studies in recent decades was on preventing mother-to-child transmission of HIV (Angell 1997; Lurie and Wolfe 1997). Peter Piot and Thomas Quinn (2013) argue for the response to the AIDS epidemic as a global health paradigm, concluding that great progress has been made in the global response to the AIDS epidemic, and that it has had a direct impact on global health as a whole. But, they caution, established "programs will require universal access, large-scale implementation, careful monitoring and evaluation, financial and technical resources, and robust commitment." As noted, it was the HIV-AIDS research program that gave rise to GPP (UNAIDS/AVAC 2011), which has been much cited and adapted to new circumstances, recently revised (UNAIDS/WHO 2021), and provided the foundation for WHO-prepared GPP guidelines for infectious disease emergencies and for COVID-19 specifically (WHO 2016a, 2020b). Folayan et al. (2019) discussed the considerations involved, noting that community engagement is necessary in an emergency, both for the success of a clinical trial (recruitment, good data, operations) and for ensuring the community understands and benefits from the research—though the latter may be more difficult during an emergency.

3.2 Fair Treatment and Support for Front-Line Workers

It is not only research partners and participants who are affected by North-South inequality. The rights and treatment of research study staff who are hired locally can raise ethical issues as well (▶ Chap. 42). It is essential to guard against the sort of paternalist condescension that can affect even the best-intentioned humanitarian, letting the concept that "we" are helping "them" define relationships rather than "we are working together to stop a disease outbreak" (Jentsch and Pilley 2003). Inequalities inevitably include large differences in opportunities (e.g., salary, benefits, and employment stability) available for research personnel from developed versus low- and middle-income countries; there have even been circumstances in which locally hired employees are expected to stay and work in insecure areas where their LMIC research partners are forbidden even to visit by the security regulations set by their home governments. Salary issues are not simple: either pay local employees based on prevailing local wages, and they receive much less than their developed-country colleagues; or pay them on an international scale, and they may receive so much more than their compatriots with similar skills that it could skew the local labor market and disproportionately induce the most talented and qualified personnel to leave the national health system (Lemay-Hébert et al. 2020).

3.3 Equity in Publication

Issues related to publication of and public attention to scientific and ethically sound results are crucial in at least two respects: (a) equitable inclusion of fellow researchers as authors, and (b) in relation to rumors and disinformation ("fake news"), which have been an enormous obstacle to controlling and ending the COVID-19 and Ebola pandemics (crossref, crossref). The latter has been called an infodemic, or a global epidemic of misinformation, one which has had severe consequences for health care and social well-being (Briand et al. 2021; WHO 2022b). As for publication fairness, the International Committee of Medical Journal Editors (ICMJE) has established a set of recommendations for the *Conduct, Reporting, Editing, and Publication of Scholarly Work in Medical Journals*, aimed at ensuring that all individuals included as authors take responsibility for what is published (ICMJE 2019). While ICMJE encourages "collaboration and co-authorship with colleagues in the locations where the research is conducted," the decision on whom to include as an author is explicitly left in the hands of the authors, who need to take collective responsibility for fairness.

Popular distrust of scientists and scientific information is multifaceted, and it is an open question how much people in one country will be better convinced of the validity of scientific results just because their compatriots are on the research team. Mistrust of science in high-income countries is rampant even though most scientific research is conducted there. In any case, both justice and the potential for more effective communication with the public are better served by equitable representation.

3.4 Work with Non-government Organizations (NGOs) Already on the Ground or with Relevant Experience

There are several highly skilled humanitarian response NGOs with broad international experience (MSF 2013), which may have established good relationships with communities in an outbreak zone before research programs have begun to work, though in some cases, e.g., eastern Democratic Republic of the Congo (DRC), the circumstances may be exceptionally difficult (MSF 2019). Emergency medical response NGOs have in the past sometimes viewed research and researchers with suspicion; they may believe that randomly controlled trials (RCTs) deprive some patients of their only possible option, or they may be skeptical about the research bringing any benefit in the course of the current emergency (► In Focus 30.1). Moreover, it may be argued that the longer-term agendas of many medical and development NGOs have been shaped in recent decades by a neoliberal paradigm that is not in the best interest of all communities, most especially the least advantaged (Keshavjee 2014). Even with these caveats, however, NGOs are fundamental for emergency response in low-income countries.

4 Nation-States and Global Response

In each country where an infectious disease emergency response is underway, there should be a country coordinating mechanism. While sovereignty inheres in national governments, in case of need an international institution, often WHO, may lead the coordination in partnership with local governments, professional associations, academia, etc., as well as all international actors involved in the response. The coordinating body tracks deployments, reduces duplication, establishes common and complementary goals, and forestalls clashes among the various response organizations (IASC 2019).

4.1 When Governments Put Their Own Interests First

One must keep in mind the possibility that perceived and often quite real urgency during an emergency may be used to circumvent ethical and human rights standards (London and Kimmelman 2020). This can present moral dilemmas to emergency response workers, especially researchers who must engage on a broad range of practical issues with national and local authorities from governments of all sorts, sometimes having to work with military and police forces who may be brutal and corrupt (Buth et al. 2018). The best preparation for such work is a thorough grounding in fundamental ethical principles in medicine and biomedical research, so that applying guidelines is not a mere formality but a methodology for thinking through the ethical dimensions of a research project. This understanding must include an appreciation for the possibility of conflict between ethical principles. For example, the need for individual informed consent can be overridden by the need to treat an unconscious patient urgently; public health contact tracing needs may conflict with the right to privacy; or the lethality of a disease can change the weighting of safety vs. efficacy of a medical countermeasure. Here again, the involvement of all stakeholders, including civil society, is of paramount importance, together with clear and culturally sensitive dissemination of information.

4.2 Protecting Nations at Risk

Optimistically speaking, the waning of the COVID-19 pandemic should be a historical moment for an intense movement to increase investment in health, housing, education, and water and sanitation, especially in the most vulnerable countries. It is urgent to establish a preparedness system that can help prevent future epidemics and respond when they occur and to strengthen and build on existing preparedness capabilities. This is a moment when it should be clear to all leaders that comprehensive preparedness is not only a humanitarian and moral imperative but also serves the self interest of all states that care about the health of their populations. Moreover, preparedness cannot be comprehensive without a strong, functional health care system (Brown et al. 2022; Fukuda-Parr et al. 2021; Nuzzo et al. 2019).

For capacity building and preparedness planning, having an up-to-date, comprehensive list of countries most at risk is useful. In January 2020, as the COVID-19 outbreak began spreading worldwide, WHO Director General Tedros Adhanom Ghebreyesus warned in his annual report to the WHO Executive Board in Geneva that the world may be dangerously ill-prepared for the next pandemic, and he urged the WHO member states to "invest in preparedness," not "panic" (WHO 2020c). He added that funding for outbreak preparedness "has remained grossly inadequate" in the past. "For too long, the world has operated on a cycle of panic and neglect. We throw money at an outbreak, and when it's over, we forget about it and do nothing to prevent the next one." This reasoning will be familiar from speeches in many previous global emergencies. However, this could be an opening for an intense movement to increase investment in health, housing, education, water, and sanitation, especially in the most vulnerable communities/countries. In

2020, WHO convened an International Independent Panel for Pandemic Preparedness and Response (2021). The panel's report was published in May 2021, and a summary of its findings and recommendations concluded that "To prepare the world for the future so that the next disease outbreak does not become a pandemic, the panel calls for a series of crucial reforms that will address gaps in high-level coordinated leadership globally and nationally, funding, access to what must become global goods, and WHO's independence, focus, and authority" (Sirleaf and Clark 2021).

4.3 International Economic Interventions Can Undermine Preparedness

As mentioned above, the challenges are many and complex, albeit not without potential solutions. Often and increasingly, the economic collapse that many nations are facing is related not only to local responsibility but also to international intervention: structural economic changes meant to strengthen economies have often led to weakened social protections, including health care (Thomson et al. 2017). A clear example was the situation in West Africa just before the Ebola outbreak in 2014. Kentikelenis et al. (2015) described the chaos of the local health sector in Sierra Leone in relation to the economic prescriptions of the International Monetary Fund (IMF), including spending cuts for structural adjustment, which affect social services including the health system. A major reason the outbreak spread so rapidly was the weakness of health systems in the region. There were many factors behind this, including a legacy of conflict and state failure. Since 1990, the IMF has provided support to Guinea, Liberia, and Sierra Leone, for 21, 7, and 19 years, respectively, and all three countries were under IMF programs when Ebola emerged. IMF lending comes with strings attached ("conditionalities") that require recipient governments to adopt policies that have been criticized for prioritizing economic objectives over investment in health and education. To keep government spending low, the IMF often requires caps on the public-sector wage bill—and thus constrains funding to hire or adequately remunerate doctors, nurses, and other health-care professionals.

Such limits are "often set without consideration of the impact on expenditures in priority areas" (IMF 2007) and have been linked to emigration of health personnel. With the implementation of such austerity, the number of public sector employees in Sierra Leone was reduced. "Between 1995–1996, the IMF required the retrenchment of 28% of government employees, and limits on wage spending continued into the 2000s" (Kentikelenis et al. 2015). During that time, community health workers decreased from 0.11/1000 population in 2004 to 0.02/1000 in 2008. Stuckler and Basu (2013) add that "it is not even clear that they have strengthened economic performance." Although the IMF says it has taken such criticism seriously and issued a new social spending strategy in 2019, its results could not be assessed during the ensuing pandemic emergency (IMF 2019).

4.4 National Sovereignty vs. Possible Global Impact

This is a crucial issue. Economic and research disparities tend to affect most intensely those countries where capacity to respond adequately to disease outbreaks is very low, where health systems are understaffed and underfinanced, and where infectious diseases may be more likely to emerge or re-emerge. This adds up to multifaceted problems. On the one hand, financial support, research project design, and experienced researchers are generally going to come from industrialized countries; one risk is that research products will either not reach or will not be affordable for those most at need in the most vulnerable countries.

On the other hand, actual research implementation will directly affect countries that are most likely already struggling with other endemic diseases (communicable and non-communicable) and in some cases may be facing socioeconomic and health system collapse. Affected countries' capacity to evaluate the ethics of proposed research may be very limited, with weak research ethics and regulatory review systems, and they may be predisposed in an emergency to accept whatever seems to provide immediate help. This situation can make it difficult to establish the kinds of relationships that would allow local populations, institutions, and governments to see themselves as equal partners in an emergency response, particularly when it comes to research. But the effort must be made, and the partnerships between foreign researchers and colleagues from the DRC during recent Ebola outbreaks shows that it can be done (Mulangu et al. 2019). It is worth re-stating that an international institution like WHO could act as a broker to deal with conflicting situations.

A substantial number of guidelines, guidance documents, and reports are already available to deal with most aspects of research ethics in outbreak and health emergency situations. However, considering that the current ethical standards for human research should be fully applicable in emergencies, it is important to expand and deepen the discussion about the ethics surrounding research and to reinforce the rights of research participants during health emergencies. This broader discussion includes the ethical standards that apply after the trials and to the right to access adequate health care for all (CIOMS 2016; Lucas 2019; WHO 2016a, 2018, 2020a; WHO AFRO 2021).

Box 2: Selected International Guidelines for Medical Research

(Listed with the date of introduction; current version in citation)

World Medical Association, 1964, *The Declaration of Helsinki, 2013* (WMA 2013)

CIOMS, 1982, *International Ethical Guidelines for Health-Related Research Involving Humans* (CIOMS 2016)

UNESCO, 2005, *Universal Declaration of Bioethics and Human Rights* (UNESCO 2005)

UNAIDS, 2007, *Good Participatory Practice Guidelines for Biomedical HIV Prevention Trials* (UNAIDS/AVAC 2011)

UNAIDS/WHO, 2007, *Ethical Considerations in Biomedical HIV Prevention Trials* (UNAIDS/WHO 2021)

WHO GPP-EP, 2016, *Good Participatory Practice Guidelines for Trials of Emerging (and Re-Emerging) Pathogens that Are Likely to Cause Severe Outbreaks in the Near Future and for Which Few or No Medical Countermeasures Exist* (WHO 2016a)

Nuffield Council on Bioethics, 2020, *Research in Global Health Emergencies: Ethical Issues* (Nuffield Council on Bioethics 2020)

WHO, 2020, *Good Participatory Practice for COVID-19 Clinical Trials: A Toolbox* (WHO 2020b)

5 Questions and Conclusion

5.1 Can We Achieve Sustainable Preparedness and Response?

Is it possible to ensure post-pandemic global, sustainable, clinical research capacity and all that it requires without tackling the social determinants of health? Preparedness includes everything that may be considered essential to all aspects of emergency research response, before, during, and after the trials. As WHO defines it, preparedness is "the ability (knowledge, capacities, and organizational systems) of governments, professional response organizations, communities, and individuals to anticipate, detect, and respond effectively to, and recover from, the impact of likely, imminent or current health emergencies, hazards, events, or conditions. It means putting in place mechanisms that will allow national authorities, multilateral organizations, and relief organizations to be aware of risks and deploy staff and resources quickly once a crisis strikes" (WHO 2017).

In its 2021 report, the Global Preparedness Monitoring Board (GPMB) notes that "hundreds of expert recommendations have been made over the last two decades, new structures have been created, but the level of ambition and action has failed to match the global need… We need a new global social contract to prevent and mitigate health emergencies" (GPMB 2021). However, as the GPMB and other world institutions focus on pandemic preparedness, there has been relatively little attention to address the social determinants of health and serious efforts to remedy conditions in the "too many places [that] lack even the most rudimentary health-care infrastructure. Communities that cannot care for a pregnant woman and her new-born child cannot protect against a disease outbreak" (GPMB 2019). It is important not to lose sight of the greatly increased risk of new, serious public health threats among people plagued by poverty and associated illnesses, malnutrition, high population density, armed conflict, population displacement, poor access to clean water and sanitation, inadequate vector control, and insufficient access to health care. Any one of these factors increases vulnerability, when combined with climate change and pressure on land, water, and air resources, they are practically a recipe for pandemics (Morand and Walther 2020).

A reasonably just world requires continuing effort to ensure every person "the enjoyment of the highest attainable standard of health ... one of the fundamental rights of every human being" as specified in the WHO Constitution (International Health Conference 1946). The need to ameliorate obscene inequalities throughout the world is urgent; responding only when these disparities become manifest in an outbreak or epidemic is neither wise nor good (Kentikelenis et al. 2015; Rull et al. 2015). In the same vein, there should be an evaluation of the real impact of all local and international money invested to tackle outbreaks and the costs of epidemics. Although estimates vary greatly, the U.S. CDC has calculated that the three countries most affected by the 2014–2016 Ebola epidemic—Guinea, Liberia, and Sierra Leone—lost an estimated US$ 2.2 billion of their combined GDP during the outbreak (CDC 2019). A recent, more comprehensive estimate places the total cost, including response expenditures, total economic costs, and lives lost and diminished, at some $53 billion (Huber et al. 2018). The losses resulting from COVID-19—more than seven million human lives and counting, and an estimated US$16 trillion (16 thousand billion)—are already immense and their impact will last for many years to come (Cutler and Summers 2020; Johns Hopkins 2022).

5.2 Conclusion

On paper, much of what is needed to ethically and scientifically respond to emerging disease outbreaks is in place. This includes, but is not limited to:

- An established international framework, such as the International Health Regulations (2005) (IHR) established to identify and respond to outbreaks, along with the WHO Health Emergencies Program and numerous international initiatives and national plans to prepare for and respond to infectious disease emergencies (Oppenheim et al. 2019; WHO 2016b).
- Several sets of established ethical guidelines directed both to "normal" situations and to health emergency response. Of course, this abundance of guidelines could be either a blessing or a source of confusion. A thorough grounding in biomedical ethics for research program designers and management will help them navigate any apparent conflicts among differing codes and guidelines.
- Since the COVID-19 pandemic entered its third year (2022), there has been an increasing number of initiatives to better prepare for future pandemics. The importance of addressing health inequities, which means tackling the social determinants of health, both in the present response and in preparedness, has been championed (among others) by WHO Director General Tedros Adhanom Ghebreyesus.

- Universal health care and pandemic preparedness and response are linked in the recently introduced WHO Universal Health and Preparedness Review process, which will feed into negotiations of the new international pandemic instrument. This is an effort to act on the concept that the availability of health care for all is inextricably linked with global pandemic preparedness (WHO 2021b, 2022c).

Though the focus of this volume is on emergency research response, and though infectious disease emergencies may affect countries at all income levels, the likelihood of novel pathogens appearing, the potential for them to spread unchecked, and their severity are usually greater in the most vulnerable countries and communities. In preparedness and response, the health, medical, and humanitarian sectors must go beyond existing ethical and research guidelines and work toward full compliance with the IHR (2005), amended at the 2024 World Health Assembly and binding for all WHO members. If they and all of us wish to improve readiness and resilience further, we must work towards goals like the 17 UN Sustainable Development Goals (◘ Fig. 1)—a blueprint for tackling global disparities. The UN describes the goals as "an urgent call for action by all countries—developed and developing—in a global partnership. They make clear that ending poverty and other deprivations must go hand in hand with strategies that improve health and education, reduce inequality, and spur economic growth—all while tackling climate change and working to preserve our oceans and forests." There are, however, substantive hurdles to their effective application, and they require the following actions:

- Ensure real international participation and adequate financing.
- Seek and ensure transparency and unbiased, clear, culturally sensitive, and timely dissemination of information.
- Establish mechanisms to curb conflicts of interest in emergency response, including political decisions resulting in vaccine hoarding and business decisions slowing total production of medical countermeasures.
- Expand the discussions on waiving patents for vaccines and medicines, especially but not exclusively for health emergencies (A patent waiver on COVID vaccines is right and fair 2021; UNESCO 2021; Usher 2020).
- Disseminate relevant information concerning national, commercial, and other interests.

In addition, action by the health, medical, and humanitarian response communities must move beyond research, medical care, and emergency assistance, and even beyond the goal of making the highest attainable standard of physical and mental health available to all. Imperative actions include confronting isolationism and xenophobia; countering anti-scientific sentiment and behavior (e.g., virus and vaccine denialism); supporting open clinical studies data; and demanding meaningful action to counteract climate change, an important driver of disease outbreaks (Watts et al. 2019). Last and most important, this joint effort must urgently address the social determinants of health that facilitate the establishment and spread of various illnesses (Braveman 2011; Galobardes et al. 2008). In other words, the international medical, health, research, and ethics communities, with all their capacity and visibility, must truly work together to tackle the gaping disparities among and within countries, including but not limited to health access. Mechanisms to mitigate with the goal of eliminating such disparities must be included in each and every discussion, guidance paper, and covenant regarding emerging infectious diseases.

Although research to develop diagnostic tools, drugs, and vaccines is essential to curb the COVID-19 pandemic, the results of the research must be transformed into real access to health care for all. The opening remarks of WHO Director General Tedros on the ethics of access to COVID-19 vaccines at WHO Executive Board in January 2021 are appropriate (WHO 2021a):

> "I need to be blunt: the world is on the brink of a catastrophic moral failure—and the

price of this failure will be paid with lives and livelihoods in the world's poorest countries. Even as they speak the language of equitable access, some countries and companies continue to prioritize bilateral deals, going around COVAX, driving up prices and attempting to jump to the front of the queue... This is wrong. Forty-four bilateral deals were signed last year, and at least 12 have already been signed this year. The situation is compounded by the fact that most manufacturers have prioritized regulatory approval in rich countries where the profits are highest, rather than submitting full dossiers to WHO."

Discussion Questions

1. On what basis and to what extent are high-income countries required to share the fruits of their research with LMICs?
2. What are the obligations of research programs to ensure their results are shared with research participants? Does the obligation extend to the community, the country of the participants, or worldwide?
3. What is the role of an individual research program in ameliorating social and political injustices in host countries?
4. What are the ethical issues involved in carrying out a research program sponsored by a high-income country in a low-income country in the following areas?
   (a) Partnerships with local scientists and institutions
   (b) Participation of civil society
   (c) Hiring local staff
   (d) Compensating research participants for their time and expenses
   (e) Health care for study participants who suffer from conditions other than the one being studied
   (f) Elimination of exploitation risks
   (g) Post-trial access to products that have shown to be safe and effective
   (h) Limits on the use of placebo, if any

References

A patent waiver on COVID vaccines is right and fair. Nature. 2021;593(7860):478. https://doi.org/10.1038/d41586-021-01242-1.

Angell M. The ethics of clinical research in the Third World. N Engl J Med. 1997;337(12):847–9. https://doi.org/10.1056/nejm199709183371209.

Baggio O, Camara CA, Prue C. Bringing community perspectives to decision-making in the Ebola response in the Democratic Republic of Congo. Humanitarian Practice Network; 2019.

Bayntun C, Houlihan C, Edmunds J. Ebola crisis: beliefs and behaviours warrant urgent attention. Lancet. 2014;384(9952):1424. https://doi.org/10.1016/s0140-6736(14)61856-0.

BBC. Ebola crisis: Liberian troops impose slum quarantine. BBC News. 2014.

Beauchamp TL, Childress JF. Principles of biomedical ethics. 8th ed. New York: Oxford University Press; 2019.

Bobbio N. The age of rights. Cambridge, UK: Polity Press; 1996.

Bottan NL, Hoffmann B, Vera-Cossio DA. The unequal impact of the coronavirus pandemic: evidence from seventeen developing countries. Washington, DC: Inter-American Development Bank; 2020.

Braveman P. Accumulating knowledge on the social determinants of health and infectious disease. Public Health Rep. 2011;126:28. https://doi.org/10.1177/00333549111260S306.

Briand SC, Cinelli M, Nguyen T, Lewis R, Prybylski D, Valensise CM, et al. Infodemics: a new challenge for public health. Cell. 2021;184(25):6010–4. https://doi.org/10.1016/j.cell.2021.10.031.

Brodeur A, Gray D, Islam A, Bhuiyan S. A literature review of the economics of COVID-19. J Econ Surv. 2021;35:1007. https://doi.org/10.1111/joes.12423.

Brown GW, Bridge G, Martini J, Um J, Williams OD, Choupe LBT, et al. The role of health systems for health security: a scoping review revealing the need for improved conceptual and practical linkages. Glob Health. 2022;18(1):51. https://doi.org/10.1186/s12992-022-00840-6.

Buth P, de Gryse B, Healy S, Hoedt V, Newell T, Pintaldi G, et al. 'He who helps the guilty, shares the crime'? INGOs, moral narcissism and complicity in wrongdoing. J Med Ethics. 2018;44(5):299–304. https://doi.org/10.1136/medethics-2017-104399.

Camus A. The plague. New York: The Modern Library; 1948.

CDC. Cost of the Ebola epidemic. Atlanta: Centers for Disease Control and Prevention (US); 2019. https://www.cdc.gov/vhf/ebola/history/2014-2016-outbreak/cost-of-ebola.html?CDC_AA_refVal=https%3A%2F%2Fwww.cdc.gov%2Fvhf%2Febola%2Foutbreaks%2F2014-west-africa%2Fcost-of-ebola.html. Accessed 13 Feb 2020.

CIOMS. International ethical guidelines for health-related research involving humans. Geneva: Council for International Organisations of Medical Sciences; 2016.

Coalition USGL. COVID-19 brief: impact on the economies of low-income countries. Washington, DC: U.S. Global Leadership Coalition; 2021. https://www.usglc.org/coronavirus/economies-of-developing-countries/. Accessed 7 June 2022.

Council of Europe. Additional protocol to the Convention on human rights and biomedicine, concerning biomedical research. 2005.

CRS. Global economic effects of COVID-19. Washington, DC: Congressional Research Service; 2021. Report No.: R46279 Contract No.: R46279.

Cutler DM, Summers LH. The COVID-19 pandemic and the $16 trillion virus. JAMA. 2020;324(15):1495–6. https://doi.org/10.1001/jama.2020.19759.

Daniels N. Equity and population health: toward a broader bioethics agenda. Hastings Cent Rep. 2006;22(4):22–36.

David PM, Le Dévédec N, Alary A. Pandemics in the age of the Anthropocene: is 'planetary health' the answer? Glob Public Health. 2021;16(8–9):1141–54. https://doi.org/10.1080/17441692.2021.1893372.

Emanuel EJ, Wendler D, Grady C. What makes clinical research in developing countries ethical? The benchmarks of ethical research. J Infect Dis. 2004;189:930–7.

Folayan MO, Allman D, Haire B, Yakubu A, Afolabi MO, Cooper J. Considerations for community engagement when conducting clinical trials during infectious disease emergencies in West Africa. Dev World Bioeth. 2019;19(2):96–105. https://doi.org/10.1111/dewb.12215.

Folke C, Polasky S, Rockström J, Galaz V, Westley F, Lamont M, et al. Our future in the Anthropocene biosphere. Ambio. 2021;50(4):834–69. https://doi.org/10.1007/s13280-021-01544-8.

Fukuda-Parr S, Buss P, Ely Yamin A. Pandemic treaty needs to start with rethinking the paradigm of global health security. BMJ Glob Health. 2021;6(6):e006392. https://doi.org/10.1136/bmjgh-2021-006392.

Galobardes B, Lynch JW, Smith GD. Is the association between childhood socioeconomic circumstances and cause-specific mortality established? Update of a systematic review. J Epidemiol Community Health. 2008;62(5):387–90. https://doi.org/10.1136/jech.2007.065508.

Gavi. Gavi, the Vaccine Alliance helps vaccinate almost half the world's children against deadly and debilitating infectious diseases. Geneva: Gavi, the Vaccine Alliance; 2022. https://www.gavi.org/our-alliance/about. Accessed 2 Mar 2022.

GPMB. A world at risk: annual report on global preparedness for health emergencies. Geneva: Global Preparedness Monitoring Board, World Health Organization; 2019.

GPMB. From worlds apart to a world prepared: Global Preparedness Monitoring Board report 2021. Geneva: Global Preparedness Monitoring Board, World Health Organization; 2021.

Greco D. Commentary 20.2: Researchers' obligations to uninfected partners in discordant couples in an HIV transmission trial in the Rakai district, Uganda. In: Lavery JV, Grady C, Wahl ER, Emanuel EJ, editors. Ethical issues in international biomedical research: a casebook. Oxford: Oxford University Press; 2007.

Greco D. The AIDS epidemic—social, scientific and economical impacts and perspectives. Dossiê Epidemias. 2008;22(64):73. https://doi.org/10.1590/S0103-40142008000300006.

Hoffman SJ, Silverberg SL. Delays in global disease outbreak responses: lessons from H1N1, Ebola, and Zika. Am J Public Health. 2018;108(3):329–33. https://doi.org/10.2105/ajph.2017.304245.

Horton R. Offline: COVID-19 is not a pandemic. Lancet. 2020;396(10255):874. https://doi.org/10.1016/s0140-6736(20)32000-6.

Huber C, Finelli L, Stevens W. The economic and social burden of the 2014 Ebola outbreak in West Africa. J Infect Dis. 2018;218(Suppl_5):S698–704. https://doi.org/10.1093/infdis/jiy213.

IASC. Humanitarian system-wide scale-up activation protocol for the control of infectious disease events. Geneva: Inter-Agency Standing Committee; 2019.

ICMJE. Recommendations for the conduct, reporting, editing, and publication of scholarly work in medical journals. International Committee of Medical Journal Editors; 2019. p. 19.

IMF. The IMF and aid to Sub-Saharan Africa. Washington, DC: International Monetary Fund, Independent Evaluation Office 2007. Report No.: ISBN: 978-1-58906-635-9.

IMF. A strategy for IMF engagement on social spending. Washington, DC: Internatonal Monetary Fund; 2019.

Independent Panel for Pandemic Preparedness & Response. COVID-19: make it the last pandemic. Independent Panel for Pandemic Preparedness & Response; 2021.

International Health Conference. Constitution of the World Health Organization. New York: United Nations; 1946.

Jentsch B, Pilley C. Research relationships between the South and the North: Cinderella and the ugly sisters? Soc Sci Med. 2003;57(10):1957–67. https://doi.org/10.1016/S0277-9536(03)00060-1.

Johns Hopkins. Coronavirus Resource Center. Baltimore, MD: Johns Hopkins University Medical Center; 2022. https://coronavirus.jhu.edu/map.html. Accessed 14 Mar 2022 2022.

Kentikelenis A, King L, McKee M, Stuckler D. The International Monetary Fund and the Ebola outbreak. Lancet Glob Health. 2015;3(2):e69–70. https://doi.org/10.1016/s2214-109x(14)70377-8.

Keshavjee S. Blind spot: how neoliberalism infiltrated global health. Oakland, CA: University of California Press; 2014.

Kutalek R, Wang S, Fallah M, Wesseh CS, Gilbert J. Ebola interventions: listen to communities.

Lancet Glob Health. 2015;3(3):e131. https://doi.org/10.1016/S2214-109X(15)70010-0.
Lemay-Hébert N, Marcelin LH, Pallage S, Cela T. The internal brain drain: foreign aid, hiring practices, and international migration. Disasters. 2020;44(4):621–40. https://doi.org/10.1111/disa.12382.
Lie RK, Emanuel E, Grady C, Wendler D. The standard of care debate: the Declaration of Helsinki versus the international consensus opinion. J Med Ethics. 2004;30(2):190–3. https://doi.org/10.1136/jme.2003.006031.
London AJ, Kimmelman J. Against pandemic research exceptionalism. Science. 2020;368(6490):476–7. https://doi.org/10.1126/science.abc1731.
Lucas B. G7 and G20 commitments on health. Brighton, UK: Institute of Development Studies; 2019.
Lundgren JD, Grund B, Barkauskas CE, Holland TL, Gottlieb RL, Sandkovsky U, et al. A neutralizing monoclonal antibody for hospitalized patients with Covid-19. N Engl J Med. 2021;384(10):905–14. https://doi.org/10.1056/NEJMoa2033130.
Lurie P, Wolfe SM. Unethical trials of interventions to reduce perinatal transmission of the human immunodeficiency virus in developing countries. N Engl J Med. 1997;337(12):853–6. https://doi.org/10.1056/nejm199709183371212.
Malmqvist E. Better to exploit than to neglect? International clinical research and the non-worseness claim. J Appl Philos. 2017;34(4):474–88. https://doi.org/10.1111/japp.12153.
Morand S, Walther BA. The accelerated infectious disease risk in the Anthropocene: more outbreaks and wider global spread. BioRxiv. 2020; https://doi.org/10.1101/2020.04.20.049866.
MSF. Involving communities: guidance document for approaching and cooperating with communities. Vienna: Médecins sans Frontières. Unit VE; 2013.
MSF. Restoring trust among communities fearful of Ebola. Vienna: Médecins sans Frontières; 2019.
Mulangu S, Dodd LE, Davey RT Jr, Tshiani Mbaya O, Proschan M, Mukadi D, et al. A randomized, controlled trial of Ebola virus disease therapeutics. N Engl J Med. 2019;381(24):2293–303. https://doi.org/10.1056/NEJMoa1910993.
National Council of Health (BR). Resolution no. 466, of 12 December 2012. Brasilia: Jusbrasil; 2012. p. 12.
Nuffield Council on Bioethics. Research in global health emergencies: ethical issues. Oxford, UK: Nuffield Council on Bioethics; 2020.
Nuzzo JB, Meyer D, Snyder M, Ravi SJ, Lapascu A, Souleles J, et al. What makes health systems resilient against infectious disease outbreaks and natural hazards? Results from a scoping review. BMC Public Health. 2019;19(1):1310. https://doi.org/10.1186/s12889-019-7707-z.
OECD. Development resource flows—total official and private flows. Paris: Organisation for Economic Co-operation and Development; 2022. https://data.oecd.org/drf/total-official-and-private-flows.htm. Accessed 14 Jan 2022.
Oppenheim B, Gallivan M, Madhav NK, Brown N, Serhiyenko V, Wolfe ND, et al. Assessing global preparedness for the next pandemic: development and application of an Epidemic Preparedness Index. BMJ Glob Health. 2019;4(1):e001157. https://doi.org/10.1136/bmjgh-2018-001157.
Our World in Data. Coronavirus (COVID-19) vaccinations. Oxford: Our World in Data; 2022. https://ourworldindata.org/covid-vaccinations. Accessed 20 May 2022.
Piot P, Quinn TC. Response to the AIDS pandemic—a global health paradigm. N Engl J Med. 2013;368(23):2210–8. https://doi.org/10.1056/NEJMra1201533.
Pratt B, Loff B. A framework to link international clinical research to the promotion of justice in global health. Bioethics. 2014;28(8):387–96. https://doi.org/10.1111/bioe.12009.
Rull M, Kickbusch I, Lauer H. Policy debate: international responses to global epidemics: Ebola and beyond. J Int Dev. 2015; https://doi.org/10.4000/poldev.2178.
Schuklenk U. The standard of care debate: against the myth of an "international consensus opinion". J Med Ethics. 2004;30(2):194–7. https://doi.org/10.1136/jme.2003.006981.
Singer M, Bulled N, Ostrach B, Mendenhall E. Syndemics and the biosocial conception of health. Lancet. 2017;389(10072):941–50. https://doi.org/10.1016/s0140-6736(17)30003-x.
Sirleaf EJ, Clark H. Report of the Independent Panel for Pandemic Preparedness and Response: making COVID-19 the last pandemic. Lancet. 2021;398(10295):101–3. https://doi.org/10.1016/s0140-6736(21)01095-3.
Stern JE. Hell in the hot zone: why a massive international effort has failed to contain the Ebola epidemic. Vanity Fair. 2014.
Stuckler D, Basu S. The body economic: why austerity kills. New York: Basic Books; 2013.
Thomson M, Kentikelenis A, Stubbs T. Structural adjustment programmes adversely affect vulnerable populations: a systematic-narrative review of their effect on child and maternal health. Public Health Rev. 2017;38(1):13. https://doi.org/10.1186/s40985-017-0059-2.
UN. The 17 goals. New York: UN Department of Economic and Social Affairs; 2021. https://sdgs.un.org/goals. Accessed 28 Sept 2021.
UNAIDS/AVAC. Good participatory practice: guidelines for biomedical HIV prevention trials. Geneva: UNAIDS (Joint United Nations Programme on HIV/AIDS); 2011.
UNAIDS/WHO. Ethical considerations in biomedical HIV prevention trials: UNAIDS/WHO guidance document. Geneva: Joint United Nations Programme on HIV/AIDS (UNAIDS); 2021. p. 70.
UNESCO. Universal declaration on bioethics and human rights. UNESCO General Conference, 33rd Session. Paris: UNESCO; 2005.

UNESCO. Joint statement of UNESCO's ethics commissions on ensuring equal access for all to vaccines and therapeutics developed to confront COVID-19: joint statement of the UNESCO International Bioethics Committee (IBC) and UNESCO World Commission for the Ethics of Science and Technology (COMEST). Paris: UNESCO; 2021.
Usher AD. South Africa and India push for COVID-19 patents ban. Lancet. 2020;396(10265):1790–1. https://doi.org/10.1016/s0140-6736(20)32581-2.
Watts N, Amann M, Arnell N, Ayeb-Karlsson S, Belesova K, Boykoff M, et al. The 2019 report of The Lancet Countdown on health and climate change: ensuring that the health of a child born today is not defined by a changing climate. Lancet. 2019;394(10211):1836–78. https://doi.org/10.1016/s0140-6736(19)32596-6.
WHO. Good participatory practice guidelines for trials of emerging (and re-emerging) pathogens that are likely to cause severe outbreaks in the near future and for which few or no medical countermeasures exist (GPP-EP). Geneva: World Health Organization; 2016a. p. 53.
WHO. International Health Regulations (2005). 3rd ed. Geneva: World Health Organzation; 2016b.
WHO. A strategic framework for emergency preparedness. Geneva: World Health Organization; 2017.
WHO. Consultation on monitored emergency use of unregistered and investigational interventions (MEURI) for Ebola virus disease (EVD). In: Notes for the record. Geneva: World Health Organization; 2018. https://www.who.int/ebola/drc-2018/notes-for-the-record-meuri-ebola.pdf. Accessed 3 Mar 2022.
WHO. About the R&D blueprint. Geneva: World Health Organization; 2020a. https://www.who.int/blueprint/about/en/. Accessed 6 Feb 2020.
WHO. Good Participatory Practice for COVID-19 clinical trials—a toolbox. Geneva: World Health Organization; 2020b.
WHO. Report of the Director-General, 146th meeting of the Executive Board. Geneva: World Health Organization; 2020c.
WHO. WHO Director-General's opening remarks at 148th session of the Executive Board. Geneva: World Health Organization; 2021a.
WHO. Universal health and preparedness review (UHPR) Member States information session. Geneva: World Health Organization; 2021b.
WHO. The access to COVID-19 tools (ACT) accelerator. Geneva: World Health Organization; 2022a. https://www.who.int/initiatives/act-accelerator. Accessed 2 Mar 2022.
WHO. Infodemic. Geneva: World Health Organization; 2022b. https://www.who.int/health-topics/infodemic#tab=tab_1. Accessed 16 Feb 2022.
WHO. Strengthening WHO preparedness for and response to health emergencies. Geneva: World Health Organization; 2022c. Report No.: Seventy-Fifth World Health Assembly A75/21. Provisional agenda item 16.2.
WHO. WHO Director-General's opening remarks at first meeting of the Intergovernmental Negotiating Body to draft and negotiate a WHO convention, agreement or other international instrument on pandemic prevention, preparedness and response. Geneva: World Health Organization; 2022d.
WHO AFRO. African Vaccine Regulatory Forum (AVAREF). Brazzaville: World Health Organization African Regional Office; 2021. https://www.afro.who.int/health-topics/immunization/avaref. Accessed 7 Jun 2022.
Wilkinson A, Parker M, Martineau F, Leach M. Engaging 'communities': anthropological insights from the West African Ebola epidemic. Philos Trans R Soc Lond Ser B Biol Sci. 2017;372(1721):20160305. https://doi.org/10.1098/rstb.2016.0305.
WMA. Declaration of Helsinki: ethical principles for medical research involving human subjects. Ferney-Voltaire, FR: World Medical Associsation; 2013.
WHO. Seventy-seventh World Health Assembly: daily update: 1 June 2024 [press release]. Geneva: World Health Organization. 2024. https://www.who.int/news/item/01-06-2024-seventy-seventh-world-healthassembly. daily update. Accessed 1 Jun 2024.

6 Meeting Regulatory Criteria and Seeking Licensure: Medicines Development Before and During Public Health Emergencies

Marco Cavaleri, Marion Gruber, Rogerio Gaspar, and Mimi Darko

Contents

Learning Track Note: This chapter appears in Learning Tracks: Clinical Research; Health Policy, Multilateral Cooperation, International Governance

E. S. Higgs and R. A. Sorenson (eds.), *Principles and Practice of Emergency Research Response*, https://doi.org/10.1007/978-3-031-48408-7_8

Learning Objectives

This chapter will help readers understand and describe:

- The role of regulatory agencies in expediting clinical development and product approvals
- Awareness of regulatory flexibilities during pandemics in order to expedite progress through clinical trials
- Advances in manufacturing methods and platform technologies enabling streamlined medical countermeasure development
- The regulatory evaluation of benefits and risks in an evolving situation, with transparent communication and close collaboration with multiple stakeholders
- Basic knowledge about
  - What preclinical and clinical studies must demonstrate and what essential product aspects they must characterize
  - Safety assessment and communication
  - Special populations
  - Appropriate design of Phase II/III studies considered sufficiently robust to meet regulatory standards for assessment of benefits and risks
  - Lessons learned from the Randomized Evaluation of COVID-19 Therapy through Randomized Trials (RECOVERY)
- Awareness of
  - Key regulatory bodies, including the International Coalition of Medicines Regulatory Authorities (ICRMA)
  - The role of regulators in the countries where emerging infectious diseases (EID) outbreaks have occurred
  - The greatest challenges in chemistry, manufacturing, and controls for MCM producers

1 Introduction

Regulatory agencies play a critical role in the national and international response to emerging and re-emerging infectious diseases (EIDs). Their responsibilities span a range of regulatory activities, from providing guidance on design of preclinical and clinical trials; assessing the data trials produce; ensuring data quality; developing chemistry, manufacturing, and controls (CMC) for medical countermeasure (MCM) production; to reviewing all data that ultimately lead to authorization or approval of MCMs—the crucial requirement for large-scale deployment of and access to therapeutic and preventive products. In other words, regulatory agencies are not just there to review data provided by clinical and other investigatory trials but to work with the many actors involved in bringing a new MCM into the pharmacopeia. Thus, there is a continuum in the regulatory appraisal of investigational agents and diagnostics from early development into initial (Phases I and II) and then to large-scale clinical trials (Phases II and III) and post-approval evidence gathering (Phase IV). One important focus, as the world considers how we can better prepare for novel and re-emerging EIDS, is what can be done to advance vaccines, therapeutics, and diagnostics against potential pandemic pathogens before a crisis strikes. This includes both virus families known to include pathogens and "pathogen X," a novel pathogen that may arise unforeseen. SARS-CoV, as an example, arose as a novel pathogen but was a member of a family, *Coronaviridae*, that was already under study because two viruses in the family had come to notice in recent years: SARS-CoV-1 and the Middle Eastern respiratory syndrome virus (MERS-CoV) in 2002 and 2012, respectively.

In the context of EID emergencies, a key question is how research can be designed and conducted during a health emergency to produce reliable evidence as expeditiously as possible to confirm or establish whether a given intervention has a positive risk-benefit balance. This chapter will describe regulatory approaches used and experiences gained in the global regulatory response to public health emergencies, using the 2014–2016 West Africa Ebola outbreak and the COVID-19 pandemic as examples.

2 Development and Licensure of Medicinal Products in Brief

Each clinical development program and regulatory licensure strategy for medicinal products being developed against an emerging or potentially emerging pathogen must be tailored to the particular investigational agent and the epidemiological context. The type and extent of preclinical and clinical studies needed to demonstrate the quality, efficacy, and safety of the product depend on its characteristics, its proposed indications, and its target population.

In general, the clinical evaluation of medicinal products during the premarketing stage occurs in discrete trial phases, i.e., Phases I, II, and III. Phase I trials are intended to provide an initial evaluation of safety and pharmacokinetics (PK), and in the case of vaccines safety and likely immunogenicity. They are typically conducted in a small number (e.g., 20–80) of closely monitored adult volunteers. Phase II studies can involve up to several hundred participants, are often randomized and well controlled, and provide further information on safety, immunogenicity for vaccines, and optimal dose. Phase III studies are large-scale trials to provide a more thorough assessment of safety as well as a definite assessment of efficacy. Efficacy should ideally be demonstrated in randomized, double-blind, controlled trials with product-specific endpoints. They may be clinical disease endpoints or, for vaccines, immune response endpoints if a biomarker has been identified as a reliable correlate of protection; in some cases, a surrogate endpoint reasonably likely to predict clinical benefit can be identified (▶ Chap. 22 and In Practice 22.1).

Safety is one of the most important considerations for evaluating MCMs such as vaccines and therapeutics. In general, when evaluating safety, one must compare the risk of the disease or condition with the risk of adverse event(s) potentially associated with the product. For products evaluated in clinical endpoint efficacy trials, a large safety database likely will emerge from a double-blind, randomized, well-controlled efficacy study. Additional controlled safety studies are often requested when the number of subjects included in the efficacy studies are deemed insufficient to provide adequate safety data. Licensure must also be supported by data demonstrating that the manufacturing process will ensure product consistency and quality and that the facility is compliant with current good manufacturing practices (EC 2011). Given the many requirements, drug and vaccine development from the discovery stage to late-stage development normally takes a rather long time, often several years or more (◘ Fig. 1).

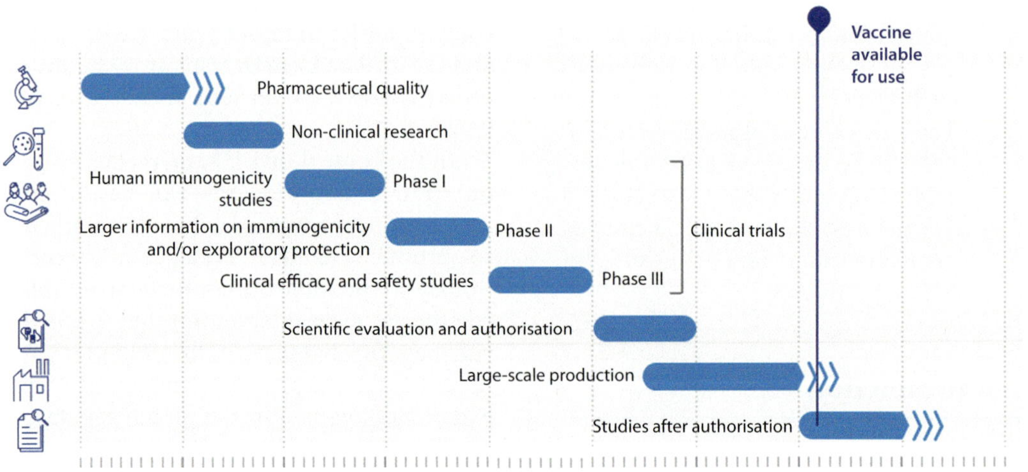

◘ **Fig. 1** Selected steps to vaccine approval and distribution (EMA 2022) (free use with attribution). This time scale can vary considerably, from the 4 years it took to develop the mumps vaccine in the 1960s to an average of 15–20 years. (Janse et al. 2021; Hilleman et al. 1968)

3 Medical Countermeasure Development During a Public Health Emergency

The Ebola outbreak in West Africa necessitated compressed product development programs to provide life-saving medicinal products in an accelerated manner. In this case, there were two preclinical vaccine candidates that could not be entered into clinical trials until over a year after the outbreak began in December 2013. The pathogen causing the outbreak was not identified until March 2014; full-scale international involvement did not begin until the World Health Organization (WHO) declared a Public Health Emergency of International Concern in August (Moon et al. 2015; Higgs et al. 2017).

As research response began, regulatory agencies engaged with each other, vaccine manufacturers, and other stakeholders to accelerate the development of MCMs (Cavaleri et al. 2016). To advance vaccine candidates, international regulators rapidly assessed product characterization data and clinical trial protocols to allow clinical trials to begin. Immunogenicity and safety data were rapidly reported and assessed, allowing initiation of Phase III clinical studies of vaccines in individuals residing in outbreak areas and collection of data supporting licensure of these products. National regulatory agencies engaged in joint reviews with WHO and West African regulators to discuss study designs, ethical considerations, and the product information requirements for international regulatory consensus on approval or authorization, thus facilitating development of trial protocols and data management plans. However, available investigational drugs and vaccine candidates were still in preclinical development at the time of the Ebola outbreak. Despite the use of compressed development programs for both vaccines and therapeutics and initiation of clinical efficacy studies, trials occurred at what turned out to be a later stage in the epidemic when Ebola disease incidence rates were dropping (Kennedy et al. 2017).

As a consequence, pivotal Phase III studies (PREVAIL and Ebola Ça Suffit!) had to be terminated before reaching statistical significance due to the waning number of Ebola infection cases (Henao-Restrepo et al. 2017; Kennedy et al. 2017). Regulators and manufacturers alike had to balance the need for rigorous and robust study designs on one side with ethical and feasibility considerations on the other, acknowledging that implementing clinical trial ethical standards is dependent on the actual situation and remains at the discretion of local ethics committees and investigators. The discussion on the role of randomized trials and inclusion of adequate controls for therapeutics clinical evaluation was particularly challenging as differing views were expressed by investigators and competent authorities. The main lesson learned was that only large, well-designed randomized studies with appropriate controls could lead to results that would be interpretable in the context of evolving epidemiology, fluctuation in morbidity and mortality, and lack of outstanding clinical efficacy.

In addition, there were other factors that hindered timely gathering of product safety and effectiveness data. These included but were not limited to lack of an appropriate infrastructure for clinical research, timely agreement on study design, the availability of adequate supply of investigational medicinal products and, importantly, lack of early product characterization and quality data to support the clinical use of the medicinal products at the intended posology (the size or frequency of a dose or doses).

The COVID-19 pandemic has provided many examples of how regulatory agencies collaborated with national and global partners in emergency response. The pandemic has been an extraordinary challenge to global health, claiming the lives of millions of people worldwide. National regulatory authorities collaborated in an unprecedented effort with product manufacturers, research scientists, epidemiologists, public health, and government officials to develop vaccines and therapeutic products against SARS-CoV, utilizing

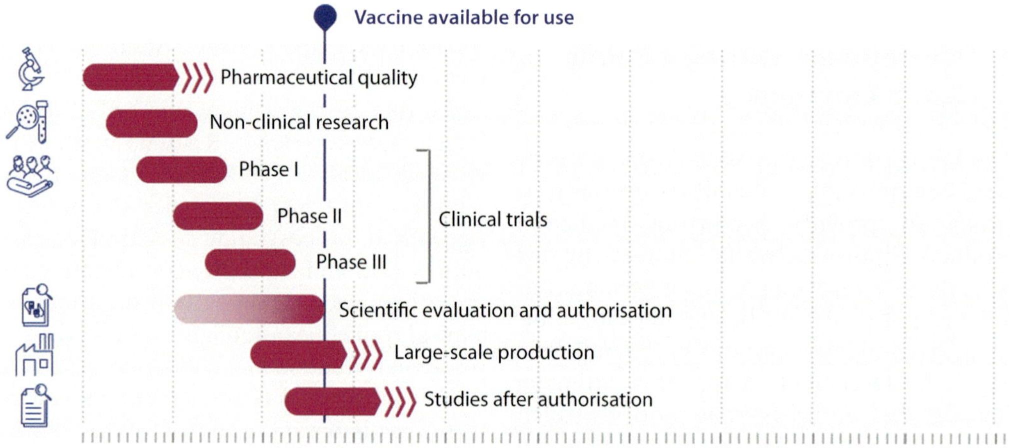

Fig. 2 Accelerated timeline for COVID-19 vaccines: note the much greater degree of overlap among steps to approval, showing they are conducted simultaneously rather than in sequence to a much greater extent than in "normal" vaccine development. (EMA 2022; free use with attribution)

both traditional and novel platforms and manufacturing technologies (Fig. 2).

Regulators worked closely with manufacturers and provided them with expedited feedback and regulatory guidance. Regulatory agencies conducted expedited reviews of manufacturing information, preclinical and clinical protocols, and clinical trials data, and provided timely advice through frequent interactions with product manufacturers. Knowledge gained from previous experience with the technology now being used to manufacture new MCMs was considered to supplement and abbreviate some of the quality testing and preclinical study requirements for initiating human clinical trials (Wagner et al. 2021). This is one example of how research requirements can be met in expedited fashion, without compromising safety or scientific rigor, to pave the way for expedited determination of safe and immunogenic doses to be used in pivotal vaccine efficacy and safety studies.

Animal models provided early indications of COVID-19 vaccine candidates providing protection from challenge with the pathogen, leading to lower levels of enhanced respiratory disease and robust T helper type 1 (T_H1)-skewed immune responses (Wang et al. 2021). For repurposed therapeutic agents, gathering sufficient proof-of-concept data to support progression to large clinical trials has proven to be more challenging than for vaccines, underscoring the need for better infrastructure for rapid and efficient preclinical testing (► Chap. 14).

Regulators agreed to the use of adaptive and/or seamless clinical trial designs for allowing for more rapid progression through the usual phases of clinical development. At the same time, they had to ensure that data were adequate and interpretable, and that respective regulatory standards were met to support authorization and ultimately licensing for both investigational life-saving COVID-19 therapeutic products and COVID-19 vaccines. Good clinical practices (GCPs) need to be maintained in clinical studies to ensure the possible use for regulatory decisions despite challenges associated with clinical research during emergencies. Investigators and sponsors need to ensure that data are collected and stored in compliance with GCPs to the extent possible and to take into account the possibility that regulators conduct inspections to verify the quality of the clinical trials. At the same time regulators understand the need to maintain flexibilities and proportionality with respect to GCP compliance in emergency settings.

These collaborative efforts enabled the timely initiation of Phase III clinical studies for some of the COVID-19 vaccine constructs, trials that produced safety and efficacy data to support widespread use of these products in millions and ultimately billions of people. For therapeutic products the fragmentation of clinical research has been a major hurdle in the initial phase of the pandemic. Sufficiently sized platform clinical trials proved to be of major value in generating the required evidence in a timely manner. A few months into the COVID-19 pandemic, there were calls from regulators to increase the efficiency of clinical trials for COVID-19 medicinal products (Eichler et al. 2020). Specific suggestions were made:

- The research community should consider whether their planned trial can become part of a larger platform trial.
- Developers of COVID-19 treatments should seek interactions with regulators as early as possible.
- Well-established public or private consortia should ramp up their activities and take on a wider role in the management of trials.
- Regulators should show flexibility in clinical trial management to address the challenges arising from the COVID-19 pandemic, while ensuring a high level of quality, efficacy, and safety of medicines.
- Ethics committees should ensure that the benefits of conducting clinical trial for COVID-19 outweigh risks and burdens to participants.
- Trial sponsors should establish infrastructure sufficient to support clinical trial conduct.
- Umbrella patient organizations and learned societies should use their influence to encourage clinical trial coordination.

In addition, regulators generated pertinent guidance documents for the development of therapeutic products and vaccines and met with their regulatory counterparts to discuss convergence of regulatory approaches to facilitate accelerated development and deployment of COVID-19 vaccines and other therapeutic products (see ▶ Sect. 5).

4 Lessons Learned and Regulatory Strategies to Prepare for Future Emergencies

Together, the Ebola and COVID-19 examples illustrate the importance of proactive data collection to enhance preparedness when an outbreak occurs. Importantly, product characterization, preclinical, and early safety and immunogenicity pharmacokinetics/pharmacodynamics clinical studies should be performed, to the extent possible, well in advance of any epidemic or pandemic public health emergency. This is one element in the logic behind the prototype pathogen approach being adopted as a research avenue for pandemic preparedness (Graham and Corbett 2020).

4.1 Chemistry, Manufacturing, and Controls and Reliance on Available Data on Platform Technologies

A timely response to an emerging pathogen may be facilitated by the availability of a well-characterized technology platform (for example, a well-characterized mRNA or adenovirus platform), where the same backbone is used with a new insert, one different from that previously used against another pathogen. In certain situations, CMC and preclinical data accrued for such a platform may support the nonclinical safety of an investigational agent directed against an emerging pathogen, allowing more streamlined regulatory decision making. It can be argued that existing knowledge of the manufacturing process and the safety database accumulated with biological medicinal products produced with existing, previously successful technology will provide supportive evidence and may alleviate some of the testing and data otherwise required. It should be well understood, however, that *efficacy* data cannot be extrapolated from one pathogen to another based on using the same platform technology. There will still be considerable scientific and regulatory challenges associated with developing and testing new medical countermeasures against EIDs, because they will likely use novel technologies and new assays to evaluate their potency.

4.2 Preclinical Studies

Non-clinical studies, including repeated toxicity and pharmacology studies to support the safe and effective use of a medicinal product to be used in an emergency, could be derived from similar vaccine or therapeutic products manufactured using proven technology. For example, for a vaccine candidate, these studies may be conducted using the same vaccine construct and technology but expressing a different antigen. Data from these studies may then be used to support use of the vaccine constructs expressing the antigen of interest in the event of a public health emergency. Different guidelines (WHO 2005) describe the type of non-clinical studies that are usually required in order to allow clinical trial initiation and to facilitate product development toward licensure.

Studies in animal models to provide evidence of proof of concept are valuable tools to support further clinical evaluation of the investigational product developed either as prophylaxis or for treatment. In situations where it is not possible to perform clinical efficacy studies, e.g., for ethical reasons or when the disease outbreak is unpredictable, pivotal studies for inferring clinical efficacy can be conducted in animal models (FDA 2021).

Even though animal challenge/protection models and studies are not a requirement to support initiation of clinical trials, data from such studies may contribute significantly to assess the benefit/risk of the product to clinical study participants and should thus be considered as an integral component of a preclinical package supporting clinical trial applications in the setting of EIDs. Regulators would expect that developers provide appropriate evidence to support the value of the chosen animal models in terms of similarity to the disease in humans, similar viral propagation, and kinetics. Differences between animals and humans in the pharmacokinetics profile for therapeutics and quality and quantity of the immune response for vaccines will need thorough consideration when supporting any dose/schedule to be used in humans.

4.3 Clinical Studies

For therapeutics for emergent diseases, a properly designed Phase II study exploring dose response and providing proof of concept of efficacy would normally be needed before moving to Phase III studies. However, this presents a challenge during epidemics, when rapid progression to confirmatory evidence generation may be vital to mitigating the consequences of the disease. Thus, in many instances, demonstration of safety and efficacy during an emergency is planned to occur through a single seamless or single-dose Phase II/III clinical study. Seamless studies may embed a Phase II or proof-of-concept phase that allows rapid decision making toward possible progression into a confirmatory larger part of the study, or Phase III.

In consideration of such aspects, development of countermeasures such as antivirals should ideally be started ahead of an epidemic or pandemic and should include studies to identify dose(s) and posology of the investigational agent that could be used during an outbreak. A good understanding of the pharmacology (pharmacokinetics and pharmacodynamics) for drugs, and immunogenicity in the target population in the case of vaccines, is needed. To achieve this goal, a combination of preclinical models and clinical studies is likely to be needed, as well as data demonstrating how findings in animal models can help build a bridge to the clinic. Adequate validation/qualification of assays to measure immune response or therapeutics concentrations in body fluids, across several tested species and in humans is expected.

In terms of dose selection, certain therapeutic agents may have generated efficacy data against other more common pathogens that could allow some level of bridging based on similarity in microbiological activity and type of disease caused, e.g., to support dose selection for treatment of plague or anthrax, clinical data for the treatment of bacterial pneumonia could provide relevant supportive evidence.

Considerations of safety and efficacy of the product in special populations such as children and pregnant women are often important, albeit difficult, areas to address ahead of a crisis. Any kind of evidence that could be collected in preparedness and to support use needs to be considered early, notwithstanding feasibility and ethical constraints related to investigation in vulnerable groups with no or limited apparent direct benefit from the investigational agent.

Randomized controlled clinical trials will remain the preferred approach and are the gold standard to generate scientifically valid data to support regulatory and other important public health policy decisions. Indeed, experience from the EVD epidemic has shown that uncontrolled or externally controlled trials failed to provide a robust basis for public health decision making, in particular, given the challenges in a reliable quantification of the rapidly changing disease epidemiology (Brueckner et al. 2018). Nevertheless, alternative options to randomized trials will need to be considered in situations where randomized controlled clinical trials are no longer feasible, e.g., unpredictable, sporadic, or reduced disease incidence; or availability/approval of other efficacious therapeutics or vaccines. In this context, it is important to accrue qualitative and quantitative data on disease epidemiology.

During the COVID-19 pandemic, randomized clinical trials have been essential to determine the benefits of new therapeutics because of the complexity of the disease, the potential effect of therapeutics at different stages of the disease and differential benefit based on patient phenotypes (e.g., with respect to inflammation and coagulation). Additionally, COVID-19 showed that even randomized trials, considered to be adequately sized based on preliminary assumptions, were not able to provide confirmation of efficacy, and only very large studies with hard clinical endpoints such as mortality could provide the required evidence, e.g. tocilizumab and RECOVERY trial (RECOVERY Collaborative Group 2021). On the other hand, very large therapeutic trials with heterogenous patient populations and varying standards of care employed have the risk of diluting any possible effect in specific patients and would not be the preferred option unless there is expectation of an overall very large treatment effect.

The COVID-19 pandemic reinforced the important principle that antivirals should be used as early as possible after initial infection and symptom onset, as this maximizes the chances of having an impact on the progression of the disease when the virus is driving pathogenesis. Moreover, it is apparent that patients unable to promptly mount an immune response—those with deficits in their immune systems—are more likely to benefit from antiviral treatment. Finding antivirals that are active on a conserved part of the virus, such as the polymerase, make them more prone to be active across different families of viruses, and therefore, better candidates for pre-outbreak trials and earlier use in the case of new emergent viruses.

Monoclonal antibodies have confirmed their antiviral potency and would be a suitable platform for future preparedness. However, promptly collecting data on resistance and neutralization evasion is critical and requires close regulatory monitoring and continuous engagement with the sponsors. For example, key mutations in the SARS-COV2 virus have completely evaded the activity of neutralizing antibodies authorized for use because they showed efficacy against viral strains previously in circulation. In these instances, regulatory authorities need to work closely with the scientific groups monitoring the impact of mutations on product potency, and to change regulatory guidance as appropriate. Denying regulatory approval due to limitations in the spectrum of antiviral activity would be controversial and might not be warranted as potential value in certain epidemiological settings cannot be excluded, e.g., approval and unchanged regulatory status of Ronapreve (casirivimab and imdevimab) and Regkirona (regdanvimab) after emergence of Omicron variant of SARS-COV2, for which there is lack of neutralization in in vitro studies, as it cannot be excluded that based on further viral evolution these products may return to being active.

With regard to vaccines, large placebo-controlled randomized studies were conducted due to high COVID-19 disease incidence that resulted in robust estimates of the level of protection and ensured fast regulatory decision making. In less than a year, the United States granted three COVID-19 vaccine candidates Emergency Use Authorization, while five vaccines initially received conditional approval in the EU. Regulators agreed on the type of endpoints that would be acceptable, while leaving individual manufacturers the ability to propose endpoints that met the criteria. Step-down pediatric studies were deferred until after results from adults were available. Vulnerable groups such as pregnant women could not be enrolled before data from preclinical studies and efficacy and safety in the general population were made available.

Balancing benefits and risks of medicines in the uncertain and dynamic conditions of an emergent epidemic is not trivial and adds to the difficulty in coming up rapidly with decisions in the interest of the public and bodies in charge of providing field response. Protection of public health means also making sure that patients and individuals are not exposed to undue risks or unfounded expectations of benefit from the new countermeasures.

4.4 Post-approval Monitoring

Post-approval monitoring of safety and effectiveness is another crucial activity under the shared responsibility of public health authorities and regulators. Rapid review of adverse events reported via pharmacovigilance systems in the course of mass vaccination campaigns has proved challenging but essential to reassure the public and ensure that the risk-benefit balance of the vaccine remains positive. In addition to pharmacovigilance reporting, active surveillance studies using healthcare systems databases and networks of specialized centers are needed to properly characterize the incidence and risk factors for any potential adverse event that could be causally linked to vaccination or administration of certain therapeutics (▶ Chap. 36).

Suspected adverse reactions should also be reported by marketing authorization holders in periodic safety update reports, which provide competent authorities with an update of the worldwide safety experience of medicinal products at defined points after authorization. Such updates include a critical evaluation of the risk-benefit balance of the product in light of new or changing information. This will determine whether further investigation should be done and if changes should be made to the marketing authorization and product information. For vaccines, the periodic safety update report also includes reports of lack of efficacy/vaccine failure, for example, as seen with pathogen variants.

When vaccination campaigns associated with emerging health threats may require rapid decision making to minimize risks, the observed-to-expected (O/E) method provides rapid signal validation and preliminary signal evaluation when there is insufficient time to review a large number of individual cases. It compares the observed number of cases of an adverse event occurring in vaccinated individuals and recorded in a data collection system (e.g., a spontaneous reporting system or an electronic health care record database) and the expected number of cases that would have naturally occurred in the same population without vaccination, estimated from available incidence rates in a non-vaccinated population. Key requirements of O/E analyses include the observed number of cases detected in a passive or active surveillance system, near real-time exposure data, appropriately stratified background incidence rates calculated on a population similar to the vaccinated population (for the expected number of cases), the definition of appropriate risk periods (where there is suspicion and/or biological plausibility that there is a vaccine-associated increased risk of experiencing the event) and sensitivity analyses around these measures. O/E analyses may require some adjustments for continuous monitoring due to inflation of type 1 error rates when multiple tests are performed.

During an emergency, the acceptability of specific risks associated with vaccination must

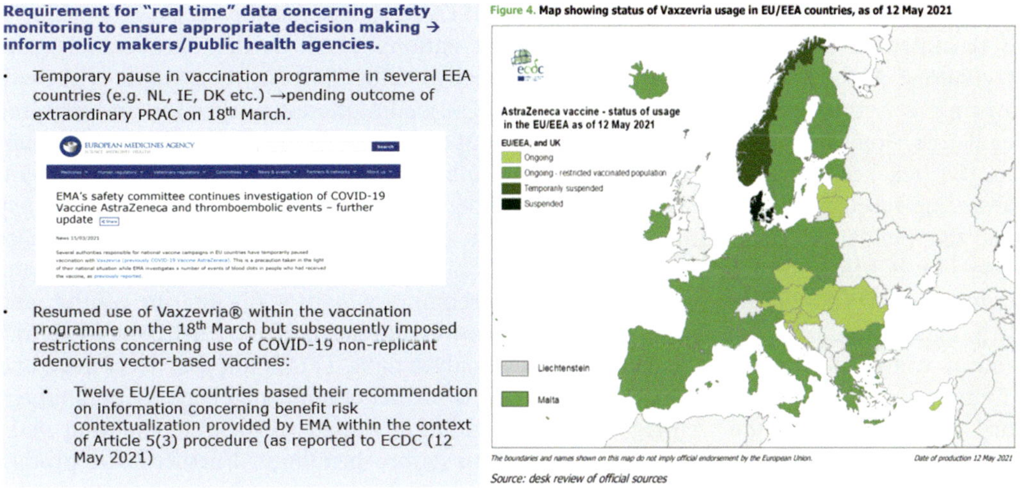

Fig. 3 Emergence of thrombosis with thrombocytopenia syndrome (TTS) cases after administrations of Vaxzevria and the impact on use in the European Union and European Economic Area before and after regulatory actions were taken by the EMA Pharmacovigilance Risk Assessment Committee. (Courtesy EMA)

be contextualized with the benefits associated with vaccination at a personal and population level and with the specificities of the emergency and public health needs. This is the case for very rare adverse events, such as thrombosis with thrombocytopenia syndrome (TTS) or myocarditis, which have been associated with some SARS-CoV vaccines (Greinacher et al. 2021). In the context of the high morbidity and mortality associated with the disease and the high expected benefits of the vaccines against severe outcomes and death, the benefit/risk ratio is still considered strongly positive. Risk contextualization is normally performed by Public Health Authorities and National Immunization Technical Advisory Groups (NITAGs), which decide on the most appropriate vaccination strategies for the specific situation at country level (Donadel et al. 2021) (Fig. 3).

5 Regulatory Communications and Stakeholder Exchange

All these aspects highlight the importance of early engagement of the product manufacturer with regulatory agencies to mutually agree on the data needed regarding product quality, nonclinical safety, and proof-of-concept studies, as well as clinical studies to determine the optimal dose and dose regimen and to demonstrate the safety and effectiveness of the product. Regulatory agencies from countries where the initial clinical studies will be conducted are likely to be more engaged in early product development discussions with developers. However, it is important to expand such interactions to a broader set of regulators to assure that there is consensus from the global regulatory community on the type of testing and clinical studies required to support licensure of products. In particular, regulators from regions where an emerging pathogen is likely to cause disease outbreaks, e.g., Lassa fever in Western Africa, should be consulted and made aware early of the development plans. As examples of international collaborations between regulators, U.S. FDA, EMA, and other regulators regularly discuss topics related to vaccines and antibacterial or antiviral agents, including advice to developers on countermeasures against emergent pathogens. WHO has also played a significant role in hosting discussion among regulators from different parts of the world and connecting them with established regional clusters of regulators, such as the African Vaccine Regulatory Forum (AVAREF).

During the COVID-19 pandemic, the role of the International Coalition of Medicines Regulatory Authorities (ICMRA) has been growing as a forum where alignment among regulators from different parts of the world can be reached on the requirements for advancing vaccines and therapeutics for tackling the pandemic. Workshops have been hosted by ICMRA to discuss vaccines development for COVID-19, from requirements for early clinical studies to design of late-stage clinical trials. In addition, regulators from around the world discussed the global regulatory response to the emergence of SARS-COV2 variants, especially Omicron. As an example, a meeting was convened at the time of Omicron spread to review available evidence for the effectiveness of the approved COVID-19 vaccines against the Omicron variant and reach alignment on the key regulatory requirements to support development of a possible adapted vaccine. Participants from the 24 members and 13 associated members and experts from WHO agreed that clinical data are needed for approving an updated vaccine and that different strategies should be considered in terms of vaccine composition. The decision to switch manufacturing to a different strain should ideally be reached at a global level and should not only be a regulatory decision, even if regulators are in the front line discussing their proposals with developers. These workshops underline the power of ICMRA's leadership in achieving alignment between regulators to expedite and streamline global development and authorization of new or modified COVID-19 vaccines against emerging coronavirus variants.

It is important to ensure optimum coordination and communication on the role of regulators in medicines approval and safety monitoring, in complement to the role of public health authorities and national committees on immunization (NITAGs). NITAGs determine the vaccination strategy at national level, as this can become especially challenging during a major crisis with high media interest in spotting and pointing out differences in the decisions made by public health decision makers in different countries. Risk communication and transparency on emerging issues during a crisis implies communicating uncertainty, highlighting the preliminary nature of interim results, and conveying the need to further collect and analyze data. This is not easy to convey, and it is further complicated because preliminary findings resonate in social media after making it into headlines. Furthermore, prompt and timely communication outside the timelines for standard regulatory procedures must sometimes be considered, as, for example, was done by EMA in the EU for ivermectin.

The rapid emergence of COVID-19 confronted health authorities, the healthcare community, and policy makers with the pressing need for an agile system to support development of in vitro diagnostics to test for the presence of the causative agent or the body's immune response to the pathogen. A more structured discussion among regulators on performance of in vitro diagnostics has emerged as an often-neglected area that would require a more coherent global discussion.

In addition to having products advance to later stage clinical development ahead of an epidemic or pandemic, approaches for granting approval even without efficacy data which could only be gathered during an epidemic have been proposed in order to facilitate early use of the product. As such an approach presents several scientific challenges, robust interaction between the scientific community, regulators, and public health authorities from different regions will be essential to define the best ways to advance regulatory science for better preparedness and response.

Box 1: International Coalition of Medicines Regulatory Authorities (ICMRA)

The mission of ICMRA is to safeguard public health by facilitating strategic leadership and greater cooperation among international medicines authorities on shared regulatory issues and challenges (Fig. 4).

Main objectives. ICMRA promotes international cooperation among medicines regulatory authorities to strengthen global dialogue, facilitate the wider exchange of reliable and comparable information, encourage greater leveraging of resources and joint work between authorities, and advocate for better informed, risk-based allocation of authorities' resources and deeper collaboration among them. The group also addresses current and emerging human medicine regulatory and safety challenges. These efforts aim to strengthen the quality, safety, and efficacy of medicinal products globally.

Main working areas. There are currently several ICMRA projects on antimicrobial resistance, communications, drug shortages, innovation, pharmacovigilance, public health response, and supply chain integrity.

COVID-19 response, emergency response. ICMRA members and WHO have closely collaborated to address the public health needs posed by the COVID-19 pandemic, looking for alignment and convergence on regulatory and scientific aspects during early stages of therapeutic and vaccine development, including clinical trials and requirements to support approvals. ICMRA provided an agile platform for rapid sharing and follow-up on safety and efficacy of vaccines and therapeutics by:

- Working to prioritize well-designed clinical trials that will provide robust and reliable results.
- Ensuring that there are meaningful and scientifically sound endpoints and safety data of sufficient duration in clinical trials.
- Sharing data between regulators in real time to facilitate multi-country approvals.
- Putting in place processes and policies utilizing the principles of regulatory agility by ICMRA members and WHO member states, providing an agile and rapid response to the global emergency.

Cooperation during the pandemic followed earlier guidance by ICMRA on standard operating procedures for regulatory cooperation during global health crises, the first systematic effort of its kind (ICMRA 2019; WHO-ICMRA 2020).

Membership and governance. ICMRA brings together 38 regulatory authorities representing all global regions, as well as WHO as a Standing Observer. ICMRA strategy recommendations and initiatives are adopted and supported by the wider membership, with an Executive Committee responsible for the overall direction and governance issues.

More information. ▶ https://www.icmra.info/drupal/

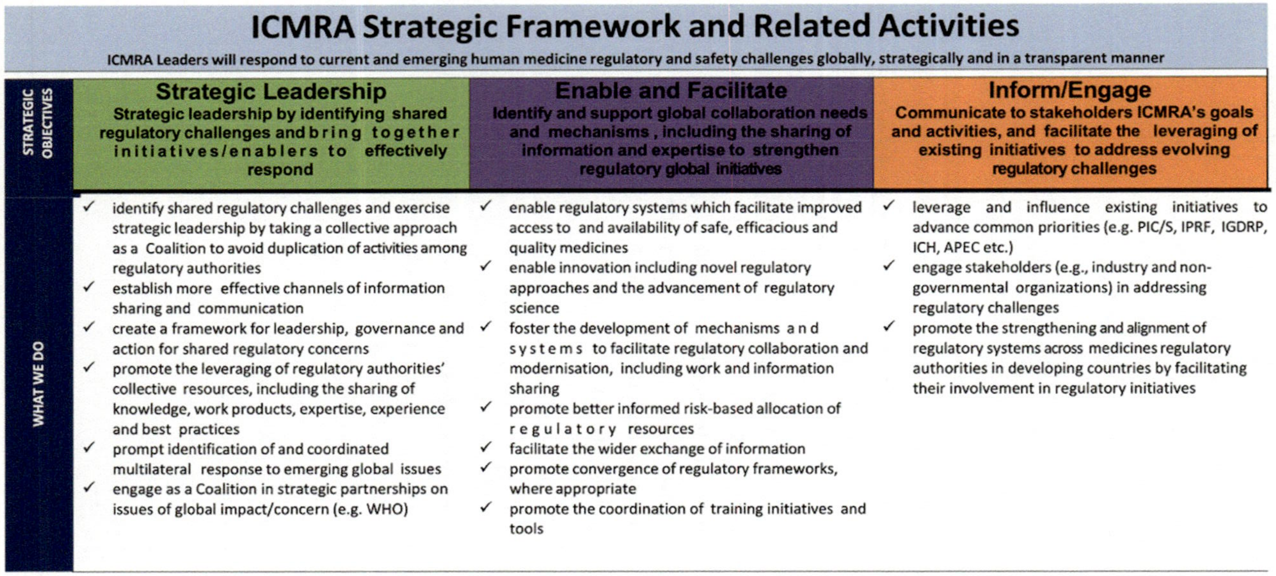

Fig. 4 ICMRA Strategic Framework

5.1 Additional Considerations on Chemistry, Manufacturing, and Controls

Beyond the conduct of preclinical and clinical studies, manufacturing scale up is a crucial area that requires intense dialogue with regulators from early in product development. Fine tuning and validation of the production process as it scales up through trial phases and into quantities needed for commercial release for consistent, high quality medicinal products is integral to meeting regulatory requirements. Early, frequent engagement, including confirmation of site readiness, is critical for rapid approvals of medicinal products, especially complex biologics like vaccines. As seen during the COVID-19 pandemic, in some cases, the CMC package, manufacturing readiness, and supply chain management dramatically lagged behind clinical development (Aars et al. 2021). In a pandemic, however, where positive interim clinical trial read-outs facilitate early approval, immature CMC packages or late supply chain planning can delay approval and supply, respectively (LaFraniere et al. 2021).

Even with promising clinical data, a certain threshold of CMC data and manufacturing readiness is required to commence review. Administrative issues, such as inaccurately translated and incorrectly structured documents, increased the review time during COVID. For life-cycle management, regular interactions facilitate streamlined, timely approvals of post-approval changes, reducing bottlenecks of this kind. The authorized COVID-19 vaccines benefited from existing CMC flexibilities to facilitate the risk-benefit evaluation, since the incomplete data package regarding risks could be supplemented with development data for similar products with a plan to file any remaining data post-approval.

For the approved COVID-19 vaccines, major objections raised during review included comparability of the commercial product to that used in clinical trials, validation of the commercial manufacturing process to demonstrate product reproducibility, and product stability data (Wagner et al. 2021). Product-specific flexibilities have been tailored to the situation: For example, experienced developers could leverage prior knowledge from similar production platforms or manufacturing experience from clinical/pilot manufacturing site(s) where commercial process validation was incomplete. Regulators regard good product understanding when demonstrated through characterization data and appropriate analytical technology as a prerequisite to a flexible process validation approach; product quality can then be reliably monitored as part of routine batch release specifications.

A host of other issues are under discussion:

- Substantial site investment by companies is done "at risk" in the pandemic, even before knowing the results of key clinical trials. This investment by companies, including third-party production sites, is critical to facilitating rapid authorization and ensuring sufficient, timely post-authorization manufacturing capacity and resilience.
- Good manufacturing practice (GMP) describes the production standard for medicines and ensures their consistent high quality. It applies both to commercial production of COVID-19 vaccines and generation of key site-specific data before vaccine authorization. Inspections to verify compliance with these standards are normally conducted (ICH 2022).
- During a pandemic, as seen with COVID-19, travel restrictions can mean that virtual inspections, extensive interactions, and reliance on inspections by trusted international partners often replaced on-site inspections by each licensing body. The validity of existing GMP certificates was also extended. Although a risk-based approach was used to permit virtual inspections, sometimes on-site inspections are still required, as with new sites and activities, where major issues highlighted justifying the early engagement on GMP to facilitate this. During the COVID-19 pandemic, however, the successful conduct of required inspections in certain places has proven to be a major bottleneck for advancing the review of biological products,

including vaccines. This has caused tangible delays in approval and demonstrated that manufacturing options and a careful choice of production facilities need to be considered as early as possible to minimize potential hurdles for GMP certification.

- Experience has demonstrated that commercial production sites and supplies of many raw materials—those for both biologics production and for packaging and distribution—are initially insufficient to satisfy the exceptional demand for vaccine in a pandemic situation. Therefore, a well-mapped plan for scale-up of production and QC testing should be formulated before initial submissions to regulators. Advance planning to prevent such delays should also be part of pandemic preparedness.

A plan allows prioritization of critical post-approval changes, understanding the need for inspection, and helps to avoid regulatory review bottlenecks. To streamline and accelerate changes further, applicants can make use of post-approval change management protocols, most optimally included in the initial marketing authorization application dossier. This way conditions and criteria for introduction of certain types of future changes can be predefined.

Timely consideration of data requirements for improvements to storage and transport conditions, packaging, formulation, and dosing can facilitate early approval.

Differing regional CMC requirements have challenged global COVID-19 vaccine development and supply. Regulatory requirements are governed by varying legal frameworks. However, opportunities for greater international collaboration including mutual reliance (for example, on determination that GMP requirements have been met) and initiatives for collaborative reviews are being explored, particularly within the context of the ICMRA, which also supports interactions between regulators and industry to further understand and exchange COVID-19 lessons learned, with the aim of continuing to ensure uninterrupted supply of medicinal products to patients. In the meantime, ad hoc interactions between regions on CMC are beneficial. Companies are encouraged to share advice received from other regions with regulators so that differences can be resolved jointly.

6 Concluding Remarks

The serious impact of public health emergencies on human life in the absence of effective therapies warrants moving forward with preclinical and clinical development and testing in the most expedited manner. Advances in manufacturing and technologies as well as clinical trial design create new opportunities for faster access to life-saving products. Of critical importance is an efficient, scientifically sound regulatory evaluation of investigational therapies during public health emergencies. Experience gained during the Ebola outbreak in West Africa and the global COVID-19 pandemic indicate that the usual phased product development approach can be accelerated by leveraging quality and preclinical data derived from studies conducted on interventions produced with the same technologies, novel clinical trial designs, and careful risk/benefit considerations that take into consideration the severity of the disease. In such emergency settings, it may be appropriate to accept greater-than-usual degrees of uncertainty and risk in order to move rapidly to clinical trials, with the goal of getting safe and effective therapies to patients sooner (Singh 2020).

To ensure that studies will meet licensure requirements, including requirements for ethical conduct, close collaboration between public health authorities, national regulatory authorities, the community, clinical investigators, and the developers is essential.

It is critical that developers and sponsors of studies with investigational agents not only engage early in development with regulators to reach agreement on the development and licensure pathway but also to continue regular interactions with regulatory agencies.

Indeed, the importance of proactive discussions with regulators has often been undervalued, even though it is of critical importance to assure the successful advancement and availability of therapies, diagnostics, and vaccines. Regulators understand the impact of their decisions and, based on the experience gained throughout a number of emergencies, continuously reflect on how to improve their efficiency and effectiveness in responding to the public health needs. In addition, the regulator's ability to successfully interact with other stakeholders, beyond the established interface with manufacturers, has proven to be paramount for achieving tangible progress in the containment of the crisis. Moreover, the nature of the emerging threats, i.e., a global pandemic or an initially localized outbreak, requires that regulators from different geographical regions come together and share views so as to strengthen the regulatory response and avoid divergent or inconsistent sets of requirements that would slow down the development and ultimately the access to these countermeasures.

Overall, each public health crisis will be different in some or many aspects and a flexible approach toward response and ways of studying the impact of medical interventions will be required. This calls for a coordinated discussion of lessons learned from the recent epidemic and pandemic to inform how clinical practice, research and development activities, clinical trials, and observational research can be rapidly and effectively implemented in any future epidemic.

? Discussion Questions

Short Questions

1. What are some of the responsibilities of regulatory agencies in research responses to emerging and re-emerging infectious diseases?
2. What issues have hindered the timely generation of safety and efficacy data adequate to meet regulatory requirements?
3. How have study designs been adapted to meet the challenges of an abbreviated timeline during a public health emergency?
4. How can information derived from preclinical studies on similar products based on the same platform be used to support the safe and effective use of a medicinal product in an emergency?
5. What special populations need to be considered when designing clinical studies for experimental medicinal products in an emergency?

Long Questions

1. Discuss actions that can be taken in advance of a pandemic to better prepare for response to novel and re-emerging pathogens with pandemic potential.
2. What are some of the challenges of balancing the need to produce reliable evidence expeditiously and meeting regulatory standards for safe conduct of trials and robust safety assessment of medical interventions?
3. Discuss the roles of ethics committees and (principal) investigators implementing trials in upholding clinical trial standards.
4. Describe some practical issues encountered for chemistry, manufacturing, and controls (CMC) by stakeholders producing medicines for pandemics.
5. What are some key lessons of recent epidemics and pandemics for regulators?

References

Aars OK, Clark M, Schwalbe N. Increasing efficiency in vaccine production: a primer for change. Vaccine X. 2021;8:100104. https://doi.org/10.1016/j.jvacx.2021.100104.

Brueckner M, Titman A, Jaki T, Rojek A, Horby P. Performance of different clinical trial designs to evaluate treatments during an epidemic. PLoS One. 2018;13(9):e0203387. https://doi.org/10.1371/journal.pone.0203387.

Cavaleri M, Thomson A, Salmonson T, Hemmings RJ. A viewpoint on European Medicines Agency experience with investigational medicinal products for Ebola. Clin Trials (London, England). 2016;13(1):101–4. https://doi.org/10.1177/1740774515619860.

Donadel M, Panero MS, Ametewee L, Shefer AM. National decision-making for the introduction of new vaccines: a systematic review, 2010–2020. Vaccine. 2021;39(14):1897–909. https://doi.org/10.1016/j.vaccine.2021.02.059.

EC. Good manufacturing practice: medicinal products for human and veterinary use. Annex 11: computerised systems, SANCO/C8/AM/sl/ares(2010)1064599. 2011.

Eichler HG, Cavaleri M, Enzmann H, Scotti F, Sepodes B, Sweeney F, Vamvakas S, Rasi G. Clinical Trials for COVID-19: can we better use the short window of opportunity? Clin Pharmacol Ther. 2020;108(4):730–3. https://doi.org/10.1002/cpt.1891. Epub 2020 Jun 12. PMID: 32407539; PMCID: PMC7272975.

EMA. COVID-19 vaccines: development, evaluation, approval and monitoring. Brussels: European

Medicines Agency; 2022. https://www.ema.europa.eu/en/human-regulatory/overview/public-health-threats/coronavirus-disease-covid-19/treatments-vaccines/vaccines-covid-19/covid-19-vaccines-development-evaluation-approval-monitoring. Accessed 7 Feb 2022.

FDA. Animal rule information. Silver Spring, MD: U.S. Food and Drug Administratrion; 2021. https://www.fda.gov/emergency-preparedness-and-response/mcm-regulatory-science/animal-rule-information. Accessed 20 Feb 2022.

Graham BS, Corbett KS. Prototype pathogen approach for pandemic preparedness: world on fire. J Clin Invest. 2020;130(7):3348–9. https://doi.org/10.1172/JCI139601.

Greinacher A, Thiele T, Warkentin TE, Weisser K, Kyrle PA, Eichinger S. Thrombotic thrombocytopenia after ChAdOx1 nCov-19 vaccination. N Engl J Med. 2021;384(22):2092–101. https://doi.org/10.1056/NEJMoa2104840.

Henao-Restrepo AM, Camacho A, Longini IM, Watson CH, Edmunds WJ, Egger M, et al. Efficacy and effectiveness of an rVSV-vectored vaccine in preventing Ebola virus disease: final results from the Guinea ring vaccination, open-label, cluster-randomised trial (Ebola Ca Suffit!). Lancet. 2017;389(10068):505–18. https://doi.org/10.1016/S0140-6736(16)32621-6.

Higgs ES, Dubey SA, Coller BAG, Simon JK, Bollinger L, Sorenson RA, et al. Accelerating vaccine development during the 2013–2016 West African Ebola virus disease outbreak. Curr Top Microbiol Immunol. 2017;411:229–61. https://doi.org/10.1007/82_2017_53.

Hilleman MR, Buynak EB, Weibel RE, Stokes J. Live, attenuated mumps-virus vaccine. N Engl J Med. 1968;278(5):227–32. https://doi.org/10.1056/NEJM196802012780501.

ICH. Quality guidelines. Geneva: International Council for Harmonisation; 2022. https://www.ich.org/page/quality-guidelines. Accessed 22 Feb 2022.

ICMRA. Framework for the involvement of health regulatory authorities in the management of global health crises. London: International Coalition of Medicines Regulatory Authorities; 2019.

Janse M, Brouwers T, Claassen E, Hermans P, van de Burgwal L. Barriers influencing vaccine development timelines, identification, causal analysis, and prioritization of key barriers by KOLs in general and Covid-19 vaccine R&D. Front Public Health. 2021;9:612541. https://doi.org/10.3389/fpubh.2021.612541.

Kennedy SB, Bolay F, Kieh M, Grandits G, Badio M, Ballou R, et al. Phase 2 placebo-controlled trial of two vaccines to prevent Ebola in Liberia. N Engl J Med. 2017;377(15):1438–47. https://doi.org/10.1056/NEJMoa1614067.

LaFraniere S, Weiland N, Gay Stolberg S. The F.D.A. tells Johnson & Johnson that about 60 million doses made at a troubled plant cannot be used. New York Times. 2021.

Moon S, Sridhar D, Pate MA, Jha AK, Clinton C, Delaunay S, et al. Will Ebola change the game? Ten essential reforms before the next pandemic. The report of the Harvard-LSHTM Independent Panel on the Global Response to Ebola. Lancet. 2015;386(10009):2204–21.

RECOVERY Collaborative Group. Tocilizumab in patients admitted to hospital with COVID-19 (RECOVERY): a randomised, controlled, open-label, platform trial. Lancet. 2021;397(10285):1637–45. https://doi.org/10.1016/s0140-6736(21)00676-0.

Singh JA. COVID-19 vaccine trials: duty of care and standard of prevention considerations. Vaccine. 2020;38(48):7578–80. https://doi.org/10.1016/j.vaccine.2020.10.012.

Wagner R, Hildt E, Grabski E, Sun Y, Meyer H, Lommel A, et al. Accelerated development of COVID-19 vaccines: technology platforms, benefits, and associated risks. Vaccines (Basel). 2021;9(7):747. https://doi.org/10.3390/vaccines9070747.

Wang S, Li L, Yan F, Gao Y, Yang S, Xia X. COVID-19 animal models and vaccines: current landscape and future prospects. Vaccines (Basel). 2021;9(10):1082. https://doi.org/10.3390/vaccines9101082.

WHO. WHO guidelines on nonclinical evaluation of vaccines. Geneva: World Health Organization; 2005.

WHO-ICMRA. WHO-ICMRA joint statement on the need for improved global regulatory alignment on COVID-19 medicines and vaccines. Geneva: World Health Organization; 2020.

7 Research, Sample, and Data Sharing During Outbreaks, Pandemics, and Beyond

Robert Fraser Terry and Katherine Littler

Contents

Learning Track Note: This chapter appears in Learning Tracks: Clinical Research; Health Policy, Multilateral Cooperation, International Governance; One Health

E. S. Higgs and R. A. Sorenson (eds.), *Principles and Practice of Emergency Research Response*, https://doi.org/10.1007/978-3-031-48408-7_9

Learning Objectives

This chapter will help readers understand and describe

- Principles, ethical issues, history, and current landscape of data sharing between scientists and nations during an EID emergency
- Search and analysis criteria for identifying a virus sequence in a database
- Why some researchers are reluctant to share high-volume data and the steps introduced by GISAID to address this
- Benefits of aggregating COVID-19 clinical data into a large, standardized data set, as ISARIC is doing
- Ethical and legal challenges of data sharing
- FAIR (findable, accessible, interoperable, and reusable) principles for data sharing
- Recommendations for coordinated data sharing during public health emergencies

1 Introduction

On March 14, 2000, the president of the United States and the prime minister of the United Kingdom made a joint statement to celebrate the release of the first draft of the human genome (White House 2000). They recognized the project as one of the most significant scientific achievements of all time and as the foundation for developing new measures to prevent, treat, and, in some cases, eliminate disease. They also applauded the decision of the scientists involved to share the raw, fundamental DNA sequence and its variants rapidly and unencumbered in the public domain (Human Genome Project information archive 1990–2003 2019). They commended the policy of open sharing as an example to other scientists to promote new discoveries and enhance the quality of life for all humankind.

The formal leaders' announcement recognized a set of principles that had been informally agreed between genomic scientists over the previous decade and set out in statements of intent that include the Bermuda Principles and Fort Lauderdale Agreement (Maxson Jones et al. 2018; Wellcome Trust 2003). These statements, which predate widespread discussions of open access to research publications, promote the concept that science is improved through the unencumbered sharing of research data and that greater efficiencies and benefits would be achieved if those data were shared in a timely, standardized manner. The Bermuda Principles also introduced the concept of "community resources," whereby a tripartite of research producers, research users, and research funders agree to produce open and accessible research resources that benefit science (Wellcome Trust 2003).

In subsequent decades, similar principles of open access to research publications and open access to the data that underly those publications have been developed, adopted, and promoted as representing good research practice. Many research funding agencies and journal editors have supported these concepts by formalizing them as requirements into their funding agreements and submission processes.

In a parallel development, as many other types of health data, not just those collected under a research protocol, became digitized in one form or another, the aggregation and sharing of those data rapidly and at marginal cost became a reality. Such data access and analysis have created a wide range of potential benefits. For example, electronic health records have enabled greater integration across different levels of a healthcare system, improving clinical care and facilitating more pragmatic advances, such as administration of invoicing to cover care costs (Kruse et al. 2018).

This rich seam of digital health data from care provision and research is seen as a valuable public health asset and a public good. These data often have commercial value, and countries consider them natural resources, contributing to their sovereign wealth. Those spending time and resources curating and analyzing data want recognition and rewards for their efforts; others raise concerns over data misuse and intrusion on privacy. A whole industry has grown up to develop software and standards to support the development of data management—there are more than 900 standards in the life sciences alone. This growth in data as a commodity plays out against a backdrop of global inequity, where richer countries have a greater capacity to set the research agenda, analyze, and exploit data. Poorer countries with limited resources and lower research capacity often object to what seems to be a one-way flow in which they are excluded from the benefits of that analysis (i.e., they are not invited to collaborate on the research or as co-authors of resulting publications). In addition, lower-income countries see themselves excluded from the very health products, such as vaccines, which may have been developed with data derived in part from their own populations.

Thus, the environment within which data sharing now operates must contend with conflicting political, legal, commercial, ethical, and technical interests. What some consider favorable for academic progress, others may see as exploitation for the benefit of populations in high-income countries. To ensure public health benefits are fully realized, progress toward a more equitable and efficient system of health data usage, reuse, and analysis will require active engagement and negotiation with all parties. However, the challenge of reaching such a global agreement highlights the absence of strong international mechanisms to create global goods with health data. While there are numerous calls from within the UN and international funding bodies for researchers and countries to "do the right thing," improving the health data system will require systems thinking (UNESCO 2021; Wellome Trust 2020; WHO 2022e).

2 The Impact of Pandemic Diseases on Health Data Sharing

So, a question arises as to whether a global threat, such as the COVID-19 pandemic that emerged in December 2019, was a strong enough incentive to overcome these national and localized interests that inhibit efficient sharing of data. Did we see changes in cooperative behavior that might unlock the current impasse? Are there examples of good practice that need to be identified and built on as we go forward?

The simple answer is that the COVID-19 pandemic has highlighted both good and poor practices. There were improvements in some areas, such as greater access to published literature through the temporary removal of subscription paywalls, even as further evidence of yawning global inequities became evident, for example, in unequal access to the health products enabled through the sharing of health data. Dr. Tedros Adhanom Ghebreyesus, the Director General of the World Health Organization (WHO), described the unequal distribution of vaccines as putting the world on the brink of a moral catastrophe (WHO 2021).

3 The Utility of Viral Sequences

With respect to data sharing, perhaps the highest-profile success in the COVID-19 pandemic has been the rapid sharing of viral sequences. The practice of sharing raw sequence data established under the Human Genome Project enabled the relatively swift attribution of the new respiratory disease that emerged from Wuhan, China, in December 2019 to a coronavirus, provisionally named 2019 nCov. Early publication of the virus genome sequence enabled the U.S. National Institutes of Allergy and Infectious Diseases (NIAID) and the German biotechnology firm BioNTech to create messenger RNA (mRNA) vaccine candidates very quickly. The achievement was based on years of research on coronaviruses, including the severe acute respiratory syndrome coronavirus 1 (SARS-CoV-1), and separate research on adapting mRNA for use in vaccines. Other vaccine candidates produced through other methods also benefited from the rapid publication of the genome. Yet it is easy to imagine scenarios in which a virus genome is not rapidly shared. The place where it emerges may not have the capacity to identify and sequence a new virus, or political leadership may decide, for any of a number of reasons, not to share the sequence, perhaps not even to admit to the presence of an outbreak or novel pathogen.

Even as preclinical and clinical work on the new vaccine candidates was beginning, by early March 2020, the new virus had been placed in the species *severe acute respiratory syndrome-related coronavirus* by taxonomists. This is the same species as severe acute respiratory syndrome coronavirus (SARS-CoV, now called SARS-CoV-1), which caused an outbreak in 2003. The 2019 nCoV virus was named SARS-CoV-2 accordingly, while the disease and pandemic caused by the new virus were subsequently called coronavirus disease 2019, or COVID-19 (Coronaviridae Study Group of the International Committee on Taxonomy of Viruses 2020).

The process of identifying a virus from its sequence requires many elements to be in place to search across hundreds of different databases. A special search function, the Basic Local Alignment Search Tool (BLAST) and related software, finds regions of similarity between biological sequences and analyzes and calculates the statistical match of a new sequence of nucleotides or protein sequences against a library of sequences stored in a wide range of databases (NIH 2022a). These databases contain sequences collected and isolated from various sources, including animal vectors (e.g., bats, mosquitoes), human subjects receiving care or participating in clinical trials, and other sources such as food, wastewater, or the environment (Alföldi and Lindblad-Toh 2013). The numerical scale of such searching and matching is vast: SARS-CoV-2 has approximately 30,000 base pairs, while a typical mammalian genome has 3 billion base pairs, making cross-species comparisons extremely complex (Albery et al. 2021). For example, the International Nucleotide Sequence Database Collaboration (INSDC) was estimated in 2018 to contain quadrillions ($>10^{15}$) of nucleotides from over 300,000 organisms and to double about every 18 months (INSDC 2021). The National Center for Biological Information (NCBI) alone had over 6,000,000 nucleotide records on SARS-CoV-2 by August 2022 (NIH 2022b).

That a BLAST search can find matches for a virus needle in such an enormous haystack within seconds illustrates the power and efficiency enabled by data sharing when it is done well. Many elements must be in place to make such a system operate, including rich metadata and a summary record that describes the data set that can be read by a computer using a specialized search engine tool via the Internet. Access to the data set must be unrestricted, and the data must be formatted against a set of standards that enables comparison and subsequent identification as a known virus, a variant, or a new virus. Anything that reduces findability, accessibility, interoperability, or reuse reduces the value or utility of the resource and the subsequent analysis and benefit it can generate. These technical requirements form the basis of the FAIR (findable, accessible, interoperable, and reusable) principles (◘ Fig. 1), which are now considered the baseline for creating useful data-sharing initiatives (Wilkinson et al. 2016). The need for holistic or systems-based approaches to develop effective data-sharing mechanisms seems clear.

FAIR Guiding Principles for sharing and reuse of health-related data for research

Findable:
F1 (meta)data are assigned a globally unique and persistent identifier F2 data are described with rich metadata (defined by R1 below)
F3 metadata clearly and explicitly include the identifier to the data it describes F4 (meta)data are registered or indexed in a searchable resource.
Accessible:
A1.0 (meta)data are retrievable by their identifier using a standardized communications protocol A1.1 the protocol is open, free and universally implementable
A1.2 the protocol allows for an authentication and authorization procedure, where necessary A2.0 metadata are accessible, even when the data are no longer available.
Interoperable:
I1 (meta)data use a formal, accessible, shared, and broadly applicable language for knowledge representation
I2 (meta)data use vocabularies that follow FAIR principles
I3 (meta)data include qualified references to other (meta)data.
Reusable:
R1.0 (meta)data are richly described with a plurality of accurate and relevant attributes R1.1 (meta)data are released with a clear and accessible data usage license
R1.2 (meta)data are associated with detailed provenance
R1.3 (meta)data meet domain-relevant community standards.

Fig. 1 The FAIR guiding principles. (Wilkinson et al. 2016)

4 Sharing Data

In using large data sets, the game changer has been Internet-enabled digital access and the computer algorithms that interrogate the data. The more automatic and open the process is, the greater the efficiency. Openness of access and reuse means data can be compared across multiple sites. Such a system builds in community-based quality assurance through the comparison of data with other data sets in other databases. Any process steps that reduce this flow, such as manual registration to access the data, review of access requests by committee, or requirements to seek agreement for each reuse by the data originator, reduce the efficiency of the process and the utility of the data. Essentially, the greater the ongoing human input required in the workflow, the less effective the process becomes.

However, this minimalist approach, while working well for sharing raw sequence data, is not universally scalable to all forms of health data. As data become more complex and include associated personal identifiers, such as medical records, sharing mechanisms must include governance arrangements that manage the related ethical and legal requirements to protect the rights and privacy of individuals. These arrangements must be coupled with positive political will and research culture to share those data and must exclude commercial interests that wish to protect the intellectual property within those data.

Experience shows that another major barrier to high-volume data sharing is the reluctance of the researchers themselves. Although data sharing is required by several research funders in their terms and conditions for grants, researchers often do not feel they are sufficiently benefitted by sharing the data. They have to spend time and funds cleaning the data and preparing it for sharing, and may be skeptical about whether the utility of the shared data for secondary analysis matches the effort required to prepare the data for sharing (i.e., the value of the secondary analysis is low). Researchers also fear that others might find errors in their data or undertake a secondary analysis that is better than the original work or, worse, contradicts the original findings.

This reluctance to share may be felt most keenly by researchers in low- and middle-income countries with lower infrastructure capacity for data management and analysis. They may have previous experience with getting what they believe is insufficient attention and credit for their research. High-capacity research teams in the Global North can absorb and analyze data from the South, leaving researchers in low- and middle-income countries feeling more like data exporters than partners in data sharing (Hate et al. 2015).

A similar picture emerges at the national level. An example of this sort of inequity was highlighted by the government of Indonesia in 2007, which felt that while it supplied data on the influenza virus H5N1 to researchers in WHO Collaborating Centers, the resulting commercial vaccines would not be available in developing countries (WHO 2007).

For data sharing during pandemics caused by influenza, Ebola, and COVID-19, the debate on openness has surfaced several times with researchers calling for a greater degree of openness in data sharing (Van Noorden 2021; Yozwiak et al. 2015).

4.1 Mechanisms for Sharing Data

One approach to address the lack of attribution and benefit sharing was developed by the Global Initiative on Sharing All Influenza Data (GISAID) launched at the World Health Assembly in 2006 (GISAID 2022). GISAID introduced several steps in both depositing and using genome sequences on its site, including (1) a registration step so that users could be identified as bona fide researchers and (2) a data access agreement (DAA) that requires use of a specific format to acknowledge data depositors in citations with a unique identifier or accession number. GISAID began with a focus on influenza, adapted its system to include COVID-19, and in November 2021 had over 5.1 million genome sequence submissions. During the COVID-19 pandemic, the GISAID resource became one of the most reliable resources for tracking the spread of COVID-19 and all its variants (Maxmen 2021). Many researchers and their governments point to the terms of the DAA as providing reassurance on control of their data when sharing on this platform (Wilkinson et al. 2016).

But GISAID's efforts to address benefit sharing through a requirement for attribution and collaboration have received criticism for reducing data openness and the ability to provide quality assurance by comparing the underlying raw sequence with other databases (Heard et al. 2022). So, in achieving one target to serve pressing public health objectives through viral monitoring, other research benefits through openly sharing data without restrictions have been reduced. In time, a comprehensive review will be needed to understand the full impact of these trade-offs and the true value of the differences in the governance arrangements for these genomic resources. For example, a meta-analysis across all the SARS-Cov-2 records in GISAID as of January 2021 indicates that the data may suffer from geographical and gender bias and poor quality of the data entered where manual entry is relied upon. The article was later retracted because it was found to violate GISAID terms of usage, another barrier to openness (Zelenova et al. 2021, 2022).

Such reduced interoperability and reuse would present a problem even within a discipline or a single domain but is seen more acutely when a multidisciplinary response is essential. In health, particularly when understanding a new and emerging disease, the value of integration is being able to make associations between the basic sequence information of a new pathogen, identification of isolates from different hosts and vectors, and the trajectory and etiology of the disease as it infects humans. This interconnectivity is demonstrated by the COVID-19 Data Portal (◘ Fig. 2) (COVID-19 data portal 2022).

Recording the pathology of a disease in patients increases the complexity and volume of the data collected by adding the physiological, biochemical, and imaging measures included in case reports, patient records, diagnostic and clinical procedures, and research protocols if applicable. The use of data linked to an identifiable person enormously complicates the need to protect patient privacy in accordance with ethical and legal frameworks, complexities further multiplied because data from different countries will

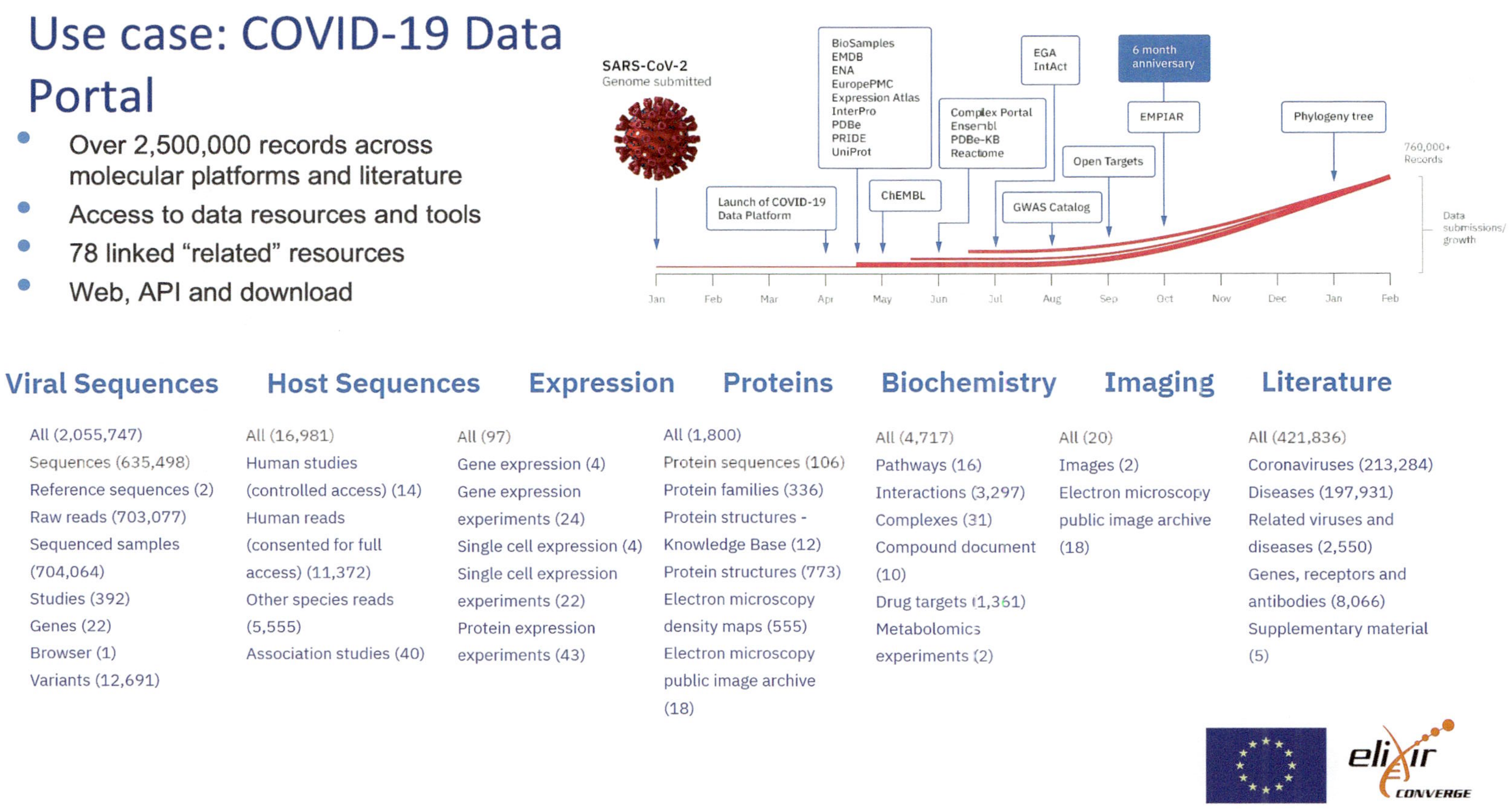

Fig. 2 Many of the applications of COVID-19 genetic data, as shown on the COVID-19 Data Portal page. (Credit: COVID-19 Data Portal [2021] and ELIXIR-CONVERGE [Horizon 2020 Project 871075])

Sharing mechanism	Research becomes transparent	Potential health benefit	Cost and sustainability
Accessible: online repository	Yes	Uncertain	Low cost, relatively easy to maintain.
Useable: repository with discoverable, well documented metadata	Yes	Possible with extensive user effort	Moderate cost, relatively easy to maintain
Useful: data are curated, standardized, and comparable across time and place; managed access	Sometimes	Great	Expensive, long-term investments needed.

Fig. 3 Benefits and costs of different levels of data sharing. (Pisani et al. 2016)

need to meet differing requirements—even without considering the format of the data submitted (Fig. 3).

Data platforms that address ethical obstacles to sharing individual patient data (IPD) have been established. For data collected on the Ebola outbreak in 2016, a platform to share resources from Guinea, Liberia, and Sierra Leone was established at the Oxford University-based Infectious Diseases Data Observatory (IDDO) (2023). Developing this resource required extensive work to create a governance mechanism through a data access committee overseen by a steering committee. Standing ethical approval was obtained from the three countries contributing data which included a number of records provided by Médecins Sans Frontières. Following public consultation, a research agenda was developed to describe the general areas of research these data could be used for and a set of standard operating procedures to manage access and create data transfer agreements. The data required extensive curation. By mid-2022, seven applications for secondary analysis had been approved, all of which included researchers from Ebola endemic countries as a condition of access. More applications are anticipated, but the platform has exhausted its initial funding. Access to the resource is free, but clearly sustainability of such resources, which require funding for governance, cannot be guaranteed with a grant-based approach to funding.

For COVID-19, the International Severe Acute Respiratory and Emerging Infection Consortium (ISARIC), also based in Oxford and in partnership with IDDO, established the COVID-19 Clinical Database for individual patient (or participant) data (IPD) of hospitalized cases (or clinical trial volunteers). This resource quickly grew to include close to 700,000 individual records from nearly 800 sites in 66 countries, of which half include records from low- and middle-income countries (ISARIC 2022). By the end of 2021, more than 50 studies had been published while others were pending. The aggregation of these data into such a large standardized data set has enabled statistically powerful research to identify different case definitions linked to age and sex, links with comorbidity, and regular reporting of clinical findings across the whole data set, which have been rapidly disseminated on the medRxiv preprint server (Baillie et al. 2022).

4.2 Rapidity vs. Equity?

A key feature of the dialogue on data and sample sharing, both in global health research and public health emergencies, is the ethical duty to share data as rapidly as possible (Modjarrad et al. 2016). In essence, the data informing the response to an outbreak becomes a global public good (Pisani et al. 2018). However, experiences from the 2014–2016 West African Ebola outbreak and the 2015–2016 Zika outbreaks have revealed that the global public good argument alone is not enough to ensure effective data sharing. Relevant policy instruments are also needed, including the further development of principles and global norms and the need for a growing body of evidence to inform appropriate and inclusive governance arrangement for data sharing (Nuffield Council on Bioethics 2020).

In a pandemic, data informing outbreak response becomes a global public good.

Box 1: Key Messages from "Beyond Open Data: Realizing the Health Benefits of Sharing Data" (Pisani et al. 2016)

- Simple accessibility of data is enough to promote research transparency, but public health gains require more complex models.
- Meaningful and equitable collaboration with local researchers and policymakers in low- and middle-income countries is needed to ensure the right research questions get asked and research results are used.
- Useful data sharing requires long-term investment in infrastructure, networks, and scientific careers, including in the data sciences.
- It is not enough to share data: we need to share governance structures, scientific questions and ideas, and interpretation.

Despite major policy advances and a growing focus on preparedness in recent years, including the ethical oversight of data sharing, significant ethical challenges remain, particularly in terms of equity (Moorthy et al. 2020; Saxena et al. 2019). As already mentioned, these include (1) continuing asymmetries between the capacities of low- and middle-income country and high-income country researchers, (2) continuing lack of credit or acknowledgment of data collectors and generators by secondary users of data, and (3) lack of benefits flowing back to communities and populations from which data was originally derived. Additionally, communities living near the origin of an outbreak may face stigmatization, compounding the need for systematic capacity development to address some of the larger inequalities (Pratt and Bull 2021).

There are still unresolved issues regarding broad consent models for data sharing and the need for additional components of the ethics and global infectious disease response ecosystem to support data-sharing policies and practices, including community engagement and the development of trustworthy relationships (Nuffield Council on Bioethics 2020). Recent analyses of data-sharing activities during epidemics and pandemics have also drawn attention to the fact that much of the ethical argument for sharing has focused on utility at the expense of other issues, particularly equity (Pratt and Bull 2021). Going forward, the scientific community must consider whether the current ethical focus of the debate is correct, and whether we are making the right ethical trade-offs in both the arguments about and the implementation of data-sharing policies and practices.

Another challenge is understanding whether and how specific populations are being excluded from the benefits of data sharing because they are not included in the original research studies or other methods of data collection and analysis, for example, pregnant and lactating women, disadvantaged populations, etc. (Pratt and Bull 2021). Such exclusions and bias could lead to the development of medical countermeasures (MCMs) that have not demonstrated their safety and efficacy in members of the excluded groups. Then the question arises whether or not members of those groups should use the MCMs in question, exacerbating preexisting inequalities. The exclusion of pregnant women from many COVID-19 vaccine trials is a case in point (Van Spall 2021). In fact, sharing data can enable an aggregation of enough participants from these excluded groups in a meta-analysis to bring them into research analysis.

4.3 Legal Frameworks

The variety of legal frameworks that operate at a national or regional level also has a significant impact on the practice of sharing health data. So, in many cases, is the lack of certainty about legal requirements. These are generally framed with the intention of protecting individual rights, such as privacy or intellectual property. As such, they tend to restrict and regulate, rather than enable greater sharing. But there are exceptions. One example is the European Union (EU) General Data Protection Regulation (GDPR), which applies to activities in EU member countries but also imposes restrictions on use of data generated in the EU anywhere in the world. However, the stated objective of GDPR includes enabling innovation as well as protecting privacy rights through the standardization of privacy laws across EU member states and special derogations that exempt use of data for research. This objective may allow research on a subject's data without consent and even for the transfer of those data to a third country without the need for additional terms and conditions (Article 6 EU GDPR "Lawfulness of processing" 2022). However, for many researchers, the interpretation of GDPR and the full implications of its implementation remain to be seen, and a version of the precautionary principle, "*Don't share; you might get caught by GDPR*" is still the primary concern (reference: EU workshop October 2021 awaiting report).

Global-level discussions have sought to determine whether an adaptation of the Nagoya protocol on access to genetic resources and the fair and equitable sharing of benefits arising from their utilization (Nagoya Protocol) to the Convention on Biological Diversity (CBD) might provide a legal basis to ensure the fair sharing of benefits that arise from the utilization of genetic resources, including pathogen samples and by extension genetic sequences.[1] This is seen as one possible solution to concerns raised by, for example, Indonesia with respect to influenza (see above), but the Protocol requires each member state to adopt its own legislative and regulatory framework to implement its provisions—something that remains a work in progress. At its World Health Assembly in May 2019, WHO member states agreed to explore this solution further (WHO 2022b). However, one challenge is that the CBD was never conceived as a rapid response mechanism to encourage data sharing. The CBD takes a considered approach on how the use of a genetic resource, which has contributed or may contribute to commercial benefits (e.g., a product and any resulting income) might be fairly distributed among the interested parties. The CBD and Nagoya Protocol reflect the stance that there is value in the genetic resource and that the sovereign owner, either a country or community, has rights over the utilization of that material. But deciding on who owns what and the value of scientific research and development (R&D) to realize a concrete benefit is not an easy or rapid process. The purpose of the Nagoya Protocol is to govern the sharing of benefits, not the rapid sharing of data—a purpose that runs counter to the concept of sharing health data as a public good with benefits to all. Some have expressed concern that even minor delays of weeks in deciding if a locally isolated influenza strain is covered by a national interpretation of the Nagoya Protocol could damage the long-standing global mechanism for selecting the flu strains required to manufacture up-to-date seasonal influenza vaccines (GISAID 2019). Concern about possible delays will grow as the ability to develop vaccines and therapies is further streamlined (Pandemic Preparedness Partnership 2021).

Certainly, much more work is needed to determine if the Nagoya Protocol can play an effective role. The need for a new pandemic treaty has been highlighted by WHO's Director General (WHO 2022f). Countries in southern Africa were among those making the strongest calls for an international agreement. Following the identification and rapid sharing by Botswana and South Africa of a new variant of COVID-19, Omicron, a number of other

1 The Nagoya Protocol itself does not specifically cover genetic sequences in the form of data, not surprisingly since at the time of drafting (2010) they had less utility than they do now.

countries imposed travel restrictions on them. While the information they shared had a short-term impact in slowing the spread of Omicron, the wider impact on the lives and economy of the region was severe and felt by many to be unjustified, since such rapid and punitive action provides a major disincentive to share such information (Mallapaty 2021).

In December 2021, a special session of the WHO World Health Assembly established an Intergovernmental Negotiating Body to draft and negotiate a WHO convention, agreement, or other international instrument on pandemic prevention, preparedness, and response (INB) (WHO 2022h); in July 2022, the INB determined it would pursue a legally binding international treaty (WHO 2022a). One element of these discussions was to establish a working group to explore the feasibility of adapting the International Health Regulations (WHO 2022d).

We conclude that to achieve optimal benefit from data sharing, a systems or holistic approach is needed to address all the political, ethical, social (e.g., research culture), technical (e.g., meeting FAIR principles), legal, and economic (e.g., funding data platforms) challenges. ◘ Table 1 summarizes how a selection of policy statements have tried to address these issues.

WHO has combined these principles into a framework for good practice in the sharing and reuse of health-related data for research. This framework combines the FAIR principles with an additional three, efficiency, ethics, and equity, which are defined as follows (GloPID-R 2018):

- *Efficient*. Any approach to data sharing should be aimed at enhancing/optimizing the quality and value of the use of those data and enabling their contribution to improving public health. Data sharing should be done as promptly and in as open a manner as possible, building on existing norms, policies, and practices and reducing unnecessary duplication and competition.
- *Ethical*. All data sharing should balance and protect the privacy of individuals and the dignity of communities while acknowledging the imperative to improve public health through the most productive use of data.
- *Equitable*. Any approach to the sharing of data should recognize and balance the needs of participants and researchers who generate and use data; other analysts who might want to reuse those data; and those communities who expect health benefits to arise from research.

Health Data Research UK undertook a comprehensive mapping of participant-level COVID-19 data-sharing platforms, registries, and meta-registries against these principles to understand how far COVID-19 data resources have been able to apply to them and whether the pandemic has provided an impetus for improvement (HDR UK 2022). The effort identified 47 registries and 21 platforms (from an examined total of 132) that collected, curated, and provided access to these data to varying degrees across all languages between May 2020 and June 2021.[2] These platforms and registries were then assessed using existing tools and algorithms to estimate FAIRness combined with a novel analysis to describe the utility of the resource (Knoppers 2014; Knoppers et al. 2011; WHO 2022c). The full data set, methods, and results are published, and only the conclusions are used here for discussion.

The Maxwell review shows how difficult it is to precisely define what the FAIR principles mean in every context, for example, when different data sets have varying levels of managed access to identifiable patient data. It also highlights the need for greater review and monitoring of the use of these data platforms and registries to assess their utility and subsequent health benefit against some agreed measures. Since this survey was completed in June

2 A platform combines big data tools and infrastructure. Major investment to continuously store, manage, and mine big data sets (e.g., OMICs, imaging data). It may contain one type of data or various specified data types. A registry is a collection of data physically stored in an assigned location, requiring a low level of investment. Data were generally entered or uploaded using the same case report form/data dictionary and focus on a particular disease, condition, or exposure. Registries were generally one type of data (HDR UK 2022).

Table 1 Summary of principles from selected health data sharing frameworks

Domain	GloPID-R[a] Principles of Sharing Data in Public Health Emergencies (GloPID-R 2018)	Health Data Research UK COVID-19 National Core Studies Data Sharing Principles (HDR UK 2022)	International Code of Conduct for Data Sharing in Genomic Research (Knoppers et al. 2011)	GA4GH Framework for Responsible Sharing of Genomic and Health-Related Data (Knoppers 2014)	CARE Principles for Indigenous Data Governance (Carroll et al. 2021)
Collaboration		Work collaboratively to actively share data to allow the scientific community to pool expertise, draw fresh insights, increase collective understanding	Share governance between funders, generators, and users of data. Encourage mechanisms for interoperability and management. Build capacity. Recognize all data generators	Dedicate education and training resources to advance data sharing and data management to improve data quality and integrity	
FAIR data (Findable, Accessible, Interoperable, and Reusable)	Accessibility. Public health emergency (PHE)-related data to be shared with minimal restrictions. Use conditions to be clearly stated. Provision and use of data with fair treatment and recognition of all. Access terms to reflect international commitments to benefits sharing	All data, code, and tools generated through studies are FAIR. Research outputs, observations, code and tools generated to be open source, rapidly and freely accessible as a public good	Accessibility. (Facilitation of data deposit and access. Databases to promote sharing for maximum value. Harmonization of procedures for deposit, access and use promotes accessibility, equity, and transparency.)		
Ethics	To build trust of all stakeholders, observe applicable ethical and legal standards: beneficence, respect for confidentiality, privacy of individuals, dignity of communities, and cultural norms	Consent. Unconsented data accessed through secure, accredited platforms or accredited in process UK Statistics Authority	Mutual respect among stakeholders based on integrity. Foresight measures to prevent harm and meet public concerns and scientific needs. Common policies, with clear sanctions for breach of requirements	Risk-Benefit Analysis. Minimize harms and maximize benefits for data providers, society, and health care systems. Security. Mitigate risk of unauthorized access, data loss, and misuse	All data sharing should protect the privacy of individuals and the dignity of communities, while respecting the need to improve public health through the most productive use of data

Community engagement	Equity. Data available to all interested parties during a public health emergency at low or no cost to ensure equal access to data needed to collaborate and collective benefits to communities affected by a PHE	Active and ongoing engagement with patients and public in design, development, and governance to ensure activities are in public interest	Accountability. Inter-agency co-operation and funding for monitoring and governance. Ongoing public engagement tailored to the database and local cultures		Equity. Data-sharing approach recognizes and balances needs of researchers generating, using, and reusing data and communities and funders expecting health benefits from research
Transparent governance	Process for sharing data and facilitating access clearly explained, outlining how and when data can be shared and defining associated data descriptors	Transparency in use of personal data. Respect individual privacy and confidentiality, complying with legal requirements and ethical guidelines	Public policies on publication, intellectual property, and industry involvement. Websites allow public feedback	Clearly defined, accessible information on purpose, procedures, and governance frameworks for data sharing	
Compliance with data protection laws		Transparent use of personal data; respect for privacy and confidentiality of individuals (repeat of above)	Security. Trust and promotion of data sharing rely on sound data management, security, oversight	Privacy, data protection, confidentiality. Compliance with privacy and data protection regulations	
Platform utility and value		Uses existing UK infrastructure and research investments as far as possible and open competitions where necessary to develop new infrastructure capability while keeping costs in check. Money by using existing infrastructure and research investments as far as possible and using open infrastructure	Accountability (systems for data sharing that respect this Framework). Track chain of data access and exchange to source. Identify and manage conflicts of interest. Implement mechanisms for complaints of data misuse; identifying, reporting and managing breaches, including appropriate sanctions	Accountability. Data sharing systems consistent with Framework. Chain of data access traces to source. Identify and manage conflicts of interest. Measures to adjudicate and correct violations	Efficiency. Data sharing modalities should improve quality and value of research and value to public health. Build on existing practice, reduce duplication and competition

(continued)

Table 1 (continued)

Domain	GloPID-R[a] Principles of Sharing Data in Public Health Emergencies (GloPID-R 2018)	Health Data Research UK COVID-19 National Core Studies Data Sharing Principles (HDR UK 2022)	International Code of Conduct for Data Sharing in Genomic Research (Knoppers et al. 2011)	GA4GH Framework for Responsible Sharing of Genomic and Health-Related Data (Knoppers 2014)	CARE Principles for Indigenous Data Governance (Carroll et al. 2021)
Quality	Appropriate data standards ensured by provider. Data users apply at least equal quality standards. All relevant metadata, methodology, assumptions, and experimental details are provided, ensuring work conducted with data considers context in which data was produced		Scientists involved in data sharing are bona fide researchers with proof of academic or other standing. Harmonization of data collection, processing, and archiving ensures scientific quality. Collaboration promotes efficiency, sustainability, and comparability	Data quality and security. Store and process data in accurate, verifiable, unbiased, current way. Enhance interoperability and replicability; preserve data searchability and integrity. Ensure feedback on data and metadata quality, security, accuracy, and reusability	

Adapted in part from Maxwell et al. (2021) (CC Attribution 4.0 International)

[a] *GloPID-R* Global Research Collaboration for Infectious Disease Preparedness; *GA4GH* Global Alliance for Genomics and Health

2021, another Internet search using the same terms has revealed that another 50 new COVID-19 data resources have come online, and it is expected this trend will continue. The analysis shows very limited interoperability between resources and large overlaps in the data, creating almost a competition between platforms and registries for data as opposed to collaboration. The utility of these resources is highly variable, and there are few metrics for assessing the return on investment. This is not to say that successes from shared data are lacking; we have noted intensive use of GISAID for viral variant tracking and the contributions to better clinical management provided by ISARIC COVID-19 clinical research resources (Maxwell et al. 2021). Early on in the pandemic, ISARIC worked with WHO to create a set of standardized electronic case report forms (eCRF) to enhance the interoperability of clinical data. While 54% (29 of 54) of platforms required data uploaded to be in a standard eCRF, only one platform was using the WHO-recommended eCRF.

In 2015, WHO called for the public disclosure of clinical trial results, and, as a follow up, in 2017 many of the major funders of trials joined forces to reiterate the importance of trial registration and the timely reporting of data (Clarke et al. 2019). An analysis of research data submitted with registered clinical trials and published in the International Clinical Trials Registry Platform in 2021 reveals a similar lack of traction between policies and their implementation (Wilkinson et al. 2019). This analysis looked at the total records for approximately 650,000 trials registered in the WHO International Clinical Trials Registry Platform (ICTRP) up to the end of January 2021. A subset of those trials related to potential pandemic diseases identified in the WHO R&D Blueprint were disaggregated (Rosnet et al. 2021).

Since 2019, all national clinical trial registries contributing to ICTRP have been required to collect intentions to share the IPD underlying a trial and methods to provide data access. Only 13% of registered trials report any intention of sharing data, with no significant difference between all registered trials and those concerned with diseases with potential to cause public health emergencies. This finding reinforces a similar 2018 analysis looking at data availability of published trial results, which found only one-third (31% or 98 out of 319 published papers, excluding case studies) included any data availability statement for the data underlying the paper. And 65% of these papers give no information on how to find or access the data. Only two clinical trials out of 58 on interventions for WHO priority pathogens provided any link in their registry entry to the background data (Terry et al. 2018).

Both these examples illustrate the gap between principles and normative guidance, as published by WHO and others, and implementation. A consortium of 160 international research funders led by Wellcome Trust, a foundation focused on health research, have tried to quantify the impact of their policies and statements to encourage greater data sharing specifically during a pandemic. Their analysis finds a similar gap between the effort to encourage data sharing and the little health data actually shared, even during an emergency (Chiarelli et al. 2022). The report highlights the importance of linking any policy statement with a commitment to monitor and evaluate its impact. Importantly, research funders must undertake regular audits to measure compliance with their intention to see more data shared and understand non-compliance. This should enable the design of more effective mechanisms for additional funding, training, or other forms of capacity building, particularly for those researchers based in low- and middle-income countries.

5 A Roadmap to Improve Data Sharing

So, what can be done to change a system containing few incentive carrots and virtually no effective sticks? In this final section, an action roadmap is presented, which must be adopted and taken forward by each stakeholder group (◘ Table 2). Each stakeholder plays a different role. However, as previously emphasized, to change the research system, a systems-based approach is necessary.

Table 2 Recommended actions for stakeholders to support coordinated data-sharing efforts for improving public health

Stakeholder	Recommended safeguards for data sharing and reuse
Funders	– Metrics to quantify return on investment in data-sharing efforts they support – Incentives beyond citation and attribution for originators sharing data – Data management and sharing plans based on good/best practice – More FAIR data (through, e.g., registration in a system with machine-readable metadata like FAIR sharing) – Registration of observational studies on a platform collecting metadata and/or assigning a digital object identifier (DOI) – Set-asides for data interoperability funding – Community-developed standards for research studies – Meta-catalogues to facilitate data reuse – Engagement with research participants and patients to understand any concerns on reuse of their data
UN and member states	– Framework recognizing data as a global public good and defining fair sharing of benefits – Consideration of how existing international agreements, such as WHO (2016) or Nagoya Protocol, might be adapted
Journal editors	– Compliance with recommendations of the International Committee of Medical Journal Editors (ICMJE 2022) – Peer review that adequately reviews the data availability statement for an article – DOI for participant-level data set and research protocol to improve study and data discoverability – Machine-readable FAIR checklist that covers issues of data availability, interoperability, and registration of metadata – Incentives for data reuse through special issues or specific collections
Regulators	– Clinical Data Interchange Standards Consortium (CDISC) standards for clinical research (CDISC 2022) – Regulatory body for observational research
Bioinformaticians, software developers, data stewards, and the open science community	– Mixed methods research on dataset availability – Standards to measure overall utility of a platform or registry – Case studies that illustrate the new knowledge and impact gained from secondary reuse of data – Connections between data-sharing infrastructures (data on one platform automatically available through others) – Open science initiatives to facilitate data reuse – Implementation of community-defined standards for reporting and reuse of data and metadata – Indicators for evaluating the FAIRness of data – Compliance with best practices for future use of data or samples consistent with international ethics guidelines
Legal advisors	– Clear guidance on data protection law (particularly re: GDPR) barriers to data access – Clear information on subnational legal barriers to implementation – Clear information on legal barriers to reuse of data for secondary purposes – Clear information on legal barriers related to the reuse of data from protected minority groups – Data protection governance that allows data subjects to assert their rights in international data sharing – Legal tools for international data transfer in emergencies – Technical and data security measures to offer data protection but also allow data sharing and use in emergencies – Collision rules when legal frameworks are inconsistent

Table 2 (continued)

Stakeholder	Recommended safeguards for data sharing and reuse
Ethics advisory bodies	– Healthcare providers, researchers, and other stakeholders aware of ethics guidelines for data sharing and reuse – Guidelines on privacy and confidentiality when sharing and reusing data – Transparency and accountability – Harmonized guidelines and consistent approach to shared ethical concerns – Community-developed recommendations for community engagement on data sharing and reuse – Community-developed governance for data sharing or data reuse-related infrastructure – Norms and standards for consent and governance arrangements acceptable to community – Section on FAIR data required for ethics submissions for observational research
Data-sharing platforms or registries	– Improved expertise on community-developed standards – Engagement with communities on data sharing – Mutual understanding of language about broad consent for future use – Measures for fair sharing of benefits for depositors and users

Adapted from Maxwell et al. (2021) (CC Attribution 4.0 International
FAIR findable, accessible, interoperable, reusable; *GDPR* General Data Protection Regulation

6 Conclusion

The COVID-19 pandemic has shown that data curated to a common standard and aggregated has tremendous power in addressing multiple public health needs. The pandemic has also highlighted that the data-sharing environment is growing organically, with limited controls on the conflicting values from political, ethical, social, technical, legal, and economic perspectives. Table 2 highlights a long wish list of recommended actions. But perhaps funders, researchers, and journals (three of the key stakeholders) have the tools to implement a more effective framework by more actively monitoring, implementing, and reporting their existing policies. If the appropriate reviews can be undertaken, the value of effective sharing could yet be realized before the next pandemic strikes. At the same time, we cannot lose sight of outstanding equity issues associated with data sharing. These challenges are likely to arouse lively debate during forthcoming consideration of polices and instruments to improve preparedness for future emerging infectious diseases (Pratt and Bull 2021).

At the time of this writing, the newly formed International Negotiating Body (INB) established by WHO member states at their Assembly in May 2022, finished its second meeting, following two rounds of public hearings (WHO 2022h). The INB concluded at that meeting that the world needed a legally binding instrument on pandemic prevention and as of early 2023 the INB was beginning to prepare a "zero draft" of or pandemic treaty for the World Health Assembly in May 2023. While the negotiations will of necessity be quite detailed and lengthy, it is a positive development that there is once again political will to focus on how to ensure fair, equitable, and timely data access and benefit sharing to create a coordinated, timely, and evidence-based pandemic response (WHO 2022g).

Discussion Questions

1. Discuss the elements that need to be in place to allow for searching across hundreds of databases to identify a virus by genomic sequence.

2. Why are some researchers reluctant to share voluminous data, particularly in low- and middle-income countries?
3. What steps did GISAID introduce, for both depositing and gaining access to genome sequences on its site, to encourage data attribution and benefit sharing?
4. ISARIC established the COVID-19 Clinical Database for individual data from hospitalized patients and clinical trial participants. What are the benefits of aggregating individuals' data into a large, standardized data set?
5. Discuss other ethical questions in data sharing (e.g., rapidity vs. equity).
6. What are some of the legal frameworks under which data sharing occurs, including WHO's merger of FAIR principles with efficiency, ethics, and equity?

Review ◘ Table 2 and choose and analyze some of the recommended stakeholder actions, their degree of difficulty, and their potential benefit for global public health and pandemic response.

References

Albery GF, Becker DJ, Brierley L, Brook CE, Christofferson RC, Cohen LE, et al. The science of the host–virus network. Nat Microbiol. 2021;6(12):1483–92. https://doi.org/10.1038/s41564-021-00999-5.

Alföldi J, Lindblad-Toh K. Comparative genomics as a tool to understand evolution and disease. Genome Res. 2013;23(7):1063–8. https://doi.org/10.1101/gr.157503.113.

Article 6 EU GDPR "Lawfulness of processing". 2022.

Baillie JK, Baruch J, Beane A, Blumberg L, Bozza FA, Broadley T, et al. ISARIC COVID-19 clinical data report issued: 27 March 2022. medRxiv. 2022; https://doi.org/10.1101/2020.07.17.20155218.

Carroll SR, Herczog E, Hudson M, et al. Operationalizing the CARE and FAIR Principles for Indigenous data futures. Sci Data 2021;8:108. https://doi.org/10.1038/s41597-021-00892-0.

Chiarelli A, Loffreda L, Cox E, Johnson R, Ferguson C, Vignola-Gagné E, et al. From intent to impact: investigating the effects of open sharing commitments. London: Wellcome Trust; 2022.

Clarke DJB, Wang L, Jones A, Wojciechowicz ML, Torre D, Jagodnik KM, et al. FAIRshake: toolkit to evaluate the FAIRness of research digital resources. Cell Syst. 2019;9(5):417–21. https://doi.org/10.1016/j.cels.2019.09.011.

Clinical Data Interchange Standards Consortium (CDISC) About CDISC | CDISC. Accessed May 2022. https://www.cdisc.org/about.

Coronaviridae Study Group of the International Committee on Taxonomy of Viruses. The species *Severe acute respiratory syndrome-related coronavirus*: classifying 2019-nCoV and naming it SARS-CoV-2. Nat Microbiol. 2020;5(4):536–44. https://doi.org/10.1038/s41564-020-0695-z.

COVID-19 data portal. European COVID-19 Data Platform. 2022. https://www.covid19dataportal.org/. Accessed 22 Aug 2022.

GISAID. GISAID's comments on the WHO report of the public health implications of implementation of the Nagoya protocol. Munich: Freunde von GISAID e.V.; 2019.

GISAID. GISAID. Munich: Freunde von GISAID e.V.; 2022. Accessed 22 Aug 2022.

GloPID-R. Principles of data sharing in public health emergencies. Global Research Collaboration for Infectious Disease Preparedness; 2018.

Hate K, Meherally S, Shah More N, Jayaraman A, Bull S, Parker M, et al. Sweat, skepticism, and uncharted territory: a qualitative study of opinions on data sharing among public health researchers and research participants in Mumbai, India. J Empir Res Hum Res Ethics. 2015;10(3):239–50. https://doi.org/10.1177/1556264615592383.

HDR UK. National core studies data sharing principles COVID-19. Health Data Research UK; 2022. https://www.hdruk.org/covid-19/covid-19-national-core-studies/ncs-data-sharing-principles/. Accessed 27 Aug 2022.

Heard E, Birney E, Apweiler R, Blomberg N, Cochrane G, Lauer K, et al. Open letter: support data sharing for COVID-19. COVID-19 Data Portal; 2022.

Human Genome Project information archive 1990–2003. U.S. Department of Energy Office of Science, Office of Biological and Environmental Research. 2019. https://web.ornl.gov/sci/techresources/Human_Genome/research/bermuda.shtml. Accessed 17 Aug 2022.

ICMJE. Recommendations for the Conduct, Reporting, Editing, and Publication of Scholarly Work in Medical Journals, 2022.

IDDO. Infectious Diseases Data Observatory. Oxford: The Infectious Diseases Data Observatory (IDDO); 2023. https://www.iddo.org/news/new-poem-celebrates-data-sharing. Accessed 27 May 2023.

INSDC. International Nucleotide Sequence Database Collaboration. Hinxton, UK: International nucleotide sequence database collaboration; 2021. https://www.insdc.org/. Accessed 9 Oct 2022.

ISARIC. COVID19 clinical research resources. Oxford: ISARIC; 2022. https://isaric.org/research/covid-19-clinical-research-resources/. Accessed 22 Aug 2022.

Knoppers BM. Framework for responsible sharing of genomic and health-related data. HUGO J.

2014;8(1):3. https://doi.org/10.1186/s11568-014-0003-1.

Knoppers BM, Harris JR, Tassé AM, Budin-Ljøsne I, Kaye J, Deschênes M, et al. Towards a data sharing Code of Conduct for international genomic research. Genome Med. 2011;3(7):46. https://doi.org/10.1186/gm262.

Kruse CS, Stein A, Thomas H, Kaur H. The use of electronic health records to support population health: a systematic review of the literature. J Med Syst. 2018;42(11):214. https://doi.org/10.1007/s10916-018-1075-6.

Mallapaty S. Omicron-variant border bans ignore the evidence, say scientists. Nature. 2021;600(7888):199. https://doi.org/10.1038/d41586-021-03608-x.

Maxmen A. One million coronavirus sequences: popular genome site hits mega milestone. Nature. 2021;593(7857):21. https://doi.org/10.1038/d41586-021-01069-w.

Maxson Jones K, Ankeny RA, Cook-Deegan R. The Bermuda triangle: the pragmatics, policies, and principles for data sharing in the history of the Human Genome Project. J Hist Biol. 2018;51(4):693–805. https://doi.org/10.1007/s10739-018-9538-7.

Maxwell L, Shreedhar P, Dauga D, McQuilton P, Terry RF, Denisiuk A, et al. FAIR, ethical, and coordinated data sharing for COVID-19 response: a review of COVID-19 data sharing platforms and registries. Zenodo. 2021; https://doi.org/10.5281/zenodo.5642635.

Modjarrad K, Moorthy VS, Millett P, Gsell PS, Roth C, Kieny MP. Developing global norms for sharing data and results during public health emergencies. PLoS Med. 2016;13(1):e1001935. https://doi.org/10.1371/journal.pmed.1001935.

Moorthy V, Henao Restrepo AM, Preziosi MP, Swaminathan S. Data sharing for novel coronavirus (COVID-19). Bull World Health Organ. 2020;98(3):150. https://doi.org/10.2471/blt.20.251561.

NIH. Basic local alignment search tool. Bethesda, MD: NIH, National Library of Medicine, National Center for Biotechnology Information; 2022a. https://blast.ncbi.nlm.nih.gov/Blast.cgi. Accessed 22 Aug 2022.

NIH. NCBI SARS-CoV-2 resources. Bethesda, MD: NIH, National Library of Medicine, National Center for Biotechnology Information; 2022b. https://www.ncbi.nlm.nih.gov/pmc/articles/PMC8184206/. Accessed 22 Aug 2022.

Nuffield Council on Bioethics. Research in global health emergencies: ethical issues. Oxford, UK: Nuffield Council on Bioethics; 2020.

Pandemic Preparedness Partnership. 100 days mission to respond to future pandemic threats: reducing the impact of future pandemics by making diagnostics, therapeutics and vaccines available within 100 days: a report to the G7. London: G7 United Kingdom; 2021.

Pisani E, Aaby P, Breugelmans JG, Carr D, Groves T, Helinski M, et al. Beyond open data: realising the health benefits of sharing data. BMJ. 2016;355:i5295. https://doi.org/10.1136/bmj.i5295.

Pisani E, Ghataure A, Merson L. Data sharing in public health emergencies: a study of current policies, practices and infrastructure supporting the sharing of data to prevent and respond to epidemic and pandemic threats. London: Wellcome Trust; 2018.

Pratt B, Bull S. Equitable data sharing in epidemics and pandemics. BMC Med Ethics. 2021;22(1):136. https://doi.org/10.1186/s12910-021-00701-8.

Rosnet T, de Lamotte F, Devignes M-D, Lefort V, Gaignard A. FAIR-checker: supporting the findability and reusability of digital life science resources. Institut Français de Bioinformatique; 2021. p. 1.

Saxena A, Horby P, Amuasi J, Aagaard N, Kohler J, Gooshki ES, et al. Ethics preparedness: facilitating ethics review during outbreaks—recommendations from an expert panel. BMC Med Ethics. 2019;20(1):29. https://doi.org/10.1186/s12910-019-0366-x.

Terry RF, Littler K, Olliaro PL. Sharing health research data—the role of funders in improving the impact. F1000Res. 2018;7:1641. https://doi.org/10.12688/f1000research.16523.2.

UNESCO. UNESCO recommendation on open science. Paris: United Nations Educational, Scientific, and Cultural Organization; 2021.

Van Noorden R. Scientists call for fully open sharing of coronavirus genome data. Nature. 2021;590(7845):195–6. https://doi.org/10.1038/d41586-021-00305-7.

Van Spall HGC. Exclusion of pregnant and lactating women from COVID-19 vaccine trials: a missed opportunity. Eur Heart J. 2021;42(28):2724–6. https://doi.org/10.1093/eurheartj/ehab103.

Wellcome Trust. Sharing data from large-scale biological research projects: a system of tripartite responsibility: report of a meeting organized by the Wellcome Trust and held on 14–15 January 2003 at Fort Lauderdale, USA. Fort Lauderdale, FL: The Wellcome Trust; 2003.

Wellome Trust. Sharing research data and findings relevant to the novel coronavirus (COVID-19) outbreak. London: Wellcome Trust; 2020.

White House. Joint statement by President Clinton and Prime Minister Tony Blair of the U.K. Washington, DC: The Executive Office of the President (US); 2000.

WHO. Indonesia to resume sharing H5N1 avian influenza virus samples following a WHO meeting in Jakarta. Jakarta: World Health Organization; 2007.

WHO. WHO Director-General's opening remarks at 148th session of the Executive Board. Geneva: World Health Organization; 2021.

WHO. Pandemic instrument should be legally binding, INB meeting concludes. Geneva: World Health Organization; 2022a.

WHO. Public health implications of implementation of the Nagoya Protocol. Geneva: World Health Organization; 2022b. https://www.who.int/initiatives/public-health-implications-of-the-nagoya-protocol. Accessed 23 Aug 2022.
WHO. Sharing and reuse of health-related data for research purposes: WHO policy and implementation guidance. Geneva: World Health Organization; 2022c.
WHO. Strengthening WHO preparedness for and response to health emergencies. Geneva: World Health Organization; 2022d. Report No.: Seventy-Fifth World Health Assembly A75/21. Provisional agenda item 16.2.
WHO. WHO data policy: WHO policy on the use and sharing of data collected by WHO in Member States outside the context of public health emergencies. Geneva: World Health Organization; 2022e. https://www.who.int/about/policies/publishing/data-policy. Accessed 22 Aug 2022.
WHO. WHO Director-General's opening remarks at first meeting of the Intergovernmental Negotiating Body to draft and negotiate a WHO convention, agreement or other international instrument on pandemic prevention, preparedness and response. Geneva: World Health Organization; 2022f.
WHO. Working draft, presented on the basis of progress achieved, for the consideration of the Intergovernmental Negotiating Body at its second meeting. Geneva: World Health Organization; 2022g.
WHO. The world together: the Intergovernmental Negotiating Body to draft and negotiate a WHO convention, agreement or other international instrument on pandemic prevention, preparedness and response. Geneva: WHO; 2022h. https://inb.who.int/. Accessed 27 Aug 2022.
World Health Organization (2016). International Health Regulations (2005), 3rd ed. World Health Organization. https://iris.who.int/handle/10665/246107.
Wilkinson MD, Dumontier M, Aalbersberg IJ, Appleton G, Axton M, Baak A, et al. The FAIR guiding principles for scientific data management and stewardship. Sci Data. 2016;3(1):160018. https://doi.org/10.1038/sdata.2016.18.
Wilkinson MD, Dumontier M, Sansone SA, da Silva B, Santos LO, Prieto M, Batista D, et al. Evaluating FAIR maturity through a scalable, automated, community-governed framework. Sci Data. 2019;6(1):174. https://doi.org/10.1038/s41597-019-0184-5.
Yozwiak NL, Schaffner SF, Sabeti PC. Data sharing: make outbreak research open access. Nature. 2015;518(7540):477–9. https://doi.org/10.1038/518477a.
Zelenova M, Ivanova A, Semyonov S, Gankin Y. Analysis of 329,942 SARS-CoV-2 records retrieved from GISAID database. Comput Biol Med. 2021;139:104981. https://doi.org/10.1016/j.compbiomed.2021.104981.
Zelenova M, Ivanova A, Semyonov S, Gankin Y. Retraction notice to "Analysis of 329,942 SARS-CoV-2 records retrieved from GISAID database" [Comput. Biol. Med. 139 (2021) 104981]. Comput Biol Med. 2022;146:105527. https://doi.org/10.1016/j.compbiomed.2022.105527.

Preparedness for Emergency Research Response

Robert A. Sorenson

Overview of Book Section III: Nothing determines response to an emergency more than the steps taken to prepare for it. It has been understood for millennia that humanity is struck by periodic pandemics, but it has been less than a century since medical science has been able to respond with much more than quarantine or palliative measures. It has been 20 years since what one might identify as the first real-time vaccine development efforts, during the SARS-CoV-1 epidemic, and less than a decade since the first rigorous clinical trials were implemented during an emergency, the West Africa Ebola outbreak of 2014–2016. Perhaps only now, after the accelerated research response to the COVID-19 pandemic, it is evident to most people that preparedness for accelerated research response is imperative.

Nahid Bhadelia et al. (► Chap. 8) address one of the paradoxes of pandemic preparedness: countries most vulnerable to outbreaks often have the least capacity to respond. Building research partnerships and capacity in low- and middle-income countries strengthens resilience against infectious disease, helps scientists refine research questions and operations, and should contribute to stronger health systems and better population health status. It gives countries and the world a head start on scientific information about emerging pathogens, and then developing, assessing, producing, and distributing effective MCMs. Building biomedical research capacity, strengthening biosurveillance, sequencing pathogens, analyzing patient data, and conducting clinical trials is not simple or cheap. It requires sustained investment by countries and international partners and progress toward universal healthcare. Lisa Hensley et al. lay out the requirements for clinical research laboratories, and how to build them in advance or when needed in an emergency (► Chap. 9).

Andrew Clements et al. (► Chap. 10) look at emerging zoonotic pathogens, the source of most human infectious diseases, focusing on how and where zoonotic pathogens circulate, pathways to emergence, potential for sustained human-to-human transmission, and gaps in our knowledge. An interlinked global surveillance and warning system could improve collection and use of information before an outbreak occurs to improve global health security. An outbreak of a novel infectious disease also requires rapid innovation in diagnostic testing to screen populations and diagnose active infection in patients. C. Taylor Gilliland et al. (► Chap. 11) describe the approach and lessons learned through the Rapid Acceleration of Diagnostics program, which dramatically reduced the time needed for development, commercialization, and implementation of new diagnostics during the COVID-19 pandemic. The program followed a new paradigm that enabled dozens of testing technologies to obtain regulatory authorization, delivered billions of tests, and catalyzed a shift toward self-testing.

Emergency preparedness includes the development of candidate vaccines for pathogens yet unknown. Karin Bok (► Chap. 12 and In Focus 12.1) reviews recent progress on several relatively novel vaccine platforms (mRNA, DNA, and vector-based) and other techniques to formulate vaccine candidates. Understanding viral structures and self-assembly, intended target proteins, and conserved but vulnerable viral epitopes, as well as immune system reactions to viral infection, is foundational to preparedness for the emergence of pathogens and rapid development of new medical countermeasures. Furthermore, establishing global mRNA supply chains, manufacturing, and fill/finish capacities promise prompt control of emerging epidemics and pandemics. The ambitious goal of delivering vaccines within 100 days after identification of a novel pathogen with pandemic potential, pursued by the Coalition for Epidemic Preparedness Innovations (► Chap. 13), will require advances in scientific research, production technology, clinical trial readiness, response organization and governance, and financing. Elizabeth Higgs cover preparedness and response for therapeutics (► Chap. 14), discussing both accelerated research programs during the COVID-**19** pandemic and organizational steps for future preparedness. Finally, Peter Horby et al. (► In Practice 14.1) describe the largest COVID-**19** treatment study, the Randomized Evaluation of COVID-**19** Therapy Trial, which within 100 days provided clear results on the safety and efficacy (or lack thereof) of three drugs and enabled life-saving changes in clinical practice.

Contents

8 Building Biomedical Research Capacity in Low- and Middle-Income Countries: Why It Matters and Some of the Barriers to Success

Nahid Bhadelia, Vasee Moorthy, Robert A. Sorenson, and Soumya Swaminathan

Contents

Learning Track Note: This chapter appears in Learning Tracks: Emergency Research Response, Research Operations (► Sect. 3); Health Policy, Multilateral Cooperation, International Governance; One Health; Preparedness; Public Health and Epidemiology

E. S. Higgs and R. A. Sorenson (eds.), *Principles and Practice of Emergency Research Response*,
https://doi.org/10.1007/978-3-031-48408-7_10

Learning Objectives

This chapter will help readers understand and describe:

- The need for research capacity to strengthen preparedness, response, and resilience against infectious disease emergencies in low- and middle-income countries
- How global maldistribution of medical research capacity hinders preparedness for public health emergencies
- The intersection of factors determining research capacity, including education, healthcare and public health systems, health financing, connections with the global scientific community, and governance
- Advantages of strong research capacity in currently underserved areas and some of the metrics used to measure research capacity and activity
- The roles of the World Health Organization (WHO) and Coalition for Epidemic Preparedness Innovations (CEPI) in developing research capacity
- Some of the requirements for and obstacles to building health research capacity in low- and middle-income countries

1 Introduction

Several chapters in this volume emphasize the central place of research in urgent response to emerging infectious diseases (EIDs). This chapter elaborates on the importance of preexisting research capacity in low- and middle-income countries (LMICs) for strengthening resilience against EID threats. Wernli et al. (2021) broadly define societal resilience as "the ability of societies to maintain their core functions while minimizing the health impact of the pandemic and other societal effects," and ◘ Fig. 2 illustrates some of the elements of resilience. As the COVID-19 pandemic has demonstrated, broadly available research capacity can contribute to resilience by helping the global research community refine the research questions that should be asked and elucidate essential scientific information about emerging pathogens more quickly and effectively (Krause et al. 2020; WHO Solidarity Trial Consortium 2021). Strong research capacity in LMICs also contributes to more equitable governance of research during outbreaks (Peters et al. 2017; Pratt and Hyder 2017). Moreover, a strong domestic research capacity could help identify, characterize, and then slow or contain the spread of a new or unfamiliar pathogen, meanwhile giving research scientists more time to understand and counteract it. Recall, for example, that the Ebola virus was not even identified as the cause of a rapidly spreading hemorrhagic fever in West Africa until 3 months after the index case in December 2013 (Olu 2016).

In 2000, the World Health Organization (WHO) Global Forum for Health Research noted that only 10% of research spending is devoted to the health problems of 90% of the world's population and remarked that "strengthening research capacity in developing countries is one of the most effective and sustainable ways of advancing health and development" (Coloma and Harris 2009; Global Forum for Health Research 1999). Several indicators are in use to measure research activity. For example, a recent review of academic publications focused on EIDs over the last two decades notes that while U.S. institutions and researchers still lead by number of contributions, a growing share of data and publications comes from Asia, Africa, and the Middle East (Sweileh 2017). Despite this increase, a disproportionate lack of researchers and research capacity still prevails in LMICs. Some regions, including many African countries, have had a slower rate of growth in the research sector than others (◘ Fig. 1) (National Academies of Sciences Engineering and Medicine 2017). Sub-Saharan Africa accounts for 11% of the world's population and 24% of the global disease burden, but the African continent produces only about 2% of the world's research by various measures (IBRD 2016; IFC 2008; Kay 2015).

African research and development increased by 50% between 2007 and 2013 but still accounts for only 1.5% of the world's total expenditure in the sector (Marsh 2016; Yozwiak et al. 2016). And yet data suggest that high biodiversity, including that of pathogens and disease vector and reservoir

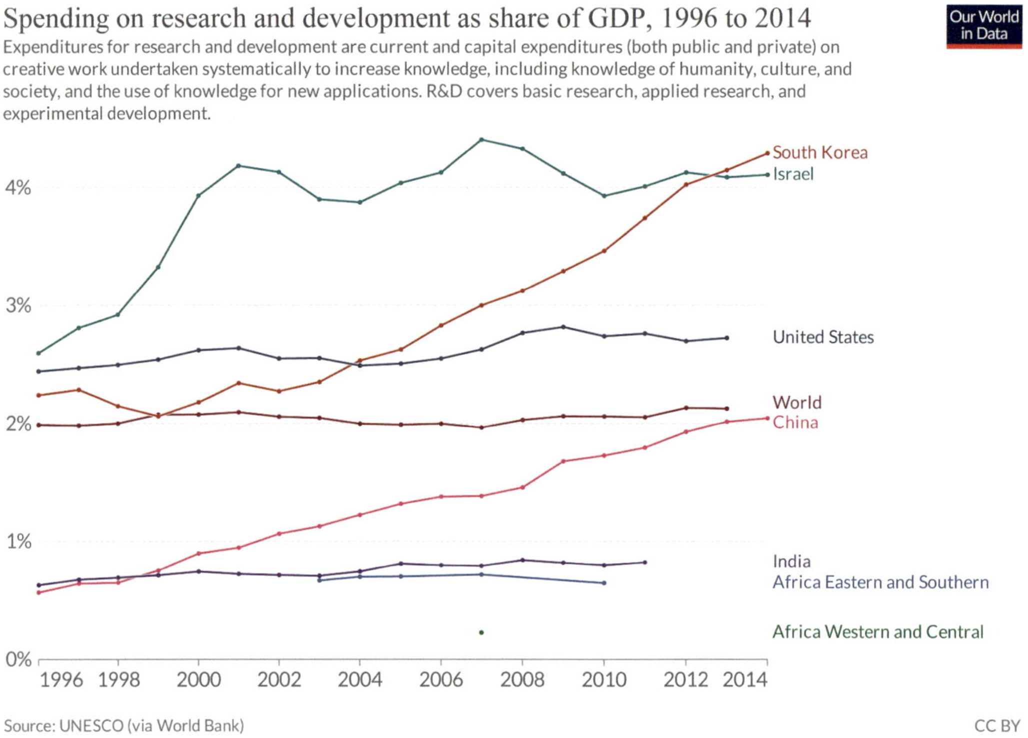

Fig. 1 Spending on research and development (R&D) as share of gross domestic product (GDP), 1996–2014. Note the single-year data point for Western and Central Africa, perhaps a more eloquent indicator than the statistics themselves. Note also that the Eastern and Southern Africa statistics include South Africa's robust biotechnology sector. (Our World in Data 2022)

species, in conjunction with fewer resources for disease control, heighten the risk for EID emergence and spread in many LMICs (Dunn et al. 2010; Jones et al. 2008; Murray et al. 2015).

To move knowledge of EIDs forward, the ad hoc importation of research machinery in outbreaks will not suffice (Yozwiak et al. 2016). The experience of the Coalition for Epidemic Preparedness Innovations (CEPI), a global collaboration for the development of vaccines for EIDs, has highlighted the importance of research capacity in vulnerable areas to conduct clinical trials, monitor adverse effects, and generate reliable data (Bernasconi et al. 2020). While clinical trial capacity is critical, upstream research—for example, understanding the natural history and epidemiology of EIDs, developing diagnostics, and building the scientific evidence base for culturally appropriate public health responses—is also heavily dependent on strong research sectors in LMICs.

In this chapter, the authors outline the importance of regional and local public health context in EID research, discuss the infrastructure and human capital necessary for building research response in LMICs, and outline the contributions such capacity can be expected to provide for research during future outbreaks. We identify the synergy between public health, healthcare system, and research capacity for EID response. Lastly, we highlight some underlying challenges to health research capacity building in LMICs.

2 Local or National Research Agendas Enable Research Capacity to Respond to Local Needs

The ultimate beneficial health impact of research relies on evidence generation, translation into policies, public health interventions, medical countermeasures (MCMs), improvements in patient care, and the consistent utilization of such interventions for those who need them. The reality in many low-income settings is that research programs and capacity funding decisions are in great measure made in high-income donor countries, and the capacity and research that follow may not be well aligned with needs on the ground (Sheikh et al. 2020).

The 2017 World Report on Health Policy and Research found that that this mismatch between funding and needs further limited the capacity of LMICs to use research evidence to inform decision-making and policy (WHO 2017b). A survey of ministries of health conducted by the Alliance for Health Policy and Systems Research for WHO found that the lack of locally relevant applied research, along with poor presentation of research findings and inadequate communication between researchers and policymakers, were the three most cited barriers to getting evidence to decision makers (WHO 2017b). The importance of "learning healthcare systems" for EID preparedness was underscored by the U.S. National Academy of Medicine's *Neglected Dimension of Health Security*, which, among other findings, identified engaging local scientists and communities in the conduct of research as critical to research response to infectious disease threats (NAM 2016). The goals of Global Health Security Agenda (GHSA) to prevent, detect, and respond to EIDs focus on several useful areas for EID response, such as capacity building in data collection and improvements in integrated laboratory disease surveillance. GHSA does not, however, include actions to improve partner country capacity for clinical research, either to improve patient care when an EID outbreak occurs or to evaluate the efficacy of MCMs (GHSA 2014, 2022; Marston et al. 2017).

To achieve genuine resilience against EIDs, low-income countries need not just funding but also achievable roadmaps and metrics to guide the improvement or establishment of functional research capacity (Eigbike 2020), and ultimately comprehensive health systems that can support both timely interventions for affected populations and career paths for healthcare professionals from the patient bedside to the research lab (Nuzzo et al. 2019). Although significant progress has been made in identifying such metrics and indicators, greater effort is needed for data collection and reporting on indicators (Eigbike 2020). A key enabler for better aligning research capacity investments with local priorities and needs is the existence of nationally coordinated, articulated visions for research and manufacturing capacity (McGregor et al. 2014). A major focus of work at WHO in this sector has been to reorient the funding environment to place an emphasis on first understanding locally identified knowledge gaps and research needs, building political support for local investment, and leveraging international donors to catalyze the transition to full local ownership of research priorities and institutions. In 2018 and 2019 WHO assisted with development of local and subregional research agendas for Lassa fever research in West Africa (WHO 2018). This included a national Lassa fever research consortium in Nigeria, co-led by Nigeria Centers for Disease Control and local researchers. Also, a regional consultation mapped out the end-to-end pathway for Lassa fever vaccine, starting with the perspective of West African scientists, regulators, and public health officials (Salami et al. 2020). These developments challenged and displaced what had once been common practice, that vaccine trials for diseases prevalent only in Africa would start in high-income countries with little or no input from African researchers or end-users in local communities.

It is increasingly understood in infectious disease research and other fields that it is critical to start product development with local public health goals, regulatory perspectives, and health system capacities in mind, and that this can only be achieved through early, bottom-up consultations. Along these lines, the Indian Council of Medical Research and the Bangladesh Institute of Epidemiology, Disease Control and Research identified local research priorities for response and preparedness plans related to Nipah virus outbreaks. Their involvement has improved not only the quality of Nipah virus research but also public health response to recent Nipah virus outbreaks (Sadanadan et al. 2018; Sahay et al. 2020).

Development of national research agendas needs to be driven through coordination and communication between ministries of health, science and technology, finance, and education, along with national research institutes, civil society, and the private sector. Collaborations between ministries of health and research institutes embedded in the health system, directed by a government-articulated vision, can lead to quicker filling of critical knowledge gaps and scaling up of solutions. WHO's Research and Development, Innovation, and Access Accelerator efforts have highlighted that much more can be done to synchronize international funding with national priorities, although many national research agenda setting exercises have already taken place. Doing so would not only better align research with health needs but also effectively accelerate the scaleup of promising innovations to progress toward the Sustainable Development Goals (UN 2021; WHO 2019b). When international donors support national research agendas, they can maximize the impact of their investments by aligning with local priorities. This can greatly increase the chances for uptake of research outputs into policy processes. More remains to be done in ensuring that national and community voices from low- and middle-income countries are well integrated into the definition of international research capacity initiatives as co-owners rather than clients.

3 Investing in Local Research Infrastructure Before Crises

Fostering resilient health capacity (Fig. 2) requires investing in *researchers* from LMICs, supporting the *research institutions* that house them, working with national governments to improve *regulatory oversight*, overcome *operational shortcomings* for programs and products, and engage vulnerable *communities* in research partnerships before crisis strikes.

3.1 Education and Training

Like their Global North counterparts, LMIC scientists are necessarily at the heart of successful research enterprises and institutions

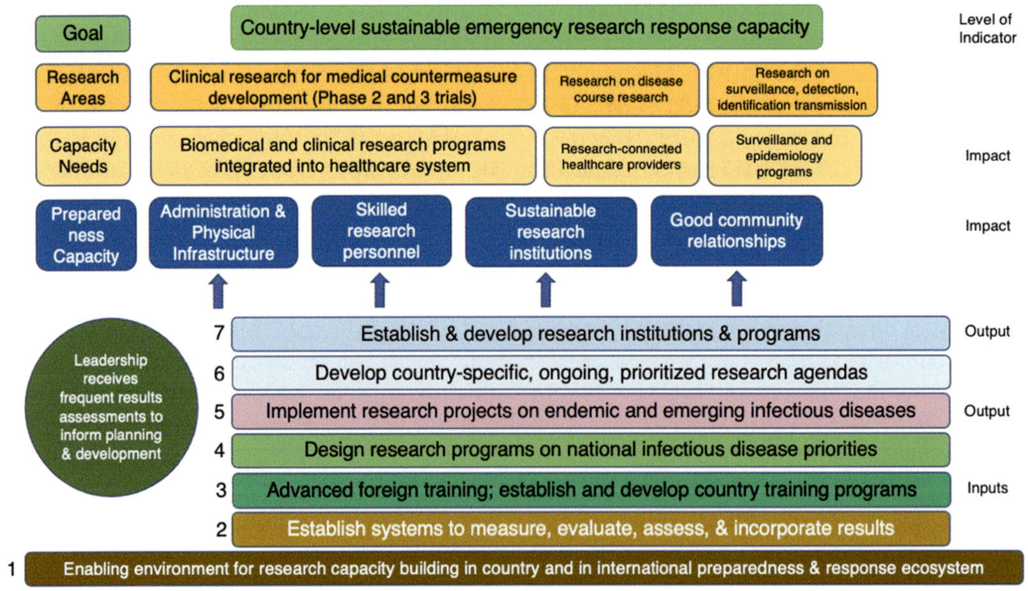

Fig. 2 Some of the many requirements for developing research capacity. (Elizabeth S. Higgs and Robert A. Sorenson, unpublished)

in the Global South. It is no surprise then that the most common research capacity-building programs to date have been those that support individual researcher training and career development. Training programs ranging from the U.S. National Institutes of Health (NIH) and NIH Fogarty International Center (FIC) fellowships and the U.S. Centers for Disease Control and Prevention (CDC) Field Epidemiology Training Program to United Nations, World Bank, and World Health Organization (WHO) programs have supported the growth of the cadre of LMIC researchers (Bridbord et al. 2019; Käser et al. 2016). The experiences of these programs demonstrate that research capacity investments in LMICs can have global benefits for surveillance, identification, and management of new pathogens and outbreaks. For example, FIC-trained researchers helped detect the Zika epidemic in Brazil and Peru (Drain et al. 2017). Similarly, research laboratories at Redeemers University in Nigeria provided the definitive diagnosis of Ebola virus disease (EVD) in the imported case from Liberia in 2014, which facilitated a rapid public health response to the outbreak (Folarin et al. 2016).

Clinicians and biomedical and social science researchers from countries where high-consequence pathogens are endemic and EIDs are likely to cause outbreaks can provide longitudinal perspectives and a more granular understanding of clinical, epidemiological, and social dimensions of these diseases. As discussed above, LMIC scientists and academic institutions also play a critical role in helping their national governments in task setting and research priority creation (Global Forum on Bioethics in Research 2015; InterAcademy Council 2015). The creation of in-country and regional scientific expertise, as well as the development of national research agendas by host countries, can facilitate more equitable and rapid agreements on clinical trials, as well as a swifter exchange of pathogen genetic materials during outbreaks. In the absence of such agreements, practices such as "parachute research," where outside investigators arrive in the country during outbreaks, work in isolation, and leave with biological samples can flourish (Doe-Anderson et al. 2016; Yozwiak et al. 2016). Having successful collaborations in place between researchers and research institutions from Global North and South can decrease the time for initiation of new research and facilitate the discovery and dissemination of critical public health information during outbreaks. For example, Nigerian, U.S., and Sierra Leonean researchers who conducted Lassa fever research via an existing partnership between the U.S.-based Viral Hemorrhagic Fever Consortium and the African Center of Excellence for Genomics of Infectious Disease, headquartered in Nigeria, were one of the first groups to produce scientific data about the Ebola strain involved in the 2014–2016 West African EVD epidemic (Yozwiak et al. 2016).

Additionally, researchers at Global South universities serve as instructors and can potentially mentor new researchers in their own countries (Lescano et al. 2019). Ongoing research at LMIC institutions generates training and grant opportunities and financial support for new scientists and research support staff. In effect, it creates a cadre of trained specialists who can pivot during outbreaks from their ongoing research to that required in an emergency, as so many scientists did worldwide after the emergence of SARS-CoV-2. A culture of research and the presence of research support infrastructure (including regulatory oversight, ethical review, and data management) can help ensure adherence to ethical standards and regulatory requirements for research during emergency settings and improve the quality of results (Ng et al. 2015).

3.2 Institutional Infrastructure

Training researchers by itself is hardly adequate for the creation of research capacity in LMICs. Despite having received advanced training, many researchers in resource-limited settings struggle to influence or implement a national research agenda and effectively compete for international funding. They are frequently hampered by a lack of institutional capacity, the power differential in global research collaborations, and international funding dynamics (Dean et al. 2015; Izugbara et al. 2017). A dearth of institutional resources for financial and administrative management of research administration, as well as ethical and regulatory review, has frequently been identified as a barrier to increasing new health research in LMICs (Rani et al. 2011). Lack of adequate administrative infrastructure leads to concerns about accountability, transparency, and efficiency in the research conducted in low-resource academic centers (Rani et al. 2011). Unfortunately, these limitations create a scenario where LMIC partners in international research consortia have less shared authority and fewer resources in funded projects, which means they receive less of the indirect cost payments (overhead) that typically support administrative infrastructure in developed countries (Mahmood et al. 2011; Pratt and Hyder 2017). An ESSENCE on Health Research (2014) report identified robust research governance structures as essential to research capacity strengthening. Without the ability to initiate and bring in new funding for local research enterprises through indirect support, LMIC researchers in global partnerships will often continue to occupy supportive rather than architectural roles (Coloma and Harris 2009). Some authors have stressed the importance of dedicated capacity-building funds to provide core funding for operations of LMIC research institutions, activities that should be ongoing before emergencies, to ensure equitable distribution of decision-making, accountability, and resources within international collaborations.

National regulatory oversight for clinical trials and drug or device evaluation also contributes to confidence from sponsors and manufacturers looking to conduct research in LMICs. However, that confidence needs to work both ways. Two important enablers for this process are effective mechanisms to solicit local regulatory input into clinical trial plans and clarity on the full line of sight through high- and low-income regulatory needs. Early engagement of national regulatory bodies with external research sponsors allows elucidation of WHO and national policy needs for data generation, as well as critical feasibility considerations that will enable implementation at a large scale in resource-poor settings. WHO's development of detailed, open-access target product profiles (TPPs) for vaccines, therapeutics, diagnostics, and medical devices can provide a degree of clarity that de-risks product development for manufacturers and funders, with a major emphasis on including all stakeholders' input and end-user perspectives. WHO has developed over 30 documents explaining TPPs for emerging and other infectious diseases (WHO 2022).

3.3 Operational Needs

Just-in-time research infrastructure creation during outbreaks faces incredible logistical impediments, which can delay or halt research during emergencies (see Part VII). The presence of experienced researchers and well-resourced research facilities in LMICs where outbreaks with high-consequence pathogens can occur overcomes many of these barriers. In many resource-limited settings, basic infrastructure challenges, such as lack of reliable water supply or power grids, inability to maintain cold chains for vaccines, medicines or samples, or poor Internet connectivity for transfer of data, can stymie research (NASEM 2017). Negotiating and resolving these challenges in the middle of an outbreak becomes a Herculean task when added to required efforts to import research equipment, recruit staff, and achieve regulatory and procedural readiness to conduct trials. Aside from providing staff with longer-term experience and proficiency in biosafety, ongoing research activities can ensure continuous investment in critical physical infrastructure and services that can serve as swing resources during emergencies. The longer-term operations of research centers in LMICs can ensure many of the logistical issues have been tackled before outbreaks occur, through both practical experience and established partnerships and relationships that can facilitate more seamless operations during emergencies. The ongoing presence of research staff and facilities also creates market demand that has the potential to improve supply chains through the development of local providers of products and services, which can decrease cost over time.

A flourishing research sector can also promote a supportive biomedical business sector in LMICs. Research instruments and laboratory equipment are generally produced in higher-income countries and imported into LMICs through purchases or donations. A 2011 study of 16 low-income countries showed that 40% of inventoried medical equipment was nonfunctional (Perry and Malkin 2011). Not many biomedical companies generally offer regional technical support in low-income countries. Currently, only 13% of medical device manufacturers are located in LMICs—countries which in many cases have no biomedical engineering training programs (DePasse et al. 2016). It is important to think through maintenance requirements and other aspects of ensuring new technology will be useful for the normal lifetime of the product in the environments for which it is bound. Long-standing research partnerships can allow time for such preplanning, the careful selection of materials, and the identification of resources to help facilitate repair. The luxury of such forethought is limited when laboratory equipment is obtained and deployed during outbreaks. Research equipment, like most medical devices, requires calibration, maintenance, repair, user training, and decommissioning, activities which require a significant investment that is best planned before outbreaks occur. Through such avenues, ongoing research programs can not only begin to establish a support base, but they can also contribute, however modestly, to economic development, trade ties, and private-sector technical knowledge.

3.4 Community Engagement

Last and most critical, trust and community engagement have always been incredibly important factors in outbreak control and have played a critical role in the two recent Ebola virus disease outbreaks (Kucharski and Piot 2014; Nguyen 2019). The new normal in global health threats from EIDs appears to be large, unexpected, rare, highly disruptive outbreaks that can become epidemics or pandemics and cause widespread social disruption (Bedford et al. 2019). We have learned during the coronavirus disease 2019 (COVID-19) pandemic that distrust of research and resulting MCMs, particularly vaccines, is by no means confined to low-resource communities. Historical and political factors, including generalized mistrust of authorities for a wide variety of reasons, lack of knowledge regarding medical science including clinical trials, and periodic outbreaks of "viral" ideas that have little or no factual basis, can all contribute to false perceptions of well-founded medical interventions (Enria et al. 2016; Mackay 1841; Tanner et al. 2015). Community involvement in trial design, execution, and oversight can help bridge some of this distrust and lead to increased participation (Dickert and Sugarman 2005). Longer-term engagement between communities of interest and research enterprises can afford additional opportunities to identify true stakeholders, understand and dispel fears and concerns, and result in better uptake of MCMs.

4 Research, Public Health, and Healthcare Capacity as Synergistic Forces for EID Response

Research cannot be separated from public health and clinical care functions associated with EID response, either during outbreaks or between them. Efforts to improve research capacity need to be intimately tied to the struggle for universal health coverage and health systems strengthening. Although not in themselves sufficient, a strong public health and healthcare system are essential for building preparedness capacity, and especially research capacity (Lal et al. 2021). The challenges faced by limited-resource areas in detecting and responding to EID outbreaks, especially in the case of a novel pathogen, are exacerbated by limitations of their public health and healthcare institutions, which are faced with the need to gather scientific knowledge about these pathogens through research-grade diagnostics and may then be called upon to evaluate novel vaccines and therapeutics through regulatory-level clinical trials. Without a strong health system to support it, research capacity is not sustainable in any country, leaving foreign partners to provide the bulk of resources for emergency research in LMICs, slowing research implementation while infrastructure systems are installed and perpetuating North–South inequality.

Scientific knowledge about the epidemiology, pathophysiology, and ecological and social factors contributing to the spread of EIDs evolves with outbreak response and with further data collection. Moreover, EID symptoms often mimic common endemic diseases, such as malaria (particularly in the early phases of the disease), and affect the same populations (WHO 2014). About half of the world's population still lacks access to essential health services, and many healthcare facilities in resource-limited settings have scant diagnostic capacity (Pai et al. 2019; WHO 2017a). Nearly 90 new human pathogens have been discovered since 1980, and more new pathogens are emerging every decade, underscoring the importance of continual surveillance, both disease specific and capable of detecting an emergent pathogen (Jones et al. 2008; Woolhouse and Gaunt 2007).

Far from those working in Geneva, Brussels, or Washington to establish adequate global surveillance for infectious diseases are communities that may or may not have access to healthcare. The delays in diagnosis and treatment that affect them can mean the progression of EID case clusters to outbreaks or epidemics. Early detection of EID cases through strong healthcare and public health infrastructure can help decrease transmission both in communities and in nosocomial settings if surveillance leads to timely isolation of patients and infection prevention and control (Hitchcock et al. 2007). Surveillance and rapid diagnosis can also improve patient outcomes through early presentation to care. At the individual patient level, confirmed laboratory diagnosis of patients with EIDs can expedite appropriate clinical care. At the population level, laboratory capacities can help determine the burden of existing infectious diseases and provide information for policy-making and resource allocation. When laboratory capacity for EIDs is linked to national public health systems and utilized in alignment with surveillance programs for endemic diseases, it can also help reveal data about coinfections and shifting disease patterns (Petersen et al. 2019). Such data about disease distribution are particularly important for the future of global health security: vector and host density and geographical spread are shifting with climate change and other social and ecological factors.

Global surveillance for influenza and novel respiratory pathogens requires widespread laboratory research capacity. In fact, WHO's 2019–2030 Global Influenza Strategy highlights the importance of research on viral characteristics and surveillance for variants/strains, diagnostics and countermeasures, and operational research for prevention, control, and MCM delivery as part of national capacities for preparedness and response against novel influenza strains (WHO 2019a). Other public health capabilities, such as data reporting and contact tracing, linked with laboratory capacity can help answer scientific questions about emerging diseases. For example, a viral genomic study paired with clinical and epidemiological data shed light on the possible sexual transmission of Ebola from an Ebola virus disease survivor over 15 months after symptom onset (Diallo et al. 2016).

The development of diagnostic assays during outbreaks with novel viruses needs to occur in near real time after pathogen identification, highlighting the importance of strong national public health laboratories (Roberts and Maslow 2018). Even for some infectious diseases that were discovered decades ago, few facile diagnostics are available, whether because the genetic diversity of the pathogen helps it elude identification or because of limited investment in development, testing, and commercialization of appropriate diagnostics (Cnops et al. 2019; Raabe and Koehler 2017). The development of diagnostic assays for many viral hemorrhagic fever pathogens, for example, requires maximum containment laboratories, most of them in high-income countries, and yet testing for the diagnostic efficacy of any new assays needs to occur where and when outbreaks of these pathogens occur—often in low-resource regions of low-income countries (Carpenter and Bhadelia 2019). LMICs need public health laboratories with the bandwidth and resources to conduct such research alongside their other functions. Technological advances such as next-generation sequencing present increasing promise for continuous surveillance, rapid diagnosis, and tracking of cases during outbreaks. Strengthening public health laboratory infrastructure and related human resources in LMICs is critical to the full realization of the promise of these technologies (Gardy and Loman 2018).

As with laboratory functions, the development of core functions in healthcare delivery can contribute to both research and public health response to EIDs. In the 2018–2020 North Kivu and Ituri EVD outbreak in the Democratic Republic of the Congo, for example, up to 18% of new cases were thought to be nosocomial in origin (Aruna et al. 2019; WHO AFRO 2019). In many LMIC healthcare settings, general infection control and prevention (IPC) remain weak due to lack of resources and training among healthcare workers (Vilar-Compte et al. 2017). Thus, in a large outbreak in a low-income country, seeking healthcare is a double-edged sword: patients receive care, which may be of doubtful efficacy with a disease like EVD, they are isolated from family and friends, and they may be at risk for transmission if proper cohorting and infection control is not followed (Weber et al. 2016).

Strong healthcare systems respond to this challenge through the designation of properly equipped spaces for patient isolation and care, investment in IPC resources and systems, and training healthcare workers to make IPC functional and effective. The existence of this basic infrastructure serves as a bedrock capacity on which clinical research can be safely and rigorously conducted, while decreasing transmission of common infectious diseases as well as the outbreak under investigation. When this is a viral hemorrhagic fever, research and clinical care both need to be conducted under a strict infection control methodology, which has usually meant restrictive personal protective equipment (▶ In Practice 40.1) (Raj et al. 2019). During viral hemorrhagic fever (VHF) outbreaks, healthcare workers in LMICs have often been asked to overcome a lack of both basic resources and training and are expected to perform at an expert level with personal protective equipment they are not accustomed to. In West Africa and in other VHF outbreaks, fear of nosocomial transmission on the part of healthcare workers limited the extent of clinical care in Ebola treatment units (ETUs), while infected people who feared the treatment units contributed to spread in the community (Roddy et al. 2011). Clinical research in VHF clinical units adds an extra level of complexity, requiring healthcare workers to spend more time at bedside and perform new activities beyond their clinical training—though they should be supplemented by research staff who can share patient care tasks, just as the clinical care workers provide research support (▶ In Practice 17.1). IPC training and experience providing care within biocontainment settings prior to outbreaks can increase healthcare worker comfort and ability to adjust to new and more complicated tasks (Hewlett et al. 2015), and of course experienced research staff are an invaluable addition to any research program in such conditions.

Centers of excellence that combine clinical care and research can increase scientific understanding of the natural history of EIDs by allowing accurate, relatively routine collection of granular data about patients. Over the longer term, such facilities can provide data for standardization of medical care and improve supportive care, which in turn allows for a more accurate perspective on the efficacy of experimental MCMs (Bhadelia et al. 2019). The Joint Mobile Emerging Diseases Incident Control Capability (JMEDICC) program, for example, has worked with Ugandan partners to establish a viral hemorrhagic fever clinical care unit in Fort Portal, Uganda. A collaboration between U.S. and Ugandan partners, including the Ugandan Ministry of Health, JMEDICC is funded by the U.S. Department of Defense. It illustrates the benefits of long-term training for healthcare workers in laboratory operations, patient care, and clinical research, offering a platform for research and clinical capacities.

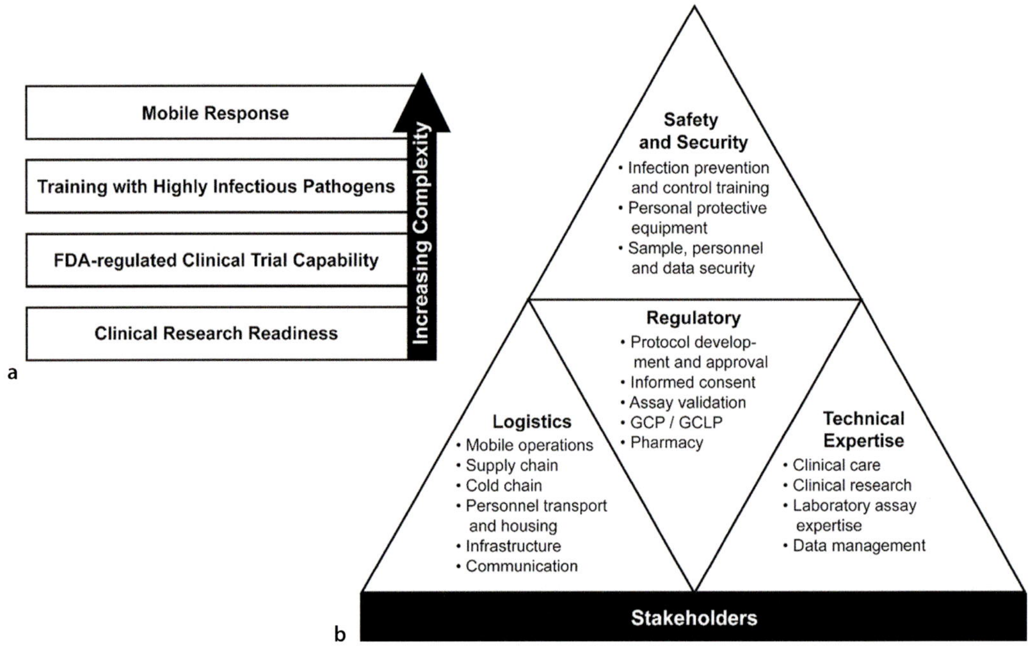

Fig. 3 JMEDICC execution schematic highlighting **a** JMEDICC approach of increasing complexity as competency is established and **b** the multifaceted nature of the project preparedness and response. *JMEDICC* Joint Mobile Emerging Disease Clinical Capability. (Naluyima et al. 2019)

Between VHF outbreaks, the collaboration conducts research on sepsis and febrile illnesses, and during outbreaks it pivots to conducting clinical research while providing high level clinical care for VHF patients. The staff is trained in conducting clinical research and patient care as well as IPC and biocontainment, along with many other skills needed for conducting a research operation (Fig. 3). Over a period of 3 years, such training has helped improve staff confidence and ability to provide high-quality care for highly communicable diseases and other endemic infections and increased capacity for clinical research. JMEDICC has worked with the Ugandan government and other response partners to receive ethical approvals and performed protocol-specific training for promising medical countermeasures against endemic VHF, allowing the organization to respond quickly and with appropriate resources and skills to new outbreaks in the area (Naluyima et al. 2019).

The value of such established clinical centers of excellence is also apparent when one examines the need for long-term follow-up of clinical research participants in outbreak research programs in resource-limited settings. For example, tracking adverse events following immunizations (AEFIs) in poor communities during the post-study period is challenging, as many participants may no longer have access to reliable medical care. In many of the Ebola vaccine trials, AEFI were recorded either when patients returned for follow up or during home visits by community health liaisons. Many LMICs do not have good national systems for tracking AEFIs in the post marketing period and "while clinical trial sponsors are responsible to put in place the safety assessment and reporting systems, there are often no national guidelines defining requirements for this safety monitoring" (Chen et al. 2015).

5 COVID-19 and Lessons for Research Capacity Strengthening

The COVID-19 pandemic painfully illustrated that lack of research and data analysis infrastructure limits our ability to answer important scientific and epidemiological questions about how the severe acute respiratory syndrome coronavirus 2 (SARS-

CoV-2) is affected populations in LMICs (Gupta et al. 2020). Where richer countries themselves continued to struggle to gather comprehensive, accurate data on COVID-19 for public policy during a crisis, in many resource-limited settings data on the pandemic, including basics like numbers of cases and deaths, were even less adequate (Tracking covid-19 excess deaths across countries 2022).

Currently, our overall understanding of COVID-19, despite worldwide research on an unprecedented scale, is limited by the very uneven distribution of that research. For example, mapping of human T cell epitopes after infection is starkly limited to populations in high-income countries (Sette and Crotty 2021). Additionally, global surveillance for new variants is woefully insufficient due to limited laboratory infrastructure to conduct viral genomic research in many parts of the world (Schmidt 2021).

Moreover, even after highly effective vaccines against SARS-CoV-2 completed clinical trials, most low-income countries have received little vaccine. Although the COVAX facility, designed to improve LMIC access to vaccines, had some success with broader distribution, it fell well short of early expectations (Goldhill 2021). Among the factors hindering something closer to universal distribution are insufficient global manufacturing capacity, lack of intellectual property rights agreements, lack of technical production know-how, and raw material supply shortages and disruptions (Asundi et al. 2021). However, efforts such as WHO's mRNA technology transfer hub have been catalysts in knowledge sharing. Many vaccine manufacturers tried to expand manufacturing through "fill and finish" plants, where products are sent in bulk for the last stage of vaccine production in Global South countries. Through regional cooperation and global commitment, countries like Senegal and Rwanda are advancing their capacity for "end to end" vaccine manufacturing, not only for COVID-19 vaccines but also potential mRNA vaccine candidates for tuberculosis and malaria (Burger 2021; Jerving 2021). The fact that vaccines and therapeutics have yet to reach many populations, especially those who might be especially affected by deleterious social determinants of health, makes it harder to get a clear picture of the effectiveness of MCMs in diverse populations.

The experience of the WHO Solidarity trial, a large global randomized controlled trial evaluating the efficacy of COVID-19 therapeutics, highlights the importance of multinational research collaboration, which can recruit diverse patient populations rapidly to answer critical clinical questions during pandemics. It also provides a framework of how diverse health systems with differing research capacity can be engaged in research through adaptive trial design and simple procedures (Krause et al. 2020; WHO Solidarity Trial Consortium 2021). The Solidarity trial has enrolled 2000 researchers from 52 countries and continues to serve as platform to answer new therapeutic questions during the COVID-19 pandemic. The COVID-19 pandemic demonstrated both the cost of not having an equitable research landscape, but also how resources can be mobilized when there is funding and the will for new methodologies for global engagement in evidence generation.

6 Systemic Challenges to LMIC Research Capacity Strengthening

Improving LMIC biomedical research capacity requires, first and foremost, an equitable approach to research in resource-limited settings and a commitment to continuous investments (Bamako call to action: research for health 2008). Coordination between funders and other partners is needed to reduce duplicative efforts for preparedness and when emergency research response is required.

A long-term funding commitment needs to include recognition by national governments of the importance of research as an integral part of a functional healthcare system and continued willingness to make the corresponding investments. At the 2008 Global Ministerial Forum on Research in Health in Bamako, Mali, 60 countries committed to the

Bamako call to action: research for health (2008). However, in many countries such investment still accounts for less than 0.5% of gross domestic product (Fosci et al. 2019). Similarly, lack of consistent, long-term investment from global funders is an important barrier to a sustainable research sector in LMICs. The public interest and governmental attention garnered during the COVID-19 pandemic can be used to energize more lasting financial commitments to this issue, particularly through platforms like the Global Preparedness Monitoring Board (Eigbike 2020).

A recent ESSENCE on Health Research report also highlighted the importance of structured efforts to facilitate shared learning and strengthen collaboration to coordinate research capacity programs in LMICs. Such efforts can reduce duplication and identify gaps to be addressed (Eigbike 2020). Lastly, research collaborations between high-income and LMIC researchers often benefit the former disproportionately in terms of academic advancement. Despite the existence of guidelines for equitable research partnerships, a devil lurks in the details of how academic institutions in high-income countries assess individual faculty members based on grants and publications, which creates an inherent disincentive to open space for LMIC research leadership (Walsh et al. 2016). Without getting into questions of whether the current incentive structure needs wholesale revision or modest reform, clearly efforts are needed by funders and institutions to make cooperation and capacity strengthening rewarding in career terms for researchers (Hedt-Gauthier et al. 2018).

7 Conclusion

The COVID pandemic has crystalized the need for global scientific solidarity. Whether by improving our ability to detect new outbreaks and new pathogens, reducing the time to emergency research implementation, maximizing our engagement with affected communities, or better reflecting national and regional research priorities, strong research capacity in LMICs and its integration into global EID outbreak response research is critical to our survival. The COVID-19 experience has the potential to provide political and social impetus toward new models of collaboration, which can improve global resilience against new threats. Whether that potential will be realized is for us to determine in the very near future.

Discussion Questions

1. Define societal resilience. Discuss some resilience elements and contributing factors.
2. In many low-income settings, research programs and capacity funding decisions are made in high-income donor countries, and the capacity and research that follow may not align well with needs on the ground. How can LMICs better align research capacity investments to local priorities and needs?
3. Fostering resilient health capacity requires, (a) investing in *researchers* from LMICs, (b) supporting the *research institutions* that house them, (c) working with national governments to improve *regulatory oversight*, (d) overcoming *operational shortcomings* for programs and products, and (e) engaging vulnerable *communities* in research partnerships before crises strike. Review ► Sect. 3, choose one or two of these requirements, and discuss their historical precedent, importance, and future directions.
4. Research should support public health and clinical care functions associated with an EID response, both between and during outbreaks. Describe some obstacles to detecting and responding to EID outbreaks in places with few resources.
5. List some needs for strengthening research capacity that became evident during the COVID-19 pandemic.
6. What are the most promising approaches for overcoming systemic challenges to LMIC research capacity strengthening?

References

Aruna A, Mbala P, Minikulu L, Mukadi D, Bulemfu D, Edidi F, et al. Ebola virus disease outbreak—Democratic Republic of the Congo, August 2018–November 2019. MMWR Suppl. 2019;68(50):1162–5. https://doi.org/10.15585/mmwr.mm6850a3.

Asundi A, O'Leary C, Bhadelia N. Global COVID-19 vaccine inequity: the scope, the impact, and the challenges. Cell Host Microbe. 2021;29(7):1036–9. https://doi.org/10.1016/j.chom.2021.06.007.

Bamako call to action: research for health. Lancet. 2008;372(9653):1855. https://doi.org/10.1016/S0140-6736(08)61789-4.

Bedford J, Farrar J, Ihekweazu C, Kang G, Koopmans M, Nkengasong J. A new twenty-first century science for effective epidemic response. Nature. 2019;575(7781):130–6. https://doi.org/10.1038/s41586-019-1717-y.

Bernasconi V, Kristiansen PA, Whelan M, Román RG, Bettis A, Yimer SA, et al. Developing vaccines against epidemic-prone emerging infectious diseases. Bundesgesundheitsblatt Gesundheitsforschung Gesundheitsschutz. 2020;63(1):65–73. https://doi.org/10.1007/s00103-019-03061-2.

Bhadelia N, Sauer L, Cieslak TJ, Davey RT, McLellan S, Uyeki TM, et al. Evaluating promising investigational medical countermeasures: recommendations in the absence of guidelines. Health Secur. 2019;17(1):46–53. https://doi.org/10.1089/hs.2018.0092.

Bridbord K, Weymouth KH, Puderbaugh A, Wolfman C, Belter CW, Breman JG, et al. Fifty years of supporting global health research at the NIH Fogarty International Center. Ann Glob Health. 2019;85(1):43. https://doi.org/10.5334/aogh.2432.

Burger L. BioNTech eyes Rwanda, Senegal for malaria, tuberculosis vaccine production. Reuters; 2021.

Carpenter S, Bhadelia N. Maximum containment infectious disease laboratories as an integral part of emergency preparedness and emergency response. In: Singh SK, Kuhn J, editors. Defense against biological attacks. 1st ed. New York: Springer; 2019. p. 125–44.

Chen RT, Shimabukuro TT, Martin DB, Zuber PL, Weibel DM, Sturkenboom M. Enhancing vaccine safety capacity globally: a lifecycle perspective. Vaccine. 2015;33(Suppl 4):D46–54. https://doi.org/10.1016/j.vaccine.2015.06.073.

Cnops L, De Smet B, Mbala-Kingebeni P, van Griensven J, Ahuka-Mundeke S, Arien KK. Where are the Ebola diagnostics from last time? Nature. 2019;565(7740):419–21. https://doi.org/10.1038/d41586-019-00212-y.

Coloma J, Harris E. From construction workers to architects: developing scientific research capacity in low-income countries. PLoS Biol. 2009;7(7):e1000156. https://doi.org/10.1371/journal.pbio.1000156.

Dean L, Njelesani J, Smith H, Bates I. Promoting sustainable research partnerships: a mixed-method evaluation of a United Kingdom–Africa capacity strengthening award scheme. Health Res Policy Syst. 2015;13:81. https://doi.org/10.1186/s12961-015-0071-2.

DePasse J, Caldwell A, Santorino D. Affordable medical technologies: bringing Value-Based Design into global health. BMJ Innov. 2016;2:2–7. https://doi.org/10.1136/bmjinnov-2015-000069.

Diallo B, Sissoko D, Loman NJ, Bah HA, Bah H, Worrell MC, et al. Resurgence of Ebola virus disease in Guinea linked to a survivor with virus persistence in seminal fluid for more than 500 days. Clin Infect Dis. 2016;63(10):1353–6. https://doi.org/10.1093/cid/ciw601.

Dickert N, Sugarman J. Ethical goals of community consultation in research. Am J Public Health. 2005;95(7):1123–7. https://doi.org/10.2105/AJPH.2004.058933.

Doe-Anderson J, Baseler B, Driscoll P, Johnson M, Lysander J, McNay L, et al. Beating the odds: successful establishment of a phase II/III clinical research trial in resource-poor Liberia during the largest-ever Ebola outbreak. Contemp Clin Trials Commun. 2016;4:68–73. https://doi.org/10.1016/j.conctc.2016.06.008.

Drain PK, Subbaraman R, Heimburger DC. Preserving the Fogarty International Center—benefits for Americans and the World. N Engl J Med. 2017;377(1):9–11. https://doi.org/10.1056/NEJMp1704690.

Dunn RR, Davies TJ, Harris NC, Gavin MC. Global drivers of human pathogen richness and prevalence. Proc Biol Sci. 2010;277(1694):2587–95. https://doi.org/10.1098/rspb.2010.0340.

Eigbike M. Health research capacity strengthening in low and middle-income countries: current situation and opportunities to leverage data for better coordination and greater impact. Geneva: Mechanism for the review of investments in health research capacity strengthening in low and middle-income countries (LMICs) convened by ESSENCE for Health Research; 2020.

Enria L, Lees S, Smout E, Mooney T, Tengbeh AF, Leigh B, et al. Power, fairness and trust: understanding and engaging with vaccine trial participants and communities in the setting up the EBOVAC-Salone vaccine trial in Sierra Leone. BMC Public Health. 2016;16(1):1140. https://doi.org/10.1186/s12889-016-3799-x.

ESSENCE on Health Research. Seven principles for strengthening research capacity in low- and middle-income countries: simple ideas in a complex world. Geneva: ESSENCE on Health Research; 2014.

Folarin OA, Ehichioya D, Schaffner SF, Winnicki SM, Wohl S, Eromon P, et al. Ebola virus epidemiology and evolution in Nigeria. J Infect Dis. 2016;214(Suppl 3):S102–9. https://doi.org/10.1093/infdis/jiw190.

Fosci M, Loffreda L, Velten L, Johnson R. Research capacity strengthening in LMICs: a rapid evidence

assessment report. London: UK Department for International Development; 2019.
Gardy JL, Loman NJ. Towards a genomics-informed, real-time, global pathogen surveillance system. Nat Rev Genet. 2018;19(1):9–20. https://doi.org/10.1038/nrg.2017.88.
GHSA. Global Health Security Agenda: action packages. Atlanta: U.S. Centers for Disease Control and Prevention; 2014. p. 26.
GHSA. Global Health Security Agenda. GHSA; 2022. https://ghsagenda.org/. Accessed 17 May 2022.
Global Forum for Health Research. Global Forum for Health Research: an overview. Geneva: Global Forum for Health Research; 1999.
Global Forum on Bioethics in Research. Meeting report: Emerging epidemic infections and experimental medical treatments. Annecy, FR: Global Forum on Bioethics in Research; 2015.
Goldhill O. 'Naively ambitious': how COVAX failed on its promise to vaccinate the world. Stat News. 2021.
Gupta M, Wahl B, Adhikari B, Bar-Zeev N, Bhandari S, Coria A, et al. The need for COVID-19 research in low- and middle-income countries. Glob Health Res Policy. 2020;5:33. https://doi.org/10.1186/s41256-020-00159-y.
Hedt-Gauthier B, Airhihenbuwa CO, Bawah AA, Burke KS, Cherian T, Connelly MT, et al. Academic promotion policies and equity in global health collaborations. Lancet. 2018;392(10158):1607–9. https://doi.org/10.1016/S0140-6736(18)32345-6.
Hewlett AL, Varkey JB, Smith PW, Ribner BS. Ebola virus disease: preparedness and infection control lessons learned from two biocontainment units. Curr Opin Infect Dis. 2015;28(4):343–8. https://doi.org/10.1097/QCO.0000000000000176.
Hitchcock P, Chamberlain A, Van Wagoner M, Inglesby TV, O'Toole T. Challenges to global surveillance and response to infectious disease outbreaks of international importance. Biosecur Bioterror. 2007;5(3):206–27. https://doi.org/10.1089/bsp.2007.0041.
IBRD. Sub-Saharan African science, technology, engineering, and mathematics research: a decade of development. Washington, DC: International Bank for Reconstruction and Development/The World Bank; 2016.
IFC. The business of health in Africa: partnering with the private sector to improve people's lives. Washington, DC: International Finance Corporation; 2008.
InterAcademy Council. Enhancing the capacity of African science academies: the final evaluation of ASADI. InterAcademy Council; 2015. Contract No.: ISBN 978 90 6984 698 9.
Izugbara CO, Kabiru CW, Amendah D, Dimbuene ZT, Donfouet HPP, Atake EH, et al. "It takes more than a fellowship program": reflections on capacity strengthening for health systems research in sub-Saharan Africa. BMC Health Serv Res. 2017;17(Suppl 2):696. https://doi.org/10.1186/s12913-017-2638-9.
Jerving S. AU launches partnership for African vaccine manufacturing. DEVEX. 2021.
Jones KE, Patel NG, Levy MA, Storeygard A, Balk D, Gittleman JL, et al. Global trends in emerging infectious diseases. Nature. 2008;451(7181):990–3. https://doi.org/10.1038/nature06536.
Käser M, Maure C, Halpaap BM, Vahedi M, Yamaka S, Launois P, et al. Research capacity strengthening in low and middle income countries—an evaluation of the WHO/TDR Career Development Fellowship Programme. PLoS Negl Trop Dis. 2016;10(5):e0004631. https://doi.org/10.1371/journal.pntd.0004631.
Kay S. Africa's leadership in biomedical research: shifting the center of gravity. Sci Transl Med. 2015;7(314):314ed13. https://doi.org/10.1126/scitranslmed.aad5529.
Krause P, Fleming TR, Longini I, Henao-Restrepo AM, Peto R, World Health Organization Solidarity Vaccines Trial Expert Group. COVID-19 vaccine trials should seek worthwhile efficacy. Lancet. 2020;396(10253):741–3. https://doi.org/10.1016/s0140-6736(20)31821-3.
Kucharski A, Piot P. Containing Ebola virus infection in West Africa. Euro Surveill. 2014;19(36):20899. https://doi.org/10.2807/1560-7917.es2014.19.36.20899.
Lal A, Erondu NA, Heymann DL, Gitahi G, Yates R. Fragmented health systems in COVID-19: rectifying the misalignment between global health security and universal health coverage. Lancet. 2021;397(10268):61–7. https://doi.org/10.1016/S0140-6736(20)32228-5.
Lescano AG, Cohen CR, Raj T, Rispel L, Garcia PJ, Zunt JR, et al. Strengthening mentoring in low- and middle-income countries to advance global health research: an overview. Am J Trop Med Hyg. 2019;100(1_Suppl):3–8. https://doi.org/10.4269/ajtmh.18-0556.
Mackay C. Extraordinary popular delusions and the madness of crowds. London: Richard Bentley; 1841.
Mahmood S, Hort K, Ahmed S, Salam M, Cravioto A. Strategies for capacity building for health research in Bangladesh: role of core funding and a common monitoring and evaluation framework. Health Res Policy Syst. 2011;9:31. https://doi.org/10.1186/1478-4505-9-31.
Marsh K. How Africa can close its continent-wide science funding gap. The Conversation. 2016.
Marston HD, Paules CI, Fauci AS. The critical role of biomedical research in pandemic preparedness. JAMA. 2017;318(18):1757–8. https://doi.org/10.1001/jama.2017.15033.
McGregor S, Henderson KJ, Kaldor JM. How are health research priorities set in low and middle income countries? A systematic review of published reports. PLoS One. 2014;9(9):e108787. https://doi.org/10.1371/journal.pone.0108787.
Murray KA, Preston N, Allen T, Zambrana-Torrelio C, Hosseini PR, Daszak P. Global biogeography of

human infectious diseases. Proc Natl Acad Sci USA. 2015;112(41):12746–51. https://doi.org/10.1073/pnas.1507442112.
Naluyima P, Kayondo W, Ritchie C, Wandege J, Kagabane S, Tumubeere L, et al. The Joint Mobile Emerging Disease Clinical Capability (JMEDICC) laboratory approach: capabilities for high-consequence pathogen clinical research. PLoS Negl Trop Dis. 2019;13(12):e0007787. https://doi.org/10.1371/journal.pntd.0007787.
NAM. The neglected dimension of global security: a framework to counter infectious disease crises. Washington, DC: National Academy of Medicine; 2016.
NASEM. Conducting clinical research during an epidemic. In: Busta ER, Mancher M, Cuff PA, McAdam K, Keusch G, editors. Integrating clinical research into epidemic response: the Ebola experience. Washington, DC: National Academices Press; 2017. p. 37–82.
National Academies of Sciences Engineering and Medicine. Strengthening capacity for response and research. In: Gerald Keusch KM, Cuff PA, Mancher M, Busta ER, editors. Integrating clinical research into epidemic response: the Ebola experience. Washington, DC: The National Academies Press; 2017. p. 342.
Ng LC, Hanlon C, Yimer G, Henderson DC, Fekadu A. Ethics in global health research: the need for balance. Lancet Glob Health. 2015;3(9):e516–7. https://doi.org/10.1016/S2214-109X(15)00095-9.
Nguyen V-K. An epidemic of suspicion—Ebola and violence in the DRC. N Engl J Med. 2019;380:1298. https://doi.org/10.1056/NEJMp1902682.
Nuzzo JB, Meyer D, Snyder M, Ravi SJ, Lapascu A, Souleles J, et al. What makes health systems resilient against infectious disease outbreaks and natural hazards? Results from a scoping review. BMC Public Health. 2019;19(1):1310. https://doi.org/10.1186/s12889-019-7707-z.
Olu OO. The Ebola virus disease outbreak in West Africa: a wake-up call to revitalize implementation of the International Health Regulations. Front Public Health. 2016;4:120. https://doi.org/10.3389/fpubh.2016.00120.
Our World in Data. Spending on research and development as share of GDP, 1996–2014. Oxford: Our World in Data; 2022. https://ourworldindata.org/grapher/research-and-development-expenditure-of-gdp?tab=chart&country=OWID_WRL~ISR~KOR~CHN~IND~USA~Africa+Western+and+Central~Africa+Eastern+and+Southern. Accessed 2 Feb 2022.
Pai M, Boehme C, Kickbusch I. Diagnostics are essential for universal health coverage to succeed. Stat News. 2019.
Perry L, Malkin R. Effectiveness of medical equipment donations to improve health systems: how much medical equipment is broken in the developing world? Med Biol Eng Comput. 2011;49(7):719–22. https://doi.org/10.1007/s11517-011-0786-3.
Peters DH, Keusch GT, Cooper J, Davis S, Lundgren J, Mello MM, et al. In search of global governance for research in epidemics. Lancet. 2017;390(10103):1632–3. https://doi.org/10.1016/S0140-6736(17)32546-1.
Petersen E, Abubakar I, Ihekweazu C, Heymann D, Ntoumi F, Blumberg L, et al. Monkeypox—enhancing public health preparedness for an emerging lethal human zoonotic epidemic threat in the wake of the smallpox post-eradication era. Int J Infect Dis. 2019;78:78–84. https://doi.org/10.1016/j.ijid.2018.11.008.
Pratt B, Hyder AA. Governance of global health research consortia: sharing sovereignty and resources within future health systems. Soc Sci Med. 2017;174:113–21. https://doi.org/10.1016/j.socscimed.2016.11.039.
Raabe V, Koehler J. Laboratory diagnosis of Lassa fever. J Clin Microbiol. 2017;55(6):1629–37. https://doi.org/10.1128/JCM.00170-17.
Raj D, Hornsey E, Perl TM. Personal protective equipment for viral hemorrhagic fevers. Curr Opin Infect Dis. 2019;32(4):337–47. https://doi.org/10.1097/QCO.0000000000000562.
Rani M, Bekedam H, Buckley BS, World Health Organization Regional Office for the Western Pacific. Improving health research governance and management in the Western Pacific: a WHO expert consultation. J Evid Based Med. 2011;4(4):204–13. https://doi.org/10.1111/j.1756-5391.2011.01161.x.
Roberts CC, Maslow JN. Assay challenges for emerging infectious diseases: the Zika experience. Vaccines (Basel). 2018;6(4):70. https://doi.org/10.3390/vaccines6040070.
Roddy P, Colebunders R, Jeffs B, Palma PP, Van Herp M, Borchert M. Filovirus hemorrhagic fever outbreak case management: a review of current and future treatment options. J Infect Dis. 2011;204(Suppl 3):S791–5. https://doi.org/10.1093/infdis/jir297.
Sadanadan R, Arunkumar G, Laserson KF, Heretik KH, Singh S, Mourya DT, et al. Towards global health security: response to the May 2018 Nipah virus outbreak linked to Pteropus bats in Kerala, India. BMJ Glob Health. 2018;3(6):e001086. https://doi.org/10.1136/bmjgh-2018-001086.
Sahay RR, Yadav PD, Gupta N, Shete AM, Radhakrishnan C, Mohan G, et al. Experiential learnings from the Nipah virus outbreaks in Kerala towards containment of infectious public health emergencies in India. Epidemiol Infect. 2020;148:e90. https://doi.org/10.1017/S0950268820000825.
Salami K, Gsell PS, Olayinka A, Maiga D, Formenty P, Smith PG, et al. Meeting report: WHO consultation on accelerating Lassa fever vaccine development in endemic countries, Dakar, 10–11 September 2019. Vaccine. 2020;38(26):4135–41. https://doi.org/10.1016/j.vaccine.2020.01.017.
Schmidt C. New coronavirus variants are urgently being tracked around the world. Sci Am. 2021.

Sette A, Crotty S. Adaptive immunity to SARS-CoV-2 and COVID-19. Cell. 2021;184(4):861–80. https://doi.org/10.1016/j.cell.2021.01.007.

Sheikh K, Agyepong I, Jhalani M, Ammar W, Hafeez A, Pyakuryal S, et al. Learning health systems: an empowering agenda for low-income and middle-income countries. Lancet. 2020;395(10223):476–7. https://doi.org/10.1016/s0140-6736(19)33134-4.

Sweileh WM. Global research trends of World Health Organization's top eight emerging pathogens. Glob Health. 2017;13(1):9. https://doi.org/10.1186/s12992-017-0233-9.

Tanner A, Kim SH, Friedman DB, Foster C, Bergeron CD. Barriers to medical research participation as perceived by clinical trial investigators: communicating with rural and African American communities. J Health Commun. 2015;20(1):88–96. https://doi.org/10.1080/10810730.2014.908985.

Tracking covid-19 excess deaths across countries. London: The Economist. 2022. https://www.economist.com/graphic-detail/coronavirus-excess-deaths-tracker. Accessed 13 Mar 2023.

UN. The 17 goals. New York: UN Department of Economic and Social Affairs; 2021. https://sdgs.un.org/goals. Accessed 28 Sept 2021.

Vilar-Compte D, Camacho-Ortiz A, Ponce-de-Leon S. Infection control in limited resources countries: challenges and priorities. Curr Infect Dis Rep. 2017;19(5):20. https://doi.org/10.1007/s11908-017-0572-y.

Walsh A, Brugha R, Byrne E. "The way the country has been carved up by researchers": ethics and power in north-south public health research. Int J Equity Health. 2016;15(1):204. https://doi.org/10.1186/s12939-016-0488-4.

Weber DJ, Rutala WA, Fischer WA, Kanamori H, Sickbert-Bennett EE. Emerging infectious diseases: focus on infection control issues for novel coronaviruses (Severe Acute Respiratory Syndrome-CoV and Middle East Respiratory Syndrome-CoV), hemorrhagic fever viruses (Lassa and Ebola), and highly pathogenic avian influenza viruses, A(H5N1) and A(H7N9). Am J Infect Control. 2016;44(5 Suppl):e91–e100. https://doi.org/10.1016/j.ajic.2015.11.018.

Wernli D, Clausin M, Antulov-Fantulin N, Berezowski J, Biller-Andorno N, Blanchet K, et al. Building a multisystemic understanding of societal resilience to the COVID-19 pandemic. BMJ Glob Health. 2021;6(7):e006794. https://doi.org/10.1136/bmjgh-2021-006794.

WHO. A brief guide to emerging infectious diseases and zoonoses. New Delhi: World Health Organization, Regional Office for South-East Asia; 2014. Report No.: ISBN 978-92-9022-458-7. Contract No.: ISBN 978-92-9022-458-7.

WHO. World Bank and WHO: Half the world lacks access to essential health services, 100 million still pushed into extreme poverty because of health expenses. Tokyo: World Health Organization; 2017a.

WHO. World report on health policy and systems research. Geneva, World Health Organization; 2017b. Contract No.: ISBN 978-92-4-151226-8.

WHO. Lassa fever research and development (R&D) roadmap (draft). Geneva: World Health Organization; 2018.

WHO. Global influenza strategy 2019–2030. WHO; 2019a. Contract No.: ISBN 978-92-4-151532-0.

WHO. SDG Global Action Plan Accelerator 5: R&D, innovation, & access: elevating national research for health priorities to achieve effective scale-up: recommendations. WHO; 2019b.

WHO. WHO target product profiles. Geneva: World Health Organization; 2022. https://www.who.int/observatories/global-observatory-on-health-research-and-development/analyses-and-syntheses/target-product-profile/who-target-product-profiles. Accessed 31 Jan 2022.

WHO AFRO. WHO and partners to help the Government boost health facility defences against Ebola in the Democratic Republic of the Congo. WHO AFRO; 2019.

WHO Solidarity Trial Consortium. Repurposed antiviral drugs for Covid-19—interim WHO Solidarity trial results. N Engl J Med. 2021;384(6):497–511. https://doi.org/10.1056/NEJMoa2023184.

Woolhouse M, Gaunt E. Ecological origins of novel human pathogens. Crit Rev Microbiol. 2007;33(4):231–42. https://doi.org/10.1080/10408410701647560.

Yozwiak NL, Happi CT, Grant DS, Schieffelin JS, Garry RF, Sabeti PC, et al. Roots, not parachutes: research collaborations combat outbreaks. Cell. 2016;166(1):5–8. https://doi.org/10.1016/j.cell.2016.06.029.

9 Laboratory Needs for Research Response

Lisa E. Hensley, John D. Klena, Jason T. DeBoer, Joel M. Montgomery, Placide Mbala, Melissa E. Moses, Katie J. Knapek, and Gene G. Olinger

Contents

Learning Track Note: This chapter appears in Learning Tracks: Clinical Research; Emergency Research Response, Research Operations; Global Health Law (► Sect. 3.3) One Health

E. S. Higgs and R. A. Sorenson (eds.), *Principles and Practice of Emergency Research Response*,
https://doi.org/10.1007/978-3-031-48408-7_11

Learning Objectives

This chapter should enable readers to understand and discuss:

- Limitations of diagnostic assays used to detect new or re-emerging pathogens in animals and the environment
  - The importance of testing samples from various sources and monitoring animal infectious diseases
- Requirements of the response or research program which determine field laboratory criteria
  - Critical elements for the adequacy of a laboratory and clinical research site
  - Determinative factors for the selection of laboratory assays and equipment for research response
- The need for regulatory management tools, expedited evaluation and approval processes, and diagnostic preparedness during an emergency outbreak in low-resource settings
- Challenges to specimen collection, transport, and storage
- The role of effective laboratory biosafety and biosecurity for preventing and controlling infection
- The critical roles of data management and effective documentation for delivering accurate patient test results, epidemiological investigation, and supporting accurate interpretation and implementation of findings from clinical studies
- Key advances in laboratory, point-of-care, and imaging diagnostic tools; applications of innovative diagnostics in outbreaks; and why multiple, versatile diagnostic technologies are important for research response
- How the lack of diagnostic capacity contributed to ongoing transmission of the Ebola virus from a small village in Guinea to the cities of West Africa
- Obstacles that may hinder the rapid deployment of laboratories to outbreak emergencies

1 Introduction

Clinical and research laboratories are indispensable elements of clinical studies to assess candidate medical countermeasures (MCMs), whether for long-duration trials or for trials meant to rapidly establish the safety and efficacy of MCMs in an infectious disease emergency. Over the last two decades, there has been increasing recognition that clinical trials can be central to meeting the goals of emergency response, that is, to (a) save lives and avert suffering, (b) accelerate the end of the outbreak, and (c) develop measures to prevent and mitigate future outbreaks (▶ Introduction 1 and Chap. 3). Not surprisingly, calls to rapidly deploy laboratory assets in response to infectious disease outbreaks or other public health emergencies have markedly increased in the last decade and continue to rise. Historically, diagnostic assays used to detect a new or re-emerging disease have been limited by a lack of commercial availability. When available, often they are highly complex, requiring specialized equipment and multiple steps, and are designed for use in CLIA-certified laboratories.[1] Deployment and scale-up of highly or even moderately complex assays are limited by available infrastructure, including trained personnel, making their use in low-resource settings challenging.

The size and infrastructure requirements for traditional clinical and research equipment and the logistical challenges associated with transporting and operating such equipment have also contributed to limiting the laboratory's role during outbreaks and the ability to support response research, particu-

1 The Clinical Laboratory Improvement Amendments (CLIA) are a U.S. legislative standard that applies not only to clinical labs in the United States, but in many instances to labs outside the United States receiving U.S. grant monies. International Standards Organization (ISO) 15189 is the prevailing standard in EU countries as well as many others around the world.

larly in low-resource and remote environments (▶ Chaps. 37 and 38). As a result, the footprint of the deployed laboratory has often been small, and the range of assays performed restricted. Technological advances have led to the development of smaller, more rapid, and more robust equipment designed to use commercially available assays that can be performed at or near the point of patient care. This equipment is designed for lower complexity assays and requires minimal operation and data processing training. The availability of assays to detect high-consequence but low-frequency pathogens and emerging diseases has increased, including assays for use near or at the point of care. These newer-generation assays often have improved sensitivity and specificity. Advances in genomic sequencing have slashed the time and cost of sequencing novel pathogens, facilitating the rapid development of candidate diagnostic assays and vaccines (▶ Chaps. 11 and 12). As these newer technologies and assays have made it to the field, the role of the laboratory has been reimagined, setting a new standard for what is possible, even in the most remote settings.

2 Who, What, Where, When, and Why

Multiple outbreak-associated factors, along with the requirements of the response or research program, define the requirements of the field laboratory. The requirements, combined with local capacities and available infrastructure, will shape the capability and capacity of the field laboratory. Often, these are described as the "Who? What? Where? When? Why?" of the laboratory response (◘ Fig. 1). Command and control in a dynamic, high-stress environment are critical. The laboratory response must be nested within the larger outbreak response efforts, requiring coordination with local and national authorities, partner agencies, and healthcare providers. Partnership requires defining *who* will be responsible for the infrastructure, supply, set-up, and operation of the laboratory response. Partners should coordinate to prevent duplication of effort or waste of limited resources and ensure that efforts are meeting host country needs. "Who" also includes the research participants and their communities.

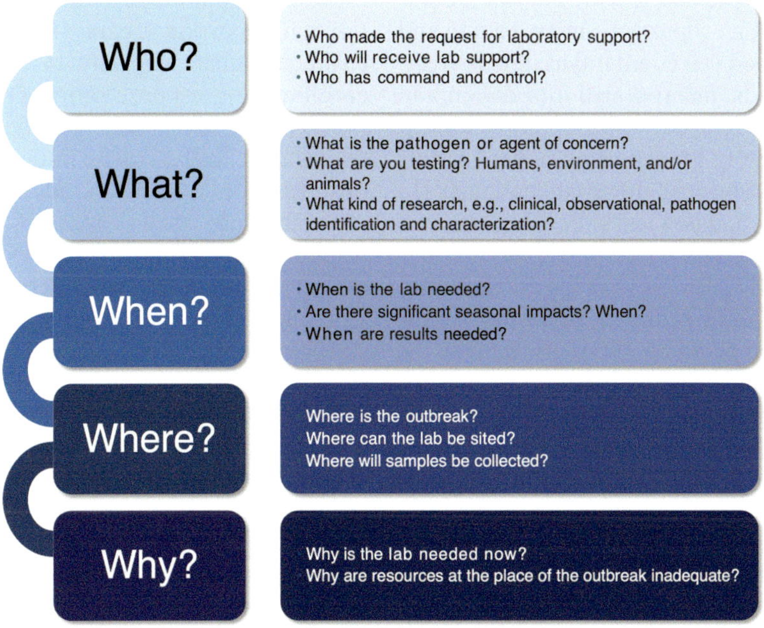

◘ **Fig. 1** Key outbreak-associated factors for field laboratories in low-resource environments. (Authors)

It is essential to recognize that the laboratory is one component of a larger response effort and must be integrated into the response framework as a whole. Many aspects of the logistical arrangements needed for a research program in a low-resource environment are described in Book Part VII.

The *what* includes the availability of assays suited to the etiological agent of the outbreak, the sample types to be tested, and the requirements for qualitative or quantitative results, which will determine equipment and assay choices. The availability, feasibility, complexity, and cost will narrow or refine selections. In some cases, especially with a novel pathogen, no assay may be available, requiring the rapid development and validation of diagnostic assays before a laboratory can be fully deployed or engaged. The agent/pathogen will drive biosafety and biosecurity needs, including personal protective equipment (PPE), inactivation and decontamination methods, and infrastructure requirements. Depending on the cause of the outbreak, vaccines, pre- and post-exposure prophylaxis, and reliable therapeutics may or may not be available. As patient care becomes a larger part of the response, the need for the laboratory to provide routine clinical laboratory results (e.g., clinical chemistry testing and complete blood cell counts) that impact treatment should be incorporated into design and deployments. To avoid downstream complications, a pathway for reporting patient results while protecting patient confidentiality (to whom, when, and how) must be delineated and strictly adhered to.

Where, when, and why are the greatest drivers of laboratory size and scope. Initial considerations when planning a response include the current size and geographical scope of the crisis and its projected trajectory. These will be overlaid with the distribution of treatment facilities, transport networks for moving samples and materials rapidly (roads, water, and air routes), and the availability of existing laboratories within the region. Several important factors must be considered when selecting a specific site for the laboratory (see ▶ Sect. 3.1). Dialogue with and input from local communities and community leaders is essential prior to laboratory deployments (▶ Chap. 18).

Time is critical in emergency response management. In the laboratory, processing time, assay run time, results reporting, and resupply times must all be planned for. Long wait times for lab results can delay access to treatment, increase the risk of transmission or exposure in quarantine facilities, and discourage patients or potential trial participants. Prolonged transport time or insufficient capacity may degrade sample quality, make results less reliable, and hinder interpretation. Geographically dispersed outbreaks may require the mobilization of multiple laboratories to minimize these variables.

The terms of reference for the laboratory must be clearly defined and prioritized at the onset of operational planning. Early engagement of the laboratory in the design of a clinical trial will help ensure the success of the protocol and the laboratory. Laboratory testing is often essential for determining suitability for enrollment of participants and reliably observing primary and secondary study endpoints. Upon finalization of the operational requirements or study design, the laboratory can identify suitable assays that will meet the needs of the study, procure necessary equipment and supplies, develop data documentation and reporting streams (▶ Chap. 35), and ensure adequate capacity to support study enrollment or response efforts. Once the laboratory is established, additional service requests are likely to arise in the course of an outbreak or research study. Building or strengthening local capacity to enhance response and promote local resilience is an ethical requirement, often a political necessity, and a practical priority for laboratory staff and operations. Local staff bring cultural and geographical knowledge, have ties with local communities, and provide continuity in cases where expatriate employees rotate in and out—the usual practice where there are hardship conditions or during prolonged response efforts (▶ Chap. 42). Early engagement of the laboratory during the planning of response efforts and research protocol development is required regardless of the resource level of the study location to prevent delays and minimize potential failures of the studies.

3 Field Laboratories

"Field" or "mobile" laboratories are terms often used interchangeably to describe a temporary structure or facility to collect, process, analyze, and report results on samples received from outbreak patients. As mentioned in the previous section, the size and scope of the laboratory will vary depending on many factors, and emergency deployment is not restricted to low-resource environments. Mobile laboratories have been used for decades in various capacities, including routine surveillance, outbreak response, and research activities (Racine and Kobinger 2019). Over time, the contents and capabilities of mobile labs have evolved to meet the specific needs of outbreak situations. Mobile laboratories for disease diagnostics typically include diagnostic instruments and equipment necessary for detecting and characterizing infectious agents, which must be matched appropriately with the mobile laboratory design. Mobile laboratories have demonstrated their efficacy in disease diagnostics through successful evaluations with simulated specimens (training) and during outbreaks (Roh et al. 2022; Xing et al. 2021). These labs offer the advantage of rapid and flexible deployment to disease transmission hotspots and austere locations, often in resource-constrained settings. Many labs have been expanded to include clinical assay support to guide case management and support response research, including clinical studies. The laboratory design can be as simple as a specimen tent and a lab in a suitcase to vehicles in a range of sizes designed to provide or deliver laboratory space, such as hardened laboratory containers that can remain functional as a laboratory well beyond a typical outbreak response (◘ Fig. 2). Regardless of the size, shape, or location of the laboratory, the same quality and safety standards should always be implemented.

3.1 Where? Site Location

The following three critical elements must be considered during the site selection process for a laboratory.

- Safety
  - Personal safety
  - Biosafety
  - Biosecurity
- Outbreak response requirements
  - Surveillance and epidemiology
    - Diagnostics
    - Pathogen identification and characterization
  - Patient treatment needs
  - Clinical research data collection and analysis
- Data quality and integrity

The laboratory should be placed where the public health response can be addressed while balancing the needs and safety of the staff. The lab must be close enough to diagnosis and treatment centers to allow samples to be transported, received, and assayed promptly, in a way that does not compromise the testing results. Where roads are unpaved or security is poor, this may mean that laboratories need to be co-located with medical care facilities (◘ Fig. 4). In situations where the outbreak that has spread over a wide geographical area there may be a need for multiple laboratories. As the outbreak evolves, the location, size, and number of laboratories may need to be adjusted. A site location matrix (◘ Fig. 3) is a useful tool for comparing the advantages and disadvantages of candidate sites.

The laboratory site must allow for the work to be conducted without compromising biosafety or data integrity. "Biosafety" refers to procedures intended to protect against infection from or release of harmful biological agents, including the ability to effectively respond to a potential laboratory exposure or accident. Ideally, the laboratory is established as early as possible in an outbreak to perform

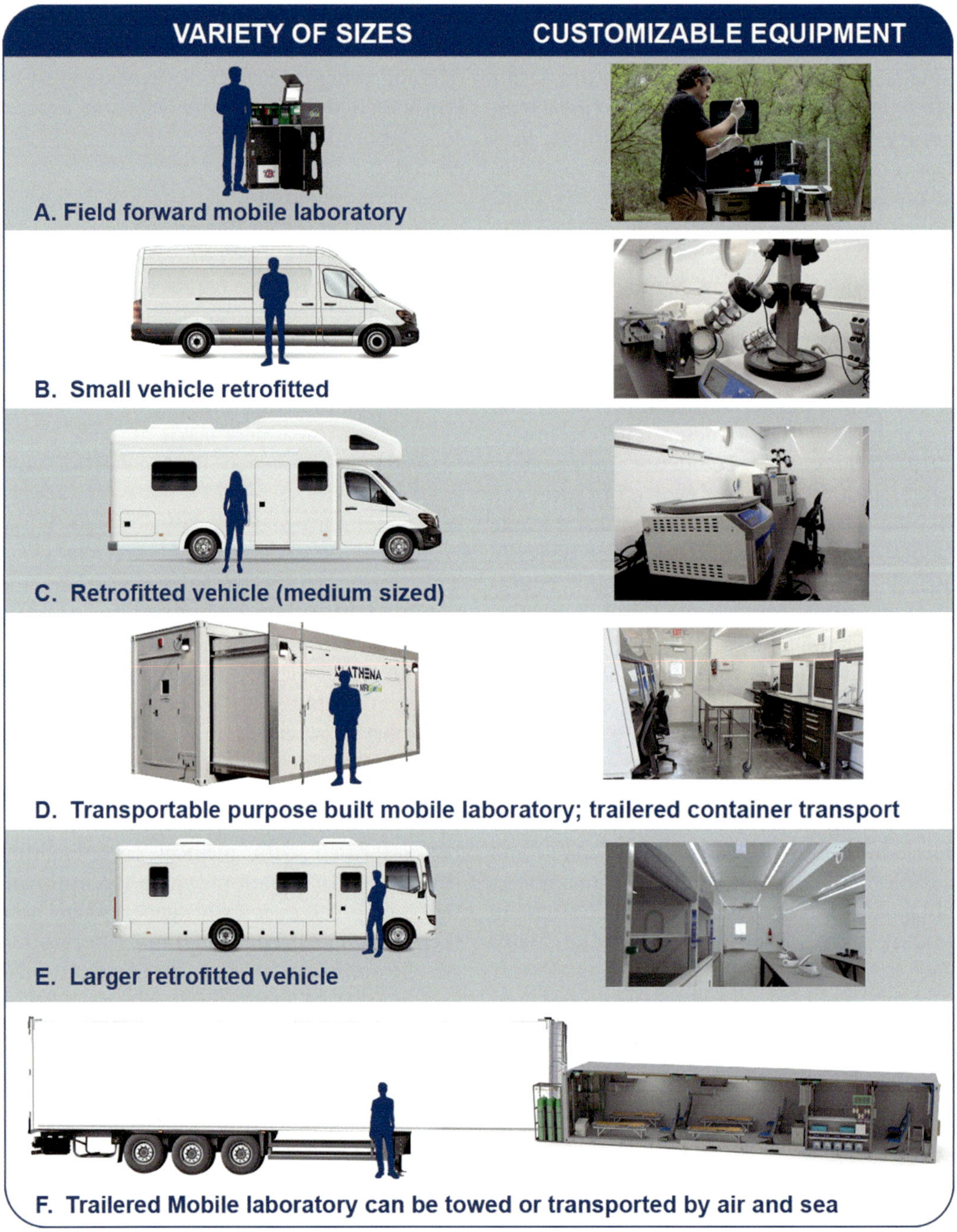

Fig. 2 Various configurations of mobile and deliverable laboratory systems. (Credit: Tina May/MRIGlobal)

diagnostics (including in some cases assisting with pathogen identification and characterization) and to support early medical response by local health systems or nongovernmental organizations (NGOs) (e.g., Médecins Sans Frontières [MSF] or Doctors Without Borders). Depending on the response activities and requirements, as well as the trajectory of the outbreak, the laboratory capacity may need to be expanded and/or specialized labs established.

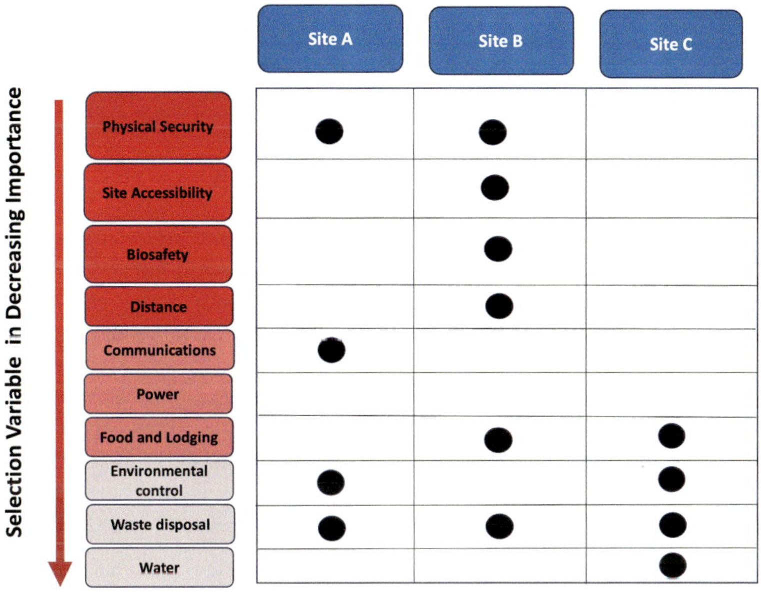

Fig. 3 A comparison matrix is a useful tool for selecting a clinical site. (Authors)

Available infrastructure may need to be renovated, or supplemented, to meet the needs of the facility. When permanent buildings are unavailable or unsuitable, tents, labs installed in vehicles or shipping containers, or temporary structures can be considered. If there are sufficient resources, construction of a new facility may also be viable. If an existing structure is repurposed or a new structure constructed, its use after the emergency should be considered: Can the structure be sustained as a medical or research laboratory? Will it have to be decontaminated? What will decontamination entail? Decisions on the location of the laboratory, construction, and disposition of the space at the end of the outbreak must be made in partnership with local officials and other partners.

The following multiple factors contribute to the suitability of a given location to host a laboratory (▶ Chaps. 32 and 40).

- Physical security (▶ Chap. 41)
- Accessibility of the site
- Logistics, including resupply chains for reagents and equipment (▶ Chap. 37)
- Availability of electronic communications (▶ Chap. 34)
- Availability, reliability, and source of electricity (▶ Chap. 39)
- Availability of clean water
- Adequate lighting and environmental control (▶ Chap. 38)
- Food and lodging for staff
- Treatment and/or evacuation of staff in case of accident, illness, or infection
- Waste disposal (solid and liquid)

Box 1: Lions, Tigers, and Wastewater: Oh My!

According to WHO, approximately 60% of all infectious diseases and 75% of emerging infectious diseases are zoonotic (WHO et al. 2019). It is not surprising during an outbreak or emergency response that the laboratory is often asked to test samples from a variety of sources. During the West Africa Ebola outbreak, there was a suspicion that the transmission was related to contact with contaminated wastewater or with a variety of local animals. Testing animal samples during outbreaks serves several purposes: identification of the source of the agent, informing transmission dynamics, monitoring and surveillance, as well as to answer basic research questions. Early detection of zoonotic pathogens in animals may allow preplacement of laboratory facilities and response efforts in advance of or shortly after spillover events occur (▶ Chap. 10).

Likewise, testing of wastewater or performing wastewater-based epidemiology (WBE) can be useful for (1) early detection of the agent in new areas, (2) population or community-based monitoring, (3) monitoring in areas of strong community resistance where people may object to providing samples, (4) identification or tracking of the source, and (5) evaluating control/intervention methods. WBE has been employed in several outbreaks, including severe acute respiratory syndrome coronavirus 2 (SARS-CoV-2) and poliovirus.

The challenge for many laboratories is being able to adapt to these requests and to have the tools to perform the testing on these alternative sample types. Samples may require different extraction methods; controls may not function across different species. Assays may not readily transfer between species, and additional validation may be required. Outbreaks affecting humans and animals will require adjustments in other areas, including community engagement and waste disposal. Many laboratories do not have the bandwidth or tools to validate a test for a new sample type or species. Veterinary diagnostic labs, if available, can help characterize the pathogen, assist with strain identification, and contribute to epidemiological monitoring.

When repurposing assays in the field it is critical to understand the limitations. For example, without being able to validate a test for a new sample type, a positive result may be helpful but a negative result cannot be interpreted. As the role of the lab continues to expand and there is greater recognition of the importance of One Health research, labs deploying in response to an outbreak should expect to see an increase in the need to test samples beyond humans.

The intended and projected workloads of the laboratory are another important variable. Is the space sufficient to address surges in workloads? Secondary sites should be identified and prepared to accommodate work surges if the primary site is insufficient. Are there political (including regional stability) and/or social factors that might impact or drive site selection? (▶ Chap. 16 and In Practice 16.1). Community engagement or good participatory practice (GPP) is essential for an ongoing, respectful dialogue with the surrounding community to address possible suspicions and misapprehensions, encourage trial recruitment, and mitigate "not in my backyard" sentiments. Every situation is unique, and in an emergency time for selecting laboratory sites is often limited. There may be no perfect site, but a matrix-based approach to identifying candidate laboratory sites may minimize challenges.

3.2 Assay and Equipment Selection

Multiple factors will drive the selection of assays and equipment, including the pathogen and clinical course of disease in patients. The first question for the laboratory is "What are you trying to measure or test for?" or more broadly, "What question are you trying to answer?" The responses combined with the required timeframe will help narrow the selection of available assays or identify where a new assay needs to be developed. Other factors will include the expected number of samples and the turnaround time desired or required. The skill of the laboratory staff must be considered. Can available staff safely and accurately perform complex assays or is there sufficient time to build personnel capacity? Is the available facility suitable for running complex assays? What is the availability of reagents and assays? Biosafety and safe handling of samples cannot be overlooked. Ideally handling of high-hazard samples should be minimized and inactivation should be performed whenever feasible.

During the coronavirus disease 2019 (COVID-19) pandemic and 2014–2016 West Africa Ebola outbreak, laboratories faced substantial challenges with shortages of reagents and disposable supplies. As travel and transport to and from the region was curtailed, shipment of supplies became even more difficult, requiring some laboratories to establish alternate means to transport supplies (i.e., staff hand-carrying large quantities of supplies) or develop capabilities to run multiple different assays for the same agent depending on availability. The need to pivot between assays complicated laboratory operations and required increased training to master additional testing protocols and devise strategies to bridge between different assays. Other factors also influence assay selection, including but not limited to the cost per assay, sample requirements (type and volume of samples), the equipment's power requirements, and the data's intended use. As cartridge and multiplex assays, which provide quantitative or semi-quantitative measurement of multiple analytes, have become more commonplace, multiplex assays are often favored as they provide more information from one test procedure. However, these assays are often more expensive and may be unaffordable or unsustainable for many countries. The use of the data will also influence the assays selected. Clinical care, clinical research, diagnostic, and surveillance needs differ. For clinical studies, what is being tested must match the protocol. Moreover, trial participants' informed consent must include the purpose of testing and analysis. Using human biological samples for purposes participants have not consented to is unethical (though it has not always been considered so) (Garrison 2013).

For more information on the importation of study products, please refer to ▶ Chap. 38. For transport and storage considerations, see ▶ Chap. 39.

3.3 Regulatory and Legal Concerns

Managing regulatory and legal requirements during an outbreak is a complex and exacting task, and even more so in low-resource settings. Generic terms like "low-resource settings" or "developing countries" should be accompanied by a deeper understanding of the local context to avoid assumptions and tailor regulatory compliance measures accordingly (van Zyl et al. 2021). Robust regulatory oversight is crucial. In a bilateral partnership, it requires understanding and meeting local, national, and international requirements. Stringent regulatory authorities will not accept evidence from noncompliant trials as evidence for authorization or licensing, but they have shown flexibility in adjusting formal requirements during public health emergencies (▶ Chap. 6).

As the size of the emergency grows, resources will be strained; low-resource settings where healthcare systems may already face capacity and accessibility constraints are especially vulnerable (Siow et al. 2020). In some environments, gaps may exist in regulatory guidance and responsible regulators may have limited capacity for oversight and guidance. Often the engagement of external experts is beneficial in these situations to augment local resources and help enhance long-term capacity (▶ Chap. 33, In Practice 33.2, and 33.3). For clinical studies with human participants, it is essential that the proposed study be reviewed and approved by all appropriate research ethics committees (also known as institutional review boards). A data and safety monitoring plan and board to implement it are also essential (▶ Chap. 23).

3.3.1 Regulatory Management Tools for Emergencies

Governments employed various regulatory management adjustments during the COVID-19 pandemic and other recent public health emergencies. Methods including rapid regulatory impact assessments, consultations with stakeholders, and international partnerships helped ensure robust, substantive regulatory oversight during the pandemic while easing administrative burdens (OECD 2020). Complying with regulatory and legal requirements in low-resource settings during outbreaks requires a multifaceted approach. Governments and regulatory bodies should leverage regulatory management tools and establish expedited evaluation processes to ensure timely access to critical medical interventions while maintaining appropriate oversight (OECD 2020; van Zyl et al. 2021).

Working in partnership with ethical review committees and regulators with greater response capacity can help countries with fewer resources perform their own due diligence more readily, for example, by reviewing collected evidence rather than gathering and compiling it de novo (► In Practice 33.3). It is also essential to consider the unique challenges and context of each low-resource setting to develop tailored and effective regulatory strategies (Siow et al. 2020; van Zyl et al. 2021).

Global disparities in healthcare tend to be especially acute in low-resource environments (van Zyl et al. 2021) (► Chap. 5). The effort to address disparities is complicated by inadequate investment in healthcare infrastructure, shortages of trained personnel, and other scarce resources. In some areas, there may be profound distrust or even fear of the healthcare system that has become entrenched through the history of that country or the experiences of some members of the population (Siow et al. 2020). Recognition of disparities and active engagement with the community is essential to ensure widespread access to healthcare for those in need and create or bolster the willingness of community members to report disease, receive treatment, and participate in clinical studies (► Chap. 18 and In Practice 18.1). Social mobilization and outreach are essential to ensure that the laboratory, treatment, and research centers are accepted by the community. Failure to engage the community can increase security risks to treatment and research sites, discourage study recruitment, hinder efforts to contain the emergency and lessen the effectiveness of participant follow-up—all of which could impact the rigor and generalizability of results. For example, failure to recruit study participants representative of the population affected by an outbreak may limit the applicability of study findings and potentially compromise the study results. The engagement of sociologists and anthropologists and the development of robust social mobilization teams are essential to ensure that messages and engagements are understandable, culturally appropriate, and effective (► Chap. 26).

3.3.2 Expedited Evaluation and Approval Processes

During public health emergencies, such as an Ebola outbreak, expedited evaluation and approval processes for diagnostic assays, medical products, and interventions are essential (van Zyl et al. 2021) in order to facilitate prompt access to safe, effective MCMs to mitigate suffering and the loss of life. For many emerging disease threats, there are limited interventions, or interventions such as candidate vaccines are still under development. Use of these early-stage products may be of great benefit but often they have not gone through clinical trials in humans to assess their safety and potential efficacy. Ideally an accelerated clinical trial is designed and implemented to determine as rapidly and definitively as possible whether the candidate product is safe and provides benefit. Advanced development of protocols that could be rapidly adapted to specific situations can help reduce the amount of time to initiate response research and respond to emergencies as effectively as possible. Preplacement of these protocols and engagement of regulatory groups in reviewing these protocols should be encouraged. As their research capacity develops, countries at risk should take ownership of the preparation and implementation of these protocols (► Chap. 8). In an emergency, such products may also be distributed under an expanded access program such as the World Health Organization (WHO) program for monitored emergency use of unregistered and experimental interventions (MEURI). Such programs cannot, however, generally provide the scientifically well-founded results required to demonstrate safety and efficacy to regulators, and in some cases could discourage enrollment in high-quality clinical trials by offering potential participants certain access to an experimental intervention rather than the uncertainty of a randomized controlled trial (WHO 2018).

3.3.3 Diagnostic Preparedness

Pathogens identified as having pandemic potential under the WHO R&D Blueprint, those causing priority diseases designated by the Coalition for Epidemic Preparedness Innovations (CEPI), and the virus families included in the NIAID-sponsored priority pathogen approach require diagnostic preparedness and may all be candidates for advanced development of diagnostics (Cassetti et al. 2022; CEPI 2023; Sigfrid et al. 2020; WHO 2023a) (▶ Chaps. 11 and 12). Identified pathogens with pandemic potential include, for example, Nipah virus, Ebola virus, Lassa virus, Crimean-Congo hemorrhagic fever virus; potential new species in virus families known to infect humans; and the specter of Disease X, an unknown and unanticipated new human infection. Diagnostic preparedness for these priority pathogens presents the following specific challenges:

- *Lack of rapid diagnostic tests*. Developing accurate and rapid diagnostic tests for newly emerging pathogens can be technically challenging and time-consuming. The identification of specific antigens or genetic markers/sequences (of the pathogen) requires extensive research and validation.
- *Limited access to diagnostic tools*. Low-resource settings often face limited access to advanced diagnostic technologies, such as PCR or sequencing platforms. The availability and affordability of these tools can be a significant constraint.
- *Diagnostic infrastructure*. Establishing and maintaining an efficient diagnostic infrastructure, including laboratories equipped with adequate biosafety and biosecurity measures, trained personnel, and quality assurance systems, is crucial but challenging in resource-limited settings.

Infectious disease emergencies present the following additional challenges to diagnostic preparedness.

- *Rapid response*. Timely response is critical during outbreaks, but developing, producing, and deploying diagnostic tests quickly enough to keep pace with a rapidly evolving situation is a demanding project. Work is underway to facilitate accelerated development (▶ Chap. 11).
- *Diagnostic capacity*. Low-resource settings often have limited diagnostic capacity, including inadequate laboratory facilities, shortages of trained personnel, insufficient supply chains for reagents and consumables, and lack of operational equipment to perform complex analysis.
- *Sample collection and transportation*. Proper collection, handling, and transportation of samples from suspected cases to diagnostic facilities can be logistically challenging, particularly in remote areas with limited infrastructure and transportation networks. Improper collection, shipping, or processing can lessen the value of the operation (▶ Chap. 39).
- *Sensitivity and specificity*. Ensuring the sensitivity and specificity of diagnostic tests is essential for accurate identification of cases during outbreaks. However, achieving both high sensitivity and specificity can be demanding, requiring extensive validation and quality control measures.
- *Integration and coordination*. Coordinating diagnostic efforts among different stakeholders, including healthcare providers, laboratories, public health agencies, and international organizations, is crucial but can be complex, particularly in emergencies when there are not yet accepted standards for identification or diagnosis. Difficulties are compounded in resource-limited settings.
- *Data documentation, management, and reporting*. Clear documentation of data is essential to allow correct identification of samples and to reliably link laboratory, epidemiological, and clinical data. Effective data management and reporting systems are necessary for real-time surveillance, monitoring, and decision-making. Poor data documentation and reporting compromise outbreak mitigation efforts and clinical studies. Setting up robust systems and ensuring their functionality can be challenging, especially in low-resource settings with limited digital infrastructure. Systems should not be overly complex, but developed to meet situational needs with available resources. As long as there is Internet connectivity, even if it is sporadic, demanding analytical work can be done in well-equipped data centers elsewhere (▶ Chap. 35).

3.4 Specimen Collection, Transport, and Storage

Specimen collection, transport, and storage during outbreaks can be daunting (Tripathi et al. 2020). Appropriate packaging of the samples is necessary to protect the safety of the laboratory staff and transportation teams and to ensure the sample can be analyzed (Fig. 4). Accurate, standardized labeling, documentation, and reporting are crucial for epidemiological monitoring and control, and to ensure samples can be properly identified and results reported. Long-distance transport can be complicated by the availability of transport vehicles, personnel, and supplies. Air transport pilots may decline any cargo if they perceive it as a risk to themselves, crew, or others. Moreover, aviation regulations may vary by location and must be considered when attempting to transport samples or materials. During the 2014–2016 West Africa Ebola outbreak, it was difficult for researchers outside the region to obtain samples of the virus and patient sera, largely because the few air transport assets operating in the region were extremely reluctant to transport the sample, no matter how well packaged (Steenhuysen 2014) (Fig. 5).

Staff with training in packaging and transport—not only the how but the why—is essential for any clinical research operation, but the task becomes harder where transportation and infrastructure are limited. Well-trained staff can pivot and adjust as needed. Training is also needed for sample collection, to ensure samples are packed with clear and adequate documentation, in packaging that will protect the sample, staff, and community, and are transported safely, efficiently, and in compliance with all regulations. All training should be documented. Importantly, refresher training should be done periodically or when breaks in procedures are identified. Transport of samples requires coordination and should only be done with the agreement and permission of the host country and in close coordination with biosafety professionals.

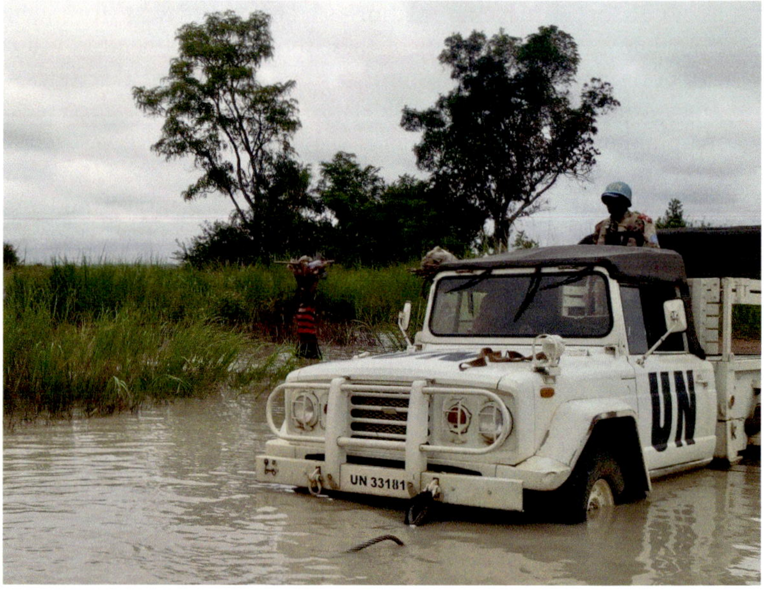

Fig. 4 A UN peacekeeping patrol in the Democratic Republic of the Congo during the rainy season. (Credit: MONUSCO Photos)

Handling and Transport of Blood Specimens Potentially Infected with Ebola Virus

1 Handling Blood Collection Tubes

STEP 1. Collect blood specimen and ensure the tops on the tube are secure

Helpful Hint 1
Check to make sure that bleach won't remove the writing on the tubes. If you aren't sure, you can always also write the name on the glove or bag or on a piece of paper and place in the first bag.

STEP 2. Disinfect collection tube by spraying with 5% bleach solution

STEP 3. Roll collection tube back and forth across a damp paper towel, if available

STEP 4. Wrap collection tube in a clean paper towels or absorbent material. (This reduces the chance of accidental freezing if using cold packs and absorb any samples that spills.)

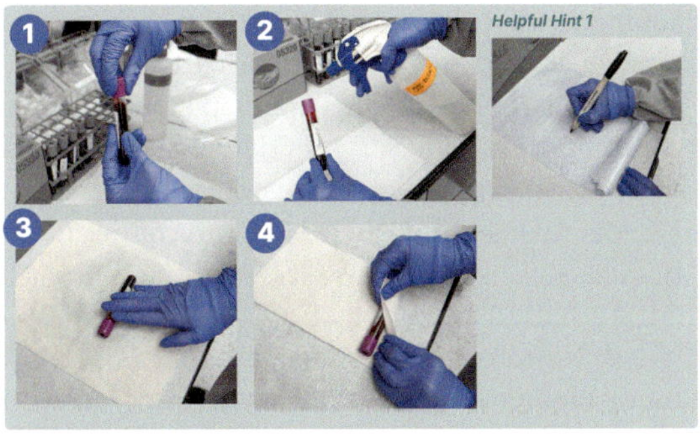

2 Preparing Collection Tubes for Transportation

STEP 1. Place wrapped tube in ziplock bag, lay flat, and press out excess air. Close bag and check seal.

Helpful Hint 2
If ziplock bags are not available, you can substitute gloves or a plastic bag that can be tied. Note gloves would be the best second option. Example: place tube with absorbent material in gloved hand, and remove and reverse glove to wrap around collection tube, and tie.

Helpful Hint 3
Check seals by inversion of the bags

STEP 2. Place the sealed bag into a second ziplock bag. Spray inside of bag or glove with bleach, and seal bag. Check the seal.

STEP 3. Place second bag into a third ziplock bag or glove. Spray inside of bag or glove with bleach, and seal bag. Check the seal.

STEP 4. Spray the outside of third bag or dunk the bag in a bucket of disinfectant. Remove the bag from the laboratory.

STEP 5. Outside the laboratory, place the wet bag inside a cleaned or deconned cooler or transport container. Ideally, container should have paper towels or an absorbent material. If sample is to be kept cold, include cooler packs.

Helpful Hint 4
If cooler is not available, use yellow/white screw-top containers for specimen transport. Any other hard-walled container will work. The goal is to protect the sample and person carrying it. If the container you use does not seal, place the container in a biohazard bag and seal.

Helpful Hint 5
If your cooler is in the lab, make sure you decontaminate the cooler.

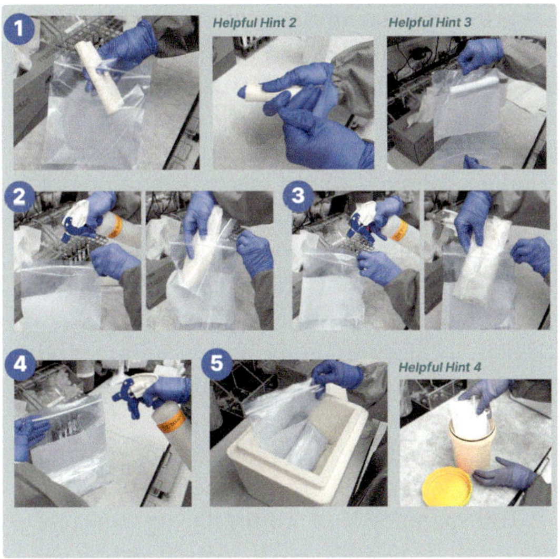

Fig. 5 Packaging an infectious disease sample for transport. (Credit: Bonnie Dighero-Kemp and the overseas support team Integrated Research Facility, Frederick MD)

3.5 Obstacles to Proper Sample Packaging and Transport

- Unreliable electrical power (Cornish et al. 2021)
- Inadequate inventory management systems for samples and records
- Failure to develop and implement a system for unique identifiers to link diagnostic, clinical, and epidemiological records
- Lack of adequate supplies and materials for collection, documentation, packaging, and shipping
- Insufficient training for packaging and transport
- Logistical challenges (i.e., roads, vehicles, fuel, etc.)
- Lack of willing and able personnel to package and transport materials

4 Implementing Effective Laboratory Biosafety and Biosecurity

The Ebola outbreaks and COVID-19 pandemic have highlighted the critical role of effective infection prevention and control (IPC) and the need for biosecurity and biosafety plans. Given the potential number and diverse characteristics of pathogens and wide geographical area at risk, there is no one-size-fits-all solution. Every country, especially ones with life-threatening endemic diseases, must have executable national and facility-based biosecurity plans that can be implemented within their capabilities.

Although the concept of biosecurity originated within the context of biological weapons prohibition, it has expanded to all sectors of the life sciences and is generally used as an encompassing term meant to protect humans, animals, and plants from biological threats (Renault et al. 2021). The U.S. Department of Health and Human Services defines biosecurity as protecting biological agents from theft, loss, or misuse (HHS 2015). International organizations such as WHO and the Food and Agriculture Organization (FAO) of the United Nations have a much broader definition of biosecurity, "a strategic and integrated approach to analyzing and managing relevant risks to human, animal and plant life and health and associated risks for the environment" (FAO 2023; WHO 2020). The overall approach must include the buy-in and support of the local populace and national government, adapted to realistic expectations of each country's current capabilities and targeted, executable solutions to identified gaps in capabilities. Major obstacles to developing and implementing biosecurity plans include lack of local community and governmental engagement and support, limited national and local infrastructure, inadequate funding, difficulty procuring material and supplies, and shortages of trained professionals.

Transparency and culturally appropriate strategies are necessary. Any perceived secrecy or untoward intentions will derail efforts and create an environment of suspicion and hostility. Without the investment of the local and national government the development and sustainment of a biocontainment or secure research facility will not succeed. The human factor is the most important and sometimes difficult to capture. Inexperienced staff, local instability, and bad actors are all variables that must be considered and addressed.

The state of local and nationwide infrastructure needs to be considered in the feasibility and scope of biosecurity blueprints. The ability of security teams to respond to a site may be hampered by weather, available working vehicles, and infrastructure. Payment of staff is also essential. As resources are stretched, are staff receiving appropriate compensation?

Continuity of electrical power has been previously addressed for storing samples and reagents, but consistent power is also necessary to ensure workers can operate safely. As biosecurity plans are put into place, the impact of a power loss must be considered. The power source, vulnerability, and quality will directly impact the safety and security of the laboratory. As laboratories become increasingly complex, back-up systems, preferably more than one, should be set up to ensure the safety of the personnel in the area, the community, and the security of the samples. These failsafe approaches may include additional generators, solar-powered battery systems, uninterrupted power sources, other engineering features, and training (▶ Chap. 39).

In the past, the WHO, philanthropic organizations, and other nations have invested in strengthening the biosecurity of less-resourced countries with varying success. The long-term success of any program depends on sustainability over time. Realistic expectations of the local and national budget allocations and partner contributions toward these programs will determine the feasibility of both near- and long-term sustainability. Many countries, due to competing priorities and low gross domestic product (GDP), cannot sustain the cost of running a biological containment facility or simply do not consider it to be a high priority for funding. When budgets are insufficient, cost cuts may include hiring less capable staff or reducing vetting of staff, reducing or halting equipment maintenance, and insufficient PPE and other supplies. Low or intermittent pay will lead to rapid staff turnover and potential nefarious actions by insiders. As biotechnology expands the potential for what can be done in a lab, and as investments continue to be made in secure laboratory infrastructure around the globe, the long-term sustainability of facilities is a prominent concern.

5 Documentation, Data Quality, and Data Management

Effective data management and maintaining data integrity are critical for clinical diagnostics to provide accurate results for the patient, to track the epidemiological evolution of an incident or outbreak, and to allow accurate interpretation and implementation of findings from clinical studies. Any shortfalls in data management and integrity can impact the quality and reliability of diagnostic information, which in turn affects decision-making response efforts and clinical trials results. Data management does not require complex commercial systems. Simple computer software and handwritten records are suitable if the data is legible and well documented—and if the records can be safely maintained. On the other hand, there are dedicated electronic clinical trial data capture and management systems that can be used free of charge and will provide the safety of multiple copies of trial data. However, these systems require careful coordination with the research project information technology team as well as considerable training for users, especially those with minimal computer skills (▶ Chaps. 34 and 35). It is essential that laboratory, epidemiological, and clinical data are well linked through common or unique identifiers, particularly in larger outbreaks and multisite research efforts.

One essential for a clinical trial is high data quality, data integrity, and security of patient data (Basit et al. 2021). Collecting accurate, reliable data during an outbreak can be hindered by various obstacles (Eck 2018). Therefore, strategies to ensure data quality, such as standardized data collection protocols and rigorous validation, become crucial. Staff should be trained in data collection, documentation, and storage. Training staff in Good Clinical Practice (GCP) (ICH 2016) and standardized data management is also useful. It is essential that data be stored safely, and that backups of data and study notebooks be maintained.

Data analysis and management play a functional role that can extend well beyond the patient-level analysis of clinical diagnostics (O'Hare et al. 2022). Analyzing data from paper and electronic health records (EHRs) can help identify dominant themes and patterns, providing valuable insights into the diagnosis and management of diseases like Ebola virus disease in its post-acute patient sequelae. There is often a need to confirm the diagnosis in patients that have long-term impacts from disease but may have very low serum levels of the virus. Robust data analysis techniques, including machine learning and data mining, can enhance diagnostic capabilities, both in the post-acute phase and in the earliest stages of infection.

Storage and management of data pose specific challenges in emergency and remote clinical diagnostic settings (Eck 2018). All too often, paper or basic spreadsheets are the only available option; these are functional but tend to require more labor for transfer to a purpose-made data storage system. The centralized or compartmentalized nature of paper records (or electronic ones in some cases) may hinder access, limiting clinicians and outbreak response teams from effectively utilizing information to improve patient care while dedicated MCMs remain in the future, for example. In areas with Internet, cellular, or satellite services, cloud-based solutions are increasingly utilized, but must be selected and configured to ensure data integrity and privacy protection. Data integrity is paramount in clinical trials, and ensuring accurate data collection, validation, and preservation are critical aspects of maintaining data integrity. Protecting the personal information of trial participants is an ethical norm and a strict legal requirement in most jurisdictions.

The implementation of next-generation sequencing (NGS) in clinical diagnostic settings offers vast opportunities for comprehensive genetic analysis (Eck 2018). However, it also presents challenges in data storage and management due to the large volume of data generated. Efficient data storage solutions and management strategies are necessary to handle the data influx and ensure its accessibility and security during an outbreak. Transmission of the data may be very slow in areas with limited communication capabilities (▶ Chap. 37).

Documentation of test control data and equipment validation is sometimes overlooked. Failure to include controls or perform routine equipment calibrations may compromise the integrity of the data. Frequently, quality assurance data such as control runs, maintenance logs, or validation materials are not archived, or archived separately and difficult to access and review. Fast-moving emergency response situations often require the use of whatever equipment is on hand or quickly procurable, and quality documentation for these instruments may be missing or limited. However, laboratories can actively address such concerns through the implementation of control samples, running calibration materials, the use of independent proficiency panels to assess performance, and clear, accessible documentation of these efforts. As an alternative to independent proficiency panels, if more than one laboratory with sufficient bandwidth is available, laboratories may exchange samples for comparison of results. When no other options are available, labs can repeat procedures with a small portion of previously tested samples and incorporate additional performance controls. Documentation of training and competency of all staff should be part of the data quality assurance package. Regardless of the strategies implemented, it is essential that laboratories not just produce results, but implement quality assurance practices to ensure overall data quality and integrity.

In summary, during an outbreak and in response research, any lapse in data quality management and integrity in clinical diagnostics can raise questions that significantly impact decision-making, response efforts, clinical studies, and post-outbreak or post-MCM-licensure data analyses. Ensuring high data quality, employing robust data analysis techniques, addressing storage and management challenges, and prioritizing data integrity is paramount. Adapting to changing conditions and handling large volumes of data are essential aspects of clinical data management during an outbreak. By addressing these challenges, healthcare systems can enhance their diagnostic capabilities and more effectively respond to public health emergencies (Fig. 6).

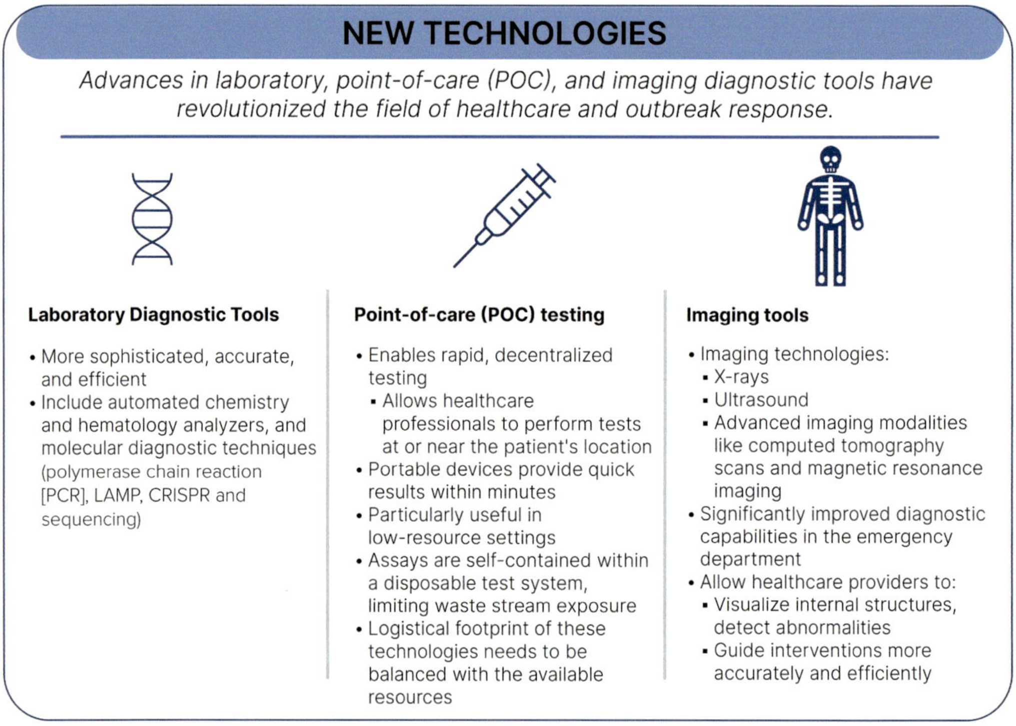

Fig. 6 Many recent innovations have made clinical laboratories, including mobile labs and labs set up urgently in emergencies, more capable than ever. Further advances can be expected. (Authors)

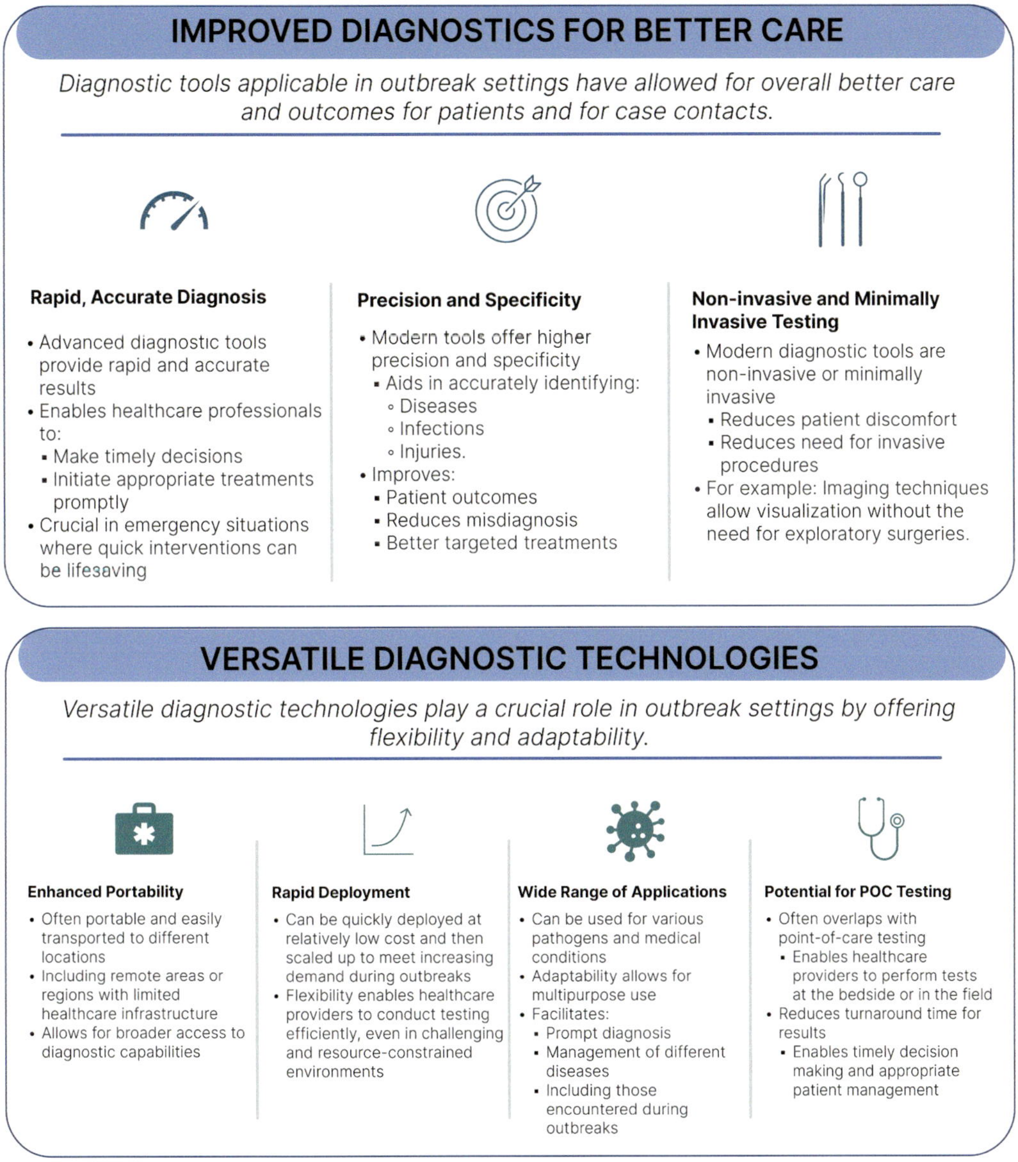

Fig. 6 (continued)

6 Case Study

As the Ebola virus spread from the rural areas of Guinea, Liberia, and Sierra Leone to population-dense urban settings (Conakry, Monrovia, and Freetown), the need to establish diagnostic capabilities reached a crisis point. In 2014, there was no or very limited diagnostic capacity to detect Ebola virus in West Africa. It was not until March 2014 that the viral disease that had appeared in Guinea in December 2013 was identified as Ebola, and until mid-April testing of suspect cases required the transport of samples to a mobile response laboratory run by the European Union in Guinea, taking hours and sometimes days.

The request for laboratory support was unique in that the Liberian Ministry of Health not only desired in-country Ebola testing to be established, but wanted that capability transferred to their national reference labora-

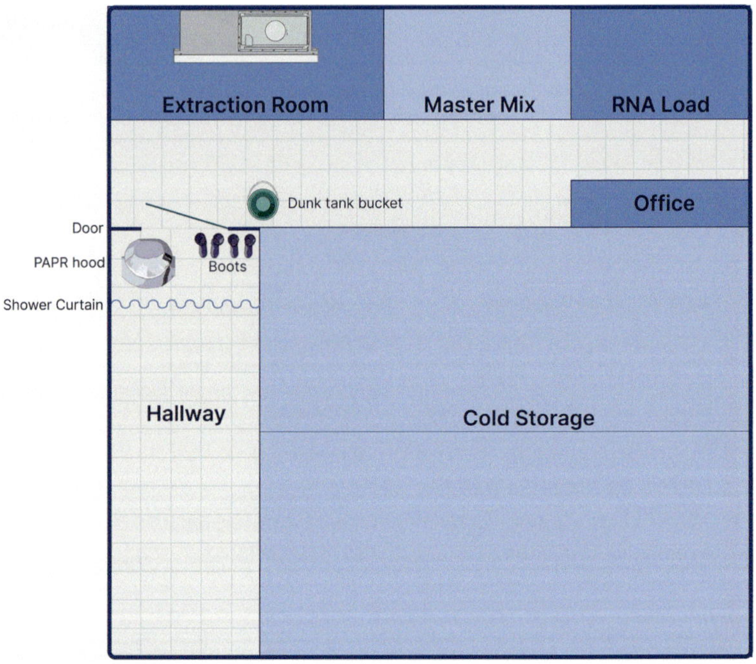

Fig. 7 Layout of PREVAIL laboratory space at the Liberian Institute of Biomedical Research. (Credit: Saraina Adams/USDA)

tory. The inclusion of training as a primary mission objective during an active outbreak adds significant work and stress to deploying teams. This stress is compounded when the previous experience and skill level of the staff to be trained is unknown or limited. The site for the laboratory was preselected at the Liberian Institute for Biomedical Research (LIBR), an aging 1970s research facility located approximately 65 miles outside of the capital. An HIV laboratory diagnostic space composed of a single room with a class II biosafety cabinet (BSC) and several small rooms was identified for the team's use. Electricity was provided by generators which ran several hours a day; power spikes were common. The facility was without running water during the dry season and water leaked through the roof and carried bat guano into the labs during the rainy season.

Due to the unknown availability of supplies in the country, all equipment and supplies were hand-carried by the team coming to the country on commercial flights. Available assays at the time were limited and there were no assays with regulatory approval. Two assays developed by the U.S. Army, EZ-1 and MGB, were selected because the Army had applied for (but not received) emergency use authorization (EUA) with the Food and Drug Administration and could provide the assays (Bettini et al. 2023; Presser et al. 2021). (The EZ1 assay did receive an EUA designation during the outbreak.) The use of two assays allowed cross-checking to increase stringency and reduce the likelihood of false positives. Samples were considered positive only if both targets were detected. If a single target was detected the sample was considered indeterminate, and repeat testing in 48 h was recommended. In addition, a standard ribonuclease P (RNaseP) assay was included to ensure sample quality. As the outbreak continued, other Ebola virus assays were developed and validated for platforms including Biofire® and Cepheid®.

The provided space consisted of four rooms and a hallway with a single-door access from the LIBR main wing hallway (Fig. 7). To ensure the highest available level of biosafety containment, the room with the biosafety cabinet was used to process all specimens from suspected cases. In the absence of engineering controls, attempts to create directional airflow were implemented by disabling air conditioning in the sample processing room, creating a temperature differential with surrounding rooms. To limit cross-contamination issues, the reagent mixture room and sample loading spaces were segregated as seen in ◘ Fig. 7. Small trash buckets and spray bottles were placed on the entry and exit areas of the space to serve as chemical disinfectant spaces (dunk tanks). Since the location lacked a vestibule area to allow for donning and doffing PPE, a curtain was used to establish an area for this function.

Appropriate PPE is based on a risk analysis intertwined with the facility design, planned procedures, and the primary containment equipment present, and focuses on the type(s) of exposures anticipated (splash, spray, touch) and the overall risk to the staff member when exposed to specific agents. PPE must be durable and appropriate for the task of preventing exposure. Powered air-purifying respirators (PAPR) were selected for multiple reasons. PAPRs have the benefit of preventing accidental contamination of mucosal membranes by staff members touching their faces or adjusting PPE; fit testing for N95s in the field was not possible and the use of PAPRs eliminated the risk posed by face shaving, as micro-abrasions create a potential portal of entry for infection.

A variety of commercial disinfectants have been identified as suitable for Ebola virus decontamination. Given the availability, local use, and effectiveness of chlorine bleach as a disinfectant in clinical settings, it was chosen as a primary method for decontaminating surfaces potentially contaminated with Ebola virus. Full-strength bleach, however, is corrosive, a contact irritant, and emits toxic fumes—not ideal in an unventilated space. A diluted bleach solution was used to reduce these hazards while killing the virus (◘ Fig. 8) (PHAC 2023; WHO 2023b). A contact time of 10 min is ideal and fresh preparations were made daily, or when high amounts of organic material (e.g., blood) were mixed with the solution. In some cases, a 5% solution of water and MicroChem Plus® was used with sensitive equipment and metal that could be damaged by bleach.

Local staff had limited prior laboratory experience. A major emphasis in training was how to safely handle samples, hazardous waste disposal (liquid and dry waste), proper biological safety cabinet use, and sample flow to prevent molecular assay contamination. Most notable was learning and practicing the principles of PPE—donning and doffing the PPE in a logical and safe manner, and how to test and care for the PAPR and disposable PPE. Staff were also trained in basic laboratory principles and techniques, such as PCR-based assays, molecular assays, reagent preparation, prevention of common contamination issues, and troubleshooting. Most importantly, they learned to interpret assay results and discussed in depth the implications of false positive or false negative results for the clinical setting. A train-the-trainer approach was used to reinforce training and ensure program sustainability.

LIBR was one of several laboratories eventually established in the region. Many of the laboratories reported common challenges. For example, consistent and reliable electricity was a primary issue. Molecular assays require uninterrupted power during the run and frequent power interruptions and surges compromise runs. In addition, variable power resulted in instrument failures and compromised reagents due to temperature fluctuations in freezers without power.

Communication was also a constant concern. Intermittent Internet, Wi-Fi, and cellular signals at the laboratory compounded problems with logistical issues and data reporting. Internet access was often down for days to weeks during the outbreak.

Waste disposal at the site was another hurdle. The plumbing often failed or was unusable. The site had a purpose-built incinerator, but it was collapsing. Fuel for burning was in short supply. Burn barrels or the use of a pit provided usable alternatives. Safe and secure storage of waste was another common issue. Bags of waste should be stored in a secure area with limited access prior to incineration or destruction.

Sample packing, identification, and quality were also problematic. Samples often arrived unpacked or simply inside a glove, posing risks to everyone from the collector to the delivery team to the laboratory workers. Sample labels were difficult to read or missing. Samples arrived frozen and in varying amounts. Educational materials were pre-

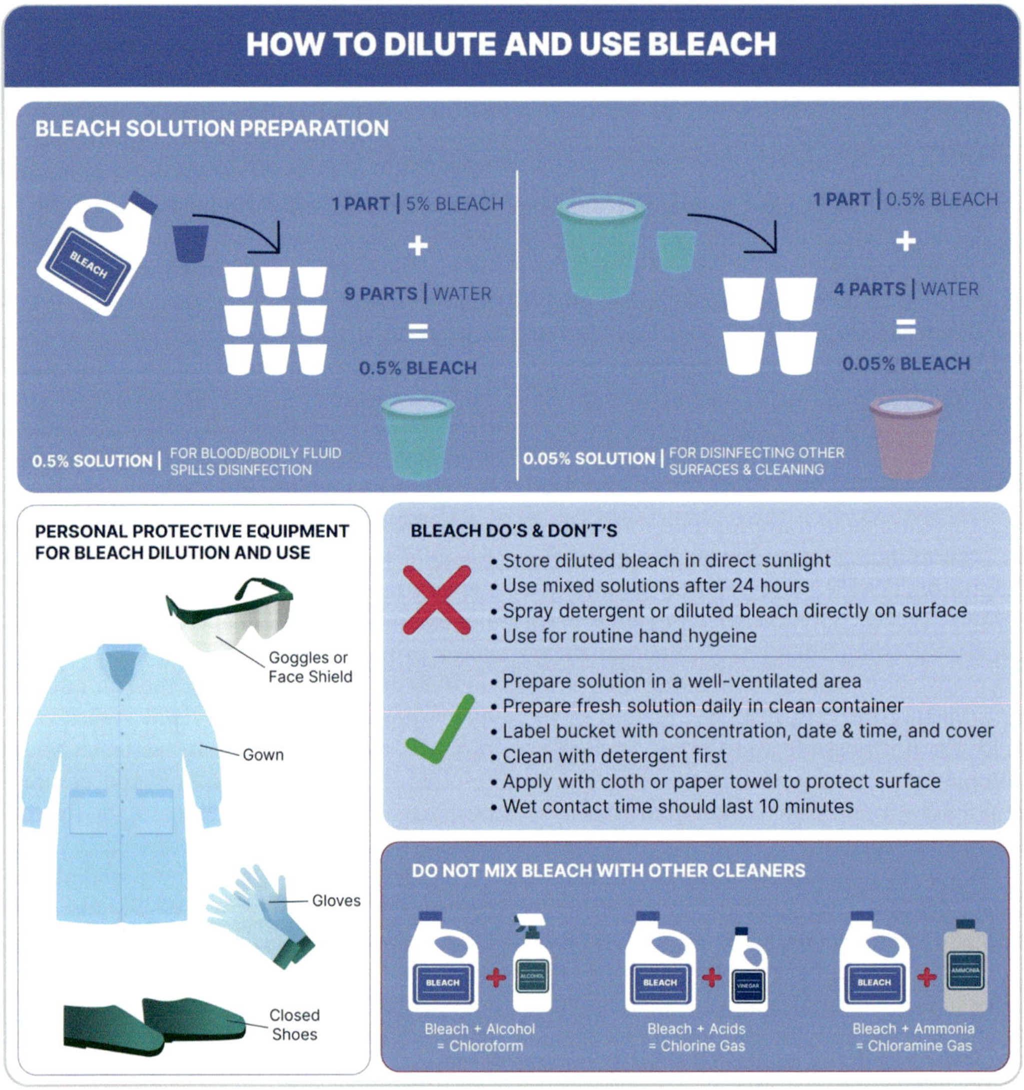

Fig. 8 Instructions for using bleach as a disinfect for Ebola virus and other pathogens. (Credit: Saraina Adams/USDA)

pared to train staff in appropriate sample collection type and labeling, and a drop-off point was established to receive and log samples and provide supplies for collection and transport as the teams needed, including data collection sheets once they were developed.

The teams that responded and worked with the national team at LIBR faced a rapidly changing situation. Sample numbers grew from the tens to the hundreds during the outbreak. Staff had to be adaptable and adjust to the challenges in the field. Training and the overall curriculum had to be adapted daily to meet the needs of the teams. The mission was an overall success, in large part due to local and international partnership and the willingness of the teams involved to be nimble and resilient.

7 Summary and Conclusion

Laboratory responses to emergencies face new, unanticipated obstacles in every outbreak. The first of these is often the logistics of transporting staff, reagents, and equipment to where they are needed. Preparedness of staff for deployment is often not just a matter of a passport and plane ticket. Visas, vaccines, and medications, to say nothing of jobs and family left behind, can delay departure.

Other delays are likely because equipment or reagents are not immediately available for rapid deployment. Since specialized laboratory equipment is often procured through special orders, prestaging or early acquisition of these items can significantly reduce the time from first detection of a new or re-emerging pathogen to deployment of lab teams. This in turn requires resources for the storage and continued maintenance of equipment as well as replenishment of supplies as they approach expiration. Depending on the location of the outbreak, there may be additional considerations, including inadequate transport options, import barriers, and customs clearance that hinder the importation of materials and supplies. National or regional instability may also limit the willingness and ability of staff to deploy to conflict areas.

As rapid deployment of laboratories has become more common, new challenges have emerged. The first is the retention or disposition of samples after an emergency. Establishment of biobanks or biorepositories is of growing interest. However, the use of retained samples raises ethical considerations. Can deidentified samples be used? Are samples collected from deceased individuals covered by human subject guidelines? Were the samples collected with informed consent, and what uses did it cover? What can be done and by whom is a growing discussion area and will be heavily driven by local human subject protection review. The cost–benefit of proposed biobanks should be considered. Maintenance of biobanks requires funds for freezers, fuel, personnel for maintaining samples, and software for inventory and biosecurity features to ensure that samples are maintained safely. The long-term retention of samples containing high-consequence pathogens is a growing global biosecurity concern. Another challenge is the blurring of the line between public health response and research and the desire to publish results and information while protecting individuals' rights and privacy. All too often, a lab is requested to run additional tests, but concerns are raised when it is unclear how the requested tests support the public health response, patient care, or clinical protocol requirements (▶ Chap. 7).

The end of the response brings other responsibilities, such as disposition of equipment, reagents, and the laboratory. Working with the local teams, decisions must be made whether to decontaminate and decommission or transfer the lab to local control. Equipment must also be managed accordingly. Broken equipment should be thoroughly decontaminated before disposal. All waste should be inactivated before disposal. Samples should be properly stored and transferred to local authorities or disposed of appropriately. Records should be transferred. If samples, equipment, or facilities are retained, trained local staff and adequate resources are essential, with some assurance provided that the lab will be sustainable. The closing or transfer of the laboratory should be well planned and highly coordinated with local officials and partners. As laboratory response capabilities continue to evolve and grow, the expectations for what laboratory teams can do will grow too, sometimes outstripping reality.

? Discussion Questions

1. Discuss the *who, what, where, when, and why* of outbreak-determined factors and requirements of the response or research program, which shape the capability and capacity of the field laboratory.
2. Define field/mobile laboratories.
3. Describe the critical elements and factors that contribute to the suitability of a given location to host a laboratory.
4. Describe the multiple factors that drive the selection of laboratory assays and equipment for research response.
5. Managing regulatory and legal requirements during an emergency outbreak is a complex and exacting task, especially in low-resource settings. Discuss the need for
   (a) Regulatory management tools
   (b) Expedited evaluation and approval processes
   (c) Diagnostic preparedness

6. What common obstacles are there to specimen collection, transport, and storage?
7. What is the role of laboratory biosafety and biosecurity?
8. Why is good data management essential to successful clinical trials?
9. What advances in laboratory, point-of-care, and imaging diagnostic tools have revolutionized healthcare and outbreak response?
10. How have improved diagnostic tools led to better care and outcomes for patients and potentially infected contacts during outbreaks?
11. How did Ebola virus transmission through chains of contact from rural areas to cities in West Africa demonstrate the need for better diagnostic capacity?

References

Basit MA, Lehmann CU, Medford RJ. Managing pandemics with health informatics: successes and challenges. Yearb Med Inform. 2021;30(1):17–25. https://doi.org/10.1055/s-0041-1726478.

Bettini A, Lapa D, Garbuglia AR. Diagnostics of Ebola virus. Front Public Health. 2023;11:1123024. https://doi.org/10.3389/fpubh.2023.1123024.

Cassetti MC, Pierson TC, Patterson LJ, Bok K, DeRocco AJ, Deschamps AM, et al. Prototype pathogen approach for vaccine and monoclonal antibody development: a critical component of the NIAID Plan for pandemic preparedness. J Infect Dis. 2022;227:1433. https://doi.org/10.1093/infdis/jiac296.

CEPI. Priority diseases. Oslo: Coalition for Epidemic Preparedness Innovations; 2023. https://cepi.net/research_dev/priority-diseases/. Accessed 5 May 2022.

Cornish NE, Anderson NL, Arambula DG, Arduino MJ, Bryan A, Burton NC, et al. Clinical laboratory biosafety gaps: lessons learned from past outbreaks reveal a path to a safer future. Clin Microbiol Rev. 2021;34(3):e0012618. https://doi.org/10.1128/CMR.00126-18.

Eck SH. Challenges in data storage and data management in a clinical diagnostic setting. J Lab Med. 2018;42(6):219–24. https://doi.org/10.1515/labmed-2018-0310.

FAO. Progressive management pathway for terrestrial animal biosecurity (FAO-PMP-TAB). Rome: Food and Agriculture Organization of the United Nations (FAO); 2023.

Garrison NA. Genomic justice for Native Americans: impact of the Havasupai case on genetic research. Sci Technol Human Values. 2013;38(2):201–23. https://doi.org/10.1177/0162243912470009.

HHS. Biosecurity. Washington, DC: U.S. Department of Health and Human Services; 2015. https://www.phe.gov/s3/BioriskManagement/biosecurity/Pages/default.aspx. Accessed 25 May 2023.

ICH. Good clinical practice: ICH harmonised guideline. Integrated addendum to ICH E6(R1): guideline for good clinical practice ICH E6(R2) ICH consensus guideline. Geneva: International Council for Harmonisation of Technical Requirements for Pharmaceuticals for Human Use (ICH); 2016.

O'Hare AM, Vig EK, Iwashyna TJ, Fox A, Taylor JS, Viglianti EM, et al. Complexity and challenges of the clinical diagnosis and management of long COVID. JAMA Netw Open. 2022;5(11):e2240332. https://doi.org/10.1001/jamanetworkopen.2022.40332.

OECD. Regulatory quality and COVID-19: the use of regulatory management tools in a time of crisis. Organization for Economic Co-operation and Development; 2020.

PHAC. Biosafety guidelines for laboratories handling specimens from patients under investigation for Ebola disease. Ottawa: Public Health Agency of Canada; 2023. https://www.canada.ca/en/public-health/services/infectious-diseases/viral-haemorrhagic-fevers/interim-biosafety-guidelines-laboratories-handling-specimens-patients-under-investigation-ebola-disease.html. Accessed 26 May 2023.

Presser LD, Coffin J, Koivogui L, Campbell A, Campbell J, Barrie F, et al. The deployment of mobile diagnostic laboratories for Ebola virus disease diagnostics in Sierra Leone and Guinea. Afr J Lab Med. 2021;10(1):1414. https://doi.org/10.4102/ajlm.v10i1.1414.

Racine T, Kobinger GP. Challenges and perspectives on the use of mobile laboratories during outbreaks and their use for vaccine evaluation. Hum Vaccin Immunother. 2019;15(10):2264–8. https://doi.org/10.1080/21645515.2019.1597595.

Renault V, Humblet MF, Saegerman C. Biosecurity concept: origins, evolution and perspectives. Animals (Basel). 2021;12(1):63. https://doi.org/10.3390/ani12010063.

Roh KH, Hong KH, Nam MH, Kim TS, Seong MW, Lee JK, et al. Guidelines for mobile laboratories for molecular diagnostic testing of COVID-19. Ann Lab Med. 2022;42(5):507–14. https://doi.org/10.3343/alm.2022.42.5.507.

Sigfrid L, Maskell K, Bannister PG, Ismail SA, Collinson S, Regmi S, et al. Addressing challenges for clinical research responses to emerging epidemics and pandemics: a scoping review. BMC Med. 2020;18(1):190. https://doi.org/10.1186/s12916-020-01624-8.

Siow WT, Liew MF, Shrestha BR, Muchtar F, See KC. Managing COVID-19 in resource-limited settings: critical care considerations. Crit Care.

2020;24(1):167. https://doi.org/10.1186/s13054-020-02890-x.
Steenhuysen J. U.S. Ebola researchers plead for access to virus samples. Reuters; 2014.
Tripathi A, Sathua K, Pachauri V, Flora SJS. Chapter 7—Collection, storage, and transportation of samples for offsite analysis. In: Flora SJS, Pachauri V, editors. Handbook on biological warfare preparedness. Academic; 2020. p. 133–49.
van Zyl C, Badenhorst M, Hanekom S, Heine M. Unravelling 'low-resource settings': a systematic scoping review with qualitative content analysis. BMJ Glob Health. 2021;6(6):e005190. https://doi.org/10.1136/bmjgh-2021-005190.
WHO. Consultation on monitored emergency use of unregistered and investigational interventions (MEURI) for Ebola virus disease (EVD). Geneva: World Health Organization; 2018. Contract No.: 25 Aug.
WHO. WHO guidance on implementing regulatory requirements for biosafety and biosecurity in biomedical laboratorie—a stepwise approach. Geneva: World Health Organization; 2020.
WHO. WHO R&D blueprint. Geneva: World Health Organization; 2023a. https://www.who.int/observatories/global-observatory-on-health-research-and-development/analyses-and-syntheses/who-r-d-blueprint/background. Accessed 19 May 2023.
WHO. Infection prevention and control guideline for Ebola and Marburg disease. Geneva: World Health Organization; 2023b. WHO/WPE/CRS/HCR/2023.1. Licence: CC BY-NC-SA 3.0 IGO.
WHO, FAO, WOAH. Taking a multisectoral, one health approach: a tripartite guide to addressing zoonotic diseases in countries. Geneva: World Health Organization, UN Food and Agriculture Organization, World Organization for Animal Health; 2019.
Xing W, Wang J, Zhao C, Wang H, Bai L, Pan L, et al. A highly automated mobile laboratory for on-site molecular diagnostics in the COVID-19 pandemic. Clin Chem. 2021;67(4):672–83. https://doi.org/10.1093/clinchem/hvab027.

10 Understanding How and Where Pathogens Emerge: Preparedness and Response for Zoonotic Diseases

Andrew Clements, Ian Mendenhall, and Daniel Schar

Contents

Learning Track Note: This chapter appears in Learning Tracks: Health Policy, Multilateral Cooperation, International Governance; One Health; Public Health and Epidemiology

Note: The views and opinions expressed in this paper are those of the authors and not necessarily the views and opinions of the United States Agency for International Development.

E. S. Higgs and R. A. Sorenson (eds.), *Principles and Practice of Emergency Research Response*,
https://doi.org/10.1007/978-3-031-48408-7_12

Learning Objectives

This chapter will help readers understand and describe:

- Zoonotic diseases that have emerged or reemerged at the wildlife–livestock–human–environment interface and some indications of potential spillover
- Zoonotic pathogen circulation, pathways to emergence in humans, and potential for sustained human-to-human transmission
- Opportunities to deploy targeted preventive measures against spillover; how pre-outbreak information bolsters global health security
- Why many zoonotic pathogen spillovers cannot be predicted or anticipated
- New data streams needed to better characterize the wildlife–livestock–human–environment interface
- Recommendations for better preparedness for and response to infectious disease emergencies

1 Introduction

This chapter will examine what we know about how and where zoonotic disease threats[1] emerge and key gaps in the information needed for preparedness, both before an outbreak and in emergency response. The mechanisms of zoonotic pathogen spillover and adaptation to humans are in many cases poorly understood and require sustained and focused research to

1. Characterize spillover mechanisms.
2. Develop interventions to reduce spillover, amplification, and onward transmission of emerging zoonoses.
3. Design and assess interventions such as diagnostics, therapeutics, and vaccines.
4. Refine surveillance targets.
5. Prepare for accelerated response where risks are greatest, ideally through local capacity building.

In this chapter, "pre-outbreak information" refers to data on known or potential zoonotic pathogens circulating in animals, humans, or blood-feeding arthropods before the first cluster of infections among people is recognized and reported (◘ Fig. 1). Spillover may also result in limited human-to-human transmission that does not sustain itself and is never detected.

1 In most usage "zoonotic" refers to pathogens like Ebola virus, some coronaviruses, and Nipah virus that are transmissible between vertebrate hosts and humans. This chapter will mostly focus on zoonotic viruses that can be transmitted from vertebrates to people by direct contact, but also includes vector-borne viruses.

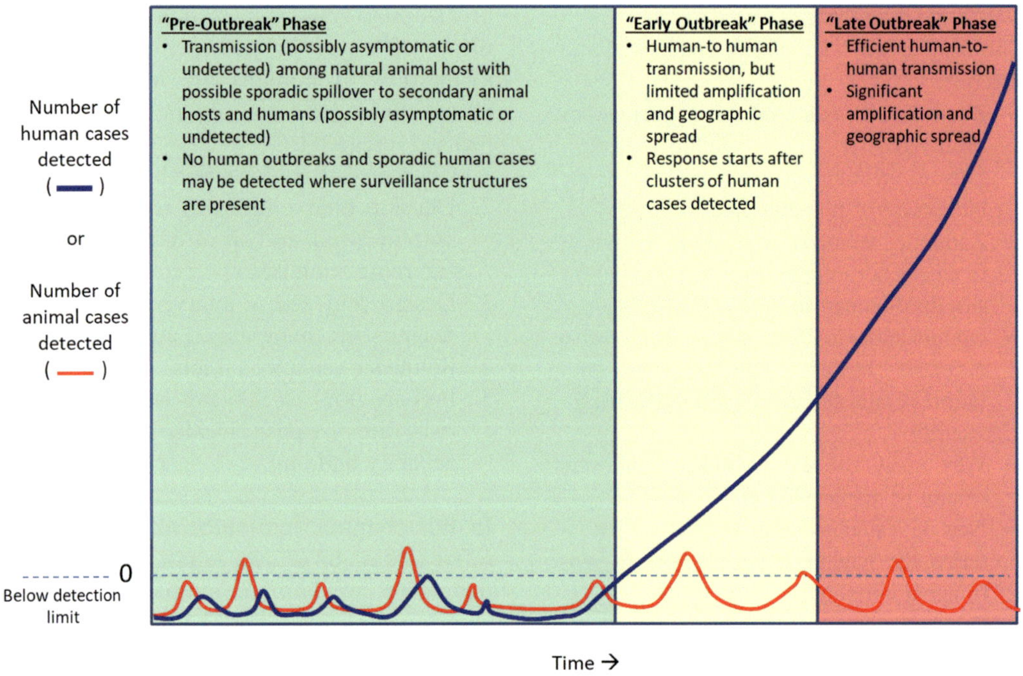

Fig. 1 Phases of human outbreaks with emerging zoonotic pathogens. (Authors)

2 Why Is Pre-outbreak Information Important?

Given the substantial impact of emerging zoonoses and the present scarcity of tools for prevention, detection, and response, along with the need to regularly update those that exist, investments in collecting and analyzing pre-outbreak information and using the results to reduce spillovers and limit their amplification and geographical spread would likely yield a high return on investment and strengthen global health security (Bernstein et al. 2022; Berry et al. 2022; World Bank 2012).

Collecting pre-outbreak information presents a unique opportunity to synthesize and distill pathogen, host, ecology, and other sources of data into actionable risk mitigation and to guide preparedness for future outbreaks in human populations. Reasons for investing in collecting pre-outbreak information are described below.

2.1 Impact of Uncontrolled Emerging Zoonoses

Novel pathogens have emerged in hominid populations over millions of years, sometimes followed by devastating epidemics or pandemics that have caused long-lasting social and economic damage, re-shaped society, and led to selection of protective genes in the human genome (Klunk et al. 2022). Since 1900, zoonotic pathogens have been responsible for at least six worldwide viral pandemics, caused by HIV, SARS-CoV-2, and influenza viruses, as well as numerous human outbreaks of highly pathogenic avian influenza, Ebola virus, Hendra virus, Marburg virus, MERS-CoV, mpox (previously known as monkeypox) virus (WHO 2022f), Nipah virus, and SARS-CoV-1 (Piret and Boivin 2021). The global health and economic impacts of some emerging threats have been enormous. For example, the 1918 influenza pandemic killed more than 50 million people

(CDC 2018a); HIV-AIDS has resulted in more than 36 million deaths (UNAIDS 2022); and the death toll of COVID-19 is more than 6.6 million people as of January 2023 (WHO 2023c). In many cases, the economic impacts of pandemics have driven people into poverty, especially in low- and middle-income countries (WBG 2022a).

By breaking down the expected costs of relatively infrequent pandemics on an annual basis, Fan et al. (2018) estimate the costs of influenza pandemics totaled approximately $500 billion annually, or about 0.6% of global income. For the COVID-19 pandemic, many economic sectors dropped by double-digit percentages in 2020 alone (Delardas et al. 2022), which is within the range of outcomes examined by Fan et al. With the rate of zoonotic pathogen emergence increasing, and climate-change related alterations at human–animal–environment interfaces, the future impact may be greater (Morand and Walther 2020). For example, one study estimated that while the probability of large epidemics varies over time, there is a 38% chance of experiencing a pandemic equivalent to COVID-19 in the next 100 years, and this may double in the coming decades (Marani et al. 2021).

2.2 Increasing Rates of Emergence and Potential Future Threats

Of the more than 1400 known human pathogens, over 60% are of zoonotic origin (Taylor et al. 2001). A retrospective study of new diseases emerging between 1940 and 2004 provides other key information:

- The rate of emergence (not merely the rate of detection) after adjusting for sampling bias has been increasing over time.
- Most new threats are viruses originating in wildlife.
- "Hot spots" for emergence are likely to be concentrated in tropical and sub-tropical regions.
- Resources for detection and response are not well distributed geographically or equally, and may be least available in low-latitude countries where the risks are greatest (Jones et al. 2008).

In addition, there are likely millions of uncharacterized viruses in mammals and birds, with roughly 700,000 of these estimated to be capable of crossing the species barrier to infect humans (Carroll et al. 2018). If new pathogens can cause asymptomatic infections, or if there is a long lag between infection and symptom onset, as with HIV, there may be "silent" (i.e., undetected) transmission in high-risk individuals.

Uncontained disease transmission among humans increases the risk of new pathogens becoming endemic in human populations and becoming established in previously uninfected animal species through spillback. Examples include SARS-CoV-2 spilling from people into multiple mammalian species and pandemic H1N1 influenza spilling from people into birds, pigs, and other mammals; spillback of mpox is also a concern (Blagrove et al. 2022; Frazzini et al. 2022; Keenliside 2013). The establishment of new animal reservoirs for zoonotic pathogens has important implications for their control and containment.

2.3 Availability of Targeted Interventions to Prevent, Detect, and Respond to Emerging Zoonoses

Many infectious diseases in humans, such as malaria, measles, and tuberculosis, have been known for centuries or millennia, and in many cases there are existing strategies and vaccines, therapeutics, and diagnostics (VTDs) to address them. However, for new and emerging zoonotic diseases, information, strategies, and tools to counter them may neither be available nor effective—particularly in acute outbreak settings where pathogen characteristics, modes of transmission, and clinical presentation may yet to have been fully elucidated. Examples of delays in the initial recognition, reporting, and implementation of interventions include the responses to HIV/AIDS, the 2014–2016 West Africa Ebola epidemic, and the current mpox public health emergency; these have resulted in thousands or millions of human infections occurring (CDC 2022a; Gallo and Montagnier 2003; WHO 2022a, b, 2023d). Even the relatively swift identification and genome sequence publication of the SARS CoV-2 virus did not prevent the outbreak from spreading worldwide because many countries were operating without critical information to inform timely, evidence-based decision-making or chose to ignore expert advice, thereby delaying action. However, the genomic sequence information was rapidly used to develop diagnostics, therapeutics, and vaccines.

2.4 Time, Focus, and Resources Are Limited Once Outbreaks Start

Research and surveillance efforts to collect missing information on emerging zoonotic diseases require a number of necessary, but time-consuming steps: building trust and establishing partnerships with affected populations, securing approvals from regulatory bodies, national and local governments, and other stakeholders, developing strategies, and training and equipping staff and institutions to do the work. It is easier to implement these steps between outbreaks because there is more time available, although funding can be a challenge unless this work has been prioritized by countries and donors. Serial episodes of pandemic response and repeated cycles of panic and neglect undermine the ability to discern patterns of spillover risk and guide interventions aimed at prevention. A prime example is the Ebola virus, which was first reported in 1976. Despite more than 30 outbreaks affecting 19 countries (nine of which occurred between 2017 and 2022) (CDC 2022b), the natural and incidental animal hosts for this family of viruses in endemic countries have not been definitively identified, although some bat species are thought to play a significant role in viral maintenance and transmission (Schuh et al. 2017). Indeed, West Africa was not considered to be at risk for Ebola until the 2014–2016 outbreak.

In an ideal world, collection of pre-outbreak information through early warning surveillance would complement outbreak prevention, detection, and response efforts. These components would be adequately funded and coordinated to maximize the chances of reducing the incidence and impact of outbreaks, epidemics, and pandemics. Pre-outbreak information would support a global early warning system to detect and respond to outbreaks by providing early information on potential public health threats and allow for targeting of surveillance at specific locations, interfaces, and species associated with spillover. At the same time, pre-outbreak information would also contribute to pre-outbreak planning to include the development of spillover prevention strategies as well as the development of VTDs (Carroll et al. 2018).

3 Pre-outbreak Information: What We Already Know About How and Where Pathogens Emerge

Information gathered over the last few decades has provided valuable—though not complete—insights into the zoonotic disease emergence process. Key points are summarized below.

3.1 The Risk Landscape Is Not Uniform: Specific Conditions Create Spillover Hot Spots

Emergence of zoonotic threats is complex and requires that humans, infectious agents, their animal hosts, and arthropod vectors such as ticks, fleas, or mosquitoes (if needed for transmission) are all present in the same place and time (Plowright et al. 2017). These interactions are part of a dynamic and continually evolving process (Hendry et al. 2017). Even when a pathogen infects humans, however, onward transmission is far from certain. Following spillover, if the infectious agent, host immune response, and population dynamics do not permit sustained human-to-human transmission, the event will likely die out. However, if the agent is capable of (or subsequently develops the capacity for) efficient human-to-human transmission in an immunologically naive population, as was the case for SARS-CoV-2, the spillover event may be followed by amplification and geographical spread, resulting in a country, regional, or global outbreak. Spillover of wildlife-hosted pathogens to people can happen directly (e.g., from wildlife to hunters or consumers) or indirectly via livestock.

If sufficient information is available on human, pathogen, animal host, and vector populations, predictive modeling can be a powerful tool to map potential spillover hot spots. As shown in ◘ Fig. 2, spillover risk for emerging zoonotic threats is predicted to be highest in forested regions in the tropics that are elevated and undergoing land-use changes, and also in areas with high wildlife biodiversity, primarily in sub-Saharan Africa, South and Southeast Asia, and East Asia (Allen et al. 2017; Jones et al. 2008). This hot spot mapping is mostly consistent with the location of spillovers of avian influenza viruses, Nipah virus, SARS-CoV-1, and SARS-CoV-2 in South and Southeastern Asia, as well as Ebola, HIV, Marburg, and Zika viruses in East and Central Africa. Regions with a high risk of spillover tend to have significant biodiverse and abundant wildlife populations (including species hosting emerging zoonotic threats), livestock production and trade with sub-optimal biosafety/biosecurity conditions, and land-use change. It is important to note that multiple spillover hot spots may be connected, existing as nodes in a transmission chain, and that the spillover potential may vary from location to location and at different times in the same location. For example, coronavirus detection rates increased as rodents in Vietnam were moved from their source along supply chains to markets (Huong et al. 2020).

While predictive model outputs are instructive and useful for framing risk profiles, it is important to recognize that they have inherent limitations, and that predictive accuracy is highly dependent upon data availability and use. Because of disparities in funding for research and surveillance, the United States and European countries often report individual human infections with Lassa virus, MERS-CoV, and mpox virus in travelers from endemic countries in Africa, Asia, and the Middle East (Allen et al. 2017). The fact that

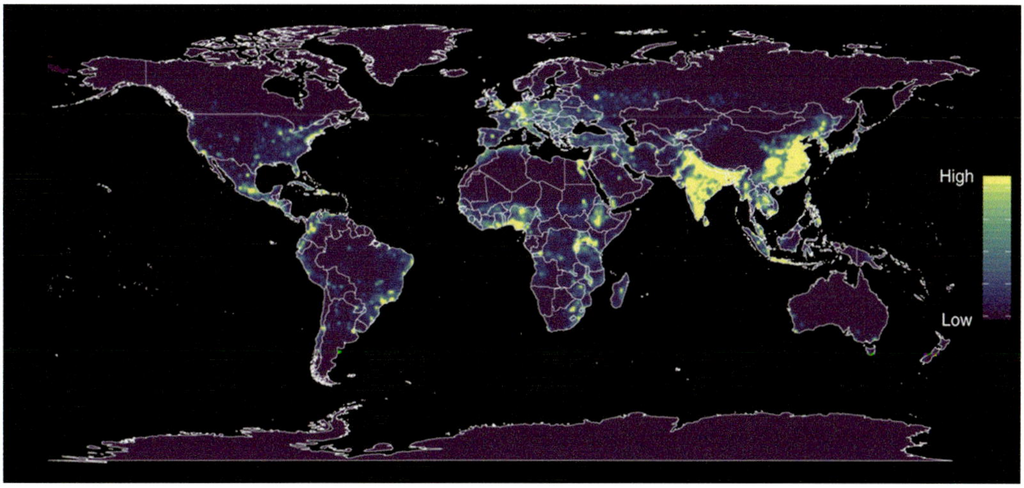

◘ **Fig. 2** Heat map of predicted relative risk distribution of zoonotic EID events, showing the estimated risk of event locations after factoring out reporting bias Hot-spots map 2.0. (Allen et al. 2017; open access)

biodiverse regions such as the Amazon that are experiencing increasing rates of land-use change do not show up as spillover hot spots suggests that zoonotic spillover risk is not captured equitably across the world (de Oliveira et al. 2022; Winck et al. 2022). This is supported by the emergence of MERS-CoV in the Arabian Peninsula, the 2009 H1N1 pandemic influenza virus in Mexico, and Lyme disease in the United States (Memish et al. 2014; Smith et al. 2009; Steere et al. 2004).

3.2 Specific Conditions and Human Behaviors at Hot Spots Affecting Spillover, Amplification, and Geographical Spread

Human behaviors and activities play an important role in the amplification, transmission, and dispersal of emerging zoonotic diseases (Lindahl and Grace 2015). The evolution and adaptation of humans have changed our exposure to the environment, while at the same time radically modifying our relationship with each other, the landscape, livestock and companion animals, wild animals, and vectors (Hendry et al. 2017; Nyhus 2016; Plowright et al. 2021). Anthropogenic environmental disruptions, including land-use change, agricultural intensification, and food production systems, drive the emergence of infectious diseases (Gibb et al. 2020; Keesing and Ostfeld 2021). The vast majority of tropical forest loss is caused by agricultural expansion; among the impacts is increasing zoonotic spillover (Pendrill et al. 2022). Within known geographical hot spot regions for spillover, specific animal–human interfaces may have increased frequency and duration of contact among humans, livestock, and wildlife (and vectors) because of agriculture and grain storage near homes (Lassa virus); raising livestock (avian influenza); mineral extraction and visiting caves (Marburg virus); collection of fruit tree sap (Nipah virus); and contact with wildlife during hunting, farming, or trade (Ebola, HIV, SARS-CoV-1, mpox) (CDC 2003; Glidden et al. 2021; Plowright et al. 2017). Other potential spillover interfaces include bats roosting in homes (Schuh et al. 2017), bat guano farming (Huong et al. 2020), and keeping primates and other wildlife as pets (Chomel et al. 2007). After spillover occurs, zoonotic pathogens can be amplified in human populations by crowded living or working conditions, congregation, inadequate infection prevention and control in healthcare facilities, and sexual behaviors, leading to geographical dispersion through travel and trade (Jones et al. 2013; Poletti et al. 2017). Shifting demographics—including a trend toward urbanization—and historically underserved and mobile populations without access to healthcare may further serve to amplify pathogen transmission among people and create routes for global dispersal. A summary of some pathogens, animal hosts, and spillover interfaces is shown in ◘ Fig. 3.

Human behavioral measures, the mainstay of early public health response to an infectious disease emergency, can also be protective in reducing spillover (Magouras et al. 2020; WHO et al. 2019). Examples include:

- Limiting contact with and consumption of animals, especially wildlife and sick animals
- Wearing protective gear when in contact with animals
- Vaccinating at-risk people (when available, e.g., rabies, yellow fever)
- Avoiding contaminated fruit
- Excluding wild animals from homes, whether as pests or pets
- Rearing livestock in biosafe and biosecure environments
- Implementing food safety measures, including boiling or pasteurizing beverages (e.g., water, milk), cooking food, and ensuring hygiene and sanitation in food preparation

Subsequent amplification and geographical spread of zoonotic pathogens in human populations can also be reduced by changing human behaviors, such as wearing masks; social distancing; infection prevention and control in healthcare facilities; vaccination (when available, e.g., influenza, COVID-19, yellow fever,

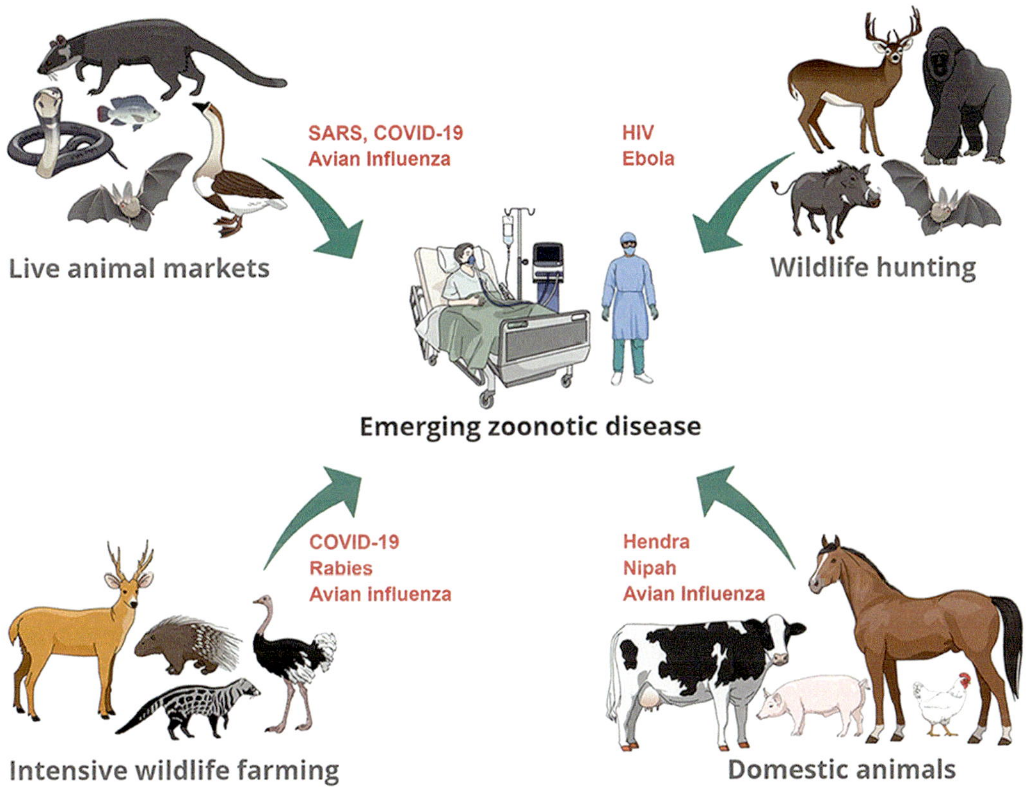

Fig. 3 Examples of zoonotic pathogens that have (re-)emerged at the animal–human–environment interface. Transmission pathways include direct contact through handling of living animals (wildlife trade, domestic animals) and preparation of slaughtered animals for consumption of meat or for traditional medicinal uses. (Magouras et al. 2020)

mpox); and pre- and post-exposure prophylaxis, partner reduction, and safe sex (Groves et al. 2021; Michie and West 2021).

3.3 Certain Animals Tend to Be Associated with Zoonotic Pathogens and Spillover Events

Numerous studies have shown that animals such as bats, rodents, nonhuman primates, and birds are more likely to be associated with zoonotic spillover than other animals (Luis et al. 2013; Olival et al. 2017). Pathogens may be widely distributed among these animal groups or limited to specific species (e.g., Marburg virus hosted by *Rousettus* bats). This is likely due to several factors, including the following:

- Their genetic relatedness to humans
- Relative abundance, density, and geographical distribution of species
- Biodiversity and loss of biodiversity in ecosystems
- The ability of some species to adapt to living in human-altered ecosystems
- Animals being farmed and traded because of their value for food and medicine or as pets

Furthermore, taxa predominating in human-altered landscapes are more likely hosts for zoonotic disease than those in undisturbed locations. The protective effects of biodiversity in mitigating disease emergence risk, possibly through a dilution effect, have also been observed (Keesing and Ostfeld 2021). Collectively, as Mollentze and Streicker (2020) note, four taxonomic groups (bats, rodents, nonhuman primates, and birds) are known to host many epidemic-prone pathogens, including pre-cursors of SARS-like coronaviruses and MERS-CoV; Ebola and Marburg viruses; avian influenza viruses; Hendra and Nipah viruses; and Hanta and Lassa viruses. In 2022, a study found that the overall rate of discovery of viruses in mammals, even those heavily sampled, is increasing or constant, illustrating that our understanding of virus diversity is still incomplete (Gibb et al. 2022).

In some animal hosts, biology and life history can result in seasonal shedding of zoonotic pathogens. For example, the reproductive pulses of bats appear to drive coronavirus shedding and filovirus and henipavirus seroprevalence patterns (Brook et al. 2019; Hayman 2015; Joffrin et al. 2022; Montecino-Latorre et al. 2020). Bird migration patterns and timing may play a role in the seasonality of avian influenza events, although not universally. In Bangladesh, little seasonality was observed in transmission within live bird markets (Berry et al. 2022; Tian et al. 2015; Wacharapluesadee et al. 2009). There is also evidence of seasonality of MERS-CoV in camels, Lassa virus in *Mastomys* rats, and Nipah virus in flying foxes in Thailand (Akhmetzhanov et al. 2019; Dudas et al. 2018; Wacharapluesadee et al. 2009). Vector-borne infectious diseases are also driven by seasonal patterns. In temperate climes, temperatures and rainfall drive the proliferation of mosquitoes and subsequent outbreaks, as seen with Rift Valley fever virus (Anyamba et al. 2009).

3.4 Some Zoonotic Pathogens Are More Capable of Spillover

Many properties are intrinsic to individual viruses or families of viruses and make them especially adept at spilling over from animals to people (Antonovics et al. 2017; Duffy et al. 2008; Finlay and McFadden 2006; Grassly and Fraser 2006; Kreuder Johnson et al. 2015). These include

- Adaptability through rapid mutation, especially for RNA viruses
- Stability in the environment
- Transmissibility via multiple routes (e.g., saliva, urine, feces, blood)
- The ability to infect multiple host species (i.e., host plasticity)
- Ability to evade or suppress host defenses

3.5 Spillover of Zoonotic Pathogens Can Change Over Time

Pathogen spillover is likely substantially more common than our current surveillance systems are able to detect (Sánchez et al. 2022) and can increase or decrease if the presence of humans, infectious agents, animal hosts, and arthropod vectors changes in response to anthropogenic, climatic, or environmental drivers (Smolinski et al. 2003). For example, spillover may decrease over time if the animal hosts for specific pathogens can no longer survive in that environment or humans change a behavior that was necessary for spillover. For example, research on Hendra virus in Australia demonstrated pathways to spillover risk where specific and actionable risk mitigation can be undertaken by changing land-use patterns (Eby et al. 2022).

On the other hand, spillover may increase if the frequency and duration of contact between people and the animal host(s) of a pathogen increases because of land-use change, climate change or other alterations in shared ecologies. These can change animal and human habitats by

- Forcing the sharing and cross-contamination of water due to limited supply
- Allowing for greater movement and mixing of species through
  - Building new roads and settlements
  - Increasing the number and species diversity of livestock and wildlife farmed and traded
- Displacing wildlife through deforestation followed by monoculture, such as palm oil plantations (Hassell et al. 2017; Morand and Lajaunie 2021; Plowright et al. 2021)

Changing habitats jeopardize wildlife health as global forest loss occurs at staggering rates, drastically reducing biodiversity (Betts et al. 2017). Loss of biodiversity tends to increase the transmission risk of zoonoses, such that zoonoses are positively correlated with the number of threatened bird and mammal species (Morand et al. 2019). Climate change can also drive the emergence of zoonoses (Betts et al. 2017). The expansion of suitable habitats for arthropod vectors can facilitate autochthonous (locally acquired) transmission of pathogens (Caminade et al. 2019), and warmer temperatures can also shorten developmental stages for arthropod vectors and decrease the intrinsic incubation period of the pathogen (Bartlow et al. 2019). Warmer temperatures can also stress animal hosts, resulting in decreasing immune function and increasing pathogen shedding that may lead to increased zoonotic disease spillover risk (Mora et al. 2022).

Within human-disrupted habitats, there are specific, synanthropic animals, such as some rat (*Rattus* spp.), mice (*Mus* spp.), and macaque (*Macaca* spp.) species that are able to take advantage of disruptions to the ecosystem, resulting in known wildlife hosts of human-shared pathogens and parasites overall comprising a greater proportion of local species richness (18–72% higher) and total abundance (21–144% higher) in sites under substantial human use (Mora et al. 2022). These species can also transport pathogens between human-modified habitats and natural habitats (McFarlane et al. 2012). They are often introduced and/or invasive, have flexible habitat and resource needs, and can rapidly adapt to changing environments including human domiciles, providing opportunities for zoonotic pathogen spillover (Hornok et al. 2015; Voigt et al. 2016).

The human population has grown from less than two billion to eight billion over the past century, with commensurate increases in livestock production, travel, trade, and land exploitation engendering more frequent contact among humans, animals, and microbes, as well as arthropod vectors (Smith et al. 2014). For example, the large-scale farming of waterfowl (e.g., ducks and geese) in Asia under sub-optimal biosecurity conditions facilitated the spread of avian influenza viruses from wild birds to high-density domestic flocks, where their amplification led to occasional spillover causing severe human infections and deaths (Liu et al. 2020; Webster and Hulse 2004).

3.6 Interventions to Reduce Spillover Risk

Even without knowing the exact mechanism by which some pathogens spill over from animals to humans, it is possible in some instances to reduce risk. For example, immunizing poultry with avian influenza (AI) vaccines specific for viral sub-types and variants can prevent or reduce infection in flocks and spillover to humans (Capua and Alexander 2006). A second approach is pathogen agnostic and involves employing good farm and market biosecurity to limit not only spillover, but also amplification and geographical spread of AI viruses and other pathogens. Good biosecurity limits pathogen spread from wildlife to poultry, from poultry to humans, and from poultry back to wild birds (Capua and Marangon 2006; Chowdhury et al. 2020; Liu et al. 2020). As mentioned above, excluding farm animals such as pigs and horses from areas with fruiting trees frequented by flying foxes can limit livestock exposure to Nipah virus and Hendra virus, respectively (Fig. 4) (Kummer and Kranz 2022).

Developing interventions to reduce spillover risk requires enough pre-outbreak information to identify the pathogen–host and transmission pathway(s). However, this information is not always collected or shared, which limits the ability of countries to prevent, prepare for, or respond to spillover events. In contrast to open-source outbreak tracking and reporting structures managed by international organizations such as the World Health Organization (WHO 2022c), the UN Food and Agriculture Organization, the World Organization for Animal Health, and the Program for Monitoring Emerging

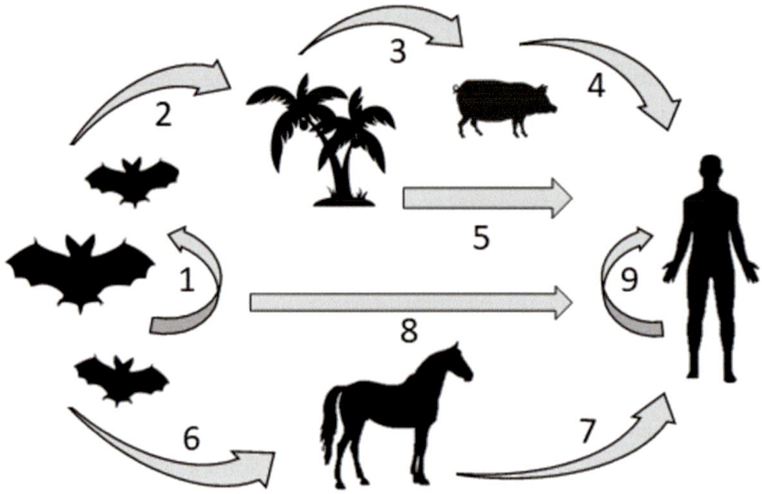

Fig. 4 Presumptive Henipavirus transmission routes: (1) from bats to bats via placental transmission, lactation, or mating; (2) fruit consumption; (3) excretion and partially eaten fruits; (4) from pig to farmer (Nipah virus Malaysia); (5) date palm consumption (Nipah Bangladesh); (6) excretion; (7) from horse to owner (Henipavirus, Nipah Philippines; Hendra virus, Australia); (8) bite, scratch, etc.; and (9) from human to human (Nipah Philippines, Nipah Bangladesh). (Kummer and Kranz 2022)

Diseases (PROMED 2022; WHO 2023a; WOAH 2022), findings from pre-outbreak research are disseminated more slowly.

4 What We Still Need to Know

While current data on zoonotic pathogen emergence have made it possible to better focus prevention, detection, and response capacities on specific locations and animal–human–environment interfaces, gaps remain in knowledge and in systems for analyzing and sharing information. Animal hosts and animal–human–environment interfaces where spillover occurs are known for some zoonotic pathogens, such as the Marburg and Nipah viruses, but considerable uncertainty remains for others, such as coronaviruses, Ebola, Lassa, and mpox viruses. In many cases, the primary animal host is uncertain. In others, the full range of animals that can serve as hosts, the specific behaviors and practices associated with spillover of each pathogen, and the frequency, duration, and dynamics of animal–human contact are unclear (Recht et al. 2020). However, research on infections in animals faces many challenges, not least the cost and scale of the programs required (Koopmans 2013).

Prioritizing resources to fill current knowledge gaps and improve data systems for reporting both ongoing research and new outbreaks should be a near-term goal for countries and the global community to enable targeted risk mitigation interventions and development of medical countermeasures (MCMs). Key gaps are summarized below.

4.1 Characterization of Risk at the Animal–Human–Environment Interface

For some zoonotic pathogens, enough information on hosts and interfaces is available to begin limiting risk. In the case of Marburg virus, demonstrated spillover routes include human contact with Egyptian fruit bats in caves or mines. Avoiding such locations or wearing protective gear may limit the risk (Adjemian et al. 2011; Timen et al. 2009). For many zoonotic pathogens, basic information is urgently needed to update risk maps and develop risk-reduction interventions, as well as diagnostics, therapeutics, and vaccines.

Missing information includes potential host species; the extent to which animals have been exposed to and carry pathogens of interest; specific practices facilitating or preventing spillover; seasonal patterns of host infections and pathogen shedding; and the capacity of specific host taxa to serve as reservoirs of additional, as-yet-unknown pathogens (Carlson et al. 2021; Roberts et al. 2021). Detection of animal host taxa and their range is still imperfect. Estimates of abundance, presence, and absence, especially for rare host taxa, may be highly variable and become more difficult as ecosystems change under pressure of human usage and climate change (Kellner and Swihart 2014). Leveraging large datasets facilitates testing of models to understand geographical hot spots for emergence, predicting the presence of host animals, the potential pathogens they may carry, which newly discovered microbes may be prone to infect humans, and how to prioritize viral research in zoonotic reservoirs (Allen et al. 2017; Becker et al. 2020; Carlson et al. 2021; Grange et al. 2021). Ideally, datasets would include the same metadata to make analyses more robust.

For Nipah virus, two spillover mechanisms have been described so far (Fig. 4). In Malaysia, the virus moved from *Pteropus* bat species, through partially eaten fruit to farmed pigs, and then to people (Chua 2003). In Bangladesh, *Pteropus* bats shed virus into date palm sap collected for human consumption (Islam et al. 2013; Rahman et al. 2012). No further spillover has been documented in Malaysia since 1999, suggesting that the bat–pig–human interface was successfully disrupted. In Bangladesh, where sporadic human infections continue to occur, with short chains of human-to-human transmission (Nikolay et al. 2019), additional work is needed to determine why uptake of effective interventions to block Nipah virus transmission is low (Khan et al. 2012; Nahar et al. 2010, 2017). Additional knowledge gaps include why the Nipah virus can be detected seasonally from *Pteropus lylei* bats in Thailand, yet no human or domestic animal cases have been reported to date (Wacharapluesadee et al. 2009, 2021a). The interface and mechanism for repeated Nipah virus spillover to people in Kerala State, India, in recent years has not yet been identified (Yadav et al. 2022).

While some information is available on animal hosts for Lassa and mpox viruses (Monath et al. 1974; Parker and Buller 2013; Ter Meulen et al. 1996; Wozniak et al. 2021), the interface(s) and mechanism(s) for spillover in West Africa are unknown, hampering efforts to develop interventions. Although the first human infection with the H5N1 avian influenza was detected more than 25 years ago, and it is well known that direct and indirect contact with infected poultry is a major risk factor, the specific nature of the contact needed for transmission has not been definitively identified (Li et al. 2019). Possibilities include inhalation of air-borne virus or physical contact with contaminated birds during farming, slaughtering, defeathering, or processing (Wan et al. 2011), each of which would potentially require different types of risk-reduction interventions.

Many zoonotic diseases spill over directly from wildlife or livestock to people, but another key interface involves wildlife contact with livestock. This mechanism allows zoonotic pathogens to spill over from wildlife to livestock and then, following amplification in these domesticated species (with or without symptoms), into humans. Examples include avian influenza viruses moving from wild birds to poultry to people (Yoon et al. 2014); Nipah virus spilling from bats to pigs and then to people, and Hendra virus starting in bats and then infecting horses and finally humans (Kessler et al. 2018). With the increasing number of livestock produced each year to feed the growing human population, the wildlife–livestock interface could grow as a source of spillover events and should be regularly monitored.

Improving characterization of animal–human–environment interfaces requires improving the sharing of existing pre-outbreak information. For existing data, country, regional, and global partners routinely produce data from research studies and outbreaks, including information on pathogens, animal hosts, and sometimes human behavior, but their release is often via publication of peer-reviewed scientific papers, which may take years. In addition, data may be unavailable to many researchers if they are published in a journal with limited access, reported in a student thesis or doctoral dissertation, or the researcher does not have the ability to conduct specialized analyses. Thus, obstacles to researchers collectively sharing, analyzing, and using pre-outbreak information in near-real time constrains the ability of countries to improve prevention, detection, and response to emerging zoonotic diseases (Kucharski 2022). The urgency of understanding SARS-CoV-2 during the COVID-19 pandemic helped lead to more streamlined processes, with increased communications between researchers and public health officials, pre-prints of articles becoming available before full peer review, subscription-only journals making their COVID-19 articles open access, and genetic sequence data quickly posted on accessible platforms such as GISAID. Such interchanges must be improved and accelerated in routine practice for the global health ecosystem to prevent more outbreaks from becoming global emergencies and ensure that tools are available for prevention and response.

Another way to improve the characterization of animal–human–environment interfaces is to add new data streams, especially regularly updated data that reflect population-level changes. Satellites can now collect near-real-time data on habitat changes and forest loss or transformation of biodiverse forests into monocultures (e.g., oil palm)—phenomena that should be prioritized for spillover surveillance (Hansen et al. 2013). Useful data streams could also come from monitoring or screening:

- Human and animal population movements
- Wildlife migration
- Wildlife and pet trade, legal and illegal
- Extractive industry operations which can
  - Destroy habitat
  - Drive consumption of wildlife ("bush meat") by workers
- Livestock production near wildlife-rich locations
- Clean water availability for people and animals
- Pathogens in wastewater or sewage

Such data can add more detail on temporal and spatial variability in host distributions, shedding of potential pathogens, and reservoir host immunological status (Plowright et al. 2017).

The global capacity for genome sequencing and analysis has advanced at a remarkable pace for several decades and has facilitated a better understanding of microbial diversity and informed epidemiological studies of outbreaks (DeLong et al. 2022; Pappalardo et al. 2016). However, gaps remain in being able to use a pathogen's genetic instructions to predict key phenotypic features such as virulence, transmissibility, host range, host-cell binding, and host immune escape—analytical tools that could revolutionize risk assessments. Genome-predictive models of microbial zoonotic and epidemic potential remain nascent (Nwadiugwu and Monteiro 2022). Better understanding of pathogen diversity and use of next-generation sequencing to identify and then detect markers of virulence and host cell receptor binding targets could help prioritize surveillance efforts and interventions for those microbes with potential pathology in humans.

As the volume of data and the complexity of analyses increase, in-country bioinformatics and other analytic capacities must be strengthened to expedite the use of biological, behavioral, and environmental data for risk assessments, forecasting, identifying interventions, and developing risk-reduction measures and VTDs. Unhindered, expedited data sharing, including genetic sequences, among sectors and between scientists in different countries is essential for successful coordination and execution of research, surveillance, laboratory detection, spillover risk reduction, outbreak response, and development of VTDs before and during outbreaks. As seen with vaccines to counter SARS-CoV-2, global capabilities for accelerated vaccine development based on genome sequence opened new possibilities for rapid deployment of interventions, but emergency development of inter-

Fig. 5 Examples of interventions against emerging zoonotic diseases

Selected Non-Pharmaceutical Interventions	Selected Medical Countermeasures (Pathogen specific or broad spectrum)
Social (physical) distancing	Vaccines
Masks and other personal protective equipment	Therapeutics: antivirals, monoclonal antibodies, antibiotics, immune-system modulators
Hand washing	Diagnostics
Heating potentially contaminated food and water	Patient care guidelines to optimize supportive care and disseminate information on MCMs
Practicing safer sex	
Minimizing contact with possible host animals	

ventions VTDs still requires the timely sharing of genetic sequences and pathogen samples (▶ Chap. 7) (Pandemic Preparedness Partnership 2021).

4.2 Developing and Assessing Safety and Efficacy of Interventions to Reduce Spillover, Amplification, and Geographical Spread

Once sufficient data about a pathogen (e.g., hosts, pathogenesis, modes of transmission, and other factors) are available, interventions to reduce spillover risk can be developed and further assessed. Interventions broadly fall into the categories of nonpharmaceutical (a.k.a. public health) and MCMs, as shown in Fig. 5.

In order to develop broad-acting VTDs against families of pathogens that infect humans, genetic diversity across the virus family will need to be assessed and research done on key shared genetic sequences, antigen mapping, and pathogenic mechanisms.

As mentioned previously, interventions such as farm and market biosecurity along with animal vaccines have been shown to lower the number of human infections with influenza viruses (Youssef et al. 2021; Zhou et al. 2018). Emerging pathogens transmitted by arthropod vectors can potentially be addressed using vector-control measures, but these are difficult and expensive to implement at scale. At present, few interventions to prevent spillover are available for viruses such as Ebola, Lassa, mpox, and Nipah that are transmitted directly from wildlife to people. For Nipah, interventions have been proposed that would be expected to be effective, but they have not been widely adopted. For example, the boiling of date palm sap before consumption kills the virus, but also changes the composition of the product and its desirability (Khan et al. 2012). Bamboo "tree skirts" to block bats from accessing collected sap from date palm trees have been shown to prevent Nipah contamination of the sap, but collectors have not adopted the practice consistently because they lack the time and resources (Nahar et al. 2010).

In conclusion, filling in some of the gaps in pre-outbreak information will allow for more precise understanding of animal–human–environment interfaces, provide vital information to improve surveillance and early warning, and develop risk-reduction interventions to minimize the chances of future spillover.

5 Pre-outbreak Information: Best Practices and Recommendations

The dynamics between spillover of zoonotic pathogens and when an outbreak is detected and identified in humans are complex and involve many sectors and disciplines. While previous efforts to establish pre-outbreak monitoring often have been a "learning-by-doing" exercise, there are some best practices that have emerged over the past few decades.

5.1 Strengthening Country Capacities Improves Detection and Response for Zoonotic Pathogens

Since spillover of emerging zoonotic pathogens can happen in any country, all nations should be able to prevent, detect, and respond to routine and emerging infectious disease threats. Regular surveillance to collect pre-outbreak information and detect unusual events should be established and linked to risk characterization and outbreak investigation (Institute of Medicine and National Research Council 2009). If regular surveillance is not in place, focused research studies can provide valuable insights, as demonstrated by community-level monitoring of SARS-CoV-2 and mpox virus in wastewater and sewage (Corpuz et al. 2020; Wolfe et al. 2022).

A strong, agile laboratory system is an important component for pre-outbreak monitoring (▶ Chap. 9). Virus detection, genetic sequencing, serology, and phylogenetic analyses provide valuable information on viral prevalence, composition, and diversity, helping to guide epidemiological investigations, target surveillance, and develop interventions. Ideally, there should be at least one highly capable laboratory facility in every country, though there are security concerns that a proliferation of biosafety level 4 facilities could present biosafety and biosecurity vulnerabilities. Laboratories must include facilities at the appropriate biosafety and security level for the work being carried out to minimize risks (Eaves 2020). Research data of this kind is also useful for generating serological tests to determine exposure and understand decay rates of antibody titers and immune escape (Andreano et al. 2021; Chia et al. 2021; Tan et al. 2020). Sensitive detection assays, such as quantitative polymerase chain reaction (qPCR), multiplex serological assays, and next-generation sequencing, can provide same-day turnaround for detection and preliminary characterization, even for use at the point of collection (Laing et al. 2021; Watsa et al. 2020). As some emerging microbes may be challenging to grow in a laboratory, models have been developed to predict the capacity for human infection (Mollentze et al. 2021). Other techniques include phylogenetic reconstruction of ancestral viruses to study adaptations that facilitate cross-species transmission, assessing immunological responses when exposing cell cultures to viral proteins, and understanding receptor binding sites to provide insight into which viruses are likely capable of infecting humans (Damas et al. 2020; Le Bert et al. 2020; Su et al. 2021; Zhao et al. 2005).

Because of the sheer volume and broad distribution of spillover interfaces, the limited staff and resources available for collecting pre-outbreak information must be deployed where spillover risk is greatest. Targeted surveillance can use currently available information on the mechanisms and relative risks of specific emerging zoonotic threats, based on factors like the size, density, and distribution of human, animal, and microbial populations; human behavior; and potentially high-risk chains of transmission that could lead to outbreaks, sustained human-to-human transmission, and geographical spread of emerging zoonotic pathogens (Alexander et al. 2018; Becker et al. 2019). An important aspect of detecting emerging threats early is understanding which human populations might be infected first and show clinical signs. Like SARS-CoV-2, some emerging zoonotic threats (e.g., H7N9 avian influenza, MERS-CoV) may be asymptomatic or mildly symptomatic in many healthy and younger individuals (Badawi and Ryoo 2016; Wang et al. 2017), highlighting the importance of monitoring comorbid or immunocompromised people. It is also critical to focus research on understanding the mechanisms of emergence of zoonotic pathogens in humans (including Ebola virus, MERS-CoV, Nipah virus, and SARS-CoV-1 and 2).

Better pre-outbreak information collection is necessary for improving prevention and preparedness for a rapid response when needed. Pre-outbreak research programs during interpandemic periods can pivot to emergency response when necessary; in the case of zoonoses, research can focus on origins and spillover mechanisms to prevent recurrence and identify similar pathogens of concern. Funding and research sparked by the SARS-CoV-1 outbreak in 2002–2003, for example, informed surveillance and development of MCMs later used to address SARS-CoV-2 (Padron-Regalado 2020; Wang et al. 2006). After the publication of the SARS-CoV-2 genetic sequence, many countries quickly tested archived or new animal samples to learn more about the hosts of SARS-CoV-2-like viruses and their geographical distribution. Related viruses were detected in some horseshoe bat species and pangolins in Cambodia, Japan, Laos, Thailand, and Vietnam (Murakami et al. 2020; Wacharapluesadee et al. 2021b). Research on viruses related to SARS-CoV-2 in these countries improves risk assessment by expanding understanding of the host range of coronaviruses that can use human ACE-2 receptors (Delaune et al. 2021; Temmam et al. 2022).

The success of early warning surveillance systems in guiding effective response efforts depends on

- Contextual information collected during pre-outbreak monitoring and research.
- Ability to rapidly detect the first signal of an unusual infectious disease event and confirm the identity of the pathogen.
- Quality and completeness of pre-outbreak and post-outbreak data.
- Speed with which the information is collected, analyzed, and shared.

The detection of Marburg virus in bats sampled in Sierra Leone in 2017–2018 provided notice of the virus's presence in West Africa and allowed countries to prepare for future spillover events (Amman et al. 2020). Both Guinea in 2021 and Ghana in 2022 were then able to contain Marburg virus outbreaks with little or no onward spread in humans (WHO 2021, 2022d). In Thailand, diagnostic capacities developed for proactive monitoring of wildlife for zoonotic viruses were quickly repurposed in January 2020 to detect SARS-CoV-2 in visitors from Wuhan, China, allowing the government to immediately implement isolation and social-distancing measures before commercial testing kits were available (Wacharapluesadee et al. 2020).

Strengthening country capacities for collecting pre-outbreak information involves planning, staffing, training, equipment and supplies, coordination, communications, and funding to support efforts that span multiple sectors and levels of government. When research is supported by external funds or technical support, these partnerships must be equitable (► Chaps. 4 and 30). Numerous tools are available for countries to assess human and institutional capacities to identify gaps in pre-outbreak monitoring and outbreak detection and response. For example, the Joint External Evaluation, developed by WHO, brings together governments and other relevant stakeholders to develop a targeted National Action Plan for Health Security. The Electronic State Parties Self-Assessment Annual Reporting Tool (e-SPAR) provides a platform to develop accountability for meeting the requirements of the (WHO 2016). It should be noted that these rating systems for country capacity are more predictive of success in containing smaller outbreaks than for pandemics such as COVID-19 (Jain et al. 2022). After-action reviews and international negotiations to improve pandemic response are ongoing (WHO 2024). Simulation exercises can also be used to evaluate planned responses to infectious disease outbreaks in order to make program and policy improvements.

5.2 Systematic Collection of Pre-outbreak Information

The ability to collect, analyze, share, and use pre-outbreak information related to emerging zoonotic diseases in a targeted way is vital to prevention, preparedness, and response. Without such initial data, a vast number of samples may have to be collected in the dark, as it were, to understand the natural history of an emerging virus. For example, a 3-year study in Guinea, Liberia, and Sierra Leone needed to test about 45,000 specimens from apparently healthy animals in order to detect Ebola Zaire in a bat from Liberia, Marburg virus in *Rousettus* bats from Sierra Leone, and a new species of Ebola (*Bombali ebolavirus*) in specific bat species in Guinea and Sierra Leone (PREDICT Consortium 2021). Along with identifying the bat species hosting these viruses, this work also indicated potential spillover interfaces (e.g., caves, homes).

Greater specificity of serosurveys to assess previous population exposure to viruses is critical for designing well-focused data collection tools and strategies (Epstein et al. 2020). Broad screening techniques have been valuable but are hampered by cross-reactivity issues (i.e., inability to distinguish between related viruses). Serological assays are becoming more refined, however, and it is now possible to distinguish exposure to SARS-CoV-2 from seasonal coronaviruses (Gilbert et al. 2013; Laing et al. 2021). One recent study from eastern Democratic Republic of the Congo used serology to detect previous exposure to Ebolaviruses (including Bombali virus) among people not otherwise known to have been infected (Goldstein et al. 2020). Other serological surveys have shown evidence for human exposure to several types of emerging zoonotic threats, including HIV, primate T-lymphotropic viruses, simian foamy viruses in primate hunters, and filoviruses in bat hunters (Dovih et al. 2019; Kurpiers et al. 2016; Wolfe et al. 2005).

But additional data on how and where pathogens emerge are of limited value if not analyzed, shared, and used to shape action by funders, policymakers, and at-risk populations. There are many obstacles to timely data sharing, as noted above, but there have been some recent advances in addressing some of the bottlenecks. For example, the researchers who detected Bombali virus in Sierra Leone rapidly presented their findings in ProMED (Archive Number: 20190408.6409703) and in a brief journal communication (Goldstein et al. 2018). In addition, the detection of Marburg virus in Sierra Leone was reported in ProMED and in brief communications in several other electronic venues more than a year in advance of peer-reviewed publication (Amman et al. 2020). Since the start of the COVID-19 pandemic, the use of data-sharing platforms such as GISAID, Our World in Data, and others, as well as preprint publication platforms, has accelerated the circulation of outbreak information and research data (Fraser et al. 2021; WHO 2022e).

5.3 Surveillance and Research Networks Improve Information Sharing, Preparedness, and Response

Cloud-based storage and sharing platforms such as GISAID[2] provide secure, rapid access for experts to analyze and assess influenza virus and SARS-CoV-2 sequence data in order to expeditiously identify and track viral variants and provide advice to policymakers and affected populations. The online availability of SARS-CoV-2 genetic sequence data in January 2020 was one of the factors that facilitated the development of diagnostic assays and safe, effective COVID-19 vaccines less than a year after the first human infections were noted (▶ Chap. 12).

Laboratories are more powerful if linked together to share data and workload. Laboratory networks may be based on a specific type of pathogen (e.g., influenza) (WHO 2023b); the surveillance data generated from both the animal and human health sectors are analyzed twice yearly to determine the composition of seasonal influenza vaccines for the human population (WHO 2023b). Other lab networks host data on multiple pathogens and may be regional or global, allowing for coordination, communications, standardization, and training before outbreaks occur (Africa CDC 2023; ECDC 2023; IAEA 2023). There have been recent discussions on further enhancing global and country surveillance by mobilizing a "coordinated network of multisector and multilateral stakeholders to collect

2 Originally the Global Initiative on Sharing Avian Influenza Data, now known simply as GISAID.

data, share insights, and respond to signals of early disease outbreaks" (Krofah et al. 2021). Though data provenance is a critical aspect of data collection, it is also critical that protocols are established and implemented that ensure data storage and sharing are safe and secure. This will minimize opportunities for the unintentional release or theft of such assets or the use of the data for harmful purposes. Safe data-sharing protocols should be developed, as they do not exist currently, so that both in-country and international partners are following similar standards.

Focused research projects such as the Centers for Research in Emerging Infectious Diseases (CREID) and the PREDICT emerging infection disease project have used a standardized surveillance and detection approach across many countries and regions to link scientists and laboratories together to generate pre-outbreak information on emerging pathogens (CREID 2022; PREDICT Consortium 2021).

5.4 Targeted Risk Reduction Interventions Work

There is evidence that when enough information on spillover dynamics is available for specific zoonotic pathogens (e.g., avian influenza viruses in Hong Kong live bird markets, Nipah virus in Malaysia), their spillover to people can be reduced (Leung et al. 2012; Nahar et al. 2017). Larger scale changes in policy (e.g., conditions on pig farms or live animal markets, vaccination of poultry) potentially yield much broader impact than efforts to change individual behaviors. Interventions to reduce spillover are generally not available for zoonotic diseases such as Ebola, Lassa fever, and mpox because information on the mechanisms of spillover is lacking. As a result, spillover events continue irregularly with the potential for any one of them escalating to a sustained outbreak, epidemic, or pandemic.

In order to support the application of spillover risk-reduction interventions, all countries should have the capacity to conduct pre-outbreak research and risk assessments across sectors to include cost–benefit analyses to aid decision-makers regarding policies and allocation of funds. Both the financial burden of inaction and the magnitude of previously hidden losses driven by "business-as-usual" must be captured and quantified to assess policy options (Schar et al. 2018). Disease emergence risks may be driven by practices that redound to the benefit of some and the detriment of others, and such economic factors must be considered in the planning and promotion of risk mitigation. Extractive industries, for example, may bring humans into new areas, destroy habitat, and pollute watercourses, all of which can drive disease emergence. The financial and quality of life burdens are distributed broadly across communities, livelihoods, and health systems, while the financial benefits may accrue to a handful of investors. Taking a whole-of-society approach to the analysis of costs and benefits helps identify equitable measures to minimize risks and promote sustainable interventions. Establishing benchmarks for low-risk industry practices paired with certification could (1) generate market-based pull incentives (e.g., premium pricing for quality-assured food products produced with minimal ecological disruption), and (2) establish a framework for corporate tax incentives (to the extent that the activities driving zoonotic risk are in the formal sector of the economy).

Given the substantial benefits to society of preventing disease outbreaks, this work should be supported financially by national and international stakeholders in both the public and private sectors. Illustrating the value of emerging disease prevention as a global public good, the promotion of avian influenza vaccination of commercial poultry through subsidized vaccines matched to currently circulating strains could be an important tool in reducing pandemic influenza risk (Wu et al. 2019). Finally, support should also go to longitudinal work to understand the dynamics of zoonoses in natural reservoirs subject to new pressures from climate and land-use change, as well as how interventions can influence current policies, business practices, and behaviors in order to reduce spillover risk.

5.5 Coordination with Other Infectious Disease Programs and Across Sectors to Improve Prevention, Detection, and Response

While infectious disease control programs and networks are often pathogen specific, it is important for existing programs to have some flexibility to adapt to a new pathogen. Every infectious disease program has experts with skills in surveillance, detection, prevention, risk communication, epidemiology, and research, among other areas. As occurred during the COVID-19 pandemic, such existing capacity can pivot to understanding and containing new threats in an emergency. For example, surveillance and laboratory systems for respiratory symptoms were able to test for SARS-CoV-2. In addition, many countries used their animal health labs to provide surge support for SARS-CoV-2 detection in human samples at the beginning of the COVID-19 pandemic or repurposed other surveillance and outbreak response structures (Drew et al. 2020; Wacharapluesadee et al. 2020). Risk communications and outreach expertise from HIV/AIDS programs were able to support interrupting person-to-person transmission of mpox virus, and, along with vaccination, appears to have helped bring the 2022 outbreak under control in Europe and North America (Kirby 2022). Successful redirection of resources to contain an outbreak of an emerging pathogen depends on the speed with which it can be accomplished as well as appropriate use of capabilities. This requires development (between outbreaks) of well-planned yet flexible preparedness and response strategies and standard operating procedures for how and when to launch an emergency research response, along with clear channels for emergency financing when necessary (▶ Chap. 28).

Given the complex interactions between emerging zoonotic pathogens, animal hosts, susceptible humans, vectors, and the environment, a multidisciplinary, collaborative, and coordinated research and response approach is required. Identifying and assessing potential hazards and having systems and procedures in place to detect, respond, and share information will prepare governments, businesses, communities, and others for future outbreaks. Some of the tools now available to facilitate multisectoral preparedness planning and response include.

- Table-top simulation exercises
- The *Tripartite Zoonoses Guide* compiled by the Food and Agriculture Organization of the United Nations (FAO), WHO, and the World Organization for Animal Health (WOAH) (WHO et al. 2019)
- One Health zoonotic disease prioritization workshops (CDC 2018b)
- Systematic incorporation of One Health perspectives, methodologies, and coordination into pandemic preparedness (NASEM 2022)
- Case studies from around the world conveying lessons from One Health programming (PREDICT Consortium 2021)

Together, these strategies, with support from global and regional partners, can assist countries in strengthening their capacities to promote preparedness and societal resilience. Preparedness planning must also try to avoid the common human error of applying the lessons of a past crisis without careful consideration of present needs.

5.6 Linking Action Plans to Resource Mapping

In most countries, strengthening surveillance, research capacity, and collection and dissemination of pre-outbreak data requires additional funding. Sustainable and innovative funding mechanisms are necessary to incentivize prevention, detection, and response. This includes access to grants or low-interest loans, especially to communities with lower resource bases and the highest spillover risk. WHO and other partners currently support countries in mapping internal and external funding sources available to support global health security National Action Plans (NAPs). These plans not only identify funding and capacity gaps but also allow prospective donors to see what their funds would support.

The World Bank has established a Pandemic Fund to finance pandemic prevention, preparedness, and response capabilities and address critical gaps in low- and middle-income countries (▶ Chap. 28) (WBG 2022b).

Several funding mechanisms have been created to improve early warning detection systems or research. The U.S. National Institutes of Health (NIH) established the Centers for Research in Emerging Infectious Diseases in 2020 to develop multidisciplinary studies into where and how zoonotic agents "emerge from wildlife and spillover to cause disease in people" (NIH 2021). These centers focus on natural reservoirs, high-risk interfaces, and urban areas, while developing diagnostics to improve detection and facilitate study of human immune responses to zoonotic pathogens. The U.S. National Science Foundation has created the Predictive Intelligence for Pandemic Prevention Development grant program to support research on infectious disease emergence through "state-of-the art forecasting, real-time monitoring, mitigation and prevention of the spread of pathogens" (NSF 2022). Other efforts include a French/European Commission program called PREZODE: PREventing ZOonotic Disease Emergence (Peyre et al. 2021) and current efforts by the U.S. Agency for International Development building upon more than a decade of support to advance viral zoonosis detection.

In the long term, all countries need sustainable funding mechanisms to maintain capacities to prevent, detect, and respond to infectious disease threats, including collection of pre-outbreak information. Given that the private sector has an interest in preventing the staffing, supply, and sales disruptions caused by epidemics and pandemics, companies should be included in discussions about financing pandemic prevention, preparedness, and response. Leveraging the resources of capital markets and environmental, social, and governance investing has facilitated the adoption of lower-risk food animal production practices (FAIRR 2022) and may have some potential to incentivize private sector-led innovation in shifting both endemic and emerging disease risk landscapes. Examples of private sector investments include the analysis of Google searches for influenza symptoms to help prioritize regional distribution of seasonal influenza vaccine in the United States (Ginsberg et al. 2009).

6 Recommendations

Despite the availability of the best practices discussed above, it is still not customary in many countries to collect and use pre-outbreak information to reduce the risk of zoonotic disease spillover and spread. To address this challenge, we recommend three broad mechanisms, each of them with suggested supporting activities. The overarching theme of these recommendations is to strengthen country's capacities to collect, analyze, and share pre-outbreak information while avoiding replacing existing capacity or building parallel systems. Equitable partnership with local and regional stakeholders from concept through design and implementation is critical. So is a risk-based approach that informs where resources and effort should be applied to provide the greatest impact. All of the suggestions below can and should be built on top of existing investments in global health security and the response to the COVID-19 pandemic.

6.1 Strengthen and Prioritize Collection of Pre-outbreak Information

Without the pre-outbreak information providing a sense of relative zoonotic disease risks, countries will be limited in their ability allocate their resources to prevent, detect, and respond to outbreaks.

6.1.1 Country Activities, Taking into Consideration the Best Practices and Gaps Previously Mentioned

- Identify and map stakeholders and potential partners, including sources of funding.
- Endorse and facilitate routine coordination and collaboration across infectious disease programs and across sectors.

- Conduct cross-sectoral risk assessments for priority zoonotic pathogens (and unknown pathogens) and identify what is needed to support risk reduction and data collection.
- Prioritize populations and animal-human-environment interfaces for routine monitoring based on cross-sectoral risk assessments.
- Strengthen surveillance and monitoring mechanisms to include routine collection of pre-outbreak information where it is most needed.
- Strengthen laboratory capacity for pathogen identification, sequencing, and further research, including emerging zoonotic diseases. Methods needed include serological studies, genetic sequencing, and rapid multiplexed assays.
- Introduce appropriate technological innovations to generate and utilize new data streams, especially genome sequencing and analysis methodologies, for example, wastewater monitoring.
- Ensure long-term funding and training for key technical support staff.

6.1.2 Regional and Global Activities, Taking into Consideration the Best Practices and Gaps Previously Mentioned

- Support regional reference lab structures that serve as common specialized resources where individual countries may not be able to support cutting-edge, expensive capacities.
- Provide technical guidance, strategies and tools, training, and financial support to improve the capacity for collection of pre-outbreak information.
- Provide back-up surge support for pathogen identification in case countries need assistance with preparedness, prevention, detection, and response.
- Provide financial support.

6.2 Strengthen In-County Data Systems and Their Linkages with International Databases

Given the wealth of data that can be generated by pre-outbreak monitoring and other biosurveillance, it is imperative that systems be in place for data collection, storage, and sharing with adequate controls to protect the rights of the data owners, including intellectual property, privacy, security, and sovereignty (► Chap. 7). Pre-outbreak information must be analyzed and shared expeditiously. Many countries have existing data systems that coordinate across different diseases and sectors, especially as a function of integrated national health systems, but they may not be optimally linked either domestically or internationally, may be slow in processing data, may not collect all information needed, and may not have adequate funding.

6.2.1 Country Activities, Taking into Consideration the Best Practices and Gaps Previously Mentioned

- Identify and map stakeholders and potential partners, including sources of funding and owners and end-users of pre-outbreak information.
- Identify and assess existing data systems that can compile and provide access to pre-outbreak information, including identifying gaps and bottlenecks.
- Update policies and regulations to facilitate linkages among existing data systems so they can routinely share essential pre-outbreak information across sectors and across borders.
- Prioritize and strengthen the capacities of existing data systems and staff to improve routine collection, analysis, and sharing of pre-outbreak information. Incorporate technological developments such as wastewater testing and more capable point-of-care diagnostics (veterinary as well as human) to increase the coverage and speed of detection.

6.2.2 Regional and Global Activities, Taking into Consideration the Best Practices and Gaps Previously Mentioned

- Develop or strengthen international standards, agreements, databases, and systems for sharing pre-outbreak information.
- Provide technical guidance, strategies and tools, training, and financial support to improve the equitable sharing of pre-outbreak information among sectors, countries, and international databases.

6.3 Distill Pre-outbreak Information into Actionable Disease Intelligence for Risk Mitigation

6.3.1 Country Activities, Taking into Consideration the Best Practices and Gaps Previously Mentioned

- Operationalize pre-outbreak information data systems to gather and synthesize diverse data across sectors for actionable disease intelligence.
- Identify and map stakeholders who can use pre-outbreak information to take action.
- Generate evidence-based risk profiles and policy recommendations tailored to local and national disease emergence risk dynamics.
- Leverage data availability and foresight analysis to identify trends informing disease early warning, pre-outbreak deployment of surveillance and response capacities, and targeted risk mitigation.
- Utilize advances in pathogen assessment and the prototype pathogen approach (Cassetti et al. 2022) to prepare for and rapidly implement MCM development, including prioritized VTDs.
- Apply findings from pre-outbreak information systems in the iterative refinement of priority surveillance targets and risk mitigation strategies.
- Use a shared lexicon to expedite scientific understanding and proactively avoid stigmatizing animals.

6.3.2 Regional and Global Activities, Taking into Consideration the Best Practices and Gaps Previously Mentioned

- Provide guidance, technical support, and funding for developing and validating risk mitigation measures.
- Assist with sharing and adapting validated risk-mitigation measures among countries.

7 Conclusion

Collection and use of pre-outbreak information is critical for much-needed improvements in country and global preparedness and response to emerging zoonotic diseases. Substantial progress has been made in collecting valuable information in advance of human-to-human transmission of zoonotic pathogens. However, there continue to be outbreaks caused by zoonotic pathogens such as Ebola virus, mpox virus, and SARS-CoV-2 that are not detected until there is sustained human-to-human transmission. These events highlight the significant risks involved in waiting for pathogens to emerge in the human population before developing and applying containment and mitigation measures. Strengthening capacity for collecting pre-outbreak information is crucial to the early warning that could be provided by effective surveillance. Investments to strengthen pre-outbreak information systems would also contribute to an interlinked global early warning system for emerging infectious disease threats.

Securing resources for in-country capacity improvements for global health security is frequently a major obstacle to pandemic prevention, preparedness, and response. Several internal and external options are potentially available for countries to support immediate needs. In the longer term, financing global health security investments must transition to normal budgetary channels in both the public and private sectors. When viewed through an economic lens, expanding surveillance and prevention capacities have produced strong returns on investment by reducing the frequency, size, and impact of infectious disease outbreaks. It is vital that financial resources available to cover global health security include the collection, analysis, sharing, and use of pre-outbreak information.

Discussion Questions

1. What zoonotic diseases have emerged or reemerged recently? Discuss the potential for future zoonotic spillover and some targeted preventive measures against pathogen flow between wildlife or livestock and humans.
2. Investments in collecting pre-outbreak information on emerging zoonoses to prevent spillover, amplification, and geographical spread can yield a high return on investment and contribute significantly to strengthening global health security.
   - (a) Why are pathogen spillovers frequently undetected, or detected only after harmful delays? Consider anthropogenic, climatic, and environmental factors when answering this question.
   - (b) Why are certain vertebrate species (e.g., bats, rodents, nonhuman primates, and birds) more likely to be associated with zoonotic spillover and crossing into humans than other animals?
   - (c) Discuss how to map potential spillover hot spots using information on where human, pathogen, animal host, vector populations, and other key factors converge.
   - (d) Describe human behavioral interventions that can prevent or reduce spillover during an early public health response to infectious disease emergencies.
3. What is needed to improve the characterization of animal–human–environment interfaces by collecting new data streams reflecting population-level changes on a regular basis?
4. What are some measures that could enhance pre-outbreak monitoring of zoonotic spillovers of pathogens and detect outbreaks in humans more promptly?
5. Name some typical interventions against emerging infectious diseases that must be available to policymakers, scientists, health systems, businesses, and communities to reduce the frequency and impact of zoonotic disease spillover.
6. Provide several broad recommendations on how countries and the international community can improve detection, prevention, and response to future epidemic and pandemic threats.

References

Adjemian J, Farnon EC, Tschioko F, Wamala JF, Byaruhanga E, Bwire GS, et al. Outbreak of Marburg hemorrhagic fever among miners in Kamwenge and Ibanda Districts, Uganda, 2007. J Infect Dis. 2011;204(Suppl 3):S796–9. https://doi.org/10.1093/infdis/jir312.

Africa Centres for Disease Control and Prevention. Laboratory systems and networks. Addis Ababa: Africa Centres for Disease Control and Prevention; 2023. https://africacdc.org/programme/laboratory-systems-and-networks/. Accessed 19 Jan 2023.

Akhmetzhanov AR, Asai Y, Nishiura H. Quantifying the seasonal drivers of transmission for Lassa fever in Nigeria. Philos Trans R Soc Lond Ser B Biol Sci. 2019;374(1775):20180268. https://doi.org/10.1098/rstb.2018.0268.

Alexander KA, Carlson CJ, Lewis BL, Getz WM, Marathe MV, Eubank SG, et al. The ecology of pathogen spillover and disease emergence at the human-wildlife-environment interface. In: Hurst CJ, editor. The connections between ecology and infectious disease. Cham: Springer International Publishing; 2018. p. 267–98.

Allen T, Murray KA, Zambrana-Torrelio C, Morse SS, Rondinini C, Di Marco M, et al. Global hotspots and correlates of emerging zoonotic diseases. Nat Commun. 2017;8(1):1124. https://doi.org/10.1038/s41467-017-00923-8.

Amman BR, Bird BH, Bakarr IA, Bangura J, Schuh AJ, Johnny J, et al. Isolation of Angola-like Marburg virus from Egyptian rousette bats from West Africa. Nat Commun. 2020;11(1):510. https://doi.org/10.1038/s41467-020-14327-8.

Andreano E, Piccini G, Licastro D, Casalino L, Johnson NV, Paciello I, et al. SARS-CoV-2 escape from a highly neutralizing COVID-19 convalescent plasma. Proc Natl Acad Sci USA. 2021;118(36):e2103154118. https://doi.org/10.1073/pnas.2103154118.

Antonovics J, Wilson AJ, Forbes MR, Hauffe HC, Kallio ER, Leggett HC, et al. The evolution of transmission mode. Philos Trans R Soc Lond Ser B Biol Sci. 2017;372(1719):20160083. https://doi.org/10.1098/rstb.2016.0083.

Anyamba A, Chretien J-P, Small J, Tucker CJ, Formenty PB, Richardson JH, et al. Prediction of a Rift Valley fever outbreak. Proc Natl Acad Sci USA. 2009;106(3):955–9. https://doi.org/10.1073/pnas.0806490106.

Badawi A, Ryoo SG. Prevalence of comorbidities in the Middle East respiratory syndrome coronavirus (MERS-CoV): a systematic review and meta-analysis. Int J Infect Dis. 2016;49:129–33. https://doi.org/10.1016/j.ijid.2016.06.015.

Bartlow AW, Manore C, Xu C, Kaufeld KA, Del Valle S, Ziemann A, et al. Forecasting zoonotic infectious disease response to climate change: mosquito vectors and a changing environment. Vet Sci. 2019; https://doi.org/10.3390/vetsci6020040.

Becker DJ, Washburne AD, Faust CL, Pulliam JRC, Mordecai EA, Lloyd-Smith JO, et al. Dynamic and integrative approaches to understanding pathogen spillover. Philos Trans R Soc Lond Ser B Biol Sci. 2019;374(1782):20190014. https://doi.org/10.1098/rstb.2019.0014.

Becker DJ, Seifert SN, Carlson CJ. Beyond infection: integrating competence into reservoir host prediction. Trends Ecol Evol. 2020;35(12):1062–5. https://doi.org/10.1016/j.tree.2020.08.014.

Bernstein AS, Ando AW, Loch-Temzelides T, Vale MM, Li BV, Li H, et al. The costs and benefits of primary prevention of zoonotic pandemics. Sci Adv. 2022;8(5):eabl4183. https://doi.org/10.1126/sciadv.abl4183.

Berry I, Rahman M, Flora MS, Shirin T, Alamgir ASM, Khan MH, et al. Seasonality of influenza and coseasonality with avian influenza in Bangladesh, 2010–19: a retrospective, time-series analysis. Lancet Glob Health. 2022;10(8):e1150–e8. https://doi.org/10.1016/s2214-109x(22)00212-1.

Betts MG, Wolf C, Ripple WJ, Phalan B, Millers KA, Duarte A, et al. Global forest loss disproportionately erodes biodiversity in intact landscapes. Nature. 2017;547(7664):441–4. https://doi.org/10.1038/nature23285.

Blagrove MSC, Pilgrim J, Kotsiri A, Hui M, Baylis M, Wardeh M. Monkeypox virus shows potential to infect a diverse range of native animal species across Europe, indicating high risk of becoming endemic in the region. bioRxiv. 2022; https://doi.org/10.1101/2022.08.13.503846.

Brook CE, Ranaivoson HC, Broder CC, Cunningham AA, Héraud JM, Peel AJ, et al. Disentangling serology to elucidate henipa- and filovirus transmission in Madagascar fruit bats. J Anim Ecol. 2019;88(7):1001–16. https://doi.org/10.1111/1365-2656.12985.

Caminade C, McIntyre KM, Jones AE. Impact of recent and future climate change on vector-borne diseases. Ann N Y Acad Sci. 2019;1436(1):157–73. https://doi.org/10.1111/nyas.13950.

Capua I, Alexander DJ. The challenge of avian influenza to the veterinary community. Avian Pathol. 2006;35(3):189–205. https://doi.org/10.1080/03079450600717174.

Capua I, Marangon S. Control of avian influenza in poultry. Emerg Infect Dis. 2006;12(9):1319–24. https://doi.org/10.3201/eid1209.060430.

Carlson CJ, Farrell MJ, Grange Z, Han BA, Mollentze N, Phelan AL, et al. The future of zoonotic risk prediction. Philos Trans R Soc Lond Ser B Biol Sci. 2021;376(1837):20200358. https://doi.org/10.1098/rstb.2020.0358.

Carroll D, Daszak P, Wolfe N, Gao G, Morel C, Morzaria S, et al. The Global Virome Project. Science. 2018;359(6378):872–4. https://doi.org/10.1126/science.aap7463.

Cassetti MC, Pierson TC, Patterson LJ, et al. Prototype pathogen approach for vaccine and monoclonal antibody development: a critical component of the NIAID Plan for pandemic preparedness. J Infect Dis. 2022.

CDC. Update: multistate outbreak of monkeypox—Illinois, Indiana, Kansas, Missouri, Ohio, and Wisconsin, 2003. MMWR Morb Mortal Wkly Rep. 2003;52(27):642–6.

CDC. History of 1918 flu pandemic. Atlanta: Centers for Disease Control and Prevention; 2018a. https://www.cdc.gov/flu/pandemic-resources/1918-commemoration/1918-pandemic-history.htm. Accessed 12 Oct 2022.

CDC. Prioritizing zoonotic diseases for multisectoral, One Health collaboration in the United States. Atlanta: Centers for Disease Control and Prevention; 2018b.

CDC. 2022 Monkeypox outbreak global map. Atlanta: Centers for Disease Control and Prevention; 2022a. https://www.cdc.gov/poxvirus/monkeypox/response/2022/world-map.html. Accessed 10 Oct 2022.

CDC. History of Ebola virus disease (EVD) outbreaks. Atlanta: Centers for Disease Control and Prevention; 2022b. https://www.cdc.gov/vhf/ebola/history/chronology.html#anchor_1526565058132. Accessed 10 Oct 2022.

Chia WN, Zhu F, Ong SWX, Young BE, Fong SW, Le Bert N, et al. Dynamics of SARS-CoV-2 neutralising antibody responses and duration of immunity: a longitudinal study. Lancet Microbe. 2021;2(6):e240–9. https://doi.org/10.1016/s2666--5247(21)00025-2.

Chomel BB, Belotto A, Meslin FX. Wildlife, exotic pets, and emerging zoonoses. Emerg Infect Dis. 2007;13(1):6–11. https://doi.org/10.3201/eid1301.060480.

Chowdhury S, Azziz-Baumgartner E, Kile JC, Hoque MA, Rahman MZ, Hossain ME, et al. Association of biosecurity and hygiene practices with environmental contamination with Influenza A viruses in live bird markets, Bangladesh. Emerg Infect Dis. 2020;26(9):2087–96. https://doi.org/10.3201/eid2609.191029.

Chua KB. Nipah virus outbreak in Malaysia. J Clin Virol. 2003;26(3):265–75. https://doi.org/10.1016/S1386-6532(02)00268-8.

Corpuz MVA, Buonerba A, Vigliotta G, Zarra T, Ballesteros F Jr, Campiglia P, et al. Viruses in wastewater: occurrence, abundance and detection methods. Sci Total Environ. 2020;745:140910. https://doi.org/10.1016/j.scitotenv.2020.140910.

CREID. Responding to emerging infectious diseases. RTI International; 2022. https://creid-network.org/. Accessed 11 Dec 2022.

Damas J, Hughes GM, Keough KC, Painter CA, Persky NS, Corbo M, et al. Broad host range of SARS-CoV-2 predicted by comparative and structural analysis of ACE2 in vertebrates. Proc Natl Acad Sci USA. 2020;117(36):22311–22. https://doi.org/10.1073/pnas.2010146117.

de Oliveira RC, Fernandes J, Gonçalves-Oliveira J, Guterres A, de Lemos ERS. Out of the shadows, into the spotlight: invisible zoonotic diseases in Brazil. Lancet Reg Health Am. 2022;8:100202. https://doi.org/10.1016/j.lana.2022.100202.

Delardas O, Kechagias KS, Pontikos PN, Giannos P. Socio-economic impacts and challenges of the coronavirus pandemic (COVID-19): an updated review. Sustainability. 2022; https://doi.org/10.3390/su14159699.

Delaune D, Hul V, Karlsson EA, Hassanin A, Ou TP, Baidaliuk A, et al. A novel SARS-CoV-2 related coronavirus in bats from Cambodia. Nat Commun. 2021;12(1):6563. https://doi.org/10.1038/s41467--021-26809-4.

DeLong JP, Al-Sammak MA, Al-Ameeli ZT, Dunigan DD, Edwards KF, Fuhrmann JJ, et al. Towards an integrative view of virus phenotypes. Nat Rev Microbiol. 2022;20(2):83–94. https://doi.org/10.1038/s41579-021-00612-w.

Dovih P, Laing ED, Chen Y, Low DHW, Ansil BR, Yang X, et al. Filovirus-reactive antibodies in humans and bats in Northeast India imply zoonotic spillover. PLoS Negl Trop Dis. 2019;13(10):e0007733. https://doi.org/10.1371/journal.pntd.0007733.

Drew DA, Nguyen LH, Steves CJ, Menni C, Freydin M, Varsavsky T, et al. Rapid implementation of mobile technology for real-time epidemiology of COVID-19. Science. 2020;368(6497):1362–7. https://doi.org/10.1126/science.abc0473.

Dudas G, Carvalho LM, Rambaut A, Bedford T. MERS-CoV spillover at the camel-human interface. Elife. 2018;7:e31257. https://doi.org/10.7554/eLife.31257.

Duffy S, Shackelton LA, Holmes EC. Rates of evolutionary change in viruses: patterns and determinants. Nat Rev Genet. 2008;9(4):267–76. https://doi.org/10.1038/nrg2323.

Eaves E. The risks of building too many bio labs. New Yorker. 2020.

Eby P, Peel AJ, Hoegh A, Madden W, Giles JR, Hudson PJ, et al. Pathogen spillover driven by rapid changes in bat ecology. Nature. 2022;613:340. https://doi.org/10.1038/s41586-022-05506-2.

ECDC. Emerging Viral Diseases-Expert Laboratory Network (EVD-LabNet). Solna, SE: European Centre for Disease Prevention and Control; 2023. https://www.ecdc.europa.eu/en/about-us/partnerships-and-networks/disease-and-laboratory-networks/evd-labnet. Accessed 19 Jan 2023.

Epstein JH, Anthony SJ, Islam A, Kilpatrick AM, Ali Khan S, Balkey MD, et al. Nipah virus dynamics in bats and implications for spillover to humans. Proc Natl Acad Sci USA. 2020;117(46):29190–201. https://doi.org/10.1073/pnas.2000429117.

FAIRR. FAIRR: the world's fastest-growing investor network focusing on ESG risks in the global food sector. London: The FAIRR Initiative; 2022. https://www.fairr.org/. Accessed 16 Oct 2022.

Fan VY, Jamison DT, Summers LH. Pandemic risk: how large are the expected losses? Bull World Health Organ. 2018;96(2):129–34. https://doi.org/10.2471/blt.17.199588.

Finlay BB, McFadden G. Anti-immunology: evasion of the host immune system by bacterial and viral pathogens. Cell. 2006;124(4):767–82. https://doi.org/10.1016/j.cell.2006.01.034.

Fraser N, Brierley L, Dey G, Polka JK, Pálfy M, Nanni F, et al. The evolving role of preprints in the dissemination of COVID-19 research and their impact on the science communication landscape. PLoS Biol. 2021;19(4):e3000959. https://doi.org/10.1371/journal.pbio.3000959.

Frazzini S, Amadori M, Turin L, Riva F. SARS CoV-2 infections in animals, two years into the pandemic. Arch Virol. 2022;167:2503. https://doi.org/10.1007/s00705-022-05609-1.

Gallo RC, Montagnier L. The discovery of HIV as the cause of AIDS. N Engl J Med. 2003;349(24):2283–5. https://doi.org/10.1056/NEJMp038194.

Gibb R, Redding DW, Chin KQ, Donnelly CA, Blackburn TM, Newbold T, et al. Zoonotic host diversity increases in human-dominated ecosystems. Nature. 2020;584(7821):398–402. https://doi.org/10.1038/s41586-020-2562-8.

Gibb R, Albery GF, Mollentze N, Eskew EA, Brierley L, Ryan SJ, et al. Mammal virus diversity estimates are unstable due to accelerating discovery effort. Biol Lett. 2022;18(1):20210427. https://doi.org/10.1098/rsbl.2021.0427.

Gilbert AT, Fooks AR, Hayman DTS, Horton DL, Müller T, Plowright R, et al. Deciphering serology to understand the ecology of infectious diseases in wildlife. EcoHealth. 2013;10(3):298–313. https://doi.org/10.1007/s10393-013-0856-0.

Ginsberg J, Mohebbi MH, Patel RS, Brammer L, Smolinski MS, Brilliant L. Detecting influenza epidemics using search engine query data. Nature. 2009;457(7232):1012–4. https://doi.org/10.1038/nature07634.

Glidden CK, Nova N, Kain MP, Lagerstrom KM, Skinner EB, Mandle L, et al. Human-mediated impacts on biodiversity and the consequences for zoonotic disease spillover. Curr Biol. 2021;31(19):R1342–r61. https://doi.org/10.1016/j.cub.2021.08.070.

Goldstein T, Anthony SJ, Gbakima A, Bird BH, Bangura J, Tremeau-Bravard A, et al. The discovery of Bombali virus adds further support for bats as hosts of ebolaviruses. Nat Microbiol. 2018;3(10):1084–9. https://doi.org/10.1038/s41564-018-0227-2.

Goldstein T, Belaganahalli MN, Syaluha EK, Lukusa JK, Greig DJ, Anthony SJ, et al. Spillover of ebolaviruses into people in eastern Democratic Republic of Congo prior to the 2018 Ebola virus disease outbreak. One Health Outlook. 2020;2(1):21. https://doi.org/10.1186/s42522-020-00028-1.

Grange ZL, Goldstein T, Johnson CK, Anthony S, Gilardi K, Daszak P, et al. Ranking the risk of animal-to-human spillover for newly discovered viruses. Proc Natl Acad Sci USA. 2021;118(15):e2002324118. https://doi.org/10.1073/pnas.2002324118.

Grassly NC, Fraser C. Seasonal infectious disease epidemiology. Proc Biol Sci. 2006;273(1600):2541–50. https://doi.org/10.1098/rspb.2006.3604.

Groves HE, Piché-Renaud PP, Peci A, Farrar DS, Buckrell S, Bancej C, et al. The impact of the COVID-19 pandemic on influenza, respiratory syncytial virus, and other seasonal respiratory virus circulation in Canada: a population-based study. Lancet Reg Health Am. 2021;1:100015. https://doi.org/10.1016/j.lana.2021.100015.

Hansen MC, Potapov PV, Moore R, Hancher M, Turubanova SA, Tyukavina A, et al. High-resolution global maps of 21st-century forest cover change. Science. 2013;342(6160):850–3. https://doi.org/10.1126/science.1244693.

Hassell JM, Begon M, Ward MJ, Fèvre EM. Urbanization and disease emergence: dynamics at the wildlife-livestock-human interface. Trends Ecol Evol. 2017;32(1):55–67. https://doi.org/10.1016/j.tree.2016.09.012.

Hayman DT. Biannual birth pulses allow filoviruses to persist in bat populations. Proc Biol Sci. 2015;282(1803):20142591. https://doi.org/10.1098/rspb.2014.2591.

Hendry AP, Gotanda KM, Svensson EI. Human influences on evolution, and the ecological and societal consequences. Philos Trans R Soc Lond Ser B Biol Sci. 2017;372(1712):20160028. https://doi.org/10.1098/rstb.2016.0028.

Hornok S, Földvári G, Rigó K, Meli ML, Gönczi E, Répási A, et al. Synanthropic rodents and their ectoparasites as carriers of a novel haemoplasma and vector-borne, zoonotic pathogens indoors. Parasites Vectors. 2015;8(1):27. https://doi.org/10.1186/s13071-014-0630-3.

Huong NQ, Nga NTT, Long NV, Luu BD, Latinne A, Pruvot M, et al. Coronavirus testing indicates transmission risk increases along wildlife supply chains for human consumption in Viet Nam, 2013–2014. PLoS One. 2020;15(8):e0237129. https://doi.org/10.1371/journal.pone.0237129.

IAEA. Zoonotic Disease Integrated Action (ZODIAC): current status and future direction. Vienna: International Atomic Energy Agency; 2023. https://www.iaea.org/newscenter/news/zoonotic-disease-integrated-action-zodiac-current-status-and-future-direction. Accessed 19 Jan 2023.

Institute of Medicine, National Research Council. Achieving an effective zoonotic disease surveillance system. In: Keusch GT, Pappaioanou M, González MC, Scott KA, Tsai P, editors. Sustaining global surveillance and response to emerging zoonotic diseases. Washington, DC: The National Academies Press; 2009. p. 338.

Islam M, Luby S, Gurley S. Developing culturally appropriate interventions to prevent person to person transmission of Nipah virus in Bangladesh: cultural epidemiology in action. In: Banwell C, Ulijaszek S, Dixon J, editors. When culture impacts health. London: Academic; 2013. p. 329–37.

Jain V, Sharp A, Neilson M, Bausch DG, Beaney T. Joint External Evaluation scores and communicable disease deaths: an ecological study on the difference between epidemics and pandemics. PLoS Glob Public Health. 2022;2(8):e0000246. https://doi.org/10.1371/journal.pgph.0000246.

Joffrin L, Hoarau AOG, Lagadec E, Torrontegi O, Köster M, Le Minter G, et al. Seasonality of coronavirus shedding in tropical bats. R Soc Open Sci. 2022;9(2):211600. https://doi.org/10.1098/rsos.211600.

Jones KE, Patel NG, Levy MA, Storeygard A, Balk D, Gittleman JL, et al. Global trends in emerging infectious diseases. Nature. 2008;451(7181):990–3. https://doi.org/10.1038/nature06536.

Jones BA, Grace D, Kock R, Alonso S, Rushton J, Said MY, et al. Zoonosis emergence linked to agricultural intensification and environmental change. Proc Natl Acad Sci USA. 2013;110(21):8399–404. https://doi.org/10.1073/pnas.1208059110.

Keenliside J. Pandemic influenza A H1N1 in swine and other animals. In: Richt JA, Webby RJ, editors. Swine Influenza. Berlin, Heidelberg, Springer; 2013. p. 259–71.

Keesing F, Ostfeld RS. Impacts of biodiversity and biodiversity loss on zoonotic diseases. Proc Natl Acad Sci USA. 2021;118(17):e2023540118. https://doi.org/10.1073/pnas.2023540118.

Kellner KF, Swihart RK. Accounting for imperfect detection in ecology: a quantitative review. PLoS One. 2014;9(10):e111436. https://doi.org/10.1371/journal.pone.0111436.

Kessler MK, Becker DJ, Peel AJ, Justice NV, Lunn T, Crowley DE, et al. Changing resource landscapes and spillover of henipaviruses. Ann N Y Acad Sci. 2018;1429(1):78–99. https://doi.org/10.1111/nyas.13910.

Khan SU, Gurley ES, Hossain MJ, Nahar N, Sharker MA, Luby SP. A randomized controlled trial of interventions to impede date palm sap contamination by bats to prevent Nipah virus transmission in Bangladesh. PLoS One. 2012;7(8):e42689. https://doi.org/10.1371/journal.pone.0042689.

Kirby T. From early alarm to gradual control of monkeypox. Lancet HIV. 2022;9:e824. https://doi.org/10.1016/S2352-3018(22)00299-5.

Klunk J, Vilgalys TP, Demeure CE, Cheng X, Shiratori M, Madej J, et al. Evolution of immune genes is associated with the Black Death. Nature. 2022;611:312. https://doi.org/10.1038/s41586-022-05349-x.

Koopmans M. Surveillance strategy for early detection of unusual infectious disease events. Curr Opin Virol. 2013;3(2):185–91. https://doi.org/10.1016/j.coviro.2013.02.003.

Kreuder Johnson C, Hitchens PL, Smiley Evans T, Goldstein T, Thomas K, Clements A, et al. Spillover and pandemic properties of zoonotic viruses with high host plasticity. Sci Rep. 2015;5:14830. https://doi.org/10.1038/srep14830.

Krofah E, Choe SH, Sud A, Degarmo A. A global early warning system for pandemics: a blueprint for coordination. Santa Monica, CA: Milken Institute; 2021.

Kucharski A. Fragmented outbreak data will lead to a repeat of COVID-19. Nature. 2022;608(7924):649. https://doi.org/10.1038/d41586-022-02268-9.

Kummer S, Kranz DC. Henipaviruses—a constant threat to livestock and humans. PLoS Negl Trop Dis. 2022;16(2):e0010157. https://doi.org/10.1371/journal.pntd.0010157.

Kurpiers LA, Schulte-Herbrüggen B, Ejotre I, Reeder DM. Bushmeat and emerging infectious diseases: lessons from Africa. In: Angelici FM, editor. Problematic wildlife: a cross-disciplinary approach. Cham: Springer International Publishing; 2016. p. 507–51.

Laing ED, Sterling SL, Richard SA, Epsi NJ, Coggins SA, Samuels EC, et al. Antigen-based multiplex strategies to discriminate SARS-CoV-2 natural and vaccine induced immunity from seasonal human coronavirus humoral responses. medRxiv. 2021; https://doi.org/10.1101/2021.02.10.21251518.

Le Bert N, Tan AT, Kunasegaran K, Tham CYL, Hafezi M, Chia A, et al. SARS-CoV-2-specific T cell immunity in cases of COVID-19 and SARS, and uninfected controls. Nature. 2020;584(7821):457–62. https://doi.org/10.1038/s41586-020-2550-z.

Leung YH, Lau EH, Zhang LJ, Guan Y, Cowling BJ, Peiris JS. Avian influenza and ban on overnight poultry storage in live poultry markets, Hong Kong. Emerg Infect Dis. 2012;18(8):1339–41. https://doi.org/10.3201/eid1808.111879.

Li YT, Linster M, Mendenhall IH, Su YCF, Smith GJD. Avian influenza viruses in humans: lessons from past outbreaks. Br Med Bull. 2019;132(1):81–95. https://doi.org/10.1093/bmb/ldz036.

Lindahl JF, Grace D. The consequences of human actions on risks for infectious diseases: a review. Infect Ecol Epidemiol. 2015;5:30048. https://doi.org/10.3402/iee.v5.30048.

Liu S, Zhuang Q, Wang S, Jiang W, Jin J, Peng C, et al. Control of avian influenza in China: strategies and lessons. Transbound Emerg Dis. 2020;67(4):1463–71. https://doi.org/10.1111/tbed.13515.

Luis AD, Hayman DT, O'Shea TJ, Cryan PM, Gilbert AT, Pulliam JR, et al. A comparison of bats and rodents as reservoirs of zoonotic viruses: are bats special? Proc Biol Sci. 2013;280(1756):20122753. https://doi.org/10.1098/rspb.2012.2753.

Magouras I, Brookes VJ, Jori F, Martin A, Pfeiffer DU, Dürr S. Emerging zoonotic diseases: should we rethink the animal-human interface? Front Vet Sci. 2020;7:582743. https://doi.org/10.3389/fvets.2020.582743.

Marani M, Katul GG, Pan WK, Parolari AJ. Intensity and frequency of extreme novel epidemics. Proc Natl Acad Sci USA. 2021;118(35):e2105482118. https://doi.org/10.1073/pnas.2105482118.

McFarlane R, Sleigh A, McMichael T. Synanthropy of wild mammals as a determinant of emerging infectious diseases in the Asian-Australasian region. EcoHealth. 2012;9(1):24–35. https://doi.org/10.1007/s10393-012-0763-9.

Memish ZA, Cotten M, Meyer B, Watson SJ, Alsahafi AJ, Al Rabeeah AA, et al. Human infection with MERS coronavirus after exposure to infected camels, Saudi Arabia, 2013. Emerg Infect Dis. 2014;20(6):1012–5. https://doi.org/10.3201/eid2006.140402.

Michie S, West R. Sustained behavior change is key to preventing and tackling future pandemics. Nat Med. 2021;27(5):749–52. https://doi.org/10.1038/s41591-021-01345-2.

Mollentze N, Streicker DG. Viral zoonotic risk is homogenous among taxonomic orders of mammalian and avian reservoir hosts. Proc Natl Acad Sci USA. 2020;117(17):9423–30. https://doi.org/10.1073/pnas.1919176117.

Mollentze N, Babayan SA, Streicker DG. Identifying and prioritizing potential human-infecting viruses from their genome sequences. PLoS Biol. 2021;19(9):e3001390. https://doi.org/10.1371/journal.pbio.3001390.

Monath TP, Newhouse VF, Kemp GE, Setzer HW, Cacciapuoti A. Lassa virus isolation from *Mastomys natalensis* rodents during an epidemic in Sierra Leone. Science. 1974;185(4147):263–5. https://doi.org/10.1126/science.185.4147.263.

Montecino-Latorre D, Goldstein T, Gilardi K, Wolking D, Van Wormer E, Kazwala R, et al. Reproduction of East-African bats may guide risk mitigation for coronavirus spillover. One Health Outlook. 2020;2(1):2. https://doi.org/10.1186/s42522-019-0008-8.

Mora C, McKenzie T, Gaw IM, Dean JM, von Hammerstein H, Knudson TA, et al. Over half of known human pathogenic diseases can be aggravated by climate change. Nat Clim Chang. 2022;12(9):869–75. https://doi.org/10.1038/s41558-022-01426-1.

Morand S, Lajaunie C. Outbreaks of vector-borne and zoonotic diseases are associated with changes in forest cover and oil palm expansion at global scale. Front Vet Sci. 2021;8:661063. https://doi.org/10.3389/fvets.2021.661063.

Morand S, Walther BA. The accelerated infectious disease risk in the Anthropocene: more outbreaks and wider global spread. BioRxiv. 2020; https://doi.org/10.1101/2020.04.20.049866.

Morand S, Blasdell K, Bordes F, Buchy P, Carcy B, Chaisiri K, et al. Changing landscapes of Southeast Asia and rodent-borne diseases: decreased diversity but increased transmission risks. Ecol Appl. 2019;29(4):e01886. https://doi.org/10.1002/eap.1886.

Murakami S, Kitamura T, Suzuki J, Sato R, Aoi T, Fujii M, et al. Detection and characterization of bat Sarbecovirus phylogenetically related to SARS-CoV-2, Japan. Emerg Infect Dis. 2020;26(12):3025–9. https://doi.org/10.3201/eid2612.203386.

Nahar N, Sultana R, Gurley ES, Hossain MJ, Luby SP. Date palm sap collection: exploring opportunities to prevent Nipah transmission. EcoHealth. 2010;7(2):196–203. https://doi.org/10.1007/s10393--010-0320-3.

Nahar N, Asaduzzaman M, Sultana R, Garcia F, Paul RC, Abedin J, et al. A large-scale behavior change intervention to prevent Nipah transmission in Bangladesh: components and costs. BMC Res Notes. 2017;10(1):225. https://doi.org/10.1186/s13104-017-2549-1.

NASEM. Systematizing the One Health approach in preparedness and response efforts for infectious disease outbreaks: proceedings of a workshop. Washington, DC: National Academies Press (US); 2022.

NIH. Centers for Research in Emerging Infectious Diseases (CREID). Bethesda, MD: National Institutes of Health; 2021. https://www.niaid.nih.gov/research/centers-research-emerging-infectious-diseases. Accessed 16 Oct 2022.

Nikolay B, Salje H, Hossain MJ, Khan A, Sazzad HMS, Rahman M, et al. Transmission of Nipah virus—14 years of investigations in Bangladesh. N Engl J Med. 2019;380(19):1804–14. https://doi.org/10.1056/NEJMoa1805376.

NSF. NSF predictive intelligence for pandemic prevention: development grant (pipp phase I). Washington, DC: National Science Foundation; 2022. https://beta.nsf.gov/events/nsf-predictive-intelligence-pandemic-prevention#:~:text=Synopsis%20of%20Program%3A,pandemics%20through%20prediction%20and%20prevention. Accessed 16 Oct 2021.

Nwadiugwu MC, Monteiro N. Applied genomics for identification of virulent biothreats and for disease outbreak surveillance. Postgrad Med J. 2022;99:403. https://doi.org/10.1136/postgradmedj-2021-139916.

Nyhus PJ. Human–wildlife conflict and coexistence. Annu Rev Environ Resour. 2016;41(1):143–71. https://doi.org/10.1146/annurev-environ-110615-085634.

Olival KJ, Hosseini PR, Zambrana-Torrelio C, Ross N, Bogich TL, Daszak P. Host and viral traits predict zoonotic spillover from mammals. Nature. 2017;546(7660):646–50. https://doi.org/10.1038/nature22975.

Padron-Regalado E. Vaccines for SARS-CoV-2: lessons from other coronavirus strains. Infect Dis Ther. 2020;9(2):255–74. https://doi.org/10.1007/s40121--020-00300-x.

Pandemic Preparedness Partnership. 100 days mission to respond to future pandemic threats: reducing the impact of future pandemics by making diagnostics, therapeutics and vaccines available within 100 days: a report to the G7. London: G7 United Kingdom; 2021.

Pappalardo M, Juliá M, Howard MJ, Rossman JS, Michaelis M, Wass MN. Conserved differences in protein sequence determine the human pathogenicity of Ebolaviruses. Sci Rep. 2016;6(1):23743. https://doi.org/10.1038/srep23743.

Parker S, Buller RM. A review of experimental and natural infections of animals with monkeypox virus between 1958 and 2012. Future Virol. 2013;8(2):129–57. https://doi.org/10.2217/fvl.12.130.

Pendrill F, Gardner TA, Meyfroidt P, Persson UM, Adams J, Azevedo T, et al. Disentangling the numbers behind agriculture-driven tropical deforestation. Science. 2022;377(6611):eabm9267. https://doi.org/10.1126/science.abm9267.

Peyre M, Vourc'h G, Lefrançois T, Martin-Prevel Y, Soussana J-F, Roche B. PREZODE: preventing zoonotic disease emergence. Lancet. 2021;397(10276):792–3. https://doi.org/10.1016/S0140-6736(21)00265-8.

Piret J, Boivin G. Pandemics throughout history. Front Microbiol. 2021;11:631736. https://doi.org/10.3389/fmicb.2020.631736.

Plowright RK, Parrish CR, McCallum H, Hudson PJ, Ko AI, Graham AL, et al. Pathways to zoonotic spillover. Nat Rev Microbiol. 2017;15(8):502–10. https://doi.org/10.1038/nrmicro.2017.45.

Plowright RK, Reaser JK, Locke H, Woodley SJ, Patz JA, Becker DJ, et al. Land use-induced spillover: a call to action to safeguard environmental, animal, and human health. Lancet Planet Health. 2021;5(4):e237–45. https://doi.org/10.1016/s2542--5196(21)00031-0.

Poletti P, Visintainer R, Lepri B, Merler S. The interplay between individual social behavior and clinical symptoms in small clustered groups. BMC Infect

Dis. 2017;17(1):521. https://doi.org/10.1186/s12879-017-2623-2.

PREDICT Consortium. PREDICT: advancing global health security at the frontiers of disease emergence. Davis, CA: PREDICT Consortium; 2021.

PROMED. PROMED-mail. Brookline, MA: International Society for Infectious Diseases; 2022. https://promedmail.org/. Accessed 12 Oct 2022.

Rahman MA, Hossain MJ, Sultana S, Homaira N, Khan SU, Rahman M, et al. Date palm sap linked to Nipah virus outbreak in Bangladesh, 2008. Vector Borne Zoonotic Dis. 2012;12(1):65–72. https://doi.org/10.1089/vbz.2011.0656.

Recht J, Schuenemann VJ, Sánchez-Villagra MR. Host diversity and origin of zoonoses: The ancient and the new. Animals. 2020;10(9):1672.

Roberts M, Dobson A, Restif O, Wells K. Challenges in modelling the dynamics of infectious diseases at the wildlife-human interface. Epidemics. 2021;37:100523. https://doi.org/10.1016/j.epidem.2021.100523.

Sánchez CA, Li H, Phelps KL, Zambrana-Torrelio C, Wang LF, Zhou P, et al. A strategy to assess spillover risk of bat SARS-related coronaviruses in Southeast Asia. Nat Commun. 2022;13(1):4380. https://doi.org/10.1038/s41467-022-31860-w.

Schar DL, Yamey GM, Machalaba CC, Karesh WB. A framework for stimulating economic investments to prevent emerging diseases. Bull World Health Organ. 2018;96(2):138–40. https://doi.org/10.2471/blt.17.199547.

Schuh AJ, Amman BR, Towner JS. Filoviruses and bats. Microbiol Aust. 2017;38(1):12–6. https://doi.org/10.1071/ma17005.

Smith GJ, Vijaykrishna D, Bahl J, Lycett SJ, Worobey M, Pybus OG, et al. Origins and evolutionary genomics of the 2009 swine-origin H1N1 influenza A epidemic. Nature. 2009;459(7250):1122–5. https://doi.org/10.1038/nature08182.

Smith KF, Goldberg M, Rosenthal S, Carlson L, Chen J, Chen C, et al. Global rise in human infectious disease outbreaks. J R Soc Interface. 2014;11(101):20140950. https://doi.org/10.1098/rsif.2014.0950.

Smolinski MS, Hamburg MA, Lederberg J. Microbial threats to health: emergence, detection, and response. Washington, DC: Naional Academies Press; 2003.

Steere AC, Coburn J, Glickstein L. The emergence of Lyme disease. J Clin Invest. 2004;113(8):1093–101. https://doi.org/10.1172/jci21681.

Su W, Harfoot R, Su YCF, DeBeauchamp J, Joseph U, Jayakumar J, et al. Ancestral sequence reconstruction pinpoints adaptations that enable avian influenza virus transmission in pigs. Nat Microbiol. 2021;6(11):1455–65. https://doi.org/10.1038/s41564-021-00976-y.

Tan CW, Chia WN, Qin X, Liu P, Chen MI, Tiu C, et al. A SARS-CoV-2 surrogate virus neutralization test based on antibody-mediated blockage of ACE2-spike protein-protein interaction. Nat Biotechnol. 2020;38(9):1073–8. https://doi.org/10.1038/s41587--020-0631-z.

Taylor LH, Latham SM, Woolhouse ME. Risk factors for human disease emergence. Philos Trans R Soc Lond Ser B Biol Sci. 2001;356(1411):983–9. https://doi.org/10.1098/rstb.2001.0888.

Temmam S, Vongphayloth K, Baquero E, Munier S, Bonomi M, Regnault B, et al. Bat coronaviruses related to SARS-CoV-2 and infectious for human cells. Nature. 2022;604(7905):330–6. https://doi.org/10.1038/s41586-022-04532-4.

Ter Meulen J, Lukashevich I, Sidibe K, Inapogui A, Marx M, Dorlemann A, et al. Hunting of peridomestic rodents and consumption of their meat as possible risk factors for rodent-to-human transmission of Lassa virus in the Republic of Guinea. Am J Trop Med Hyg. 1996;55(6):661–6. https://doi.org/10.4269/ajtmh.1996.55.661.

Tian H, Zhou S, Dong L, Van Boeckel TP, Cui Y, Newman SH, et al. Avian influenza H5N1 viral and bird migration networks in Asia. Proc Natl Acad Sci U S A. 2015;112(1):172–7. https://doi.org/10.1073/pnas.1405216112.

Timen A, Koopmans MP, Vossen AC, van Doornum GJ, Günther S, van den Berkmortel F, et al. Response to imported case of Marburg hemorrhagic fever, the Netherlands. Emerg Infect Dis. 2009;15(8):1171–5. https://doi.org/10.3201/eid1508.090015.

UNAIDS. Fact sheet. Geneva: UNAIDS; 2022.

Voigt CC, Phelps KL, Aguirre LF, Corrie Schoeman M, Vanitharani J, Zubaid A. Bats and buildings: the conservation of synanthropic bats. In: Voigt CC, Kingston T, editors. Bats in the anthropocene: conservation of bats in a changing world. Cham: Springer International Publishing; 2016. p. 427–62.

Wacharapluesadee S, Boongird K, Wanghongsa S, Ratanasetyuth N, Supavonwong P, Saengsen D, et al. A longitudinal study of the prevalence of Nipah virus in *Pteropus lylei* bats in Thailand: evidence for seasonal preference in disease transmission. Vector Borne Zoonotic Dis. 2009;10(2):183–90. https://doi.org/10.1089/vbz.2008.0105.

Wacharapluesadee S, Buathong R, Iamsirithawon S, Chaifoo W, Ponpinit T, Ruchisrisarod C, et al. Identification of a novel pathogen using family-wide PCR: initial confirmation of COVID-19 in Thailand. Front Public Health. 2020;8:555013. https://doi.org/10.3389/fpubh.2020.555013.

Wacharapluesadee S, Ghai S, Duengkae P, Manee-Orn P, Thanapongtharm W, Saraya AW, et al. Two decades of one health surveillance of Nipah virus in Thailand. One Health Outlook. 2021a;3(1):12. https://doi.org/10.1186/s42522-021-00044-9.

Wacharapluesadee S, Tan CW, Maneeorn P, Duengkae P, Zhu F, Joyjinda Y, et al. Evidence for SARS-CoV-2 related coronaviruses circulating in bats and pangolins in Southeast Asia. Nat Commun. 2021b;12(1):972. https://doi.org/10.1038/s41467--021-21240-1.

Wan XF, Dong L, Lan Y, Long LP, Xu C, Zou S, et al. Indications that live poultry markets are a major source of human H5N1 influenza virus infection in China. J Virol. 2011;85(24):13432–8. https://doi.org/10.1128/jvi.05266-11.

Wang LF, Shi Z, Zhang S, Field H, Daszak P, Eaton BT. Review of bats and SARS. Emerg Infect Dis. 2006;12(12):1834–40. https://doi.org/10.3201/eid1212.060401.

Wang X, Jiang H, Wu P, Uyeki TM, Feng L, Lai S, et al. Epidemiology of avian influenza A H7N9 virus in human beings across five epidemics in mainland China, 2013–17: an epidemiological study of laboratory-confirmed case series. Lancet Infect Dis. 2017;17(8):822–32. https://doi.org/10.1016/s1473--3099(17)30323-7.

Watsa M, Erkenswick GA, Pomerantz A, Prost S. Portable sequencing as a teaching tool in conservation and biodiversity research. PLoS Biol. 2020;18(4):e3000667. https://doi.org/10.1371/journal.pbio.3000667.

WBG. Finance for an equitable recovery. World Development Report. Washington, DC: World Bank Group; 2022a.

WBG. Pandemic fund. Washington, DC: World Bank Group; 2022b. https://www.worldbank.org/en/programs/financial-intermediary-fund-for-pandemic-prevention-preparedness-and-response-ppr-fif. Accessed 22 Nov 2022.

Webster RG, Hulse DJ. Microbial adaptation and change: avian influenza. Rev Sci Tech. 2004;23(2):453–65. https://doi.org/10.20506/rst.23.2.1493.

WHO. International Health Regulations (2005). 3rd ed. Geneva: World Health Organization; 2016. 74 p.

WHO. Marburg virus disease—Guinea. Disease Outbreak News; 2021.

WHO. Ebola: North Kivu/Ituri, Democratic Republic of the Congo, August 2018–June 2020. Geneva: World Health Organization; 2022a. https://www.who.int/emergencies/situations/Ebola-2019-drc-. Accessed 10 Oct 2022.

WHO. Ebola: West Africa, March 2014–2016. Geneva: World Health Organization; 2022b. https://www.who.int/emergencies/situations/ebola-outbreak-2014-2016-West-Africa. Accessed 10 Oct 2022.

WHO. Epidemic intelligence from open sources (EIOS): zero impact from health threats. Geneva: World Health Organization; 2022c. https://www.who.int/initiatives/eios. Accessed 11 Dec 2022.

WHO. Marburg virus—Ghana. Disease Outbreak News; 2022d.

WHO. Mitigating the COVID-19 outbreak through global data sharing. 2022e. https://www.who.int/teams/health-care-readiness/covid-19/data-platform/mitigating-the-covid-19-outbreak-through-global-data-sharing. Accessed 13 Oct 2022.

WHO. WHO recommends new name for monkeypox disease. Geneva: World Health Organization; 2022f.

WHO. International Negotiating Body Geneva: World Health Organization; 2024 [updated 1 Jun 2024]. Available from: https://inb.who.int.

WHO. Disease outbreak news. Geneva: World Health Organization; 2023a. https://www.who.int/emergencies/disease-outbreak-news. Accessed 17 Jan 2023.

WHO. Global Influenza Surveillance and Response System (GISRS). Geneva: World Health Organization; 2023b. https://www.who.int/initiatives/global-influenza-surveillance-and-response-system. Accessed 28 May 2023.

WHO. WHO coronavirus (COVID-19) dashboard. Geneva: World Health Organization; 2023c. https://covid19.who.int. Accessed 28 May 2023.

WHO. WHO coronavirus (COVID-19) dashboard. Geneva: World Health Organization; 2023d. https://covid19.who.int/. Accessed 10 Jan 2023.

WHO, FAO, WOAH. Taking a multisectoral, one health approach: a tripartite guide to addressing zoonotic diseases in countries. Geneva: World Health Organization, UN Food and Agriculture Organization, World Organization for Animal Health; 2019.

Winck GR, Raimundo RLG, Fernandes-Ferreira H, Bueno MG, D'Andrea PS, Rocha FL, et al. Socioecological vulnerability and the risk of zoonotic disease emergence in Brazil. Sci Adv. 2022;8(26):eabo5774. https://doi.org/10.1126/sciadv.abo5774.

WOAH. World Animal Health Information System: WAHIS Portal: animal health data. Paris: World Organisation for Animal Health; 2022. https://www.woah.org/en/what-we-do/animal-health-and--welfare/disease-data-collection/world-animal-health-information-system/. Accessed 12 Oct 2022.

Wolfe ND, Heneine W, Carr JK, Garcia AD, Shanmugam V, Tamoufe U, et al. Emergence of unique primate T-lymphotropic viruses among central African bushmeat hunters. Proc Natl Acad Sci USA. 2005;102(22):7994–9. https://doi.org/10.1073/pnas.0501734102.

Wolfe MK, Duong D, Hughes B, Chan-Herur V, White BJ, Boehm AB. Detection of monkeypox viral DNA in a routine wastewater monitoring program. medRxiv. 2022; https://doi.org/10.1101/2022.07.25.22278043.

World Bank. People, pathogens and our planet: the economics of One Health. Washington, DC: World Bank; 2012. Report No.: 69145-GLB.

Wozniak DM, Riesle-Sbarbaro SA, Kirchoff N, Hansen-Kant K, Wahlbrink A, Stern A, et al. Inoculation route-dependent Lassa virus dissemination and shedding dynamics in the natural reservoir—Mastomys natalensis. Emerg Microbes Infect. 2021;10(1):2313–25. https://doi.org/10.1080/22221751.2021.2008773.

Wu J, Ke C, Lau EHY, Song Y, Cheng KL, Zou L, et al. Influenza H5/H7 virus vaccination in poultry and reduction of zoonotic infections, Guangdong Province, China, 2017–18. Emerg Infect Dis. 2019;25(1):116–8. https://doi.org/10.3201/eid2501.181259.

Yadav PD, Sahay RR, Balakrishnan A, Mohandas S, Radhakrishnan C, Gokhale MD, et al. Nipah virus outbreak in Kerala State, India amidst of COVID-19 pandemic. Front Public Health. 2022;10:818545. https://doi.org/10.3389/fpubh.2022.818545.

Yoon SW, Webby RJ, Webster RG. Evolution and ecology of influenza A viruses. Curr Top Microbiol Immunol. 2014;385:359–75. https://doi.org/10.1007/82_2014_396.

Youssef DM, Wieland B, Knight GM, Lines J, Naylor NR. The effectiveness of biosecurity interventions in reducing the transmission of bacteria from livestock to humans at the farm level: a systematic literature review. Zoonoses Public Health. 2021;68(6):549–62. https://doi.org/10.1111/zph.12807.

Zhao P, Cao J, Zhao LJ, Qin ZL, Ke JS, Pan W, et al. Immune responses against SARS-coronavirus nucleocapsid protein induced by DNA vaccine. Virology. 2005;331(1):128–35. https://doi.org/10.1016/j.virol.2004.10.016.

Zhou X, Wang Y, Liu H, Guo F, Doi SA, Smith C, et al. Effectiveness of market-level biosecurity at reducing exposure of poultry and humans to avian influenza: a systematic review and meta-analysis. J Infect Dis. 2018;218(12):1861–75. https://doi.org/10.1093/infdis/jiy400.

11 Accelerating Diagnostic Innovation for Pandemic Control

C. Taylor Gilliland, William Heetderks, Krishna Juluru, Anthony Kirilusha, Tiffani B. Lash, Todd Merchak, Felicia Qashu, Douglas M. Sheeley, Mark Snyder, Andrew Weitz, Michael Wolfson, and Bruce Tromberg

Contents

Learning Track Note: This chapter appears in Learning Tracks: Preparedness

E. S. Higgs and R. A. Sorenson (eds.), *Principles and Practice of Emergency Research Response*,
https://doi.org/10.1007/978-3-031-48408-7_13

Learning Objectives

This chapter will help readers understand and describe:

- How government research and development institutes can catalyze diagnostic innovation to meet the needs of an infectious disease emergency caused by a novel pathogen
- Elements of the RADx Tech program that could serve as examples in future response to EID outbreaks
- Barriers to the development and deployment of point-of-care testing (POC) and over-the-counter (OTC) tests during the COVID-19 pandemic
- Steps to take now to improve diagnostic readiness for the next pandemic

1 Introduction

1.1 Background on Testing Technologies for Diagnosing Acute SARS-CoV-2 Infection

Testing is an essential component of the public health response to an emerging infectious disease for

- Mitigating pathogen transmission
- Characterizing the pathogen and pathogenesis
- Enabling contact tracing and quarantine of infected persons
- Informing clinical and public health decision making
- Enabling identification of infection for enrollment in clinical trials
- Ascertaining endpoints in vaccine and/or therapeutic clinical trials
- Providing a pathway to safe return to work, school, and leisure

The COVID-19 pandemic provided a stark illustration of challenges to the development and distribution of tests to detect the novel SARS-CoV-2 virus. In the beginning, viral testing was conducted exclusively in centralized, high-complexity clinical laboratories by order of a healthcare provider, leading to massive shortages of tests and slow return of results. This, coupled with early missteps in expanding capacity and approving new tests, hindered the ability of public health systems to control viral spread. However, the pandemic also generated an unprecedented R&D investment in diagnostic innovation that will likely have lasting benefits for how existing and emerging diseases are detected, treated, and controlled. This chapter will provide an overview of how the U.S. National Institutes of Health (NIH) built a national program to accelerate innovation in COVID-19 diagnostic testing and convey some lessons learned from the experience that may be applicable to future efforts in pandemic control.

This chapter will focus exclusively on testing for acute or active viral infection (viral tests), rather than tests to measure prior infection (antibody or serology tests). While antibody tests are critical for understanding the epidemiology of SARS-CoV-2 and monitoring levels of acquired or vaccine-induced immunity in individuals or populations, they are not suitable for the diagnosis of acute viral infection or for tracking community transmission since human antibodies to the virus may not be detectable for weeks after initial exposure. Among viral tests, there are generally three primary purposes (HHS 2020); a fourth use for testing arose as tests became increasingly available.

1. *Diagnostic testing* to confirm or support a clinical diagnosis of viral infection in symptomatic individuals and inform treatment, enrollment in or endpoint for clinical trials, and implement preventive measures to contain further spread.
2. *Contact tracing testing* to trace, test, and monitor persons who may have been in contact with infected individuals.
3. *Surveillance testing* to enable public health authorities to assess and manage risks associated with the infectious disease, guide implementation of control measures, detect and control outbreaks, and monitor epidemiological trends.

	Molecular	Antigen
Point of Care	Mesa Biotech/ThermoFisher, Visby Medical 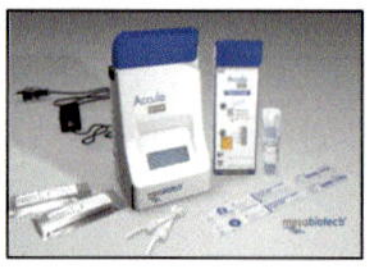 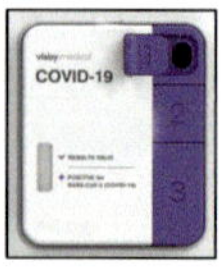	Quidel 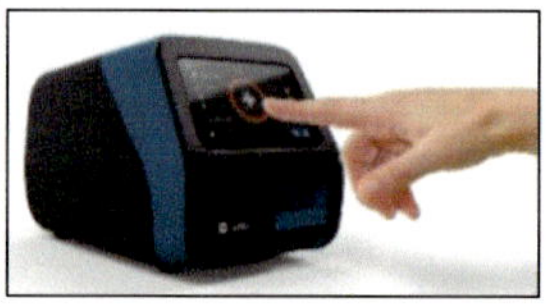
Self-test / At home, work, etc.	Detect 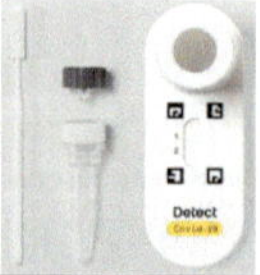	Quidel, Ellume 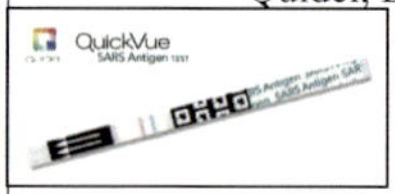 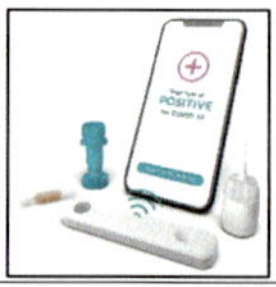

Fig. 1 Examples of SARS-CoV-2 molecular and antigen testing technologies developed with NIH support via the Rapid Acceleration of Diagnostics Technology initiative. (Courtesy ThermoFisher, Quidel, Detect, Acula)

4. *Managing exposure risk.* As diagnostic innovation continued through the pandemic and tests for home use became increasingly available, a fourth primary purpose arose: enabling individuals and families to test for potential infection and reduce the risk they could expose and infect others.

There are three primary environments (discussed further in ▶ Sect. 1.2) in which each of these viral testing strategies can be implemented:

1. In central reference laboratories in the commercial diagnostic, hospital, academic, or public health sectors
2. At the point of care (POC), such as in a physician's office, urgent care facility, or worksite clinic
3. At one's home, workplace, or other nonmedical location

The primary purpose of the test as well as its intended use environment will help determine the choice of underlying detection technology, as well as the requirements for test usability, performance (sensitivity, specificity, time to result), cost, and accessibility. Viral tests typically involve the collection of a sample from the nose, nasopharynx, or mouth and can largely be grouped into two categories based on whether they assess for the presence of viral genetic material or antigens. Nucleic acid amplification tests (NAATs), also referred to as molecular tests, specifically amplify and detect viral ribonucleic acid sequences from the SARS-CoV-2 genome, with amplification driven by either the reverse transcription polymerase chain reaction (RT-PCR) or a variety of isothermal amplification methods. Antigen tests, on the other hand, typically detect the presence of a specific viral protein through antibody–antigen interactions that are coupled to some type of measurable signal, often in the form of visible light or fluorescence. ◘ Figure 1 provides examples of SARS-CoV-2 diagnostic technologies for molecular and antigen tests that can be used either at POC or at home and that were developed with NIH support.

1.2 Implementation of Testing Technologies

Research and development of new diagnostic technologies require appropriate implementation and rigorous commercialization plans. To facilitate implementation, diagnostic testing tools and playbooks can guide health officials, employers, community organizations, and the public on testing modalities for specific use cases and/or settings. This section describes the implementation of diagnostics in the three primary environments: labs, at the point of care, and at home for self-testing (see

Fig. 3), as well as considerations distinguishing disease diagnosis from screening.

1.2.1 Lab-Based Testing

Lab-based diagnostics can be performed by clinical, hospital, or research laboratories that are certified and accredited to perform moderate to highly complex tests and report individual results (FDA 2021a). These labs can offer testing of individual or pooled samples to detect targeted antigens or nucleic acid sequences with high sensitivity (>95% for molecular assays that involve RT-PCR or next-generation sequencing). Lab-based testing can scale to thousands or hundreds of thousands of tests per day with innovations in the pre-analytical and analytical processes, such as bar coding of samples for quick accessioning and automated equipment interoperating with laboratory information management systems.

While labs can process diagnostic assays relatively quickly (e.g., less than an hour for viral antigen tests, 4–6 h for molecular tests/NAATs), sample shipment and accessioning for offsite laboratories can increase the turnaround time for lab-based tests to 12–24 h or more. A hub and spoke model, with multiple sample collection sites feeding into one or more testing hubs, can minimize turnaround times. The hub and spoke model can also provide testing support over a larger area and can be used to mitigate issues with supplies or capacity at a single lab by sending samples to another hub.

Various approaches to sample collection can be used to support lab-based testing, depending on the requirements for sample stability over time and transport options. Samples can be collected by health providers and then sent to the lab for processing through partnerships between labs and patient care facilities or local health departments. Lab-based assays can also be validated for use with samples collected by the patients themselves using a home collection kit. Assays may require biospecimens to be stored in saline, buffer solutions, or viral transport media, but maintaining biospecimens on dry swabs may also be an option, if validated with the lab-based assay.

Box 1: Clinical Laboratory Improvement Amendments (CLIA)

The U.S. Food and Drug Administration (FDA) , as authorized by CLIA, categorizes diagnostic tests by the complexity of their testing methodology—from the least to the most complex: waived tests, moderate complexity tests, and high complexity tests. CLIA categorization is determined after the FDA has cleared or approved a marketing submission or upon request for legally marketed devices. Under CLIA, laboratories performing only waived tests are subject to minimal regulation. Waived tests may also include any tests approved or cleared for home use by untrained individuals. Laboratories performing moderate- or high-complexity tests are subject to specific laboratory standards governing certification, personnel, proficiency testing, patient test management, quality assurance, quality control, and inspections (FDA 2021a).

1.2.2 Point-of-Care (POC) Testing

Diagnostics implemented in the POC setting include tests performed on-site under a Clinical Laboratory Improvement Amendments (CLIA) (▶ Box 1) certificate of waiver at public health clinics, urgent care centers, physicians' offices, pharmacies, retail clinics, emergency departments, and hospital labs. POC tests, often based on qualitative detection of an antigen or nucleic acid sequence, generally require less expensive, less complex equipment or instrumentation, and may have similar or somewhat limited detec-

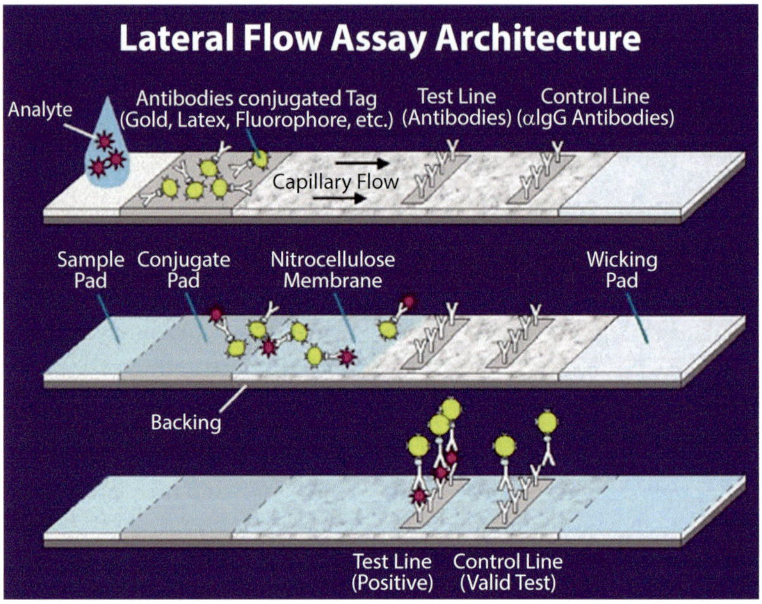

Fig. 2 Diagram describing the architecture of a generic lateral flow immunochromatographic assay. (NASA, public domain [▶ https://commons.wikimedia.org/wiki/File:Lateral_Flow_Assay.jpg])

tion thresholds compared to lab-based assays. Examples include lateral flow assays (Fig. 2) with a visual or instrument reader, loop-mediated isothermal amplification instruments, and sample in, result out RT-PCR platforms. With results typically available within 30 min, POC tests facilitate timely clinical decision-making for infected patients.

1.2.3 Self-Testing

Self-tests are diagnostic tests that can be used at home and other nonlaboratory settings—offices, schools, sporting events, airports, etc.—where individuals perform the test themselves. Self-tests may detect antigens or nucleic acid sequences but are most commonly noninstrumented, antigen-based rapid lateral flow assays, similar to home pregnancy tests.

Over-the-counter (OTC) tests require end-users to use and interpret the results themselves, thus requiring usability data to support their reliability. Home use tests requiring a prescription may be supervised or verified by a healthcare provider (e.g., through telehealth services). OTC tests can increase testing accessibility since they are available online, at retail stores, or via government distribution, potentially at no cost to the individual.

Packaged with quick-read instructions, self-tests may also have an associated digital app, which can reduce the incidence of errors or invalid results. A digital app can also enable reporting of an OTC result to public health departments. Individuals testing positive with OTC tests are advised to follow up with a clinical provider, to confirm a diagnosis, inform clinical care, and for public health reporting.

1.2.4 Asymptomatic Screening

Diagnostic tests may also be used for asymptomatic screening. When asymptomatic transmission is common for a given pathogen, as it is for SARS-CoV-2, community screening may be an important tool to identify infections and prevent further transmission. Screening programs may also be implemented by businesses, communities, and schools to reduce asymptomatic spread within a subpopulation, or to control access to sports, social, or entertainment venues.

Repeated or serial testing (e.g., 2–3 times per week) with rapid self or POC tests can increase the likelihood of identifying an asymptomatic positive case during an early stage of infection and enabling safety measures such as quarantine to protect others from being infected. Serial testing by schools of those who have been in close contact with a positive case can avert the need for precautionary quarantine of everyone exposed, reducing the burden of remote learning for quarantined students.

1.3 Overview of the NIH Rapid Acceleration of Diagnostics (RADx) Initiative

Early in the COVID-19 pandemic, only nucleic acid amplification tests (NAATs) were available to diagnose acute infection with SARS-CoV-2. While highly sensitive and accurate, NAATs are generally conducted in centralized, high-complexity laboratories with strict regulatory requirements and skilled technicians. Given the time required for both transport and testing, test results generally were not available until days or even weeks after sample collection, greatly limiting their utility in preventing transmission. Supply chain limitations for common consumables such as pipette tips and nucleic acid extraction reagents led to additional delays. The need for alternative tests that could be used more widely and return results much faster was evident. A coordinated testing strategy had to have the following components:

- Public–private partnerships to accelerate innovation in diagnostic technology
- Increased manufacturing capacity and better supply chain management to enable sustainable domestic production
- Robust, secure data collection and utilization systems
- Methods for ensuring testing access for underserved populations to address health disparities

In response to the demand for greatly increased testing, NIH launched the Rapid Acceleration of Diagnostics (RADx) initiative in April 2020 to support the development, production scale-up, and deployment of accurate, rapid tests across the country (NIH 2022c) (Fig. 3).

The emergence of COVID-19 illuminated some of the challenges a society faces when it relies on a hospital- and office-based healthcare model to address a rapidly spreading infectious disease. In particular, it highlighted the immediate need for a dynamic, distributed, and accessible diagnostic testing ecosystem. NIH's RADx Initiative was established as an integrated, holistic approach to these challenges through four initial programs to speed inno-

Fig. 3 Comparison of lab-based POC and self/at-home tests across multiple parameters. (Authors)

	Lab-based	Point of Care (POC)	Self / At-home
Test Type	Molecular (primarily)	Molecular, Antigen	Antigen (primarily)
Sensitivity	> 95%	> 90%	> 80%
Specificity	> 95%	> 90%	> 90%
Limit of Detection (copies/mL)	$> 10^2$	$> 10^2$ (molecular); $> 10^3$ (antigen)	$> 10^3$
Time to Result	24-48 hours longer if testing volume exceeds capacity	~ 30 – 60 min	~ 15 – 30 min
Cost per Result	$$$	$$	$
Results Reporting	Integrated with public health reporting infrastructure to automatically provide test result	May be integrated with public health reporting or may require healthcare provider to manually report test result	Typically requires user to voluntarily report test result to a public health agency or the test manufacturer

vation in technologies for COVID-19 testing and build an equitable national testing infrastructure (NIH 2022c) and others that followed.

- RADx Tech aims to identify and accelerate the development, scale-up, and deployment of innovative POC and at-home testing technologies.
- RADx Advanced Technology Platforms (RADx ATP) supports the scale-up of more advanced technologies that can achieve immediate, substantial increases in testing capacity.
- RADx Underserved Populations (RADx UP) establishes community-engaged implementation projects to improve access to testing in underserved and vulnerable populations.
- RADx rad (shorthand for radical) focuses on innovative testing methods that have a slightly longer horizon to technology maturation.
- Two additional RADx programs were established later on:
  - The RADx Independent Test Assessment Program (RADx ITAP) provides federal resources for test validation and regulatory prioritization to qualifying manufacturers in order to increase the availability of high-quality OTC COVID-19 tests to the public.
  - The RADx Mobile Application Reporting through Standards (RADx MARS) program promotes a standards-based approach to reporting COVID-19 self-test results with application to future reporting of remote diagnostics.

1.3.1 RADx Tech

RADx Tech is a fast-track technology development program led by the National Institute of Biomedical Imaging and Bioengineering (NIBIB) that leverages the NIH Point of Care Technology Research Network (POCTRN) and partnerships across relevant federal agencies to speed innovation in the development, commercialization, and implementation of technologies for COVID-19 testing. The program's innovation funnel approach (Fig. 4) was designed to compress the customary diagnostic technology development timeline from years to months. As with many other aspects

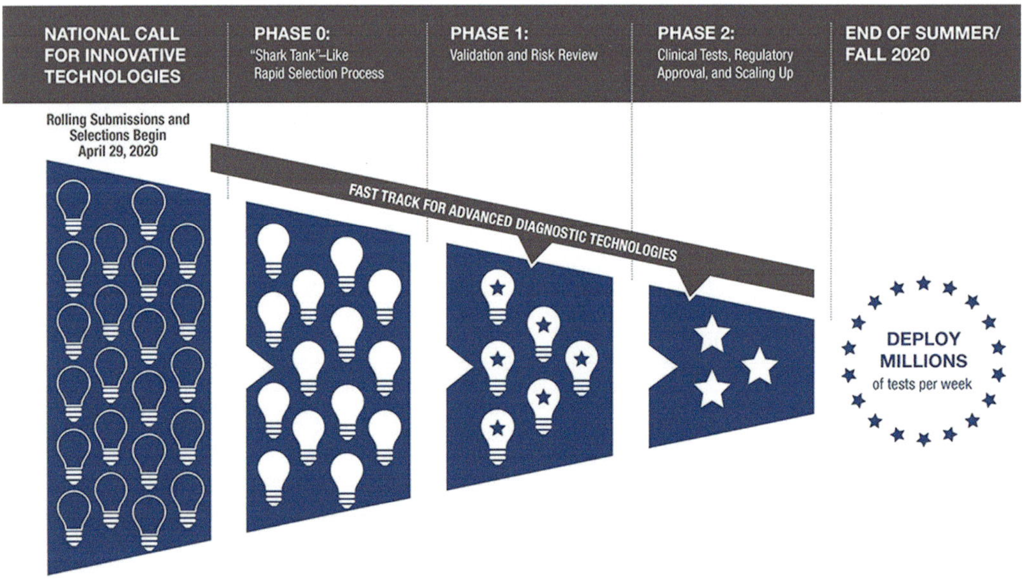

Fig. 4 NIH Rapid Acceleration of Diagnostics (RADx) Initiative for COVID-19 Technology Development Funnel. (@NIHDirector 2020; NIH, public domain)

of expedited research response to public health emergencies, the approach has been employing expert teams in parallel rather than in sequence to address technical, regulatory, clinical, and commercialization requirements and to support the validation, de-risking, scale-up, manufacturing, and deployment of novel tests. The RADx Tech program (along with RADx ATP) represents a new paradigm by which the NIH, and the federal government writ large, can catalyze medical technology development during a public health emergency. A more detailed description of the components and operation of the RADx Tech program is provided in ▶ Sect. 2.

1.3.2 The RADx Advanced Technology Platforms (RADx ATP)

The RADx Advanced Technology Platforms (RADx ATP) program was established to increase POC testing capacity by identifying existing and late-stage testing platforms for COVID-19 that can potentially achieve rapid scale-up and broader distribution relatively quickly. The program focuses on validating throughput and then improving and/or scaling up applicable technologies, including high-throughput platforms. As with RADx Tech, test and platform developers were evaluated, and then selected projects accelerated using the innovation funnel methodology. Developers that met RADx ATP criteria quickly advanced to Phase 2 of the program following the Phase 0 "deep dive." In contrast to RADx Tech, RADx ATP primarily supported testing technologies that had received or were close to U.S. Food and Drug Administration (FDA) authorization and could be produced in rapidly expanding quantity. Another goal was to establish or expand regional testing hubs and help expand testing to areas with underserved populations. Close collaboration and open communication with the Biomedical Advanced Research and Development Authority (BARDA), Department of Defense (DoD), and FDA were critical to minimize duplication of effort and ensure the tests developed and sold were ready for public use.

1.3.3 RADx UP

COVID-19 has disproportionally affected underserved and vulnerable populations. The RADx Underserved Populations (RADx UP) program was established with the overarching goals of (1) understanding the factors associated with disparities in COVID-19 morbidity and mortality for underserved and vulnerable populations who are disproportionately affected by the COVID-19 pandemic, and (2) laying the foundation for strategies to reduce those disparities. RADx UP funded a diverse cohort of community projects across the United States to assess and expand COVID-19 testing for populations including African Americans, Native Americans, and Alaska Natives; those in nursing homes, jails, and prisons; rural areas and underserved urban areas; pregnant women; and the homeless. Specifically, the program established multiple clinical research sites to evaluate testing methods in varying populations, places, and settings; encouraged collaboration between the program sites and the community to meet their needs; and developed strategies to apply technological advances in real-world settings, such as the "Say Yes! COVID Test" and Return to School testing initiatives.

For example, the Say Yes! COVID Test program (◘ Fig. 5), implemented in collabo-

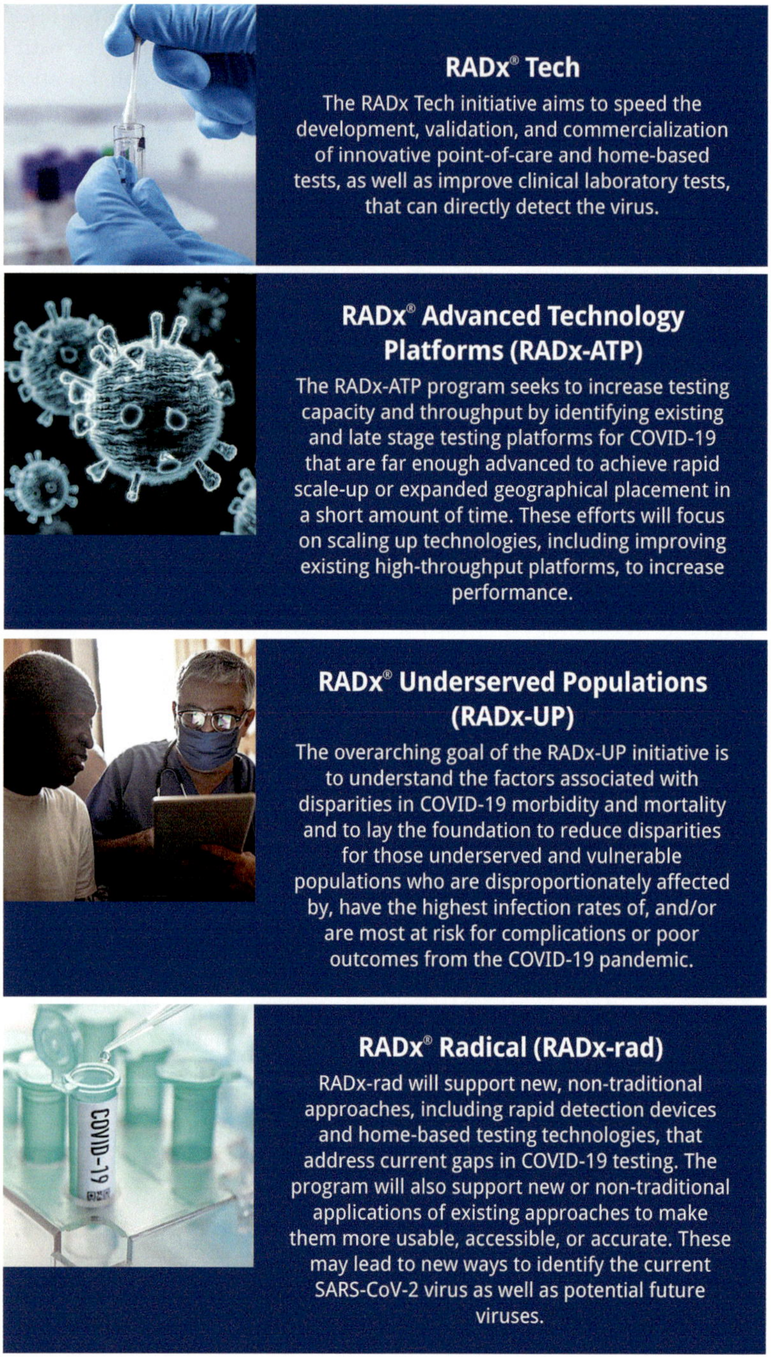

Fig. 5 Overview of the foundational RADx programs established by NIH to speed innovation in the development, commercialization, and implementation of technologies for COVID-19. (NIH, public domain, from ▶ https://www.nih.gov/research-training/medical-research-initiatives/radx/radx-programs)

ration with state health departments and the U.S. Centers for Disease Control and Prevention (CDC), provided select communities and public health departments access to free, rapid antigen tests for at-home use to determine whether frequent self-administered COVID-19 testing helps reduce community transmission. The Safe Return to School Diagnostic Testing Initiative (► Box 2) funded projects in multiple states to determine the best strategies combining frequent testing protocols and proven safety measures to enable students and staff in vulnerable and underserved communities to return to school (NIBIB 2021).

> **Box 2: Safe Return to School Diagnostic Testing Initiative**
> The RADx-UP program funded projects at ten institutions across eight states to build evidence on safely returning students, teachers, and support staff to in-person school in areas with vulnerable and underserved populations. The projects evaluated both at-home COVID-19 testing and pooled, in-school testing approaches using either antigen or molecular tests to analyze nasal swabs or saliva samples. While ongoing at the time of this publication, the studies have already demonstrated methods to overcome logistical and operational barriers in forming school–academic–public health partnerships during a pandemic and implementing robust diagnostic testing programs at K-12 schools to help reduce educational and health disparities.

1.3.4 RADx-Rad

RADx Radical (RADx-rad) was established to support new, nontraditional approaches, including rapid detection devices and home-based testing technologies, that address current gaps in COVID-19 testing. The program also supported novel applications of existing approaches to make them more usable, accessible, or accurate, which may lead to new ways to identify the SARS-CoV-2 virus as well as potential future viruses. Many of the technologies supported by RADx-rad are unique approaches, including community wastewater analysis, next-generation sequencing analytical platforms, and testing technologies coupled with artificial intelligence systems. Once sufficiently matured and demonstrated to have commercialization promise, select technologies supported by RADx-rad were encouraged to apply for the RADx Tech program to further accelerate their development, validation, and market entry.

1.3.5 RADx ITAP

The RADx Independent Test Assessment Program (RADx ITAP) was established by NIBIB in partnership with the FDA in order to accelerate regulatory review of OTC COVID-19 tests for the public (POCTRN 2022a). NIH provides dedicated RADx ITAP resources for independent laboratory validation, clinical studies, and streamlined data collection in support of FDA emergency use authorization (EUA) applications. For test manufacturers that can scale up quickly and meet the FDA's performance and quality standards, the FDA will use the information from RADx ITAP to accelerate the EUA review process.

1.3.6 RADx MARS

At-home and self-administered SARS-CoV-2 tests, unlike diagnostic tests in laboratories, are not routinely reported or included in health statistics. The RADx Mobile Application Reporting through Standards (RADx MARS) program was established by NIBIB in partnership with the U.S. Department of Health and Human Services (HHS) Office of the National Coordinator for Health Information Technology (ONC) to accommodate the increased use of at-home testing by enabling results reporting. RADx MARS assists diagnostic manufacturers that provide a compan-

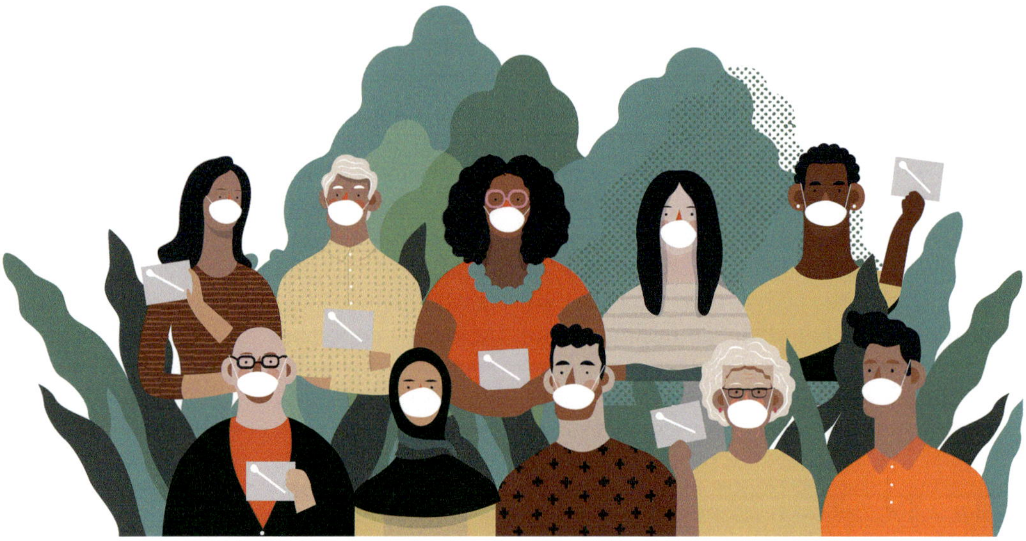

Fig. 6 Online caption at Say Yes! COVID Test: Help us learn more about the different ways to test for COVID-19 at home!

ion mobile application or website to implement standardized results reporting based on two principles: (1) encoding of results and associated data in a healthcare industry-standard format, and (2) identifying one (or a few) destination(s) where these results can be sent and subsequently re-transmitted to appropriate state, federal, and related health systems (Fig. 6).

2 The RADx Tech Program

2.1 Overview of Program Design and Operation

Named to recall the World War II-era program at the Massachusetts Institute of Technology Radiation Laboratory (Rad Lab) that developed radar (Collins 2020), the RADx Tech program was launched in April 2020 by NIBIB to swiftly develop and bring to market millions of diagnostic tests for SARS-CoV-2. Central to the design, implementation, and management of RADx Tech is the NIH Point of Care Technology Research Network (POCTRN 2022b), which was well established prior to the pandemic and uses a partnership model to improve clinical care by developing POC test devices, assessing clinical needs, training technology developers, and providing administrative support. Described as "a competitive shark tank" by U.S. Senator Lamar Alexander, who co-sponsored funding legislation (Senate testimony on new tests for COVID-19 2020), RADx Tech leverages POCTRN and harnesses the strengths of the U.S. government, academic, and private sectors to rapidly vet, fund, support, and bring new tests to market. While other programs under the RADx umbrella focused on early-stage technologies, laboratory-based tests, and supporting underserved populations, RADx Tech initially focused on new POC tests with some support for at-home tests (Tromberg et al. 2020). This focus evolved with time due to real-world test usage studies (Dempsey et al. 2021), the needs of public health agencies, and the proliferation of SARS-CoV-2 variants.

Innovators from across the business, academic, nonprofit, and other sectors with promising COVID-19 diagnostic devices or testing platforms were invited to submit a detailed proposal describing their product and development plans. Proposals were reviewed by an external panel of experts for feasibility based on technical, clinical, regula-

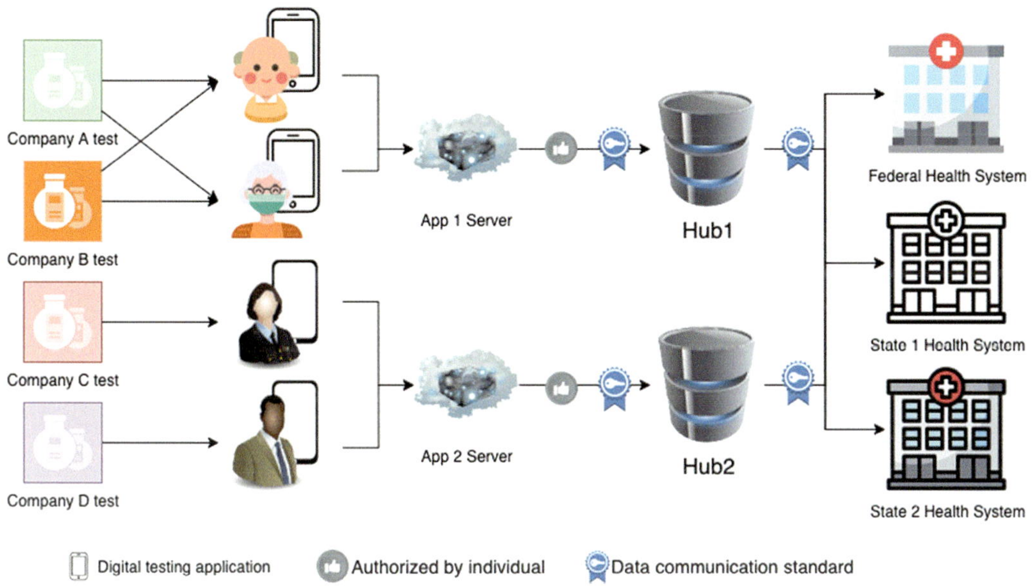

Fig. 7 How results from a self-administered test are sent to public health systems. The workflow supports tests developed by different manufacturers. Results are first captured in a mobile application (app) that accompanies a specific test. The App creates a healthcare data communication standards-based message that it sends to a third-party hub. The hub then relays the message to the appropriate public health system(s). (NIH, public domain, from ▶ https://www.nibib.nih.gov/covid-19/radx-tech-program/mars)

tory, and commercialization criteria (Fig. 7). Qualifying proposals advanced to the "deep dive" stage (Phase 0) for work package (WP) development and were assigned a team of healthcare commercialization and content experts to assess the proposal and identify risk factors that could impede progress. Milestones indicating risk resolution and further progress were assigned. Projects with the greatest potential to increase national testing capacity and fill key gaps in the testing ecosystem were advanced to the next phase (Phase 1) and were provided financial resources via a grant subaward from a POCTRN center; expert advisors; and in-kind technical, clinical, and business support to address high-risk barriers to development success. Sufficiently de-risked projects were issued substantial contract awards by NIBIB in the final phase (Phase 2) to support the full range of activities needed for large-scale distribution to the public, including manufacturing. As of September 2022, the RADx Tech innovation funnel (includes RADx ATP and RADx ITAP) has enabled 35 novel technologies to obtain FDA emergency use authorization, delivering a cumulative five billion additional COVID-19 tests and test products to the market, including the first over-the-counter test for at-home use. The following sections will provide an overview of the program design and operations of RADx Tech; for further information, Schachter and Parrish (2021) published an extensive description of the program's components as a special section in the *IEEE Open Journal of Engineering in Medicine and Biology*.

2.2 The Innovation Funnel

The RADx Tech selection methodology is referred to as the innovation funnel (Fig. 7) because the multistage review process, designed to quickly eliminate unlikely prospects and provide deep, intensive evaluation of likely prospects prior to funding, resulted in a narrowing pipeline ending with the deployment of highly competitive products. The funnel was open for a broad assortment

Category	Criteria
Technical	Can the technology be developed to the highest levels of analytical performance (e.g., sensitivity, specificity, dynamic range, limit of detection, reliability, accuracy, speed, and throughput) as well as operational performance, such as patient- and user-friendly design, alternative sampling strategies (saliva, exhaled breath, etc.), optimization of swab materials and test reagents, mobile-device integration, increased accessibility, and home use? Do these technical and design advances help expand national testing capacity and provide clear advantages over current approaches?
Clinical	Is the proposal a realistic approach to increasing SARS-CoV-2 testing? Can it be rapidly integrated into the healthcare system?
Commercial	Assuming the technology works as anticipated, can it be implemented and produced economically at scale?
Regulatory	Are there feasible plans to perform the studies required for FDA Emergency Use Authorization (EUA) and subsequent FDA clearance?

Fig. 8 RADx Tech project review criteria

of technologies at various stages of maturity from any sponsoring organization. One key principle was that there is strength in diversity, and that RADx Tech would explore the best exemplar of each approach to detecting the SARS-CoV-2 virus.

The 700-plus proposals received by August 11, 2020, when the submissions window initially closed, were reviewed by NIH staff, scientific consultants, and industry experts using a defined set of evaluation criteria (Fig. 8) with the goal of rapidly enabling commercialization (NIH 2022b). As these proposals went through multiple evaluation steps, the numbers narrowed: 140 (20%) from this initial cohort were invited to participate in the "deep dive" process (Phase 0) where reviewers met with the test developer to quickly vet the technology, the team, and the commercialization potential. Fewer than one-third of the 140 projects then advanced to Phase 1: a detailed evaluation of risks, steps required for commercialization, and needed funding. NIBIB funded more than 30 of these work package-1 (WP1) projects in Phase 1, designed to de-risk (i.e., identify risk factors that could impede development and deployment of the proposed technology) the technology and manufacturing process and to obtain regulatory authorization. A handful of proposals were immediately ready for the next stage of support. These, along with successful WP1 projects, were awarded work package-2 (WP2) contracts, for example, to scale up production or broaden their usability, such as taking a POC authorized product and getting over-the-counter authorization. NIBIB reopened the innovation funnel for new applications in July 2021 and, as of November 2021, has awarded more than 45 WP2 contracts in Phase 2, with a cumulative value of almost $700M (NIH 2022a).

Not all projects were successful. While the failure rate of WP1 to WP2 transitions was relatively low, the number of WP2 projects that failed to meet their milestones on time has been relatively high. Due to the ongoing pandemic, NIBIB has made several difficult decisions to discontinue support for projects that met technical milestones but not commercialization goals.

As part of the ongoing evaluation of each funded WP1 and WP2 project, NIH program managers and the RADx network of expert advisors and consultants meet weekly and even daily with the test developer to assess progress. A dedicated team of scientific, technical, and industrial experts provides coaching to get the product from concept to full-scale production and implementation. In addition to deep involvement with the test developer, RADx Tech supported an independent validation process that subjected each product to bench testing, analytical testing, evaluation with clinical samples, and ultimately clinical evaluation against a "gold standard" reverse transcriptase-polymerase chain reaction (RT-PCR) assay. For over-the-counter use, products also underwent human factors evaluation to assess the ability of users to perform the test and read the results accurately. As virus variants evolved and became epidemiologically relevant, tests were also required to undergo evaluation for their ability to detect these new variant strains. The end goal of this independent validation was to ensure that each product met the FDA's EUA requirements and could provide documentation of device performance. Within a year, the test developers supported by RADx were producing 17 million POC and at-home tests per month.

2.3 Test Validation

Independent verification of the test performance data provided by the developer was a critical component of Phase 1 (WP1) of RADx Tech and enabled NIBIB to make more informed decisions on whether to continue funding the project. It would also prove instrumental in assessing the impact of SARS-CoV-2 variants on the efficacy of rapid antigen tests (Frediani et al. 2021) and in establishing standards for evaluating diagnostic technologies that would go on to become the foundation for RADx ITAP. The Test Verification Core (TVC) was rapidly initiated at the Atlanta Center for Microsystems Engineered Point of Care Technologies, a partnership between Emory University, Georgia Institute of Technology, and Children's Healthcare of Atlanta, to serve as the national test validation hub, providing impartial assessment of the design and performance of diagnostic tests.

The organization, operation, and technical assessments conducted by the TVC are described in detail elsewhere (Nehl et al. 2021). Briefly, a multi-institutional and transdisciplinary team was assembled along the following workstreams: laboratory and clinical device evaluation to understand the sensitivity, specificity, and cross-reactivity of candidate devices in controlled and community settings and compared to RT-PCR tests; regulatory expertise to identify and overcome barriers to device approval and distribution; usability testing by patients and others to identify and overcome device limitations; and engineering assessment to evaluate robustness of design including human factors, manufacturability, shipment and storage requirements, and scalability. This comprehensive test assessment program required extensive laboratory resources, comprising biosafety level 2 and 3 facilities, biobanks of COVID-19 positive and negative patient specimens, community-based collection, and engineering design and human factors assessment labs.

2.4 Clinical Studies

While the Test Verification Core (TVC) provided a detailed assessment of diagnostic tests largely under controlled laboratory conditions, RADx Tech established the Clinical Studies Core (CSC) to evaluate COVID-19 tests in real-world situations and generate clinical data for regulatory authorization. The CSC was created by the Center for Advancing Point of Care Technologies (CAPCaT) in Heart, Lung, Blood, and Sleep Diseases, a POCTRN technology hub at the University of Massachusetts Lowell and the University of Massachusetts Medical School, with contributions from other POCTRN centers at Northwestern, Emory, and Johns Hopkins Universities. The primary objective of the CSC was to design and implement diagnostic device clinical studies to evaluate test performance and usability across diverse use-case populations and settings.

Gibson et al. (2021) describe in detail how the CSC built and maintained clinical studies infrastructure and platform trial designs that could be rapidly adapted for clinical trials of each testing technology entering RADx Tech Phase 2. This included a master protocol, consent form, digital study platform, data management system, single institutional review board (research ethics review committee) with study site reliance agreements, community engagement mechanisms, and multisite partnerships. The infrastructure and core design enabled standardization while accommodating the diverse testing methods and test environments under study. Further accelerating the studies was the Eureka digital research platform through which trials were executed (Eureka 2022). Supported by NIH and developed at the University of California San

Francisco, Eureka engaged study participants through a web-based interface or mobile app to assess their eligibility for the study, obtain their consent to participate, and complete digital surveys on their interpretations of test results and assessments of device usability. Taken together, the CSC's efforts to streamline studies significantly reduced the time and costs of trials and enabled successful products to get to market faster.

2.5 Regulatory Review and Emergency Use Authorization

Before a medical device, including in vitro diagnostics such as COVID-19 tests, can be marketed in the United States, clinical studies are generally needed to demonstrate to the FDA that the device is safe and effective. Following the January 31, 2020, declaration by the Secretary of Health and Human Services of a national public health emergency in response to COVID-19, the FDA exercised its authority to waive some of these requirements and issue emergency use authorization (EUA) for medical devices that had not gone through the entire traditional approval or clearance process. However, test developers were still required to provide sufficient evidence to validate analytical and clinical function of the diagnostic device. The FDA requires rigorous data because unreliable COVID-19 tests could harm individual and public health (FDA 2021b). False positive results can lead to unnecessary quarantine, resources wasted on contact tracing and testing, and delay in accurate diagnosis and appropriate treatment. False negatives could mean patients do not get the treatment they need, even as they potentially spread the disease to others.

To help test developers and manufacturers design their clinical studies, the FDA provides EUA templates that lay out clear protocols and guidelines to follow as one pathway to authorization (FDA 2022). In broad terms, the FDA asks developers to demonstrate that a COVID-19 test meets analytical and clinical criteria in a randomized, blinded clinical study that compares test results with paired reference samples. The analytical study typically includes an assessment of the limit of detection (LOD) (i.e., test sensitivity), cross-reactivity with other pathogens (i.e., test specificity), and flex studies to check that the test will function properly despite minor product or sample variations—the sort of assessment that usually precedes a full clinical study.

The clinical study must demonstrate that an in vitro diagnostic device does what it claims for the population it is intended to serve. Test developers must consider whether the intended population will include children, whether the test distinguishes between levels of infection, whether it is intended only for symptomatic individuals or also for asymptomatic screening, and of course the use environment. For POC and at-home tests, developers must demonstrate that the intended user can successfully run the test "first time out of the box" using only the provided instructions. Usability testing is generally conducted in parallel with the clinical study to accelerate the timeline to regulatory review submission.

With the high opportunity cost of delaying test development during the COVID-19 pandemic, the RADx Tech program sought to accelerate regulatory authorization by conducting some of the analytical, clinical, and usability studies in parallel. While this puts investment at greater risk compared to the traditional sequential approach, it accelerated market entry for tests that met regulatory standards. Coordination between NIH and FDA throughout the RADx initiative was critical to efficient analytical and clinical study design and implementation.

2.6 Deployment: Supply Chain, Manufacturing, and Distribution

In anticipation of FDA emergency use authorization of a RADx Tech-supported test, NIBIB invested considerable effort and funds to enable test developers to produce tests in high volume immediately upon authorization. It is rare for a medical product to launch with a high production volume; typically, there is a "beta" period after the product has been approved when marketing strategies are developed, supply chains are built, and consistent product quality is assured. Sometimes the production is paired with storage to ensure wide availability after the post-approval steps are complete. These are not options during a pandemic when tests are needed at scale immediately.

Most of the RADx Tech-supported developers had little experience launching new products, while supply chains, manufacturing, and distribution have not normally been within the purview of NIH. Therefore, a team of commercialization, procurement, logistics, and supply chain experts was incorporated into the RADx network as a Deployment Core to provide test developers in Phase 1 and Phase 2 of the program with coordinated infrastructure to enable market entry. Consultative services provided by the Deployment Core included, but were not limited to, procurement and supply chain, manufacturing and development, logistics, distribution, quality management, regulatory, recruiting, reimbursement, market research, and verification/validation (Walsh et al. 2021). Critical to the success of the Deployment Core were close partnerships and collaborations with the HHS Assistant Secretary for Preparedness and Response (ASPR),[1] the Biomedical Advanced Research and Development Authority (BARDA), and multiple components of the Department of Defense, including the U.S. Air Force Acquisition COVID-19 Task Force.

The deployment challenges were compounded by pandemic-related supply chain constraints, labor shortages, and competition for scarce resources. Prior to the formation of the HHS Testing and Diagnostics Working Group, the Deployment Core developed projections of raw material needs, potential suppliers, and market rates. These projections were used to build forecasts for critical components of COVID-19 diagnostic tests, such as nasal swabs, nitrocellulose membranes for lateral flow assays, automated manufacturing equipment, pipette tips for high-throughput assays, sample collection vials, and sterilization and packaging equipment. These forecasts, combined with other Deployment Core outputs, informed RADx Tech programmatic and funding decisions to support additional technologies that used alternative materials or sample collection methods. Strategic, albeit limited implementation of Defense Production Act (DPA) authority to prioritize government contracts with suppliers also helped reduce supply chain limitations. For example, RADx Tech has relied on DPA authorities to support procurement of pressure sensors, fluid flow sensors, microcontrollers, and automation equipment for test developers in its portfolio.

The Deployment Core also developed educational tools to inform the public about available tests and how to use them in a variety of settings. A continually updated online guide (on when to perform testing in various environments, situations, and using different kinds of diagnostic technologies) is a key source for public information (When to test 2022). Built in collaboration with the MIT Institute for Data, Systems, and Society, ► WhenToTest.org provides science-based guidance for individuals and organizations on mitigation and testing strategies, and how to combine COVID-19 prevention and containment with the latest testing strategies to minimize the spread of the virus in specific environments (Walsh et al. 2021). Based on individual user input on contacts with others or their organization's mitigation strategies, level of compliance, and community prevalence of COVID-19, the underlying mathematical model provides recommendations and guidance for developing and implementing a specialized testing strategy.

2.7 Digital Health Infrastructure and Tools

Reflecting the potential of digital health technologies to augment COVID-19 testing, a key

1 Now the Administration for Strategic Preparedness and Response.

element of the RADx Tech program was development and evaluation of digital health tools. These fall into four categories, each with the potential to guide individuals through the pandemic in specific but synergistic ways.

2.7.1 Wearables

Wearables for monitoring and detection, including smartwatches, fitness trackers, and other wearable sensors, can continuously monitor physiological signals as individuals go about their lives. Sensor data can be analyzed with statistical or deep learning models to detect anomalies or changes in signals from baseline, a potential indicator of deteriorating health or disease. This approach has been used to detect COVID-19 onset from smartwatch data prior to appearance of symptoms (Mishra et al. 2020). While this strategy has shown promise, it currently suffers from relatively low detection sensitivity and specificity. A practical application of this technology may therefore be to alert individuals of suspected COVID-19 and encourage them to get tested, rather than trying to make a diagnosis from smartwatch data alone.

2.7.2 Digital Contact Tracing and Exposure Notification Systems

Digital Contact Tracing and Exposure Notification Systems, such as the one developed by Apple and Google (2022), were among the widely known mobile health technologies emerging during the COVID-19 pandemic. This smartphone-based technology causes phones that come near each other to exchange anonymous key codes via Bluetooth or other wireless communication protocols; if a phone owner later tests positive, it can trigger a notification to all other phones that were nearby in the preceding days, alerting those notified to get tested. This novel digital approach supplements manual contact tracing, which is resource intensive. However, digital contact tracing has yet to achieve widespread adoption largely due to concerns about privacy, security, and trust (GAO 2021). Future efforts are needed to demonstrate the effectiveness of digital contact tracing tools and better educate the public about their value.

2.7.3 Proof-of-Health Status Technologies

While contact tracing is useful when an individual tests positive, other digital health technologies can offer value to people who test negative. Proof-of-health-status technologies, also known as testing or vaccine passports, can provide a digital record of an individual's test result or vaccination history. Several solutions have emerged during the COVID-19 pandemic that leverage advances in cryptography and blockchain to provide securely identified certification of health status while protecting individual privacy. As with digital contact tracing technologies, public adoption has been limited due to politicization and concerns over security and privacy. Nevertheless, some practical solutions have emerged. For example, through a partnership between the identity verification provider CLEAR and the at-home test manufacturer Lucira Health, the Golden State Warriors NBA team leveraged testing passports to ensure that unvaccinated fans tested negative for SARS-CoV-2 before entering the stadium (NBA 2021).

2.7.4 Smartphone Companion Testing Apps

As self-administered tests became more prevalent during the COVID-19 pandemic, so did the availability of *smartphone companion testing apps*. These apps are generally designed to assist users with test administration, either through on-screen instructions or by connecting users with a live telehealth proctor. Another important feature of these apps enables individuals to share their test results with state and federal health systems. In some cases, the apps can even interpret test results; for example, by analyzing a photograph of the test strip.

2.7.5 Combined Technologies

While each of the above technologies can serve a unique role in guiding individuals through pandemic life, their greatest impact can be achieved by combining them into an integrated system. Consider a person who feels healthy, but whose smartwatch generates an alert about suspected COVID-19 onset. The person self-administers a COVID-19 test

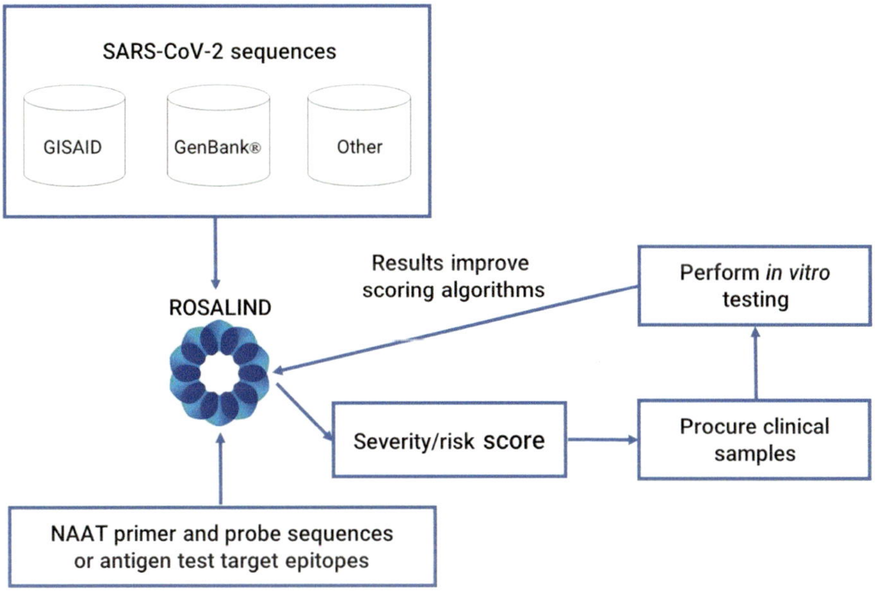

Fig. 9 RADx Variant Task Force program for assessing the impact of variants on SARS-CoV-2 molecular and antigen tests. (Creager et al. 2021; CC BY 4.0)

at home under the guidance of a smartphone app. The app interprets the test result as being positive, shares the result with the state public health department, and leverages digital contact tracing to automatically notify other phones that were in close proximity in recent days. Two weeks pass, and the person recovers from COVID-19 and self-administers another test that yields a negative result. The testing app issues a digital testing passport, allowing the person to board a plane for vacation. While this scenario is not currently possible, it may be an element of future pandemic response.

2.8 Monitoring and Anticipating Viral Variants

The emergence of the COVID-19 Delta variant in 2021 underscored the importance of ongoing monitoring and quality control of test sensitivity. The NIH, CDC, and FDA developed a collaborative strategy to address this challenge. The CDC established a nationwide genomic surveillance program, engaging multiple high-throughput laboratories to perform whole-genome sequencing on up to 100,000 SARS-CoV-2 samples per week. The NIH and the FDA jointly created the RADx Variants Task Force (VTF), which brought together RADx Tech's test verification and bioinformatics cores and the FDA's Center for Devices and Radiological Health. The mission of the VTF was to ensure that testing technologies supported by RADx Tech would accurately and comprehensively detect SARS-CoV-2 variants. This was a critical aspect of nationwide access to an array of effective COVID-19 tests.

The VTF carried out its work through a combination of computational and laboratory approaches. The computational aspect centered on continuous processing of viral genomes deposited into the global genetic database GISAID[2] and public sequence databases to track the distribution of viral lineages and identify lineage-specific mutations (Fig. 9). These mutations were compared to known primer probes of molecular tests and known epitopes of antigen tests to evaluate whether loss of affinity or signal was likely.

2 Originally called the Global Initiative on Sharing Avian Influenza Data.

All tests computationally identified as being at risk for loss of sensitivity were referred to the Test Verification Core for laboratory follow up.

The laboratory component of the VTF effort relied on collection of viral samples from partner laboratories. Only samples that were fully characterized through whole-genome sequencing were collected. The emphasis was on samples of variants that could lead to loss of sensitivity, although a representative library of SARS-CoV-2 lineages was maintained whenever possible. Existing tests computationally shown to be at risk for sensitivity loss were evaluated against variants in a laboratory setting, with the outcome guiding potential adjustment of either the test or the accompanying label. Experts from the FDA participated in the design and evaluation of both computational and laboratory metrics, enabling test developers to use the VTF data as part of their EUA or other regulatory submission. Administration officials overseeing pandemic response were briefed when emerging SARS-CoV-2 variants seemed likely to reduce the sensitivity of any test when used in a meaningful new market, as well as on the outcome of ensuing validation or remediation.

3 Summary of Key Lessons Learned

The RADx Tech Program has demonstrated the value of active NIH engagement across scientific, technical, operational, and commercial boundaries during a health emergency. RADx Tech compressed the timeline and increased the success rate for innovative biomedical technology development and commercialization. The urgency of the pandemic and declaration of a public health emergency provided the opportunity to speed up program implementation, fund at-risk activities in parallel with de-risking work, explicitly support product development and commercialization through direct partnerships with experienced industry consultants, and collaborate freely and intensively with other government agencies and departments. Shared, urgent goals in a public health crisis underscored the value of combining complementary capabilities from government, industry, and academia to solve interdisciplinary challenges. These experiences will likely have a lasting impact on how NIH, and by extension the U.S. Government (USG), approaches biomedical technology development.

3.1 Scientific and Technological

Investment in diverse diagnostic platforms is essential to ensuring that different use cases can be met successfully. RADx Tech supported a diverse portfolio of diagnostic assays and platform technologies; these ranged from hand-held RT-PCR devices with isothermal amplification to CRISPR-based (clustered regularly interspaced short palindromic repeats) assays to lateral flow assays utilizing quantum dot technology, to name a few. Multiplexed platforms, analyte concentration reagents that increase assay sensitivity, and injection-molded plastic nasal swabs are additional innovations developed with RADx Tech support. By spreading its investments across a variety of detection approaches targeting diverse viral genomic sequences and antigens, the potential that SARS-CoV-2 variants could evade tests across the diagnostic portfolio was reduced. Similarly, the impact of supply chain disruptions was diminished when tests utilized different components, from buffers to reagent enzymes to swab types. This scientific and technological heterogeneity was a critical design component of RADx Tech's approach to accelerating diagnostic innovation, and has had the secondary benefit of supporting many small businesses and diversifying the program's positive economic impact.

Another scientific and technological advance was the establishment of VTF with experimental analysis from the Test Verification Core (TVC). Building diagnostic resilience against the arrival of SARS-CoV-2 variants required resources to monitor their emergence and measure impact on test performance. The VTF and TVC built their sample collection, inventory, and storage management capabilities and assay protocols to analyze test sensitivity quickly and quantitatively as variants emerged. Again, the diversity of molecular and viral tests receiving RADx Tech support was critical as the ability to adapt testing technologies to viral variants is not uniform across diagnostic platforms. Rapid antigen tests tend to design robustness against variants into the initial selection of antibody/antigen pairs but require laboratory or real-world analysis to demonstrate continued accuracy, while nucleic acid amplification-based tests can more rapidly be modified with new primers that identify mutated sequences based on computational analysis of binding affinity.

Overall, the technologies accelerated through the innovation funnel are likely catalyzing a fundamental shift in the diagnostic testing ecosystem, away from the dominance of laboratory assays to further integration of rapid POC and at-home tests powered by cutting-edge analytical science and digital health technologies. The acceptability of and demand for access to facile, on-demand testing is growing, and continued diagnostic innovation will be needed to meet that demand. This is a story that continues to unfold, and the relevance of in vitro diagnostic testing, both in a health crisis and in the larger context of healthcare and personalized medicine going forward, was captured in a recent *Nature Biotechnology* editorial stating, "[the] combination of RADx technologies, together with structural changes to healthcare during the pandemic, has the potential to radically change diagnostics, opening up the point of care (POC), at-home and community testing settings" (Radical solutions 2021).

3.2 Operational

A critical programmatic tool NIH has used to bring scientific discoveries into the clinic to positively impact human health is public–private partnerships. NIH has a substantial record of achievement in supporting research that leads to the development of technologies for basic science and clinical applications. However, NIH has traditionally not provided active support for development and commercialization activities that follow the research phase of technology development. That work has historically been regarded as the province of industry, though the significant challenges of moving technologies from laboratory prototype to commercial product are many. While NIH encourages the licensing and commercialization of products originating in agency-funded research, direct support for commercialization has been limited.

RADx Tech, building on the POCTRN operational model and further expanding industry partnerships, provides a roadmap for NIH success in the acceleration of technology development, preparation for regulatory submissions, and commercialization of impactful health technologies. The success of RADx Tech demonstrates that urgency and willingness to step beyond the traditional NIH approach to technology development can significantly accelerate the transition from concept to proven product. Engaging a large cadre of consultants with significant industry experience proved critical. This includes leadership for rapidly growing companies, navigating a complex, rapidly evolving regulatory process, and solving problems in supply chain, cash flow, marketing, and sales, among other tasks. The availability of experts with practical experience and a network of industry contacts has been essential. Industry insiders have been able to establish connections, build trust, and mentor emerging companies. Under a typical industry-funded development pathway, it usually takes 5–7 years to get a new medical device cleared by the FDA. RADx Tech has proven that with an all-hands-on deck approach and the investment of sufficient resources this can be reduced to as little as 12 months.

For a program like RADx Tech to be successful, it requires decision-making that extends beyond technical and scientific assessment. Investment decisions must also consider the capabilities of the company and its ability to execute the plans proposed. RADx Tech includes mechanisms to evaluate that larger picture. The team has had to learn to recognize warning signs of failure and be willing to move on when a diagnostic in development does not meet its performance metrics. Test developers supported by RADx Tech face many hurdles, and not every company with an attractive technology platform has been able to fully act on the regulatory guidance and production assistance developed through the program. A clear-eyed appreciation that not every project will succeed must be tempered with the patience to see a promising project through the crises that are inherent in development and commercialization—problems different from the routine setbacks that scientists encounter in their research.

New collaborative arrangements with industry partners were not the only operational innovation; the success of the RADx Tech program would not have been possible without active partnerships across government. The urgency of addressing a global pandemic gave formal and informal networks among departments and operating divisions new importance and legitimacy. Those networks have addressed problems as diverse as expediting the movement of research materials through ports of entry, finding alternative suppliers for critical parts, developing novel approaches to rapid approval of tests already available outside the United States without diminishing the rigor of the regulatory review process, and ensuring that support for test development by different agencies is complementary rather than duplicative.

Government agencies have innovated together not just to accelerate processes but to improve them and increase confidence in outcomes. Sustaining these collaborative networks going forward has the potential to institutionalize a level of communication and cooperation that will not only impact ongoing technology development but also provide a warm base for action in subsequent public health crises.

RADx Tech has also leveraged the public health emergency-authorized flexibilities in federal procurement to award Phase 2 and other contracts at a rate commensurate with urgency of expanding COVID-19 testing while ensuring proper stewardship of federal funds. Prior to the pandemic, most large NIH contracts required an average of a full year to go from initial solicitation to final award. RADx Tech staff reduced this timeline down to a range of 10 days to 4 weeks. Another unique capability utilized by the program were "letter contracts," which support efforts with loosely defined objectives that are not guaranteed to achieve their deliverables or may not even be needed by the time the deliverable is completed. A key element has been to balance the need to act swiftly and decisively while maintaining good practices for government procurement. An important lesson as the country emerges from the pandemic will be to maintain the degree of flexibility appropriate for inherently risky activities like technology development directed at a moving target.

The approaches outlined above can be applied to other opportunities no less urgent but with a narrower impact than the COVID-19 pandemic, such as diseases with similar or worse consequences but affecting fewer individuals, building on NIH investments in the development of therapies for understudied and rare diseases.

3.3 Regulatory

The RADx Tech program has provided an opportunity to better understand how agencies with complementary missions such as NIH and FDA can collaborate while maintaining their autonomous decision authority. Facile communication between agencies has allowed NIH and the RADx Tech program to support participating test developers more effectively. It has also ensured that FDA has the necessary information for expedited review and issuance of EUAs. One example is the bi-weekly meetings that have shared awareness of trends, cross-cutting issues, and specific product issues among trusted interlocutors. A good example of what can result is the "universal" protocol RADx Tech developed with the FDA for clinical product evaluation, a protocol that provides more consistency in regulatory submissions for different products and reduces review time.

In the current healthcare regulatory paradigm, it is not the responsibility of the U.S. government to validate an individual product or monitor its market performance. Currently, the FDA does not have authorization or appropriations to build analytical software or perform independent laboratory or clinical validation of performance and safety data submitted by test developers. In response, RADx Tech utilized the resources it had available to experimentally validate data from diagnostic products not associated with government-funded programs and build extensive analytical software to collect, manage, and store this data.

Initially, little effort was put into verifying shelf life, though as the pandemic progressed it became apparent that waves of infection would continue, and shelf life would be an important criterion. Given the relative immaturity of most POC and OTC technologies, the FDA has required "real-time" shelf-life evaluation, where sample products must sit on a shelf in typical storage conditions for the entire duration of the shelf-life claim being sought in order to demonstrate its viability.

Although genome sequences fulfill many functions that required physical samples until recently, this is not true of diagnostic validation. In the current state of uncertainty about sample sharing in international law, cross-border sample acquisition has rarely been possible during the last few years (Halabi 2019). This leaves diagnostic validation weeks behind the emergence of new variant strains since the strain must first spread to the United States, be detected domestically, sequenced, and sent to NIBIB or other labs in sufficient quantity to validate the performance of both authorized and pending products. In addition, during a lull in SARS-CoV-2 transmission, it became very difficult to collect enough positive samples domestically to support EUA claims.

3.4 Manufacturing and Supply Chain

The unpredictable ups and downs of the pandemic have led to further volatility in the changing diagnostic market, complicating a highly competitive and fragile supply chain for test components. It has been an iterative process to learn which supply chain items have a long manufacturing ramp-up that cannot be accelerated, and which can. This introduces additional risk, as items that require a long time to produce may be highly customized and usable only for one product—one that may have failed by the time the component is ready. Automated manufacturing equipment has been a perpetual challenge as it is expensive, usually highly customized, specific to a product, cannot be built quickly, and must be ordered and paid for before the product has been validated.

This led to a very challenging situation in the fall of 2021 as various market forces collided. The demand for COVID-19 testing had decreased compared to the previous summer, and most testing companies did not project enough long-term demand to maintain manufacturing capacity. Meanwhile, the global economy had begun to return to catch up on a year-long backlog in the supply chain. When the emergence of the Delta variant sparked demand for additional testing, there was intense competition across all market segments for commodity items such as semiconductor chips and other electronic components. Given the volatile behavior of the diagnostics market, most suppliers gave preference to their steady nondiagnostic customers. This left most POC and high-end OTC diagnostic products in short supply.

Talent and human resources have also been a severe constraint at various junctures. Many products went through an initial phase of production by manual or semi-automated assembly, both of which require short-term technicians to be hired and trained quickly. For lab-based tests, this shortage is even more critical given the training and certifications required. As one industry member put it, skilled and trained labor "cannot be stockpiled."

There has been constant tension between leveraging foreign manufacturing capacity to ramp up quickly versus the more sustained investment to build domestic capacity. Domestic manufacturing is ultimately more responsive to national needs and addresses national security concerns. However, domestic production costs are higher, which affects price, public access to testing, and long-term market competitiveness.

The key lesson learned, however, is that if the federal government wishes small businesses to build and develop new products quickly for a market that had not previously existed, then the government needs to provide key resources. For example, a half dozen industry experts were brought on board to coordinate RADx Tech supply chain activities. They provided a single RADx Tech point of contact with suppliers to support multiple products, and a small team to monitor ongoing and potential supply constraints.

3.5 Implementation

A key chicken-and-egg problem for RADx has been bringing new companies with new products to a new market. In several cases, it has been challenging to garner enough attention to get these small businesses over the hump. For example, a new medical product might need the same swab as an established diagnostic manufacturer. As there has never been an oversupply of swabs, the small company is usually unable to get the swabs they need for a comparative clinical evaluation prior to entering the market to compete with the established company.

On another note, the Centers for Medicare & Medicaid Services (CMS) has not been deeply involved in RADx activities, since Congress mandated that they pay for all *diagnostic* tests. The lack of reimbursement for anything other than *medical* diagnosis has put a massive crimp in national surveillance and early detection. While CDC and state departments of health have funded some efforts, other organizations (e.g., schools and businesses) must be subsidized (e.g., the joint DoD and HHS Operation Expanded Testing) or make difficult business decisions about whether to pay for testing as a proactive measure to detect and avoid COVID-19 transmission. Moreover, day-care and pre-kindergarten settings, falling outside of the usual K-12 structure, have been a blind spot in testing policy and economics.

Another difficulty has been ensuring that all test results are reported to a public health authority. Since reporting is not required by the FDA or CMS and costs time and money, there is little incentive for reporting. This is particularly critical for cost-sensitive POC and OTC tests. But it goes both ways. On several occasions, county-scale efforts to distribute tests with reporting built in were rebuffed by the local department of health as they lacked data processing capacity. Logistics for transporting finished products from the site of manufacture to the end-user has been an underdeveloped component of the national strategy, particularly as logistics may account for up to two-thirds of the cost of a test. This was compounded for some time starting in the fall of 2021 by the severe backlog of ships waiting to unload at seaports.

Finally, the national testing strategy has primarily been reactive to changing conditions. While vaccines and therapeutics have been supported proactively through deployment and implementation, emphasis and resources have been provided to testing only as need arises. Further, perceptions regarding the need for and value of testing have fluctuated as diagnostics (relative to vaccines and therapeutics) grows into its role in that triad. Given the months-long ramp-up time to manufacture new tests and get them to market, testing capacity has frequently lagged demand. This on-demand approach has led to some very high-profile and unfortunate situations where manufacturers have ceased production or eliminated their capacity (Fink 2021). As the nation prepares for SARS-CoV-2 to become an endemic disease with new waves as variants emerge, and as global health attention shifts to negotiating a preparedness instrument for the next pandemic (WHO 2022), it is incumbent upon us to ensure that diagnostics does not become the weak leg of the disease response tripod.

3.6 Digital Health Technologies

Digital health platforms should empower individuals to manage their healthcare data, make better-informed decisions for themselves and their families, facilitate communication with their healthcare providers, and support public health response when needed. With home-use diagnostics, data may be generated and collected in disparate systems. For example, an individual may use one device to collect heart rate data, a separate device to check blood pressure, and a third device to monitor blood oxygenation. Platforms that aggregate these data are needed and will be central to the digital health connectivity of the future. Systems such as Apple Health are early entrants into this market, and others are being developed. These platforms must adhere to principles of patient accessibility, patient control, and patient empowerment (Layman 2020). The public would be best served with a choice of such platforms that compete for market share by providing the best services for the best value, yet they must provide data to a unified healthcare platform for advanced applications to be developed to provide personal guidance to patients.

To support such data aggregation, devices need to collect, store, and transmit diagnostic data in standard formats. This will enable the data generated by tests and devices of different manufacturers to be stored in a variety of personal health records. The standards must also allow exchange of information between an individual and other electronic health records, including public health systems. Such communications should be bidirectional, allowing a diabetic patient, for example, to share results of home blood glucose tests with their primary care physician, and allowing that same patient to obtain electronic copies of lab results residing in the physician's electronic medical record. Results of home COVID-19 tests sent to public health departments could help inform state and federal responses to a public health emergency. Health Level Seven International Version 2 (HL7v2) has been a tried and tested communications standard for decades, one that continues to evolve and adapt to meet new requirements such as remote diagnostics. The Fast Healthcare Interoperability Resource (FHIR) is an emerging communications standard compatible with HL7 that may be well suited for the mobile applications associated with remote diagnostics but requires wider adoption and development to reach its full potential.

Discussion Questions

1. How can government research and development institutions best design and implement programs to catalyze diagnostic innovation in the face of an infectious disease emergency?
2. What are some attributes of the RADx Tech program that provide lessons for future infectious disease outbreaks? What elements of RADx Tech could be improved?
3. Note some barriers to the development and deployment of POC and OTC tests during the COVID-19 pandemic. Consider issues in various domains, for example, scientific, technological, clinical, regulatory, and commercial. Propose an approach to overcoming one or more barriers in the future.
4. How might the proliferation and utilization of self-tests for at-home SARS-CoV-2 testing affect how we detect and diagnose other diseases, both infectious and noncommunicable, moving forward?

References

@NIHDirector. NIH RADx initiative for COVID-19. Twitter. 2020.

Apple, Google. Privacy-preserving contact tracing. 2022. https://covid19.apple.com/contacttracing. Accessed 1 Jun 2022.

Collins FS. Rising to the COVID-19 challenge: rapid acceleration of diagnostics (RADx). NIH Director's blog. Bethesda, MD: U.S. National Institutes of Health; 2020.

Creager RS, Blackwood J, Pribyl T, Bassit LC, Rao A, Greenleaf M, et al. RADx Variant Task Force program for assessing the impact of variants on SARS-CoV-2 molecular and antigen tests. IEEE Open J Eng Med Biol. 2021;2:286–90. https://doi.org/10.1109/OJEMB.2021.3116490.

Dempsey M, Tessier P, Collins J, Caro E. The RADx Tech deep dive and work package 1 process. IEEE Open J Eng Med Biol. 2021;2:131–7. https://doi.org/10.1109/ojemb.2021.3070827.

Eureka. About Eureka. San Francisco: Eureka; 2022. https://info.eurekaplatform.org/team/. Accessed 1 Jun 2022.

FDA. Clinical laboratory improvement amendments (CLIA). In: IVD regulatory assistance. Silver Spring, MD: U.S. Food and Drug Administration; 2021a. https://www.fda.gov/medical-devices/ivd--regulatory-assistance/clinical-laboratory--improvement-amendments-clia. Accessed 31 May 2022.

FDA. Policy for coronavirus disease-2019 tests during the public health emergency (revised): guidance for developers and Food and Drug Administration staff. Silver Spring, MD: U.S. Food and Drug Administration; 2021b.

FDA. In vitro diagnostics EUAs. Silver Spring, MD: U.S. Food and Drug Administration; 2022. https://www.fda.gov/medical-devices/coronavirus-disease--2019-covid-19-emergency-use-authorizations-medical-devices/in-vitro-diagnostics-euas. Accessed 1 Jun 2022.

Fink S. Maker of popular Covid test told factory to destroy inventory. New York Times. 2021.

Frediani JK, Levy JM, Rao A, Bassit L, Figueroa J, Vos MB, et al. Multidisciplinary assessment of the Abbott BinaxNOW SARS-CoV-2 point-of-care antigen test in the context of emerging viral variants and self-administration. Sci Rep. 2021;11(1):14604. https://doi.org/10.1038/s41598-021-94055-1.

GAO. Exposure notification: benefits and challenges of smartphone applications to augment contact tracing. Washington, DC: United States Government Accountability Office; 2021. Contract No.: GAO-21-104622.

Gibson L, Fahey N, Hafer N, Buchholz B, Dunlap D, Murphy R, et al. The RADx Tech clinical studies core: a model for academic based clinical studies. IEEE Open J Eng Med Biol. 2021;2:152–7. https://doi.org/10.1109/ojemb.2021.3070830.

Halabi S. Viral sovereignty, intellectual property, and the changing global system for sharing pathogens for infectious disease research. Ann Health Law. 2019;28:101.

HHS. Report to Congress: COVID-19 strategic testing plan. Washington, DC: U.S. Department of Health and Human Services; 2020.

Layman EJ. Ethical issues and the electronic health record. Health Care Manag (Frederick). 2020;39(4):150–61. https://doi.org/10.1097/hcm.0000000000000302.

Mishra T, Wang M, Metwally AA, Bogu GK, Brooks AW, Bahmani A, et al. Pre-symptomatic detection of COVID-19 from smartwatch data. Nat Biomed Eng. 2020;4(12):1208–20. https://doi.org/10.1038/s41551-020-00640-6.

NBA. Warriors to welcome fans back to Chase Center beginning April 23. New York: National Basketball Association; 2021.

Nehl EJ, Heilman SS, Ku D, Gottfried DS, Farmer S, Mannino R, et al. The RADx Tech test verification core and the ACME POCT in the evaluation of COVID-19 testing devices: a model for progress and change. IEEE Open J Eng Med Biol. 2021;2:142–51. https://doi.org/10.1109/OJEMB.2021.3070825.

NIBIB. NIH-funded COVID-19 testing initiative aims to safely return children to in-person school: new RADx-UP research effort combines testing and safety measures in underserved populations. Bethesda, MD: NIH; 2021.

NIH. RADx® Tech and ATP programs: phase 2 awards. Bethesda, MD: U.S. National Institutes of Health; 2022a. https://www.nibib.nih.gov/covid-19/radx--tech-program/radx-tech-phase2-awards. Accessed 31 May 2022.

NIH. RADx® Tech/ATP/ITAP dashboard. Bethesda, MD: U.S. National Institutes of Health; 2022b. https://www.nibib.nih.gov/covid-19/radx-tech--program/radx-tech-dashboard. Accessed 1 Jun 2022.

NIH. Rapid acceleration of diagnostics (RADX). 2022c. https://www.nih.gov/research-training/medical--research-initiatives/radx. Accessed 1 Sept 2022.

POCTRN. Independent test assessment program. Bethesda, MD: Point of Care Technology Research Network; 2022a. https://www.poctrn.org/itap. Accessed 31 May 2022.

POCTRN. Welcome to the Point of Care Technology Research Network. Bethesda, MD: Point of Care Technology Research Network; 2022b. https://www.poctrn.org/itap. Accessed 31 May 2022.

Radical solutions. Nat Biotechnol. 2021;39(4):391. https://doi.org/10.1038/s41587-021-00908-5.

Schachter SC, Parrish JA. RADx(SM) tech: a new paradigm for MedTech development overview of this special section. IEEE Open J Eng Med Biol. 2021;2:118. https://doi.org/10.1109/ojemb.2021.3070826.

Senate testimony on new tests for COVID-19. U.S. Senate Health, Education, Labor and Pensions Committee; 2020.

Tromberg BJ, Schwetz TA, Pérez-Stable EJ, Hodes RJ, Woychik RP, Bright RA, et al. Rapid scaling up of Covid-19 diagnostic testing in the United States: the NIH RADx initiative. N Engl J Med. 2020;383(11):1071. https://doi.org/10.1056/NEJMsr2022263.

Walsh B, Hosoi A, Kingsley M, Moreira S, Ramakrishnan S, Tessier P, et al. The RADx Tech deployment core: a model for academic/government based support of large-scale manufacturing and implementation of medical technologies. IEEE Open J Eng Med Biol. 2021;2:158–62. https://doi.org/10.1109/ojemb.2021.3070822.

When to test. Do I need to get tested? Boston: Consortia for Improving Medicine with Innovation & Technology; 2022. https://whentotest.org/. Accessed 6 Sep 2022.

WHO. WHO Director-General's opening remarks at first meeting of the Intergovernmental Negotiating Body to draft and negotiate a WHO convention, agreement or other international instrument on pandemic prevention, preparedness and response. Geneva: World Health Organization; 2022.

12 Vaccine Candidates for Novel Pathogens

Karin Bok

Contents

Learning Track Note: This chapter appears in Learning Tracks: Clinical Research; Preparedness

E. S. Higgs and R. A. Sorenson (eds.), *Principles and Practice of Emergency Research Response*,
https://doi.org/10.1007/978-3-031-48408-7_14

Learning Objectives

This chapter will help readers understand and describe:

- How advances in virology have helped inform initial medical countermeasure (MCM) development
- Why nucleic acid and viral vector vaccines are advantageous for responding to a public health emergency
- How preparedness facilitated success in COVID-19 emergency vaccine development; roles of basic virology, structure solving, and engineering in vaccine design
- Nine essential elements for MCM development
- Prototype approach to MCM development for preparedness against pathogen families and future unknown viral challenges

1 Introduction

Novel vaccine platform technologies and adjuvants have been explored and advanced in the last few decades to both tackle challenging viral diseases lacking prevention measures, such as respiratory syncytial virus (RSV) and Ebola (GSK 2020), and to improve on the performance of existing vaccines (*Varicella zoster*, i.e., chickenpox/shingles), which were developed using more traditional approaches (FDA 2017). Basic scientific breakthroughs in understanding fundamentals in virology, such as viral assembly and viral structure characterization, as well as delivery, such as nanoparticle design, atomic-level engineering, and formulation with innovative adjuvants, represent part of the progress toward improved humoral and cellular immune responses to the most advanced medical counter measure (MCM) candidates (Mascola and Fauci 2020). Additionally, advances in formulation and manufacturing technology have contributed to shortening the reaction time to an emergency outbreak and to developing safe, efficacious MCMs for rapid deployment in emergency situations, ideally with a one-dose schedule, rapid onset of immunity, and easily achievable cold chain requirements (Pardi et al. 2020). Nucleic acid and viral vector vaccines are especially advantageous platform choices to respond to an emergency since they trigger both antibody-mediated and cell-mediated immunity while having potential for simplified or standardized manufacturing at mass scale (Soleimanpour and Yaghoubi 2021).

This chapter will review the latest breakthroughs in vaccinology enabling highly efficacious MCMs, the evolution of novel genetic platform use during emergency outbreaks, and key roadblocks in the race to deploy countermeasures for timely impact against epidemics. and the groundbreaking designs and manufacturing technologies currently being implemented to combat SARS-CoV-2.

2 Novel Vaccine and Immune System Research Approaches Used in Previous Emergency Responses

2.1 2002 Severe Acute Respiratory Syndrome Coronavirus (SARS-CoV) Outbreak

Several SARS-CoV (or SARS-CoV-1) vaccine candidates were in development in 2002–2004 at the time of the first recent coronavirus outbreak. They included protein subunit, virus-like particle, DNA, viral vector, whole-inactivated, and live-attenuated vaccines (Li et al. 2020). A SARS-CoV vaccine (VRC-SRSDNA015-00-VP) produced with a DNA platform is one of the candidates that has been developed furthest to date; it was found to be safe, well tolerated, and immunogenic in healthy adults during early clinical testing (Martin et al. 2008). The design and development of a coronavirus vaccine using a fast genetic platform was the first attempt by scientists at the Vaccine Research Center (VRC), National Institute of Allergy and Infectious Diseases (NIAID), to respond to an emergency using an accelerated timeline. The VRC scientists encoded the gene for the full spike protein of SARS-CoV in a DNA platform vaccine candidate, which was shown to be immunogenic and efficacious in pre-clinical challenge studies in mice (Yang et al. 2004). Amid the international emergency response to SARS, the DNA platform offered a more advanced and rapid manufacturing option than more traditional cell-based manufacturing methods tested previously, but it still took approximately 20 months from the design decision and selection of the target sequence to the day of product administration in the first-in-human clinical study (Martin et al. 2008).

Although DNA vaccines have clear manufacturing advantages compared to traditional vaccine production technologies (Liu 2011), efficient delivery of sufficient DNA to the cell nucleus requires specialized immunization devices (e.g. Biojector 2000® Needle-Free Injection Management System™), and may necessitate much larger amounts of active material than other vaccine technologies. Typically doses in milligrams have been used in DNA vaccine clinical studies compared to dosing in the microgram range for protein-subunit and mRNA vaccines. In the end, VRC-SRSDNA015-00-VP was found to be immunogenic in most trial participants (21–49 years old), with varying levels of neutralizing antibodies and duration of immune response. The vaccine was not further developed or ever deployed because public health control measures had contained the outbreak by the time early clinical studies concluded. Nevertheless, the experience of responding to an emergent outbreak highlighted the need to incentivize preparedness activities, further improve manufacturing times, and address other gaps in the response plan (Anderson et al. 2004).

2.2 2014–2016 West African Ebola Outbreak

Ebola outbreaks with mortality rates up to 90% have been sporadically reported since the disease was first identified in 1976 (Lambe et al. 2017; WHO Ebola Response Team et al. 2014). On August 8, 2014, the World Health Organization (WHO) declared an Ebola Zaire outbreak in West Africa to be a Public Health Emergency of International Concern (PHEIC) for the first time since the identification of the virus (CDC 2021; WHO 2014). The outbreak had begun in December 2013 but was not identified as Ebola—which had not previously been seen in West Africa—until March 2014. The largest Ebola Zaire outbreak ever recorded, it launched an unprecedented international collaborative emergency research response that included developing vaccines and other MCMs to prevent disease, mitigate morbidity and mortality, and control transmission in affected countries. Two vaccine candidates were advanced to respond to the outbreak at the time: (a) a vesicular stomatitis virus-based, replication-competent prototype, rVSV-ZEBOV, and (b) a chimpanzee adenovirus-based nonreplicating vaccine ChAd3-EBO-Z, both aiming to deliver the intact Ebola Zaire surface glycoprotein (GP) intracellularly, using recombinant viral vectors as vehicles (De Santis et al. 2016; Henao-Restrepo et al. 2017; Kennedy et al. 2017). This strategy, reflecting the need for a rapid response, selected existing candidates that had accumulated enough preclinical evidence and early clinical data to be safely and quickly advanced to Phase I–II trials. The platform offered certain advantages for the containment of Ebola virus disease (EVD); for example, using viral vector vehicles for vaccines presented the opportunity to standardize and accelerate manufacturing of a known vector adaptable to insertion of genetic material based on other pathogens; the potential for one-dose regimen vaccines, a key characteristic for quick disease prevention through widespread vaccination and to minimize logistical challenges; lastly, they elicit both humoral and CD8+ T-cell immune responses, believed to be correlated with EVD protection based on experimental infection of vaccinated nonhuman primates (Sullivan et al. 2011). This was evident even though no viral vector-based vaccines had been licensed for humans at the time, making them a new class of product without accumulated real-world data.

Viral vector vehicles for vaccines presented the opportunity to standardize and accelerate manufacturing of a known vector adaptable to insertion of genetic material based on other pathogens.

A Phase II study (PREVAIL 1) was rapidly launched to generate initial safety and immunogenicity data in the target population of West Africa, which evaluated comparatively the two most promising candidates, rVSV-ZEBOV and ChAd3-EBO-Z (Kennedy et al. 2017). Both vaccines presented an acceptable safety profile and elicited immune responses that were largely maintained through 12 months. This trial highlighted the importance of gathering safety and immunogenicity data on the target population since endpoints varied among different African populations, effectively enabling the subsequent pivotal clinical study.

rVSV-ZEBOV was tested using a novel clinical trial design: a ring vaccination, cluster-randomized controlled trial conducted in Guinea and Sierra Leone, called *Ebola Ça Suffit!*, while the outbreak was still ongoing, and it was found to be highly efficacious at preventing disease (Henao-Restrepo et al. 2017). However, neither clinical trials, nor advancement to licensure, nor manufacturing was rapid enough to play a major role in containing the 2014–2016 outbreak. The vaccine was later deployed as an emergency countermeasure in a large Ebola outbreak in 2018–2020 in the Democratic Republic of the Congo (DRC) (WHO 2018b), before achieving commercial licensure by regulatory authorities in 2019, after the 2018 Ebola Zaire outbreak had been contained with the help of the vaccine and additional MCMs (EMA 2019; FDA 2019). As of June 2022, the vaccine (brand name Ervebo) was again deployed in the emergency response to contain a renewed outbreak in the northeastern DRC (IFRC 2021).

The progress of Ebola MCMs availability highlights some of the obstacles to timely containment of emergent infectious diseases with preventive or treatment measures, even with an accelerated research program and rapid manufacturing methods. Planning for preclinical and clinical research as an integral part of outbreak response would increase the odds that enough data could be gathered for licensure before an outbreak ends (NASEM 2017). In the case of Ebola Zaire, it took the re-emergence of the virus in subsequent outbreaks to advance MCMs to the final stage.

◘ Figure 1 illustrates two examples of different scenarios and key roadblocks when responding to emergency situations. The first example (◘ Fig. 1A, above the arrow) is the 2018–2020 epidemic of Ebola Zaire, that is, a previously known pathogen with MCMs on the shelf ready to be deployed. The candidate therapeutics still had to navigate several critical checkpoints (completing enrollment of timely Phase I trials and identification of a licensing partner willing to sponsor the product, among others) (Gaudinski et al. 2019; Newswire 2018; WHO 2018a), sometimes at risk of not being further advanced. Four candidates were eventually selected for an international collaborative clinical study, the PALM trial (*Pamoja Tulinde Maisha*, "Together Save Lives" in Swahili) (Mulangu et al. 2019).

The PALM trial concluded that two of four early-stage MCMs (REGN-EB3 and mAb114) were efficacious at reducing mortality from EVD, in comparison to the ZMapp control (Mulangu et al. 2019). Carefully reviewing and understanding previous emergency responses contributes to improved and thoughtful preparedness activities with higher chances of success in the next research response. It is clear from the Ebola emergency response that key factors such as global emergency response needs, capacity, and policy need to be balanced with national efforts to boost research and manufacturing capacity and promote innovation of vaccine candidates.

The study and approval pathway of mAb-114 (now branded Ebanga) contrasts with the accelerated timeline of another countermeasure designed by VRC scientists, mRNA-1273 (◘ Fig. 1B; below the arrow), deployed in response to a global pandemic. SARS-CoV-2 mRNA vaccines' rapid development, clinical trials, and emergency use authorization are detailed in other sections of this chapter and ► Chap. 15.

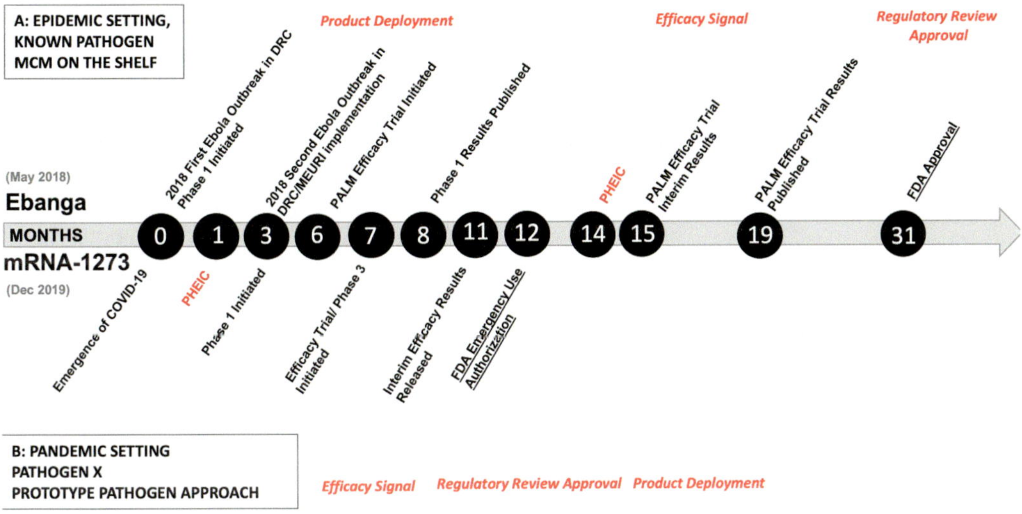

Fig. 1 A, B Highlights of critical events during emergency responses leading to the deployment and approval of medical countermeasures (MCMs) designed at the VRC. (Karin Bok)

3 The Importance of Preparedness and Innovation in Vaccine Design for Novel Pathogens

3.1 The Fundamental Role of Basic Virology, Structure Solving, and Engineering in Vaccine Design

One emergency response approach to novel pathogens is the rapid design and deployment of vaccine candidates chosen because they can be expeditiously produced using long-established vaccine technologies and made available at mass scale by utilizing established vaccine manufacturing capacity (Hotez and Bottazzi 2021). Advancing only vaccine platforms chosen in this way is not optimal for the design and development of potentially highly efficacious vaccines while also minimizing anticipated safety risks—especially important when moving quickly to population-scale deployment. A careful study of virus target proteins, informed by virology and immunology, along with deliberative, structure-based vaccine design approaches that incorporate understanding of host immunity, is essential to the success of new MCMs (McLellan et al. 2013; Nabel 2013).

A platform or manufacturing capacity-based approach may not yield MCMs with optimized efficacy and safety (WHO 2021). This has been the case with traditional-design SARS-CoV-2 inactivated vaccine candidates, which have been shown to have lower efficacy and effectiveness than more novel vaccine prototypes utilizing modern platforms and delivering antigens purposely designed to bypass viral mechanisms to evade the host immune system and elicit robust immune responses (Tregoning et al. 2021). Basic understanding of virus structure and self-assembly, the structure and function of the intended target proteins, and identification of vulnerable epitopes conserved across virus genera or families is foundational to preparing for the emergence of novel or variant pathogens (Corbett et al. 2020). This process yields high-quality proteins that are the cornerstone of promising vaccine design, effective treatments, and diagnostic tests and immunoassays (Graham 2020).

Confronted with SARS-CoV-2 as it spread around the globe, scientists acted on knowledge accumulated about related coronaviruses and the progress in protein manipulation gained by studying other, more or less distantly related viruses to design MCMs for response (Fig. 2). Indeed, the resources

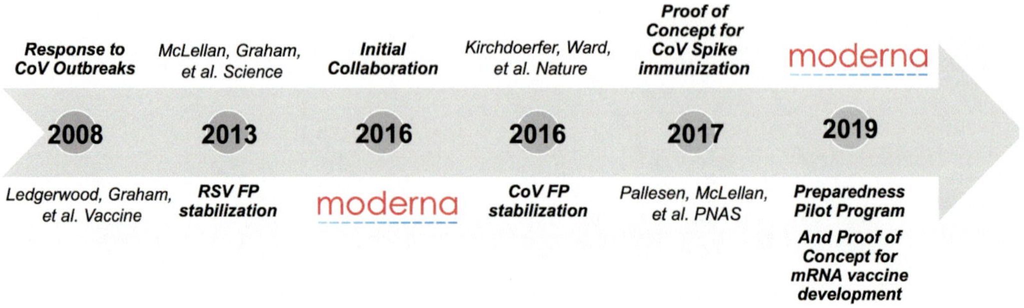

Fig. 2 Critical events in the preparedness stage leading to the success in the response to the COVID-19 emergency. (Karin Bok)

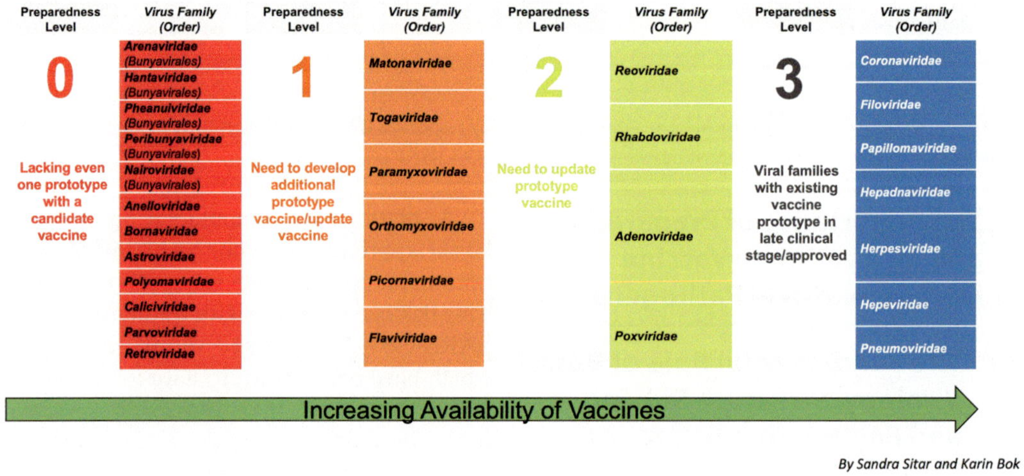

Fig. 3 Prototype pathogen approach to preparedness (virus families not prioritized). (Sandra Sitar and Karin Bok)

dedicated to another global epidemic, HIV/AIDS, benefited the whole field of virology and ushered in a new era of vaccinology (Vasan and Pitisuttithum 2021). The struggle to develop an efficacious HIV vaccine resulted in ancillary scientific advances central to the response to COVID-19. Focusing research resources on the detailed investigation and engineering of the structure of the HIV-1 envelope protein, for example, and the characterization of common potent broad neutralizing epitopes led to the first proof of concept for the prevention of HIV infection by a broadly neutralizing monoclonal antibody—decades after HIV was first identified (Corey et al. 2021). The investment and effort dedicated to HIV research also led to advances in vaccinology for other class I fusion proteins like RSV. The proof of concept of immunization with a pre-stabilized fusion protein validating this strategy was a breakthrough in vaccine design (Crank et al. 2019).

Figure 2 illustrates that success in the design of highly efficacious SARS-CoV-2 vaccines is due in part to more than a decade studying and understanding alternative approaches to countering related infectious pathogens, and to attempting MCM development against a *Coronaviridae* family prototype (SARS-CoV-1 and MERS-CoV). We were more prepared for the emergence of a new coronavirus than we would have been for the emergence of a virus from another viral family for which we have not yet accumulated enough understanding to rapidly advance to clinical testing (Fig. 3). Thus, our post-coronavirus pandemic preparedness strategy should focus on coordinating global resources to address the knowledge gaps in virus families with the potential to infect humans (◘ Fig. 3) and developing vaccine prototypes against known threats. These prototypes would then be ready for late-stage clinical testing, and the knowledge of virus structure and target proteins would leave us better prepared for the emergence of currently unknown viruses. U.S. government scientists have proposed a model Prototype Pathogen Preparedness Plan (P4) to maximize preparedness by accumulating knowledge on less studied pathogen families and eventually transitioning strategies developed through targeting known virus families to unknown challenges; this concept has been incorporated into current U.S. government preparedness planning (Cassetti et al. 2022; Graham and Sullivan 2018; NIAID 2021; White House 2021).

3.2 Preparedness Strategies and the Prototype Pathogen Approach

The initial emergence or re-emergence of viral infectious diseases and their global reach depends on the biology of the virus (respiratory diseases are much more likely to spread rapidly and more difficult to contain), availability of animal or human reservoir, possibility of zoonotic or vector-borne transmission, and serostatus of the affected populations, among other factors. Ideally, scientists can rely on basic virology and immunology, established and well-tested vaccinology approaches, and early-stage clinical development of medical countermeasures to aid in accelerating the response to emerging pathogens (Bok et al. 2021). Translational science (turning observations in the laboratory, clinic, and community into interventions that improve health) starts with successively improving versions of a vaccine prototype being tested for safety, immunogenicity, and efficacy in animal model challenge experiments, with either the target virus or an adapted version (Pallesen et al. 2017). An iterative process of improving vaccine prototypes begins with design proposals and advances through pre-clinical testing, process development, pilot manufacturing, and regulatory strategy, building toward the stages of clinical testing, emergency authorization or licensing, and deployment in an expedited response (◘ Fig. 4). This kind of process is also essential for generating reagents, optimizing immune assays, and

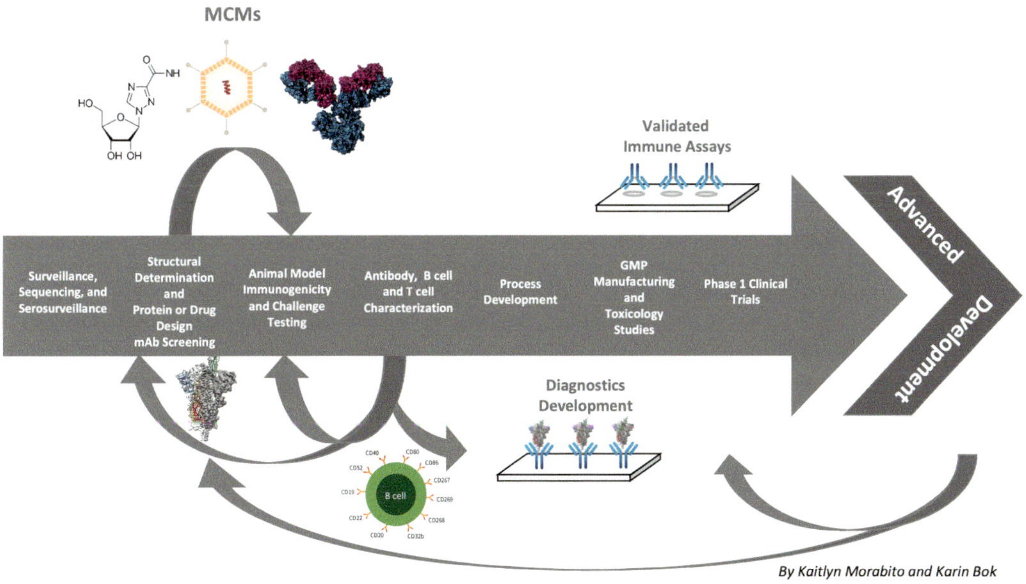

◘ **Fig. 4** Prototype pathogen approach to MCM development for preparedness. (Kaitlyn Morabito and Karin Bok)

Vaccine Characteristic	Minimal Attribute	Preferred Attribute
Indication	For prevention of severe disease	For prevention of infection and symptomatic disease
Targets (Breadth)	Circulating target pathogen	Target pathogen; variant-proof
Efficacy	~70% efficacy across all targets	>90% efficacy across all targets
Safety	Vaccine benefits outweigh safety risks (i.e. extremely rare SAEs associated with vaccination)	Highly favorable benefit/risk profile (i.e. only mild, transient adverse events related to vaccination)
Dose Regimen	No more than 2 doses in primary series	Single-dose primary series
Desired Immunity	Systemic, humoral immunity	Systemic and mucosal, humoral and cellular immunity (depending on pathogen)
Durability of Immune Response	>9 months from primary series	>12 months from primary series
Manufacturing	Process development, release, and scale up under 12 months	Process development, release, and scale up under 6 months
Storage	Stable at −18 °C	Temperature stable, only refrigeration required

Fig. 5 Target product profile of ideal emergency response vaccine. (Adapted with permission from Kevin Carlton)

establishing animal models and other pathogen-specific tools needed for the development of candidate MCMs (Corbett et al. 2020; Monrad et al. 2021).

In the launch of a new MCM development program, the ideal candidates incorporate critical, innovative safety and immunogenicity features into their designs, with attributes clearly delineated on a thoughtful target product profile (Fig. 5). In addition, the development strategy must consider how to adapt new technology to manufacturing, formulation, and delivery, and eventually scaling up to commercial manufacturing and mass delivery and administration. The prototype countermeasure would preferably be advanced to at least early clinical testing for safety and indications of immunogenicity; pilot-scale, clinical-grade material would be stored on the shelf ready to be further advanced (CEPI 2021).

This is the optimal preparedness scenario for the emergence of a virus previously identified as having pandemic potential, such as Ebola, Nipah, or enterovirus D68 viruses. On the other hand, when preparing to respond to unknown pathogens with pandemic potential, such as novel viruses transmitted through zoonotic events or arthropod vectors, or when responding to viruses with little accumulated scientific knowledge, our best approach is to rely on a prototype pathogen preparedness method (Graham and Sullivan 2018). Just as the design of MCMs against SARS-CoV-2 was based on previous information obtained by studying other members of the family *Coronaviridae*, such as SARS-CoV and MERS-CoV, the knowledge accumulated while developing a prototype against another virus family could be transitioned into the development of MCMs against related viruses in the same family or group (Corbett et al. 2020).

There are about 30 virus families known to infect humans, and they could be classified into preparedness levels (Fig. 3) based on key criteria, such as availability of any MCM or early-stage prototype, transmission route, and zoonotic reservoirs, among others. Figure 3 is not meant to classify virus families by priority for MCM development, but rather to summarize the state of knowledge for each family and provide an overall understanding of which families are the least studied to date in terms of vaccine development. The P4 plan main objective is to select at least 30 viruses, classified in order of urgency and priority, including at least one from each family, and develop new or technologically more advanced (for families with existing countermeasures which require updating) prevention, treatment, and diagnostic tools. These would then be ready to enter clinical trials or deploy in an emergency, or be quickly adapted to design, develop, and deploy countermeasures against related emerging pathogens. This is a commonsense approach that attempts to best utilize restricted resources (funding and scientific discovery/development capacity) to be maximally prepared for eventual outbreaks or pandemics caused by known or as yet unknown threats (Pathogen X).

Discussion Questions

1. List the breakthroughs in virology that have helped improve the immune response to advanced MCM candidates.
2. Discuss the reasons why nucleic acid and viral vector vaccines are especially advantageous for responding to an emergency viral epidemic.
3. Broadly, compare and discuss two examples of different scenarios and key roadblocks when responding to emergency situations. (Hint: refer to Fig. 1.)
4. Discuss the critical events in the preparedness stage leading to the success in the response to the COVID-19 emergency, emphasizing the role of basic virology, structure solving, and engineering in vaccine design.
5. List nine essential elements for MCM development.
6. After the design of highly efficacious SARS-CoV-2 vaccines, we were more prepared for the emergence of a new coronavirus than for the emergence of a virus from another viral family for which we have not yet accumulated enough understanding to rapidly advance to clinical testing. Describe a prototype approach to MCM development for preparedness against less studied pathogen families and future unknown viral challenges.

References

Anderson RM, Fraser C, Ghani AC, Donnelly CA, Riley S, Ferguson NM, et al. Epidemiology, transmission dynamics and control of SARS: the 2002–2003 epidemic. Philos Trans R Soc Lond Ser B Biol Sci. 2004;359(1447):1091–105. https://doi.org/10.1098/rstb.2004.1490.

Bok K, Sitar S, Graham BS, Mascola JR. Accelerated COVID-19 vaccine development: milestones, lessons, and prospects. Immunity. 2021;54(8):1636–51. https://doi.org/10.1016/j.immuni.2021.07.017.

Cassetti MC, Pierson TC, Patterson LJ, Bok K, DeRocco AJ, Deschamps AM, et al. Prototype pathogen approach for vaccine and monoclonal antibody development: a critical component of the NIAID Plan for pandemic preparedness. J Infect Dis. 2022;227:1433. https://doi.org/10.1093/infdis/jiac296.

CDC. History of Ebola virus disease (EVD) outbreaks. Atlanta, GA: U.S. Centers for Disease Control and Prevention; 2021. https://www.cdc.gov/vhf/ebola/history/chronology.html. Accessed 17 Oct 2021.

CEPI. The urgency of now: turning the tide against epidemic and pandemic infectious diseases. CEPI; 2021.

Corbett KS, Edwards DK, Leist SR, Abiona OM, Boyoglu-Barnum S, Gillespie RA, et al. SARS-CoV-2 mRNA vaccine design enabled by prototype pathogen preparedness. Nature. 2020;586(7830):567–71. https://doi.org/10.1038/s41586-020-2622-0.

Corey L, Gilbert PB, Juraska M, Montefiori DC, Morris L, Karuna ST, et al. Two randomized trials of neutralizing antibodies to prevent HIV-1 acquisition. N Engl J Med. 2021;384(11):1003–14. https://doi.org/10.1056/NEJMoa2031738.

Crank MC, Ruckwardt TJ, Chen M, Morabito KM, Phung E, Costner PJ, et al. A proof of concept for structure-based vaccine design targeting RSV in humans. Science. 2019;365(6452):505–9. https://doi.org/10.1126/science.aav9033.

De Santis O, Audran R, Pothin E, Warpelin-Decrausaz L, Vallotton L, Wuerzner G, et al. Safety and immunogenicity of a chimpanzee adenovirus-vectored Ebola vaccine in healthy adults: a randomised, double-blind, placebo-controlled, dose-finding, phase 1/2a study. Lancet Infect Dis. 2016;16(3):311–20. https://doi.org/10.1016/S1473-3099(15)00486-7.

EMA. First vaccine to protect against Ebola. EMA; 2019.

FDA. SHINGRIX. Silver Spring, MD: U.S. Food and Drug Adminisration; 2017. https://www.fda.gov/vaccines-blood-biologics/vaccines/shingrix. Accessed 21 Oct 2021.

FDA. ERVEBO. 2019. https://www.fda.gov/vaccines-blood-biologics/ervebo. Accessed 17 Oct 2021.

Gaudinski MR, Coates EE, Novik L, Widge A, Houser KV, Burch E, et al. Safety, tolerability, pharmacokinetics, and immunogenicity of the therapeutic monoclonal antibody mAb114 targeting Ebola virus glycoprotein (VRC 608): an open-label phase 1 study. Lancet. 2019;393(10174):889–98. https://doi.org/10.1016/S0140-6736(19)30036-4.

Graham BS. Rapid COVID-19 vaccine development. Science. 2020;368(6494):945–6. https://doi.org/10.1126/science.abb8923.

Graham BS, Sullivan NJ. Emerging viral diseases from a vaccinology perspective: preparing for the next pandemic. Nat Immunol. 2018;19(1):20–8. https://doi.org/10.1038/s41590-017-0007-9.

GSK. A phase III double-blind study to assess safety and efficacy of an RSV maternal unadjuvanted vaccine, in pregnant women and infants born to vaccinated mothers (GRACE). Bethesda, MD: National Library of Medicine; 2020. https://clinicaltrials.gov/ct2/show/NCT04605159. Accessed 21 Oct 2021.

Henao-Restrepo AM, Camacho A, Longini IM, Watson CH, Edmunds WJ, Egger M, et al. Efficacy and effectiveness of an rVSV-vectored vaccine in preventing Ebola virus disease: final results from the Guinea ring vaccination, open-label, cluster-randomised trial (Ebola Ca Suffit!). Lancet. 2017;389(10068):505–18. https://doi.org/10.1016/S0140-6736(16)32621-6.

Hotez PJ, Bottazzi ME. Whole inactivated virus and protein-based COVID-19 vaccines. Annu Rev Med. 2021;73:55. https://doi.org/10.1146/annurev-med-042420-113212.

IFRC. Emergency plan of action (EPoA) DRC: Ebola virus disease outbreak. Geneva: International Federation of Red Cross and Red Crescent Societies; 2021. p. 18.

Kennedy SB, Bolay F, Kieh M, Grandits G, Badio M, Ballou R, et al. Phase 2 placebo-controlled trial of two vaccines to prevent Ebola in Liberia. N Engl J Med. 2017;377(15):1438–47. https://doi.org/10.1056/NEJMoa1614067.

Lambe T, Bowyer G, Ewer KJ. A review of phase I trials of Ebola virus vaccines: what can we learn from the race to develop novel vaccines? Philos Trans R Soc Lond Ser B Biol Sci. 2017;372(1721):20160295. https://doi.org/10.1098/rstb.2016.0295.

Li YD, Chi WY, Su JH, Ferrall L, Hung CF, Wu TC. Coronavirus vaccine development: from SARS and MERS to COVID-19. J Biomed Sci. 2020;27(1):104. https://doi.org/10.1186/s12929-020-00695-2.

Liu MA. DNA vaccines: an historical perspective and view to the future. Immunol Rev. 2011;239(1):62–84. https://doi.org/10.1111/j.1600-065X.2010.00980.x.

Martin JE, Louder MK, Holman LA, Gordon IJ, Enama ME, Larkin BD, et al. A SARS DNA vaccine induces neutralizing antibody and cellular immune responses in healthy adults in a phase I clinical trial. Vaccine. 2008;26(50):6338–43. https://doi.org/10.1016/j.vaccine.2008.09.026.

Mascola JR, Fauci AS. Novel vaccine technologies for the 21st century. Nat Rev Immunol. 2020;20(2):87–8. https://doi.org/10.1038/s41577-019-0243-3.

McLellan JS, Chen M, Joyce MG, Sastry M, Stewart-Jones GB, Yang Y, et al. Structure-based design of a fusion glycoprotein vaccine for respiratory syncytial virus. Science. 2013;342(6158):592–8. https://doi.org/10.1126/science.1243283.

Monrad JT, Sandbrink JB, Cherian NG. Promoting versatile vaccine development for emerging pandemics. npj Vaccines. 2021;6(1):26. https://doi.org/10.1038/s41541-021-00290-y.

Mulangu S, Dodd LE, Davey RT Jr, Tshiani Mbaya O, Proschan M, Mukadi D, et al. A randomized, controlled trial of Ebola virus disease therapeutics. N Engl J Med. 2019;381(24):2293–303. https://doi.org/10.1056/NEJMoa1910993.

Nabel GJ. Designing tomorrow's vaccines. N Engl J Med. 2013;368(6):551–60. https://doi.org/10.1056/NEJMra1204186.

NASEM. Integrating clinical research into epidemic response: the Ebola experience. Washington, DC: National Academies of Sciences Engineering and Medicine Publications, The National Academies Press; 2017.

Newswire P. Ridgeback Biotherapeutics LP announces licensing of mAb114, an experimental Ebola treatment, from the National Institute of Allergy and Infectious Diseases. 2018. https://www.prnewswire.com/news-releases/ridgeback-biotherapeutics-lp-announces-licensing-of-mab114-an-experimental-ebola-treatment-from-the-national-institute-of-allergy-and-infectious-diseases-300765146.html.

NIAID. Antiviral program for pandemics. 2021. https://www.niaid.nih.gov/research/antivirals. Accessed 27 Jul 2021.

Pallesen J, Wang N, Corbett KS, Wrapp D, Kirchdoerfer RN, Turner HL, et al. Immunogenicity and structures of a rationally designed prefusion MERS-CoV spike antigen. Proc Natl Acad Sci USA. 2017;114(35):E7348–57. https://doi.org/10.1073/pnas.1707304114.

Pardi N, Hogan MJ, Weissman D. Recent advances in mRNA vaccine technology. Curr Opin Immunol. 2020;65:14–20. https://doi.org/10.1016/j.coi.2020.01.008.

Soleimanpour S, Yaghoubi A. COVID-19 vaccine: where are we now and where should we go? Expert Rev Vaccines. 2021;20(1):23–44. https://doi.org/10.1080/14760584.2021.1875824.

Sullivan NJ, Hensley L, Asiedu C, Geisbert TW, Stanley D, Johnson J, et al. CD8+ cellular immunity mediates rAd5 vaccine protection against Ebola virus infection of nonhuman primates. Nat Med. 2011;17(9):1128–31. https://doi.org/10.1038/nm.2447.

Tregoning JS, Flight KE, Higham SL, Wang Z, Pierce BF. Progress of the COVID-19 vaccine effort: viruses, vaccines and variants versus efficacy, effectiveness and escape. Nat Rev Immunol. 2021;21:626. https://doi.org/10.1038/s41577-021-00592-1.

Vasan S, Pitisuttithum P. Vaccine development lessons between HIV and COVID-19. Lancet Infect Dis. 2021;21(6):759–61. https://doi.org/10.1016/S1473-3099(21)00274-7.

White House. American pandemic preparedness: transforming our capabilities. Washington, DC: White House; 2021.

WHO. Statement on the 1st meeting of the IHR Emergency Committee on the 2014 Ebola outbreak in West Africa. Geneva: World Health Organization; 2014.

WHO. Notes for the record: Consultation on monitored emergency use of unregistered and investigational interventions (MEURI) for Ebola virus disease (EVD). Geneva: World Health Organization; 2018a. p. 6.

WHO. WHO supports Ebola vaccination of high risk populations in the Democratic Republic of the Congo. 2018b. https://www.who.int/news/item/21-05-2018-who-supports-ebola-vaccination-of-high-risk-populations-in-the-democratic-republic-of-the-congo.

WHO. Interim recommendations for use of the inactivated COVID-19 vaccine, CoronaVac, developed by Sinovac. 2021. Contract No.: WHO reference number: WHO/2019-nCoV/vaccines/SAGE_recommendation/Sinovac-CoronaVac/2021.1.

WHO Ebola Response Team, Aylward B, Barboza P, Bawo L, Bertherat E, Bilivogui P, et al. Ebola virus disease in West Africa—the first 9 months of the epidemic and forward projections. N Engl J Med. 2014;371(16):1481–95. https://doi.org/10.1056/NEJMoa1411100.

Yang ZY, Kong WP, Huang Y, Roberts A, Murphy BR, Subbarao K, et al. A DNA vaccine induces SARS coronavirus neutralization and protective immunity in mice. Nature. 2004;428(6982):561–4. https://doi.org/10.1038/nature02463.

12.1 In Focus: Novel Manufacturing Platforms for Pandemic Preparedness and Emergency Response

Karin Bok

Contents

Learning Track Note: This chapter appears in Learning Tracks: Clinical Research; Preparedness

E. S. Higgs and R. A. Sorenson (eds.), *Principles and Practice of Emergency Research Response*,
https://doi.org/10.1007/978-3-031-48408-7_15

Learning Objectives

This chapter will help readers understand and describe:

- The development of viral vectors as candidates for antigen delivery
- How vaccine delivery using an mRNA technology platform was advanced to overcome key roadblocks related to its stability, translation efficiency, activation of the innate immune response, and delivery of the intact mRNA molecule
- Novel vaccine designs and manufacturing platforms advanced during the COVID-19 pandemic
- The advantages of the mRNA platform
- The circumstances in which the mRNA platform may not be the ideal choice and mRNA research questions that are still being investigated

1 Overview of Genetic Platforms

Novel manufacturing platforms for vaccine design have emerged in the past few decades to meet the challenge posed by infectious diseases that have been difficult to prevent or foresee, and to aid in the rapid response to emerging pathogens. Gene-based platforms (mRNA, DNA, or vector based) are excellent tools for delivery of a well-designed vaccine antigen, which will induce potent humoral and cellular immune responses while avoiding vaccine-associated safety concerns observed with some pathogens such as dengue or respiratory syncytial virus (RSV) (Graham 2020). mRNA-based vaccines can induce both humoral and cellular immunity but may avoid some of the limitations of vector-based platforms, such as anti-vector immunity, or potential risks associated with DNA vaccines like integration into the host cell genome. The manufacture of vector-based vaccines is also easily standardized and scaled up, and this platform is amenable to one-dose vaccine schedules.

1.1 Viral Vectors

Research using recombinant vaccinia viruses as vaccine delivery vehicles for inserted genetic sequences from target viruses (e.g., hepatitis B) ushered in a new era of vaccinology in the mid-1980s (Moss et al. 1984). Many viral vectors have been explored as candidates for gene therapy, cancer treatment, and vaccines (Ramezanpour et al. 2016). Viral vectors were the first vaccine platform technology pursued by scientists and manufacturers, mainly to overcome the challenges of growing wild-type or attenuated viruses to produce inactivated or live-attenuated vaccines, respectively (Ulmer et al. 2006), and to take advantage of stimulating CD8+ T-cell and antibody responses, which might result in efficacious vaccines against challenging diseases lacking prevention measures.

The only viral-vector-based vaccine approved by the U.S. Food and Drug Administration (FDA) is a recombinant live-attenuated replication competent vesicular stomatitis virus (VSV)-based Ebola vaccine, Ervebo (FDA 2019). VSV is an enveloped bullet-shaped virus from the rhabdovirus family with an 11-kb negative-sense RNA genome (Fields et al. 2007). VSV-based vaccines induce robust cellular and humoral immunity against the antigen of interest and grow to high titers in cell lines validated for manufacturing (e.g., Vero cells). Because of its RNA genome, it also lacks a DNA intermediate during viral replication, which might improve its overall safety profile (Humphreys and Sebastian 2018). Replicating viral vector vaccines also have the ability to reach beyond the site of inoculation to other organs or tissues, where resident immunity might improve protection against disease. However, precisely because VSV-based vaccines replicate in this way, certain localized rare adverse events have been described, which are not found in platforms using replication-deficient virus vectors (Agnandji et al. 2016).

Adenovirus vectors are a replication-deficient platform and one of the most stud-

PLATFORM	SPONSOR	VACCINE PLATFORM	TARGET PROTEIN	DOSING REGIMEN	CURRENT STATUS
Nucleic Acid	Pfizer / BioNTech	mRNA	•Prefusion stabilized (S-2P) •Transmembrane anchored full length spike protein	2 doses / 21 days apart	Licensed by FDA
	Moderna	mRNA	•Prefusion stabilized (S-2P) •Transmembrane anchored full length spike protein	2 doses / 28 days apart	Licensed by FDA
Viral Vector	AstraZeneca / Oxford	Chimpanzee Adenovirus Vector	•Transmembrane anchored spike protein	2 doses / 28 days apart	Phase III
	Janssen	Human Adenovirus Vector (26)	•Prefusion stabilized (S-2P) •Transmembrane anchored full length spike protein	1 dose	EUA

Fig. 1 Genetic platform vaccines supported by USG in response to the SARS-CoV-2 pandemic (Karin Bok)

ied clinically (Ramezanpour et al. 2016), with many different serotypes having been explored as candidate platforms for vaccines against infectious diseases. Adenoviruses are nonenveloped icosahedral viruses with 30–40 kb linear DNA genomes. The antigen of interest is most often inserted to replace the adenovirus envelope (E1) gene, rendering the virus replication deficient. Adenovirus vectors can accommodate genetic inserts of up to 7 kb (Fields et al. 2007). The advance of adenoviruses as vaccine vectors has relied on two major improvements: circumventing human seroprevalence against certain adenovirus types (Mennechet et al. 2019) and enhancing vaccine-specific immunogenicity (Morris et al. 2016). Relying on less prevalent human adenovirus genotypes or using adenoviruses of nonhuman origin (chimpanzee and gorilla) has helped overcome preexisting immunity against the adenovirus vector in humans, in which those seropositive for the adenovirus vector being used have lower neutralizing antibody titers and a reduction in antigen-specific immunogenicity in clinical trials (Pine et al. 2011). Moreover, different adenovirus serotypes, regardless of seroprevalence levels, were shown to induce varying immunogenicity profiles, including differences in resulting antibody titer, phenotype, function, and duration of cellular immune response (Tan et al. 2013). Interestingly, research has shown that a robust and durable CD8+ T-cell immune response after adenovirus-based vaccination is directly correlated with higher levels of antigen expression detected over longer periods of time. Such studies provide useful criteria for selecting available human and simian adenovirus serotypes for vaccine applications, based not only on seroprevalence data and the efficiency of growing the vector to high in vitro titers, but also on the potency of the virus vector and its ability to induce appropriate levels of immunity (Quinn et al. 2015). Although adenovirus type 5 had been initially proposed as a potent vaccine vehicle, and therefore advanced to large clinical trials, it has since been replaced by serotypes with less seroprevalence in the human population (Mennechet et al. 2019). Some studies have described adenovirus type 3 of chimpanzee origin (ChAd3) as a comparable potent adenovirus vector for vaccine delivery (Quinn et al. 2015; Stanley et al. 2014). Given the extensive history of testing adenoviruses as vehicles for vaccine delivery and the possibility of utilizing one-dose schedules, which are extremely advantageous for immunizing an entire population in record time, it was not surprising that the U.S. government response to the pandemic included two candidates that utilized adenovirus vectors in their design (Fig. 1).

1.2 mRNA and DNA

Although both DNA and RNA proof-of-concept transfection (inserting RNA or DNA into cells) and translation experiments were published concomitantly, initially DNA immunization was advanced more rapidly, given the concerns about whether mRNA molecules had the stability needed to deliver

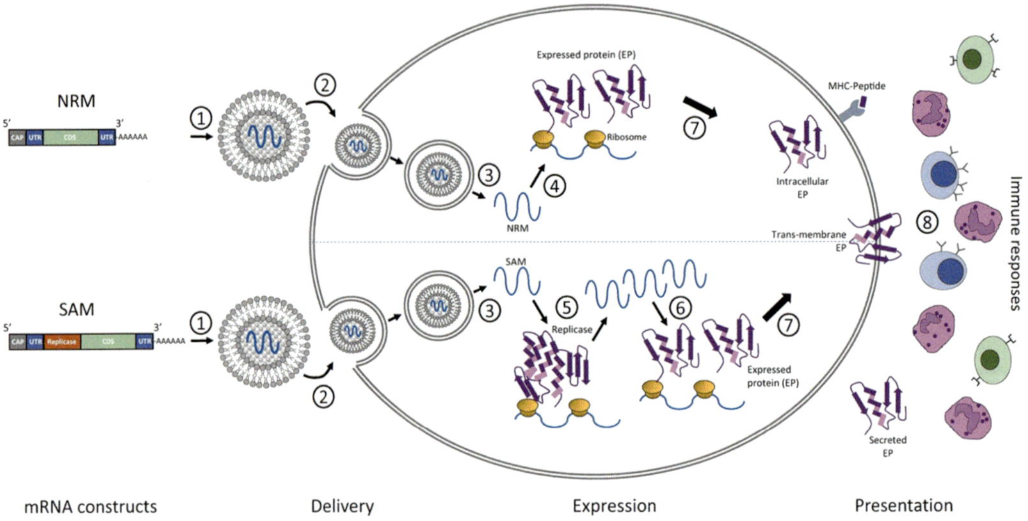

Fig. 2 Two types of mRNA constructs, nonreplicating mRNA (NRM) and self-amplifying mRNA (SAM) (Jackson et al. 2020)

immunogens (Tombácz et al. 2021; Wolff et al. 1990).

The possibility of simplified, synthetic manufacturing combined with the stimulation of cytotoxic T-lymphocytes was the rationale for advancing the DNA platform, promising accelerated timelines for responding to emergencies with more sophisticated immunogens. The most appealing characteristics of this new class of vaccines were their ability to induce humoral, CD4+, and CD8+ T cells, as well as innate immune responses, while avoiding drawbacks from other classes of platform vaccines, such as immunity to the delivery vector or some of the safety concerns that have been described for vector vaccines (Iavarone et al. 2017). The DNA platform has been proposed as a vaccine candidate against numerous infectious disease targets, some have advanced to late clinical testing, and several have been licensed for veterinary use (Kutzler and Weiner 2008). However, the DNA platform has not yet been licensed for use in humans by U.S. or European regulatory authorities and is not currently being deployed to combat the SARS-CoV-2 pandemic globally (WHO 2021b).

By contrast, two types of mRNA technologies are being studied and advanced to prevent infectious diseases: (a) nonreplicating and (b) self-amplifying mRNA platforms (Fig. 2) (Jackson et al. 2020; Liu 2019). mRNA constitutes the smallest vector able to deliver the gene of interest destined to be translated in the cytosol and presented to the immune response by antigen presenting cells. The design of the mRNA molecule typically includes untranslated 5′ and 3′ regions (UTRs), an open-reading frame encoding the vaccine target to be translated, a 5′ cap and a poly(A) tail. Self-amplifying versions of mRNA also incorporate an RNA-dependent polymerase that enables intracellular RNA replication and increased expression of the protein of interest (Pardi et al. 2018).

Over the three decades following the first successful attempt at a transfection experiment, vaccine delivery using mRNA technology was advanced to overcome key roadblocks related to its stability, translation efficiency, activation of the innate immune response, and delivery of the intact mRNA molecule. Several modifications were found to be advantageous and to promote increasing levels of protein production. The addition of synthetic caps, poly(A) tails, and 5′ and 3′ UTRs stabilize the mRNA molecule, while nucleoside modifications alter the inflammatory profile of synthetic mRNA (Kariko et al. 2005). The degree to which vaccines delivered via mRNA stimulate the innate immune response must be carefully considered: mRNA vaccines can be

Infectious Disease	Sponsor	Name	Target	Dose and Schedule	Status	Study ID
CMV	Moderna	mRNA-1647	Pentameric Complex/Glycoprotein B	50mg,100mg,150mg; day 1, day 56 and day 168	Phase II	NCT04232280
Zika	Moderna	mRNA-1893	Pr, M, E	2X 30mg or 100 mg; 28 days apart	Phase II	NCT04917861
Influenza	Moderna	mRNA-1010	influenza A H1N1, H3N2 and influenza B Yamagata and Victoria	TBD; single dose	Phase I-II	NCT04956575
Influenza	Sanofi	SP0273	A/H3N2 strain	TBD; single dose	Phase I-II	TBA
SARS-CoV-2	Moderna	mRNA-1273	Spike (Pre-stabilized)	2X 100mg; 28 days apart	EUA approved	NCT04470427
SARS-CoV-2	Moderna	mRNA-1273.211	Spike (Pre-stabilized)	2X 100mg; 28 days apart	Phase II-III	NCT04927065
SARS-CoV-2	Pfizer-Biointech	BNT162b2	Spike (Pre-stabilized)	2X 30mg; 21 days apart	BLA Licensed	NCT04368728
SARS-CoV-2	Pfizer-Biointech	BNT162b2 B.1.351	Spike (Pre-stabilized)	2X 30mg; 21 days apart	Phase II-III	NCT0471355 3
SARS-CoV-2	Curevac	CVnCoV	Spike	2X 12mg; 28 days apart	Phase III	NCT04674189

Fig. 3 mRNA vaccines in advanced clinical stage or approved for infectious diseases (author)

self-adjuvanted, in effect, by enabling the engagement of pattern recognition receptors or inducing a robust type I interferon response and promoting the expansion of CD8+ T cells (Pardi et al. 2020). However, they are also capable of triggering innate antiviral responses and pro-inflammatory signals that may lead to excess degradation of the RNA molecule or increased local or systemic reactogenicity. Modifying the signature nucleotide of the RNA molecule by replacing the original uridine with a functional but less reactive pseudouridine moderates the innate immune response to the mRNA delivery and optimizes the translation levels of the target protein (Maruggi et al. 2019). Codon usage also affects the efficiency of translation. Common modifications include replacing rare codons from the virus with more abundant synonymous ones and enriching the guanine–cytosine content of the sequence. This modification will enhance translation but might result in drawbacks, such as the formation of undesirable tertiary structures that should be evaluated in the design phase of the final vaccine sequence. The final mRNA molecule should also be carefully purified to eliminate undesirable side products of the in vitro transcription reaction, especially double-stranded RNA, which has a powerful pathogen-associated molecular pattern and will evoke a robust antiviral response, upregulating molecules that will interfere with adequate translation and promoting the degradation of mRNA (Rosa et al. 2021).

One major obstacle to advancing mRNA technology into the pharmaceutical space has been the unavailability of efficient delivery methods. RNA is a large, highly negatively charged molecule with little chance of penetrating a cell membrane with negative potential by itself (Kowalzik et al. 2021). Several methods have been proposed to overcome this obstacle (many derived from the well-studied small interfering RNA technology field), and lipid nanoparticles (LNPs) have become the most commonly used method to deliver mRNA into the cytoplasm (Hou et al. 2021; Kowalski et al. 2019).

Once the technology had been optimized, mRNA vaccine candidates showed that they could elicit robust humoral and cellular immune responses with low doses and schedules comparable to traditional protein-based vaccines (Corbett et al. 2020b; Vogel et al. 2021). Several mRNA vaccines against infectious diseases are in advanced clinical testing or have been approved for combating the SARS-CoV-2 pandemic (Figs. 1 and 3). Commercial manufacturers have demonstrated that the cell-free in vitro transcription process is efficient, fast, and easily scalable, making mRNA vaccine platforms extremely suitable and adaptable to respond to emergencies (Pfizer 2020).

Formulation of the final mRNA candidates is an area of continuing progress. Buffers and other additives have been tested in order to improve the stability and storage conditions of the final product, which has required shipment and storage at −70° C, complicating distribution, especially in remote areas without access to the necessary equipment (FDA 2021). Currently mRNA vaccines are stored at regular freezing temperatures, or even 4 °C for short-term storage, and some candidate vaccines are already being tested with lyophilized formulations, which can easily be transported and stored for increasing periods of time (Moderna 2021).

2 Novel Vaccine Designs and Manufacturing Platforms Advanced During the COVID-19 Pandemic

The vaccine candidates utilizing rapid and adaptable platforms and supported by the U.S. government to prevent COVID-19 are summarized in ◘ Fig. 1. While adjuvanted, protein-based vaccines have been licensed and approved for use against other viral pathogens, and SARS-CoV-2 vaccines using this technology are likely to complete the development phase, the U.S. government also supported two novel genetic programmable platforms that could potentially be manufactured in large quantities in a much shorter period, accelerating not only the potential start of large clinical trials, but also allowing manufacturing scale-up to meet the demands of the U.S. and global populations relatively rapidly (Bok et al. 2021).

Adenovirus-based vaccines had undergone extensive clinical trials (Humphreys and Sebastian 2018) and had been shown to be efficacious in preventing infectious disease in humans (Henao-Restrepo et al. 2017). Two adenovirus vector-based vaccines were approved by trusted international regulatory authorities (EMA 2020; FDA 2019). Two adenovirus vector vaccines against SARS-CoV-2 were widely authorized for emergency use in humans after phase III clinical trials: a human adenovirus-26 containing an innovative pre-stabilized coronavirus spike design (Ad26, Janssen-Johnson & Johnson) and a chimpanzee adenovirus never approved as a vaccine platform before (ChAdOx1, modified from *Pan troglodytes* Y25, Oxford in collaboration with Astra Zeneca) (COVID-19 vaccine tracker 2022; Mercado et al. 2020; van Doremalen et al. 2020). Several modified coronavirus spike inserts included in the Ad26 candidate were extensively studied in preclinical evaluations before selecting the final prototype encoding a prefusion stabilized spike immunogen, which induced robust immune responses and provided near-complete protection against SARS-CoV-2 challenge in rhesus macaques with only one dose (Mercado et al. 2020). The spike sequence cloned into the ChAdOx1 candidate consisted of the full-length, trans-membrane anchored, wild-type sequence, that is, it was not modified to "lock" the spike protein in its prefusion conformation as with the mRNA vaccines or J&J candidate (Watanabe et al. 2021); it was also shown to be immunogenic and protective against SARS-CoV-2 challenge in a macaque model (van Doremalen et al. 2020).

The most novel platform advanced as an accelerated response to the SARS-CoV-2 pandemic was mRNA. This technology was in earlier stages of development than the adenovirus-based candidates. However, mRNA also had extensive clinical experience, and the technology had progressed to provide the potential for full scale-up to hundreds of millions of doses; meanwhile, several infectious disease vaccine candidates were already being tested preclinically or in early clinical stages (Zhang et al. 2019). Two mRNA vaccines with very similar designs were selected to prevent COVID-19. The final design of mRNA-1273 (Moderna) was finalized only a few days after the first SARS-CoV-2 sequence was publicly available (Corbett et al. 2020a). Its design relied on more than a decade's worth of research evaluating structure-guided vaccine design, in addition to comparable MERS-CoV vaccine prototypes that had been found immunogenic in mice (Pallesen et al. 2017).

Initially, two mRNA vaccine prototypes were sponsored by the BioNTech/Pfizer collaborative effort, BNT162b2 and BNT162b; they were tested in phase I clinical trials to determine the final candidate to advance to late-stage clinical testing (Mulligan et al. 2020; Walsh et al. 2020a, b).

The final designs of both mRNA and J&J vaccine candidates sponsored by Moderna, Pfizer, and Johnson & Johnson included key modifications to the SARS-CoV-2 full-length spike sequence that enabled exposure of neutralizing epitopes while accounting for the possibility of Vaccine Associated Enhanced Respiratory Disease (VAERD), as reviewed by Graham (2020) and Munoz et al. (2021). The targeted design and platform selected for these candidates were vital. Early during the pandemic, in the absence of clinical and immunological data for the prevention of COVID-19 utilizing vaccines, these vaccine candidates aimed to induce higher rates of neutralizing antibodies than vaccine designs utilizing the unmodified spike sequence while stimulating a CD4+ T-helper 1-biased immune response, which had been identified as the preferred strategy to avoid potential and unknown negative vaccine-related safety outcomes (Acosta et al. 2015). Both mRNA vaccine candidates selected by the U.S. government (Pfizer's clinical study was not supported by the U.S. government) were advanced to late clinical stage testing in record time, only 6 months after the emergence of SARS-CoV-2. Moreover, they showed the highest efficacy values in phase III trials of any COVID-19 vaccine studied worldwide (◘ Fig. 2 ▶ Chap. 14 represents the mRNA-1273 timeline) (Higdon et al. 2021). While the efficacy values and trial results of U.S. government-supported vaccines have been reviewed elsewhere (Bok et al. 2021), both mRNA candidates were shown to prevent COVID-19 infection with about 95% efficacy, and both clinical trial and real-world effectiveness data suggested that these vaccines are also efficacious at preventing asymptomatic infections or that breakthrough cases presented with lower virus quantities (measured by CT values)[1] in vaccinated individuals compared to unvaccinated individuals (Fowlkes et al. 2021; Tregoning et al. 2021). This was an outstanding accomplishment by an accelerated response to a pandemic, in part due to a combination of pivotal technological advances with years of accumulated knowledge on coronavirus and related viruses.

Efficacy trials were designed to be independent but harmonized phase III vaccine trials with closely aligned primary endpoints (e.g., prevention of symptomatic COVID-19). In addition, NIH established a common independent data safety and monitoring board (DSMB) staffed with expert clinicians and statisticians from government and academia to oversee the trials (Corey et al. 2020). Operation Warp Speed, the accelerated U.S. vaccine development program, also began a process to establish a core set of validated assays to measure vaccine-induced antibody responses as well as a biostatistical group to evaluate the data (Koup et al. 2021). Thus, each trial would have a common set of immune measurements from which to assess potential immune correlates of protection and facilitate cross-protocol comparisons.

While efficacy studies found that the vaccines were safe and effective in trial volunteers, continuing monitoring and surveillance is essential to confirm effectiveness and assure safety with real-world evidence (IVAC 2021). Vaccine safety is monitored throughout the development, deployment, and commercialization of authorized or licensed vaccines (Plotkin et al. 2020). When a vaccine or drug is administered to a global population, powerful passive and active safety surveillance systems are essential for early detection of rare adverse events signals, which are expected with the use of any medication. Several adverse event signals have been confirmed in association with COVID-19 vaccination, though these are very rare cases that are always outweighed by the benefits of receiving a vaccine. Rare cases of anaphylaxis have been associated with genetic platforms (Janssen, Pfizer, and Moderna). Adenovirus-based vaccines have been associated with Guillain–Barré syndrome and thrombosis with thrombocytopenia syndrome. Both mRNA vaccines have been linked to rare cases of myocarditis, especially in young male

1 Cycle threshold value: the total number of cycles required for a polymerase chain reaction (PCR) test to exceed the threshold for a result positive result. Baselines CT values are specific to each test platform, and generally range from about 15 to 45 cycles.

vaccinees (CDC 2021b). The safety surveillance systems in place in the United States and many other countries, in combination with sponsors' pharmacovigilance plans, continue to provide robust data for regulators and policy advisors to make recommendations about the use of vaccines based on scientific evidence, always prioritizing public health and individual safety.

At the time of drafting of this chapter, scientists are actively reviewing data and evaluating the durability of the immune response for authorized or licensed vaccines. Several sources of data indicate that immunity from mRNA vaccines wanes between 6 and 8 months after vaccination, and that antibody levels can be boosted to higher levels than peak geometric mean titer (GMT) levels initially observed after the second dose by adding a third dose to the schedule of any mRNA vaccine (El Sahly et al. 2021; Pfizer 2021; Thomas et al. 2021). The combination of waning immunity and emergence of evolutionarily distinct SARS-CoV-2 variants has fueled a new wave of COVID-19 cases all over the world, even in highly vaccinated countries such as Israel (Bar-On et al. 2021). Effectiveness of the coronavirus vaccines against symptomatic disease has decreased over time, and in some cases their effectiveness against hospitalizations and severe disease has also waned (El Sahly et al. 2021). The CDC has already recommended that third doses of Pfizer, Moderna, and Janssen vaccines be administered to people over 65 years of age and others at increased risk (CDC 2021a). Ongoing testing and surveillance efforts will determine if these vaccines need to be updated to match circulating variants or if additional doses will be required in the future to sustain the prevention of disease.

3 The Future of the mRNA Vaccine Platform for Preparedness

The first successful mRNA vaccines ever deployed to prevent disease in a human population became a reality 30 years after the first report of the proof of concept that in vitro transcribed mRNA led to readily detectable expression of an introduced protein in an animal model (Wolff et al. 1990). The technology to deliver an mRNA-based vaccine advanced slowly after that initial demonstration, given concerns about the instability of the mRNA molecule, the reactogenicity elicited by stimulating the innate immune response, and lack of a straightforward and efficient method for delivering translatable mRNA into the cell. Fast forward several decades and the mRNA platform has clear advantages over traditional manufacturing methods and even over other genetic platforms (DNA and virus vector):

1. mRNA has one of the most favorable safety profiles among genetic platforms since it naturally degrades and cannot integrate itself into the cellular genome. Also, additional safety modifications can be integrated during design.
2. Efficacy can also be modulated and enhanced by optimizing translation efficiency.
3. It can be administered repeatedly since mRNA constitutes the smallest genetic vector, precluding immune reaction to the platform (as can occur with viral vector vaccines).
4. Cell-free manufacture of mRNA not only allows for accelerated production, but is highly scalable, standardizable, and requires reduced manufacturing footprints. This enables individual facilities to manufacture multiple products with minimal adaptations in their equipment, processes, and formulation (Jackson et al. 2020; Pardi et al. 2018).

The advantages of this platform, when combined with thoughtful target engineering, careful design, and understanding of the host immune system, make it an attractive alternative not only for pandemic preparedness and emergency response applications, but very likely for a new generation of vaccines addressing unmet medical needs and improving on existing vaccines (Fig. 3).

mRNA might also play a role in updating current vaccines, leveraging not only scientific but also logistical advantages. In September 2021, Sanofi announced plans for their phase I/II trial on a monovalent mRNA influenza vaccine, with plans to test a quadrivalent version in the near future. A new mRNA-based influenza vaccine candidate might not only prove to be more effective but might also allow for later decision-making on annual influenza strain selections, decreasing the chances of deploying vaccines that will not match strains circulating that season (Sanofi 2021; WHO 2021c).

However, the mRNA platform may not be the ideal choice to target certain viruses that benefit from other approaches, such as live-attenuated vaccine candidates delivered through the natural route of infection, or for pathogens that are dependent on proteases for post-translation protein processing, as with the family *Picornaviridae* (Baggen et al. 2018; Kulkarni et al. 2017). In this case, the mRNA would need to deliver the coding sequence for a virus protease in addition to the target antigen, which might raise safety concerns. We should also keep in mind that traditional manufacturing technologies will still play the primary role in global vaccine manufacturing as the most prolific global vaccine providers continue to utilize existing resources, that is, established Good Manufacturing Practice facilities to provide the world with life-saving immunizations as part of longstanding international vaccination plans (EC 2011; Serum Institute of India 2021).

As with any groundbreaking new technology, important research questions are still being investigated. Future studies will further knowledge of both pathogen-specific mRNA vaccines and the platform in general. Alternative routes of delivery are still being tested, which might provide resident tissue immunity and improve effectiveness and performance of certain vaccines. New routes of vaccine delivery include nasal, intradermal, and intravenous, among others (Broos et al. 2016; Gan et al. 2019; Phua et al. 2014).

The importance of and interplay between antibody and cellular immunity in the prevention of disease or transmission is also still a fruitful research area. Correlates of protection studies indicate that humoral immunity plays an important role in preventing symptomatic disease, but also clearly indicate that cellular immunity needs to be better understood (Corbett et al. 2021; Feng et al. 2021; Koup et al. 2021). Moreover, the mechanism of action by which mRNA vaccines cause certain adverse events also needs further investigation (Rosenblum et al. 2021). Detailed understanding of the immunization process might allow for further modification of both the vaccine itself and optimization of the immunization schedule to avoid undesirable rare consequences and improve efficacy and/or durability of protection.

Finally, international health and infectious disease-focused organizations have now proposed aggressive "Apollo Mission" or "100 Day Mission" preparedness plans to improve on the lessons learned from the coronavirus pandemic and compress the timelines to achieve global access to lifesaving vaccines. There is no doubt mRNA vaccines will be fundamental to achieving these ambitious goals (Pandemic Preparedness Partnership 2021; White House 2021). But if mRNA is to be an important tool for future pandemic preparedness, global access and especially availability of mRNA manufacturing in low- and middle-income countries will be an essential capability to develop and support over time (WHO 2021a, 2022). Expanding worldwide mRNA manufacturing and fill and finish capacity, together with establishing a solid global supply chain, are essential if we want to control epidemics and pandemics in a timely manner and promote equal access to health interventions.

Discussion Questions

1. Discuss the development of viral vectors as candidates for gene therapy.
2. Discuss how vaccine delivery using mRNA technology was advanced to overcome key roadblocks related to its stability, translation efficiency, activation of the innate immune response, and delivery of the intact mRNA molecule.
3. Discuss novel, groundbreaking vaccine designs and manufacturing platforms advanced during the COVID-19 pandemic.
4. The mRNA platform has four clear advantages (conducive to emergency response applications, improvement of

existing vaccines, and development of new ones) over traditional manufacturing methods and even over other genetic platforms (DNA and virus vector). Discuss these advantages.
5. The mRNA platform may not be the ideal choice in all circumstances. Discuss these circumstances and mRNA research questions that are still being investigated.

Acknowledgments I am very grateful to Dr. Nancy Sullivan, Dr. John Mascola, and Sandra Sitar for thoughtful suggestions and review.

References

Acosta PL, Caballero MT, Polack FP. Brief history and characterization of enhanced respiratory syncytial virus disease. Clin Vaccine Immunol. 2015;23(3):189–95. https://doi.org/10.1128/CVI.00609-15.

Agnandji ST, Huttner A, Zinser ME, Njuguna P, Dahlke C, Fernandes JF, et al. Phase 1 trials of rVSV Ebola vaccine in Africa and Europe. N Engl J Med. 2016;374(17):1647–60. https://doi.org/10.1056/NEJMoa1502924.

Baggen J, Thibaut HJ, Strating J, van Kuppeveld FJM. The life cycle of non-polio enteroviruses and how to target it. Nat Rev Microbiol. 2018;16(6):368–81. https://doi.org/10.1038/s41579-018-0005-4.

Bar-On YM, Goldberg Y, Mandel M, Bodenheimer O, Freedman L, Kalkstein N, et al. Protection of BNT162b2 vaccine booster against Covid-19 in Israel. N Engl J Med. 2021;385:1393. https://doi.org/10.1056/NEJMoa2114255.

Bok K, Sitar S, Graham BS, Mascola JR. Accelerated COVID-19 vaccine development: milestones, lessons, and prospects. Immunity. 2021;54(8):1636–51. https://doi.org/10.1016/j.immuni.2021.07.017.

Broos K, Van der Jeught K, Puttemans J, Goyvaerts C, Heirman C, Dewitte H, et al. Particle-mediated intravenous delivery of antigen mRNA results in strong antigen-specific T-cell responses despite the induction of type I interferon. Mol Ther Nucleic Acids. 2016;5(6):e326. https://doi.org/10.1038/mtna.2016.38.

CDC. CDC statement on ACIP booster recommendations. Atlanta, GA: U.S. Centers for Disease Control and Prevention; 2021a. https://www.cdc.gov/media/releases/2021/p0924-booster-recommendations-.html. Accessed 17 Oct 2021.

CDC. COVID-19 vaccine safety technical (VaST) work group reports. Atlanta, GA: U.S. Centers for Disease Control and Prevention; 2021b. https://www.cdc.gov/vaccines/acip/work-groups-vast/index.html?CDC_AA_refVal=https%3A%2F%2Fwww.cdc.gov%2Fvaccines%2Facip%2Fwork-groups-vast%2Ftechnical-report.html. Accessed 24 Oct 2021.

Corbett KS, Edwards DK, Leist SR, Abiona OM, Boyoglu-Barnum S, Gillespie RA, et al. SARS-CoV-2 mRNA vaccine design enabled by prototype pathogen preparedness. Nature. 2020a;586(7830):567–71. https://doi.org/10.1038/s41586-020-2622-0.

Corbett KS, Flynn B, Foulds KE, Francica JR, Boyoglu-Barnum S, Werner AP, et al. Evaluation of the mRNA-1273 vaccine against SARS-CoV-2 in non-human primates. N Engl J Med. 2020b;383(16):1544–55. https://doi.org/10.1056/NEJMoa2024671.

Corbett KS, Nason MC, Flach B, Gagne M, O'Connell S, Johnston TS, et al. Immune correlates of protection by mRNA-1273 vaccine against SARS-CoV-2 in nonhuman primates. Science. 2021;373(6561):eabj0299. https://doi.org/10.1126/science.abj0299.

Corey L, Mascola JR, Fauci AS, Collins FS. A strategic approach to COVID-19 vaccine R&D. Science. 2020;368(6494):948–50. https://doi.org/10.1126/science.abc5312.

COVID-19 vaccine tracker. Rockville, MD: Regulatory Affairs Professionals Society. 2022. https://www.raps.org/news-and-articles/news-articles/2020/3/covid-19-vaccine-tracker. Accessed 20 May 2022.

EC. EudraLex: the rules governing medicinal products in the European Union, volume 4: good manufacturing practice: medicinal products for human and veterinary use, annex 11: computerised systems. Brussels: European Commission, Health and Consumers Directorate-General; 2011.

El Sahly HM, Baden LR, Essink B, Doblecki-Lewis S, Martin JM, Anderson EJ, et al. Efficacy of the mRNA-1273 SARS-CoV-2 vaccine at completion of blinded phase. N Engl J Med. 2021;385:1774. https://doi.org/10.1056/NEJMoa2113017.

EMA. New vaccine for prevention of Ebola virus disease recommended for approval in the European Union. Amsterdam: European Medicines Agency; 2020.

FDA. ERVEBO. 2019. https://www.fda.gov/vaccines-blood-biologics/ervebo. Accessed 17 Oct 2021.

FDA. FDA authorizes longer time for refrigerator storage of thawed Pfizer-BioNTech COVID-19 vaccine prior to dilution, making vaccine more widely available. Silver Spring, MD: U.S. Food and Drug Administration; 2021.

Feng S, Phillips DJ, White T, Sayal H, Aley PK, Bibi S, et al. Correlates of protection against symptomatic and asymptomatic SARS-CoV-2 infection. Nat Med. 2021;27:2032. https://doi.org/10.1038/s41591-021-01540-1.

Fields BN, Knipe DM, Howley PM. Fields virology. 5th ed. Philadelphia: Wolters Kluwer Health/Lippincott Williams & Wilkins; 2007.

Fowlkes A, Gaglani M, Groover K, Thiese MS, Tyner H, Ellingson K, et al. Effectiveness of COVID-19 vaccines in preventing SARS-CoV-2 infection among frontline workers before and during B.1.617.2 (Delta) variant predominance—eight U.S. locations, December 2020–August 2021. MMWR Morb Mortal Wkly Rep. 2021;70(34):1167–9. https://doi.org/10.15585/mmwr.mm7034e4.

Gan LM, Lagerstrom-Fermer M, Carlsson LG, Arfvidsson C, Egnell AC, Rudvik A, et al. Intradermal delivery of modified mRNA encoding VEGF-A in patients with type 2 diabetes. Nat Commun. 2019;10(1):871. https://doi.org/10.1038/s41467-019-08852-4.

Graham BS. Rapid COVID-19 vaccine development. Science. 2020;368(6494):945–6. https://doi.org/10.1126/science.abb8923.

Henao-Restrepo AM, Camacho A, Longini IM, Watson CH, Edmunds WJ, Egger M, et al. Efficacy and effectiveness of an rVSV-vectored vaccine in preventing Ebola virus disease: final results from the Guinea ring vaccination, open-label, cluster-randomised trial (Ebola Ca Suffit!). Lancet. 2017;389(10068):505–18. https://doi.org/10.1016/S0140-6736(16)32621-6.

Higdon MM, Wahl B, Jones CB, Rosen JG, Truelove SA, Baidya A, et al. A systematic review of COVID-19 vaccine efficacy and effectiveness against SARS-CoV-2 infection and disease. medRxiv. 2021; https://doi.org/10.1101/2021.09.17.21263549.

Hou X, Zaks T, Langer R, Dong Y. Lipid nanoparticles for mRNA delivery. Nat Rev Mater. 2021;6:1078–94. https://doi.org/10.1038/s41578-021-00358-0.

Humphreys IR, Sebastian S. Novel viral vectors in infectious diseases. Immunology. 2018;153(1):1–9. https://doi.org/10.1111/imm.12829.

Iavarone C, O'Hagan DT, Yu D, Delahaye NF, Ulmer JB. Mechanism of action of mRNA-based vaccines. Expert Rev Vaccines. 2017;16(9):871–81. https://doi.org/10.1080/14760584.2017.1355245.

IVAC. View-hub resource library. Baltimore, MD: International Vaccine Access Center (IVAC), Johns Hopkins Bloomberg School of Public; 2021. https://view-hub.org/resources. Accessed 24 Oct 2021.

Jackson NAC, Kester KE, Casimiro D, Gurunathan S, DeRosa F. The promise of mRNA vaccines: a biotech and industrial perspective. NPJ Vaccines. 2020;5:11. https://doi.org/10.1038/s41541-020-0159-8.

Kariko K, Buckstein M, Ni H, Weissman D. Suppression of RNA recognition by Toll-like receptors: the impact of nucleoside modification and the evolutionary origin of RNA. Immunity. 2005;23(2):165–75. https://doi.org/10.1016/j.immuni.2005.06.008.

Koup RA, Donis RO, Gilbert PB, Li AW, Shah NA, Houchens CR. A government-led effort to identify correlates of protection for COVID-19 vaccines. Nat Med. 2021;27(9):1493–4. https://doi.org/10.1038/s41591-021-01484-6.

Kowalski PS, Rudra A, Miao L, Anderson DG. Delivering the messenger: advances in technologies for therapeutic mRNA delivery. Mol Ther. 2019;27(4):710–28. https://doi.org/10.1016/j.ymthe.2019.02.012.

Kowalzik F, Schreiner D, Jensen C, Teschner D, Gehring S, Zepp F. mRNA-based vaccines. Vaccines (Basel). 2021;9(4):390. https://doi.org/10.3390/vaccines9040390.

Kulkarni PS, Desai S, Tewari T, Kawade A, Goyal N, Garg BS, et al. A randomized phase III clinical trial to assess the efficacy of a bovine-human reassortant pentavalent rotavirus vaccine in Indian infants. Vaccine. 2017;35(45):6228–37. https://doi.org/10.1016/j.vaccine.2017.09.014.

Kutzler MA, Weiner DB. DNA vaccines: ready for prime time? Nat Rev Genet. 2008;9(10):776–88. https://doi.org/10.1038/nrg2432.

Liu MA. A comparison of plasmid DNA and mRNA as vaccine technologies. Vaccines (Basel). 2019;7(2):37. https://doi.org/10.3390/vaccines7020037.

Maruggi G, Zhang C, Li J, Ulmer JB, Yu D. mRNA as a transformative technology for vaccine development to control infectious diseases. Mol Ther. 2019;27(4):757–72. https://doi.org/10.1016/j.ymthe.2019.01.020.

Mennechet FJD, Paris O, Ouoba AR, Salazar Arenas S, Sirima SB, Takoudjou Dzomo GR, et al. A review of 65 years of human adenovirus seroprevalence. Expert Rev Vaccines. 2019;18(6):597–613. https://doi.org/10.1080/14760584.2019.1588113.

Mercado NB, Zahn R, Wegmann F, Loos C, Chandrashekar A, Yu J, et al. Single-shot Ad26 vaccine protects against SARS-CoV-2 in rhesus macaques. Nature. 2020;586(7830):583–8. https://doi.org/10.1038/s41586-020-2607-z.

Moderna. Moderna's other vaccines: CMV vaccine (mRNA-1647). PowerPoint presentation. Cambridge, MA: Moderna; 2021.

Morris SJ, Sebastian S, Spencer AJ, Gilbert SC. Simian adenoviruses as vaccine vectors. Future Virol. 2016;11(9):649–59. https://doi.org/10.2217/fvl-2016-0070.

Moss B, Smith GL, Gerin JL, Purcell RH. Live recombinant vaccinia virus protects chimpanzees against hepatitis B. Nature. 1984;311(5981):67–9. https://doi.org/10.1038/311067a0.

Mulligan MJ, Lyke KE, Kitchin N, Absalon J, Gurtman A, Lockhart S, et al. Phase I/II study of COVID-19 RNA vaccine BNT162b1 in adults. Nature. 2020;586(7830):589–93. https://doi.org/10.1038/s41586-020-2639-4.

Munoz FM, Cramer JP, Dekker CL, Dudley MZ, Graham BS, Gurwith M, et al. Vaccine-associated enhanced disease: case definition and guidelines for data collection, analysis, and presentation of immunization safety data. Vaccine. 2021;39(22):3053–66. https://doi.org/10.1016/j.vaccine.2021.01.055.

Pallesen J, Wang N, Corbett KS, Wrapp D, Kirchdoerfer RN, Turner HL, et al. Immunogenicity and structures of a rationally designed prefusion MERS-CoV spike antigen. Proc Natl Acad Sci USA. 2017;114(35):E7348–E57. https://doi.org/10.1073/pnas.1707304114.

Pandemic Preparedness Partnership. 100 days mission to respond to future pandemic threats: reducing the impact of future pandemics by making diagnostics, therapeutics and vaccines available within 100 days: a report to the G7. London: G7 United Kingdom; 2021.

Pardi N, Hogan MJ, Porter FW, Weissman D. mRNA vaccines—a new era in vaccinology. Nat Rev Drug Discov. 2018;17(4):261–79. https://doi.org/10.1038/nrd.2017.243.

Pardi N, Hogan MJ, Weissman D. Recent advances in mRNA vaccine technology. Curr Opin Immunol. 2020;65:14–20. https://doi.org/10.1016/j.coi.2020.01.008.

Pfizer. Pfizer-Biontech COVID-19 vaccine (BNT162, PF-07302048) Vaccines and Related Biological Products Advisory Committee briefing document. Pfizer Biontech; 2020.

Pfizer. Evaluation of a booster dose (third dose). New York: Pfizer; 2021.

Phua KK, Staats HF, Leong KW, Nair SK. Intranasal mRNA nanoparticle vaccination induces prophylactic and therapeutic anti-tumor immunity. Sci Rep. 2014;4:5128. https://doi.org/10.1038/srep05128.

Pine SO, Kublin JG, Hammer SM, Borgerding J, Huang Y, Casimiro DR, et al. Pre-existing adenovirus immunity modifies a complex mixed Th1 and Th2 cytokine response to an Ad5/HIV-1 vaccine candidate in humans. PLoS One. 2011;6(4):e18526. https://doi.org/10.1371/journal.pone.0018526.

Plotkin SA, Offit PA, DeStefano F, Larson HJ, Arora NK, Zuber PLF, et al. The science of vaccine safety: summary of meeting at Wellcome Trust. Vaccine. 2020;38(8):1869–80. https://doi.org/10.1016/j.vaccine.2020.01.024.

Quinn KM, Zak DE, Costa A, Yamamoto A, Kastenmuller K, Hill BJ, et al. Antigen expression determines adenoviral vaccine potency independent of IFN and STING signaling. J Clin Invest. 2015;125(3):1129–46. https://doi.org/10.1172/JCI78280.

Ramezanpour B, Haan I, Osterhaus A, Claassen E. Vector-based genetically modified vaccines: exploiting Jenner's legacy. Vaccine. 2016;34(50):6436–48. https://doi.org/10.1016/j.vaccine.2016.06.059.

Rosa SS, Prazeres DMF, Azevedo AM, Marques MPC. mRNA vaccines manufacturing: challenges and bottlenecks. Vaccine. 2021;39(16):2190–200. https://doi.org/10.1016/j.vaccine.2021.03.038.

Rosenblum HG, Hadler SC, Moulia D, Shimabukuro TT, Su JR, Tepper NK, et al. Use of COVID-19 vaccines after reports of adverse events among adult recipients of Janssen (Johnson & Johnson) and mRNA COVID-19 vaccines (Pfizer-BioNTech and Moderna): update from the Advisory Committee on Immunization Practices—United States, July 2021. MMWR Morb Mortal Wkly Rep. 2021;70(32):1094–9. https://doi.org/10.15585/mmwr.mm7032e4.

Sanofi. Sanofi announces positive Phase 1/2 study interim results for its first mRNA-based vaccine candidate. Sanofi; 2021.

Serum Institute of India. About us: serum protection from birth onwards. Pune, India: Serum Institute of India Pvt. Ltd.; 2021. https://www.seruminstitute.com/about_us.php. Accessed 24 Oct 2021.

Stanley DA, Honko AN, Asiedu C, Trefry JC, Lau-Kilby AW, Johnson JC, et al. Chimpanzee adenovirus vaccine generates acute and durable protective immunity against ebolavirus challenge. Nat Med. 2014;20(10):1126–9. https://doi.org/10.1038/nm.3702.

Tan WG, Jin HT, West EE, Penaloza-MacMaster P, Wieland A, Zilliox MJ, et al. Comparative analysis of simian immunodeficiency virus gag-specific effector and memory CD8+ T cells induced by different adenovirus vectors. J Virol. 2013;87(3):1359–72. https://doi.org/10.1128/JVI.02055-12.

Thomas SJ, Moreira ED Jr, Kitchin N, Absalon J, Gurtman A, Lockhart S, et al. Safety and efficacy of the BNT162b2 mRNA Covid-19 vaccine through 6 months. N Engl J Med. 2021;385:1761. https://doi.org/10.1056/NEJMoa2110345.

Tombácz I, Weissman D, Pardi N. Vaccination with messenger RNA: a promising alternative to DNA vaccination. In: Sobieszczyk ME, editor. DNA vaccines, Methods in molecular biology, vol. 2197. New York: Humana; 2021.

Tregoning JS, Flight KE, Higham SL, Wang Z, Pierce BF. Progress of the COVID-19 vaccine effort: viruses, vaccines and variants versus efficacy, effectiveness and escape. Nat Rev Immunol. 2021;21:626. https://doi.org/10.1038/s41577-021-00592-1.

Ulmer JB, Valley U, Rappuoli R. Vaccine manufacturing: challenges and solutions. Nat Biotechnol. 2006;24(11):1377–83. https://doi.org/10.1038/nbt1261.

van Doremalen N, Lambe T, Spencer A, Belij-Rammerstorfer S, Purushotham JN, Port JR, et al. ChAdOx1 nCoV-19 vaccine prevents SARS-CoV-2 pneumonia in rhesus macaques. Nature. 2020;586(7830):578–82. https://doi.org/10.1038/s41586-020-2608-y.

Vogel AB, Kanevsky I, Che Y, Swanson KA, Muik A, Vormehr M, et al. BNT162b vaccines protect rhesus macaques from SARS-CoV-2. Nature. 2021;592(7853):283–9. https://doi.org/10.1038/s41586-021-03275-y.

Walsh EE, Frenck R, Falsey AR, Kitchin N, Absalon J, Gurtman A, et al. RNA-based COVID-19 vaccine BNT162b2 selected for a pivotal efficacy study. medRxiv. 2020a; https://doi.org/10.1101/2020.08.17.20176651.

Walsh EE, Frenck RW Jr, Falsey AR, Kitchin N, Absalon J, Gurtman A, et al. Safety and immunogenicity of two RNA-based Covid-19 vaccine candidates. N Engl J Med. 2020b;383(25):2439–50. https://doi.org/10.1056/NEJMoa2027906.

Watanabe Y, Mendonça L, Allen ER, Howe A, Lee M, Allen JD, et al. Native-like SARS-CoV-2 spike glycoprotein expressed by ChAdOx1 nCoV-19/AZD1222 vaccine. ACS Cent Sci. 2021;7(4):594–602. https://doi.org/10.1021/acscentsci.1c00080.

White House. American pandemic preparedness: transforming our capabilities. Washington, DC: White House; 2021.

WHO. Leaders make urgent call to accelerate vaccination globally and in Africa. Geneva: World Health Organization; 2021a.

WHO. Status of COVID-19 Vaccines within WHO EUL/PQ evaluation process. 2021b. https://extranet.who.int/pqweb/sites/default/files/documents/Status_COVID_VAX_19August2021.pdf.

WHO. World Health Organization recommendations for composition of influenza vaccines. Geneva: World Health Organization; 2021c. https://www.fludb.org/brc/vaccineRecommend.spg?decorator=influenza. Accessed 24 Oct 2021.

WHO. The mRNA vaccine technology transfer hub. Geneva: World Health Organization; 2022. https://www.who.int/initiatives/the-mrna-vaccine-technology-transfer-hub#:~:text=The%20mRNA%20vaccine%20technology%20transfer%20hub&text=Announced%20on%2021%20June%202021,the%20mRNA%20vaccine%20technology%20hub. Accessed 13 Dec 2022.

Wolff JA, Malone RW, Williams P, Chong W, Acsadi G, Jani A, et al. Direct gene transfer into mouse muscle in vivo. Science. 1990;247(4949 Pt 1):1465–8. https://doi.org/10.1126/science.1690918.

Zhang C, Maruggi G, Shan H, Li J. Advances in mRNA vaccines for infectious diseases. Front Immunol. 2019;10:594. https://doi.org/10.3389/fimmu.2019.00594.

13 Accelerating Vaccine Development: The 100 Days Mission

Aishani Aatresh, Nicole Lurie, and Richard Hatchett

Contents

Learning Track Note: This chapter appears in Learning Tracks: Emergency Research Response, Research Operations; Health Policy, Multilateral Cooperation, International Governance; Preparedness

E. S. Higgs and R. A. Sorenson (eds.), *Principles and Practice of Emergency Research Response*,
https://doi.org/10.1007/978-3-031-48408-7_16

Learning Objectives

This chapter will help readers understand and describe:

- The genesis and goals of the 100 Days Mission.
- Timelines for vaccine development against a novel pathogen.
- Why research is needed in an infectious disease emergency.
- Major systems and operational innovations that might speed vaccine development.
- Some measures to accelerate vaccine development without relaxing safety and efficacy standards.
- The means of ensuring faster, more equitable distribution of rapidly developed and authorized/approved vaccines in an emergency, compared to the COVID-19 pandemic.

1 Introduction

CEPI was created in the aftermath of the 2014–2016 Ebola epidemic in West Africa, when a vaccine that had undergone early development but been neglected was advanced further, assessed in clinical trials, and found to be safe and effective. CEPI's founders decided that the world would be better protected against potentially dangerous but rare pathogens if vaccines against them could be developed in advance of potential outbreaks through Phase II clinical trials and evaluated through further clinical trials in the event of an outbreak.

As a coalition of public, private, philanthropic, and civil society organizations, CEPI aims to accelerate the development of vaccines against emerging epidemic threats and enable access to these vaccines for people who need them during outbreaks. Initially focusing on five priority pathogens from the World Health Organization (WHO) Research and Development (R&D) Blueprint (WHO 2023c),[1] CEPI worked toward developing vaccines projected to provide health, social, and economic benefits for vulnerable populations—especially where market potential was too limited to provide a strong commercial incentive for their development and clinical assessment (CEPI 2021a). Part of CEPI's mission to develop vaccines to prevent future epidemics in the absence of market incentives therefore involves building the capacity to advance vaccine development *during* emerging outbreaks. That, in turn, requires support for high-quality infectious disease research for preparedness—research capacity that can pivot to emergency response when and where it is needed (▶ Chaps. 27 and 28) (Hatchett and Lurie 2019; World Bank 2018).

1.1 The Importance of Research During an Outbreak Response

CEPI was barely 3 years old when the WHO declared coronavirus disease 2019 (COVID-19) a global pandemic in March 2020. Conceptualizing research as a key component of response—not merely research for preparedness or "peacetime" vaccine development—had been a key tenet of CEPI's activities since its inception and continued to guide CEPI's work as soon as the severe acute respiratory coronavirus 2 (SARS-CoV-2) causing COVID-19 was identified. CEPI built on existing partnerships from its Middle East respiratory syndrome coronavirus (MERS-CoV) and rapid response platform programs and mobilized quickly to support vaccine development, clinical trials, and several syntheses of data and real-world evidence. Ultimately, CEPI's development efforts contributed to the authorization of eight vaccines. Recognizing that R&D alone would be insufficient to quell a pandemic, CEPI joined with WHO, UNICEF, and Gavi, the Vaccine Alliance, to form COVAX—the "vaccines pillar" of the Access to COVID-19 Tools Accelerator (ACT-A), designed to facilitate broad access to a large portfolio of vaccine candidates (CEPI 2022b). CEPI also supported several studies that helped establish key scientific reference standards, including correlates of protection and immunobridging approaches to regulatory authorization.

1 Middle East respiratory syndrome coronavirus, Nipah virus, chikungunya virus, Lassa virus, and Rift Valley fever virus.

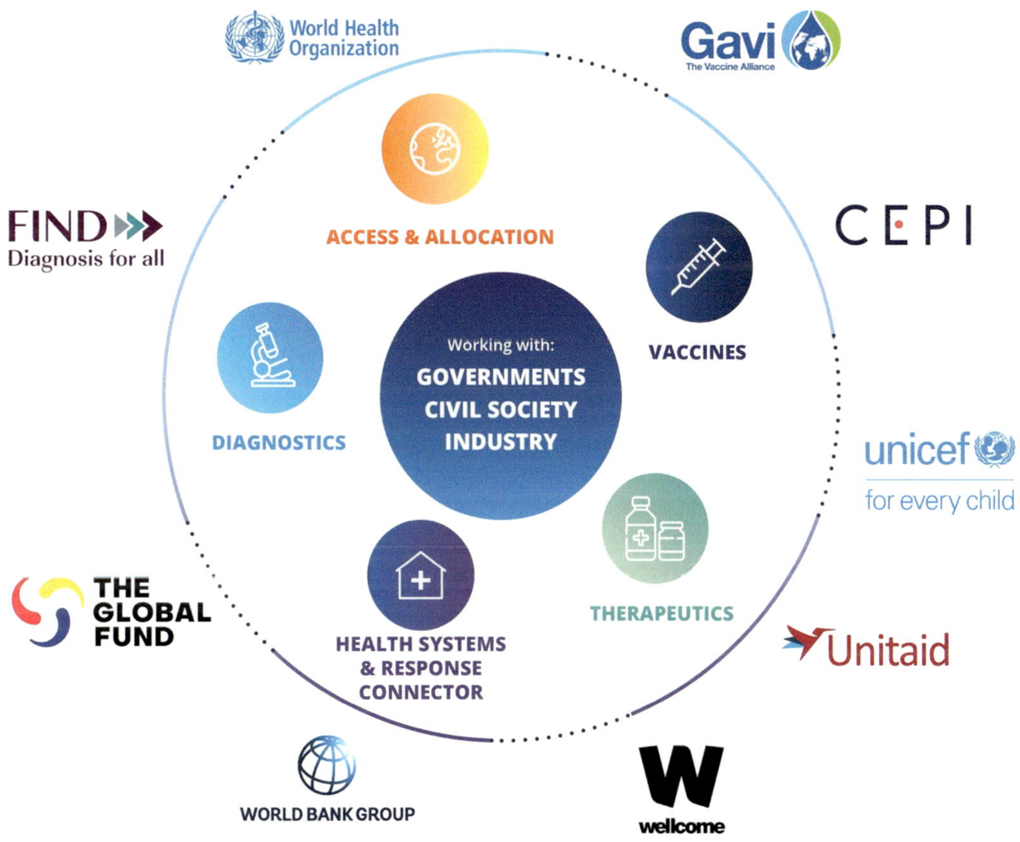

Fig. 1 The major goals and partners of ACT-A. (Access to COVID-19 Tools Accelerator) (CEPI)

Additional research funded after early-stage mobilization focused on problems such as fractional dosing, mix-and-match doses from more than one producer, efficacy in immunocompromised populations, cold chain innovations, and broadly protective coronavirus vaccines. Whether filling evidence gaps or driving technological innovation to increase access (Rodgers 2020), especially in low- and middle-income country settings, CEPI's efforts throughout the pandemic all featured research as a key instrument for response (▶ Chap. 3 and Case Study 25.1) (Fig. 1).

Outbreaks of *Sudan ebolavirus* and the Marburg virus in Uganda (late 2022) and Equatorial Guinea (early 2023) demonstrated the ongoing needs and challenges for research response. Doses of investigational vaccines for the Sudan virus were available in bulk form, but 79 days passed from the time the outbreak was declared for them to be filled and finished and arrive in Uganda. While this was faster than previous vaccine research responses to epidemics, the outbreak ended before a trial could be launched. Beyond vaccine availability, other barriers included an incomplete protocol and lacking regulatory authorization in country (Samarasekera 2023). Both outbreaks highlighted enduring complexities of launching a trial in the early stages of a response, but they have equally exemplified the importance of thinking about preparedness and response as a continuum, rather than binary aspects of different research agendas. In other words, outbreak response is outbreak preparedness, and research should always be part of it.

2 The 100 Days Mission

Outbreak response as outbreak preparedness is a natural follow-on to more familiar maxims about the importance of preparedness for rapid, effective action amid an emerging crisis.

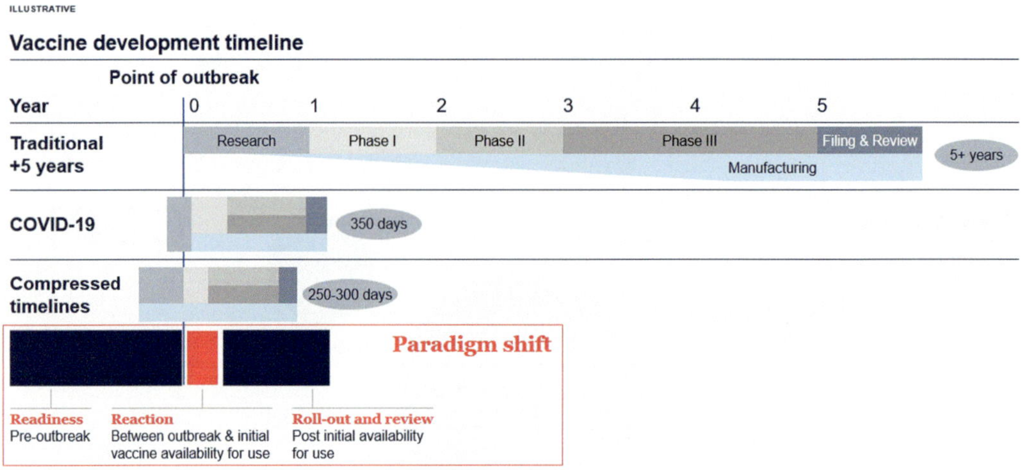

Fig. 2 Meeting the 100 Days Mission will require a paradigm shift in the vaccine development process. (CEPI)

Preparedness and response are often portrayed as two separate stages. However, the bidirectional relationship outlined in this chapter indicates that a more fluid and integrated understanding of these categories lends itself to an evolved paradigm of emergencies—one that more carefully considers how what has been done in the past can and should inform the future.

The development and authorization of novel vaccines against SARS-CoV-2 in less than a year was a technoscientific triumph, especially as part of a global response to the COVID-19 pandemic that was inadequate in many other respects. The first vaccine received emergency authorization in record time, 326 days from the date the SARS-CoV-2 genetic sequence was posted. By that time, however, more than 60 million people had been infected and over 1.5 million had died (WHO 2023b).

Developing a novel vaccine in less than a year was not merely the result of a rapid response upon the declaration of a pandemic. Decades of research into betacoronaviruses and mRNA vaccine platforms, as well as the deep experience of national biomedical institutions and well-oiled partnerships across the pharmaceutical sector, set the stage for this achievement (▶ Chap. 12). An analysis of innovations in vaccine development for COVID-19 suggests that if all possible innovations were used for the next pandemic, the time to vaccine authorization possibly might decrease further, but at most by 25% to approximately 250 days (CEPI 2022c). If we want to curtail outbreaks before they become pandemics, we must go faster. In other words, the world needs a paradigm shift for how it approaches vaccine research and development in both preparedness and response phases (Fig. 2).

In 2021, CEPI called for such a paradigm shift, articulating a 100 Days Mission (100DM): Vaccines should be ready for initial authorization and manufacturing at scale within 100 days of recognition of pathogen with pandemic potential, when appropriate. From a research perspective, this goal is structured around five key areas in the R&D life cycle:

1. Prototype vaccines for representative pathogens across viral families.
2. Biomarkers for protective and robust immune responses.
3. Global capabilities for early characterization of pathogens and outbreaks.[2]
4. Rapid manufacture and validation of experimental vaccines.
5. Ready clinical trial infrastructure that can spring into action to test experimental vaccines.

2 Surveillance and pathogen identification are beyond the scope of this chapter. It is a key enabler for CEPI's work but not directly in its purview. See ▶ Sect. 2.5.

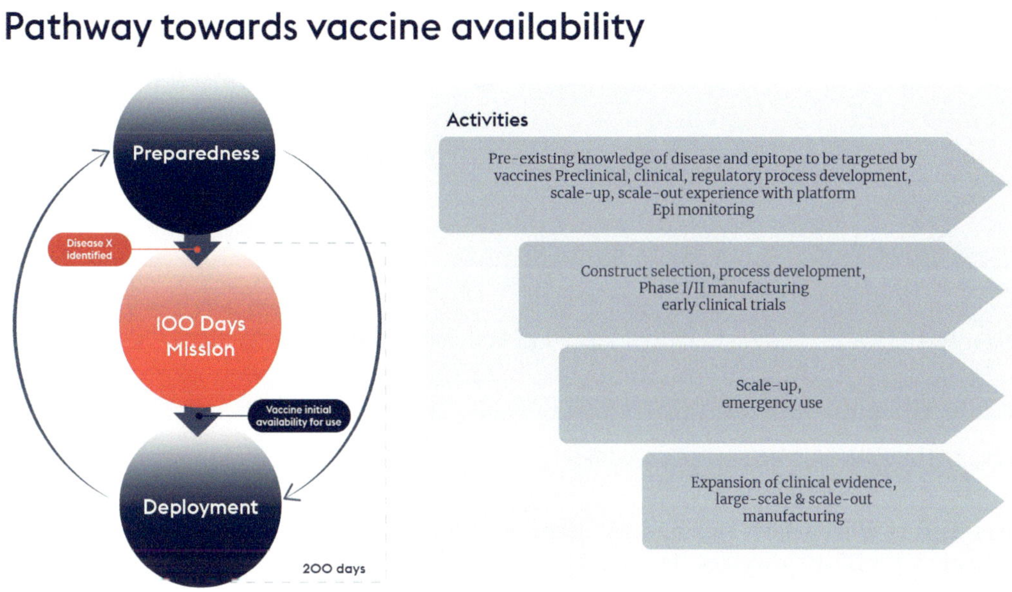

Fig. 3 Approaching outbreak response as outbreak preparedness, depicted through CEPI's activities to accelerate vaccine development. (CEPI)

The 100 Days Mission has since been adopted in multiple international arenas, including the Group of Seven (G7), Group of Twenty (G20), and the United States (U.S.) government, while more informally serving as a catalyst for improved outbreak countermeasure development and additional improvements in the "Second 100 Days" (CEPI 2022a, d; IFPMA 2021; IPP Secretariat 2023; Pandemic Institute 2023; UK.gov 2021; White House 2021).

There are two key elements of the paradigm shift implicated in achieving CEPI's 100DM that go beyond a call for "more" or "better" preparedness.[3] First, transformations in a series of overlapping processes—not just the existence of a vaccine candidate—are necessary to accelerate vaccine development and deployment. Second, "false alarms"—the outbreaks that fizzle out before becoming pandemics—and the data generated from them are important motivators, practice runs, and accelerators of speed, scale, and equitable access in pandemic responses (Fig. 3). When preparedness and response for pandemics rest on preparedness for and responses to smaller outbreaks, readiness becomes a dynamic and iterative effort wherein a series of research-driven innovations shrink timelines for the essential stages of vaccine development. Below, we briefly review key elements of such research for response.

3 There are various other definitions of the 100 Days Mission that start the clock differently or aim to reach a different endpoint (i.e., 100 days from an emergency declaration, as opposed to CEPI's definition of 100 days for the identification of a pathogen of pandemic potential). Note that the 100 days defined by CEPI are only intended to work towards initial authorization for vaccines, not immediate widespread use or other medical countermeasures for which feasibility constraints are different.

2.1 Rapid Response Platforms and Vaccine Libraries

One of CEPI's early goals was to develop platforms that could be used to rapidly make a vaccine in the event of an outbreak of a new or unknown disease, often referenced as Disease X. "Rapid response platforms" broadly refer to systems or technologies that use the same basic components but can be adapted for use against different pathogens by inserting new genetic or protein sequences. The most familiar example of such a system in the wake of COVID-19 is the mRNA plat-

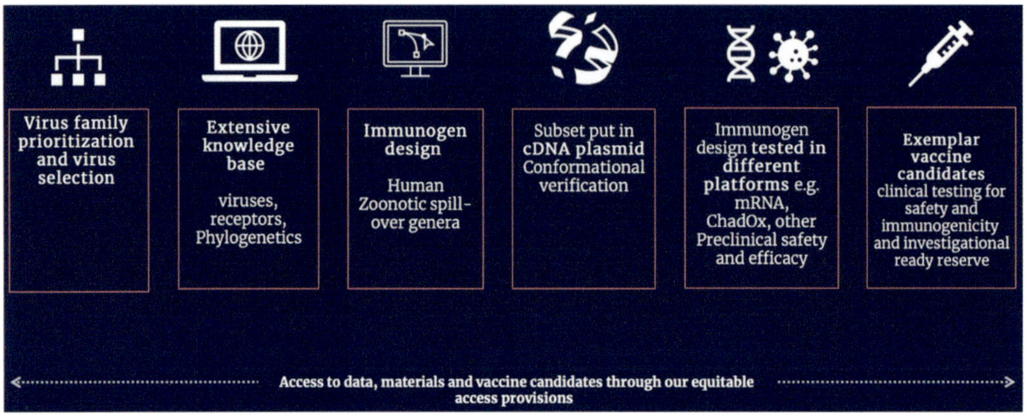

Fig. 4 Components of a vaccine library. (CEPI)

form used by Pfizer-BioNTech and Moderna for their COVID-19 vaccines, but there are other types of platforms and associated manufacturing processes that can be readied for rapid use against novel pathogens.

There are 26 families of viruses known to infect humans. Developing "prototype vaccines" against representative pathogens from viral families with the greatest pandemic potential would not only add to the often-limited toolkit for known pathogens—furthering possible ways to contribute to outbreak responses and further vaccine research—but also greatly improve our ability to respond to a novel pathogen from the given family. Creating a library of prototype vaccines for known pathogens on select rapid response platforms would provide platform-specific experience that could then be rapidly adapted to a new pathogen, such that a new sequence could be inserted in the well-characterized platform. Tested prototype vaccine candidates might also prove useful in their existing form if *in vitro* and *in vivo* data indicate that sufficient cross-protection may be elicited against a novel target. Such advances could permit preclinical work, initial human safety trials, manufacturing scale-up, and other accelerated stages of vaccine development to unfold in parallel. The precise sequence of steps and the extent to which they could be done simultaneously, rather than sequentially, would be governed by experience and judgement (Cassetti et al. 2022).

The various steps along the way to developing and determining inputs for prototype vaccines on rapid response platforms are technical milestones in their own right. Whether assembling the technical repertoire of host viral receptors and immunogen designs or expressing vaccine candidates as plasmids, steps that facilitate platform development and validation also bring together experts and build an increasingly robust foundation for preparedness and response (Fig. 4).

More broadly, rapid response platforms and vaccine libraries contribute to the 100DM by establishing an accessible knowledge base that catalyzes advances in parallel streams of medical countermeasure R&D. For example, as regulatory authorities gain experience with and gather data on a platform as it is used for vaccines, they will likely become more comfortable moving new vaccines or immunoprophylactics (e.g., monoclonal antibodies or antibody "cocktails") into clinical trials with adapted requirements, analogous to the annual approval of seasonal influenza vaccines produced on a very well-understood platform.

Despite the promise of rapid response platforms and vaccine libraries for a more integrated approach to preparedness and response, considerable challenges still remain beyond immediate technical concerns. Many of the vaccine constructs developed through a prototype or pan-family approach cannot be evaluated for real-world effectiveness in the absence of ongoing pathogen transmission. The research response of assessing candidates in rigorous clinical trials when it becomes epidemiologically feasible will require well-coordinated mobilization in an emerging outbreak—something that has often fallen short. The required investments of time, money, and scientific expertise to support innovation and infrastructure are considerable. At least some of the vaccines developed will likely never be used to counter pathogens; there are few commercial incentives to develop vaccines against diseases which may or may not ever become a serious concern, adding to the political complexity of such an endeavor. Intensive engagement with regulatory authorities will be required to evaluate where and how platform data can be used effectively to accelerate vaccine development. Even with extensive predictive efforts and ongoing research, prioritization across and within viral families will be necessary, requiring decisions in the face of insurmountable uncertainty. Ownership and sharing provisions around information, data, and constructs may in some contexts be highly contested. Carefully considering these and other such obstacles will be important to inform the best possible approaches to this channel of vaccine R&D.

2.2 Meeting Scientific Needs for the 100 Days Mission

Well-characterized assays, biomarkers, and correlates of protection are integral to the development of prototype vaccines and the rapid response platforms on which they will be made. CEPI's ambition is to support a globally distributed scientific infrastructure with the ability to collect and characterize biologic samples early in an outbreak, especially to develop animal models for testing candidate vaccines and to use advanced laboratory methods for assessing elicited immune responses. These advances work hand-in-hand with technical innovations for upstream problems such as antigen selection—for example, using artificial intelligence to optimize molecular design before preclinical testing can increase probabilities of success (CEPI 2023). CEPI continues to develop an animal model network and a clinical laboratory network with these goals in mind. These networks will support vaccine development while contributing to scientific opportunities and capacity building for regions that have typically been put at a disadvantage in these domains (► Chap. 14).

2.3 Manufacturing

Optimizing manufacturing to capitalize on the modularity offered by vaccine platform technologies is critical for response speed. Ready production capacity is important for scaling to initial investigational doses within the 100DM and then to the "second 100 days" and beyond, when delivery to large populations around the globe becomes an urgent priority. Crisis-ready scaling capacity could be facilitated by maintaining a global network of "warm" manufacturing facilities that routinely produce vaccines for national or regional use, with the ability to switch to emergency production with short notice. These facilities could change their output within days or weeks to produce vaccines in response to an outbreak.

For both economic and technical sustainability, these efforts require funding the creation and maintenance of a global network of facilities that cover multiple vaccine platforms, including mRNA, viral vector, and protein subunit vaccines. Numerous funders are supporting the establishment of expanded vaccine manufacturing, particularly in Africa. Vaccine factories cannot be quickly activated from dormancy to full production and need to be funded by markets in inter-epidemic periods for long-term operational sustainability. Brick and mortar facilities offer limited value without skilled and experienced personnel, quality systems, supply chain resilience, and other critical human and technical infrastructure. CEPI is supporting a network of "go-to" manufacturing facilities that produce vaccines on a regular basis and can be called upon to rapidly manufacture candidate vaccines, or to support rapid pandemic-scale manufacturing when needed. Among others, Plotkin et al.

(2017) have outlined some of the major challenges and requirements for vaccine manufacturing, and Kumraj et al. (2022) have presented some important proposals for expanding capacity in developing countries.

2.4 Clinical Trials

Developing vaccine candidates in advance and expanding response-ready manufacturing capabilities to produce them at scale are only as useful as the global response ecosystem's ability to assess vaccine safety and efficacy. The world's experience with betacoronaviruses through the twenty-first century exemplifies a possible new approach to regulatory approval for vaccines against novel pathogens. Knowledge from SARS-CoV-1 and MERS-CoV vaccine candidates helped accelerate SARS-CoV-2 development and clinical studies, while regulatory guidance across jurisdictions throughout the pandemic has facilitated rapid adaptation of COVID-19 vaccines to emerging variants (EMA 2023). With additional experience in other contexts, regulators could plausibly approve initial, carefully monitored use of a vaccine against an emerging pathogen based on fewer but extremely well-supported assessments, akin to how seasonal influenza vaccines are approved now.

However, evolving regulatory pathways—and improved local regulatory expertise—can only be effective if the infrastructure for emergency clinical trials exists in the first place. These studies must generate comprehensive data in time to accelerate vaccine development during an emergency and contribute to equitable access for vaccines. Bolstering capacity to run clinical trials closer to the point of need is one major component of such efforts. This allows for important research improvements, including simultaneous testing of multiple vaccines and trials in areas with higher disease prevalence (▶ Chap. 22). CEPI has recognized the foundational importance of the following three initiatives for its 100DM goals in the clinical and regulatory spheres and has begun working on some elements of them (CEPI 2021b, 2022c):

1. A global clinical trial network that is sustainable during interpandemic periods and conducts rigorous research which meets the needs of target populations, based on considerations similar to those outlined above for manufacturing.
2. A global clinical laboratory network for faster data readout, facilitated by rapid access to samples and standardized analyses.
3. National clinical trial volunteer registries to accelerate study enrollment and initiation.

These approaches to clinical trials and regulatory authorization are contingent on several key technical and procedural standards being established in "peacetime," then tested and refined through smaller crises. This includes developing accessible master files to build on prior knowledge and aid in robust protocol development while reducing administrative overhead (EFPIA et al. 2023), aligning regulatory standards across jurisdictions, and assembling and coordinating global clinical trial networks to assess vaccines in and for the populations that need them. Meanwhile, in silico models can help predict the likelihood of vaccine candidate success and inform choices of lead candidates and dosing levels.

As with any widespread attempt at harmonizing preparedness across jurisdictions, establishing and maintaining common systems across clinical trial sites, laboratories, and healthcare facilities globally would face political, ethical, and operational obstacles. Furthermore, sustaining this infrastructure during interpandemic periods requires business models that satisfy routine demand and generate revenue to keep the trial sites and laboratories active. There are several governance risks associated with collecting and managing information compiled by national registries. Other important considerations include personal data and confidentiality legislation, historically justified anxieties about studies in people that assess novel biomedical technologies and undefined threats, and limited trial registration within sub-populations that may be especially vulnerable to particular

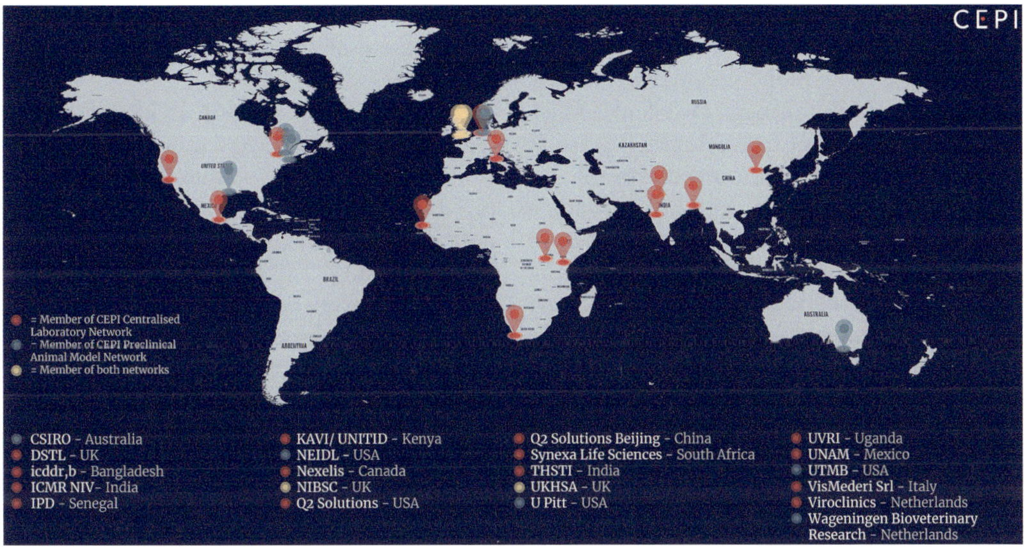

Fig. 5 CEPI's animal model and clinical research partnerships. (CEPI)

infectious diseases of concern. Cultivating a shared awareness of essential protections for patients, trial participants, communities, and citizens will help ensure standards are not compromised in the name of accelerated clinical studies (▶ Chaps. 4 and 18) (Fig. 5).

2.5 Engineering an Enabling Ecosystem

This brief overview of some core considerations for a holistic and more interconnected approach to preparedness and response—moving closer to making CEPI's 100DM a reality—focuses primarily on efforts directed toward vaccines. However, expeditiously and equitably developing vaccines would be functionally impossible without an array of other vital infrastructure. While these other components of pandemic preparedness and response are beyond CEPI's primary mandate, CEPI cannot be successful in its 100DM without them. Many were absent or insufficient before and throughout the COVID-19 pandemic, and lessons learned from ACT-A provide an important starting point for improved preparedness and response. Organizations across the global health ecosystem can continue to collaborate to realize these goals. Some of the broader considerations include, but are not limited to:

- Improved and expanded biosurveillance capacity (genomic, serological, etc.) to accurately detect an emerging infectious disease event early. Simply having a primary health care system where sick people can come and hope to be diagnosed and eventually treated is also essential but far from universal (▶ Chaps. 8 and 10).
- Stronger information sharing norms and provisions so what is (un)known about such an event can be communicated in a timely manner across various public health actors (▶ Chap. 7).
- Early epidemiological and clinical observation studies to establish key parameters (e.g., R_0, case fatality rate) and elucidate disease characteristics (e.g., mode of transmission, burden of asymptomatic disease, relationship between symptoms and transmission, pathophysiology, disease course). These must continue through an outbreak, given that quantities and dynamics can change over time—to say nothing of pathogen variants (▶ Chaps. 19 and 21).
- Swift, effective use of non-pharmaceutical interventions (e.g., contact tracing, social distancing) where applicable to suppress disease transmission.

- Accelerated development of advanced diagnostics and therapeutics, along with readiness to rapidly create and deploy them for a new pathogen (▶ Chap. 11).
- Improved medical technologies for use in lower or differently resourced settings.
- Strengthened delivery capacity (including cold chain infrastructure) to ensure access to vaccines for populations around the world. Development of vaccine platforms that are robust to temperature variations would be similarly helpful (▶ Chaps. 37 and 39).
- Engagement with communities, local and national governments, and regional organizations to design intervention strategies shaped by cultural norms and population needs (▶ Chap. 18, In Practices 18.1, and 18.2).
- Refinement of regulatory standards specific to the intended use case of and context for a medical countermeasure (▶ Chap. 6).
- Mechanisms to continue monitoring safety and efficacy as vaccines are rolled out (▶ Chap. 36).

Relatedly, no amount of preparedness can translate into an effective response, and in turn further preparedness, without clarity about when and how to mobilize. Mapping out which signals from early in an outbreak would activate pre-identified "no-regrets" levers across partners helps enable a coordinated research response to start in time to mitigate the ongoing outbreak and prevent future ones. "No-regrets" actions are those that an organization or country can and is willing to take once a certain condition is met, even if an outbreak does not then grow into a Public Health Emergency of International Concern (PHEIC). These can include mobilizing funding, collecting samples, activating clinical trials and manufacturing networks, or deploying personnel. One of the reasons research-based responses inform preparedness is that it justifies a willingness to take at-risk actions. Even when the payoff in a single instance is uncertain, a research response means that risk-benefit ratios favor acting to deploy and improve long-term preparedness efforts. Equally, having pre-determined "off-ramps" to know when to disengage ensures that research efforts are keyed as closely as possible to risk-tolerance thresholds.

The 100 Days Mission is less about the exact number of days and more about aiming toward much faster vaccine development in the event of an outbreak with pandemic potential. Coalescing around a goal starts a clock on every aspect of a response, which then informs key feasibility considerations in preparedness efforts and structures "lessons learned" to implement during future emerging outbreaks. It is also important to note that every research response is different. As such, preparedness efforts cannot be too rigidly dictated too rigidly by what has happened in the past. As the adage among epidemiologists emphasizes, "If you've seen one epidemic, you've seen one epidemic." Some assumptions will be tested and found wanting, and there will be oversights—things which we could not know or prepare for, or ought to have known and prepared for. However, we do know more than enough about outbreaks and epidemics to develop basic working checklists that ensure a coherent response—checklists which should be updated after each outbreak. This only further emphasizes that we must not squander the lessons learned over time, sometimes at a great cost, and that we must act on the cumulative experience and knowledge we have (◘ Fig. 5).

3 Systems Equity

The stark inequity in vaccine distribution and access across the globe has been one of the major features of the COVID-19 pandemic. Despite the best efforts of COVAX and ACT-A, many low- and middle-income countries did not have enough access to usable vaccines when they wanted and needed them—when supply was limited. Many high-income countries purchased a vast share of *future* available doses before low- and middle-income countries even began conversations about procurement. The highly coveted mRNA vaccines were difficult to transport and use in settings with limited cold-chain transport and storage capabilities. Variants of increased severity or transmissibility and limited supplies of medical countermeasures sometimes resulted in export controls that further sequestered vaccines, other countermeasures, and ancillary resources. However, by mid- to late 2023, there was a surplus of available vaccine doses as well as funding to purchase them, but very limited demand long after the height of the pandemic (Martuscelli 2023; Rigby 2023).

Speed and scale in outbreak response are often described as being at odds with equity. Conventional wisdom suggests a "moonshot" like the 100DM implies a high-tech race in which high-income countries compete to be the fastest to develop "their vaccines," thus systematically discounting the lives and needs of those outside of a select few countries. In practice, a national government's first responsibility is to its own citizens, and few politicians would be faulted for aiming to fulfill this responsibility. However, speed, scale, and equity are inseparable for CEPI. At the core of its 100DM is a belief that scarcity is the enemy of equity—that developing and delivering new epidemic vaccines at speed and scale enables *and* is enabled by greater global equity. The value chain of vaccine research, development, and delivery needs to be configured from the outset to produce equity as a "natural" output by overcoming the stumbling block of scarcity and cannot be pursued by any one actor alone. CEPI terms this approach "systems equity"—a way for the world to rethink its approach to pandemic preparedness and response, to put equity first rather than relegating it to an afterthought.

Factors historically delaying vaccine development, thus exacerbating inequitable access to vaccines and hindering pandemic responses more generally, have involved inadequate or absent:

- Coordination and clarity of roles.
- Research capacity where needed in outbreak settings, such as qualified clinical research programs in developing countries.
- Established financing mechanisms for R&D, at-risk manufacturing, and procurement so that funds are available when needed and low- and middle-income countries are not last in line.
- Operational infrastructure, legal provisions, and political agreements to better enable global access to vaccines, diagnostics, therapeutics, and critical equipment.

Focusing on these elements from the outset proved important to address problems with vaccine access throughout the COVID-19 pandemic. They continue to guide CEPI's broader approach to operationalizing systems equity. Maintaining an emphasis on the various competencies needed for a research-driven response—even outside of WHO-declared PHEICs—has also allowed CEPI to significantly advance vaccine candidates for its priority pathogens. This work has focused on settings where disease circulates but has been historically neglected, such that there are often no late-stage or licensed vaccines. To date, CEPI has advanced the first-ever Phase III trial for a chikungunya vaccine candidate and the first in-human Phase I trials for a Nipah vaccine candidate (CEPI 2020a, 2021c; Schneider et al. 2023). Several Lassa fever vaccine candidates are also in advanced stages of clinical development. CEPI's Enable research program to assess the burden of Lassa fever across West Africa is designed to further inform late-stage trial design while drawing on and bolstering local research capacity (CEPI 2020b). Such studies are underway to evaluate vaccine safety and efficacy in populations regularly affected by these diseases, rather than for relatively high-income travelers—as has historically been the case in other R&D efforts. Systems equity involves not only understanding and addressing disease in context through pathogen-specific interventions but also developing more general-purpose tools to make any intervention more feasible and effective. To this end, partners have been funded to advance more thermostable mRNA platforms to increase usability across settings. Manufacturing partnerships with L'Institut Pasteur de Dakar and Aspen in Africa are laying the foundation for CEPI's global manufacturing network and are crucial for increasing the share of vaccines manufactured in Africa, for Africa.

These examples demonstrate the foundational importance of researchers across the world finding roles to play anywhere along the spectrum of vaccine R&D and within the broader health ecosystem. This is equity in action—building regional capacity and developing locally driven vaccines to lay the foundation for moving away from scarcity. Through this model of systems equity, rapid, research-driven responses to emerging local outbreaks and longstanding endemic diseases begin to replace historically slow and inequitable global responses. The networks that CEPI is building to enhance manufacturing, clinical trials, animal models, and clinical labs aim to bring researchers from across the globe together around these goals.

4 International Coordination

It is important to acknowledge the obvious point that research alone cannot accomplish the 100DM and engender systems equity. Although CEPI's approach to research targets diseases and indications for which market incentives have failed, there are still additional political and economic questions to address beyond scarcity or expanded research collaborations alone. With major implications for preparedness and response, these issues include:

1. How to ensure vaccines developed in these novel contexts will be purchased and sold at affordable prices without leading to price gouging or high-income countries purchasing even greater shares of vaccine doses.
2. What is required to ensure technological innovations will be broadly and more rapidly shared.
3. How to account for intraregional and interregional heterogeneity.
4. How access and benefit sharing provisions or alternative equity-related mechanisms will be developed, negotiated, and enforced in multichannel markets for vaccine doses and funding.

Such considerations are beyond the scope of what CEPI or any one organization can take up alone. They raise broader questions for cross-partner deliberation about what success entails for an outbreak research response, including how equity gets defined and how to make decisions on some of these issues while the prospective Pandemic Accord remains under deliberation through the Intergovernmental Negotiating Body (INB) at the WHO (2023a).

More broadly, systems equity is only one core tenet of an emergency vaccine research response. The 100DM cannot be achieved without coordination across local, regional, and international partners. While increased local capacity and institutional expertise for vaccine R&D are important steps toward accelerating and improving research and response, there are crucial roles to be played by international partners to support efforts in regions and countries. Such coordination and collaboration are important to ensure that these efforts are productively contributing to global public health instead of potentially exacerbating forms of protectionist fragmentation and discord often produced during infectious disease emergencies.

Some of these questions have become more concrete through negotiations in international political fora, which primarily involve sovereign nations, that address issues such as access and benefit sharing, the definition of a pandemic, the role of zoonotic surveillance and spillover, and intellectual property regulations. These spaces for deliberation include, among others:

- The INB to draft and negotiate a convention, agreement or other international instrument for pandemic prevention, preparedness and response under the Constitution of the World Health Organization
- The Group of 20 (G20)
- The Group of Seven (G7)
- The Johannesburg Process for a Medical Countermeasures Network or Platform
- The September 2023 United Nations High-Level Meeting on Pandemic Prevention, Preparedness and Response

As negotiations evolve and geopolitical actors agree on new norms for pandemic preparedness and response, operational questions about how organizations work together, on what, and when—especially when each has a different primary focus and governance structure—remain alongside other more traditional nation-based political questions. It will be vital to develop international mechanisms to address technical, operational, and political challenges in a practical and coordinated way, learning from prior outbreaks through critical reflection and building on them with pragmatic but bold commitments for a healthier future.

5 Conclusion

Using the framework of the 100 Days Mission, this chapter presents CEPI's approach to emergency vaccine research as a form of outbreak preparedness and response and outlines key components to support these efforts. Accelerating vaccine development for future pandemics involves early preparatory activities, such as epidemiological research and regulatory-standard harmonization, that can precede outbreaks. It also requires a holistic or cyclical understanding of preparedness and response that emphasizes how each advances the other. As argued previously, "The knowledge that is generated through well-designed, effectively executed research in anticipation of, in the midst of, and after an emergency is critical to our future capacity to better achieve the overarching goals of preparedness and response: preventing injury, illness, disability, and death and supporting recovery" (Lurie et al. 2013). Beginning with specific ends in mind and building from what each of these goals may entail informs both inter-epidemic and crisis-time research. Reaching consensus around what research should be done and what it will take to achieve a goal like the 100DM means accounting for a broad range of considerations from different groups. It demands close engagement with researchers, policymakers, and the public to better understand community and country needs and to implement research that fits these specifications—and not solely in terms of vaccine hesitancy, though that too is important. Pandemics may be global events in one sense, but they are still experienced and understood differently by people across the world. Research-based response and preparedness is one important way to ensure that disease can be managed in an attentive, context-specific manner but within a broader, coordinated framework—working towards eventually preventing the next pandemic from ever growing beyond a small outbreak.

Discussion Questions

1. What is the goal of the 100 Days Mission?
2. What is the current timeline for developing a vaccine against a novel pathogen if no major, unanticipated obstacles arise?
3. What are the main systems and operational innovations that might accelerate vaccine development?
4. Does an infectious disease emergency spreading rapidly around the world, like COVID-19, justify relaxing vaccine safety and efficacy standards? Why or why not? What if a disease with much higher mortality, like SARS, caused the emergency?
5. How can vaccine development be accelerated without relaxing safety and efficacy standards?
6. Do countries or companies that contributed the most to developing and producing vaccines in an emergency have a right to preferential access to protect their own populations or seek the highest return on their investment, respectively?
7. What measures are available to ensure faster, more equitable distribution of rapidly developed vaccines in an emer-

gency, compared to the COVID-19 pandemic? What are the pros and cons of some these possibilities?

References

Cassetti MC, Pierson TC, Patterson LJ, Bok K, DeRocco AJ, Deschamps AM, et al. Prototype pathogen approach for vaccine and monoclonal antibody development: a critical component of the NIAID Plan for pandemic preparedness. J Infect Dis. 2022;227:1433. https://doi.org/10.1093/infdis/jiac296.

CEPI. CEPI-funded Nipah virus vaccine candidate first to reach phase 1 clinical trial. Oslo, Norway: Coalition for Epidemic Preparedness Innovations; 2020a.

CEPI. Largest-ever Lassa fever research programme launches in West Africa. Oslo, Norway: Coalition for Epidemic Preparedness Innovations (CEPI); 2020b.

CEPI. CEPI 2.0 program document. Oslo, Norway: Coalition for Epidemic Preparedness Innovations (CEPI); 2021a.

CEPI. CEPI and IVI collaborate on clinical research to expand access to COVID-19 vaccines in Africa. Oslo, Norway: Coalition for Epidemic Preparedness Innovations (CEPI); 2021b.

CEPI. Nipah virus: the deadly illness without a vaccine. Oslo, Norway: Coalition for Epidemic Preparedness Innovations (CEPI); 2021c.

CEPI. CEPI, UK government, and life sciences industry unite around 100 days mission. Oslo, Norway: Coalition for Epidemic Preparedness Innovations (CEPI); 2022a.

CEPI. COVAX: CEPI's response to COVID-19. Oslo, Norway: CEPI; 2022b. https://cepi.net/covax/. Accessed 9 Nov 2022.

CEPI. Delivering pandemic vaccines in 100 days—what will it take? Oslo, Norway: Coalition for Epidemic Preparedness Innovations (CEPI); 2022c.

CEPI. Global community comes together in support of 100 Days Mission and pledges over $1.5 billion for CEPI's pandemic-busting plan. Oslo, Norway: Coalition for Epidemic Preparedenss Initiatives (CEPI); 2022d.

CEPI. Using AI to speed up vaccine development against disease X. Oslo, Norway: Coalition for Epidemic Preparedenss Initiatives (CEPI); 2023.

EFPIA, CEPI, VE. Expanding master files for human medicinal products in the EU/EEA. Brussels: EFPIA, CEPI, VE; 2023.

EMA. Global regulators agree on way forward to adapt COVID-19 vaccines to emerging variants. Amsterdam: European Medicines Agency; 2023.

Hatchett R, Lurie N. Outbreak response as an essential component of vaccine development. Lancet Infect Dis. 2019;19(11):e399–403. https://doi.org/10.1016/s1473-3099(19)30305-6.

IFPMA. Biopharmaceutical industry collaborates on the implementation of the G7 100 Days Mission to improve readiness for future pandemics. Geneva: International Federation of Pharmaceutical Manufacturers and Associations (IFPMA); 2021.

IPP Secretariat. 100 Days Mission. London: Wellcome Trust; 2023. https://ippsecretariat.org. Accessed 2 Sept 2023.

Kumraj G, Pathak S, Shah S, Majumder P, Jain J, Bhati D, et al. Capacity building for vaccine manufacturing across developing countries: the way forward. Hum Vaccine Immunother. 2022;18(1):2020529. https://doi.org/10.1080/21645515.2021.2020529.

Lurie N, Manolio T, Patterson AP, Collins F, Frieden T. Research as a part of public health emergency response. N Engl J Med. 2013;368(13):1251–5. https://doi.org/10.1056/nejmsb1209510.

Martuscelli C. Germany on track to bin 200M COVID-19 vaccine doses. Politico Europe; 2023.

Pandemic Institute. The UK pandemic sciences network. Liverpool, UK: The Pandemic Institute; 2023. https://www.thepandemicinstitute.org. Accessed 2 Sept 2023.

Plotkin S, Robinson JM, Cunningham G, Iqbal R, Larsen S. The complexity and cost of vaccine manufacturing—an overview. Vaccine. 2017;35(33):4064–71. https://doi.org/10.1016/j.vaccine.2017.06.003.

Rigby J. COVID-19 vaccine scheme for poorest has $2.6 billion left to spend as pandemic recedes. Reuters; 2023.

Rodgers J. How CEPI-funded research is supporting the COVID-19 vaccine rollout. Oslo, Norway: Coalition for Epidemic Preparedness Innovations (CEPI); 2020.

Samarasekera U. Solidarity against Ebola: an update. Lancet Microbe. 2023;4(3):e139. https://doi.org/10.1016/S2666-5247(23)00035-6.

Schneider M, Narciso-Abraham M, Hadl S, McMahon R, Toepfer S, Fuchs U, et al. Safety and immunogenicity of a single-shot live-attenuated chikungunya vaccine: a double-blind, multicentre, randomised, placebo-controlled, phase 3 trial. Lancet. 2023;401(10394):2138–47. https://doi.org/10.1016/S0140-6736(23)00641-4.

UK.gov. COVID-19 response—Spring 2021. London: UK Government; 2021. https://www.gov.uk/government/publications/covid-19-response-spring-2021/

covid-19-response-spring-2021. Accessed 2 Sept 2023.

White House. American pandemic preparedness: transforming our capabilities. Washington, DC: White House; 2021.

WHO. International negotiating body. Geneva: World Health Organization; 2023a. https://inb.who.int. Accessed 8 Sept 2023.

WHO. WHO coronavirus (COVID-19) dashboard. Geneva: World Health Organization; 2023b. https://covid19.who.int. Accessed 8 Sept 2023.

WHO. WHO R&D blueprint. Geneva: World Health Organization; 2023c. https://www.who.int/observatories/global-observatory-on-health-research-and-development/analyses-and-syntheses/who-r-d-blueprint/background. Accessed 28 Aug 2023.

World Bank. Money and microbes: strengthening clinical research capacity to prevent epidemics. Washington, DC: World Bank Group; 2018.

14 Accelerating Development of Therapeutics for Preparedness, Response, and a More Secure World

Elizabeth S. Higgs

Contents

Learning Track Note: This chapter appears in Learning Tracks: Clinical Research; Preparedness

E. S. Higgs and R. A. Sorenson (eds.), *Principles and Practice of Emergency Research Response*, https://doi.org/10.1007/978-3-031-48408-7_17

Learning Objectives

This chapter will help readers understand and describe:

- The overall therapeutics development process and steps for acceleration from bench to bedside
- The optimal achievable therapeutics preparedness state to develop, assess in clinical trials, and distribute new authorized or licensed medical countermeasures (MCMs) in time to affect epidemics or pandemics
- How market failures hinder an ideal therapeutics preparedness state
- Regulatory reforms to accelerate preclinical development and reduce reliance on animal models
- The G7 Therapeutics and Vaccines Clinical Trials Charter and WHA Resolution 75.8 and what prompted them
- Some innovations in clinical trial design and execution
- The benefits of large-scale, well-designed randomized clinical studies structured by a master protocol:
  - Advantages of global master protocols
  - Platform approaches to curating clinical research priorities
  - Ways to increase clinical trial flexibility
  - Why populations that have been underrepresented in past clinical research need to be included
  - Advantages of a global clinical research network
- The need for innovations in global regulatory coordination for health emergencies
- How social value created by research should be available to all populations who may benefit from it
- The importance of multitasking to advance accelerated therapeutic development during an emergency
- The importance of implementing Good Participatory Practice (GPP) guidelines during accelerated therapeutics development for a health emergency
- The role of clinical practice guidelines in the context of accelerated therapeutics development, scale-up, and use in a health emergency

1 Introduction

Research to develop therapeutics is essential to pandemic preparedness and emergency response. In an ideal preparedness state, safe, effective therapeutics, along with knowledge of how to use them and scale production as needed would be available for all known pathogens of epidemic and pandemic potential. A more practical but still ambitious goal is to have candidate therapeutics available for one or more member species of all viral families with epidemic and/or pandemic potential. When used appropriately, effective therapeutics mitigate morbidity, minimize mortality, reduce disease severity and hospitalization, and prevent new infections in all segments of the population, including frontline health workers and vulnerable populations. In an ideal preparedness state, we would understand the pathogen natural history, know which populations are likely to be disproportionally affected by a pathogen and therefore most likely to benefit from therapeutics, and we would have safety and efficacy data for these populations. Special populations include infants, children, pregnant women, the elderly, immunocompromised individuals, and those with multiple comorbidities and underlying medical conditions.

The need for accelerated development of therapeutics aligns with the *100 Days Mission* goal, established by the G7 health leadership in June 2021 and adopted by the Coalition for Epidemic Preparedness Innovations (CEPI), the U.S. Government (USG), the World Health Organization (WHO), the United Kingdom (UK), and many other governments and multilaterals (Kelland 2023; Pandemic Preparedness Partnership 2021; White House 2022). The premise is that the faster we can develop safe, effective vaccines, therapeutics, and diagnostics (VTDs) for an escalating infectious disease outbreak, the more likely we will save lives and contain the outbreak. For all the VTDs, focused preparedness work is needed to accelerate development in interpandemic periods and enable immediate, efficient, accelerated research response to outbreaks, epidemics, and pandemics.

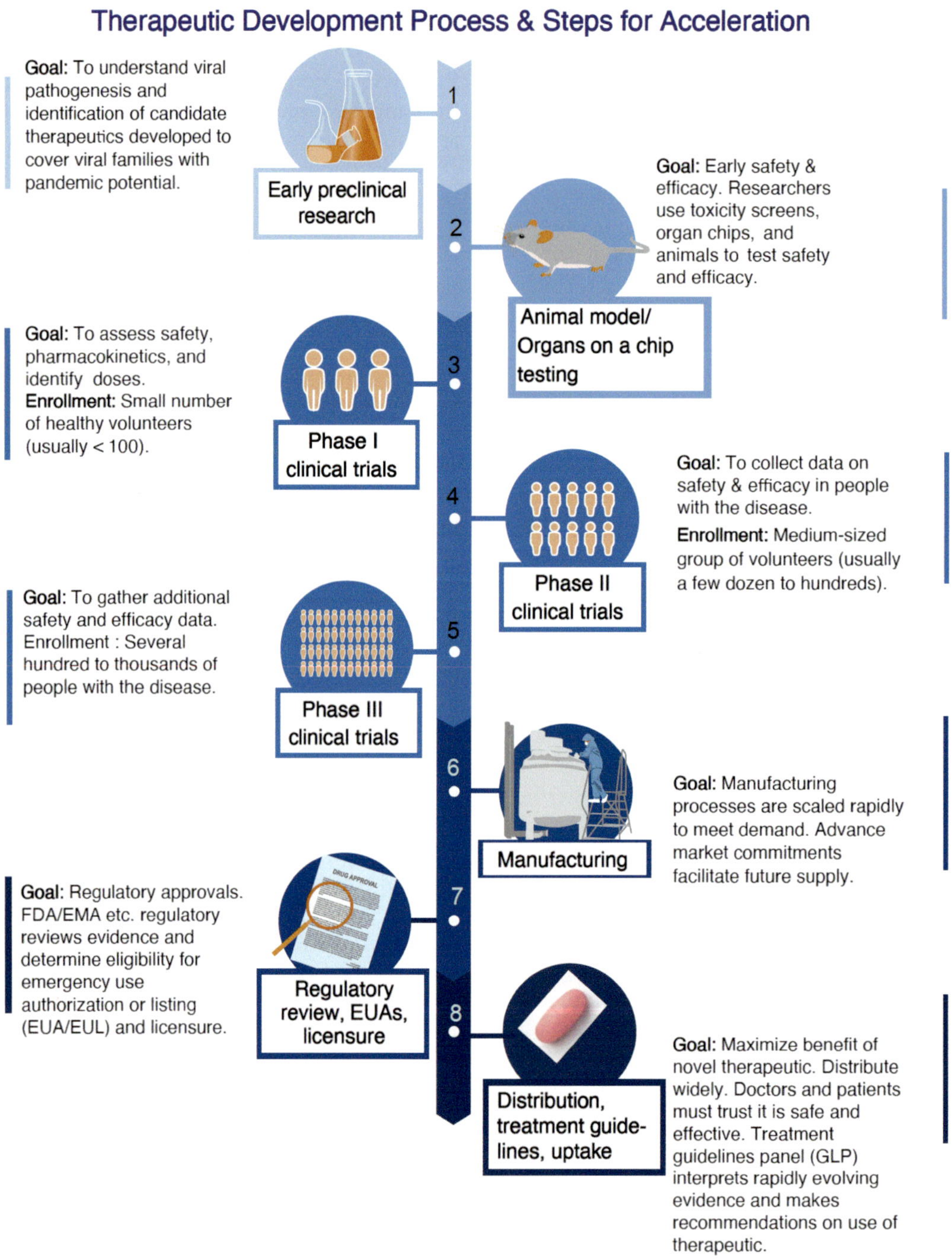

Fig. 1 Therapeutics Development Process and Steps for Acceleration. (Author, loosely based on a figure in a public domain U.S. Government Accountability Office report (GAO 2023))

Accelerated development of therapeutics refers to the process of expediting end-to-end development, regulatory authorization or approval, manufacturing, and delivery. Acceleration can be accomplished at every stage of the "bench to bedside" process (Fig. 1), including increased funding for early drug development; streamlining clinical trials; strengthening coordinated global clinical trial capacity and infrastructure; coordinating global clinical trials; ongoing advancement of clinical research in interpandemic periods; and increased collaboration between governments, academia, NGOs, and the private sector. Innovations in manufacturing to enable rapid scale-up of production, along with innovations in distribution and delivery to patients, are also essential. The primary goal of accelerated therapeutics development is to bring safe, effective treatments and prophylaxis as quickly as possible to patients and those who could be infected in health emergencies, particularly for pathogens which cause life-threatening disease or debilitating long-term conditions.

While scientific innovation and clinical research to validate safety and efficacy are essential to accelerated therapeutics development, population confidence and beliefs about research and development and the resulting products can make or break their social acceptance and use, and thus their impact on an outbreak. Clearly, if the target population refuses to use a medical countermeasure (MCM) it cannot save lives or contain outbreaks (▶ Chap. 18). In contrast, population confidence in therapeutics safety and efficacy offers secondary benefits to the pandemic response by reducing fear, encouraging early care seeking by both exposed and infected individuals, potentially reducing the time of infectivity, and encouraging the use of prophylactic agents. Empowering people to be treated outside of hospitals reduces fear as well as stress on the health care system, minimizing disruption and interruptions to care for others. Access to pre- and post-exposure prophylaxis reduces risks to healthcare workers, enabling better patient care. This is especially important with highly transmissible pathogens such as respiratory viruses and high-mortality ones like filoviruses. Finally, promoting VTD confidence among high-risk populations encourages uptake and helps protect the most vulnerable, such as pregnant women (Zika), essential workers, the elderly in nursing homes, etc. An underappreciated aspect of therapeutics preparedness is the engagement of intended users of putative therapeutics in the research process. Now, just as during the coronavirus disease 2019 (COVID-19) pandemic, much remains to be done to prepare to deliver on the full promise of therapeutics in outbreaks, epidemics, and pandemics.

Three essential principles for accelerated therapeutics preparedness and research response are relevant for all segments of the therapeutics development pipeline: (1) be prepared to respond, (2) multitask (run processes in parallel rather than in sequence) to accelerate research and development in an emergency, and (3) collaborate and synergize, e.g., include multiple voices throughout the process. Before turning to these three principles and how they can be implemented, an overview of the traditional therapeutic development pathway and how it could be reimagined is warranted.

2 Accelerated Therapeutics Development: The Traditional Pipeline Re-envisioned

The development timeline for therapeutics has commonly stretched over a decade or more, culminating if successful in regulatory licensure and followed by promotion to health care providers. Clearly this is much too slow for a public health emergency, especially since the experience of the past decade has demonstrated that VTDs can be developed much more quickly and that clinical trials can be implemented even in unstable conditions in fragile states (▶ Chap. 16) (Mulangu et al. 2019). The preparedness vision for therapeutics development must begin with the end in mind—safe, effective therapies available to all who can benefit from them. A global health security approach to accelerated therapeutics development should therefore be envisioned as a "bench to bedside" process, beginning with the identification of candidate therapeutics and ending with adequate manufacturing to enable uptake at scale by all those who need a safe and effective medicine. Preparedness must also include public education to promote a better understanding of the research and development process, from individuals participating in trials to their communities and countries, as a partial antidote to the disinformation and misinformation that has so bedeviled the COVID-19 response (van der Linden 2022).

2.1 Faster Steps

Measures to accelerate each step in the process can be taken during preparedness (interpandemic periods) as well as during an emergency research response to outbreaks, epidemics, and pandemics. If pandemic preparedness is properly implemented, therapeutics candidates for even novel pathogens in a high-risk family of viruses with pandemic potential will be available. These therapeutics candidates will have been investigated through Phase IIa clinical trials, producing preliminary conclusions about safety and potential efficacy. Candidates can then be rapidly screened for in vitro efficacy against novel pathogen X from known virus family Y.[1] Generally, the therapeutics development process can be broken into eight steps from bench to bedside (◘ Fig. 1):

2.1.1 Identification and Creation of Therapeutic Candidates

Identification and creation of therapeutic candidates involve basic research on both pathogens and how pathogens interact with human physiology to identify therapeutic targets. Reflection on the advances in human immunodeficiency virus (HIV) therapeutics over the past 20+ years reveals the critical importance of understanding viral pathogenesis and fully exploiting virologic mechanisms as therapeutic targets. Innovative approaches to identifying therapeutic candidates have expanded beyond screening compound libraries in vitro to rational drug design leveraging three-dimensional imaging, artificial intelligence, and machine learning. Hopefully, preparedness will enable us to have a "stable" of putative therapeutic candidates, including biologics, ready for screening when there is a zoonotic transmission event which causes human disease with novel pathogen X.

2.1.2 Preclinical Toxicity and Efficacy Studies

Preclinical toxicity and efficacy studies are no longer limited to animal models. Advances in in vitro technologies like "organs on a chip" (see ▶ Sect. 6.1 below) can facilitate early assessments of safety and efficacy, as well as characterize disease pathogenesis.

2.1.3 Human Drug Trials Are Traditionally Conducted Sequentially in Phases I, II, III, and IV

Human drug trials are traditionally conducted sequentially in Phases I, II, III, and IV, often at separate sites or clinical trial networks with a temporal gap between phases and separate trials of therapeutics for different indications. However, innovation in clinical trial design and infrastructure to prepare for emergencies can close these gaps and allow investigators to plan trials that overlap so that early Phase II trials can begin when Phase I trials are providing their first solid results.

2.1.4 Phase I Trials

Phase I trials provide a preliminary assessment of safety and dosage ranging should be conducted in interpandemic periods for multiple candidate therapeutics for each viral family that infects humans in a broad range of populations. Traditionally, Phase I studies have been conducted in developed countries, in part to avoid the perception of exploitation of populations in low- and middle-income countries (LMICs). In an emergency, however, this paternalistic approach does not serve as an expedited response when knowledge and acceptance of safety, tolerability, and pharmacokinetics is needed in the population for whom the product will be used.

2.1.5 Phase II Studies

Phase II studies provide additional data on safety, tolerability, and early signals of efficacy for the disease of interest in the populations infected, as well as additional information on

1 Most efforts to date are focused on viruses as the most frequent cause of outbreaks, but the approach applies in principle to other pathogens like bacteria and fungi.

dosing and duration. Phase II studies are often divided into Phase IIa and Phase IIb. Phase IIa studies focus on dosing, pharmacokinetics and pharmacodynamics, and/or specific sub-populations such as children, HIV+ persons, elderly, etc. Phase IIb trials focus on safety and efficacy at the selected dose. Phase II studies may rapidly enable Phase III study initiation in health emergencies. In this scenario, the study is designated Phase IIb/III or sometimes just Phase III. The importance of both dose and duration has often been underestimated, particularly during health emergencies. Though studies are still pending and data are inconclusive at the time of this writing, the short half-life of Paxlovid® and the prescribed 5-day course may be related to the many reports of clinical and virologic rebound in severe acute respiratory syndrome coronavirus 2 (SARS-CoV-2), at a rate yet to be determined (Akinosoglou et al. 2022). However, it is clear that biphasic illness occurs in persons with COVID-19 cases even without treatment. Regardless of etiology, concern over rebound among physicians and patients is thought to be contributing to the underutilization of Paxlovid®, which is 89% effective in preventing progression of disease and death and quite safe (McGarry et al. 2023). Promising therapeutics that have completed Phase IIa trials should be available in sufficient quantities, with up-to-date stability data, to allow for rapid initiation of Phase IIb/III studies in an outbreak.

2.1.6 Phase III Studies

Phase III studies provide additional safety and efficacy data on a larger group of participants with the disease of interest. One or two well-designed and implemented studies should be adequate for licensure. Moreover, innovation in trial design for use in health emergencies allows Phases II and III to merge into one protocol.

2.1.7 Manufacturing Innovation, Production Locations, and Capacity to Scale Up

Manufacturing innovation, production locations, and capacity to scale up have been highlighted during the COVID-19 pandemic. Progress in these areas is closely tied to demands for equity of access to the medical and social benefits of clinical trials. Equity of access must be balanced by the principle of utility; that is, when VTDs are scarce, they should be allocated and distributed to provide the greatest benefit. In response to the need for greater equity in access to therapeutics and other pandemic countermeasures, innovation and investment in manufacturing capacity for both biologics and small molecules are essential to ensuring all those who can benefit have access.

2.1.8 Regulatory Review

Regulatory review is the standard process of assessing data quality and strength to determine whether a product is safe and effective for a given indication. Normally, this results in approval or denial of a license to market the product, but emergency use authorization or its equivalent is an option available to regulatory agencies when warranted. The COVID-19 pandemic revealed the need during health emergencies for both greater global cooperation and accelerated, flexible processes that do not compromise safety or efficacy in the regulatory review of clinical trials (► Chap. 6).

2.1.9 Access to an Approved Therapeutic Is a Multistep Process

Even when a product receives an emergency use authorization, manufacturing must be scaled up, and products must be distributed, prescribed by physicians, and accepted by patients. Treatment guideline panels play a critical role in evaluating evolving clinical trial data to help provide treatment and clinical care guidance in a health emergency (► Chap. 20). As evidence quality and strength can be variable, especially in an emergency, physicians need confidence to prescribe therapies with an appropriate balance of risk and benefit. Not all countries will approve or recommend the same therapies. For example, the antiviral remdesivir was the first licensed COVID-19 therapy in the United States but was not recommended by the WHO Treatment

Guidelines (Beigel et al. 2020; WHO 2020; WHO Solidarity Trial Consortium 2022). Finally, patient uptake/demand for novel therapeutics hinges upon confidence in the research process (Trogen et al. 2020; Wilson et al. 2021). As noted frequently in this volume, demonstrating actionable evidence through rigorous clinical trials is not the final goal. Countries, health systems, physicians, and patients must accept and use the novel therapeutic to mitigate morbidity and mortality. That requires confidence in the research process based on effective communication among researchers, the populace, and decision-makers.

3 Vision for Preparedness: What Does Success Look Like?

Preparedness to advance MCMs through emergency research response is in its relative infancy. Until very recently, the vision for an ideal preparedness state was neglected, largely because it was not believed feasible to develop, assess in clinical trials, and distribute a new MCM in time to change the course of an epidemic or pandemic. Even in 2023, as tools for scientific discovery become ever more powerful, the pipeline for candidate therapeutics for pathogens with pandemic potential and high-risk viral families is extremely limited. Together, the political and scientific research community can do better. Going from the current paucity of licensed and candidate therapeutics for pathogens with pandemic potential to real therapeutic preparedness will require a new vision, sustained investments, global focus, innovation, and a process to address market failures. Being prepared is multifaceted and involves all parts of the therapeutic development pipeline, as well as improving research systems to counter endemic challenges and remain in readiness to conduct high-quality clinical research in emergencies. Proper preparation promotes efficiency, guards against poor performance and costly delays, and encourages research stakeholders and potentially affected populations to begin to work together well in advance of health emergencies.

In the wake of the COVID-19 pandemic, there are promising national, multilateral, and global steps towards envisioning and enabling a more ideal therapeutics preparedness state inclusive of equity, collaboration, and strengthening of global clinical trials (G7 2021; GLOPID-R 2023; White House 2022; WHO 2022b).

Analogous to the popular phrase "lab to jab" referring to vaccines, the therapeutics vision should be thought of as "bench to bedside" (◘ Fig. 1). An ideal state of preparedness would support interpandemic preclinical and clinical research to advance therapeutics candidates as far as possible in the development pipeline, even in the absence of active, human-to-human transmission of the pathogens they are designed to counter. Sometimes, as with influenza or respiratory syncytial virus (RSV), endemic pathogens provide the opportunity to leverage ongoing human transmission and disease to advance candidate therapeutics through Phase III trials, licensing, and stockpiling.

In the absence of endemic disease, the prototype pathogen approach to generating candidate VTDs for viruses with pandemic potential has been widely accepted as a preparedness strategy (Cassetti et al. 2022; Ford et al. 2023) (▶ Chap. 12). In a nutshell, the prototype pathogen approach leverages the fact that viruses within families have similar properties. Thus, if a new virus X emerges within a taxonomic family Y, it is likely to share properties with other Y viruses. The goal, then, is to select a known pathogen within a viral family and to develop a generalizable MCM approach that shows applicability against other viruses in the same viral family, based on the postulate that this will include novel viruses that may emerge from that family in the future (◘ Fig. 2). By developing candidate VTDs for the prototype pathogen during interpandemic times, this approach readies VTD candidates for imme-

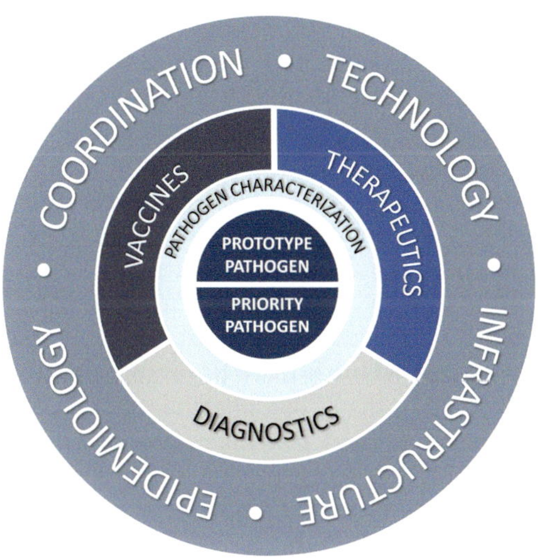

Fig. 2 NIAID's Pandemic Preparedness Plan (NIAID, USG public domain) (▶ https://www.niaid.nih.gov/sites/default/files/pandemic-preparedness-plan.pdf)

diate research response to outbreaks caused by novel pathogens, as long as they fall into a known virus family. Other things being equal, this head start on research response should considerably shorten timelines for regulatory authorization and manufacturing.

The target end state for therapeutics preparedness is to have licensed, approved therapeutics for at least one prototype pathogen from each high-risk viral family with pandemic potential and for all known pathogens with pandemic potential, along with adequate stockpiles or ability to quickly scale up to protect all segments of the population. We are a long way from this level of preparedness. A step in this direction would be to assess candidate therapeutics through clinical trial Phase IIa for all known pathogens with pandemic potential, with adequate product available for immediate later-stage trials in an outbreak. In many circumstances, demonstration of human efficacy is not possible until an outbreak occurs (NASEM 2017a). Even when a therapeutic is approved under the U.S. Food and Drug Administration (FDA) Animal Rule (United States only), it should not be assumed that it will be safe and effective when used to treat the disease in humans (FDA 2023). Candidate therapeutics, both direct-acting agents and biologics, should be ready "on the shelf" in sufficient quantities for rapid, large-scale clinical trials.

4 Applying the Lessons of Past Therapeutics Development and Use

It is important to apply what we have learned from past therapeutics development to future research responses to infectious disease pathogens. For example, RNA viruses, such as coronaviruses, mutate with greater frequency than DNA viruses, yet DNA viruses such as mpox clade 1 evolution to clade 1b demonstrates adaptations as well. Thus, for both RNA and DNA viruses to prevent therapeutic resistance, therapeutics that target more than one part of the virus lifecycle are needed (Robson et al. 2020), as with the therapeutic approach to HIV-acquired immunodeficiency syndrome (AIDS). Therapeutic monoclonal antibodies targeting single immune epitopes are vulnerable to immune escape and loss of efficacy as increasing population immunity exerts adaptive pressure on viral mutations unless the targeted epitope is highly conserved. In the course of the COVID-19 pandemic, the neutralization efficacy of hard-won anti-SARS-CoV-2 monoclonal antibody therapy products was lost, one by one, as viral evolution produced new strains. Future preparedness and response efforts need to anticipate viral evolution and resistance, and greater attention should be focused on strategies to prevent resistance, including targeting conserved epitopes, combining monoclonal antibodies with differing target epitopes, combining biologics with direct-acting antiviral agents, etc.

It is equally important to build on past success in therapeutic strategies. For example, the experience of using immune-system modulators in COVID-19 must be remembered and should be better understood. After decades of failed randomized clinical trials assessing the efficacy of immunomodulators in adult respiratory distress syndrome (ARDS), it came as a pleasant surprise to many ARDS experts that immunomodulation by the existing generic steroid dexamethasone provided up to 40% mortality benefit in sicker COVID-19 patients (Kalil et al. 2020; RECOVERY Collaborative Group 2020; Wolfe et al. 2022). In other diseases, steroids have contributed to excess mortality. It is likely that host (immune system) targeted therapeutics may be life-saving during specific stages of a disease process, e.g., steroids in severe COVID-19, while harmful in others, e.g., steroids in early stage COVID-19. Whenever a novel disease arises, thorough natural history studies are essential to understand disease pathogenesis, characterize comorbidities that alter the risk of disease progression and severity, and categorize clinical stages of the disease that might call for different types of interventions (▶ Chap. 19).

5 Rectifying Market Failures to Foster Therapeutic Preparedness

In addition to a new vision for therapeutics preparedness, adequate resourcing for therapeutics development for pandemic pathogens is needed. Historically, market forces have dominated and driven therapeutics development. Neither therapeutics for pathogens with pandemic potential nor therapeutics for pathogens disproportionately impacting the world's poorest countries have fared well in a market-driven therapeutics economy (Viergever 2013). While many pharmaceutical companies invest in neglected diseases, these investments contribute little to profit margins. It is tempting to disparage pharmaceutical companies for lack of investment in these areas, but many are for-profit organizations with boards and investors holding them accountable. More thought is needed to ensure global engagement of research innovators regardless of their origin. Even in their most commercially motivated investments, pharmaceutical companies drive a great deal of therapeutic invention, as evidenced by the rapid development of the mRNA vaccine technology. Meanwhile, innovative public-private partnerships work to advance non-commercial research, negotiate affordable prices and fund life-saving childhood vaccinations and other interventions in low-income countries. Among many, three leaders in this area are Gavi, the Vaccine Alliance, the Bill & Melinda Gates Foundation, and PATH.

Box 1: Gavi, the Vaccine Alliance

Gavi's mission is to protect people's health throughout their lives by increasing equitable and sustainable use of vaccines, especially to vaccinate the world's poorest children. Gavi calculates that it has prevented some 16 million future deaths (Gavi 2022). GAVI leverages the comparative advantages of its public and private partners (◘ Fig. 3), blending public institutions' scientific and technical expertise with the production capacity and business acumen of private industry. Since they deliver over half the world's childhood vaccines, they can negotiate a much lower price by pooling demand and guaranteeing the purchase of vaccines, securing long-term funding to bring vaccines to the poorest countries while de-risking vaccine development (Gavi 2023).

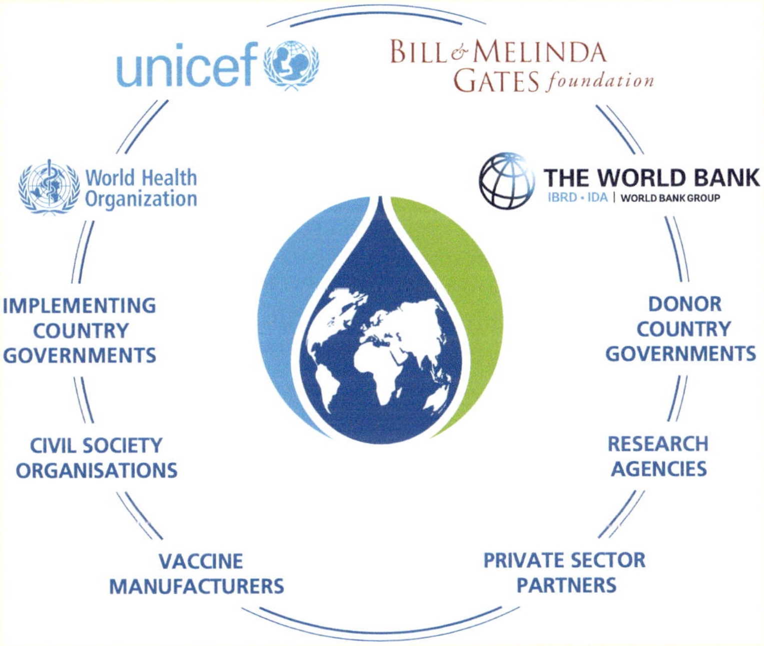

Fig. 3 Graphic from Gavi, the Vaccine Alliance, showing the diverse partners it works with to bring vaccines to those who need them, with a strong focus on the needs of children in the world's lowest-income countries. (Courtesy Gavi)

During the COVID-19 pandemic, Gavi, the Vaccine Alliance; the Gates Foundation; and WHO started the Access to COVID-19 Tools Accelerator (ACT-A), based on the Gavi model, to provide equitable access to vaccines (COVAX), therapeutics, and diagnostics to countries unable to purchase and/or acquire their own (WHO 2022a). The ACT-A for therapeutics focused on the delivery of basic COVID-19 treatments: oxygen, dexamethasone, and antivirals once they were recommended in the WHO therapeutic guidelines. Certainly, therapeutic preparedness must address end-to-end equity issues as well. From this perspective, pandemics are a great equalizer—ignoring zoonotic pathogens in LMICs is a risk for all nations, rich and poor (► Chap. 10). The development and distribution of therapeutics must be determined by need and not restricted to national boundaries or wealthier countries alone.

Governments, international organizations, foundations, and others are moving to fill the market gap for MCMs that do not offer sufficient commercial return on investment. Following SARS-1 and concerns about highly pathogenic H5N1 influenza in Asia, the U.S. government established the Biomedical Advanced Research and Development Authority (BARDA) in 2006 to advance MCMs for emerging and reemerging infectious diseases and other bioincidents, e.g., accidental release of pathogens from laboratories or bioterrorism. The Coalition for Epidemic Preparedness Innovations (CEPI) was established following the 2014–2016 West African Ebola outbreak (► Chap. 13). The European Commission established the Health Emergency Preparedness and Response Authority (HERA) as a new directorate in September 2021 in response to the COVID-19 pandemic to ensure that medicines, vaccines, and other MCMs are rapidly developed, manufactured, and made readily available (EC 2024) inside and outside the EU. Ensuring additional support for MCM product pipelines of pathogens with pandemic potential is critical.

6 Innovate to Accelerate

Envisioning and incentivizing resources for an ideal therapeutics preparedness state is in the interest of everyone, but success will also require a great deal of scientific innovation, public and private partnerships, multilateral cooperation, and strategic thinking. Some of the major building blocks:

- Sustainable global clinical trial networks conducting rigorous research on countermeasures for endemic pathogens and pathogen families with pandemic potential, prepared to pivot to novel pathogens—or known pathogens with new features—when they emerge
- National and international funding and partnerships for expanding clinical trial networks and building the infrastructure—both physical and human resources—for the years before new research capacity can sustain itself
- Global consultation and coordination to minimize trials unlikely to produce regulatory-level results, as well as to synergize, accelerate, and avoid duplication of efforts in well-designed and conducted trials
- Trust that global efforts to reduce infectious disease threats are not just a cover for commercial gain or nefarious conspiracies

6.1 Innovation in Preclinical Pipeline

Innovation is needed throughout the therapeutics development pipelines—preclinical, clinical, manufacturing, and delivery. COVID-19 has spawned a great deal of scientific innovation across the therapeutics pipeline. Leveraging machine learning and artificial intelligence (AI) to predict drug targets, predicting the activity of small molecules based on 3D molecular and chemical structures, and modelling pharmacokinetics and pharmacodynamics, etc., are among the innovations that are in use and being further developed to accelerate discovery and development of small molecules and biologics (Borkotoky et al. 2022).

There are also many innovative efforts underway to accelerate preclinical development and get more accurate initial assessments of whether therapeutic products will be safe and effective in humans, with less reliance on animal models. For decades animal models have been the gold standard for selecting therapeutics to move into human studies. Because certainty about how closely animal models mimic human physiology or pathophysiology is elusive, animal results can be misleading—"Mice lie and monkeys exaggerate"—David Weiner, quoted by Paul Offit (2017). Reducing animal suffering in scientific research to the indispensable minimum is also a driving force here (NIH 2023).

Several innovations are in development as alternatives to animal models. They are designed to mimic biological systems (the respiratory, liver, or gastrointestinal system, for example) and how human disease affects them. Potentially these innovations can more accurately replicate therapeutic toxicity and efficacy in human disease than animal models. Such approaches include 3D cell culture, organoids, and "organs on a chip" (OoC). By combining advances in tissue engineering and microfabrication, organs-on-chips systems are designed to mimic human physiology and provide predictive indications of candidate therapeutics' effects on various organ systems, elucidating disease states, pharmacokinetics, and pharmacodynamics. Linking several OoCs together can model the way human organs interact in the body, although the human body on a chip is still some way off (Fig. 4).

Regulatory agencies, including the U.S. Food and Drug Administration (FDA), have indicated a willingness to leverage alternatives to animal models to advance therapeutics candidates in human clinical studies. The FDA Modernization Act 2.0, passed in December 2022, specifies four advanced technologies, including cell-based assays, OoC and microphysiologic systems, computer modeling, and other methods based on human biology (Han 2023). Computer modeling is meant to simulate physiologic systems in silico, and the complementary use of machine learning can inform target identification, pharmacokinetics, toxicity testing, clinical trial design, and pharmacogenomics. However, overreliance on modeling is unwise since no model can precisely replicate what it models. By signaling its willingness to consider methods other than

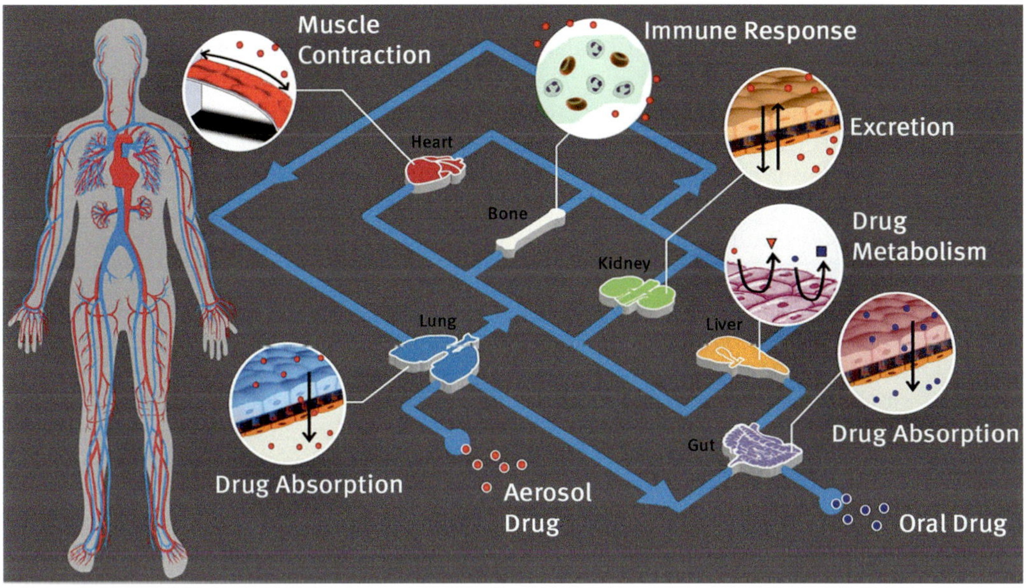

Fig. 4 An illustration from a video at ▶ https://wyss.harvard.edu/technology/human-organs-on-chips/ (or ▶ https://vimeo.com/116674365), showing how organs on a chip can be linked to simulate the interactions of bodily systems. Further information is on the website. (Credit: Wyss Institute at Harvard University)

animal models—methods that may become both faster and more predictive of therapeutics in human disease—the FDA has motivated additional innovation in this area, which should accelerate and multiply the novel agents going into the development pipelines for pathogens with pandemic potential.

6.2 Innovation in Clinical Development

The traditional clinical development process often assessed a single therapeutics candidate through pharmaceutical trials at multiple individual research sites. Clinical research networks focused on specific diseases such as HIV/AIDS, or specific populations such as children, have advantages in specialized expertise. Still, these networks are often unlinked to others and stand up temporary clinical research capacity that is not sustained. Adequate pandemic preparedness requires networks and capacity that are developed, sustained, and connected with other networks and the worldwide research ecosystem. A similar dynamic occurs with research sponsored by pharmaceutical companies; there can be a tremendous amount of uncoordinated redundancy as companies seek to assess similar products in multiple profit-driven trials. Of course, clinical research infrastructure, including personnel, is minimal or lacking in many LMICs at greatest risk for zoonotic outbreaks (▶ Chap. 8).

The optimal strategy for pandemic preparedness is to contain outbreaks at their source and prevent them from ever becoming pandemics. Along with biosurveillance and pathogen identification, the strategy requires active clinical research capacity operating close to hotspots at high risk for zoonotic outbreaks (▶ Chap. 10). Governments must be able to mobilize that capacity quickly to respond to outbreaks, calling on global partners as needed and available.

If prevention at the point of origin fails and the outbreak becomes an epidemic or pandemic, regional or global clinical trial infrastructure must be able to initiate further trials that can recruit diverse and special populations as trial participants. While the goal of well-distributed, responsive clinical trials is a vital element of the global call for equity in clinical trials capacity, there is a great deal of groundwork to be done before the capacity to design and conduct scientifically and ethically rigorous clinical trials can be assured in the many countries that currently lack such capacity. Moving too quickly could result in clinical trials that do not meet Good Clinical Practice standards (ICH 2016) or comply with international human subject protections, such as those developed by the Council of International Organisations of Medical Sciences (CIOMS 2016). Flawed trials that are unlikely to produce results regulators can use for decision-making are arguably ipso facto unethical, wasting scarce clinical research resources and putting trial participants at risk with no compensating benefits (Emanuel et al. 2000).

6.3 Coordinating Emergency Clinical Research

Another challenge to research response in health emergencies has been the lack of a unified, prioritized research agenda to coordinate strategic alignment of limited resources to support high-quality clinical trials that result in actionable evidence. Most clinical trials during the COVID-19 pandemic, especially in its earliest months, were underpowered, under-resourced, and often poorly designed (Bugin and Woodcock 2021). In response to these challenges, the G7 produced the G7 Therapeutics and Vaccines Clinical Trials Charter (G7 2021) (▶ Box 2). Following its June 2021 publication, and with particular reference to point 1, the UK co-sponsored a resolution with Argentina and Peru at the 70-fifth World Health Assembly in May 2022. After negotiation, it was approved as WHA Resolution 75.8, "Strengthening Clinical Trials to Provide High-Quality Evidence on Health Interventions and to Improve Research Quality and Coordination" (WHO 2022b). Likewise the Global Research Collaboration for Infectious Disease Preparedness (GloPID-R), a consortium of global funding organizations, has invested in enhancing preparedness to implement accelerated research response to new or reemerging infectious diseases (▶ Chap. 29). In support of the G7 Charter, GloPID-R developed a Global Clinical Trial Networks and Funders Working Group (◘ Fig. 5).

Building on such conceptual agreements about the need for reliable clinical trials with actionable evidence, an evolving paradigm shift in health security emphasizes that continuously operating high-quality clinical research programs need to be embedded in functional health systems that support medi-

Box 2: G7 Therapeutics and Vaccines Clinical Trials Charter

1. To avoid the proliferation of trials that do not contribute to valid or actionable scientific evidence, we will prioritize support for randomized controlled trials that address key public health and clinical needs, are well designed and sufficiently sized to generate reliable evidence, are consistent with good clinical practices and ethical principles and engage our citizens to strengthen confidence in science…
2. To avoid unnecessary duplication and produce valid and actionable evidence more efficiently, we will coordinate emergency and preparedness research agendas…
3. To enable timely availability of actionable information from multi-country clinical trials and to increase the comparability of data, we will work with G7 regulators, ethics institutions and committees to achieve greater harmonization and to streamline the regulatory process to act more proportionately to risk…
4. To ensure that we act as quickly as possible in response to positive and negative data results from clinical trials, we will accelerate the sharing of data and results so that therapeutics proven to be effective and safe can be approved by regulatory bodies, incorporated into clinical practice guidelines and recommended for use in routine practice…

5. To ensure that health and research systems can respond quickly and effectively to existing and emerging threats, we will make preparedness, high quality, ethical research, and randomized controlled trials part of normal practice within our healthcare and research systems. We will support the development of the global infrastructure needed to allow rapid set-up, coordinated delivery of trials, and sharing of emerging findings...
6. To expeditiously advance the development and testing of vaccines, as well as the investigation of correlates of protection and therapeutics, we will agree that as soon as novel pathogens or viral variants appear and become accessible to a G7 country, the G7 will rapidly share testing methods, reference standards and testing materials (as they relate to the virus strain) with any other G7 country and beyond, via an open material transfer agreement...
7. To make vaccine development faster, we will work to develop a framework to coordinate testing methodology and share testing materials, wherever possible, in response to pandemic threats. Where this is not possible, we will seek ways to compare the results of vaccine assessments in clinical trials...

Note: the material deleted from the text refers to implementation of the stated goals. Full text ▶ here.

cal research in addition to primary, secondary, and tertiary care. The desired end state of a global research system includes "warm base" global clinical trials infrastructure conducting ongoing regulatory-level research. Non-emergency, interpandemic research should focus on (a) endemic pathogens of high public health importance to the locations where research is conducted and (b) research guided by the prototype pathogen approach or similar prioritization rubrics in preparation for outbreaks with pandemic potential. Such research benefits research participants and their communities when successful and thus helps build community and national support for clinical research. No less important, it ensures operational preparedness to pivot to emergency research on candidate MCMs when outbreaks with pandemic potential occur. This will normally require switching to a new trial protocol, but most of the elements needed for clinical research will already be in place (◻ Fig. 6), obviating the need for a scramble to set up infrastructure and train personnel as in the Ebola trials in West Africa and the Democratic Republic of the Congo (DRC) in 2014–2016 and 2018–2020, respectively (▶ Chaps. 17 and 32, In Practice 17.1).

An operating global "warm-base" clinical trial infrastructure will have much improved proximity to (a) endemic diseases for which VTD are in development and (b) geographic hotspots where zoonotic outbreaks are most likely. Warm-base research should focus on advancing VTDs for pathogens of global health importance, especially malaria, tuberculosis, neglected tropical diseases, and viruses that can infect but are not easily transmitted among humans. Global support for creating warm-base global clinical trial infrastructure would improve equity, advance understanding of diseases with a high global health burden and candidate VTDs, and build rigorous, regulatory-level clinical research capacity where it is now lacking. For hard-eyed developed-country budgeteers, it would erect a robust defense against outbreaks becoming epidemics or pandemics that could threaten their own countries and cause incalculable damage to the world economy and population.

There are many challenges, including financing, global cooperation, and regulatory harmonization, to ensure that emergency research response protocols are coordinated among countries and can produce results that regulators can rely on. Moreover, some pathogens, like HIV, TB, and malaria, have stubbornly resisted the development of essential MCMs. Even a greatly improved emergency research response infrastructure cannot guarantee successful MCM development against

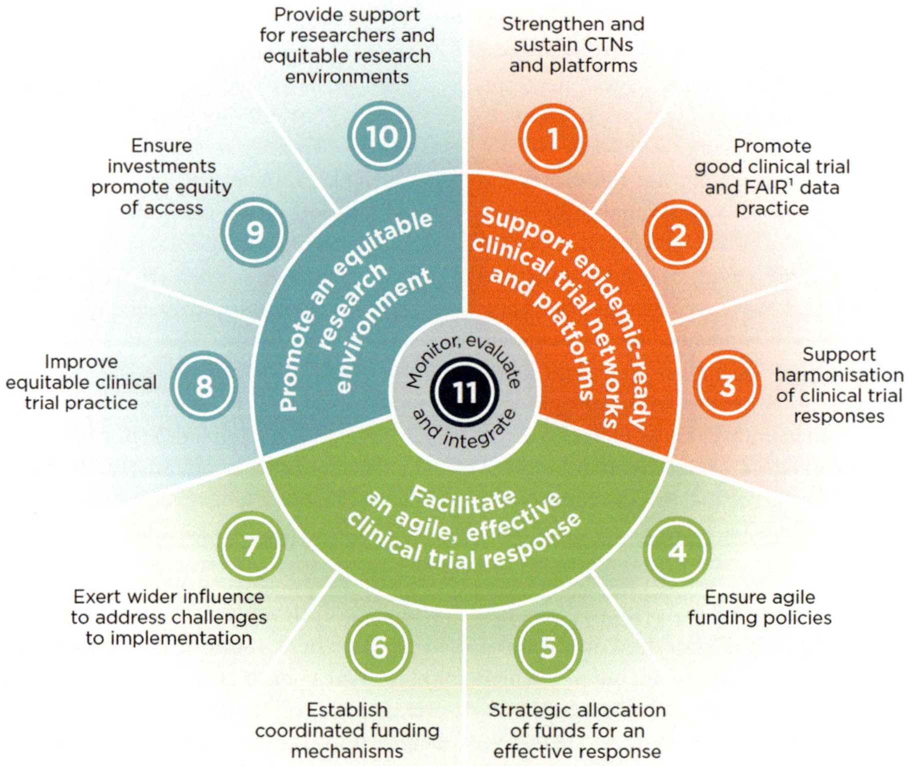

GOAL: Support epidemic-ready clinical trial networks and platforms

Principle (1) Strengthen and sustain strategic clinical trial networks and platforms

Principle (2) Promote a culture of good clinical trial practice including FAIR[1] data practices

Principle (3) Support harmonisation of clinical trial responses

GOAL: Facilitate an agile, effective clinical trial response

Principle (4) Ensure agile funding policies

Principle (5) Strategic allocation of funds for an effective response

Principle (6) Establish coordinated funding mechanisms

Principle (7) Exert wider influence to address challenges to trial implementation

GOAL: Promote an equitable research environment

Principle (8) Improve equitable clinical trial practice

Principle (9) Ensure investments promote equity of access

Principle (10) Provide support for researchers and an equitable research environment

Cross-cutting principle

Principle (11) Monitor, evaluate and integrate

Fig. 5 The three goals and 11 accompanying principles of the Living Roadmap for Clinical Trials Coordination (GLOPID-R 2023). *FAIR*: findability, accessibility, interoperability, and reuse of digital assets; *CTN* clinical trial network(s)

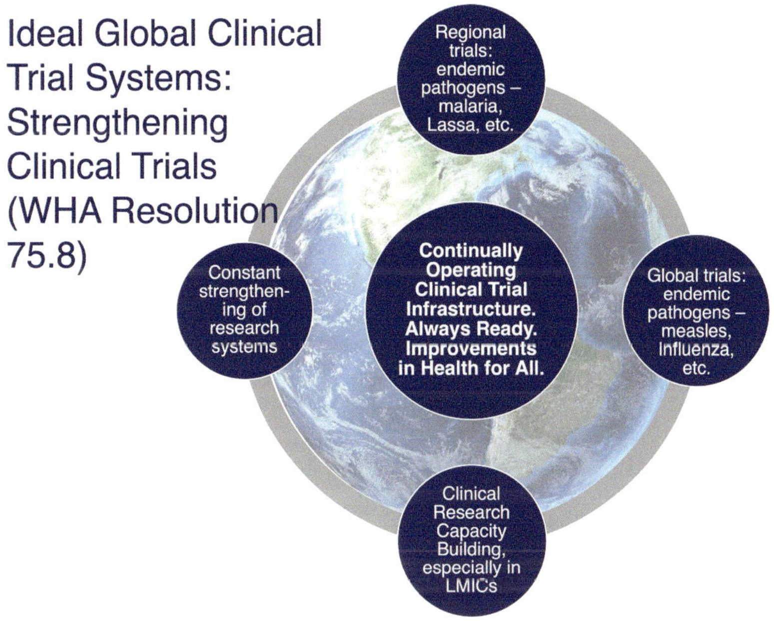

Fig. 6 Major elements of a fully functional global clinical trials ecosystem that could provide high-quality evidence on health interventions and improve research quality and coordination in both interpandemic intervals and public health emergencies. Such a vision is consistent with WHA Resolution 75.8, "Strengthening clinical trials to provide high-quality evidence on health interventions and to improve research quality and coordination." (Figure: Elizabeth S. Higgs)

the next novel pathogen if it proves similarly resistant to prevention and/or treatment. All that said, a coordinated, well-resourced, operational global system for surveillance, pathogen identification, and clinical research is an investment that will bring rich returns over time, not only in lives saved and pandemics prevented but in better health for all and prevention of the economic shocks that undermined livelihoods during the COVID-19 and other pandemics. Achieving this vision requires broad support that has often been hard to come by, but the case is compelling. Disparate countries should be able to support master protocols, stringent regulatory review, sharing of data and samples, etc. After the COVID-19 experience, many countries will insist on better future access to newly developed MCMs, and that needs to be ensured in the production phase that follows Phase III clinical trials. But we need to pull together to resolve shortfalls and overcome obstacles. The stakes are life and death, and the prospects of success are better than ever and can be better still.

6.4 Innovations in Clinical Trial Designs and Approaches

Necessity is still the mother of invention! During the 2014–2016 West Africa Ebola outbreak, there were vigorous disagreements about essential clinical trial design elements like randomization, concurrent controls, and placebos. The debates continue, as they should, but there is a growing consensus that scientific and ethical norms do not change during an outbreak, epidemic, or health emergency. Alongside innovations in clinical trial design, randomized controlled trials remain the prima facie standard for robust results (▶ In Practice 4.1 and Chap. 22). Human trial participant protection is not suddenly optional (▶ Chaps. 4 and 5). Regulatory authorities and data and safety monitoring boards (DSMB) maintain their vigilance against adverse events in patients (▶ Chaps. 6, 23, and 36). An intensive review by the U.S. National Academies of Sciences, Engineering and Medicine of the clinical research that took place during the 2014–2016

West African Ebola outbreak also endorsed the conclusion that randomized controlled trials are the most ethical way to allocate limited resources and the fastest means of obtaining safety and efficacy data on candidate therapeutics and vaccines (NASEM 2017b). The research response to the 2014–2016 Ebola outbreak demonstrated that scientifically rigorous, ethical clinical trials could be implemented in least-developed countries with minimal infrastructure (Kennedy et al. 2016). A few years later, the PAmoja TuLinde Maisha (PALM ["together save lives" in Swahili]) therapeutics trial in the DRC demonstrated that clinical trials could be conducted to the highest standards even when armed conflict among criminal gangs, militias, and security forces was added to the mix (Mulangu et al. 2019). The data these trials provided for licensing vaccines and therapeutics for Ebola led to the first approved treatments and vaccines for Ebola virus disease (EMA 2019, 2020; FDA 2019, 2020a, b).

There is now a growing list of innovative approaches to clinical trial design and execution as research is recognized as an essential element of preparedness and response to health emergencies.

The Randomised Evaluation of Covid-19 Therapy (RECOVERY) trial employed the approach shown in the third row of ◘ Table 1 during COVID-19 (► In Practice 14.1). The pragmatic clinical trial design with a simple primary endpoint (mortality), embedded as a national priority in the UK National Health Service, made critical early contributions to identifying therapeutics suitable for hospitalized COVID-19 patients by demonstrating a significant mortality benefit of dexamethasone in patients receiving invasive mechanical ventilation in hospital (RECOVERY Collaborative Group 2020). The result surprised many intensivists and pulmonary critical care specialists, since trials using immunosuppressants for ARDS had been negative for over 15 years. Despite the absence of a placebo group and the ability of unblinded physicians to select randomization arms for their patients, the number of patients enrolled made the result statistically compelling.

6.5 Appropriate Trials During Emergencies

The COVID-19 pandemic highlighted the need for large-scale, well-designed randomized clinical studies structured by a master protocol. The intent of global master protocols was to rapidly accelerate the development of safe, efficacious, novel prophylactics and treatments against SARS-CoV-2 infection. A master protocol incorporates easily adaptable trial designs into existing infrastructure to evaluate multiple agents simultaneously or sequentially. Agents can be selected for evaluation in different populations. Agent prioritization should be based on the estimated likelihood of positive clinical outcomes (Buchman et al. 2021; LaVange et al. 2021). Other criteria for ranking agents to move into clinical trials should include biologic, logistical, and safety considerations, as well as manufacturing capacity and supply chains.

A master protocol reduces the time taken to design and complete studies, enabling global comparisons to generate evidence to determine the relative effectiveness of treatments generalizable to a broad global population. Platform trials are multi-arm, enduring clinical trials that allow comparison between multiple investigational agents and allow trial arms to be dropped or added mid-trial to improve efficiency and stop giving agents that appear to be ineffective or unsafe to patients. Two interesting platform approaches in curating priorities for clinical research are exemplified by the Accelerating COVID-19 Therapeutic Interventions and Vaccines (ACTIV) and RECOVERY clinical trials.

6.5.1 The Accelerating COVID-19 Therapeutic Interventions and Vaccines (ACTIV) Partnership

Accelerating COVID-19 Therapeutic Interventions and Vaccines (ACTIV) was a public-private partnership created to accelerate the development of SARS-CoV-2 vaccines, therapeutics, and diagnostics

Table 1 Trial design elements, their relevance to epidemiologic characteristics, advantages, and examples (Elizabeth S. Higgs)

Design element	Relevant epidemiologic characteristics	Example pathogens for design element	Advantages	Example trial using a design element
Designed as multi-outbreak, multi-country, multi-arm trials continuous across outbreaks; investigational products plus standard of care (SOC) vs. placebo plus SOC	Unpredictable diseases with droplet and contact transmission; multiple countries	Filoviruses, Nipah virus	Data accrual across outbreaks to reach meaningful sample size; enables dropping and adding arms for efficacy and safety signals; can incorporate safe, effective agents into the standard of care while continuing trials	PALM 1 (Mulangu et al. 2019)
Global master platform protocols, with embedded multiple trials using similar patient populations and endpoints	Anticipated large number of cases, with discordant epidemiologic waves in different locations; aerosolized transmission	COVID-19, influenza	Continual enrollment, early stopping for futility and/or lack of efficacy, ability to start multiple trials under one protocol familiar to sites, ethics committees, DSMBs, and regulators	TICO (NIH 2021); STRIVE (NIH 2022)
Utilization of national health system (NHS) for nationally prioritized clinical research; pragmatic trials with randomization and a placebo arm but without blinding	Anticipation of a large number of cases across the population or a smaller number of cases within specific patient populations	Mpox, COVID-19	NHS-wide recruitment meant rapid accrual, larger numbers, and thus utilization of less frequent endpoints such as mortality; useful in health emergencies; numbers allow for enrollment in trials of specialized population groups, e.g. mpox in MSM and HIV community	RECOVERY (RECOVERY trial 2023)
Real-time review by the DMSB of safety and efficacy data for adding or dropping arms once a safety, efficacy, or futility endpoint is reached	Trials are enrolling quickly, and trial integrity requires maintaining the blind while enhancing safety and efficiency	Ebola virus, COVID-19	Efficiency allows an early drop of ineffective agents; effective agents are incorporated into the standard of care and outbreak response	PALM (Mulangu et al. 2019), Ebola Ça Suffit! ring trial (Henao-Restrepo et al. 2017)

(▶ Chap. 15). The ACTIV Therapeutics Working Group was tasked with developing master platform protocols and a rigorous system to analyze preclinical and clinical data to select candidate investigational products for the master protocol. The working group, composed of both government and industry scientists, selected networks (and networks of networks) to design and implement multiple platform protocols for outpatients and inpatients, focused on both host and viral targets. Interim analyses by a data and safety monitoring board (DSMB) of accumulating data throughout the study determine whether agents demonstrate either futility or lack of safety and should be discontinued, preserving resources for more promising agents.

Agents demonstrating early evidence of efficacy can proceed to larger, confirmatory studies or to regulatory submission if there are sufficient data (◘ Fig. 7). Platform efficiencies include the ability to share or pool placebo control arms for comparison to multiple agents and the use of intermediate efficacy, futility, and safety assessments so only the most promising agents go forward into full enrollment, while fewer promising candidates are rejected early. This helps minimize overlapping or redundant work on parallel protocols. The adaptive elements of stopping treatment arms based on unfavorable or very favorable interim monitoring results increase the efficiency of the master protocol trial design. However, outcome-adaptive randomization may be statistically inefficient compared to trials with equal randomization and can result in a lack of interpretability (Korn and Freidlin 2017).

6.5.2 The RECOVERY Trial

The RECOVERY trial was an investigator-initiated, nationally prioritized, individually randomized, open-label, controlled trial to evaluate the efficacy and safety of a range of putative treatments in patients hospitalized with COVID-19 (▶ In Practice 14.1 and 15.1). Most eligible patients were randomly

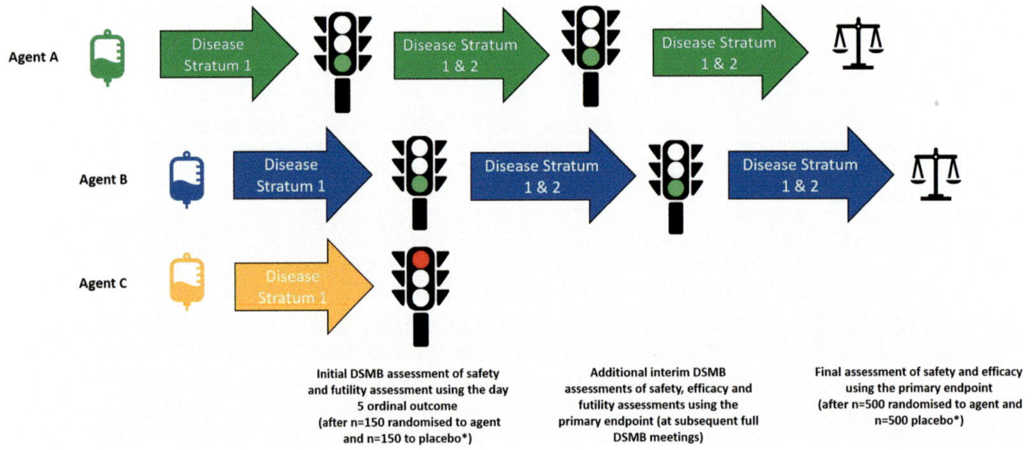

◘ **Fig. 7** Agent entry and progression through the TICO (Therapeutics for Inpatients with COVID-19) study. The TICO study allows for multiple agents to be studied concurrently and for agents to enter the study at different times. In the theoretical scenario presented in this figure, Agent (a) is the only agent available for randomization at the beginning of the study. Later, Agent (b) and Agent (c) enter the study, and new participants can be randomized to all three agents (and placebo). Agent (a) completes recruitment in Disease Stratum 1, and, after the initial futility assessment by the independent DSMB (using the day 5 ordinal outcome), the agent is approved to also include those in Disease Stratum 2 (i.e., those with end organ disease, including requirements for invasive mechanical ventilation or extracorporeal membrane oxygenation [ECMO]). Agents (b) and (c) enter the study at the same time, but after Agent (a), both progress to the initial futility assessment. However, only Agent (b) receives DSMB approval to proceed, and randomization to Agent (c) ceases. Agents (a) and (b) continue to recruit in both disease stratum 1 and 2 and undergo additional interim safety, efficacy, and futility assessments (using the primary endpoint) at subsequent full DSMB meetings before undergoing a final review of safety and efficacy (using the primary endpoint) when recruitment is complete (graphically represented by the image of scales). The placebo group may be shared across multiple agents (not graphically represented). (Figure and caption (adapted) from Murray et al. (2021))

allocated between the standard of care with no additional treatment and one of several active treatment arms. However, the treating physician could allocate patients to a particular treatment arm. New treatment arms were subsequently added to assess agent efficacy in different patient populations and novel interventions. RECOVERY benefited from a clinical research network embedded within the National Health Service (NHS) and run by NHS staff in England. The trial was also coordinated with the health services in Northern Ireland, Scotland, and Wales, enabling UK-wide deployment of a randomized controlled trial protocol across a very large hospital network, allowing tens of thousands of patients to participate across various health settings, including community hospitals. The RECOVERY trial did not have prespecified rules of when therapies should be added or removed, as is common in platform trials. The study relied on its DSMB to advise when to stop enrollment for efficacy or futility. Based on the mortality endpoint, the study design did not include enough information on pathophysiology, such as biomarkers that could inform future novel mechanistic approaches to COVID-19 therapeutics. This is a tradeoff between a simple, large pragmatic trial and smaller trials with more intensive patient sampling and visits. Both are needed in the context of a health emergency and a novel pathogen.

6.5.3 Great Flexibility Is Needed for Conducting Clinical Trials During a Pandemic

A move toward decentralized clinical trials in multiple locations may improve the adaptability of clinical design and should provide additional data for improving the design of adaptable platform trials. One big advantage of this approach is that adequately powered trials are essential for making important discoveries. They should be completed in time for the findings to help control the outbreak or pandemic that requires an emergency research response. A well-designed study that enrolls thousands of patients can answer vital questions with confidence more quickly than a smaller one. Larger studies can also characterize comorbidities since they are more likely to have statistically useful numbers with particular comorbidities. However, these studies require complex logistics and may be prohibitive in cost. They require both design simplicity and a pragmatic approach and cannot screen as many of the most promising drugs as smaller studies. Smaller studies with more intensive analysis of participants' responses to the disease and interventions can provide a better understanding of pathophysiology, viral persistence, viral clearance, and disease-specific considerations in certain patient populations. Promising interventions that reflect the specific needs of the patient population and are readily implementable are then prioritized.

6.5.4 Populations That Have Been Underrepresented in Past Clinical Research

Populations that have been underrepresented in past clinical research may have been excluded to protect them from risk since they were adjudged more vulnerable, e.g. pregnant woman, children, neonates, or populations who live in places where clinical trials were few and far between. However, these populations need to be included to assess whether they can safely use and benefit from the products that emerge from research. Including special populatoins may require different infrastructure or novel approaches to ensure participant follow-up and safety monitoring. These populations include also vulnerable individuals at risk of severe disease, e.g. older adults who may benefit from pre-exposure or post-exposure prophylaxis. One novel approach to reach remote, rural, populations without access to research sites for evaluatoin of the efficacy and safety of repurposed agents for patients not requiring hospitalization is "no-touch" trials, such as ACTIV 6 (NCT04885530). ACTIV 6 included necessary rigorous elements of research, such as randomization and placebo controls while using creative outreach to rapidly enroll COVID-19 patients who might not be interested in participating in research if required to physically present to a clinic or research site. ACTIV 6 was particularly important in addressing popular misconceptions that certain agents like ivermectin were effective for COVID-19 (Naggie et al. 2023). ACTIV 6 was able to rapidly demonstrate a lack of efficacy for a variety of repurposed agents thought by some segments of the population to be effective. The ACTIV 6 trials produced robust evidence to counter these misbeliefs, and patient populations and physicians could be guided to alternative, effective therapies. It is especially important to dissuade outpatients at high risk for progression to hospitalization from using ineffective and sometimes dangerous drugs, such as older patients and those with comorbidities such as diabetes, obesity, hypertension, etc. No-touch trials are particularly attractive for the enrollment of diverse racial and ethnic groups living where access to medical and research facilities may be limited.

Pregnant and lactating women, children, and infants should not be overlooked as they often have been, including in the major COVID-19 vaccine trials in 2020 (Beigi et al. 2021). Rather, they should be considered vulnerable people who also need treatments and prophylactics and should be included in research studies from the outset. A retrospective look at various pandemics and epidemics will show that certain populations are at higher risk for severe disease in each pandemic. In the 1918 "Spanish" influenza, for example, young adults had especially high mortality, while older adults were less severely affected (van Wijhe et al. 2018). Children and pregnant women have additional mortality in Ebola virus disease (Gomes et al. 2017). In COVID-19, older adults experienced a sharply higher incidence of morbidity and mortality than younger people, while children were much less likely to suffer severe disease. In the 2009 H1N1 influenza pandemic, obesity was noted for the first time to increase risk of severe influenza alongside other known comorbidities. At the outset of a new epidemic or pandemic it is not known which demographic and health characteristics are risk factors for severity. It is critical to evaluate the first several hundred patients to ascertain high risk groups (Simonsen et al. 2018). The inclusion of children in healthcare research remains important to ensure that evidence can be generated about how best to address their health needs. The risk and benefit assessment of clinical interventions derived from adult trials cannot be readily extrapolated to children. Pediatric studies should be conducted in parallel with adult efficacy trials rather than delaying them until adult efficacy is established.

6.5.5 A Large Global Network

A large global network is essential for rapid recruitment and generalizable results in an emergency, especially since case rates during epidemics and pandemics fluctuate spatially and temporally in unpredictable ways; severity, for example, may vary with population genetics and/or immunity. A broad range of clinical sites across multiple countries results in a demographically diverse study population, ensuring any beneficial treatments identified through clinical trials have broad applicability. An efficient global research ecosystem established through a master protocol can be leveraged through existing infrastructure and establishing standardized practice. The need for standardized practice and reporting may come across obstacles in the form of regulatory and ethical review processes of the country in which trials take place—processes with which they must comply. Varying regional and national regulatory requirements can thus present a major challenge to a nimble, efficient clinical trial ecosystem operating in multiple countries. Establishing large-scale national and international clinical trial infrastructure with standards and master protocols accepted by all trial sites and relevant authorities in each country is a major step toward real global readiness for expeditious clinical research that can provide rapid, effective clinical impact on a global scale.

7 Regulatory Innovation

Global platform protocol trials require interactions with many regulatory agencies. Many national regulators use the rigorous standards of the International Council for Harmonisation of Technical Requirements for Pharmaceuticals for Human Use (ICH) as clinical trial requirements (ICH 2023). Nevertheless, during COVID-19 every country required an individual regulatory review and approval. For example, ACTIV protocols began with FDA approval, which varied in approval time from weeks to months. After ACTIV received FDA concurrence that a protocol was safe to implement, regulatory approvals in other countries were sought, although ACTIV made efforts to obtain accelerated approval from the European Medicines Agency (EMA). Then, despite EMA approvals, each European Union country had to provide its own approval. In the case of ACTIV 3, sponsors varied by country and were facilitated by the University of Minnesota, working with WHO International Coordination Centers. Due to this slow, sequential process, recruitment for the trial had already closed by the time the protocol received regulatory and ethical approval in some countries. Given the effort, paperwork, and time spent reviewing the protocol by many persons and organizations, this was enormously frustrating to investigators.

This kind of sequential approval process slows the start of any large global trial enormously. Global goals calling for safe and effective vaccines and therapeutics within 100 days are aspirational but will be impossible under the current fragmented global regulatory system. To make a rapid research response possible, better collaboration among national and regional regulatory agencies is imperative. Discussions and efforts are underway to overcome these roadblocks with much-needed innovations in regulatory coordination (Califf 2023; EMA 2023).

8 Manufacturing and Delivery in Therapeutics Preparedness and Response

Ensuring that the social value created by research is available to all populations who may benefit—in this case from novel interventions in a health emergency—requires focused innovation and investment in manufacturing, allocation, distribution, and "last-mile" delivery to people. There are many discussions and initiatives being generated in 2023 with the end goal of improving MCM production and distribution, since the global community has made the production at scale and more equitable delivery of MCMs in a health emergency a high priority. Whether it is considered integral to the research response or the next step after the research response, this is a complex ecosystem with many entities interacting and not always having the same goals, so nothing should be assumed. A pandemic can immobilize economies, transport, workforce, and so on, challenging the best-laid plans for manufacturing and delivery. There are ways to anticipate and manage at least some of the likely bottlenecks:

- Government-subsidized, "at-risk" manufacturing of MCMs before they complete trials, with the understanding they will not be used unless cleared by regulators, but manufacturers will not bear the cost of production
- Advance marketing agreements to de-risk development costs, incentivize pharmaceutical companies, and compress the time needed for delivery and use of novel products
- International understandings or commitments by producing countries and firms that they will set aside a specified portion of pandemic MCMs for global rather than national needs

Stockouts should be anticipated in health emergencies. One of the goals of the prototype pathogen approach is to stockpile adequate supplies of candidate therapeutics that have been assessed through clinical trial Phase IIa. These will initially be needed only in the moderate quantities needed for large-scale safety and efficacy studies, generally less than 100,000 courses. Another approach being pursued following the pandemic is to develop manufacturing capacity globally, making it more likely that adequate supplies of products can be made available on all continents (Farlow et al. 2023).

9 Multitasking

Response to an outbreak sparked by a pathogen with pandemic potential should begin early, since that is the best hope of preventing a pandemic. Confirmation of such an outbreak, especially identifying a new pathogen, defines the moment to pivot the clinical research capacity to emergency research response. When that occurs, speed is paramount. Business as usual is not sufficient. Lives are at stake from the disease outbreak, and many more are at risk if the pathogen spreads to cause an epidemic or pandemic. Moreover, as we have seen during COVID-19 and in smaller epidemics like Ebola in West Africa, infectious disease events can severely harm healthcare systems, depriving people of treatment for other diseases and for accidents (Lal et al. 2021; Nuzzo et al. 2019). Essential economic functions aside from health care, such as food and energy production and distribution, education, and the service sector, can be shut down to a greater or lesser degree. Loss of income and curtailed social interaction threaten social cohesion.

The standard pharmaceutical development timeline is designed to reduce the risk of wasting resources on products that will not work. That timeline, as we have seen, is inadequate to the demands of a public health emergency. Research response accepts enhanced risk—risk to investments, not to research participants, patients, or the public—to accelerate research and development. For a disease that is not new but causes periodic, deadly outbreaks, like Ebola, the emergency research response may be the only opportunity to assess the safety and efficacy of MCMs that must be tested against circulating diseases. Even during an emergency caused by a novel pathogen, like SARS-CoV-1 in 2002–2003, public health measures may end the emergency before clinical trials can begin, certainly trials on a traditional timeline (Finlay et al. 2004; Muller et al. 2004). In a global pandemic with daily death tolls in the thousands or tens of thousands, the need for urgency is self-evident.

Accelerating therapeutics development during an emergency involves collapsing several steps into one. All eight steps in the therapeutics development pipeline (◘ Fig. 1) can be concomitantly accelerated, with innovations in each step enhancing an enabling environment and performing steps in parallel rather than in sequence. The research response goals are to contain outbreaks at their source, reduce direct mortality and morbidity, *and* prevent severe dysfunction in essential social systems (▶ Chap. 3). These three goals should drive the emergency research response.

A strategic research agenda is essential and should be agreed upon as soon as the necessary information about the pathogen and disease is in hand, but subject to change to accommodate new findings. In a localized outbreak or epidemic, the host country where the outbreak takes place has the primary leadership role. Clear leadership over the research response will include pivoting to domestic clinical research infrastructure responsive to host country leadership. Ideally clinical research capacity is adequate, with ongoing regulatory-level trials, and linked to a global clinical trial network, which can quickly bring resources and additional expertise to the outbreak at hand. Having agreements on research conduct and logistics in place with the host government beforehand helps minimize legal and policy obstacles. Clarity on leadership roles and responsibilities will avert disagreements and confusion. Without such clarity and well-meaning research responses, endeavors can engender chaos, with multiple research groups implementing underpowered studies, resulting in confusion in the community without producing actionable results. Like wars, life-threatening emergencies require command, control, communications, and intelligence (scientific findings in this case). Advance preparation empowers and informs country leadership. Existing research capacity, operational regulatory and ethics boards, and emergency planning help a country transition quickly to ongoing dialogue with the affected communities and society members.

If preparedness is effective, all eight steps of the development pathway (◘ Fig. 1) can move concurrently towards research response. In the case of a novel pathogen, it will likely be from a known viral family. If current aspirations are realized, candidates who have been through Phase IIa dose-finding clinical studies will be available. Anticipated pathogen mutations, immune escape, and resistance will be accounted for in study designs. Primed global clinical trial capacity responsive to host country priorities can rapidly adapt or write protocols. Regulatory agencies, ethics boards, and communities anticipating emergencies will implement preapproved procedures. Previously engaged communities and advisory boards can assist with communications, social mobilization, and community engagement. When research systems, preparedness, clarity of leadership and governance, and inclusion of many voices have been well thought through, planned, and preferably exercised in simulations, research response can be executed calmly and swiftly. Prepared manufacturing capacity can begin advanced manufacturing with confidence that it will not suffer financially if its product is not useful. Following the eight steps in ◘ Fig. 1 in a strict sequence is not an option when an emergency ensues. Public-private partnerships will be important to realize this vision, to ensure coordinated innovation between public and private sectors and to contribute to a strong global clinical trial infrastructure.

10 Listen to Many Voices

Accelerating the development of therapeutics from "bench to bedside" requires the inclusion of many voices to achieve an envisioned state of therapeutics preparedness. The inclusivity of stakeholders (all those who affect or are affected by the research) will have a profound impact on research progress, outcomes, and impact. The impact of even safe and effective products can be limited by poor uptake; hesitancy or mistrust can mean the difference between acceptance and use or rejection of therapeutics, frequently a matter of life and death. Usage of Paxlovid, a highly effective antiviral protease inhibitor developed for COVID-19, has been variable by region and population in the United States, with physicians hesitant to prescribe it or not well informed about its efficacy, and many patients reluctant to take it. In a utilization analysis, Paxlovid usage correlated with state vaccination rates, indicating that antiviral usage hesitancy correlated with vaccine hesitancy (Murphy et al. 2022). It has been postulated that mortality rates in some nation-states, e.g., high mortality in Bulgaria vs. low mortality in Denmark, are related to popular acceptance of vaccines and therapeutics (Matveeva and Shabalina 2023). The need to include many voices cannot be overstressed; this means genuine dialogue between researchers, public health officials, practicing healthcare providers, and other stakeholders, formalized as Good Participatory Practice principles and practice (▶ Chap. 18). Biomedical researchers should *not* view GPP simply as an aid to recruitment. Inclusivity of many voices spans the spectrum from bench to bedside to surrounding communities.

Implementation of GPP is practiced especially well in the HIV/AIDS research community, where the GPP principles originated. At-risk communities are already invested in research, and those now living with HIV have been able to do so thanks to the therapeutics developed since the disease appeared in 1981. Trials enroll quickly, HIV-positive individuals are represented on protocol teams, and they facilitate recruitment, advocate for research funding and scientific progress, and eagerly expect therapeutic advances from the research they advocate. In the COVID-19 response, despite the demonstrated success of GPP in other circumstances, efforts to include communities in the research were largely limited to recruitment efforts. The integration of research into the NHS in the UK has enabled broader inclusion and awareness of research by both patients and physicians.

In general, early inclusion of communities engenders greater confidence in research results in both doctors and patients, resulting in greater uptake and greater benefit in curtailing infectious disease. Implemented to the extent possible, preparation, multitasking, and inclusivity enable rapid, coordinated action to accelerate therapeutics development and uptake when a crisis occurs—starting with plans, resources, systems, and qualified people in place to act. Preparedness therapeutics research should integrate communities into the entire research process. Ultimately the impact of MCMs on an outbreak, epidemic, or pandemic is contingent on their being used. Neglecting good participatory practice during preparedness will hamper research response. In response to a health emergency, the leadership should resist the temptation to put off GPP during a crisis or health emergency. Communication, dialogue, and engagement of communities are more important in a crisis than under normal circumstances when participation in research and trust in research results is essential.

11 Summary

Bench to bedside, equitable access to safe, effective products, and leveraging therapeutics for treatment, prevention, and prophylaxis will contribute to health security and mitigate the morbidity and mortality from future emerging and reemerging infectious diseases. These goals are attainable, even for novel pathogen X. Yet global health security remains an unrealized vision. A strong global research and health system supported by a political and scientific alliance is a work in progress. Ensuring therapeutics preparedness for both known and unknown pathogens with pandemic potential is possible, but a clear vision of what the therapeutics preparedness state should be is an essential first step. With such a vision informing innovation in all steps of the bench-to-bedside development pathway, improvement from the current status quo is not a speculative venture but an achievable goal—assuming the scientific, political, and financial sectors work to bring it to fruition.

Discussion Questions

1. What are the steps in the therapeutics development process from bench to bedside?
2. What is needed to attain an ideal therapeutics preparedness state? What would such preparedness be able to provide?
3. Provide examples of applying what we have learned from past therapeutics development to future research responses to infectious disease pathogens.
4. Neither therapeutics for pathogens with pandemic potential nor therapeutics for pathogens disproportionately impacting the poorest countries have fared well in a market-driven therapeutics economy. How can this be remedied? What are some of the efforts now underway?
5. What innovations are being developed to accelerate preclinical development by enabling faster, more accurate initial assessments of whether therapeutic products will be safe and effective in humans, with less reliance on animal models?
6. What can innovation in clinical development contribute to pandemic preparedness?
7. The COVID-19 pandemic highlighted the need for large-scale, well-designed randomized clinical studies structured by a master protocol.
   (a) Describe the advantages of global master protocols.
   (b) Name two interesting platform approaches to emergency clinical trials.
   (c) Why do populations that have been underrepresented in past clinical research need to be included?
   (d) Describe some advantages of an operational global clinical research network.
8. What are some ways to guard against delays in regulatory review?
9. What measures are now under consideration to ensure that the social value created by research is available to all populations who may benefit from novel interventions in a health emergency?
10. Discuss how to multitask therapeutics development during an emergency.
11. Why is it important to implement Good Participatory Practice (GPP) principles even in an emergency?

References

Akinosoglou K, Schinas G, Gogos C. Oral antiviral treatment for COVID-19: a comprehensive review on nirmatrelvir/ritonavir. Viruses. 2022;14(11):2540.

Beigel JH, Tomashek KM, Dodd LE, Mehta AK, Zingman BS, Kalil AC, et al. Remdesivir for the treatment of Covid-19—final report. N Engl J Med. 2020;383(19):1813–26. https://doi.org/10.1056/NEJMoa2007764.

Beigi RH, Krubiner C, Jamieson DJ, Lyerly AD, Hughes B, Riley L, et al. The need for inclusion of pregnant women in COVID-19 vaccine trials. Vaccine. 2021;39(6):868–70. https://doi.org/10.1016/j.vaccine.2020.12.074.

Borkotoky S, Joshi A, Kaushik V, Jha AN. Chapter 6. Machine learning and artificial intelligence in therapeutics and drug development life cycle. In: Juber A, Badruddeen, Mohammad A, Mohammad Irfan K, editors. Drug development life cycle. Rijeka, HR: IntechOpen; 2022.

Buchman T, Draghia-Akli R, Adam S, Aggarwal N, Fessel J, Higgs E, et al. Accelerating coronavirus disease 2019 therapeutic interventions and vaccines—selecting compounds for clinical evaluation in coronavirus disease 2019 clinical trials. Crit Care Med. 2021;49:1963. https://doi.org/10.1097/CCM.0000000000005295.

Bugin K, Woodcock J. Trends in COVID-19 therapeutic clinical trials. Nat Rev Drug Discov. 2021;20:254. https://doi.org/10.1038/d41573-021-00037-3.

Califf RM. Now is the time to fix the evidence generation system. Clini Trials (London, England). 2023;20(1):3–12. https://doi.org/10.1177/17407745221147689.

Cassetti MC, Pierson TC, Patterson LJ, Bok K, DeRocco AJ, Deschamps AM, et al. Prototype pathogen approach for vaccine and monoclonal antibody development: a critical component of the NIAID plan for pandemic preparedness. J Infect Dis. 2022;227:1433. https://doi.org/10.1093/infdis/jiac296.

CIOMS. International ethical guidelines for health-related research involving humans. Geneva: Council for International Organisations of Medical Sciences; 2016.

EC. Paredness and Response (HERA) Brussels: European Commission; 2024 [updated 14 Aug 2024]. Available from: https://health.ec.europa.eu/health-emergency-preparedness-and-response-hera_en.

EMA. First vaccine to protect against Ebola. 2019.

EMA. New vaccine for prevention of Ebola virus disease recommended for approval in the European Union. Amsterdam: European Medicines Agency; 2020.

EMA. Report of the EMA/ETF workshop on lessons learned on clinical trials in public health emergencies. Contract No.: EMA/340269/2023. Amsterdam: European Medicines Agency; 2023.

Emanuel EJ, Wendler D, Grady C. What makes clinical research ethical? JAMA J Am Med Assoc. 2000;283(20):2701–11. https://doi.org/10.1001/jama.283.20.2701.

Farlow A, Torreele E, Gray G, Ruxrungtham K, Rees H, Prasad S, et al. The future of epidemic and pandemic vaccines to serve global public health needs. Vaccine. 2023;11(3):690.

FDA. ERVEBO. 2019. https://www.fda.gov/vaccines-blood-biologics/ervebo. Accessed 17 Oct 2021.

FDA. FDA Approves First Treatment for Ebola Virus. Washington, DC: U.S. Food and Drug Administration; 2020a.

FDA. FDA approves treatment for Ebola Virus. Washington, DC: U.S. Food and Drug Administration; 2020b.

FDA. Animal rule information. Silver Spring, MD: U.S. Food and Drug Administratrion; 2023. https://www.fda.gov/emergency-preparedness-and-response/mcm-regulatory-science/animal-rule-information. Accessed 13 Sept 2023.

Finlay BB, See RH, Brunham RC. Rapid response research to emerging infectious diseases: lessons from SARS. Nat Rev Microbiol. 2004;2(7):602–7. https://doi.org/10.1038/nrmicro930.

Ford A, Hwang A, Mo AX, Baqar S, Touchette N, Deal C, et al. Meeting summary: global vaccine and immunization research forum, 2021. Vaccine. 2023;41(11):1799–807. https://doi.org/10.1016/j.vaccine.2023.02.028.

G7. G7 therapeutics and vaccines clinical trials charter. In: Care HaS, editor. London: HMG Government (UK); 2021.

GAO. Regenerative medicine: therapeutic applications, challenges, and policy options. Contract No.: GAO-23-105430. Washington, DC: United States Government Accountability Office; 2023.

Gavi. Anual progress report 2021. Geneva: Gavi, the Vaccine Alliance; 2022.

Gavi. Gavi, the Vaccine Alliance helps vaccinate almost half the world's children against deadly and debilitating infectious diseases. Geneva: Gavi, the Vaccine Alliance; 2023. https://www.gavi.org/our-alliance/about. Accessed 18 July 2023.

GLOPID-R. GloPID-R funders living roadmap for clinical trial coordination. Oxford: Global Research Collaboration for Infectious Disease Preparedness (GloPID-R) Group CTNaFW; 2023.

Gomes MF, de la Fuente-Núñez V, Saxena A, Kuesel AC. Protected to death: systematic exclusion of pregnant women from Ebola virus disease trials. Reprod Health. 2017;14(3):172. https://doi.org/10.1186/s12978-017-0430-2.

Han JJ. FDA modernization act 2.0 allows for alternatives to animal testing. Artif Organs. 2023;47(3):449–50. https://doi.org/10.1111/aor.14503.

Henao-Restrepo AM, Camacho A, Longini IM, Watson CH, Edmunds WJ, Egger M, et al. Efficacy and effectiveness of an rVSV-vectored vaccine in preventing Ebola virus disease: final results from the Guinea ring vaccination, open-label, cluster-randomised trial (Ebola Ca Suffit!). Lancet. 2017;389(10068):505–18. https://doi.org/10.1016/S0140-6736(16)32621-6.

ICH. Good clinical practice: ICH harmonised guideline. Integrated addendum to ICH E6(R1): guideline for good clinical practice ICH E6(R2) ICH consensus guideline. Geneva: International Council for Harmonisation of Technical Requirements for Pharmaceuticals for Human Use (ICH); 2016.

ICH. Mission: harmonisation for better health. Geneva: International Council for Harmonisation of Technical Requirements for Pharmaceuticals for Human Use; 2023. https://www.ich.org/page/mission. Accessed 20 July 2023.

Kalil AC, Patterson TF, Mehta AK, Tomashek KM, Wolfe CR, Ghazaryan V, et al. Baricitinib plus Remdesivir for hospitalized adults with Covid-19. N Engl J Med. 2020;384(9):795–807. https://doi.org/10.1056/NEJMoa2031994.

Kelland K. Disease x—the 100 days mission to end pandemics. Kingston upon Thames, Surrey, UK: Canbury Press; 2023.

Kennedy SB, Neaton JD, Lane HC, Kieh MWS, Massaquoi MBF, Touchette NA, et al. Implementation of an Ebola virus disease vaccine clinical trial during the Ebola epidemic in Liberia: design, procedures, and challenges. Clin Trials (London, England). 2016;13(1):49–56. https://doi.org/10.1177/1740774515621037.

Korn EL, Freidlin B. Adaptive clinical trials: advantages and disadvantages of various adaptive design elements. J Natl Cancer Inst. 2017;109(6). https://doi.org/10.1093/jnci/djx013.

Lal A, Erondu NA, Heymann DL, Gitahi G, Yates R. Fragmented health systems in COVID-19: rectifying the misalignment between global health security and universal health coverage. Lancet. 2021;397(10268):61–7. https://doi.org/10.1016/S0140-6736(20)32228-5.

LaVange L, Adam SJ, Currier JS, Higgs ES, Reineck LA, Hughes EA, et al. Accelerating COVID-19 therapeutic interventions and vaccines (ACTIV): designing master protocols for evaluation of candidate COVID-19 therapeutics. Ann Intern Med. 2021;174:1293. https://doi.org/10.7326/m21-1269.

Matveeva O, Shabalina SA. Comparison of vaccination and booster rates and their impact on excess mortality during the COVID-19 pandemic in European countries. Front Immunol. 2023:14. https://doi.org/10.3389/fimmu.2023.1151311.

McGarry BE, Sommers BD, Wilcock AD, Grabowski DC, Barnett ML. Monoclonal antibody and oral antiviral treatment of SARS-CoV-2 infection in US nursing homes. JAMA. 2023;330:561. https://doi.org/10.1001/jama.2023.12945.

Mulangu S, Dodd LE, Davey RT Jr, Tshiani Mbaya O, Proschan M, Mukadi D, et al. A randomized, controlled trial of Ebola virus disease therapeutics. N Engl J Med. 2019;381(24):2293–303. https://doi.org/10.1056/NEJMoa1910993.

Muller MP, McGeer A, Straus SE, Hawryluck L, Gold WL. Clinical trials and novel pathogens: lessons learned from SARS. Emerg Infect Dis. 2004;10(3):389–94. https://doi.org/10.3201/eid1003.030702.

Murphy SJ, Samson LW, Sommers BD. COVID-19 antivirals utilization: geographic and demographic patterns of treatment in 2022. Washington, DC: U.S. Department of Health and Human Services, Office of the Assistant Secretary for Planning and Evaluation; 2022.

Murray DD, Babiker AG, Baker JV, Barkauskas CE, Brown SM, Chang CC, et al. Design and implementation of an international, multi-arm, multi-stage platform master protocol for trials of novel SARS-CoV-2 antiviral agents: therapeutics for inpatients with COVID-19 (TICO/ACTIV-3). Clin Trials. 2021;19(1):52–61. https://doi.org/10.1177/17407745211049829.

Naggie S, Boulware DR, Lindsell CJ, Stewart TG, Slandzicki AJ, Lim SC, et al. Effect of higher-dose ivermectin for 6 days vs placebo on time to sustained recovery in outpatients with COVID-19: a randomized clinical trial. JAMA. 2023;329(11):888–97. https://doi.org/10.1001/jama.2023.1650.

NASEM. Conducting clinical research during an epidemic. In: Keusch G, McAdam K, Cuff P, Mancher M, Busta E, editors. Integrating clinical research into epidemic response: the Ebola experience. Washington, DC: The National Academies Press; 2017a. p. 342.

NASEM. Integrating clinical research into epidemic response: the Ebola experience. Washington, DC: National Academies of Sciences Engineering and Medicine Publications, The National Academies Press; 2017b.

NIH. ACTIV-3: therapeutics for inpatients with COVID-19 (TICO). In: ClinicalTrials.gov. Bethesda, MD: National Institutes of Health; 2021. https://clinicaltrials.gov/ct2/show/NCT04501978. Accessed 20 Feb 2023.

NIH. Strategies and treatments for respiratory infections & viral emergencies (STRIVE). In: ClinicalTrials.gov. Bethesda, MD: National Institutes of Health; 2022. https://clinicaltrials.gov/ct2/show/NCT04969250. Accessed 20 Feb 2023.

NIH. Office of Laboratory Animal Welfare. Bethesda, MD: National Institutes of Health; 2023. https://olaw.nih.gov. Accessed 18 July 2023.

Nuzzo JB, Meyer D, Snyder M, Ravi SJ, Lapascu A, Souleles J, et al. What makes health systems resilient against infectious disease outbreaks and natural hazards? Results from a scoping review. BMC public health. 2019;19(1):1310. https://doi.org/10.1186/s12889-019-7707-z.

Offit P. Pandora's box: seven stories of science gone wrong. National Geographic: Washington, DC; 2017.

Pandemic Preparedness Partnership. 100 days mission to respond to future pandemic threats: reducing the impact of future pandemics by making diagnostics, therapeutics and vaccines available within 100 days: a report to the G7. London: G7 United Kingdom 2021; 2021.

RECOVERY Collaborative Group. Dexamethasone in Hospitalized Patients with Covid-19. N Engl J Med. 2020;384(8):693–704. https://doi.org/10.1056/NEJMoa2021436.

RECOVERY trial. UK Research and Innovation. 2023. https://www.ukri.org/news-and-events/tackling-the-impact-of-covid-19/vaccines-and-treatments/recovery-trial-identifies-covid-19-treatments/. Accessed 13 Sept 2023.

Robson F, Khan KS, Le TK, Paris C, Demirbag S, Barfuss P, et al. Coronavirus RNA proofreading: molecular basis and therapeutic targeting. Mol Cell. 2020;80(6):1136–8. https://doi.org/10.1016/j.molcel.2020.11.048.

Simonsen L, Higgs E, Taylor RJ. Clinical research networks are key to accurate and timely assessment of pandemic clinical severity. Lancet Glob Health. 2018;6(9):e956–e7. https://doi.org/10.1016/S2214-109X(18)30304-8.

Trogen B, Oshinsky D, Caplan A. Adverse consequences of rushing a SARS-CoV-2 vaccine: implications for public trust. JAMA. 2020;323(24):2460–1. https://doi.org/10.1001/jama.2020.8917.

van der Linden S. Misinformation: susceptibility, spread, and interventions to immunize the public. Nat Med. 2022;28(3):460–7. https://doi.org/10.1038/s41591-022-01713-6.

van Wijhe M, Ingholt MM, Andreasen V, Simonsen L. Loose ends in the epidemiology of the 1918 pandemic: explaining the extreme mortality risk in young adults. Am J Epidemiol. 2018;187(12):2503–10. https://doi.org/10.1093/aje/kwy148.

Viergever RF. The mismatch between the health research and development (R&D) that is needed and the R&D that is undertaken: an overview of the problem, the causes, and solutions. Glob Health Action. 2013;6(1):22450. https://doi.org/10.3402/gha.v6i0.22450.

White House. National biodefense strategy and implementation plan for countering biological threats, enhancing pandemic preparedness, and achieving global health security. In: President EOot, editor. Washington, DC: White House; 2022.

WHO. WHO recommends against the use of remdesivir in COVID-19 patients. Geneva: World Health Organization; 2020.

WHO. ACT-Accelerator outcomes report, 2020–2022 (incorporating Q3 update). Geneva: World Health Organization; 2022a.

WHO. Strengthening clinical trials to provide high-quality evidence on health interventions and to improve research quality and coordination. WHA 75.8. Geneva: World Health Organization. 2022b.

WHO Solidarity Trial Consortium. Remdesivir and three other drugs for hospitalised patients with COVID-19: final results of the WHO Solidarity randomised trial and updated meta-analyses. Lancet. 2022;399(10339):1941–53. https://doi.org/10.1016/S0140-6736(22)00519-0.

Wilson B, Wright K, Taylor R, Higgs E. Beyond recruitment: good participatory practice enhances the impact of research in a pandemic. Nat Med. 2021;27(3):369–71. https://doi.org/10.1038/s41591-021-01271-3.

Wolfe CR, Tomashek KM, Patterson TF, Gomez CA, Marconi VC, Jain MK, et al. Baricitinib versus dexamethasone for adults hospitalised with COVID-19 (ACTT-4): a randomised, double-blind, double placebo-controlled trial. Lancet Resp Med. 2022;10(9):888–99. https://doi.org/10.1016/S2213-2600(22)00088-1.

14.1 In Practice: RECOVERY Trial

Peter Horby, Leon Peto, and Martin Landray

Contents

Learning Track Note: This chapter appears in Learning Tracks: Clinical Research

E. S. Higgs and R. A. Sorenson (eds.), *Principles and Practice of Emergency Research Response*,
https://doi.org/10.1007/978-3-031-48408-7_18

Learning Objectives

This chapter will help readers understand and describe:

- The principles guiding the design of the Randomised Evaluation of COVID-19 Therapy Trial (RECOVERY)
- Elements essential to the implementation of the trial
- The potential benefits of streamlined point-of-care clinical trials in low- and middle-income settings

1 Introduction

Clinical trials of therapeutics are challenging even at the best of times, and, until recently, the barriers to high-quality clinical trials during health emergencies have seemed almost insurmountable. The routine burden of trial design, financing, ethical and regulatory approvals, contracting, drug supply, information and technology (IT) systems, training, etc., are compounded by extreme time pressures, political and operational constraints, and unpredictability.

At least 3000 coronavirus disease 2019 (COVID-19) treatment trials, evaluating hundreds of different therapies, have been planned since the start of the pandemic, and over 500 have reported results, but nearly all have been too small to provide answers clear enough to guide clinical practice or direct future research. As a result, we have been dependent on relatively few large trials to produce most of the reliable data on COVID-19 treatment. The RECOVERY Trial (Randomised Evaluation of COVID-19 Therapy) is the largest. At the time of writing, it had enrolled over 48,500 patients and produced clear answers on 11 therapies (RECOVERY trial 2023).

2 Early Foundations for COVID-19 Trials

2.1 Randomized Controlled Trials

The International Severe Acute Respiratory and Emerging Infections Consortium (ISARIC) is a global, grass-roots federation of clinical research networks established in 2009 to improve clinical research for epidemic and pandemic infectious diseases (ISARIC 2020). Through ISARIC, trusted peer-to-peer relationships have been established that allowed a rapid, collaborative response to the emergence of the severe acute respiratory syndrome coronavirus 2 (SARS-CoV-2). In the early days of 2020, clinical researchers within ISARIC worked together, utilizing experience with Middle East respiratory syndrome coronavirus (MERS-CoV) in Saudi Arabia, to support the rapid launch of therapeutic trials in COVID-19 in China. These included the very first randomized controlled trial in COVID-19 (Cao et al. 2020) and the very first placebo-controlled randomized trial (Wang et al. 2020). The rapid containment of COVID-19 in China meant that these trials did not achieve sufficient enrollment to provide definitive answers. Still, they did establish expectations for the rigorous study of therapeutics in COVID-19. As COVID-19 spread globally, the experience and achievements of these early trials in China informed the decision to fund and support the RECOVERY trial (◘ Fig. 1).

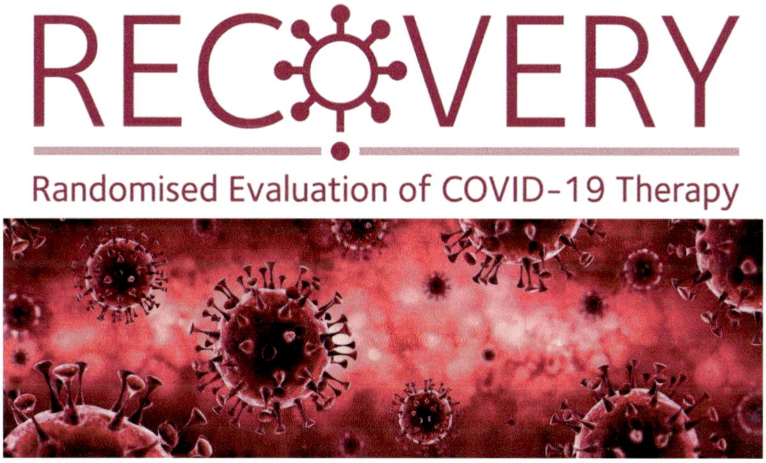

Fig. 1 Recovery logo and representation of SARS-CoV-2. (Nuffield Dept of Medicine, Oxford)

3 Principles

The design of RECOVERY was predicated on the recognition that most treatment effects are modest (perhaps reducing risk only by about one quarter), but such effect sizes on important outcomes would be very worthwhile, for example, a reduction of "only" 15–20% in the risk of death in patients hospitalized with COVID-19. A few principles were followed to reliably identify or rule out such treatment effects in the context of the pandemic.

- It needed to be ***randomized*** to ensure systematic errors (biases), such as those introduced when patient characteristics influence the treatment they receive, were substantially smaller than the treatment effect to be measured. RECOVERY initially compared multiple treatment arms with a shared control group and latterly used factorial randomization, in which patients are randomized to active treatment or usual care independently for each of the suitable study treatments. These features have meant that each patient contributed to an average of two treatment comparisons, doubling the effective size of the trial.
- It needed to be ***large*** to ensure systematic errors were substantially smaller than the treatment effect to be measured. Many trials, especially for diseases that are hard to study, apply various techniques to reduce the required sample size. These techniques include unrealistic effect sizes (such as a 50% reduction in mortality) or surrogate measures for meaningful clinical endpoints. COVID-19 was a pandemic of an acute viral illness with mortality concentrated in older patients with comorbidities: case numbers were unlikely to be limiting factors and "miracle" drugs resulting in large reductions in mortality were also unlikely. In the context of a pandemic likely to infect a large proportion of the world's population, modest effect sizes, such as a 20% reduction in mortality, could have a huge overall benefit. As such, a large trial was both desirable and feasible.
- It needed to be ***quick***. Therapeutics for epidemic infections can only be fully evaluated during an epidemic. The pandemic was moving very quickly, and previous experiences with the initial outbreak in Wuhan and other epidemic infections have shown that speed is of the essence if the infection wave is to be caught and sufficient patients enrolled to provide reliable answers.
- It needed to be ***simple***. Given the need for speed and scale, coupled with enormous impending stresses on the healthcare system and healthcare workers, simplicity was a necessity. The trial was designed to have minimal impact on frontline healthcare staff. Simplicity was achieved by simultaneously going back to first principles and fully utilizing new opportunities, such as data linkage. Due to the impracticality of

implementing a placebo-controlled design for multiple agents across hundreds of sites quickly, the objective and easily measurable clinical endpoint of survival was chosen.

Eligibility criteria were simple and trial processes (including paperwork) were minimized. The protocol was deliberately flexible so that it was suitable for a wide range of settings, allowing:

- A broad range of patients to be enrolled in large numbers, including children and pregnant women
- Randomization between only those treatment arms that are *both* available at the study-site hospital *and* not believed by the enrolling doctor to be contraindicated (e.g., by co-morbid conditions or concomitant medications)
- Treatment arms to be added or removed according to the emerging evidence
- Additional sub-studies could be added to provide more detailed information on side effects or sub-categorization of patient types, but these were not the primary objective and were not required for participation

4 Implementation

RECOVERY was established at unprecedented speed. The first draft of the protocol was available on March 10, 2020, it was submitted for regulatory and ethics review on March 13, received both approvals on March 17, and enrolled the first patient on March 19. Consequently, RECOVERY fully captured the first wave of COVID-19 in the UK, with the first 1000 patients recruited within 2 weeks and over 10,000 within 2 months. We have estimated that a delay of 2 weeks (starting recruitment on 8 April) would have missed the first 2500 recruitments and delayed the final dexamethasone results by 4 months (from mid-June to mid-October) (Fig. 2).

4.1 Infrastructure and Implementation

The RECOVERY trial captured the entire first wave of infections in the UK and enrolled more than 500 patients per day across about 175 clinical sites at its peak. This achievement owed much to the simplicity of design but also to the unique UK health research infra-

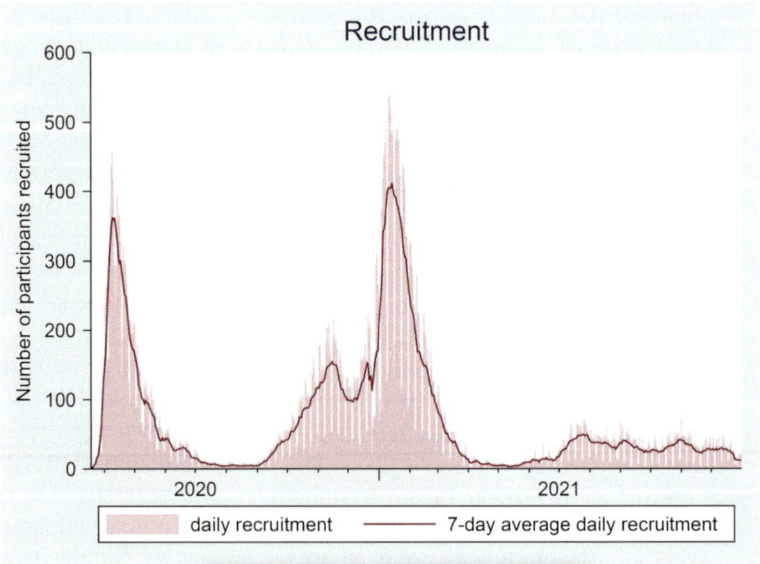

Fig. 2 RECOVERY trial recruitment over time. (Authors)

structure and environment. Four critical elements were:

1. *A national, publicly funded healthcare system*, the National Health Service (NHS). This national, standardized infrastructure enabled some key efficiencies. A single ethical committee could provide approval that was accepted by all NHS hospitals, without needing individual, site-level ethical approval. Due to similarities in contractual and legal structures, a single standard clinical trial agreement was acceptable to all sites.
2. *A national, publicly funded health research infrastructure*, the National Institutes of Health Research (NIHR): The NIHR was established in 2006 to create a health research infrastructure within the NHS. It is funded by the UK Government. The NIHR supports clinical research nurses and other vital resources for research delivery within the NHS. In 2012, in response to the poor research response to the 2009 influenza pandemic, the NIHR created a portfolio of hibernating studies that were given the status of "Urgent Public Health" (UPH) studies. This status was reenacted in 2020 and a process was initiated to designate *Urgent Public Health Research Studies for COVID*-19 (Ustianowski and Harman 2022). The designation was via an application to the NIHR Urgent Public Health Group. UPH-designated studies were prioritized for support by the NIHR infrastructure and staff. These fast-tracked, prioritized COVID-19 studies placed the UK at the forefront of global efforts to establish effective treatments against the disease.
3. *Centralized leadership through Chief Medical Officers* (CMOs): The UK has four CMOs, one for each constituent nation (England, Wales, Scotland, and Northern Ireland). These four CMOs communicated with one another at least weekly during the pandemic and supported a coordinated response, including health research. RECOVERY was designated as a national priority clinical trial. On April 1, 2020 the four CMOs, along with the NHS National Medical Director, sent a joint letter to all NHS hospitals asking that "*every effort is made to enroll COVID-19 patients in the national priority clinical trials*." The letter further stated, "*While it is for every individual clinician to make prescribing decisions, we strongly discourage the use of off-licence treatments outside of a trial, where participation in a trial is possible. The use of treatments outside of a trial, where participation was possible, is a wasted opportunity to create information that will benefit others. The evidence will be used to inform treatment decisions and benefit patients in the immediate future*."[1]
4. *A national, standardized digital health records system—NHS Digital*: Using linkage to national healthcare and viral statistics records for the measurement of trial outcomes reduces the need for data collection by local teams and improves the completeness of follow-up, improving the reliability of study outcomes. This also allows low-cost, long-term follow-up.

5 Impact and International Expansion

Within just over 100 days of opening, RECOVERY provided clear results that enabled three changes in global clinical practice: hydroxychloroquine, dexamethasone, and lopinavir-ritonavir. The results of RECOVERY had a major impact on global COVID-19 treatment guidelines and have been accepted by multiple regulatory authorities, including the U.S. Food and Drug Administration.

The early success of RECOVERY led to requests to open the trial outside the UK. While the healthcare systems in most other countries do not have the advantages of the UK, the international expansion of RECOVERY, particularly to low- and middle-income settings, is a test case for the

1 ► https://www.cas.mhra.gov.uk/ViewandAcknowledgment/ViewAlert.aspx?AlertID=103012.

wider use of streamlined clinical trial designs to fast-track improvement in healthcare globally. Successful expansion outside of the UK was demonstrated by the evaluation of higher dose dexamethasone in COVID-19, where more than half of the participants were recruited from low- and middle-income settings (RECOVERY Collaborative Group 2023).

Streamlined point-of-care clinical trials offer many benefits, but ensuring the acceptability of the results to regulatory authorities is critical (Califf et al. 2022). Proportionate risk adaptations were necessary in order to implement RECOVERY quickly and widely, and they have proven largely acceptable to regulators who have provided market authorization for new treatments for COVID-19 based on the results of RECOVERY.

Discussion Questions

1. What are the guiding principles in the design of the RECOVERY trial?
2. Provide examples illustrative of the inherent flexibility of RECOVERY.
3. Describe the critical elements that facilitated the implementation of the RECOVERY trial.
4. How would one conduct similar studies outside the United Kingdom?

References

Califf RM, Cavazzoni P, Woodcock J. Benefits of streamlined point-of-care trial designs: lessons learned from the UK RECOVERY study. JAMA Intern Med. 2022;182(12):1243–4. https://doi.org/10.1001/jamainternmed.2022.4810.

Cao B, Wang Y, Wen D, Liu W, Wang J, Fan G, et al. A trial of lopinavir-ritonavir in adults hospitalized with severe Covid-19. N Engl J Med. 2020;382(19):1787–99. https://doi.org/10.1056/NEJMoa2001282.

ISARIC. International Severe Acute Respiratory and emerging Infection Consortium. Oxford, UK: International Severe Acute Respiratory and Emerging Infection Consortium; 2020. https://isaric.org/. Accessed 14 July 2022.

RECOVERY trial. UK Research and Innovation. 2023. https://www.ukri.org/news-and-events/tackling-the-impact-of-covid-19/vaccines-and-treatments/recovery-trial-identifies-covid-19-treatments/. Accessed 13 Sept 2023.

RECOVERY Collaborative Group. Higher dose corticosteroids in patients admitted to hospital with COVID-19 who are hypoxic but not requiring ventilatory support (RECOVERY): a randomised, controlled, open-label, platform trial. Lancet. 2023;401(10387):1499–507.

Ustianowski A, Harman T. How the NIHR mobilised and adapted the UK research landscape to deliver COVID-19 studies. NIHR Blog: NIHR; 2022.

Wang Y, Zhang D, Du G, Du R, Zhao J, Jin Y, et al. Remdesivir in adults with severe COVID-19: a randomised, double-blind, placebo-controlled, multicentre trial. Lancet. 2020;395(10236):1569–78. https://doi.org/10.1016/s0140-6736(20)31022-9.

Research Response

Mosoka P. Fallah

Overview of Book Section IV: Several aspects of research response to infectious disease emergencies are described, providing both a review of recent experience and principles for improvement.

David Wholley et al. (► Chap. 15) explain the origins and organization of Accelerating COVID-19 Therapeutic Interventions and Vaccines (ACTIV), a U.S. public-private partnership created in response to COVID-19. ACTIV implemented a national research agenda for systematic, rigorous development of MCMs, culminating in well-designed clinical trials and emergency use authorization of several therapeutic agents, including direct acting antivirals and biologics. While ACTIV organized research in a country with an extremely diverse health system, Nick Lemoine et al. (► In Practice 15.1) describe the advantages of a unified health system for integrating research into infectious disease emergency response, and how they leveraged the UK National Health System to conduct prompt, rigorous research that produced safety and efficacy data on therapeutics, informed public health policy, and shaped patient care practice.

Rigorous research on response to an outbreak may well be most needed where it is hardest to implement. Rebecca Katz et al. (► Chap. 16) illustrate how conflict and state fragility can undermine population resistance to infectious disease while hindering response and suggest systemic changes to improve global preparedness. Carol Han et al. (► In Practice 16.1) highlight the work of the USAID Bureau for Humanitarian Assistance and its partners in responding to health emergencies in fragile states, where a humanitarian disaster may precede an outbreak and help it spread, or the outbreak may engender a humanitarian emergency. Mosoka Fallah (► Chap. 17) gives us a detailed picture of how the Liberian and U.S. governments worked together to implement an urgent research program in response to the 2014–2016 West Africa Ebola outbreak, cooperating in a low-income country still recovering from civil conflict. Their PREVAIL partnership demonstrated that a rigorous and ethical research response can be conducted even when most of the requirements are not immediately available. Experience during the 2014–2016 outbreak helped Richard Kojan and his colleagues at ALIMA (► In Practice 17.1) learn how effective clinical research and patient care could be carried out together, each building on and improving the other. They applied their experience during the 2018–2020 Ebola outbreak in the eastern Democratic Republic of the Congo, providing patient care and working with research staff to implement a successful Ebola therapeutics trial.

Clinical research response requires meaningful, equitable partnerships with all those who can affect or will be affected by clinical trials. Whether it is called good participatory practice (GPP) or social mobilization, communications, and community engagement (SMC), there are many reasons why respectful dialogue with the community is an indispensable part of research in an emergency, no matter how urgent the many other demands on the research team's time. Robert Sorenson et al. (► Chap. 18) provide an account of GPP in practice, while Michelle Andrasik and colleagues (► In Practice 18.1) focus on engagement between researchers and communities when there is no present emergency. Rhys O'Neill and David Cyprian (► In Practice 18.2) describe how they adapted social analytics techniques to support Ebola virus disease research response in Liberia and the eastern DRC. Ian Crozier (► Chap. 19) explains a vital but often low-profile area of infectious disease research—elucidating the natural history of a disease, including mechanisms of infection, pathology, and patient immune response—information vital to developing MCMs and clinical practice guidelines (CPGs) during public health emergencies. Donna Jacobsen et al. (► Chap. 20) explain how natural history and other emerging evidence are turned into CPGs that provide timely, useful guidance vital to good clinical care for patients, both before and after MCMs begin to become available.

Contents

15 ACTIV: A U.S. Public-Private Partnership Responds to COVID-19

David Wholley, Francis S. Collins, and Paul Stoffels

Contents

Learning Track Note: This chapter appears in Learning Tracks: Clinical Research

E. S. Higgs and R. A. Sorenson (eds.), *Principles and Practice of Emergency Research Response*,
https://doi.org/10.1007/978-3-031-48408-7_19

Learning Objectives

This chapter will help readers understand and describe:

- The purpose, scope, and organization of ACTIV, the public-private partnership devoted to Accelerating COVID-19 Therapeutic Interventions and Vaccines
- The need for close collaboration between government and private companies and what challenges the COVID-19 pandemic posed to the fulfillment of ACTIV's mission
- ACTIV studies conducted and compounds evaluated
- Key successes and lessons learned, including what features of the ACTIV response to COVID-19 are useful lessons for a future pandemic

1 The ACTIV Mission Begins

The call came on a Saturday in late March of 2020. Nearly 100,000 cases of coronavirus disease 2019 (COVID-19) had been reported in the United States, with about a thousand confirmed deaths (CDC 2020), and the scale of the threat posed by the pandemic was becoming ever more evident. The urgent need for a focused research effort by the U.S. government (USG) to reduce morbidity and mortality and slow the growth of the pandemic had become all too apparent. The scale of the public health emergency required innovative, expedited research, leveraging both public and private scientific capabilities and resources. Though early development of vaccines—which was to become the defining success of the U.S. response to the virus—was underway, it would be mid-May before Operation Warp Speed would be established to fully coordinate funding and logistics for vaccine trials, and many scientific and regulatory questions as to the conduct of these trials remained to be answered. The situation in therapeutics was considerably less promising.

Hundreds of preclinical and human clinical studies of potential treatments had already begun at biopharmaceutical companies, academic institutions, and government laboratories across the world. They would number in the thousands by August 2020. But the vast majority of these clinical studies—about 95% by Food and Drug Administration (FDA) estimates (Bugin and Woodcock 2021)—were small, non-randomized, underpowered efforts, often driven by individual investigators, that lacked the rigor and scale to deliver credible results. More than a few of these were duplicative—including several hundred studies being conducted on hydroxychloroquine (Pearson 2021).

A collaborative effort by both government and the private sector to accelerate research on therapeutics and vaccines, leveraging the resources for scientific innovation and research of the U.S. government, academia, and the private sector in well-planned trials, promised a better way forward. ACTIV was to become the closest thing the United States had to a national research agenda for therapeutic countermeasures to COVID-19, coordinating well-designed trials that could come to well-founded conclusions on the efficacy or futility of particular therapies. As Bugin and Woodcock (2021) point out, "a therapeutic trial ecosystem should possess two key capabilities … a robust screening mechanism … [and] a system to rapidly and efficiently generate definitive, highly actionable information on safety, efficacy and target population, of a quality that would be deemed acceptable by regulators." There was no such system in place in the United States in April 2020.

NIH Director Francis Collins had made the urgent weekend call to the Foundation for the National Institutes of Health (FNIH), created by Congress to facilitate innovative research that supports the NIH mission. Collins said it was time to launch a public-private research partnership in record time that could coordinate and synergize the emergency research response to COVID-19.

Urgent action on this scale required the ability to take advantage of existing resources wherever possible, including personal relationships and structures formed in previous biomedical research partnerships. Fortunately, several successful models for such a partnership were available, particularly the Accelerating Medicines Partnership (AMP) (NIH 2014), which had brought together government, academic, and pharmaceutical company scientists over the previous 6 years to tackle the characterization of disease pathways and drug targets in Alzheimer's, diabetes, and other major diseases. Taking advantage of extensive U.S. government funds already being pledged to combat the pandemic and expanding on the AMP model, the scientific leaders of four government agencies (ultimately eight), 12 biopharmaceutical companies (ultimately 20), and several nonprofit organizations rapidly assembled for an April 3 teleconference to agree on the strategy and structure for a similarly focused research response to the pandemic.

The ACTIV leadership (▣ Fig. 1) also conducted a significant campaign of outreach to other research response initiatives. Several of these were established prior to ACTIV: 12 pharmaceutical companies had formed the COVID Research and Development (R&D) Alliance in March 2020 (COVID R&D Alliance 2021), launching their own effort to identify assets that could be repurposed for ongoing trials. The Bill & Melinda Gates Foundation also launched its COVID-19 Therapeutics Accelerator to consider global testing of repurposed drugs (Suzman 2020). Representatives from both efforts were immediately incorporated into ACTIV. In addition, ACTIV leadership shared information and research strategies early on with the leaders of the UK's COVID-19 research efforts.

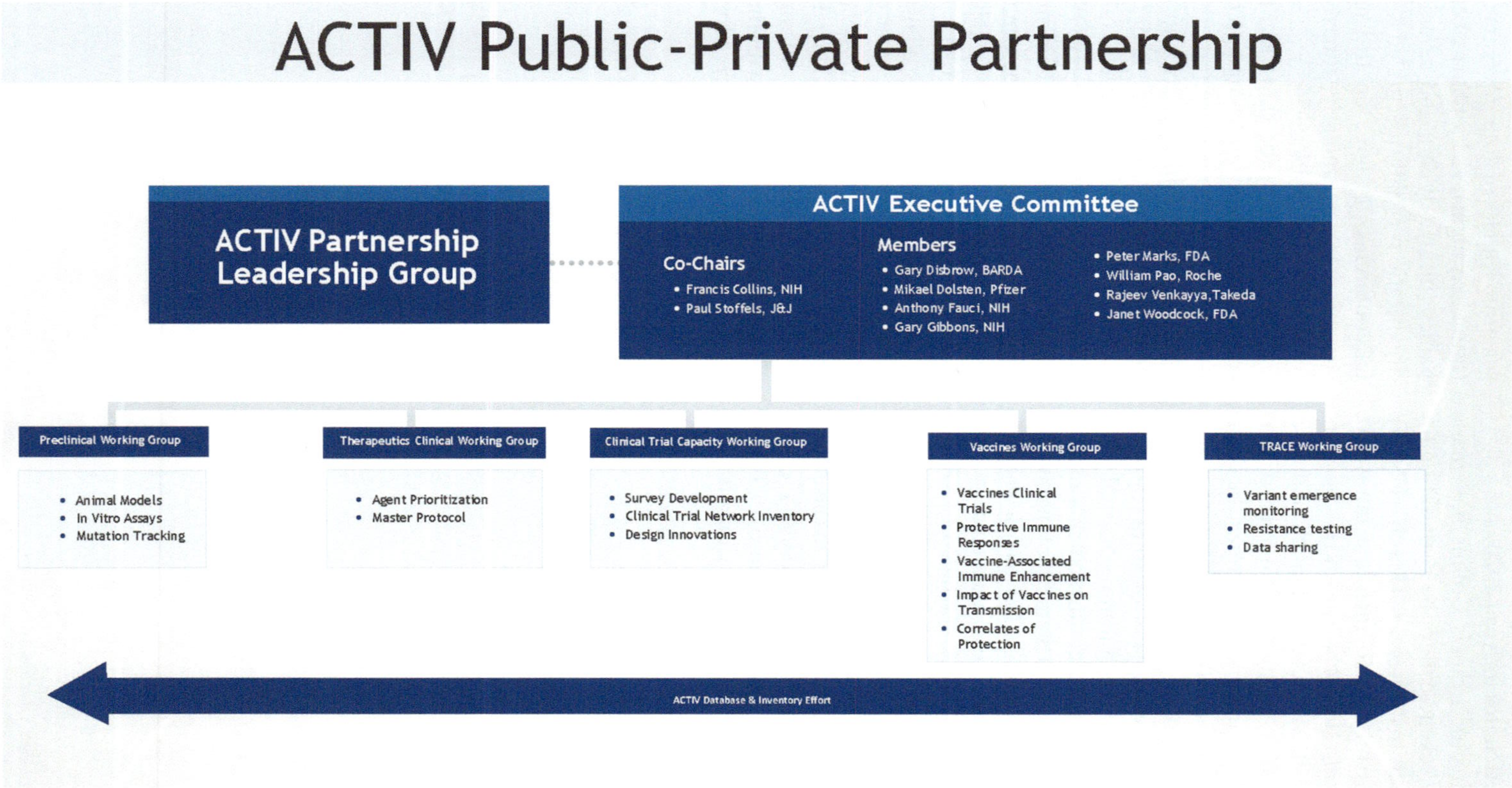

Fig. 1 Structure of ACTIV partnership. (NIH)

2 Working Groups

The ACTIV leadership quickly decided to focus on four major objectives and to assemble corresponding Working Groups (WGs) to execute them: a Therapeutics-Clinical WG, Clinical Trial Capacity WG, Preclinical WG, and Vaccines WG (Fig. 2). The leaders of the partner organizations asked over 100 scientists to join the ACTIV scientific team. They represented a broad range of disciplines, including virology, immunology, structural biology, pharmacology, toxicology, biostatistics, clinical trial management, and bioinformatics. Each WG was to be co-chaired by one senior scientist from NIH and one from a company (NIH 2021a). Seizing on an unparalleled spirit of openness and collaboration, the group also decided to share all their know-how and data, including much that would normally have been deemed proprietary, openly and promptly among all participants. The NIH Director sent personal invitations to serve on the Working Groups directly to each WG nominee within the following week. The partnership, called ACTIV (Accelerating COVID-19 Therapeutic Interventions and Vaccines), was formally launched and fully operational by April 17 (Collins and Stoffels 2020).

2.1 Preclinical Working Group

2.1.1 Charge

The Preclinical WG (PCWG) was charged with standardizing and sharing preclinical evaluation resources and methods and accelerating testing of candidate therapies and vaccines to support entry into clinical trials. Its focus was on

- Establishing a centralized process and repository for harmonizing and sharing methods and evaluating animal models
- Extending access to high-throughput screening facilities, especially in biosafety level 3 (BSL-3) labs
- Increasing access to validated animal models
- Enhancing comparison of approaches to identify informative assays
- Generating a process to assess viral variant effects on vaccines and therapeutics (NIH 2020c)

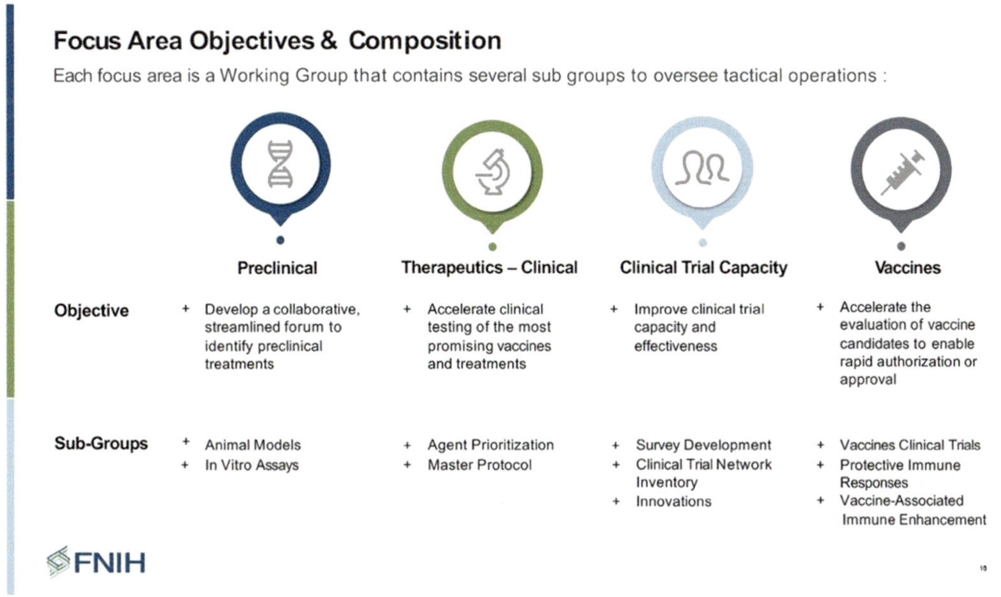

Fig. 2 Another view of the focus areas that defined the working groups. (By permission of FNIH (FNIH 2020))

COVID-19 posed numerous obstacles to preclinical research, which the ACTIV PCWG sought to address. To take one example, by April 2020 there was already a shortage of animals most relevant to SARS CoV-2 research, especially nonhuman primate (NHP) species, such as African green monkeys and rhesus macaques—shortages resulting both from demand for their use in the burgeoning number of COVID-19 research studies and from cross-border restrictions on animal transport imposed during the pandemic. Working closely with the leadership of NIH and its seven National Primate Research Centers, the PCWG developed a National Strategy for NHP Research designed to steward the remaining supply of primates and centrally coordinate studies that required their use, including the creation of a master protocol design for NHP studies (Coronavirus Vaccine and Treatment Evaluation Network 2020).

In parallel, the WG developed a master inventory of both in-vitro and in-vivo research resources for use by the partnership, established standard operating procedures (SOPs) for accelerating preclinical agent development in response to pandemics (Grobler et al. 2020), published a review of appropriate animal models (Hewitt et al. 2020) and two online "field guides" to help researchers use animal models in COVID-19 medical countermeasure development (NIH 2020a), and created a public database for sharing preclinical data generated by NIH- and company-funded studies via the National Center for Advancing Translational Sciences (NCATS) Open Science Portal (NIH/NCATS 2020b). The PCWG also posted a set of fact sheets on preclinical testing resources on the Portal (NIH/NCATS 2020a), using it to power a matchmaking process that paired resources and potential funding sources with the sponsors of agents that had been prioritized in collaboration with the TCWG.

As the pandemic progressed, the rise of viral variants and their potential to increase the transmission of severe acute respiratory syndrome coronavirus 2 (SARS-CoV-2) and to blunt the effectiveness of vaccines and therapeutics became a critical obstacle to attempts to end the pandemic. In February 2021 the PCWG established a specific initiative to help monitor the global emergence and circulation of SARS-CoV-2 mutations. This initiative, dubbed TRACE (Tracking Resistance and Coronavirus Evolution), brought together the resources of the NIH National Center for Advancing Translation, the National Library of Medicine and National Center for Biotechnological Information, and a number of ACTIV biopharmaceutical company partners to collect initial sequence data and cross reference them against databases of experimentally or clinically characterized variants at CDC and elsewhere (NIH 2021c). TRACE characterized variants that it had prioritized using both in vitro and in vivo analysis. Results were shared publicly on a weekly basis with the entire scientific community. TRACE was coordinated with surveillance and testing efforts at other U.S. government agencies. As the tasks that comprised the original mission of the PCWG were completed and its focus turned wholly to variants, the PCWG as an entity was essentially replaced by TRACE in August 2021.

2.2 Therapeutics Clinical Working Group

2.2.1 Charge

Prioritize therapeutic agents for testing within an adaptive master protocol strategy that will be jointly designed by the partnership and quickly launched in networks identified by the Clinical Trial Capacity Working Group (NIH 2020d).

2.2.2 Screening Candidate Therapeutics

The most pressing need in responding to the pandemic was to establish a systematic approach to evaluating possible COVID-19 therapeutics, with the first task being to select which out of hundreds of potential drug candidates should be advanced for clinical trials or preclinical testing. The ACTIV Therapeutics-Clinical WG (TCWG) assembled an *Agent Prioritization Subgroup* (◘ Fig. 3) that developed and then continually refined a rapid, robust process for identifying potential candidates, assembling uniform dossiers of relevant data, and conducting a systematic, unbiased evaluation of each agent (Buchman et al. 2021). ACTIV deliberately cast a wide net: the subgroup considered antiviral agents, neutralizing antibodies, immunomodulators, and symptomatic/supportive therapies, such as antithrombotics and host-targeted agents; it aimed these at different target populations, including outpatients and inpatients infected with SARS-CoV-2.

The first wave of agent prioritization, which was focused on identifying existing, already approved candidates, was necessarily opportunistic. An initial candidate list of some 450 agents was assembled using a mixture of public databases of potential COVID-19 treatments that had begun to appear by mid-April 2020, and additional lists were solicited from several collaborators. Some 170 of these agents were either fully approved or had been submitted to the FDA for Investigational New Drug (IND) authorization to go into human trials. These agents were deemed by the subgroup as potentially ready for clinical testing in COVID-19 patients and were then assigned to a small team of reviewers for further triage. Besides examining safety and efficacy data and the availability of enough active pharmaceutical ingredients for both a clinical trial and eventual treatment of large patient populations post approval, reviewers made an extensive effort to determine whether there were already sufficiently robust trials of a given agent underway so that additional trials would not be duplicative. The 39 agents that emerged from triage went through a blinded, formal scoring process by individual reviewers using preestablished criteria and then a final evaluation in common by the entire Subgroup, resulting in the selection of three immunomodulators and three antithrombotic agents for the first set of clinical trials. This initial wave was completed in 3 weeks (Buchman et al. 2021).

Agents that were not selected were not simply discarded but often deferred for additional evaluation later, as more data on the

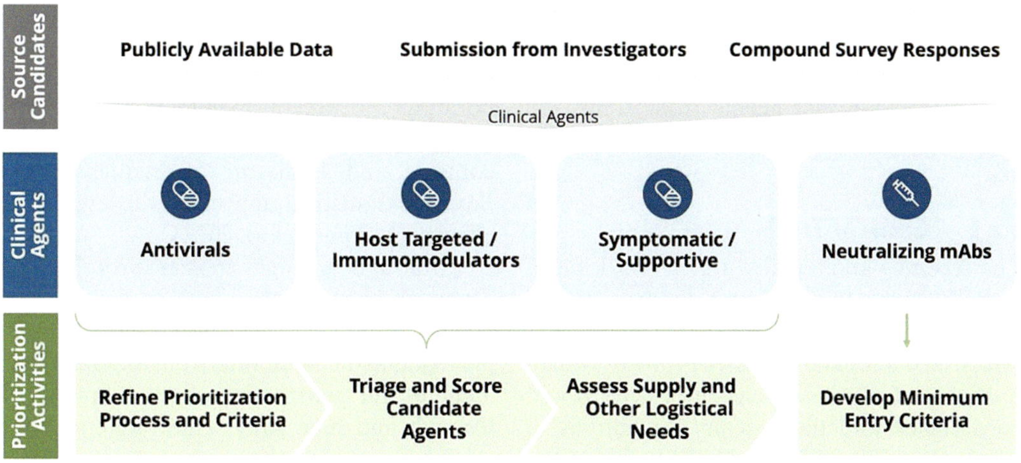

◘ **Fig. 3** An overview of the sources used to identify agents for prioritization in the ACTIV master protocols. The clinical therapeutics fall into four categories (antivirals, immunomodulators, supportive therapies, and neutralizing antibodies). The activities of the prioritization team also included refining the process and criteria, scoring the candidates, and assessing logistical needs. (NIH 2020d)

agents became available. (None of the antiviral agents considered in the first wave of evaluation were prioritized, for example, largely due to insufficient or conflicting preclinical or early clinical SARS-CoV-2 data at the time.) A second and third wave of prioritization efforts focused respectively on neutralizing antibodies and other novel agents in development or not adequately evaluated in the first wave. Several innovations were quickly added to the evaluation process for these later waves. ACTIV launched a public online survey portal to encourage the global scientific community to nominate additional agents and to provide a more automated means of collecting and disseminating the related drug data packages to reviewers (NIH 2021b). The review panels were supplemented with additional expertise to support evaluations of specific classes of agents; both scoring criteria and ways of categorizing outcomes were further refined. Because many of the nominated agents were at an earlier stage of drug development and required further preclinical investigation, the TCWG prioritization team began coordinating its evaluations with a similar team established by the Preclinical WG which could connect sponsors with the most promising early-stage therapies with appropriate preclinical research resources to advance them towards the clinic. Between mid-April 2020 and the beginning of 2022, the TCWG evaluated more than 800 agents from some 250 sources and moved 33 into ACTIV clinical trials.

2.2.3 Clinical Trials

The second—and equally urgent—task faced by ACTIV was to implement rigorous clinical trials to test these therapies. The TCWG established a separate *Master Protocol Design Subgroup* of experts to select how trials would be designed and the specific populations in which they should be conducted. Given the large number of potential candidate drugs in multiple classes to be tested and the need to test them in diverse populations exposed to COVID-19, traditional single-drug trials were judged early on to be infeasible. Instead, the group turned to an intense effort to rapidly design a set of master protocol trials. Although master protocols typically take longer to plan and launch than single-drug trials, they have the significant advantage of allowing multiple drugs at different stages of development to be tested simultaneously using a single overarching protocol (LaVange et al. 2021). They can also accommodate a streamlined regulatory approval framework encompassing both Phase II interim evaluations of safety and efficacy and Phase III registrational designs, with shared controls in many cases. Drugs may be dropped for futility or safety reasons and replaced relatively quickly with new candidates (Woodcock and LaVange 2017).

Consulting frequently with the FDA, an integrated team of pharmaceutical company, academic, and government statisticians examined protocols from existing COVID-19 trials, including ACTT, REMAP-CAP, and I-SPY COVID as input to designing each ACTIV trial (Beigel et al. 2020; I-SPY COVID-19 trial 2020; REMAP-CAP Investigators et al. 2021). They carefully selected and aligned endpoints across multiple protocols using the then-current (albeit rapidly evolving) understanding of COVID-19. They ensured each trial would be adequately powered while being executed with maximum speed and efficiency. Randomized, double-blind designs were chosen for all of the trial arms (except for ACTIV-4A, an inpatient trial of anticoagulants, which used a pragmatic design), incorporating the use of matching placebo and standard of care (where feasible), common controls, and a mixture of frequentist and Bayesian statistical approaches to evaluating efficacy (LaVange et al. 2021).

Although a single master protocol can often take more than a year to develop and launch, ACTIV launched a total of ten master protocols in the 14 months from the announcement of the partnership in mid-April 2020 through mid-June 2021. These were grouped and designated with numbers according to when protocol planning was initiated. A total of 33 distinct therapies were tested in these trials over the next 2 years.

By mid-2022, ACTIV had completed testing on 29 agents (■ Table 1) and generated significant findings on their efficacy in specific patient populations. Six of these showed com-

Table 1 Summary table of therapeutic agents studied in ACTIV trials (NIH)

Therapeutic, company	Class, administration	New/repurposed (R)	Timing/result
ACTIV-1 Inpatient Phase 3			
Orencia® (abatacept), BMS	Immune modulator, intravenous	R	Ended 2Q 2022/showed efficacy in reducing mortality
Remicade® (infliximab), Janssen	Immune modulator, intravenous	R	Ended 2Q 2022/showed efficacy in reducing mortality
Cenicriviroc, AbbVie	Immune modulator, oral	New	Ended Q3 2021/failed interim analysis
ACTIV-2 Outpatient Phase 2/3			
Tixagevimab/Cilgavimab (AZD7442), AstraZeneca	mAb cocktail, intramuscular	New	Ended Q4 2021 due to company decision
Tixagevimab/Cilgavimab (AZD7442), AstraZeneca	mAb cocktail, intravenous	New	Ended Q1 2022/awaiting topline results
Amubarvimab/Romlusevimab (Brii-196 and Brii-198), Brii Biosciences	mAb cocktail, intravenous	New	Ended Q3 2021/efficacy shown/EUA filed
Bamlanivimab (LY-CoV555), Eli Lilly	mAb single, intravenous	New	Ended Q4 2020/efficacy shown/EUA granted
Camostat Mesylate, Sagent	Antiviral, oral	R	Ended Q3 2021/graduation criteria unmet
SNG001 IFN-beta, Synairgen	Immune modulator, inhaled	R	Ended Q1 2022 due to operational futility
SAB-185, SAb Biotherapeutics	Polyclonal antibodies, intravenous	New	Passed interim analysis; ended Q1 2022 due to operational futility
BMS-9986414 and BMS 986413 (also known as C135-LS/C144-LS), Rockefeller/BMS	mAb cocktail, subcutaneous	New	Ended Q1 2022/graduation criteria unmet
ACTIV-3 Inpatient and Critical Care Phase 3			
Inpatients			
Tixagevimab/Cilgavimab (AZD7442), AstraZeneca	mAb cocktail, intravenous	New	Ended Q3 2021/showed efficacy in reducing mortality
Amubarvimab/Romlusevimab (Brii-196 and Brii-198), Brii Biosciences	mAb cocktail, intravenous	New	Ended Q1 2021/graduation criteria unmet

(continued)

Table 1 (continued)

Therapeutic, company	Class, administration	New/repurposed (R)	Timing/result
Bamlanivimab (LY-CoV555), Eli Lilly	mAb single, intravenous	New	Ended Q1 2021/graduation criteria unmet
Soratinib (VIR-7831), GSK-VIR	mAb single, intravenous	New	Ended Q1 2021/graduation criteria unmet
Ensovibep (MP0420), Molecular Partners-Novartis	DARPins®[a], intravenous	New	Ended Q4 2021/graduation criteria unmet
PF-07304814, Pfizer	Protease inhibitor, intravenous	New	Ended Q3 2021 due to company decision
Critical Care (ACTIV 3B)			
Zyesami™ (aviptadil acetate), NeuroRX and **Veklury® (remdesivir),** Gilead	Immune modulator/antiviral, intravenous	R	Zyesami arm ended due to futility 2Q 2022; Veklury arm closed due to operational futility Q2 2022
ACTIV-4 Outpatient, Inpatient, and Convalescent Phase 3			
Outpatients (ACTIV 4B)			
Eliquis® (apixaban), BMS/Pfizer	Anticoagulant, oral	R	Ended Q4 2021 due to operational futility (awaiting results)
Aspirin, BMS/Pfizer	Antiplatelet, oral	R	Ended Q4 2021 due to operational futility (awaiting results)
Inpatients (ACTIV 4A)			
Un-fractionated heparin	Anticoagulant, intravenous	R	Ended Q1 2021/efficacy shown
Low molecular weight heparin	Anticoagulant, injection	R	Ended Q3 2021/efficacy shown
Therapeutic heparin and P2Y12 inhibitors	Anticoagulant, intravenous and oral	R	Ended Q2 2021/failed interim analysis
Prophylactic heparin and P2Y12 inhibitors	Anticoagulant, intravenous and oral	R	Ended Q2 2022/passed interim analysis/ awaiting topline results
Crizanlizumab, Novartis	mAb single, intravenous	R	Projected to complete Q1 2023
SGLT2 inhibitors, various	Sodium/glucose cotransporter-2 inhibitors	R	Projected to complete Q1 2023

(continued)

Table 1 (continued)

Therapeutic, company	**Class, administration**	**New/repurposed (R)**	**Timing/result**
Inpatients (ACTIV 4HT)			
TXA127, constant therapeutics	Mas receptor agonist, intravenous	New	Ended Q2 2022/failed interim analysis
TRV027, Trevena	AT1R b-arrestin agonist, intravenous	New	Ended Q2 2022/failed interim analysis
Fostamatinib, Rigel	Immune modulator, oral	R	Projected to complete Q44 2022
Convalescent (ACTIV 4-C)			
Eliquis® (apixaban), BMS/Pfizer	Anticoagulant, oral	R	Passed interim analysis/ended due to operational futility Q2 2022
ACTIV-5 Inpatient Phase 2			
Skyrizi™ (risankizumab), AbbVie/Boehringer Ingelheim	Immune modulator, intravenous	R	Ended Q4 2021/awaiting topline results
Lenzilumab, Humanigen	Immune modulator, intravenous	New	Ended Q4 2021/awaiting topline results
Danicopan, Alexion	Factor D inhibitor, oral	New	Ended Q1 2022/awaiting topline results
ACTIV-6, Outpatient Phase 3, Repurposed Drugs			
Ivermectin 400mcg, Ingenous	Immune modulator/antiviral, oral	R	Ended Q2 2022/failed to show efficacy
Ivermectin 600mcg, Ingenous	Immune modulator/antiviral, oral	R	Projected to complete Q3 2022
Fluvoxamine, Apotex	Immune modulator, oral	R	Enrollment completed Q2 2022/awaiting topline results
Fluticasone, GSK	Immune modulator, inhaled	R	Ended Q2 2022/failed to show efficacy

[a] A multi-targeted direct acting antiviral therapeutic candidate

pelling evidence of benefit. ACTIV-1 showed that hospitalized patients taking either of two immune modulators, infliximab (Remicade) and abatacept (Orencia), experienced substantial improvement in mortality and in clinical status at 28 days over those taking a placebo. Two monoclonal antibodies—bamlanivimab and a cocktail of Brii 196/198—were proven to be effective in outpatients in the ACTIV-2 study, although they failed to show significant benefit in hospitalized patients receiving remdesivir. Lilly applied for and received an emergency use authorization (EUA) for bamlanivimab; Brii applied for an EUA for the 196/198 mAb cocktail based on the data from ACTIV-2 (Brii Biosciences 2021). In addition, the monoclonal antibody cocktail from AstraZeneca, AZD7442 (Evusheld, a combination of tixagevimab and cilgavimab), was shown to be effective in ACTIV-2 with a benefit in all-cause mortality in hospitalized patients being treated with remdesivir (ACTIV-3 TICO Study Group 2022). Combined with data from two non-ACTIV studies, REMAP-CAP and ATTAC, the ACTIV-4A trial found therapeutic dose anticoagulation superior to prophylactic dose in reducing the need for vital organ support in moderately ill hospitalized patients. In contrast, full-dose anticoagulation did not reduce the need for organ support in severely ill (ICU) patients. Just as important for clinical practice, 15 agents were shown to be ineffective against COVID-19. These and other results from the ACTIV trials were subsequently incorporated into the NIH's COVID-19 treatment guidelines.

Having achieved their stated aims—and in response to the changing nature of the pandemic—the ACTIV-1, ACTIV-2, ACTIV-3, ACTIV-3B, ACTIV-4B, ACTIV-4C, and ACTIV 5 studies closed to enrollment in early 2022. Additional results are expected from the remaining protocols.

2.3 Clinical Trial Capacity Working Group

2.3.1 Charge

Develop an inventory of clinical trial capacity, including networks from NIH Institutes and Centers and clinical research organizations (also known as contract research organizations or CROs), that will serve as potential settings in which to implement effective COVID-19 clinical trials. The working group completed its charge as of July 31, 2020.

2.3.2 Clinical Trials in Early 2020

The environment for launching clinical trials in the first months of the COVID-19 pandemic was daunting. SARS-CoV-2 infections spread rapidly and unevenly across different geographies: many hospitals that could serve as potential trial sites were overwhelmed with admissions one month and experienced steep declines in case counts the next. Hospitals were not only coping with unpredictable surges of patients, but they were also figuring out how best to treat a new and sometimes enigmatic disease. Competition for investigators and other trial staff with the many existing COVID-19 studies posed a particular challenge. The need to engage multiple existing trial networks—especially the large networks already established by NIH—was clear, but these would have to be supplemented with additional sites and resources from CROs, Site Management Organizations (SMOs), and other networks to accrue a sufficient number of patients quickly enough to address the shifting course of the pandemic. NIH lacked even a single comprehensive database of the sites available in its own networks, much less those in external networks, and the need to understand which specific sites had both the capability and available capacity to conduct additional studies was urgent.

2.3.3 The ACTIV Clinical Trial Capacity WG (CTCWG)

The ACTIV CTCWG was formed explicitly to address the challenge of launching trials amidst a global crisis. Working closely with the TCWG, it conducted an international survey of potential COVID-19 clinical trial networks and sites to assess site capabilities and readiness to conduct additional trials and continuously shared the results with the master protocol design teams. By August, the CTCWG had collected data from 63 different trial networks and 39 CROs and SMOs, including data on 725 distinct trial sites. These data were combined with geographic mapping, COVID-19 disease incidence data, and visualization capabilities into a unique geotracking tool that has enabled the ACTIV Therapeutics and Vaccines Clinical Trial Working Groups to choose the most effective networks and sites to support ACTIV master protocols and associated trials. As of mid-2022, the ACTIV clinical trials had collectively enrolled more than 21,000 patients using more than 620 sites across the U.S. and internationally. The companies represented in ACTIV also generously shared with all ACTIV WGs a compendium of their strategies for enhancing the conduct of trials during a pandemic, including specific trial strategies for deploying virtual, digital, and online technology solutions.

2.3.4 Clinical Trial Innovations and Resources

The working group created a reference guide for novel clinical trial innovations along with a resource map of available solutions to help enable the safe and efficient conduct of ACTIV clinical trials under the unique conditions imposed by the COVID-19 pandemic. Working group members worked with healthcare professionals conducting clinical trials sponsored by ACTIV and its partners to identify useful solutions for ACTIV clinical trials (NIH 2020b).

2.4 Vaccines Working Group

2.4.1 Charge

Accelerate the evaluation of vaccine candidates by supporting harmonized clinical efficacy trials and a parallel effort to generate biomarkers and other evidence for more rapid approval/authorization (NIH 2021d).

2.4.2 Harmonized Clinical Trials

With NIH and BARDA actively planning to conduct COVID-19 vaccine trials soon after the SARS-CoV-2 virus was characterized, a forum was urgently needed to review and decide a number of critical scientific, regulatory, and policy questions. The Vaccines Working Group (VWG) included high-level representation from NIH, the FDA, the European Medicines Agency (EMA), and leading academic and industry experts. Ten pharmaceutical companies were represented, including five COVID-19 vaccine developers that advanced candidates to Phase III trials: AstraZeneca, Janssen, Moderna, Novavax, and Pfizer. The ability of several of these vaccine developers to combine access to trial sites established by NIH across the globe with implementation at their own sites helped make these trials successful.

Among its first accomplishments, the VWG developed harmonized protocols with common symptomatic endpoints for the vaccine efficacy trials funded through the Biomedical Advanced Research and Development Authority (BARDA) and NIH and established the needed scale for Phase III testing to compare trial results. Correlates of protection could be analyzed across all trials (Corey et al. 2020). The working group analyzed potential regulatory pathways for vaccine introduction, including criteria for EUA of vaccines and evidence to support accelerated vaccine approval. Two manuscripts published by the VWG addressed complex, controversial scientific issues with profound public health implications: the scientific and operational challenges of developing controlled human infection trials (Deming et al. 2020) and the potential threat posed by immune-associated disease enhancement (Haynes et al. 2020). The working group also examined approaches to evaluating vaccine safety and efficacy in pregnant and pediatric populations; proposed ways to evaluate the impact of vaccines on transmission; assessed the implications of vaccine efficacy for future trials; and recommended approaches to evaluating the use of vaccines in immunocompromised patients.

2.5 ACTIV-Associated Efforts

NIH carried on many of its own COVID-19 research efforts in addition to the ACTIV Partnership. Although they benefited from the scientific policy work of the VWG, the operations of the USG's trials of SARS-CoV-2 vaccines were carried out by NIAID in collaboration with BARDA and Operation Warp Speed. NIH also sponsored and conducted a number of trials of various therapies outside of the ACTIV partnership. In many cases these benefited from the resources and knowledge established by the ACTIV WGs, as well as from strategic scientific perspectives contributed by the ACTIV Leadership Team, and became known as "ACTIV-Associated Trials" (◘ Table 2). On the other hand, the efforts to develop diagnostics for COVID-19 were managed by a separate NIH initiative, RAD-X (NIH 2021d), which is fully described elsewhere in this volume (▶ Chap. 11).

Table 2 Summary table of therapeutic agents studied in ACTIV-associated trials (NIH)

ACTIV-Associated					
Adaptive COVID-19 Treatment Trial (ACTT) Inpatient					
Gilead	Veklury® (remdesivir)	Antiviral	Intravenous	Repurposed	Ended
Gilead/Eli Lilly	Veklury® (remdesivir) and Olumiant® (baricitinib)	Antiviral/anti-inflammatory	Intravenous/Oral	Repurposed	Ended
Gilead/Merck KGaA	Veklury® (remdesivir) and Rebif® (IFN-beta)	Antiviral/immune modulator	Injection	Repurposed	Ended
Gilead/Eli Lilly/other	Veklury® (remdesivir) and Olumiant® (baricitinib) or dexamethasone	Antiviral/anti-inflammatory/immune modulator	Intravenous/oral	Repurposed	▶ Ended
Inpatient Treatment with Anti-Coronavirus Immunoglobulin (ITAC)					
Gilead/other	Veklury® (remdesivir) and hyperimmune intravenous immunoglobulin (hIVIG)	Antiviral	Intravenous	N/A	Q3 2021
Convalescent Plasma in Outpatients with COVID-19 (C3PO)					
Other	Convalescent plasma	Convalescent plasma	Intravenous	N/A	▶ Ended
Convalescent Plasma to Limit COVID-19 Complications in Hospitalized Patients (CONTAIN COVID-19)					
Other	Convalescent plasma	Convalescent plasma	Intravenous	N/A	Q2 2021
Passive Immunity Trial of Our Nation (PassItOn) Inpatient					
Other	Convalescent plasma	Convalescent plasma	Intravenous	N/A	Q2 2021

3 Organizing ACTIV

Making all of this happen in the context of a public health emergency required considerable organization and intensive communication. A Leadership Team, consisting of the heads of NIH and several of its Institutes, senior leadership from the other government agencies and nonprofits involved, and global heads of research and development from each company was established following the first ACTIV meeting in April 2020. In June, a subset of the team, the Executive Committee, convened to ensure nimble, timely decision-making. Co-chaired by NIH Director Francis Collins and Paul Stoffels, Chief Scientific Officer of Johnson & Johnson, these two groups met every 2 weeks, guided overall strategy, liaised with other COVID-19 research efforts, and provided specific direction to the Working Groups. Senior leadership remained fully engaged throughout. Although the companies contributed drugs for the trials as well as expertise, Operation Warp Speed (OWS) provided funding through NIH to support preclinical testing and clinical testing of therapeutics (Slaoui et al. 2020); its Therapeutics Head, Janet Woodcock, served as a key member of the ACTIV Executive Committee. Once OWS was formally established in mid-May 2020, liaisons from its operations were added to all the ACTIV WGs. The WGs, their sub-teams, and the groups leading each of the ACTIV clinical trial protocols met at least weekly and often more frequently, and the NIH Director convened a daily "war room" meeting involving FNIH and NIH research staff working on all aspects of the pandemic response to monitor operations and address obstacles in real time.

Ensuring the participation of diverse populations in both the vaccine and therapeutic trials, especially in minority and underserved communities, was a particular focus of ACTIV and ACTIV-related research efforts. NIH senior leadership, including NIH Director Collins and NIAID Director Anthony S. Fauci and their staffs, frequently met leaders of the major vaccine companies throughout the summer and fall of 2020 to emphasize the importance of including racial and ethnic groups disproportionately affected by the virus. In therapeutics, the ACTIV clinical trial leads teamed up with two government-led efforts to boost minority enrollment: (1) the NIH Community Engagement Alliance Against COVID-19 Disparities (CEAL) community outreach initiative and (2) HHS's online information portal, Combat Covid. As of June 2021, the participation rate of people of color in the major vaccine trials ranged between 26 and 37%—a big improvement over original projections, if still somewhat below the national proportion of people of color in the U.S. population. The participation rate of people of color across all ACTIV therapeutics trials averaged 53%.

Given all these efforts, it was not uncommon for ACTIV to generate 40 or 50 hour-long weekly meetings. Most of the ACTIV scientists were volunteers, and many continued to perform their normal responsibilities in parallel with supporting the partnership. Strong, persistent, and centralized project management was therefore essential. This was provided by four senior program management staff at FNIH under the leadership of David Wholley, supported by eight to ten project managers from Deloitte Consulting under contract to FNIH, who constituted the Central Project Management office that planned agendas, ran meetings, provided documentation and communications support, followed up on critical action items, and helped troubleshoot problems on a daily basis in an atmosphere of rapid, constant change. This team and the coherence it provided to ACTIV were critical to success.

4 Conclusions

Not everything worked, of course; there were many lessons learned from ACTIV that should inform future pandemic responses. As effective as ACTIV was in coordinating a national research response to COVID-19, particularly in therapeutics, it could not singlehandedly overcome the lack of a single, nationally coordinated system in the U.S. for conducting clinical research (Angus et al. 2021). Despite the example set by ACTIV master protocols, ACTIV continued to compete with other trials for patients. Some of these were of sufficient quality to provide actionable data for regulators, but others, many of them continuing studies by individual investigators or institutions, were inadequately powered or designed. U.S. hospitals proved to be completely unprepared to cope with the enormous surge in COVID-19 patients (UCSF 2021), resulting in critical shortages of supplies, staff, and resources to conduct many needed trials despite considerable efforts by OWS and the ACTIV trial teams to address the problem. Although CTCWG and other efforts succeeded in bringing a number of smaller hospitals into the effort, the hybrid networks put together to conduct the ACTIV master protocols were largely reliant on larger academic medical centers. They had difficulty recruiting trial sites from smaller community hospitals where many COVID patients were being treated (McNay et al. 2021). Although ACTIV was able to accelerate the process of contracting with sites and networks, it was still largely subject to prevailing policies and processes established by individual government and private sector entities before the pandemic. Standardized, streamlined contracting templates for national health emergencies would have been helpful.

Some commentators maintained that ACTIV and other U.S. government initiatives overemphasized the clinical development of vaccines, neutralizing antibodies, and intravenous therapies at the expense of novel oral or inhaled antiviral drug candidates (Zimmer 2021). The reality is that through mid-2021 only a few of the latter had adequate safety or efficacy data to enter clinical testing, and those few were identified for testing either in ACTIV protocols or advanced into company trials. In June 2021, the White House announced the Antiviral Program for Pandemics (NIAID 2021), a \$3.2 billion effort to further accelerate the development of antiviral therapies for SARS-CoV-2 and other viruses with pandemic potential, which included additional funding for preclinical development of promising antivirals. Efforts such as these to create a robust pipeline of qualified, early-stage candidates for antiviral therapies will be critical to prepare for future pandemics.

Given the scope and depth of its accomplishments and the speed with which they were executed, ACTIV remains a model for how national research efforts may be governed effectively in the setting of a public health emergency. While organization and focus were important, the most critical reason for ACTIV's success ultimately lay in the willingness of the many individuals involved, including senior leaders, to share their expertise and dedicate countless hours of their time to the urgent pursuit of common goals without regard for commercial gain, personal credit, or institutional agendas. Perhaps the greatest lesson to be learned is the need to maintain the kind of relationships and organizational infrastructures exemplified by ACTIV to deploy a similarly effective response to the next—perhaps inevitable—pandemic.

Discussion Questions

1. What aspects of the COVID-19 pandemic created the need for close collaboration between government and private companies?
2. What challenges did the consequences of the pandemic pose to the fulfillment of ACTIV's mission?
3. What was unique about the ACTIV partnership compared to other responses to global health threats?
4. What features of the ACTIV response to COVID-19 would be important to replicate in responding to a future pandemic? Beyond what ACTIV has done, are there additional steps that should be taken? What are they?

References

ACTIV-3 Therapeutics for inpatients with COVID-19 (TICO) Study Group. Lancet. 2022;10:972. https://doi.org/10.1016/S2213-2600(22)00215-6.

Angus DC, Gordon AC, Bauchner H. Emerging lessons from COVID-19 for the US clinical research enterprise. JAMA. 2021;325:1159. https://doi.org/10.1001/jama.2021.3284.

Beigel JH, Tomashek KM, Dodd LE, Mehta AK, Zingman BS, Kalil AC, et al. Remdesivir for the treatment of Covid-19—final report. N Engl J Med. 2020;383(19):1813–26. https://doi.org/10.1056/NEJMoa2007764.

Buchman T, Draghia-Akli R, Adam S, Aggarwal N, Fessel J, Higgs E, et al. Accelerating coronavirus disease 2019 therapeutic interventions and vaccines—selecting compounds for clinical evaluation in coronavirus disease 2019 clinical trials. Crit Care Med. 2021;49:1963–73. https://doi.org/10.1097/CCM.0000000000005295.

Bugin K, Woodcock J. Trends in COVID-19 therapeutic clinical trials. Nat Rev Drug Discov. 2021;20:254. https://doi.org/10.1038/d41573-021-00037-3.

CDC. Previous U.S. COVID-19 dase data. 2020. https://www.cdc.gov/coronavirus/2019-ncov/covid-data/previouscases.html#anchor_1598477381. Accessed 26 July 2021.

Collins FS, Stoffels P. Accelerating COVID-19 Therapeutic Interventions and Vaccines (ACTIV): an unprecedented partnership for unprecedented times. JAMA. 2020;323(24):2455–7. https://doi.org/10.1001/jama.2020.8920.

Corey L, Mascola JR, Fauci AS, Collins FS. A strategic approach to COVID-19 vaccine R&D. Science. 2020;368(6494):948–50. https://doi.org/10.1126/science.abc5312.

Coronavirus Vaccine & Treatment Evaluation Network. Nonhuman primate field guide: considerations for the use of primate models for SARS-CoV-2 treatments and vaccines. 2020.

COVID R&D Alliance. Accelerating research, advancing hope. 2021. https://www.covidrdalliance.com/. Accessed 24 June 2022.

Deming ME, Michael NL, Robb M, Cohen MS, Neuzil KM. Accelerating development of SARS-CoV-2 vaccines: the role for controlled human infection models. N Engl J Med. 2020;383:e63. https://doi.org/10.1056/NEJMp2020076.

FNIH. ACTIV clinical and preclinical candidate compound portal submissions. ACTIV WGs; 2020. https://fnih.org/our-programs/activ/about2020.

Grobler JA, Anderson AS, Fernandes P, Diamond MS, Colvis CM, Menetski JP, et al. Accelerated preclinical paths to support rapid development of COVID-19 therapeutics. Cell Host Microbe. 2020;28(5):638–45. https://doi.org/10.1016/j.chom.2020.09.017.

Haynes BF, Corey L, Fernandes P, Gilbert PB, Hotez PJ, Rao S, et al. Prospects for a safe COVID-19 vaccine. Sci Transl Med. 2020;12(568):eabe0948. https://doi.org/10.1126/scitranslmed.abe0948.

Hewitt JA, Lutz C, Florence WC, Pitt MLM, Rao S, Rappaport J, et al. ACTIVating Resources for the COVID-19 Pandemic: In Vivo Models for Vaccines and Therapeutics. Cell Host Microbe. 2020;28(5):646–59. https://doi.org/10.1016/j.chom.2020.09.016.

I-SPY COVID-19 trial. 2020. https://clinicaltrials.gov/ct2/show/NCT04488081. Accessed 26 July 2021.

LaVange L, Adam SJ, Currier JS, Higgs ES, Reineck LA, Hughes EA, et al. Accelerating COVID-19 therapeutic interventions and vaccines (ACTIV): designing master protocols for evaluation of candidate COVID-19 therapeutics. Ann Intern Med. 2021;174:1293. https://doi.org/10.7326/m21-1269.

McNay LA, Arnoczy G, Martell M, Mock P, Wright ME, Simpson S, et al. Community-based hospitals: new partners for government-sponsored clinical research during public health emergencies. Vaccine. 2021;39(42):6183–5. https://doi.org/10.1016/j.vaccine.2021.09.008.

NIAID. Antiviral program for pandemics. 2021. https://www.niaid.nih.gov/research/antivirals. Accessed 27 July 2021.

NIH. Accelerating Medicines Partnership (AMP). 2014. https://www.nih.gov/research-training/accelerating-medicines-partnership-amp. Accessed 11 Oct 2021.

NIH. Animal models. In: Open datab portal. 2020a. https://opendata.ncats.nih.gov/covid19/animal. Accessed 27 July 2021.

NIH. Clinical trial capacity working group. Bethesda (MD). 2020b. https://www.nih.gov/research-training/medical-research-initiatives/activ/clinical-trial-capacity-working-group. Accessed 21 Aug 2021.

NIH. Preclinical working group. National Institutes of Health, Bethesda (MD). 2020c. https://www.nih.gov/research-training/medical-research-initiatives/activ/preclinical-working-group. Accessed 21 Aug 2021 2021.

NIH. Therapeutics clinical working group. Bethesda, MD: Natinal Institutes of Health. 2020d. https://www.nih.gov/research-training/medical-research-initiatives/activ/therapeutics-clinical-working-group. Accessed 21 Aug 2021.

NIH. Accelerating COVID-19 therapeutic interventions and vaccines (ACTIV) governance. Bethesda, MD: National Institutes of Health; 2021a. https://www.nih.gov/research-training/medical-research-initiatives/activ/governance. Accessed 26 July 2021.

NIH. ACTIV COVID-19 clinical & preclinical candidate compound portal. 2021b. https://redcap.ncats.nih.gov/redcap/surveys/index.php?s=DAE87WPTE7. Accessed 26 July 2021.

NIH. Tracking resistance and coronavirus evolution (TRACE). Bethesda, MD: NIH. 2021c. https://www.nih.gov/research-training/medical-research-initiatives/activ/tracking-resistance-coronavirus-evolution-trace. Accessed 11 Oct 2021.

NIH. Vaccines working group. 2021d. https://www.nih.gov/research-training/medical-research-initiatives/activ/vaccines-working-group. Accessed 11 Oct 2021.

NIH/NCATS. Animal models. In: COVID-19 OpenData portal. Bethesda, MD: National Institures of

Health; 2020a. https://opendata.ncats.nih.gov/covid19/animal. Accessed 27 July 2021.
NIH/NCATS. COVID-19 OpenData portal. 2020b. https://ncats.nih.gov/expertise/covid19-open-data-portal. Accessed 27 July 2021.
Pearson H. How COVID broke the evidence pipeline. Nature. 2021;593:182–6.
REMAP-CAP Investigators, Gordon AC, Mouncey PR, Al-Beidh F, Rowan KM, Nichol AD, et al. Interleukin-6 receptor antagonists in critically ill patients with Covid-19. N Engl J Med. 2021;384(16):1491–502. https://doi.org/10.1056/NEJMoa2100433.
Slaoui M, Greene SE, Woodcock J. Bridging the gap at warp speed: delivering options for preventing and treating Covid-19. N Engl J Med. 2020;383(20):1899–901. https://doi.org/10.1056/NEJMp2028535.
Suzman M. Announcing the COVID-19 therapeutics accelerator. Seattle, WA: Bill & Melissa Gates Foundation; 2020. https://www.gatesfoundation.org/ideas/articles/coronavirus-mark-suzman-therapeutics. Accessed 30 July 2021.
UCSF Institute for Global Health Sciences. The United States response to COVID-19: a case study of the first year. 2021.
Woodcock J, LaVange LM. Master protocols to study multiple therapies, multiple diseases, or both. N Engl J Med. 2017;377(1):62–70. https://doi.org/10.1056/NEJMra1510062.
Zimmer C. How the search for Covid-19 treatments faltered while vaccines sped ahead. New York Times. 2021.

15.1 In Practice: Leveraging an Integrated National Health System for Research Response—The UK National Institute for Health Research Respiratory Translational Research Collaboration

Nick R. Lemoine, Patrick F. Chinnery, and Charlotte H. Taylor

Contents

Learning Track Note: This chapter appears in Learning Tracks: Clinical Research

E. S. Higgs and R. A. Sorenson (eds.), *Principles and Practice of Emergency Research Response*,
https://doi.org/10.1007/978-3-031-48408-7_20

Learning Objectives

This chapter will help readers understand and describe:

- Advantages conferred on a study by an Urgent Public Health (UPH) designation in the UK
- Performance monitoring measures developed by researchers to implement their UPH study
- How the UK COVID Therapeutics Advisory Panel and Open Submission Systems contributed to assembling a portfolio of UK platform studies
- Roles of the Therapeutics Taskforce
- UK successes in mitigating the COVID-19 pandemic

1 Introduction

1.1 UK Healthcare Landscape

The United Kingdom (UK) comprises England, Scotland, Wales, and Northern Ireland. Since 1999, powers for health have been devolved from the Westminster UK Parliament to the constituent countries of the UK: to the Scottish Parliament, Welsh Assembly, and Northern Ireland Assembly, while the UK Parliament also governs England. The National Health Service (NHS), established in 1948, operates across the UK. It is one of the most comprehensive health systems worldwide, providing free care at the point of delivery to over 66 million people from cradle to grave. NHS services are provided in primary, community, and acute settings.

The National Institute for Health and Care Research (NIHR) mission is to improve the health and well-being of the nation through research. The NIHR was established in 2006 under the UK government health research strategy Best Research for Best Health (UK Dept of Health 2006). The goal was to create a health research system in which the NHS supported outstanding researchers, working in world-class facilities and conducting leading-edge research focused on the needs of patients and the public. Within 10 years, the NIHR was acknowledged for transforming research and development in and for the NHS and the people it serves (Bell 2016; Davies et al. 2016; Hanney and González-Block 2016; Morgan Jones et al. 2016). The remit of the NIHR has since grown; it funds and supports the delivery and development of vital clinical research both in the NHS and across the wider health and social care environment.

The NIHR Clinical Research Network (CRN) has regional networks in place across England and collaborates with the Devolved Administrations (DAs) of Scotland, Wales, and Northern Ireland to ensure a UK-wide approach to clinical research. These networks enable the CRN to deliver novel and innovative trials and ensure the NHS and wider workforce have the knowledge and skills to respond rapidly and deliver the next generation of clinical trials (▫ Fig. 1).

1.2 Challenges

At the outset of the coronavirus disease 2019 (COVID-19) pandemic, the UK experienced, as did most other countries, unprecedented challenges to effectively slowing the spread of the virus and preventing loss of life. The outbreak and spread of COVID-19 represented a global public health crisis without parallel in recent years. Resources that had already been stretched across the UK research and healthcare systems were further reduced due to staff sickness and redeployment within healthcare. The devolved nature of healthcare in the UK risked fragmentation of approach across the four nations. Global "just in time" supply chains and UK domestic processes were not designed for the scale, pace, and dynamism of treating a novel, easily transmissible respiratory virus causing a pandemic. The novelty of the virus and the highly variable course of the disease meant there was significant uncertainty regarding which treatments might be effective at treating patients suffering from COVID-19 and should therefore be explored further through clinical research.

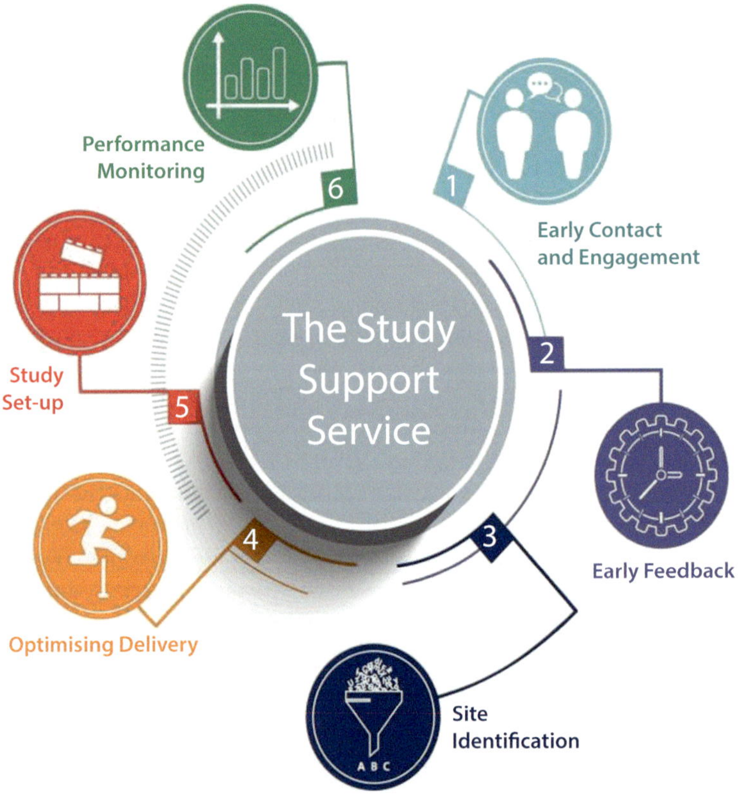

Fig. 1 The NIHR study support service delivers across the UK. (NIHR Study Support Service)

1.3 UK Approach

The UK treated research as a crucial and prioritized component of the COVID-19 response right from the start of the pandemic. The UK government relied on the NIHR and the existing research and healthcare infrastructure, using existing NIHR and NHS systems, structures, and expertise to ensure quality of research while moving forward quickly. The integrated nature of the UK system allowed the Chief Medical Officers of the four nations to guide the prioritization of resources across the system and focus efforts on the therapeutics most likely to be effective. Taking a UK-wide approach prevented fragmentation of research efforts between countries, enabling limited resources to be focused on priority areas and speeding up the generation of trial data. There was an early emphasis on confining experimental treatments to clinical trials rather than going straight to emergency use in patients (Coltart and Collet-Fenson 2021).

2 Urgent Public Health Research

2.1 Research Prioritization

Since 2014, the CRN has had Urgent Public Health (UPH) processes in place for the rapid setup and delivery of research on unexpected and severe infections with the potential to cause widespread disease in the UK. These processes are enacted according to the instructions of the Department for Health and Social Care (DHSC) in the event of a declared outbreak. In response to the spread of COVID-19, a key first step was the national endorsement of a unified portfolio by the Chief Medical Officers for England, Scotland, Wales, and Northern Ireland, focusing attention on a single common goal of identifying safe and effective treatments for COVID-19.

In January 2020, on the instruction of the DHSC, the CRN implemented UK-wide UPH processes to expedite the rapid opening of the International Severe Acute Respiratory and Emerging Infection Consortium (ISARIC) Clinical Characterization Protocol United Kingdom (CCP-UK) study. The study, led by Calum Semple, collects data and samples to characterize infectious diseases with the potential to engender public health problems. This study remains on the CRN Portfolio so that it can be activated as and when needed.

Within weeks of the initial UPH implementation, the Chief Medical Officer (CMO) for England instructed NIHR to scale up UPH processes and lead a UK-wide offer to oversee the identification, funding, and delivery of COVID-19 studies. This included a prioritization process to ensure resources were directed towards the highest-priority clinical research studies. Studies prioritized under this system were deemed "UPH designated," the advantages of which are discussed below. Responding to this instruction required the various parts of the NIHR and the Devolved Administrations to work together to build a coherent, joined-up approach to the task. CRN developed new processes, infrastructure, communication channels, and operations to identify and deliver UPH research, whilst NIHR joined with UK Research and Innovation (UKRI) to set up a rapid response funding stream, enabling high quality research to be funded and delivered at speed.

To facilitate the identification of studies, a single point of entry (the UPH Portal) for all clinical research studies wishing to be considered for UPH designation and/or to apply for rapid response funding from the joint NIHR & UKRI funding call was established. Applications included details on study protocols, evidence of funding (or a rapid response funding application), drug and testing kit requirements (to ensure stocks were available), as well as patient population requirements and likely study setting, e.g., primary, secondary or community based (to ensure infrastructure was in place to deliver the study). In a matter of days, UK researchers submitted applications in their hundreds (◘ Fig. 2) for research to be set up at hospitals and GP Practices, as well as at schools and in care homes across the UK.

The requirement to translate research findings into improved outcomes for patients within a short period of time was built into the research design. Ideally, treatments were required to be readily available and easily deployable within the existing healthcare capabilities and structures in the NHS.

Prior to prioritization decisions, applications underwent a thorough feasibility assessment to ensure the research study was deliverable in the current climate. Prioritized studies were required to provide evidence to help guide the national response and reach the population's highest-risk groups. With dedication and commitment from cross-specialty clinical and academic experts, methodologists, and relevant government institutions,

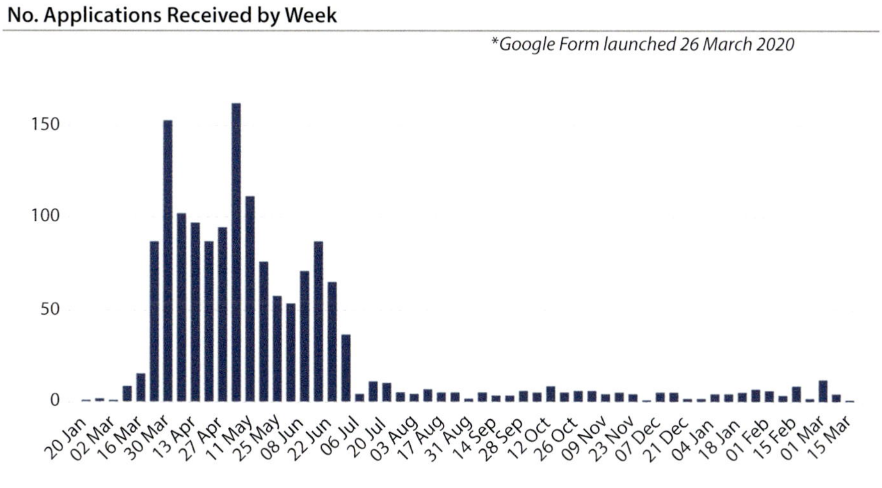

◘ **Fig. 2** Graph showing the number of applications received to the UPH Portal. (NIHR)

the Urgent Public Health Group and NIHR Rapid Response Review Panel were formed to support the critical review of studies at pace. A key ethos of NIHR is to involve patients and the public at every stage of the research pathway. Consistent with this principle, public representatives were included on both panels, and a specific public representative review was facilitated as part of the process.

The multidisciplinary UPH Group, chaired by Nick Lemoine, the Medical Director of the NIHR Clinical Research Network, convened as often as needed (often multiple times per week) to review the triaged applications for UPH designation and provide recommendations to DHSC. UPH recommendations were formally reviewed and ratified by the CMOs for implementation across the four nations. Over 1500 submissions were reviewed, and 101 applications were designated as priority studies.

It is important to note that commercial organizations were also required to submit their studies, ensuring equity of access to the resources available. The CRN Business Development and Marketing team holds a number of life science companies as key customer accounts and was able to clearly communicate the UPH process in advance of formal submissions. This early engagement also enabled early protocol development discussions to ensure the study was deliverable in the context of the COVID-19 impact on NHS and social care services. Further engagement with Life Sciences came via the various UK Taskforces set up by the UK Government, including the Vaccine Taskforce to secure COVID-19 vaccines for the UK and globally, if and when they became available, as well as the companion Therapeutics Taskforce. This included the need to support the swift delivery of large-scale studies across the UK to provide the evidence needed for authorizations. NIHR set up collaborative groups across the UK to enable this activity, which required regional infrastructure to be mobilized to provide novel approaches that ensured full recruitment to large-scale studies within a few months.

2.2 The Advantages of UPH Designation

Once identified as a UPH study, a study became eligible for expedited study setup and was deemed a priority for NHS, CRN, and DA research delivery resources. The Health Research Authority (HRA) and Medicines and Healthcare Products Regulatory Agency (MHRA) created prioritized processes to review COVID-19 research and amendments to ensure the study started as quickly as possible. This resulted in approvals being granted within an average of 8 days, compared to a median of 49 days to approval pre-pandemic. In parallel to this review, the CRN and DAs supported the rapid setup of studies at sites across the UK, liaising with the Chief Investigator (Principal Investigator) and the study team to ensure a study-wide action plan and approach was developed. Sites conducted capacity and capability assessments and governance was put in place as quickly as possible.

Finally, the NIHR communications and engagement teams highlighted UPH studies on a dedicated website and facilitated social media messaging around recruitment. This included highlighting good news stories to ensure UPH research stayed in the public eye. The team also developed the vaccine patient registry and enhanced the Be Part of Research registry (Be Part of Research 2022) to encourage more people to sign up for research participation in advance of trials being available. Far more people signed up for research than would usually be expected, and studies were able to recruit at pace by using the registries to identify eligible participants.

One of the first studies, the Randomised Evaluation of COVID-19 Therapy (RECOVERY) trial (▶ In Practice 14.1), jointly funded by NIHR and UKRI, was UPH designated on March 11, 2020, and within a week had been set up at hospitals across the UK, recruiting its first participant just 8 days after being badged as a UPH trial and continuing to recruit at unprecedented pace and scale (◘ Fig. 3).

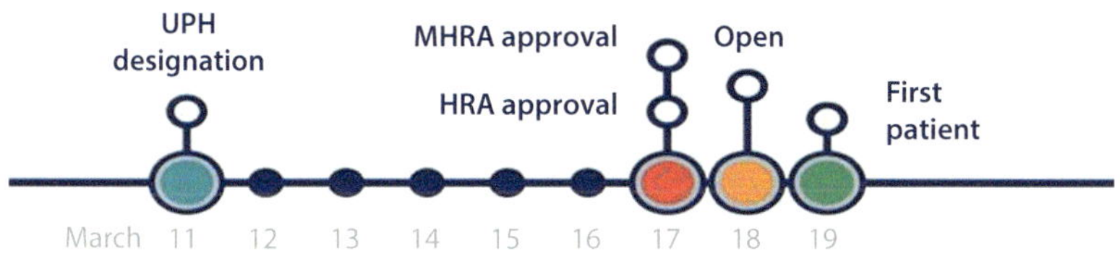

Fig. 3 The approval and setup of the RECOVERY Trial platform study in UK sites. (NIHR)

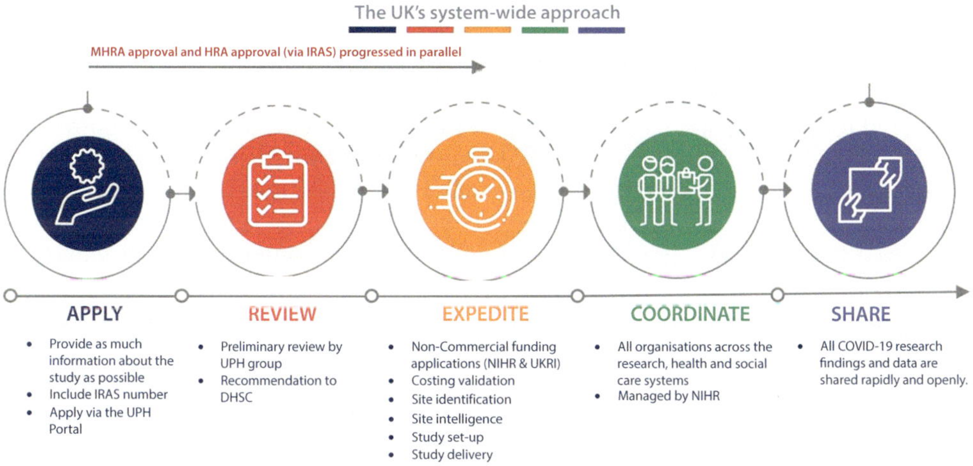

Fig. 4 The Urgent Public Health research process from submission to study dissemination. (NIHR)

2.3 Delivery of Urgent Public Health Research

Following the rapid setup of studies, the CRN developed enhanced performance monitoring services to help researchers deliver their UPH study. Public Health England, Public Health Scotland, and Public Health Wales shared strategic intelligence with the NIHR to enable the implementation and delivery of studies at locations of high disease prevalence and need and enable patients across the whole UK to participate in research. The inclusion of COVID-19 cases, hospital admissions, and deaths in NIHR data systems, alongside clinical intelligence, was fundamental to facilitating study placement and creating recruitment strategies.

Frequent engagement with chief investigators, Local Clinical Research Networks (LCRNs), Devolved Administrations, and study teams enabled troubleshooting to address delivery challenges in NHS and local authority sites. In addition, close working links with the Devolved Administrations ensured that systemic issues were dealt with on a UK-wide basis rather than in single nations.

The UPH Group provided a forum along with nominated individual "Clinical Links" (i.e., UPH Group members who could rapidly address blockages in study delivery and mobilize appropriate NIHR resources) to help studies address and resolve strategic clinical issues related to study delivery, including through mobilizing appropriate resources from NIHR. New approaches were developed to harness the expertise, data, and intelligence needed to provide thematic and strategic oversight of the research portfolio, including study setting (such as community, hospital, or care home), study design, and disease severity in study participants. Consideration was given to common problems and shared observations to learn from challenges or successes within those particular groupings. The process outlined in Fig. 4 ensured that any lessons learned could be rapidly circulated across the Network and Devolved Administrations to support effective delivery of the UPH Portfolio.

3 Platform Trials

The UK assembled a portfolio of platform trials spanning from first-in-human (Phase I) through pivotal (Phase III) trials informing clinical practice. The UPH prioritization process minimized competition between trial platforms, thus ensuring a coherent, unified approach linked to access to national resources, including the NIHR clinical research network for trial recruitment and delivery. The best early example of this was the RECOVERY trial. It also led to the rationalization of multiple Phase II platforms initially recruited from hospitals across the country, with some overlap of sites and competition to recruit within individual sites. This led to a confusing picture for a brief period, making trial delivery more challenging. However, the rationalization of the study platforms to form a single integrated network resolved these issues and enhanced the recruitment and trial delivery rate. A second key attribute was embedding Phase III trials within the National Health Service and empowering local clinicians to become co-investigators, with a light touch approach to recruitment and consent following online training. This also enabled frontline staff to participate in clinical trial activity, with many recognized formally as "associate investigators." This had a major impact on trial recruitment, particularly in non-academic centers not traditionally involved in delivering research of this type.

3.1 UK COVID-19 Therapeutics Advisory Panel

The single nationally coordinated delivery of trials required an impartial, scientifically driven process for identifying and prioritizing the drugs to be tested through the National Trial Platforms. To achieve this, the UK Covid Therapeutics Advisory Panel (UK-CTAP) was established, which made recommendations to the Chief Medical Officer to the UK Government and his deputies, and to individual trial investigators as to which drugs to test and in which patients. This ensured that recommendations were made on purely scientific grounds, enabling complementary strategies to be tackled in parallel as a balanced portfolio without duplicated effort. The approach was based on three layers of scrutiny to mitigate against conscious and sub-conscious bias (▫ Fig. 5). UK-CTAP recommendations were made by a group of clinicians and scientists with relevant expertise in clinical trial delivery and the pathophysiology of COVID-19, but who were not directly involved in the trials themselves.

The panel considered nominations made through an open web portal. Candidate drugs could be nominated by anyone, including academics, clinicians, members of the pharmaceutical industry, and the general public. An expert scientific due diligence team triaged the submissions and constructed detailed, unbiased scientific briefing documents for the candidate drugs. This required careful collation and validation of publicly available data, proprietary data that was commercially sensitive, and unpublished data collected from trials worldwide. The team was in regular dialogue with similar operations globally, including the National Institutes for Health in the United States, the European Clinical Research Infrastructure Network (ECRIN) in the European Union, and the World Health Organization, with which they shared all information. Evidence was gathered on the mode of action of the drug, what was known about the pathogenesis of COVID-19 at the time, pharmacokinetics, pharmacodynamics, the side effect profile, likely toxicity in COVID-19 patients, and drug availability and deliverability within the National Health Service.

UK-CTAP commissioned expert subgroups focused on complementary mecha-

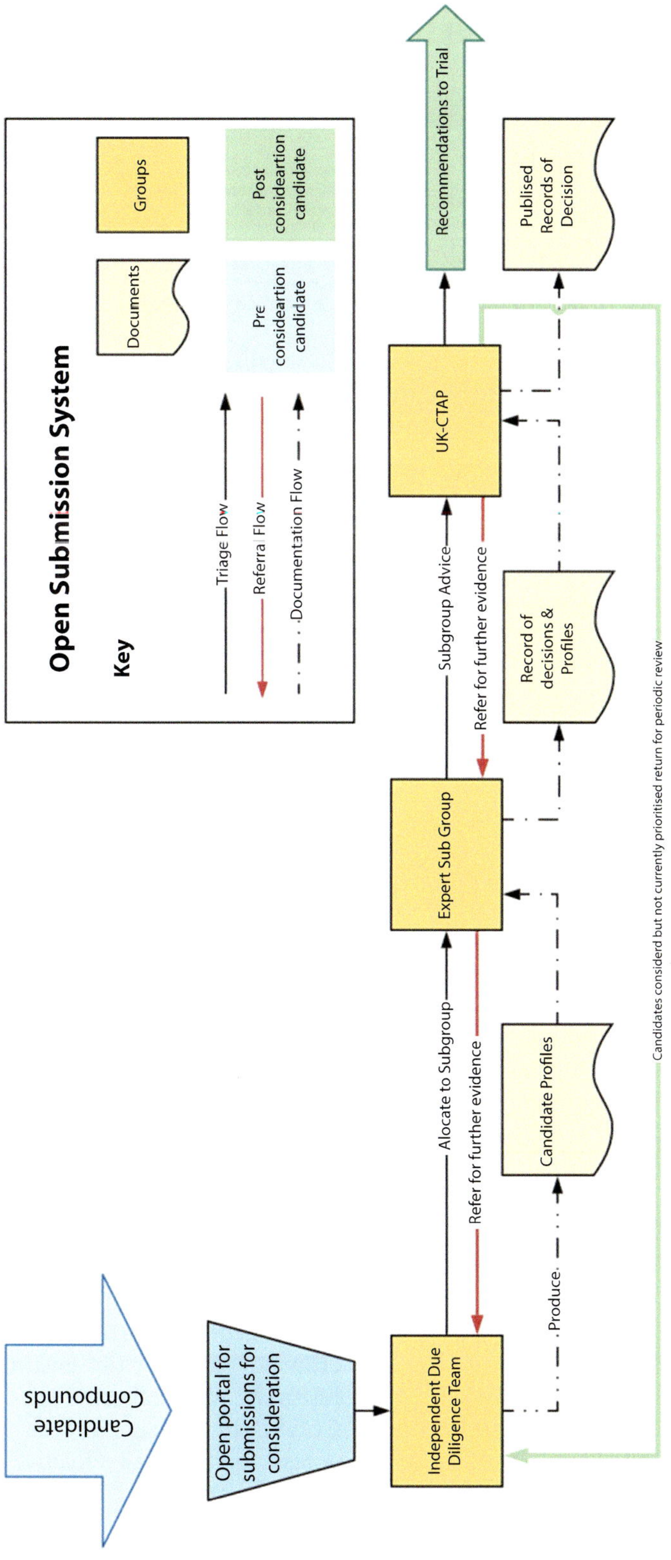

Fig. 5 The Open Submission System approach based on three layers of scrutiny to mitigate against conscious and sub-conscious bias. (Authors)

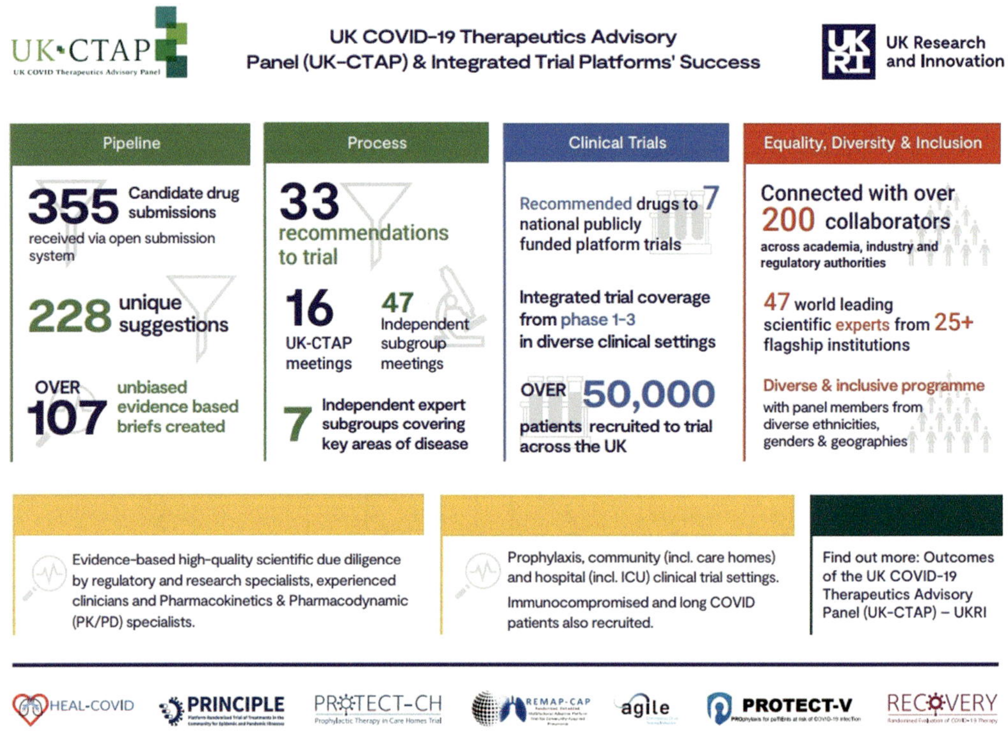

Fig. 6 Summary of CTAP's activities over 12 months. (UK-CTAP/Patrick Chinnery)

nisms relevant to COVID-19. These groups were chaired by full members of UK-CTAP and, following deliberations, made recommendations for each candidate drug. These recommendations were considered in detail by the main UK-CTAP panel to ensure a balanced portfolio of drugs with different mechanisms across the trial platforms. UK-CTAP worked at pace, making recommendations for trial inclusion within 48 h of their deliberations. Of critical importance, UK-CTAP did not accept or reject candidates but prioritized the current understanding of disease pathology. The committee revisited candidates frequently based on emerging data, allowing them to be re-presented as candidates for the trials if new, compelling data supported their inclusion. All UK-CTAP meetings and the specialist sub-group meetings were held by video-link, often out of hours given the urgency to reach a decision and often involving clinicians busy with frontline clinical duties. A summary of UK-CTAP's activities over 12 months is shown in Fig. 6.

4 Establishment of a Therapeutics Taskforce

Finding safe and effective treatments for COVID-19 was recognized immediately by the UK Government as a high priority for the COVID-19 response. Accordingly the ▶ Therapeutics Taskforce, led by the Department for Health and Social Care, was established in April 2020 to coordinate government efforts to ensure high-quality research was delivered at pace so that COVID-19 patients in the UK could get access to safe and effective treatments as soon as possible. The Taskforce provided a supporting structure for the approach to COVID-19 research established by the NIHR and agreed upon by the UK Chief Medical Officers, creating a joined-up, end-to-end system for the seamless identification, trialing, and ultimately deployment of effective treatments to the UK population.

The Taskforce played many roles in coordinating this end-to-end system. One constant objective was to ensure that the nationally prioritized clinical trial platforms established through the Urgent Public Health process were able to recruit patients as rapidly as possible and produce urgent results on the safety and efficacy of treatment candidates. Alongside the research support structures put in place by the NIHR, the Therapeutics Taskforce was able to leverage its centralized position to use ministers (including the Prime Minister) to speak about therapeutics research at televised press conferences and send letters signed by the UK CMOs to groups of healthcare professionals to encourage continued (and enhanced) engagement in supporting research. Such interventions greatly raised public awareness of clinical research and kept up momentum from patients and healthcare professionals to continue supporting these research efforts.

The Therapeutics Taskforce also played an important role in highlighting and championing research into COVID-19 treatments within the government. The Taskforce consistently engaged with other government departments and arms-length bodies (public bodies established with a degree of autonomy from the government) to represent the needs of those delivering research on the ground to ensure the successful deployment of effective treatments to UK patients. On a macro scale, this included—crucially—the alignment of COVID-19 treatment planning with wider policy issues with clear interdependencies on research, such as ensuring that COVID-19 testing programs could operate widely and early enough in the onset of symptoms to facilitate effective early treatment, or to make clear that participants in clinical research were exempt from certain lockdown restrictions, so COVID-19 and other clinical trials could continue when in-person visits were required.

4.1 UK-Wide Approach

As noted above, healthcare is devolved to the countries of the UK. From the start of 2020 the four nations and four CMOs decided to take a UK-wide approach to COVID-19 research and treatment, as reflected in the UK-wide remit of the Therapeutics Taskforce. This was a vital decision for the scale of impact the UK achieved for several reasons: it prevented fragmentation of resources that would have made larger clinical trials less feasible, focusing resources on the prioritized treatments; provided the ability to draw on diverse clinical and academic expertise from across the four nations; and importantly ensured that the research reflected population diversity both within and across the four nation and supported equity of access to treatment across the UK.

4.2 Procurement and Preparing for Roll-Out

Proactive steps were taken to translate clinical research into UK patient outcomes as quickly as possible, including the decision to procure potential COVID-19 treatments in spring 2020 while launching clinical trials well before trial results were known. The global "just-in-time" medicine supply chains and limited global supply meant that intense competition for existing treatments was anticipated once they were shown to be effective in treating COVID-19. At the time of procurement decisions, there was huge uncertainty about the trajectory of the COVID-19 pandemic, including the scale and duration of potential peaks of infection. Clinical and scientific experts provided scientifically informed opinions to officials to inform each procurement approach. Strategic cross-government leadership provided by the Therapeutics Taskforce, engaging all relevant government departments as well as delivery partners, such as the new UK Health Security Agency and the NHS, ensured that this process was robust and fast paced.

4.3 Research to Access Pathway for Investigational Drugs for COVID-19 (RAPID C-19)

The RAPID C-19 initiative (Fig. 7) was set up in spring 2020 to respond to the need to synthesize the emerging evidence; review huge

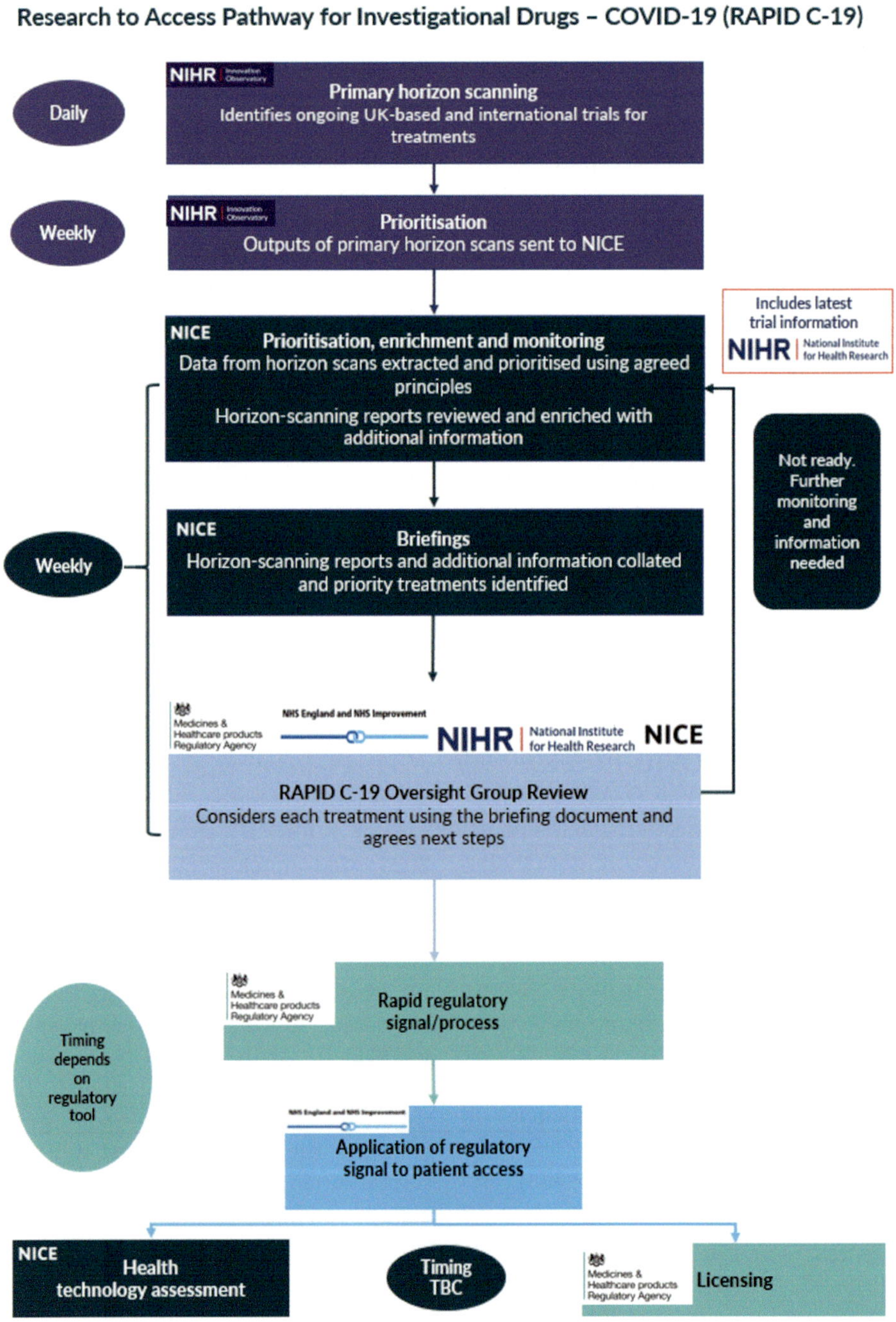

Fig. 7 The RAPID C-19 initiative set up in spring 2020. (Rapid C-19)

amounts of data at speed; and support patient access to medicines to treat COVID-19 in a pandemic. RAPID C-19 is a collaboration between the key agencies in the UK involved in the development of access pathways for therapeutics, including the regulatory authority (MHRA), research funders (NIHR), evidence assessors (the National Institute for Health and Care Excellence, or NICE), clinical commissioning (NHS England and Improvement, or NHSE&I), and the Devolved Administrations counterparts. The group has met frequently to review and consider the latest evidence from trials in the UK and around the world. The collaborative involvement aims to avoid duplication of effort and support the goal of providing timely advice on emerging evidence for COVID-19 treatments. A key achievement of RAPID C-19 has been its ability to facilitate patient access to treatments within about 10–15 days of significant trials reporting positive signals, compared with the normal timeframe of about 9 months for policy development in a non-pandemic setting in England, thanks to acceleration or waiver of some stages of the process during the pandemic emergency. The most notable of these has been dexamethasone, where the clinical access policy for NHS patients was published within hours of the RECOVERY trial, reporting major clinical benefits for its use in hospitalized patients receiving supplemental oxygen.

5 Conclusion

The UK led the world in COVID-19 research, informing government policy and providing the NHS and social care with the tools needed to prevent and treat COVID-19. The processes adopted facilitated the recruitment of over one million clinical study participants at pace over the year across the entire health and social care network. This recruitment resulted in the world's largest hospital-based study (The RECOVERY trial 2022), the UK's largest ever community-based interventional study (Fig. 8), the PRINCIPLE trial, and the UK contributing the highest number of participants globally to multinational studies such as REMAP-CAP (REMAP-CAP response to COVID-19 pandemic 2021). Finally, fast-track links to ▶ NICE enabled evidence from UPH-designated studies to be reviewed to inform evidence-based guidelines.

The research activities and outcomes attracted global interest, with the success of

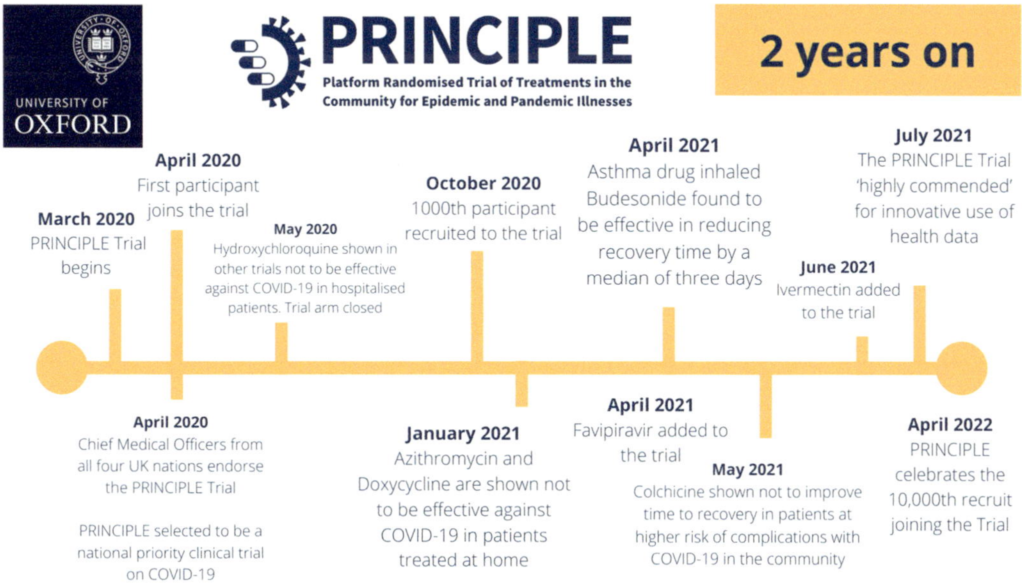

Fig. 8 Two years of achievements in the PRINCIPLE trial. (Nuffield Dept of Med)

the national response featuring in international media and journals—a testimony to the NIHR, NHS, and wider health and social care environment. This achievement would not have been possible without the dedication and commitment of the research workforce and the million people who gave their time to participate and continue to give their time. Within months of the first NIHR-supported UPH study's opening, UK researchers had published evidence to establish the world's first proven treatments for patients with COVID-19, such as dexamethasone, which is estimated to have saved at least 22,000 COVID-19 patients in the UK and one million patients globally by March 2021 (NHS England 2021; RECOVERY Collaborative Group 2020). NIHR also supported the development of the breakthrough Oxford-AstraZeneca vaccine.

With the COVID-19 outbreak continuing to be prominent in our lives, the success of the UK-wide research response has helped save millions of lives around the world and continues to support critical COVID-19 research to enable treatments and vaccines for all.

Discussion Questions

1. Once identified as a UPH study, a study received priority for expedited study setup. What other advantages did UPH designation provide?
2. What enhanced performance monitoring services were developed to help researchers deliver their UPH study?
3. The UK assembled a portfolio of platform trials spanning from first-in-human (Phase I) through safety and efficacy (Phase III) trials to inform decisions on clinical practice. Discuss how the single, nationally coordinated delivery of trials was made possible through the UK Covid Therapeutics Advisory Panel (UK-CTAP). How did the Open Submission Systems contribute to these efforts?
4. The Therapeutics Taskforce was established to coordinate government efforts to ensure high-quality research would be delivered at pace so that COVID-19 patients in the UK could get access to safe and effective treatments as soon as possible. Discuss the various roles of the Therapeutics Taskforce, including those related to the RAPID C-19 initiative.
5. Summarize successes achieved by the UK in overcoming unprecedented challenges to tackle the spread of the COVID-19 virus and prevent loss of life.

References

Be Part of Research. National Health Service, UK. 2022. https://bepartofresearch.nihr.ac.uk/. Accessed 26 Oct 2022.

Bell J. 10 years of the UK's National Institute for Health Research. Lancet. 2016;387(10032):1978–9. https://doi.org/10.1016/s0140-6736(16)30479-2.

Coltart CEM, Collet-Fenson LB. Future developments in the prevention, diagnosis and treatment of COVID-19. Best Pract Res Clin Obstet Gynaecol. 2021;73:56–80. https://doi.org/10.1016/j.bpobgyn.2021.03.012.

Davies SC, Walley T, Smye S, Cotterill L, Whitty CJ. The NIHR at 10: transforming clinical research. Clin Med (Lond). 2016;16(6):501–2. https://doi.org/10.7861/clinmedicine.16-6-501.

Hanney SR, González-Block MA. Building health research systems: WHO is generating global perspectives, and who's celebrating national successes? Health Res Policy Syst. 2016;14(1):90. https://doi.org/10.1186/s12961-016-0160-x.

Morgan Jones M, Kamenetzky A, Manville C, Ghiga I, MacLure C, Harte E, et al. The National Institute for Health Research at 10 years: an impact synthesis: 100 impact case studies. Santa Monica, CA: RAND Corporation; 2016.

NHS England. COVID treatment developed in the NHS saves a million lives. England: NHS England; 2021.

RECOVERY Collaborative Group. Dexamethasone in hospitalized patients with Covid-19. N Engl J Med. 2020;384(8):693–704. https://doi.org/10.1056/NEJMoa2021436.

REMAP-CAP response to COVID-19 pandemic. 2021. https://www.remapcap.org/coronavirus. Accessed 27 June 2022.

The RECOVERY trial. UK Research and Innovation. 2022. https://www.ukri.org/news-and-events/tackling-the-impact-of-covid-19/vaccines-and-treatments/recovery-trial-identifies-covid-19-treatments/. Accessed 14 July 2022.

UK Dept of Health. Best research for best health: a new national health research strategy. London: Department of Health; 2006.

16 Challenges for Emergency Research Response and Preparedness in Fragile, Weak, and Failed Nation States

Rebecca Katz, Alexandra L. Phelan, and Cyrus Shahpar

Contents

The future? How can I talk about the future when
I don't even know if we are going to eat today?
—Jean-Claude, displaced person in the
Central African Republic (MSF 2022)

Learning Track Note: This chapter appears in Learning Tracks: Clinical Research; Emergency Research Response, Response Operations; Health Policy, Multilateral Cooperation, International Governance; Preparedness; Research ethics; Social Science Response Research

E. S. Higgs and R. A. Sorenson (eds.), *Principles and Practice of Emergency Research Response*, https://doi.org/10.1007/978-3-031-48408-7_21

Learning Objectives

This chapter should enable readers to understand and discuss:

- How conflict and fragility impact public health and undermine infectious disease outbreak prevention, detection, and response
- How outbreaks, epidemics, and pandemics can exacerbate state fragility and weakness
- How public health services can deliver effective interventions
- Advantages and disadvantages of calling upon the military and/or security services for pandemic response assistance in states with under-resourced health systems
- Ethical standards that international organizations should follow in countries where protocols and enforcement bodies to regulate infectious disease research are under-resourced
- When emergency research should not be conducted
- Risks posed by governance reform to fragile and weakened states and how the perspectives of these states can be incorporated into international law and governance reform

1 Introduction

Starting in the 1980s, public health officials worked in partnership with political leaders to call humanitarian ceasefires to permit urgent public health interventions. "Days of tranquility" were implemented in more than a dozen countries to pause fighting in order to vaccinate children against polio, measles, and other vaccine-preventable diseases and provide humanitarian aid. Decades later, when the COVID-19 pandemic emerged, the United Nations Security Council (UNSC) passed a resolution that called for an immediate cessation to hostilities around the world and asked all parties to armed conflicts to suspend hostilities for 90 days in order to enable the delivery of humanitarian assistance necessary to combat the pandemic (UNSC 2020). Seven months later, the UNSC recognized that the call for an immediate cessation of hostilities had not actually stopped armed conflicts and again called for ceasefires to help mitigate effects of the pandemic and enable vaccine distribution (UNSC 2021). In both of these resolutions, the Security Council acknowledged that not only would armed conflict and instability exacerbate the pandemic but that the "pandemic can exacerbate the adverse humanitarian impact of armed conflicts" (UNSC 2021).

While the COVID-19 pandemic underscored just how interconnected the world is and the importance of global solidarity, by many measures, the world is becoming increasingly complex and subject to conflict. The Institute for Economics & Peace Global Peace Index deteriorated by 3.78% during the decade before the COVID-19 pandemic, driven mostly by terrorism and internal conflicts (IEP 2019). The 2023 Index found that political stability deteriorated by 0.42%, the ninth consecutive year of a fall in the Index, with 79 countries losing ground and 82 improving (IEP 2023). According to a 2018 International Committee of the Red Cross (ICRC) report, "more armed groups have emerged in the last 7 years than in the previous 70," meaning about half of all current civil conflicts are so chaotic and fractious that they involve ten or more armed groups (ICRC 2018). The Armed Conflict Location and Events Dataset also shows that from 2018 to 2022, most of the 46 countries and territories on its Conflict Severity Index were "experiencing sustained or escalating levels of severe violence" (ACLED 2023). In many countries, low-intensity sub-state conflicts persist without an end in sight, while larger-scale conflicts continue or may restart in Ukraine, Ethiopia, and between Armenia and Azerbaijan (ICG 2023). Additionally, inequality, discrimination, and a lack of sufficient access to care, food, water, and sanitation have led to humanitarian crises even in the absence of armed conflict, a situation exacerbated in many parts of the world by climate change and the COVID-19 pandemic.

As conflict and fragility spread around the world, it becomes more likely that infectious disease events will emerge or be exacerbated in these areas of instability. In order for the global health community to effectively respond to new disease emergencies and protect population health, we must first understand the evolving threats and how conflict and fragility impact public health and disease outbreaks. In this chapter, we review the link between fragile states' increased risk for infectious disease outbreaks, and particular factors exacerbating fragility and infectious disease risk. We then explore challenges in preventing, detecting, and responding to emerging infectious diseases in complex environments and understanding and addressing imbalances in political power and perception. Finally, we discuss pathways for global governance with proposed recommendations for future action.

2 Fragile States and Infectious Disease Risk

2.1 The State and Fragility

Despite the growth of international institutions and global governance, the nation state remains one of the primary political entities that impact peoples' daily lives, including their health. As the United Nations General Assembly has recognized, "[g]overnments retain the primary role and responsibility for ensuring the survival, livelihood and dignity of their citizens" (UNGA 2012). States vary in their resources, capacities, and commitment to deliver public goods to the people who live in them and may be differentiated between strong and weak states or failing or failed states, based on the success with which a state can deliver public goods. This notion is underscored by the role of governments in responding to the COVID-19 pandemic. In particular, the provision of security, defined to encompass all elements of human security, is a public good critical to the status of a state and its continued legitimacy. Without security, the provision of other public goods, such as healthcare, public health, education, and infrastructure, becomes exceedingly difficult or impossible. Human security encompasses health security, economic security, food security, environmental security, personal security, community security, and political security. This framing "recognizes the interlinkages between peace, development and human rights, and equally considers civil, political, economic, social, and cultural rights" (UNGA 2012). Where a state fails to provide the elements requisite for ensuring human security, it weakens, and may become fragile, or even disintegrate to a point where it collapses and fails (Rotberg 2003).

2.2 Enhanced Likelihood of Infectious Disease Outbreaks in Fragile States

The health status of a population is a reflection of the economic, political, and social status of a country or community. The conditions leading to fragile states also make them more vulnerable to infectious disease outbreaks. A simple model for infectious disease causation is the epidemiologic triad, which outlines how a pathogenic agent, susceptible host, and the environment interact to produce disease (▶ In Focus 21.1) (CDC 2012). In comparison to a stable state, a fragile state has more underlying vulnerabilities, which can result in increased disease transmission (◘ Figs. 1, 2, and 3). Typically, less is known about the diversity and pathogenicity of both endemic and novel infectious pathogens in fragile states, since surveillance and laboratory testing systems, as well as locally conducted scientific research into diseases affecting the population, are likely to be weak or absent in fragile states. Coordination between the animal, environmental, and human health sectors may be lacking. In addition, routine testing for antimicrobial resistance, and policies on appropriate use of antimicrobials, may be sporadic or non-existent.

Hosts (both humans and livestock) residing in a fragile state are generally more vulnerable to infectious diseases, in part since greater

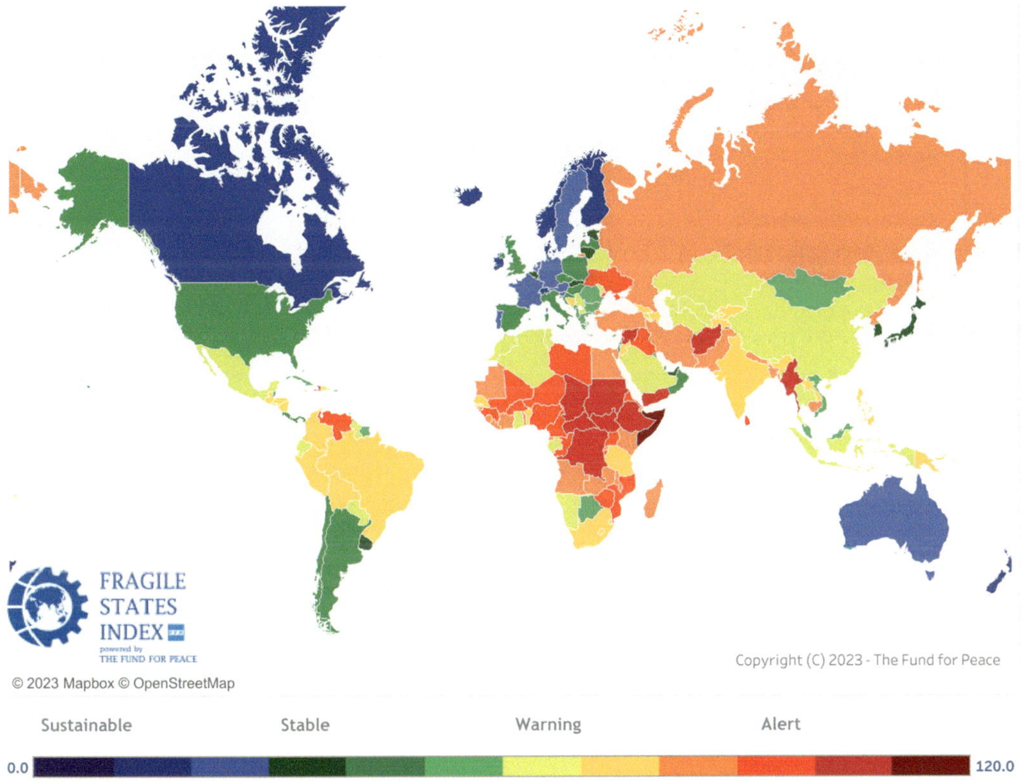

Fig. 1 Fragility in the World 2023. Fragile State Index. (Fund for Peace 2023)

animal-human interaction can lead to zoonotic infection. Humans may be vulnerable through more widespread high-risk sexual practices, unimproved water and sanitation hindering hygiene, less access to regular healthcare and lower baseline vaccination coverage, higher rates of undernutrition and malnutrition, and a higher proportion of children and pregnant women (Weiss and McMichael 2004). Environmental factors also disproportionately affect those in fragile states. In these settings, overcrowding—particularly among displaced populations—can lead to increased disease transmission. Basic healthcare services and water, sanitation, and hygiene are often lacking, which can lead to spread of diarrheal diseases and nosocomial infections. One example is the Democratic Republic of the Congo (DRC), which has long been classified as a fragile state by the Fund for Peace (2022) and the World Bank (2022). In the 2018–2020 Ebola virus disease (EVD) outbreak in DRC, nearly 18% of all EVD cases were nosocomial, leading to ongoing transmission and an unacceptable level of healthcare worker infections (Schnirring 2019). The lack of basic health services can lead to infectious cases going unrecognized or untreated, leading to ongoing disease transmission and making the outbreak more difficult to control (Fig. 4).

A critical capability needed to manage population-level infectious disease threats is early detection and control of cases. In fragile states, this may be one of many factors impeding a country's ability to effectively manage outbreaks. Economic insecurity often results in weak health system infrastructure and a lack of basic systems to find, stop, and prevent disease outbreaks. A review of detection of disease outbreaks in 22 fragile states from 2000 to 2010 showed that there were long delays from onset to detection (median 29 days) and from detection to response

FY23 List of Fragile and Conflict-affected Situations

CONFLICT	INSTITUTIONAL AND SOCIAL FRAGILITY
Afghanistan	Burundi
Burkina Faso	Chad
Cameroon	Comoros
Central African Republic	Congo, Republic of
Congo, Democratic Republic of	Eritrea
Ethiopia	Guinea-Bissau
Iraq	Haiti
Mali	Kosovo
Mozambique	Lebanon
Myanmar	Libya
Niger	Marshall Islands
Nigeria	Micronesia, Federated States of
Somalia	Papua New Guinea
South Sudan	Solomon Islands
Syrian Arab Republic	Sudan
Ukraine	Timor-Leste
Yemen, Republic of	Tuvalu
	Venezuela, RB
	West Bank and Gaza (territory)
	Zimbabwe

Fig. 2 World Bank list of fragile and conflict-affected situations (FCS). The World Bank publishes an annual list of fragile and conflict-affected situations, distinguishing between countries based on the nature and severity of issues they face. (World Bank 2022)

(investigation, confirmation, declaration, control) (Bruckner and Checchi 2011). This led the investigators to conclude that epidemic surveillance and control appear to be insufficiently timely in fragile states. According to 2019 pre-pandemic assessments of emergency preparedness by the World Health Organization (WHO) Global Preparedness Monitoring Board, most countries in Africa had little-to-no capacity in critical areas such as emergency response operations, a robust health workforce, disease surveillance, and laboratory networks; only 64 of 182 countries reporting worldwide were at the highest or second-highest preparedness level (GPMB 2019a, b). In lower-income countries, current capacity tends to be even further depleted from the COVID-19 pandemic. The health sector is often under-resourced in domestic budgets, leading to inadequate basic medical and public health services. Physical insecurity can also drive infectious disease spread, by making prevention (e.g. vaccine programs) and treatment (e.g. care facilities and medications inaccessible to populations and by making it harder to reach them with proper risk communications and outreach. Effective response can also be limited in insecure areas, as was evident in the 2018–2020 EVD outbreak in the Democratic Republic of the Congo, where intentional attacks on response teams and treatment and research facilities led to interruptions in critical activities including case management, contact tracing, and treatment; despite the dangers, both successful clinical trials and an emergency vaccination campaign that reached more than 300,000 people were conducted during the outbreak (Mulangu et al. 2019; WHO 2020b), and the PALM study was completed demonstrating successful Ebola therapeutics for the first time (► In Practice 17.1) (Mulangu et al. 2019). A review of the timing of conflict and disease transmission in this outbreak found that both the rapidity of case isolation and the population-level effectiveness of vaccination

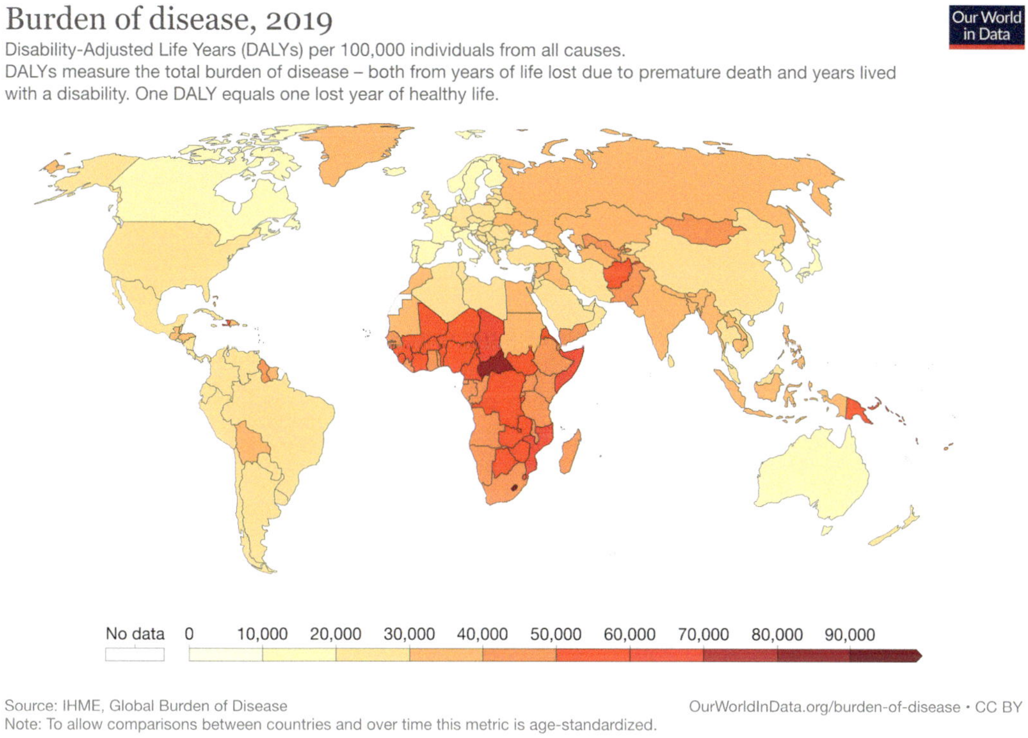

Fig. 3 Note the correlation between the fragile states map above and this map showing countries that suffer the greatest loss of disability-adjusted years of life to disease (not necessarily infectious disease). (Roser et al. 2021)

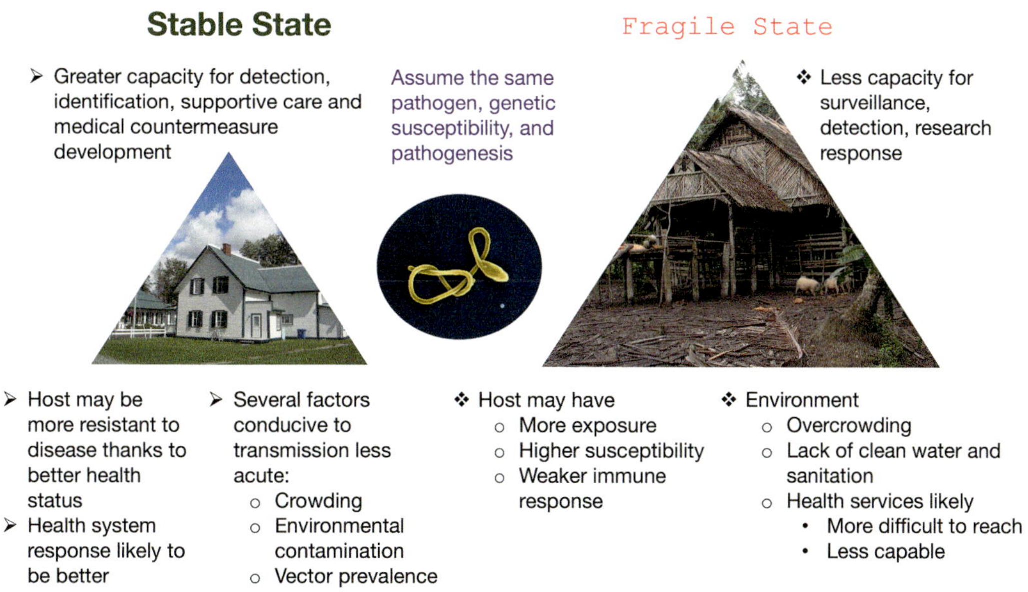

Fig. 4 Differences in epidemiologic triads between stable and fragile states. (Authors)

varied notably as a result of preceding unrest and subsequent impact of conflict events. Furthermore, conflict events were found to reverse an otherwise declining phase of the epidemic trajectory (Wells et al. 2019). Political instability can impact all facets of a health system, from leadership in ministries of health to the viability of health programs requiring sustained commitment and support. External partners supporting the health system are also more likely to cease programs in times of political instability. In countries with pockets of resistance to government authority, mistrust of government can severely limit a country's ability to control disease outbreaks (Nguyen 2019).

2.3 Insecurity Exacerbates Disease Emergence and Transmission

2.3.1 Displaced Populations

Insecurity, including conflict and violence, can lead to the displacement of populations within countries or across borders. The conditions and locations in which internally displaced populations or refugees live can facilitate the emergence and spread of infectious disease. Fleeing war in the 1980s, Afghan refugees residing in camps in Pakistan experienced over 150,000 cases of malaria each year and were inaccurately blamed for facilitating the spread of malaria to Pakistan (Baer et al. 2013; Rowland and Nosten 2016; Suleman 1988). The camps were situated next to standing water in farmland and rice fields; and following the success of malaria eradication programs in Afghanistan before the war, refugees had no immunity. Displaced populations in camps also experience overcrowding, inadequate hygiene and sanitation facilities, limited resources dedicated to public health programs, inadequate housing to protect from vector-borne disease, and particular vulnerabilities arising from potential malnutrition, stress, and other health consequences of escaping conflict. Displaced or isolated populations are also particularly vulnerable to cultural, language, and health literacy barriers to effective disease prevention and care.

Box 1

Irregular—and often official government—forces may show flagrant disregard for international humanitarian law. Direct, purposeful, and indiscriminate attacks on civilians, civilian infrastructure, and humanitarian aid, including healthcare workers and hospitals, are increasingly normalized. International law has required protection for medical personnel and facilities in times of conflict since the First Geneva Convention in 1864. Yet the deliberate destruction of hospitals and harassment and murder of healthcare workers as a tactic has been documented in 23 current armed conflicts around the globe. Dr. John Hamre, CEO of the Center for Strategic and International Studies, has noted that "the Geneva Conventions were not designed to deal with irregular combat," so incentives to adhere to such norms may be absent in most modern conflicts (Morrison et al. 2017).

In 2016, the UNSC adopted Resolution 2286, condemning deliberate attacks against medical facilities, equipment, and personnel in conflict situations, largely in response to the targeted airstrikes on hospitals and the murder of over 800 healthcare workers in the Syrian Civil War (UNSC 2016). In January 2018, the WHO also rolled out the Surveillance System for Attacks on Healthcare (SSA), to collect standardized, publicly available data on such attacks (WHO 2024). Neither of these efforts has led to an abatement in these attacks, in Syria or elsewhere. In Syria, medical buildings stopped displaying the red cross insignia, individuals avoided healthcare facilities out of fear, and by 2018, some 38% of individuals providing clinical care had received no formal training at all. While these efforts did bring these issues international attention, they have "yet to translate into effective protection of health care on the ground" (Rae 2018).

2.3.2 By the Numbers: Fragile States and Health Emergency Grades

The Fragile States Index, developed by the Fund for Peace, classifies and ranks states based on their level of fragility, using a conflict assessment framework comprising indicators for cohesion, economics, political, and social factors (Fund for Peace 2023). In December 2019, just prior to the start of the COVID-19 pandemic, every state among the ten most fragile states was also classified as having a graded health emergency under the WHO's Emergency Response Framework (see ◘ Fig. 5). The five most fragile states—Yemen, Somalia, South Sudan, Syria, and the Democratic Republic of the Congo—all had Grade 3 health emergencies, the highest level under the WHO Emergency Response Framework, that is, an emergency requiring a maximal WHO response (WHO 2017). In addition, these fragile states are among the least prepared for health emergencies according to the Prevent Epidemics ReadyScore, which assigns a preparedness score out of 100 based on objective assessments done by WHO and partners (Prevent Epidemics 2023). As expected, these fragile states continue to experience a variety of infectious disease outbreaks based on recent reports from WHO (WHO AFRO 2023; WHO EMRO 2023) (▶ In Practice 16.1).

2.4 Force Multipliers of Fragility and Infectious Disease

Increasingly, states that do not meet the typical criteria for classification as fragile and conflict-affected are experiencing fragility arising from societal, economic, political, environmental, or security instability. The Organization for Economic Cooperation and Development has found that almost half the states meeting fragile state criteria are middle-income countries. The World Bank estimates that by 2030, up to two thirds of the world's extreme poor will live in states experiencing fragility, conflict, and violence (World Bank 2023).

The causes of conflict are complex, and while more data and analysis are needed to understand interactions, it is reasonable to suspect that the impacts of climate change on

◘ **Fig. 5** Cross comparison of health emergency states and fragility grades. (Fund for Peace 2023; Prevent Epidemics 2023; WHO 2019) (Table by authors)

2022 Fragile States Index	WHO ERF	ReadyScore	Sample of reported disease outbreaks 2017-2019
1. Yemen	Grade 3	unknown	cholera, dengue, diphtheria
2. Somalia	Grade 3	29	cholera, VDPV
3. Syria	Grade 3	unknown	cutaneous leishmaniasis, VDPV
4. South Sudan	Grade 3	30	hepatitis E, measles, rift valley fever,
5. Central African Republic	Grade 2	26	mpox, VPDV
6. Democratic Republic of Congo	Grade 3	35	Ebola virus disease, measles, VDPV
7. Sudan	Grade 2	57	chikungunya, cholera, dengue
8. Afghanistan	Grade 2	38	Crimean Congo hemorrhagic fever, polio
9. Chad	Grade 1	29	cholera, measles
10. Myanmar	Grade 2	40	cholera, typhoid

natural resources, human security, and societal stability may exacerbate conflict in fragile settings (Scheffran et al. 2012). Furthermore, these impacts, as well as any impacts of adaptation and mitigation responses to climate change, may extend beyond currently fragile states. As noted in a G7-commissioned report on climate and conflict, "[e]ven seemingly stable states can be pushed towards instability" given the interaction of climate change with other social, economic, and environmental pressures (Berlin Climate and Security Conference 2019).

3 Challenges of Preventing, Detecting, and Responding to EIDs in Complex Environments: Ebola in the Democratic Republic of the Congo and Cholera in Yemen

3.1 Ebola in the DRC

In August 2018, an Ebola outbreak in the North Kivu region of the DRC brought together two major threats to international security: an area destabilized by complex, violent insurgency was hit by a deadly infectious disease outbreak. Four years after the Ebola crisis in West Africa, the global health community was relatively well prepared to deal with an Ebola threat: they were armed with logistical lessons learned, a profound motivation to avoid a repeat crisis, and a supply of an experimental Ebola vaccine and candidate therapeutics. However, the outbreak was exceptionally difficult to bring under control, largely due to armed clashes in the resource-rich region and societal distrust of central authorities that extends to incoming health workers. The movement of public health workers and supplies was severely impeded; many organizations had to barter for safe passage rights from multiple local militant groups. Even so, violence against public health and healthcare workers was a reality in this conflict, including targeted attacks on Red Cross volunteers trying to safely handle infected bodies and Médecins Sans Frontières (MSF) Ebola treatment units that were burned (MSF 2019; Nguyen 2019). The PALM Ebola treatment trial was embedded in the Ebola treatment units, and the conduct of the study was challenged and stalled repeatedly due to attacks on treatment centers and laboratory spaces. MSF decided to retrieve staff from the emergency leaving the WHO and DRC responders to staff and run some of the Ebola treatment units. Due to a highly transient population and limited mobility of public health workers, tried-and-true vaccine distribution and disease tracking strategies, notably contact tracing, were difficult if not impossible in some locations. A vast amount of misinformation also exacerbated heavy distrust for international public health and healthcare workers among local populations, whose lives were being threatened by far more than just Ebola. Armed convoys that might be necessary to protect Ebola responders from the threat of armed violence often worsened their image among the locals.

Despite difficulties and high mortality among those infected with Ebola, the as-yet unlicensed RVSV vaccine candidate that had been in trials in West Africa a few years earlier was administered to more than 300,000 people during the outbreak via a compassionate use protocol, with the accumulated data leading to its later licensure by the U.S. Food and Drug Administration (FDA) in 2019. In addition, a multi-armed clinical trial of therapeutics successfully demonstrated that two of the four therapeutic agents under investigation were clearly superior to the other two, so much so that the trial was stopped early so all trials participants could receive the more efficacious therapeutics. Those two therapeutics were also licensed by FDA (FDA 2019a, b, 2020a, b; Henao-Restrepo et al. 2017; Kennedy et al. 2016; Mulangu et al. 2019; Wells et al. 2019). The outbreak was a challenging test for conducting emergency clinical research, but the research produced lifesaving, licensed products for future Ebola outbreaks.

3.2 Civil War in Yemen

The Yemeni Civil War, which began in 2015, has also led to a severe ongoing humanitarian crisis. In addition to the violence, a devastating famine and a cholera outbreak have caused widespread preventable deaths, especially among vulnerable populations such as children. There were over 2.5 million suspected cases of cholera, making it the largest recorded outbreak of the disease in history (WHO EMRO 2023). Because of the conflict and resulting disordered environment, over 3900 people died of a preventable and treatable disease. "Everybody – international and Yemeni health workers – is focusing on emergency health provision because of the massive numbers of war wounded," meaning that the collapsing healthcare system could not even begin to detect and prevent the spread of infectious disease (Gavlak 2015; Kennedy et al. 2017).

In the DRC and Yemen, treatable diseases continue to cause significant mortality as of 2023. As we have seen in the current COVID-19 pandemic, if a novel infectious pathogen such as SARS-CoV-2 emerges, which can overwhelm both stable and fragile health systems and societies, the results can be globally catastrophic. The international community must be prepared to take decisive precautionary action to prevent such a global pandemic before it occurs, irrespective of where it starts and spreads to. Delayed identification of the new pathogen and intervention, delays much more likely in a fragile state, can result in the spread of the outbreak and ongoing pathogen evolution, leading to a continuing, sometimes acute global threat. More effective norms and agreements to protect health workers, facilities, and supplies in modern, irregular conflicts and keep public health infrastructure, particularly disease surveillance and response systems, functioning even amidst armed conflicts are vital.

Furthermore, both crises have led to significant numbers of refugees and internally displaced persons, engendering another set of health challenges, including poor living conditions, lack of resources, psychological trauma, and exposure to new pathogens for which they have no immunity (Abbas et al. 2018). This poses a risk both to displaced individuals and to their destination countries. The current experience of migrants from the Northern Triangle region of Central America to the U.S. southern border follows this pattern of armed conflict begetting an insecure situation producing refugees and internally displaced persons, leading to health consequences that affect individuals from multiple countries (Cheatham 2021).

4 Historical Injustice: Understanding and Addressing Imbalances in Political Power and Perception

The reality that protecting the health, security, and economies of developed countries is the primary driver of research funding and outbreak response perpetuates historical and continuing injustices in global health. The COVID-19 pandemic starkly demonstrated how assumptions about preparedness and response capacities can lead to insufficient national responses in developing countries, which may in turn impact the health and security of all nations. Despite this, and despite many efforts to level the playing field, the focus on problems of and threats to developed countries is likely to persist while they disproportionately possess the financial, technical, and political capital necessary for research and outbreak response (Farmer 1996). For example, efforts to address global vaccine inequity during the COVID-19 pandemic have included not only arguments about global health justice and equity but also practical concerns about preventing the emergence of variants that may have a direct impact on global populations and influence vaccine distribution in developing countries (Riaz et al. 2021).

Even so, research in responses to infectious disease epidemics before COVID-19, particularly the 2014–2016 Ebola outbreak in West Africa, the Zika outbreak, and the 2018–2020 Ebola outbreak in the northeastern DRC, reflected an ongoing shift in international research approaches away from responders and researchers "parachuting in," as in past emerging infectious disease outbreaks, toward more inclusive efforts to form local and regional partnerships and conduct effective social and community outreach (▶ Chap. 18). The COVID-19 pandemic, which occurred everywhere and curtailed international travel, by necessity curtailed parachuting.

Notable legal, policy, and operational changes have arisen in the international realm in response to concerns about old approaches, which could not only replicate historic injustices but undermine local trust and the success of response efforts. A broad range of international treaties contains binding obligations on developed nations to provide international assistance to and collaborate with developing countries, including capacity building, technology transfer, and financial support. These obligations are particularly relevant in fragile states with multiple priorities, demands, and vulnerabilities.

In weakened or fragile states, implementing or enforcing legal and policy arrangements for research, including sovereignty over genetic resources, may be deprioritized or constrained by already limited resources. This imparts a particular ethical duty on researchers operating in constrained states. In addition, states with obligations to provide international assistance and cooperation under a range of international laws, including the International Health Regulations, the Biological Weapons Convention, the Nagoya Protocol, and human rights treaties, may be hesitant to conduct capacity building where economic, social, or political disruption in fragile states may undermine the sustainability of such measures. These are challenges that states and non-state actors must consider in a non-paternalistic manner, in consultation with local communities where possible.

In addition, the entry into force of the Nagoya Protocol on Access to Genetic Resources and the Fair and Equitable Sharing of Benefits Arising from their Use (hereafter "Nagoya Protocol") in 2014 seeks to redress historical exploitation for research through access and benefit sharing of genetic resources. The status of domestic implementation of the Nagoya Protocol varies significantly between countries, adding complexity to the legal landscape for accessing genetic resources and the sharing of benefits arising from their use (Ljungqvist et al. 2024). However, researchers operating in or with partners in fragile settings need to be aware of the principles that underpin the treaty and the opportunities and obstacles that may result for public health systems.

4.1 International Obligations for Capacity Building

Building capacities for research and outbreak detection and response is a crucial component of protecting public health and meeting obligations under international law. However, while there is significant focus on the obligation of states to build these capacities and significant aid-based programming for capacity building, developed countries are sometimes hesitant to recognize their legal *obligations* expressed in a number of treaties (◘ Fig. 6) to support developing or resource constrained states in building these capacities (▶ Chap. 8). Furthermore, building capacities to conduct emerging infectious disease research is increasingly framed as part of reducing emerging infectious disease threats to the health and security of developed countries, that is, part of a (developed) state's duty to protect the health of its own citizens. While this framing of global health security may facilitate funding and investment, it may also risk masking humanitarian and ethical duties, as well as obligations under international law, of developed states to mobilize financial, political, and technical resources for capacity building.

For fragile or weakened states, capacity building is particularly important, with unique challenges for each state depending on the political, economic, technical, or social constraints that they face. Whether a fragile state is in the process of deteriorating, in post-conflict transition, a state of arrested development or in the process of early recovery will impact where and how capacity building may

Capacity Building Category	Biological Weapons Convention (1975) (see Box 5 below)	International Covenant on Economic, Social and Cultural Rights (1976)	International Health Regulations (2005) (see Box 4 below)	Nagoya Protocol (2014)
International assistance and cooperation	Article VII – provide support or assistance upon request to any party exposed to danger as a result of a violation of BWC	Article 2(1) – provide international assistance and co-operation, especially economic or technical, to realize rights, including the right to health and right to science, globally. Article 12 – right to health Article 15(b) – right to science	Article 44 – undertake to collaborate with each other: (1)(a) detection, assessment, and response to events; (1)(d) formulation of proposed laws and policies	Article 22 Capacity (NB: these obligations are in addition to any specific benefit-sharing agreed to under Mutually Agreed Terms, or a specialized international instrument)
Technology Transfer	Article X (fullest possible exchange of technology for peaceful purposes)	Article 2(1) – international assistance and cooperation Article 12 – right to science Article 15(b) – right to science	Article 44 (1)(b) – provision or facilitation of technical cooperation and logistical support	Article 23 – Technology Transfer, Collaboration, and Cooperation
Financing	–	–	Article 44 (1)(e) – mobilization of financial resources	Article 25 Financial Mechanism

Fig. 6 Selected international cooperation and assistance obligations. (Authors)

improve public health (Brinkerhoff 2007). Progress toward stability for fragile states, which is essential for sustainable capacity building, is also variable and contingent. As a result, states and other funding bodies may hesitate to invest in capacity building where economic, social, or political disruption may threaten the sustainability of capacity building measures or be seen to do so.

As set out in Fig. 6, there is a range of international treaties that impose capacity-building obligations relevant to research and outbreaks, including general international assistance, collaboration, and cooperation duties, technology transfer, and financing obligations. In each of the treaties listed, there is particular recognition of the obligation on developed countries to engage in international assistance and collaboration for developing countries in the prevention, detection, and response to outbreaks, whether naturally occurring or deliberate, as well as for the conduct of research more broadly, including as part of the realization of both the human right to health and the right to science.

Capacity building for research and outbreak response cannot occur in isolation from broader systems capacities for governance and security. This in turn affects implementation of core principles of capacity building, including prioritization based on community needs, ensuring systems are responsive and acceptable to communities, and participatory governance. In such situations, states and non-state actors assisting in outbreak response may see a "trade off between the exercise of capacity and building it" (Brinkerhoff 2007). This is particularly the case in public health emergencies, where both internal and external pressures for outside institutions to substitute for weakened or absent local capacities may undermine longer-term efforts to build research capabilities or strengthen health systems. These circumstances also risk removing country or sub-national governments from primary ownership of outbreak detection and response efforts, further entrenching the inequities that have led to the need for legal and governance responses such as access and benefit sharing.

There is a range of pathways and obligations for states to engage in assistance, collaboration, capacity building, technology transfer, and financing with fragile states (▶ Chap. 29). These duties are not simply charity but legally binding obligations, with fragile states the most vulnerable to disease outbreaks and compounded vulnerabilities or exploitation through research, even unintentionally. For emerging infection diseases, such assistance is also in the self-interest and duty

Box 2: Obligations Under the International Health Regulations (2005) for Collaboration and Assistance

Article 44 Collaboration and assistance

1. States Parties shall undertake to collaborate with each other, to the extent possible, in:
   - (a) the detection and assessment of, and response to, events as provided under these Regulations;
   - (b) the provision or facilitation of technical cooperation and logistical support, particularly in the development, strengthening and maintenance of the public health capacities required under these Regulations;
   - (c) the mobilization of financial resources to facilitate implementation of their obligations under these Regulations; and
   - (d) the formulation of proposed laws and other legal and administrative provisions for the implementation of these Regulations.
2. WHO shall collaborate with States Parties, upon request, to the extent possible, in:
   - (a) the evaluation and assessment of their public health capacities in order to facilitate the effective implementation of these Regulations;
   - (b) the provision or facilitation of technical cooperation and logistical support to States Parties; and
   - (c) the mobilization of financial resources to support developing countries in building, strengthening and maintaining the capacities provided for in Annex 1.
3. Collaboration under this Article may be implemented through multiple channels, including bilaterally, through regional networks and the WHO regional offices, and through intergovernmental organizations and international bodies (WHO 2016).

of developed countries to protect their own populations against infectious disease threats.

Box 3: Obligations Under the BWC for Collaboration and Assistance (*Convention on the Prohibition of the Development, Production, and Stockpiling of Bacteriological (Biological) and Toxin Weapons and on Their Destruction,* 1975)

Article VII

Each State Party to this Convention undertakes to provide or support assistance, in accordance with the United Nations Charter, to any Party to the Convention which so requests, if the Security Council decides that such Party has been exposed to danger as a result of violation of the Convention (BWC 1975).

4.2 Viral Sovereignty in Fragile Settings

As a general principle of international law, states have sovereignty over the resources within their territory. Since the Convention on Biological Diversity (CBD) entered into force (became binding on states that ratified it) in 1993, this includes genetic resources, and while this is not expressly stated, genetic resources have been interpreted by many states to include pathogens (UN 1992). In 2014, the Nagoya Protocol entered into force as a supplementary agreement to the CBD, providing the principles and elements for states to implement domestic legislation governing access to their genetic resources, which most states have interpreted as including pathogens. In accordance with the Nagoya Protocol, states may adopt legislation requiring their prior informed consent to access resources and the negotiation of mutually agreed terms, which may include the fair and equitable sharing of benefits that arise from the use of the resources (CBD 2011). As a result, the Nagoya Protocol seeks to rectify dual issues: both the terms of accessing pathogens and benefit sharing seen in the past, where researchers would either physically take or seek access to pathogens (even for public health purposes where local detection or response capacities were limited), while not equitably sharing the benefits of use of those resources, such as scientific publications, conferences, intellectual property rights, or commercial products made using genetic resources, such as vaccines.

Recognizing "the importance of ensuring access to human pathogens for public health preparedness and response purposes" (Preamble), the Nagoya Protocol requires parties to take health emergencies into special consideration in developing or implementing domestic legislation (Article 8[b]). This includes facilitating more rapid access to pathogens or distribution of benefits, particularly for developing countries. For fragile settings, whether expressly included in law or not, this imperative is arguably extended and expanded.

Given its relatively recent entry into force and varying state interpretations, priorities, and capacity, progress on domestic implementation of the Nagoya Protocol is inconsistent between states. Some states have comprehensive laws that expressly consider pathogens (EU 2014), while others have not yet incorporated the agreement domestically or expressly imposed access and benefit-sharing obligations for pathogens. This diversity of approaches and lack of legal certainty can be a barrier and require researchers to conduct appropriate due diligence to ensure that they comply with domestic laws. Additional uncertainties arise in the case of a rapidly spreading pandemic virus, especially when its presumed country of origin is far from eager to admit that the virus first emerged on its territory, or in a future case where the country of origin is indeterminable (Humphries et al. 2021).

These challenges are likely exacerbated in weakened or fragile states, where implementation of new laws or enforcing existing laws for genetic resources may not be a priority in view of limited financial and technical resources. Moreover, public health threats that require urgent international collaboration and assistance may require pathogen sharing for outbreak detection and response. Such dynamics reinforce the importance of trust, equity, and justice at all stages of the outbreak response. Researchers have an ethical duty not to exploit partners in the absence of domestic legislation or enforcement governing access and benefit sharing. This means adhering to international norms underpinning access and benefit-sharing regimes. This is particularly true where failure to do so risks undermining trust in research and outbreak response more broadly. Researchers need to guard against potential, actual, or perceived exploitation of weakened governance systems for the benefit of researchers from wealthy states, even where the research may be perceived to ultimately have potential benefits for affected communities. The idea that researchers and research sponsors must ensure that research participants and their communities or nations receive benefits on the basis of their participation, often at some risk to themselves, is also widely accepted and gaining currency (▶ Chap. 5). Research approaches that are consistent with providing commensurate benefits to research participants, with providing the most effective broad infectious disease response, and compliance with the Nagoya Protocol are a potential opportunity to repair mistrust and build local capacities.

Without proactive effort, there is a risk that the nuanced negotiations that occurred prior to the pandemic around finding common solutions to access to genetic resources, the need to rapidly share outbreak information, and the equitable sharing of benefits, such as vaccines, may be significantly disrupted and undone. At the same time, international discussions on post-pandemic recovery—including amendments to the International Health Regulations (2005) approved in 2024 and negotiations for a new international agreement on pandemic preparedness and response (pandemic treaty)—have focused on the obligations of countries to rapidly share information. This has included the suggested adoption of compliance measures such as investigations. Penalizing delayed information sharing may in fact result in more delay of reporting or information sharing and, for fragile settings, would be especially punitive and inappropriate. Indeed, South Africa was in effect punished for prompt reporting of the Omicron variant of SARS-CoV-2 in November 2021 when many countries imposed travel restrictions; though the intent was to prevent spread of the variant, the restrictions were hardly an incentive for prompt sequence sharing (Chutel 2021). Given discussions around the inclusion of sequence data under the Nagoya Protocol, and in light of global vaccine inequity, there is a risk that finding common solutions that benefit both public health research and equity will be especially difficult. This could discourage research, capacity building, and collaborations until resolution or clarity is reached, which may disproportionately impact fragile or weakened states (▶ Chap. 7).

5 Pathways for Global Governance

The trend in recent decades has been toward an increasing number of both infectious disease events and complex humanitarian crises emerging in failed and weak states, sometimes in tandem, as we have seen. Addressing the challenges of infectious disease events will require a multitude of steps, although there are no simple answers. Given the global impacts of the COVID-19 pandemic, there is a risk that the perspectives and experiences of fragile and weakened states may be sidelined, and explicit efforts should be taken to include fragile state experiences in any international legal and governance reform.

5.1 Strengthening the Health-Security Interface

Integrating health and security professionals (including defense, law enforcement, and national security/foreign policy experts) involved in research and response to infectious diseases in complex environments is imperative for trust-building, information-sharing, and laying a foundation for cooperation in crises. A multilateral approach to achieving this is through support of existing WHO efforts to build and strengthen the WHO Health Emergencies Programme. Active discussions are underway to consider how to strengthen this program in the post-pandemic environment. This support could include increased staffing, as well as policy reforms to specifically identify and develop response capacity and standard operating procedures for future outbreaks in nonpermissive environments, where insecurity means health providers are under threat. WHO can also more fully develop plans and certification processes for emergency medical teams specifically trained to operate in fragile states and complex environments, building on experiences and lessons identified in Iraq and Palestine (WHO 2020a).

WHO does not have the personnel or resources to sustain long-term deployment to outbreaks in nonpermissive environments without major implications for other areas of operation. Additionally, WHO currently has neither the mandate nor the resources nor the expertise to lead in a public health emergency that is deliberate in origin (i.e., bioterrorism, biological warfare). A better-resourced WHO, along with another high-level entity in the United Nations system—whether an existing or new department—with the mandate to govern such complex responses would improve global response capacity in this area (Cameron et al. 2019).

National, regional, and international public health response teams must also adapt to the increasingly complex environments in which disease outbreaks occur. Scientific training and skills must be augmented by training in operationally challenging and often insecure environments. Adapting basic disease prevention and control efforts to limited-resource settings and considering the political, cultural, and social aspects of interventions, including emergency clinical research, from design to implementation are increasingly understood as essential to effective response (▶ Chap. 26). The proper role of security forces engaged in public health response is another complex question; at a minimum, they should be trained in humanitarian principles such as impartiality and neutrality to ensure effective coordination and cooperation across sectors.

5.2 Risk Assessment and Information Sharing

The creation of standardized frameworks to assess and manage risk in nonpermissive environments could help governments make tough but appropriate calls with regard to deployment of public health professionals. Epidemiologists regularly engage in formalized processes of risk assessment during disease outbreaks, considering a variety of factors relevant to public health. Nonpermissive environments introduce additional factors to this calculation. With the expertise of security and foreign policy experts, in addition to input from epidemiologists, other experienced emergency response personnel, and global health leaders, existing epidemiological risk assessment and management tools can be adapted to include relevant security considerations, including troop movements and guidance on engaging with subnational governance figures.

A transparent mechanism of information-sharing among potentially hostile actors can protect epidemiological information essential for response but risky to share publicly. For example, news that a political figure was infected with a disease could serve propaganda ends for one side in a conflict. Disclosure that a medical NGO was the source of such sensitive information might have violent repercussions. An internationally recognized tool to share pertinent health information, with safeguards to protect the identities of patients and reporting parties, might allow previously unattainable levels of surveillance in nonpermissive environments.

5.3 Ethical Challenges

Often fragile states lack the ability to sufficiently monitor research ethics in their countries. Much needed research is conducted by outside entities, including the humanitarian community. In the DRC Ebola outbreak, international researchers, partnering with Congolese Ministry of Health officials, had to manage a clinical trials of experimental vaccines and therapeutics in extraordinary circumstances, including a skeptical host population and limited infrastructure (Farrar 2018). Lack of access and security challenges can compromise methodologies, so researchers and regulators must be flexible in their demands, while still upholding high scientific and ethical standards, and support national governments in promotion of the highest research standards possible (▶ Chap. 33, In Practice 33.2 and 33.3) (Ford et al. 2009).

5.4 Participation in Global Governance Reform

Global governance reforms to research spurred by the COVID-19 pandemic—including amendments to the IHR or negotiation of a new pandemic treaty—must proactively incorporate the perspectives of fragile and weakened states. This includes undertaking practical measures to ensure representatives from fragile states can be active negotiating partners during negotiations so that their perspectives are heard and incorporated into future governance regimes. In substance, law reform that seeks to impose obligations on countries must be developed in a manner that recognizes resource-constrained settings and self-determined priority setting. Differentiated responsibilities and capacity-building obligations on high-income countries are an opportunity to build in such recognition.

Negotiations must also facilitate civil society participation and input, particularly where civil society serves as implementers, such as provision of primary healthcare and outbreak response. Fundamentally, international reform efforts must not contribute to fragility or facilitate research practices that undermine the self-determination and rights of peoples in fragile and conflict affected settings.

Discussion Questions

1. How did the COVID-19 pandemic exacerbate fragility and weakness in some states?
2. What is the potential role of security forces (military and police) in implementing public health interventions?
3. What are the risks in using security forces for public health goals, whether in fragile states or elsewhere? How can the risks be mitigated?
4. In countries where protocols and enforcement bodies to regulate infectious disease research are inadequate, what standards should international organizations follow to ensure ethical practice?
5. Is there a point at which research should not be conducted due to the fragility of the situation or lack of oversight?
6. What are the risks that governance reform in light of the COVID-19 pandemic might pose to fragile and weakened states?
7. How can the perspectives of fragile and weakened states be better incorporated into international law and governance reform?

Acknowledgments The authors thank Aurora Johnson for contributions to earlier work/drafts and Jessica Lin for editing and administrative assistance with the chapter.

References

Abbas M, Aloudat T, Bartolomei J, Carballo M, Durieux-Paillard S, Gabus L, et al. Migrant and refugee populations: a public health and policy perspective on a continuing global crisis. Antimicrob Resist Infect Control. 2018;7(1):113. https://doi.org/10.1186/s13756-018-0403-4.

ACLED. Armed conflict and violent events data project. Armed Conflict and Violent Events Data Project. 2023. https://acleddata.com/. Accessed 1 June 2023.

Baer B, Ball A, Nygren-Krug H, Rietveld A, Weil D. Human rights-based approaches to HIV, tuberculosis, and malaria. In: Zuniga JM, Marks SP, Gostin LO, editors. Advancing the human right to health. Oxford: Oxford University Press; 2013. p. 245–60.

Berlin Climate and Security Conference. Climate-related security risks require foreign policy leadership from around the world. In: Berlin climate change and security conference. 2019.

Brinkerhoff DW. Capacity development in fragile states. Contract No.: Discussion paper No 58D. Maastricht: European Centre for Development Policy Management Centre européen de gestion des politiques de développement; 2007.

Bruckner C, Checchi F. Detection of infectious disease outbreaks in twenty-two fragile states, 2000-2010: a systematic review. Confl Heal. 2011;5:13. https://doi.org/10.1186/1752-1505-5-13.

BWC. Convention on the prohibition of the development, production and stockpiling of bacteriological (biological) and toxin weapons and on their destruction. New York: United Nations; 1975.

Cameron E, Katz R, Konyndyk J, Nalabandian M. A spreading plague: lessons and recommendations for responding to a deliberate biological event. Wahington, DC: Nuclear Threat Initiative; 2019.

CBD. Nagoya protocol on access to genetic resources and the fair and equitable sharing of benefits arising from their utilization. Montreal: Secretariat of the Convention on Biological Diversity; 2011.

CDC. Principles of epidemiology in public health practice, third edition: an introduction to applied epidemiology and biostatistics. Atlanta: U.S. Centers for Disease Control and Prevention; 2012.

Cheatham A. Central America's turbulent northern triangle. Council on Foreign Relations; 2021.

Chutel L. After detecting the omicron variant, South Africa feels 'punished' by global travel bans. New York Times. 2021.

EU. Regulation (EU) no 511/2014 of the European Parliament and of the Council of 16 April 2014 on compliance measures for users from the Nagoya protocol on access to genetic resources and the fair and equitable sharing of benefits arising from their utilization in the union, 511/2014. 2014.

Farmer P. Social inequalities and emerging infectious diseases. Emerg Infect Dis. 1996;2(4):259–69. https://doi.org/10.3201/eid0204.960402.

Farrar J. It isn't crazy to conduct an Ebola clinical trial in a war zone—it's necessary. Stat. 2018.

FDA. ERVEBO. 2019a. https://www.fda.gov/vaccines-blood-biologics/ervebo. Accessed 17 Oct 2021.

FDA. First FDA-approved vaccine for the prevention of Ebola virus disease, marking a critical milestone in public health preparedness and response. Washington, DC: U.S. Food and Drug Administration; 2019b.

FDA. FDA approves first treatment for Ebola virus. Washington, DC: U.S. Food and Drug Administration; 2020a.

FDA. FDA approves treatment for Ebola virus. Washington, DC: U.S. Food and Drug Administration; 2020b.

Ford N, Mills EJ, Zachariah R, Upshur R. Ethics of conducting research in conflict settings. Confl Heal. 2009;3:7. https://doi.org/10.1186/1752-1505-3-7.

Fund for Peace. Fragile states index annual report 2022. Washington. DC: Fund for Peace; 2022. https://fragilestatesindex.org/. Accessed 2 Oct 2022.

Fund for Peace. Fragile states index. Washington. DC: Fund for Peace; 2023. https://fragilestatesindex.org. Accessed 31 May 2023.

Gavlak D. Health system in Yemen close to collapse. Bull World Health Organ. 2015;93(10):670–1. https://doi.org/10.2471/blt.15.021015.

GPMB. Thematic paper on the status of country preparedness capacities. Background report commissioned by the Global Preparedness Monitoring Board (GPMB). Geneva: Global Preparedness and Monitoring Board; 2019a.

GPMB. A world at risk: annual report on global preparedness for health emergencies. Geneva: Global Preparedness Monitoring Board World Health Organization; 2019b.

Henao-Restrepo AM, Camacho A, Longini IM, Watson CH, Edmunds WJ, Egger M, et al. Efficacy and effectiveness of an rVSV-vectored vaccine in preventing Ebola virus disease: final results from the Guinea ring vaccination, open-label, cluster-randomised trial (Ebola Ca Suffit!). Lancet. 2017;389(10068):505–18. https://doi.org/10.1016/S0140-6736(16)32621-6.

Humphries F, Rourke M, Berry T, Englezos E, Lawson C. COVID-19 tests the limits of biodiversity laws in a health crisis: rethinking "country of origin" for virus access and benefit-sharing. J Law Med. 2021;28(3):684–706.

ICG. 10 conflicts to watch in 2023. 2023.

ICRC. The roots of restraint in war. 2018.

IEP. Global peace index 2019: measuring peace in a complex world. Annual Report. Sydney: Institute for Economics & Peace; 2019.

IEP. Global peace index 2023: measuring peace in a complex world. Sydney: Institute for Economics & Peace; 2023.

Kennedy SB, Neaton JD, Lane HC, Kieh MWS, Massaquoi MBF, Touchette NA, et al. Implementation of an Ebola virus disease vaccine clinical trial during the Ebola epidemic in Liberia: design, procedures, and challenges. Clin Trials (London, England). 2016;13(1):49–56. https://doi.org/10.1177/1740774515621037.

Kennedy J, Harmer A, McCoy D. The political determinants of the cholera outbreak in Yemen. Lancet Glob Health. 2017;5(10):e970–e1. https://doi.org/10.1016/S2214-109X(17)30332-7.

Ljungqvist G, Weets C, Stevens T, Robertson H, Zimmerman R, Graeden E, Katz R. Global Patterns in Access and Benefit-Sharing: A Comprehensive Review of National Policies preprint available here: medRxiv 2024.07.12.24310347. https://doi.org/10.1101/2024.07.12.24310347.

Morrison JS, Kenny J, Franz P. The new barbarianism. Center for Strategic and International Studies; 2017. p. 58.

MSF. MSF shuts down Ebola treatment center following violent attack. 2019.

MSF. Violence and displacement in Ippy mirror people's daily reality in CAR Geneva: Médecins Sans Frontières; 2022 [Updated 23 May 2022]. Available from: https://www.msf.org/violence-and-displacement-ippy-mirror-people%E2%80%99s-daily-reality-car.

Mulangu S, Dodd LE, Davey RT Jr, Tshiani Mbaya O, Proschan M, Mukadi D, et al. A randomized, controlled trial of Ebola virus disease therapeutics. N Engl J Med. 2019;381(24):2293–303. https://doi.org/10.1056/NEJMoa1910993.

Nguyen V-K. An epidemic of suspicion—Ebola and violence in the DRC. N Engl J Med. 2019;380:1298. https://doi.org/10.1056/NEJMp1902682.

Prevent Epidemics. Resolve to save lives, New York. 2023. https://preventepidemics.org/. Accessed 2 June 2023.

Rae M. Syrian American Medical Society [Internet]. Washington (DC): Syrian American Medical Society. 2018. [Cited 2021]. Available from: https://www.sams-usa.net/2018/10/19/the-impactsof-attacks-on-healthcare-in-syria/.

Riaz MMA, Ahmad U, Mohan A, Dos Santos Costa AC, Khan H, Babar MS, et al. Global impact of vaccine nationalism during COVID-19 pandemic. Trop Med Health. 2021;49(1):101. https://doi.org/10.1186/s41182-021-00394-0.

Roser M, Ritchie H, Spooner F. Global burden of disease. Our World in Data; 2021.

Rotberg RI. Failed states, collapsed states, weak states: Causes and indicators. In: Rotberg RI, editor. State failure and state weakness in a time of terror. Wahington, DC: World Peace Foundation/Brookings Institution Press; 2003. p. 25.

Rowland M, Nosten F. Malaria epidemiology and control in refugee camps and complex emergencies. Ann Trop Med Parasitol. 2016;95(8):741–54. https://doi.org/10.1080/00034983.2001.11813694.

Scheffran J, Brzoska M, Kominek J, Link PM, Schilling J. Climate change and violent conflict. Science. 2012;336(6083):869–71. https://doi.org/10.1126/science.1221339.

Schnirring L. With Ebola cases rising, officials launch new infection control steps. CIDRAP News; 2019.

Suleman M. Malaria in Afghan refugees in Pakistan. Trans R Soc Trop Med Hyg. 1988;82(1):44–7. https://doi.org/10.1016/0035-9203(88)90257-x.

UN. Convention on biological diversity. New York: United Nations; 1992.

UNGA. Follow-up to paragraph 143 on human security of the 2005 world summit outcome: resolution adopted by the general assembly. New York: United Nations; 2012.

UNSC. Resolution 2286 (2016). New York: United Nations Security Council; 2016. p. S/RES 2286 (016).
UNSC. Resolution 2532 (2020). New York: United Nations Security Council; 2020. p. S/RES 2532 (020).
UNSC. Resolution 2565 (2021). New York: United Nations Security Council; 2021. p. S/RES 2565 (021).
Weiss RA, McMichael AJ. Social and envrionmental risk factors in the emergence of infectious diseases. Nat. Med 2004;10(12 Suppl):S70–6. https://doi.org/10.1038/nm1150.
Wells CR, Pandey A, Parpia AS, Fitzpatrick MC, Meyers LA, Singer BH, et al. Ebola vaccination in the Democratic Republic of the Congo. Proc Natl Acad Sci U S A. 2019;116(20):10178–83. https://doi.org/10.1073/pnas.1817329116.
WHO. International Health Regulations (2005). 3rd ed. Geneva: World Health Organization; 2016.
WHO. Emergency response framework – 2nd ed. Geneva: World Health Organization; 2017.
WHO. WHO's work in emergencies: prepare, prevent, detect and respond: annual report 2018. World Health Organization; 2019.
WHO. Emergency medical teams initiative. World Health Organization, Geneva. 2020a. https://extranet.who.int/emt/. Accessed 15 Sept 2022.
WHO. Ending an Ebola outbreak in a conflict zone. Geneva: World Health Organization; 2020b. https://storymaps.arcgis.com/stories/813561c780d44af38c57730418cd96cd. Accessed 7 Dec 2020.
WHO AFRO. Outbreaks and emergencies bulletin. 2023.
WHO EMRO. Epidemic and pandemic-prone diseases: information resources: weekly epidemiological monitor. Cairo: WHO Eastern Mediterranean Regional Office; 2023. http://www.emro.who.int/pandemic-epidemic-diseases/information-resources/weekly-epidemiological-monitor.html. Accessed 2 June 2023.
World Bank. Fragile and conflict-affected situations, FY23. Washington, DC: World Bank; 2022.
World Bank. Fragility, conflict, and violence. Washington, DC: World Bank; 2023. https://www.worldbank.org/en/topic/fragilityconflictviolence. Accessed 2 June 2023.
WHO. Surveillance System for Attacks on Healthcare (SSA) Geneva: World Health Organization; 2024 [updated 26 Jul 2024]. Available from: https://extranet.who.int/ssa/Index.aspx#:~:text=Launched%20in%20December%202019%2C%20the%20Surveillance%20System%20for,of%20primary%20data%20about%20attacks%20on%20health%20care.

16.1 In Practice: Responding to an Infectious Disease Outbreak amid a Humanitarian Emergency

Elizabeth Ross, Emily Rasinski, Carol Han, and Francesco Paganini

Contents

Learning Track Note: This chapter appears in Learning Tracks: Emergency Research Response, Response Operations; Research ethics; Social Science Response Research

E. S. Higgs and R. A. Sorenson (eds.), *Principles and Practice of Emergency Research Response*,
https://doi.org/10.1007/978-3-031-48408-7_22

Learning Objectives

This chapter will help readers understand and describe:

- The roles of USAID in responding to humanitarian crises that arise from infectious disease outbreaks
- The humanitarian principles that underlie BHA's core values and how these values guide their actions
- The responsibilities of a USAID Disaster Assistance Response Team (DART) in coordinating the U.S. Government's response to humanitarian crises
- How the prevailing humanitarian crisis in the northeast DRC complicated emergency response to the Ebola outbreak there in 2018–2020
- How and why USAID expanded its humanitarian response to respond to health needs aside from Ebola virus disease
- Important aspects of BHA's response to the Ebola outbreak in North Kivu and Ituri
  - Factors that contributed to a lack of community engagement in this response
  - Five strategic priorities in the response to the northeastern DRC Ebola outbreak
  - How USAID addressed distrust and misconceptions about Ebola virus disease

1 Introduction

When the Government of the Democratic Republic of the Congo (DRC) designated Ebola Outbreak 10 in North Kivu on August 1, 2018, the country was already in the throes of an ongoing humanitarian crisis. Approximately 5.5 million people in the DRC were displaced from their homes, and decades-long armed conflicts and popular disaffection from the government in Kinshasa created a complicated environment that left affected communities hard to reach and wary of outside aid workers and response efforts (Maxmen 2019).

Armed attacks on Ebola response teams and health facilities slowed response efforts. Distrust from communities that had been marginalized or exploited for decades left fertile ground for mistrust of all authorities, feeding misconceptions about the disease and emergency responders, including beliefs that Ebola was created to wipe out populations, extort money from people, or prevent participation in elections. In eastern DRC, where thousands are killed yearly by violence and thousands more die from easily preventable diseases, seeing the international community rapidly ramp up resources to combat Ebola sowed distrust and misconceptions about the disease.

"Geographically, our teams had limited ability to travel to the areas that were hit hardest by the outbreak because of the ongoing violence that has plagued these communities for decades," Dr. Jolene Nakao, a former United States Agency for International Development (USAID) health advisor, explained. "There were also cultural differences, as well as complicated dynamics between the communities in the affected regions and the Government of the DRC" (interview by authors).

Even before the Ebola outbreak, more than 3.4 million people in North Kivu and Ituri provinces needed humanitarian aid. The outbreak further tested international humanitarian emergency response, even with technological innovation and widespread emergency use of a new vaccine carried out by the World Health Organization (WHO) and an assortment of partners, including the DRC Government (Cohen 2018).

More than two and a half years later, the outbreak was declared over with the help of USAID's Bureau for Humanitarian Assistance (BHA), the Centers for Disease Control and Prevention (CDC), WHO, and others, but not without reaching a grim milestone. Having spread to two other provinces in the DRC, it had become the second-worst Ebola outbreak in history, leaving 2280 people dead (WHO 2020).

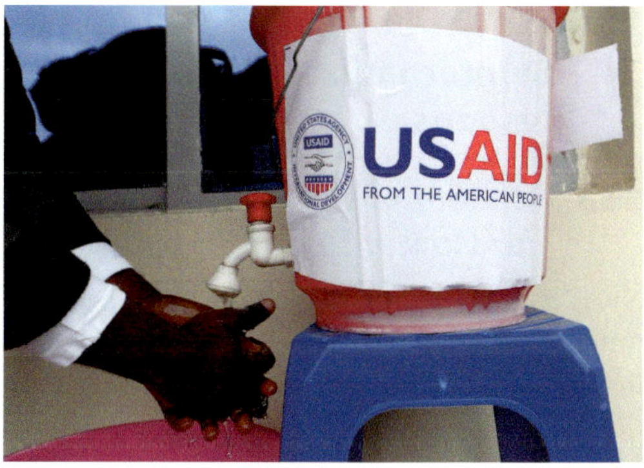

Fig. 1 To help stop the spread of the Ebola virus, USAID supported water, sanitation, and hygiene programs, as well as social mobilization programs that provided guidance to local communities on how to protect themselves from the Ebola virus disease. (Courtesy USAID)

"In the beginning, there was a lot of confusion about whether this was a health crisis or a humanitarian crisis," USAID Health Advisor Sonia Walia explained. "In reality, it was both, and both sides needed to be addressed" (interview by authors) (Fig. 1).

USAID's humanitarian experts had responded for the first time to an emergency primarily caused by a large-scale infectious disease outbreak in 2010, when cholera in Haiti ravaged communities already reeling from a catastrophic earthquake; the next time they responded was in 2014, when the West Africa Ebola epidemic required a multisectoral, multinational global response in three countries that ranked among the world's least developed but were not considered to be in a humanitarian emergency before the outbreak. The DRC outbreak, as noted, exacerbated an existing humanitarian and civil conflict emergency. Coronavirus disease 2019 (COVID-19) has since then struck the whole world, with greater or lesser intensity, in a brief period if not quite simultaneously. As scientists from many disciplines look to the future, they agree that populations everywhere—most acutely in countries with the least resources—face a future with increased pressures arising from climate change and environmental degradation, bringing novel and re-emerging infectious disease outbreaks as one of the likely consequences (Folke et al. 2021; Morand and Walther 2020). USAID and fellow humanitarian response workers are acutely aware of this probable future and are working hard to learn from the immediate past and plan for an uncertain future.

2 USAID and the U.S. Government's Role in Health Crises

The United States—in close cooperation with its international partners—prevents, detects, and responds to infectious disease threats at home and abroad. USAID plays a critical role in coordinating the U.S. Government's global health security efforts with other departments and agencies, donors, and multilateral organizations, as well as through our long-standing partnerships with developing countries. USAID partners with the Department of State, the Department of Health and Human Services (HHS), the Centers for Disease Control and Prevention (CDC), the National Institutes of Health (NIH), and other departments and agencies to respond to infectious disease-related crises. USAID is also a leading partner in implementing the Global Health Security Agenda (GHSA), an international initiative launched in 2014 to advance health security priorities multilaterally, bilaterally, and domestically (GHSA 2022). The GHSA brings together countries, international and nongovernmental organizations, and the private sector to work toward common goals for global health security. USAID's Global Health Bureau works to strengthen the capacities of partner countries to reduce the risk and impact of emerging infectious disease threats and outbreaks by ensuring the necessary systems and knowledge are in place to prevent avoidable outbreaks; detect threats early; and respond rapidly and effectively when outbreaks occur.

USAID's Bureau for Humanitarian Assistance (BHA) is the lead U.S. federal coordinator for international disaster assistance. BHA takes a holistic look at humanitarian aid and assists before, during, and after crises, from readiness and response to relief and recovery. This includes life-saving humanitarian assistance—food, water, shelter, emergency healthcare, sanitation and hygiene, and critical nutrition services—for the world's most vulnerable and hardest-to-reach people.

BHA responds to natural disasters like earthquakes, cyclones, droughts, and complex or anthropogenic disasters, such as the ongoing conflict in Syria. When appropriate, BHA can also respond to international health emergencies that occur during or become a humanitarian crisis. Examples include the 2014–2016 West Africa Ebola outbreak, the 2018–2020 DRC Ebola "Outbreak 10," and global disruptions during the COVID-19 pandemic. In these contexts, BHA's focus extends beyond the health crisis to address the possible humanitarian impacts.

Other U.S. Government agencies focused on global health, especially CDC and NIH, also work to detect, prevent, and respond to infectious disease outbreaks, along with many others worldwide, including nongovernmental organizations (NGOs), other governments, and international organizations, especially WHO. Many of them are poised to respond to outbreaks well before they become humanitarian crises requiring disaster assistance. Still, in a case like DRC Outbreak 10 where the humanitarian situation was already dire, or the West Africa outbreaks, BHA can bring vital organizational and logistical capabilities to the scene.

2.1 USAID's Leadership on International Disaster Response

2.1.1 History of the USAID Bureau for Humanitarian Assistance

Special Coordinator Designation: The 1975 amendment to the Foreign Assistance Act authorized the U.S. President to designate a "Special Coordinator for International Disaster Assistance," a role assigned to the Administrator of USAID. However, no country or organization can effectively or efficiently respond to a large-scale disaster alone. To provide effective humanitarian assistance, the U.S. Government must coordinate closely with key actors in the international humanitarian architecture. These include United Nations (UN) agencies and offices, NGOs, other government donors, and the Red Cross and Red Crescent movement.

2.1.2 BHA Guiding Framework

Core Values: BHA's humanitarian action is guided by a set of core values inspired by fundamental humanitarian principles.

Needs-Based Assistance: BHA is first and foremost focused on people who have been affected by disasters. The Foreign Assistance Act directs the President to "ensure that the assistance provided by the United States shall, to the greatest extent possible, reach those most in need." Consistent with this legislative requirement, BHA strives to provide assistance based on need. BHA ensures that people who are more vulnerable to disasters due to age, gender, disability, or other factors can equally benefit from assistance provided to the community.

Box 1: Humanitarian Principles Guiding Humanitarian Action

Humanitarian organizations are guided by four overarching principles:

Humanity. Human suffering must be addressed wherever it is found. The purpose of humanitarian action is to protect life and health and ensure respect for human beings.

Neutrality. Humanitarian actors must not take sides in hostilities or engage in political, racial, religious, or ideological controversies.

Impartiality. Humanitarian action must be carried out based on need alone, giving priority to the most urgent cases of distress and making no distinctions based on nationality, race, gender, religious belief, class, or political opinions.

Operational Independence. Humanitarian action should be autonomous from political, economic, military, or other objectives that any actor may hold with regard to areas where humanitarian action is being implemented.

These principles were first stated in this form by the International Committee of the Red Cross (ICRC) in 1921, when the organization proclaimed that its action in conflict situations was based on impartiality and political, religious, and economic independence. Humanitarian organizations who remain impartial, independent, and neutral more often gain the trust and acceptance of local populations, local and national authorities, and parties to a conflict, without which humanitarian access is difficult, if not impossible, to negotiate (ICRC 1996).

Commitment to People Affected by Disasters: BHA believes that people affected by a disaster should be at the center of the response and, as such, should be actively involved from start to finish, including in the design of programs. Recognizing that the affected communities and governments are the first responders in most disasters, BHA seeks, whenever possible, to build upon country capacities at all levels to prepare for and respond to emergencies.

Commitment to Transparency and Accountability: BHA seeks to be transparent and accountable to the American people who fund our work through their taxes, the affected populations we serve, and the partners we work with daily. BHA strives to apply industry best practices in monitoring, evaluation, and reporting to ensure that it meets its accountability and learning responsibilities.

Professionalism and Integrity: BHA strives to conduct itself professionally, making decisions based on technical knowledge and supporting program quality and continued innovation. BHA also seeks to conduct itself with integrity in its interactions with all parts of the humanitarian community as well as the local population.

Adaptability and Flexibility: The community's needs and the resources available to respond can change very quickly after a disaster or during a conflict. As a part of its commitment to placing the needs of those affected first, BHA places a high value on remaining flexible and adaptable to the changing situation during a response.

2.1.3 USAID Disaster Assistance Response Team (DART)

Activating and deploying a DART enables BHA to provide full-time, focused attention to a disaster response on the ground. A DART is a team of disaster response specialists coordinating U.S. Government assistance in response to an international disaster.

A DART can be mobilized quickly, often within 24 h. The DART is supported by a counterpart Response Management Team (RMT) in Washington, DC. The DART coordinates field-based U.S. Government engagement in the response and the provision of humanitarian assistance by determining the strategy and field-level approach to humanitarian relief. This strategy will include the sectors and geographic areas most in need of U.S. assistance; the placement and use of resources (commodities, personnel, and equipment); and the identification of program priorities and qualified implementing partners. In so doing, the DART seeks to address challenges and issues encountered in the affected country or region.

The DART's activities vary depending on the type, size, complexity, and location of the disaster. The DART assesses disaster impacts and humanitarian needs, reports on the disaster situation, and recommends follow-up actions, including the targeting and implementation of U.S. relief assistance and suggested funding levels. Based on these assessments, the DART helps develop and implement a U.S. Government response strategy and provides an operational presence capable of carrying out activities such as:

- Providing technical assistance
- Coordinating the movement and consignment of relief commodities
- Analyzing the existing capacity of the affected country's infrastructure and participating relief agencies to ensure an appropriate, efficient response
- Reviewing and recommending approval for relief program proposals
- Coordinating relief efforts with the affected country, other donors, relief agencies, and other U.S. Government entities, including the U.S. military

3 DRC Ebola Outbreak 10 (2018–2020)

Ebola virus disease is zoonotic and is likely carried by bats, though this has not been conclusively demonstrated (Caron et al. 2018). There have been periodic outbreaks of Ebola virus disease (EVD) in humans throughout the DRC and sporadically elsewhere in Central Africa since the disease was first identified in an outbreak in 1976.

On August 1, 2018, the Government of the DRC declared its country's tenth Ebola outbreak after four cases were confirmed in North Kivu province—an area where no previous outbreaks had been identified. Two weeks later, a case was found in neighboring Ituri Province—also a region that had no known previous Ebola outbreaks. The spread in these two provinces in northeast DRC aroused particular concern because of their high population density, high population mobility, and porous borders with adjacent countries such as Uganda. In addition, the northeast region of the DRC has been affected by deep-seated unrest and violent conflict for many decades, with conflict becoming more active in the two Ebola-affected provinces in 2017 (Wells et al. 2019).

Box 2: The UN Infectious Disease Response Scale-Up Declaration Protocol

The UN General Assembly created the Inter-Agency Standing Committee (IASC) in 1991 to serve as the highest-level humanitarian coordination forum, convening executive heads of 18 UN and non-UN organizations, including WHO and the United Nations Children's Fund (UNICEF).

The aim of the IASC is "to ensure coherence of preparedness and response efforts, formulate policy, and agree on priorities for strengthened humanitarian action." The Emergency Relief Coordinator (ERC) chairs the IASC to facilitate preparedness and effectiveness of the international community's response to humanitarian crises triggered by natural disasters, conflicts, and infectious disease events.

For a sudden-onset emergency or when an ongoing humanitarian emergency deteriorates, the IASC will consider activating a Humanitarian System-Wide Scale-Up. An IASC scale-up activation is based on an analysis of five criteria: scale, complexity, urgency, capacity, and risk of failure to deliver effectively and at scale to affected communities. The activation scale-up determination is made by the ERC following the prescribed consultation and decision-making processes between the IASC Principals, the relevant Resident Coordinator/Humanitarian Coordinator, and the Emergency Directors Group (EDG). If a Scale-Up is activated, it is a time-bound—maximum 6 month—mobilization that ensures sufficient capacities and resources are deployed for enhanced leadership and response operations, along with evaluation and deactivation procedures.

The IASC Infectious Disease Scale-Up Protocol, established in April 2019, builds on these scale-up procedures to specifically address the evolution of an infectious disease event, including the roles of WHO, its Director-General, and WHO Member States under the International Health Regulations. The protocol also underscores the importance of non-IASC organizations in responding to infectious disease events.

By November 2018, the outbreak, which had spread to a third province, became the biggest Ebola outbreak in the DRC's history and the second-largest Ebola outbreak known, behind only the 2014–2016 West Africa epidemic that killed more than 11,000 people (Fig. 2).

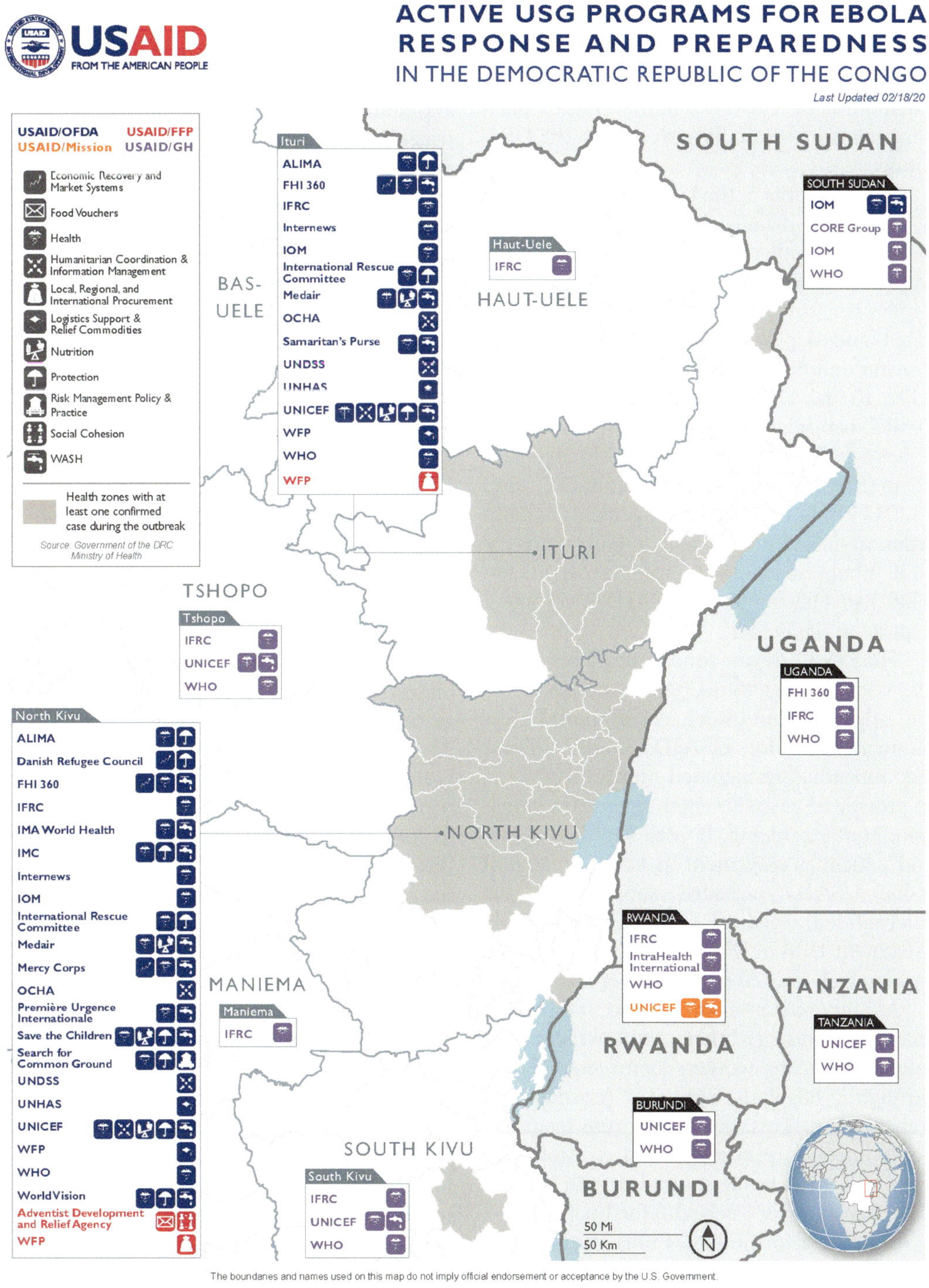

Fig. 2 Response to DRC Ebola outbreak by USAID and implementing partners. (Courtesy USAID)

3.1 BHA's Ebola Response in the DRC

In mid-August 2018, USAID deployed a senior infectious disease advisor to the DRC to assess the response, including major gaps, challenges, and potential need for the response capabilities of USAID's humanitarian partners, many of whom have worked in the DRC for decades.

On September 5, the U.S. Chargé d'affaires in Kinshasa officially declared a disaster due to the magnitude of the outbreak, paving the way for a larger U.S. response. In late September 2018, the U.S. Government activated and deployed a DART made up of disaster and health experts from USAID and CDC to the DRC. To coordinate with the DART, two teams were set up in the United States—a USAID Response Management Team (RMT) based in Washington, D.C., and a CDC Ebola Incident Management Team in Atlanta. USAID also had a liaison to the CDC Ebola Incident Management Team, and CDC had a liaison to the USAID RMT and a deputy on the DART.

The DART began conducting assessments and coordinating with Ebola response actors and other humanitarian agencies to make recommendations for USAID funding. These recommendations included supporting NGOs to provide disease surveillance, case investigation, contact tracing, border health security, and patient management in Ebola treatment units. USAID provided support for the International Medical Corps 20-bed Ebola Treatment Unit in Makeke village, Mabalako town, which opened in September 2018.

As the response progressed, additional challenges presented themselves. At alarming rates, healthcare workers contracted Ebola through hospital-acquired (nosocomial) transmission. This was largely due to inadequate infection prevention and control measures (IPC) and water, sanitation, and hygiene (WASH) standards at health facilities.

"This is also the first Ebola outbreak to occur in North Kivu, which had limited health infrastructure to begin with, and there was limited capacity for health care providers to rapidly detect cases and protect themselves," said Dr. Linda Mobula-Shufelt, a former USAID health advisor. "As a result, many health care providers have unfortunately contracted Ebola."

To help mitigate this spread, USAID began funding partners to help strengthen IPC measures and train healthcare workers and staff on best practices in case detection, triage, patient screening, and waste management. Over the first year of the response, USAID supported IPC measures in more than 360 health facilities across more than 20 health zones in eastern DRC.

After cases were confirmed in Goma, a city of approximately 600,000 people near the DRC's border with Rwanda, USAID's Bureau of Global Health began supporting preparedness efforts there, as well as in provinces adjacent to the outbreak zone and the bordering countries of Rwanda, South Sudan, and Uganda.

In coordination with USAID, and in addition to public health and medical treatment efforts, a vaccination program under a WHO Emergency Use Assessment and Listing (EUAL) procedure started in August 2018 with frontline healthcare workers and ultimately vaccinated more than 300,000 people at risk through a ring strategy (▶ In Focus 22.1), whereby contacts of those who had been affected along with contacts of these contacts received the vaccine. This is believed to have contributed to ending Outbreak 10. Based on earlier research in West Africa and the results of the monitored vaccination campaign in DRC, the vaccine was later approved by the U.S. Food and Drug Administration (FDA) (FDA 2019a, b; WHO 2018a, b, 2019a, b, 2020).

Also in the context of the humanitarian emergency, the DRC National Biomedical Research Institute and NIH spearheaded a successful trial of therapeutic agents for Ebola patients during the outbreak (▶ In Practice 17.1). The study ended early when it demonstrated that two of the four investigational therapeutics being administered were superior to the other two; the two efficacious treatments also received regulatory approval (FDA 2020a, b; Mulangu et al. 2019).

3.2 Challenges to the International Ebola Response

The DRC had been facing decades of humanitarian crisis brought on by multiple local and international conflicts. Continued violence was driving people from their homes and disrupted access to markets, agriculture, schools, health services, and livelihoods. There were reports of horrific violence against civilians, including executions, detentions, arrests of children, use of child soldiers, and sexual violence.

"Conflict is the biggest barrier to fighting the disease," noted Dr. Mobula-Shufelt. "The ongoing fighting has limited access to Ebola hotspots and prevented teams from conducting key interventions, like tracing contacts, vaccinating patients, and case investigation."

Misinformation about Ebola and the Ebola response was rampant. Many communities did not understand or agree with the outsized international attention on the outbreak, following the far more deadly impact from years of violence that had garnered significantly less global attention and the presence of other long-standing public health issues, such as measles.

"In the DRC, there are a lot of misunderstandings about the disease," said Dr. Mobula-Shufelt. "During a previous outbreak in Équateur Province, communities believed Ebola was caused by witchcraft. Right now, communities in North Kivu and Ituri believe Ebola was started as a way to wipe out the population in Beni. They also believe that politicians are spreading false information about the outbreak as a way to gain political support for the upcoming elections. There's also a high level of community reticence and mistrust towards responders" (interview by authors).

3.3 Scaling Up the Response

After nearly a year of fighting Ebola as strictly a health crisis, public health officials conceded that their battle plan was failing. They proposed a comprehensive new strategy for containing the virus that reframed the epidemic as a regional humanitarian crisis, not simply a health emergency.

On May 30, 2019, the IASC Principals, on the recommendation of the Director-General of WHO and the IASC Emergency Directors Group, unanimously agreed on the need to activate the newly established IASC "Humanitarian System-Wide Scale-Up Activation Protocol for the Control of Infectious Disease Events" for Ebola Outbreak 10. In accordance with the protocol, UN Under-Secretary General and Emergency Response Coordinator (ERC) Mark Lowcock carried out the recommendation and formally activated the scale-up, focused on health zones in the DRC provinces of Ituri and North and South Kivu, where Ebola transmission was occurring and likely to continue; there was the option of including other areas should the disease spread (IASC 2021).

IASC Principals determined that the scale-up activation for the DRC Ebola Outbreak 10 should focus on the following five strategic priorities:

1. Strengthened political engagement to create an enabling environment for the response
2. Strengthened multisectoral humanitarian coordination that fosters greater community engagement
3. Timely and sustainable financing, monitoring, and reporting on the use of funds in collaboration with the World Bank and key donors
4. Enhancing the public health response, working with the Ministry of Health
5. Leadership for a contingency cell in Goma and redoubled preparedness efforts in other countries (Burundi, South Sudan, Rwanda, and Uganda)

The decision to activate a UN scale-up, the first time the protocol was used since it was established in April 2019, followed 9 months of public health response to the outbreak, when all indicators were deteriorating, and risk of geographic spread was high. Approximately 30 security incidents—including attacks on treatment centers and healthcare workers—have slowed the Ebola response since February 2019. Confirmed Ebola cases were continuing at a high level, and other public health indicators, such as rates of effective patient isolation and healthcare worker infections, had severely deteriorated.

Up to this point, the coordination between the primary health actors—WHO, the DRC Government and the Ministry of Health—with the broader humanitarian community was minimal and at times confrontational (Crawford and Holloway 2021). The attempt to treat the Ebola outbreak in isolation from the broader humanitarian context resulted in the underutilization of humanitarian medical providers, who not only had the technical skills to address the outbreak but many of whose staff had relationships within the community. Exacerbating tensions was the fact that many of the DRC Ministry of Health staff working on the Ebola response were brought in from the capital, Kinshasa, displacing local, trusted health personnel. The lack of familiarity with these new entities had knock-on negative effects on community relationships, as new health actors were not trusted by local communities and sometimes resorted to using escorts to reach affected areas. Furthermore, these newcomers were not experienced in negotiating for unimpeded humanitarian access, resulting in problematic engagements with armed groups (► Chap. 18, In Practice 18.1).

All of this contributed to a lack of community engagement, which is essential for successful research in a low-resource area, especially one where the motives of outsiders have often been mixed, if not exploitative. As the outbreak occurred within an ongoing complex humanitarian emergency, understanding the local context and incorporating community feedback into all strategies was essential to turn the tide. In early 2019, the United States and other lead response donors urged the UN to take swift action and reset the international response, emphasizing adopting a community-based strategy. The humanitarian scale-up provided for leadership and multi-sector strategies aimed at strengthening the outbreak response through greater community engagement and coordination with the Government of the DRC.

USAID expanded its response to include programs that addressed needs other than stopping the Ebola outbreak and provided a more comprehensive approach for affected communities. These activities included providing primary health care and treating and preventing endemic diseases like malaria and measles, which caused more mortality and morbidity than Ebola virus disease. Most significantly, USAID's expansion of its Ebola response allowed partners to provide services that—while not directly addressing Ebola prevention, containment, and treatment—reflected community priorities and helped build community trust. By supporting the provision of latrines, potable water, and vocational training programs, for example, USAID addressed humanitarian needs that the community found more urgent and felt had a more significant impact on their well-being.

To address rampant distrust and misconceptions about the disease, USAID also ramped up community mobilization programs that sought to raise awareness and acceptance of the disease through outreach activities and improved communication with affected community members. USAID partners worked with local community members—including Ebola survivors, religious leaders, youth groups, and women's groups—to be a part of the response and help deliver Ebola prevention messages to their own communities. USAID also funded radio shows, public service announcements, news and rumor-control bulletins, and trained journalists to provide more accurate information about the disease. USAID sponsored more than 100,000 radio broadcasts designed to educate communities on Ebola risk and prevention techniques.

While it is difficult to measure whether all of these activities improved community acceptance of Ebola given the dynamic factors of the response, members of USAID's disaster response team say these approaches helped "move the dial" on community perceptions (► In Practice 18.2).

"The criticality of community engagement is the largest lesson, but it's not a new one," explained Dr. Jolene Nakao, former USAID Health Advisor. "It is something that should run through and through everything we do as humanitarians and in international aid at large. All humanitarian action needs to be led and driven by the affected communities. Empowerment cannot be just a development catchphrase. This response reminds us all of the centrality of this" (interview by authors).

3.4 The End of Outbreak 10 and Looking Ahead to Future Health Crises

On June 25, 2020, the DRC declared an end to the outbreak in eastern DRC. However, only weeks earlier, on June 1, 2020, the DRC Ministry of Health declared a new outbreak in Équateur Province in northwestern DRC, one that was not connected to the epidemic in eastern DRC (WHO 2020). The emergence of COVID-19 in 2020 further complicated the response to this new outbreak, diverting attention and resources and creating new obstacles to keeping frontline workers safe.

In response, USAID shifted its efforts to focus on the new outbreak in Équateur Province while continuing to support post-outbreak efforts in eastern DRC. From an administrative perspective, the inherent flexibility intentionally built into USAID's humanitarian grants was critical in allowing partners to effectively shift their programs both programmatically and geographically. Many grants were structured in such a way that USAID could rapidly deploy funding without bureaucratic modifications, allowing the agency to pivot its response westward to address the new outbreak. This included monitoring and providing follow-up care to the survivors in eastern DRC, as the virus can persist in body fluids in some survivors for an extended period, as well as continued community engagement and education to minimize the risk of transmission from survivors and mitigate stigmatization. After 6 months, on December 31, 2020, USAID stood down its response to Ebola in the DRC. This marked the first time in more than 2 years that the DRC was Ebola-free.

Subsequent outbreaks of Ebola in the DRC were successfully addressed by USAID's Bureau for Global Health, USAID's DRC Mission, and other partners without requiring a humanitarian response. USAID continues to maintain staff within the DRC focused on the ongoing humanitarian crises and the U.S. Government's investments in the country's health systems, water infrastructure, and global health security, and will continue to help the DRC as it confronts new health challenges.

Discussion Questions

1. Discuss the roles of USAID and the U.S. Government when responding to infectious disease outbreak health crises.
2. BHA's humanitarian action is guided by a set of core values inspired by fundamental principles.
   (a) Discuss the humanitarian principles that inspire BHA's core values.
   (b) Discuss the core values that guide BHA actions.
3. Activating and deploying a DART enables BHA to provide full-time, focused attention to a disaster response on the ground. DART activities vary depending on the type, size, complexity, and location of the disaster. Discuss some of these activities.
4. Highlight important aspects of BHA's Ebola Outbreak 10 response in the DRC.
5. Discuss how the DRC humanitarian crisis increased challenges to the international Ebola response.
6. What factors contributed to a lack of community engagement and proved to be a significant barrier to fighting the Ebola Outbreak 10?
7. What were the five strategic priorities on which the Scale-Up activation for the DRC Ebola Outbreak 10 focused?
8. Discuss how USAID expanded its humanitarian response to include programs that addressed health needs other than Ebola and provided a more comprehensive health approach for affected communities.
9. How did USAID address rampant distrust and misconceptions about the Ebola disease?

10. Discuss how USAID shifted its efforts to focus on the new outbreak in Équateur Province while continuing to support post-outbreak efforts in eastern DRC although the emergence of COVID-19 complicated the response.

References

Caron A, Bourgarel M, Cappelle J, Liégeois F, De Nys H, Roger F. Ebola virus maintenance: if not (only) bats, what else? Viruses. 2018. https://doi.org/10.3390/v10100549.

Crawford N, Holloway K. The Democratic Republic of Congo's 10th Ebola response: lessons on international leadership and coordination. London: Overseas Development Institute. Institute OD; 2021.

FDA. ERVEBO. 2019a. https://www.fda.gov/vaccines-blood-biologics/ervebo. Accessed 17 Oct 2021.

FDA. First FDA-approved vaccine for the prevention of Ebola virus disease, marking a critical milestone in public health preparedness and response. Washington, DC: U.S. Food and Drug Administration; 2019b.

FDA. FDA approves first treatment for Ebola virus. Washington, DC: U.S. Food and Drug Administration; 2020a.

FDA. FDA approves treatment for Ebola virus. Washinfton, DC: U.S. Food and Drug Administration; 2020b.

Folke C, Polasky S, Rockström J, Galaz V, Westley F, Lamont M, et al. Our future in the Anthropocene biosphere. Ambio. 2021;50(4):834–69. https://doi.org/10.1007/s13280-021-01544-8.

GHSA. Global Health Security Agenda. 2022. https://ghsagenda.org/. Accessed 17 May 2022.

IASC. IASC humanitarian system-wide scale-up activations and deactivations. Geneva: Inter-Agency Standing Committee; 2021. https://interagencystandingcommittee.org/iasc-transformative-agenda/iasc-humanitarian-system-wide-scale-activations-and-deactivations. Accessed 12 July 2021.

ICRC. The fundamental principles of the Red Cross and Red Crescent. Contract No.: ref. 0513. Geneva: International Committee of the Red Cross; 1996.

Maxmen A. Science under fire: Ebola researchers fight to test drugs and vaccines in a war zone. Nature. 2019;572(7767):16–7. https://doi.org/10.1038/d41586-019-02258-4.

Morand S, Walther BA. The accelerated infectious disease risk in the Anthropocene: more outbreaks and wider global spread. BioRxiv. 2020. https://doi.org/10.1101/2020.04.20.049866.

Mulangu S, Dodd LE, Davey RT Jr, Tshiani Mbaya O, Proschan M, Mukadi D, et al. A randomized, controlled trial of Ebola virus disease therapeutics. N Engl J Med. 2019;381(24):2293–303. https://doi.org/10.1056/NEJMoa1910993.

Wells C, Pandey A, Ndeffo Mbah M, Gaüzère B, Malvy D, Singer B, et al. The exacerbation of Ebola outbreaks by conflict in the Democratic Republic of the Congo, Proceedings of the National Academy of Sciences of the United States of America (PNAS). 2019. https://doi.org/10.1073/pnas.1913980116.

WHO. Consultation on monitored emergency use of unregistered and investigational interventions (MEURI) for Ebola virus disease (EVD). Contract No.: 25 Aug. Geneva: World Health Organization; 2018a.

WHO. WHO supports Ebola vaccination of high risk populations in the Democratic Republic of the Congo. 2018b. https://www.who.int/news/item/21-05-2018-who-supports-ebola-vaccination-of-high-risk-populations-in-the-democratic-republic-of-the-congo.

WHO. Preliminary results on the efficacy of rVSV-ZEBOV-GP Ebola vaccine using the ring vaccination strategy in the control of an Ebola outbreak in the Democratic Republic of the Congo: an example of integration of research into epidemic response. 2019a.

WHO. WHO prequalifies Ebola vaccine, paving the way for its use in high-risk countries.pdf. Geneva: World Health Organizaion; 2019b.

WHO. Ebola—African Region (AFRO), Democratic Republic of the Congo. Disease Outbreak News; 2020.

17 Integrating Clinical Research into Ebola Response: Liberia Case Study

Mosoka P. Fallah

Contents

Learning Track Note: This chapter appears in Learning Tracks: Clinical Research; Emergency Research Response, Research Operations; Research Ethics; Social Science Response Research

E. S. Higgs and R. A. Sorenson (eds.), *Principles and Practice of Emergency Research Response*,
https://doi.org/10.1007/978-3-031-48408-7_23

Learning Objectives

This chapter will help readers understand and describe:

- How the U.S.-Liberia partnership PREVAIL managed and coordinated research efforts during the 2014–2016 Ebola outbreak
- How the West African Ebola experience has influenced subsequent response to EID emergencies and can inform future EID response preparedness
- Prerequisites for an effective response to the emergence of a new pathogen
- Requirements for maintaining the capacity to conduct such a response
- Benefits of an operational, clinical research capacity absent an EID emergency
- Ways to improve capacity to detect, contain, and develop medical countermeasures for a newly emergent disease

1 Introduction

The clinical research carried out in West Africa during the 2014–2016 Ebola outbreak helped create broad acceptance of expedited clinical research as an integral part of emergency infectious disease response. In retrospect it was a milestone on the path to the worldwide research response that followed the emergence of severe acute respiratory system coronavirus-2 (SARS-CoV-2). As global attention turned to the Ebola outbreak in late 2014, many responders were skeptical about the value of clinical research during an acute emerging or re-emerging infectious disease (EID) emergency. Some response organizers were reluctant to make resources available for clinical research, while others even questioned the morality of carrying out randomly controlled trials while so many were dying (Adebamowo et al. 2014; London et al. 2018). Many were skeptical about whether a rigorous, logistically complex research program could be implemented in time to affect the course of the outbreak in countries with little existing research capacity (NASEM 2017a). In the event, the clinical research on Ebola in West Africa demonstrated two things: that ethical, scientifically sound clinical research can be implemented successfully in a low-resource environment and that the global community must be better prepared to embark on such research quickly whenever and wherever dangerous new pathogens arise (NASEM 2017b). The West Africa research paved the way for subsequent research in the Democratic Republic of the Congo (DRC) which generated data for licensure of the rVSVDG-ZEBOV vaccine by the U.S. Food and Drug Administration (FDA), an approval recommendation by the European Medicines Agency (EMA), and World Health Organization (WHO) prequalification, as well as FDA approval of two therapies for Ebola based on data gathered in a separate trial in the DRC (Ollmann Saphire 2020; WHO 2019b) (◘ Fig. 1).

We have seen with SARS-CoV-2 the profound results of a new pathogen sweeping through the human population, and we have all the more reason to be prepared to detect, identify, and prevent a newly emergent pathogen from spreading beyond its point of origin, wherever that may be. Of course, SARS-CoV-2 first appeared in China, a country with formidable technical and scientific prowess, but it spread worldwide regardless. The high toll of COVID-19 in human morbidity and mortality around the world, including in the most prosperous countries, has cast a harsh light on the dangers of complacency in preparedness and missteps in response (Osterholm and Olshanker 2020).

The rapid research response to Ebola in several least-developed countries, including

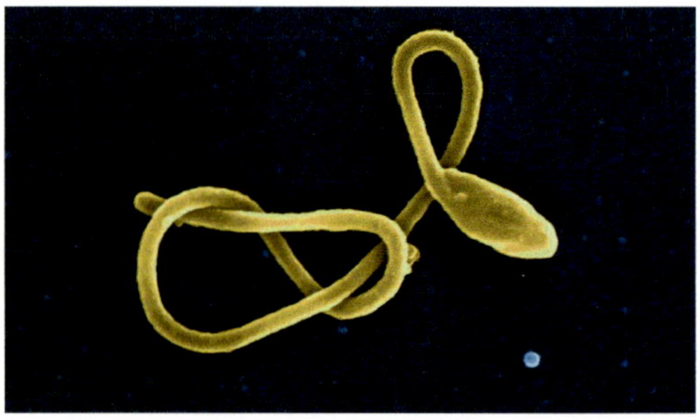

◘ **Fig. 1** Photomicrograph of the Ebola virus. (Photo: NIAID) (Public domain)

Guinea, Liberia, and Sierra Leone, starting in 2014, and the research carried out during subsequent Ebola outbreaks in the DRC, demonstrated that expedited clinical research can be done just about anywhere, but also that preparedness and pre-existing capacity matter. Since we cannot predict where the next outbreak of potential global concern will arise, we need to be prepared everywhere. When an outbreak hits a country that lacks public health preparedness and research infrastructure, the disease can more easily spread unchecked and even undetected, with accompanying human suffering and death. Especially in a fragile state (▶ Chap. 16), the outbreak can grow into a complex disaster threatening economic activity, development, and societal stability. The more cases accumulate in any country or region, the greater the chances of the disease spreading further: a pathogen spreading in Liberia today could be anywhere in the world tomorrow.

When the 2003 severe acute respiratory syndrome (SARS) outbreak spread from China to Hanoi, Singapore, and Toronto before being brought under control, it—along with the continuing threat of highly pathogenic H5N1 avian influenza and the U.S. anthrax attacks in 2001—was a major impetus in motivating completion of a revised version of the International Health Regulations (IHR) (2005) (Tucker 2005; WHO 2016). The World Health Assembly resolution adopting the IHR urged all member states to meet their own obligations and to "provide support to developing countries … in the building, strengthening and maintenance of the public health capacities" required. However, the capacity to effectively implement the IHR has remained inadequate in many countries, and the world was once again rudely awakened in 2014 to the real global threat of epidemic diseases leaving the shores—or really, the airports—of poor countries like Liberia, Sierra Leone, and Guinea. Not only was the Ebola virus not identified for months, but the declaration of a Public Health Emergency of International Concern in August 2014 seemed far later than indicated to many observers (Wenham 2017). Then, when faced with SARS-CoV-2 a few years later, many countries rated highest on evaluations of their IHR capacities did not cope very well (WHO 2019a; Yong 2020).

2 Ebola Comes to West Africa

When the Ebola outbreak that apparently originated in the tiny village of Meliandou, Géckédou town in Guinea, crossed into neighboring Liberia and Sierra Leone at the end of 2013 or the start of 2014, there was no laboratory in any of the three countries that could rapidly test patient samples and identify the Ebola virus. In the event it was nearly four months before the mysterious ailment was identified as Ebola, which had not been previously known to occur in West Africa (Coltart et al. 2017). While samples from Liberia still had to be ferried by canoe to Conakry, Guinea, for testing, Ebola was rapidly creeping into the densely populated city of Monrovia. In Monrovia, patients brought the infection into hospitals lacking basic infection prevention and control (IPC); these hospitals became amplification zones that spread the disease across the country and potentially worldwide. Redemption Hospital in New Kru Town, Monrovia (◘ Fig. 2) thus amplified the disease in June 2014 and left many health workers dead in its wake, including the Ugandan surgeon Samuel Muhumuza Mutooro (McCartney 2014). Health workers took Ebola with them to other hospitals and their families and homes. It killed many people at Tandapolee Clinic and then appeared at Cynthia Nelson Clinic, taking a heavy toll on the nurses and their families (Onishi 2014). When an Ebola chain of infection from Nzerekore, Guinea, reached Liberia in 2016, after Liberia had been pronounced Ebola-free, Redemption Hospital was better prepared; the response stopped the chain of infections in its tracks after samples were taken and sent to the newly established Eternal Love Winning Africa Hospital (ELWA) testing center for identification (de Wit et al. 2016). The result came back in hours and the ready response team quickly identified the cases and their contacts.

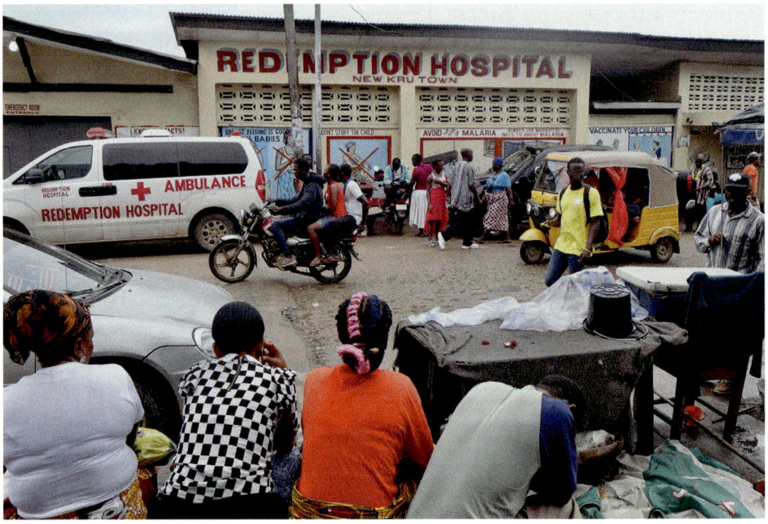

Fig. 2 Redemption Hospital in New Kru Town, Monrovia, Liberia. (Photo: Robert A. Sorenson)

Events in West Africa in 2014 were a harbinger of what we have seen since the start of 2020. This time, thanks to a virus that could be spread by the asymptomatic infected without direct contact, helped along by an inadequate public health response in many of the wealthiest nations, the outbreak became a global pandemic. The next new pathogen with human pandemic potential is likely to arise in a country with far less scientific and medical capacity than China, posing the risk of spreading undetected for a longer time.

3 Emergency Research Response to Ebola

Clinical research on Ebola medical countermeasures (MCMs) implemented in 2014–2016 produced preliminary results for the ZMapp experimental therapy (now superseded by more effective therapies) and rVSV-ZEBOV investigational vaccine by 2016. Advances in patient care measures also improved survival rates among EVD patients (Kiiza et al. 2020). Widespread use of the rVSV-ZEBOV vaccine in contacts and contacts of contacts of those infected in Guinea likely contributed to ending the spread of the Ebola virus there, and the vaccine was later used to good effect in the DRC (Henao-Restrepo et al. 2017; Wells et al. 2019b). This is an example of how even research that does not meet its initial goals can contribute to stopping outbreaks, and it highlights the necessity of preparing to implement a research agenda from the outset of an infectious disease emergency (Fig. 3).

The 2014–2016 Ebola outbreak in West Africa may turn out to be the last time in current history that many responders doubted the value of clinical research as a component of response to a rapidly spreading infectious disease outbreak. Ebola had been an episodic, self-limiting infectious disease largely restricted to remote areas of Central Africa, and though vaccine and therapeutic candidates had been created, investors did not believe the market would repay the costs of full clinical trials for these MCMs, nor did governments see Ebola as a sufficient threat to support such trials (Lakoff 2017). Investment in the rVSVDG-ZEBOV candidate vaccine developed by scientists from Public Health Canada was limited; some additional research on Ebola vaccines followed the 9/11 and anthrax attacks in the United States, based on bioterrorism concerns, and produced the ChAd3-EBO Z vaccine candidate, but neither went into full-scale clinical trials (Feldmann et al. 2018).

While the Ebola virus phenotype does not seen to have changed significantly before or during the West Africa epidemic, the new setting allowed it to spread rapidly among much larger populations, populations living

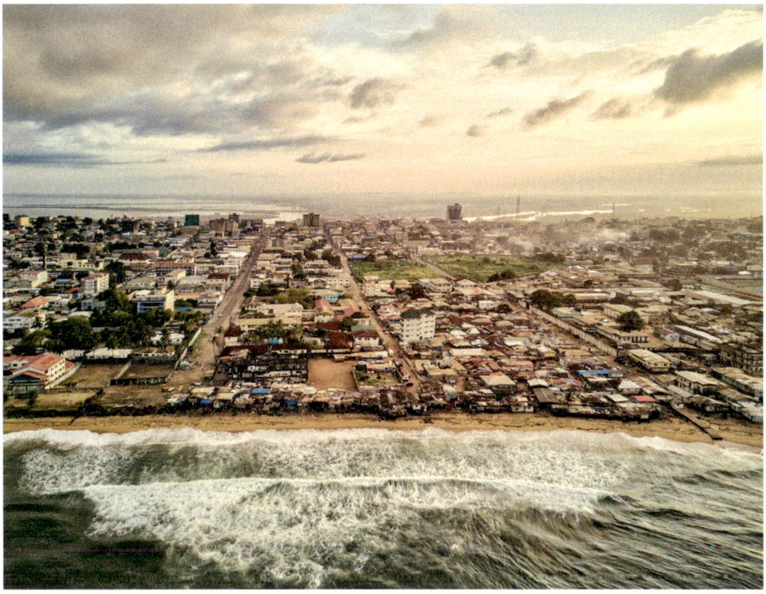

Fig. 3 Monrovia from the air. It was when Ebola reached West African capital cities with airports that it was first perceived as a global rather than a local threat. (Photo: Matt Kirchoff)

in cities with airports where infected people could embark for Europe and connecting flights around the world (Holmes et al. 2016). Global response was slow and generally ineffective until infected people began to arrive elsewhere (Otu et al. 2018), making it clear to all that this outbreak was not merely local. If the 1918 influenza outbreak could spread worldwide in less than a year and kill around 50 million people in 1918, the world in 2014 had become a global village with fast mass air travel. Ebola soon made its way to Europe and the United States, where few people were infected, but public reaction was intense (Towers et al. 2015). Global concerns kicked off intensified efforts to accelerate clinical trials for vaccines and therapies to counter the spread of the disease and treat those infected.

4 Rapid Research Implementation and Capacity Building

The absence of research infrastructure in the countries hit by the Ebola outbreak in 2014, combined with the urgency of getting research results during the explosive outbreak, meant a paradigm shift to building research capacity while conducting the research program to inform a response targeted at reducing morbidity and mortality and ending the current outbreak, rather than gathering data for future conclusions and application (Lane et al. 2016) (► Chap. 8). The Liberia experience showed it was possible to initiate research on an Ebola vaccine and the therapeutic monoclonal antibody ZMapp (NASEM 2017b). With hindsight, the go-ahead for pursuing a research response should have been given well before initial discussions between the Liberian Ministry of Health and the U.S. National Institutes of Health began in October 2014. Even when the program got underway, and despite strong Liberian and U.S. governmental support for starting the research as soon as possible, a number of factors led to delay: limited knowledge and understanding about clinical research in Liberia among both health care personnel and the general public; absence of basic research infrastructure, tools, and personnel; and challenges with electrical power, clean water, and physical facilities. It took until February 2015 to get the research program fully operational with the launch of the first trial. The protocol had called for Phase II and III trials of two experimental vaccine candidates, both expressing the surface Ebola virus glycoprotein through a recombinant virus. These were a recombinant vesicular stomatitis virus (rVSVDG-ZEBOV) and a recombinant

DNA chimpanzee adenovirus type 3 (rChAd3-EBO Z) (Higgs et al. 2017). By this time, however, public health measures were coming close to ending the outbreak, and the vaccine candidates remained in Phase II clinical trials since the number of newly infected people was insufficient for a planned Phase III trial (Doe-Anderson et al. 2016).

The same phenomenon would be seen in a therapeutic trial with the monoclonal antibody ZMapp (Prevail II Writing Group 2016). In spite of trial distribution across multiple sites in four countries (Liberia, Sierra Leone, Guinea, and the United States), there were never enough participants for the study to achieve adequate statistical power (Thielman et al. 2016). After taking thousands of lives, the epidemic had retired from the field before the new weapons against it could be honed. An earlier start to the research program and pre-outbreak investment in clinical research capacity in Liberia could have led to a quicker start and opportunities not only to determine the efficacy of MCM candidates but also to end the outbreak more quickly and avert much death and suffering. Greater readiness among outbreak response planners and personnel to integrate assessment of clinical research needs and then implement needed research would also have helped advance the start date of the studies.

The scientific, humanitarian, and medical world thus learned an important lesson: research had to be a core component of preparedness and response for the world to be protected from the next epidemic. The U.S. National Academy of Medicine gathered a team to study the situation across the affected countries, interviewed former patients and community leaders as well as experts, and published a report that was a clarion call for research to form a core component of preparedness and response to emerging and re-emerging infectious disease outbreaks (NASEM 2017b).

4.1 Missed Opportunities

Before the outbreak was finally identified as Ebola in March 2014, there were many missed opportunities for rapid response interventions in both epidemiological and clinical research (CDC 2016; Coltart et al. 2017). Initial public messaging seems to have conveyed to already distrustful communities that Ebola was a death sentence and that nothing could be done. With no cure or vaccine, a fearful and angry public spread rumors that the government had concocted an incurable disease or, equally implausibly, that the disease did not exist at all (Fassassi 2015). The U.S. Ambassador to Liberia highlighted the dire situation of an epidemic in the absence of medical countermeasures. Liberians were flocking to the U.S. Embassy, saying they would take anything to end the outbreak. In the face of such desperate requests for therapeutics or prophylaxis, the research infrastructure in Liberia was inadequate to implement a trial that could provide scientific evidence for large-scale use of any investigational new drugs (IND) or candidate vaccines, and it would take several months to build needed capacity. By the time a functional Ebola vaccine research program was underway, the perceived threat had receded, and case numbers were falling. Now mistrust, rumors, and suspicions about the vaccine research program began to circulate instead (Kobayashi et al. 2015).

4.2 Partnership for Research on Ebola Vaccine in Liberia (PREVAIL)

NIH and the Liberian Ministry of Health embarked on addressing inadequate research infrastructure for the assessment of MCMs against Ebola or a future outbreak through a structured partnership named the Partnership for Research on Ebola Vaccine in Liberia (PREVAIL). While its immediate goal was to carry out clinical research on Ebola MCMs, it also helped lay the foundations for a sustainable research platform built by Liberian and American scientists, one that could carry out various studies (see ◘ Fig. 4). Ultimately capacity built in connection with PREVAIL was brought to bear during the COVID-19

Fig. 4 Selected studies conducted on Ebola vaccines and therapeutics. (Author)

Trial	Enrollment start date	Location	Purpose
PREVAIL 1	Feb 2015	Liberia	Assess the safety and efficacy of two experimental vaccines against Ebola.
PREVAIL 2	March 2015	Liberia	Evaluate Mapp Biopharmaceutical's antibody-based Ebola treatment ZMapp.
Ebola Ça Suffit	April 2015	Guinea	Assess the safety and efficacy of the rVSV-ZEBOV vaccine against Ebola.
PREVAIL 3	June 2015	Liberia	Better understand long-term health consequences of EVD and determine if survivors develop immunity that could protect them from future Ebola infection.
PREVAIL 4	July 2016	Liberia, Guinea	Examine whether the experimental drug GS-5734 can eliminate Ebola viral RNA from semen in male survivors.
PREVAIL 5 (PREVAC)	April 2017	Guinea, Liberia, Sierra Leone, Mali	Evaluate three vaccination strategies to see which regimens hold the most promise in protecting people from Ebola virus disease.
PREVAIL 6	November 2017	Liberia	Examine how a person's genes might affect their response to Ebola.
PREVAIL 7	September 2017	Liberia	Evaluate the safety of removing cataracts and persistence Ebola virus fragments in the eyes.
PALM	November 2018	DRC	Compare mortality among EVD patients who receive one of three investigational Ebola drugs with a control group.

pandemic. In cooperation with the Liberian health system, including vertical programs like the National Malaria Control Program, the National AIDS Control Program, and the National Policy and Strategic Plan on Health Promotion (Ministry of Health Liberia 2016; National AIDS Control Program 2022; National Malaria Control Program 2021) and local Liberian scientists, as well as funders who provided grants for training, laboratory equipment, and reagents, the human and the capital infrastructure are being built for a rapid clinical response to a future outbreak. The social mobilization, communications, and community engagement (SMC) efforts connected with these research programs help build health research literacy across the country among varying stakeholders, so that distrust toward clinical research is reduced in case of future programs (▶ Chap. 18).

By September 2014, Liberia was accounting for over 50% of Ebola cases and deaths in West Africa, spurring the Liberian Health Minister to appeal directly to the U.S. Secretary of Health and Human Services to initiate clinical research for rapid investigation of vaccines that could prevent the outbreak from spreading further, as well as therapeutics that would mitigate mortality among those infected with the deadly Ebola virus (Doe-Anderson et al. 2016).

The U.S. National Institute of Allergy and Infectious Diseases (NIAID) deployed one of its senior scientists, Deputy Director for Clinical Research and Special Projects H. Clifford Lane, to Liberia to lay the groundwork for the research program. He respected the autonomy of Liberian health officials in deciding whether to accept or reject candidate vaccines and therapeutics. Further, he allowed them to commit themselves to exploring clinical research to support the response. This led to the formation of the Partnership for Research on Ebola Vaccines in Liberia (PREVAIL), with members from both Liberia and the United States, and its continuing research program. This partnership first agreed on these foundational response research goals:

1. Mitigate morbidity and mortality.
2. Accelerate the end of the outbreak.
3. Generate regulatory-level data for medical countermeasures.
4. Improve outbreak response to prevent or mitigate future outbreaks.

4.3 Research Response to Mitigate Morbidity and Mortality

In response to a rapidly spreading infectious disease, like the 2014–2016 Ebola outbreak in West Africa and subsequent Ebola outbreaks in the DRC, and more recently the emergence of SARS-CoV-2, it is crucial to implement a research program that, if successful, will cause the epidemic curve to plateau and then decline. An outbreak that continues to grow in the face of a visible response undermines trust in the responders. This tends to further fuel resistance, denial, and, in the case of Ebola, reluctance to send infected people to Ebola treatment centers and insistence on conducting unmodified traditional burials in secret rather than following safety guidelines. As a result, more people are exposed to the disease, increasing the regional or global risk of disease transmission.

Conducting research on promising candidate vaccines and therapies before an outbreak is a crucial preparedness strategy, allowing for expedited research response to infectious disease outbreaks. This was a major goal of the Coalition for Epidemic Preparedness Initiatives and the NIAID Prototype Pathogen Approach to preparedness, both established after the West Africa Ebola outbreak (Cassetti et al. 2022; CEPI 2022a). The challenge in the case of the West Africa Ebola outbreak was that, while there were candidate vaccines and therapeutics, they were not advanced enough in the development pipeline for either compassionate use or Phase III trials (except for ZMapp). Coupled with the lack of research capacity in the affected counties, this slowed the start of trials even as the window of opportunity for efficacy trials was closing as infection rates fell during the first half of 2015.

Nevertheless, the execution of the Phase II Ebola vaccine trials in Liberia and the ZMapp trials in Liberia, Guinea, Sierra Leone, and the United States produced some data on the MCM candidates for use in subsequent outbreaks. The Phase II Ebola vaccine trial in Liberia helped lay the groundwork for Guinea's Ebola Ça Suffit ring vaccine trial (Henao-Restrepo et al. 2017). The experience of conducting emergency trials in Liberia and Guinea, as well as the results, paved the way for further trials during the DRC outbreaks—whereupon the rVSVDG-ZEBOV vaccine became an accepted response tool in the containment of Ebola in the DRC, and ultimately a vaccine licensed by FDA, recommended for approval by the EMA, and prequalified by WHO (Higgs et al. 2017; Ollmann Saphire 2020; WHO 2019b).

In the same vein, the findings from the ZMapp trials demonstrated that even though ZMapp did not show statistically significant efficacy, it may have increased survivorship among Ebola patients. It thus set the stage for the use of the ZMapp and three other treatment candidates in the 2018 DRC Ebola outbreak (Mulangu et al. 2019; Prevail II Writing Group 2016). This trial, known as the PALM trial (▶ In Practice 17.1) (for *Pamoja Tulinde Maisha*, or "together save lives" in Swahili), demonstrated that two of the four candidate therapeutics investigated were significantly superior to the other two, so much so that two arms of the trial (including ZMapp) were terminated early to enroll all the participants in one of the two superior arms. The PALM trial was implemented and reached these conclusions during an outbreak in an even less accessible and less secure location than the trial locations in West Africa—in the DRC provinces of West Kivu and Ituri, against a background of armed conflict that continued during the outbreak (Mulangu et al. 2019; Wells et al. 2019a).

4.4 Accelerating the End of the Outbreak

The DRC studies demonstrated that research response, in the right circumstances, can accelerate the end of an outbreak. This had been prefigured in Guinea as well, where the last stubborn cases of Ebola were transmitted through traditional religious practices people were reluctant to change. Given the complexities hindering traditional response strategies like contact tracing, isolation, and containment, the rVSVDG-ZEBOV vaccine that was first tested for safety and immunogenicity in the Liberian outbreak was used in Guinea in a ring trial design that had been chosen for both cultural acceptability and its potential to help stop the epidemic (▶ In Focus 22.1). Publications from that trial indicated that the ring vaccination research contributed to ending the outbreak in Guinea (Henao-Restrepo et al. 2017). The same is true of the outbreak (DRC Outbreak 10) that began in the eastern DRC in August 2018 and ended in June 2020: over 300,000 doses of the rVSVDG-ZEBOV vaccine contributed to ending the outbreak, while the two leading therapeutics candidates in the PALM trial, MAb114 and REGN-EB3, helped hundreds of patients and pointed toward avenues for future research (Mulangu et al. 2019; WHO 2020).

4.5 Generating Regulatory-Level Data for Medical Countermeasures (MCM)

One of the arguments against randomized controlled trials (RCTs) in developing countries, like Liberia and the DRC, has been the lack of basic infrastructure—such as internet connectivity, electricity, and passable roads—would prevent the generation of high-quality, regulatory-level data. The notion that generating regulatory-level data is incompatible with using investigational vaccines and therapies to reduce morbidity and mortality has also generated controversy (Adebamowo et al. 2014). In fact, clinical research as a response strategy is in vain unless it can meet international standards by generating regulatory-level data. These data will be very important in two main ways: (1) in ensuring that the data safety monitoring board has high-quality data to make decisions about the candidates (▶ Chap. 23), as was done with the therapeutics in the PALM trial in the DRC and (2) the regulatory-level data will be essential to the licensure process with the various regulatory agencies, like FDA, EMA, and WHO (▶ Chap. 6).

4.6 Essential Components of a Rapid Response Research Agenda

Many of the hot spots for outbreaks of diseases with epidemic potential have either no or wholly inadequate research capabilities to rapidly integrate research into a traditional public health response without outside assistance. It is thus a top pandemic preparedness priority to consider the requirements for a rapid research agenda in the event of an outbreak, one with the goals stated for PREVAIL:

1. Mitigate morbidity and mortality.
2. Accelerate the end of the outbreak.
3. Generate regulatory-level data for medical countermeasures.
4. Improve outbreak response to prevent or mitigate future outbreaks.

Goals 1 and 2 are essential to the primary global health security goal of localizing infectious disease outbreaks and preventing them from becoming epidemics or pandemics.

There are at least three essential requirements to make such a research response work:

1. An immediate assessment of research requirements and potential results
2. Integration into a functional Incident Management System (IMS)
3. Planning for research response tailored to the characteristics and circumstances of individual outbreaks

4.6.1 Immediate Assessment of Research Needs for the Outbreak and Implementation Requirements

In the case of Ebola in West Africa, there was a clear need for clinical research on the existing vaccine candidates and the ZMapp investigational therapeutic. However, there was considerable debate about whether an RCT was the proper research methodology in the emergency (WHO 2014a, b, c). But if clinical research was to proceed, it was urgent for the team to identify one or more clinical research sites in a major hospital or health center catering to a catchment area population suitable for study enrollment. Embedding the site in a hospital is also useful, so some of the existing resources can be leveraged. Another requirement is political willingness at the level of the hospital, community, and local authorities to allow research to be conducted.

A list of hospitals and health centers was developed for Montserrado and Bong Counties, Liberia (▶ Chap. 40). Team members visited the sites to evaluate basic infrastructure like electricity, physical space, and the need for construction or renovation. John F. Kennedy (JFK) Medical Center, Redemption Hospital, and Duport Road Health Center were selected in Montserrado County, CH Rennie Hospital in Margibi County and Phebe Hospital in Bong County. Priority was given to JFK, Liberia's teaching hospital serving hundreds of thousands of people. However, distrust and miscommunication about clinical research among some medical professionals at JFK led to pushback from the hospital administration. Given the urgent state of affairs, Redemption Hospital was selected as the first site to roll out the vaccine study. Duport Road and CH Rennie would be renovated subsequently. Once sites were identified, multiple stakeholder meetings were held with government officials and local community members. This was necessary for buy-in and support because the country was naïve to clinical research during an outbreak. This was closely followed by massive renovation to operationalize a modern site and urgent procurement and import of equipment like generators, laboratory-grade refrigerator/freezer units, laboratory and pharmacy equipment and supplies, and personal protective equipment (PPE), as well as improvements in plumbing, ventilation, and so on. Such operational requirements are covered in detail in the final section of this book.

4.6.2 Integration into Incident Management System

In the three most heavily Ebola-affected countries, an incident management system (IMS) was set up, modeled after the IMS of the U.S. Centers for Disease Control and Prevention (CDC), to coordinate and facilitate a sound, rapid decision-action-feedback loop based on available data (CDC 2016). By the time the team from NIAID visited Liberia in October 2014 to discuss clinical trials of investigational vaccines and therapeutics as an innovative outbreak response strategy, there was a well-functioning IMS in place. The IMS was responsible for coordinating and directing the entire response to the outbreak, with response pillars ranging from epi-surveillance to psychosocial support to case management. To further accelerate the research, the position of deputy incident manager for research was created by the government of Liberia to ensure the full support needed to accelerate the research response. The IMS research pillar was first tried in Liberia, and it became a key component of the response in the DRC during the 2018–2020 Ebola outbreak in North Kivu and Ituri.

4.6.3 Improving Outbreak Response to Prevent, Stop, or Mitigate Future Outbreaks

When adequate, high-quality data are generated during an outbreak to validate MCMs and other measures against a subsequent outbreak, it speeds and strengthens future response and containment. Even in the short term, such effects were seen in Liberia in the re-infection episodes that followed the official end of the Ebola outbreak in Liberia, according to WHO criteria, on May 9, 2015. There were three subsequent resurgences of Ebola: in June and November 2015 and in April 2016. The first outbreak led to the rapid use of ZMapp with improved results and only one death of an infected person, an individual who reported to the Ebola treatment unit very late in the course of the disease. The second incidence led to one death and saw the first use of the rVSVDG-ZEBOV vaccine as an outbreak response strategy. The third and final outbreak in 2016 saw the combined use of the rVSVDG-ZEBOV vaccine and ZMapp; the outbreak ended rapidly with 100% survival rate from the Ebola treatment units (ETU). These three instances, unlike the initial phases of the outbreak, further validated the imperative to employ research tools in response to infectious disease emergencies, complementing more traditional, public health-oriented outbreak response strategies.

5 Sustaining Research Capacity, Planning for Research Response

One thing we have learned from the Ebola experience and from subsequent outbreaks, including the COVID-19 pandemic, is that both research capacity and careful, coordinated use of research resources are essential to an effective outbreak response. In terms of capacity, the U.S. government, largely through NIAID, has continued several research programs in Liberia, helping the country build a research platform as a preparedness and response asset. Other U.S. government partners include the CDC, the Agency for International Development, and the Department of Defense. Among other international initiatives that followed the Ebola experience were the founding at the 2017 World Economic Forum in Davos of the Coalition for Epidemic Preparedness Initiatives (CEPI), the WHO Health Emergencies Programme, World Bank Group initiatives for funding research in LMICs, and many others. The COVID-19 pandemic will leave no doubt about the value of a rapid research response to emerging infectious diseases. However, it is important not to lose sight of the fact that pathogens are still likely to emerge in developing countries where population growth and ecological disruption produce changes in the human-livestock-wildlife interface at an increasing rate—a risk factor for new pathogens to cross into humans, or for pathogens formerly seen in one region to emerge in a new one, as with Ebola in West Africa (Morens et al. 2004; Randolph et al. 2020). In addition, vaccines and therapeutics for diseases that are endemic in poor countries do not generally have the market potential to spur pharmaceutical companies to fund research and development of related MCMs, leaving it largely up to governments, academics, and foundations to take the lead in developing such MCMs (CEPI 2022b).

Over the last several years, we have seen with increasing frequency both new pathogens like SARS-CoV(1), Middle East respiratory syndrome coronavirus (MERS-CoV), SARS-CoV-2, Nipah virus, and previously known pathogens like Ebola and Zika in new places (Randolph et al. 2020). Moreover, other diseases that have been neglected due to the lack of economic incentive to develop MCMs are now becoming more widespread, among them Lassa Fever in West Africa and South Asia (Balogun et al. 2020). Mpox (formerly called monkeypox) was previously confined largely to tropical rainforest areas of central and west Africa but grew rapidly worldwide starting in May 2022, with more than 85,000 cases reported in countries that had not historically reported the disease, the vast majority from May to December 2022 (CDC 2022; Mathieu et al. 2023). WHO Director-General Tedros Adhanom Ghebreyesus declared the outbreak a Public Health Emergency of International Concern on July 23, 2022 (WHO 2022). Hence, it is vital that research response be agile, nimble, and adaptable to each outbreak. For instance, while Ebola and Lassa virus both cause viral hemorrhagic fevers, their levels of virulence and mode of transmission are different. Research on countermeasures against these two viral hemorrhagic fevers would require slightly different research responses. Vector-borne diseases like Zika require somewhat different methodologies.

In the event of an outbreak with an unknown cause, the first and most important requirement is to rapidly identify and characterize the pathogen. Thus, a multiplex, pathogen-agnostic or broad-spectrum diagnostic platform is a vital research measure for response. In Liberia alone, there are three million fever cases per annum and only about 50% of them are diagnosed, usually as malaria or typhoid; the rest are treated symptomatically. Thus, an acute febrile illness surveillance project jointly conducted by the CDC, the Liberian Ministry of Health, and the National Public Health Institute of Liberia at two health facilities has revealed co-infection of malaria and other diseases as well as pathogens less commonly encountered in Liberia, like dengue. Once these pathogens are identified, the challenge is to determine whether there are existing MCMs and, if not, whether there are candidates in development and at what stage, including different stages of licensure or prequalification. Thus, the initial research aspect of the response should include consistent determination of the pathogens and the available MCMs, whether approved or investigational. This is essential information for determining how and whether an outbreak can be countered to mitigate morbidity and mortality.

For planning purposes, WHO and CEPI postulated a "disease X" that could be lurking undiscovered to strike an unprepared human race at any time. In many ways, COVID-19 can be seen as the postulated disease X, but if so, we need to be prepared for disease Y (Iserson 2020). We have more and better tools to do so than ever before, but we still need political leadership, scientific coordination, and global solidarity to make them work.

Discussion Questions

1. What are the requirements for an effective response to the emergence of a new pathogen?
2. What would be required to establish and sustain the requirements for such a response in developing countries?
3. Aside from improved response when necessary, what are some of the other benefits of being prepared to identify and respond to a novel or re-emerging pathogen?
4. Note some potential measures for improving capacity to detect, contain, and develop medical countermeasures for a newly emergent disease.

Disclaimer The views expressed are those of the author and should not be construed to represent the positions of the Africa Centres for Disease Control and Prevention (Africa CDC).

References

Adebamowo C, Bah-Sow O, Binka F, Bruzzone R, Caplan A, Delfraissy J-F, et al. Randomised controlled trials for Ebola: practical and ethical issues. Lancet. 2014;384(9952):1423–4. https://doi.org/10.1016/S0140-6736(14)61734-7.

Balogun OO, Akande OW, Hamer DH. Lassa fever: an evolving emergency in West Africa. Am J Trop Med Hyg. 2020;104:466. https://doi.org/10.4269/ajtmh.20-0487.

Cassetti MC, Pierson TC, Patterson LJ, Bok K, DeRocco AJ, Deschamps AM, et al. Prototype pathogen approach for vaccine and monoclonal antibody development: a critical component of the NIAID plan for pandemic preparedness. J Infect Dis. 2022;227:1433. https://doi.org/10.1093/infdis/jiac296.

CDC. CDC's response to the 2014–2016 Ebola epidemic—West Africa and United States. MMWR Suppl. 2016;65(3):12.

CDC. 2022 monkeypox outbreak global map. Atlanta, GA: U.S. Centers for Disease Control and Prevention; 2022. https://www.cdc.gov/poxvirus/monkeypox/response/2022/world-map.html. Accessed 25 July 2022.

CEPI. Who we are. Oslo: Coalition for Epidemic Preparedness Innovations (CEPI); 2022a. https://cepi.net/about/whoweare/. Accessed 25 July 2022.

CEPI. A world in which epidemics and pandemics are no longer a threat to humanity. Oslo: Coalition for Epidemic Preparedness Innovations; 2022b. https://cepi.net/about/whyweexist/. Accessed 14 Nov 2022.

Coltart CE, Lindsey B, Ghinai I, Johnson AM, Heymann DL. The Ebola outbreak, 2013-2016: old lessons for new epidemics. Philos Trans R Soc Lond Ser B Biol Sci. 2017;372(1721) https://doi.org/10.1098/rstb.2016.0297.

de Wit E, Rosenke K, Fischer RJ, Marzi A, Prescott J, Bushmaker T, et al. Ebola laboratory response at the eternal love winning Africa campus, Monrovia, Liberia, 2014-2015. J Infect Dis. 2016;214(suppl 3):S169–S76. https://doi.org/10.1093/infdis/jiw216.

Doe-Anderson J, Baseler B, Driscoll P, Johnson M, Lysander J, McNay L, et al. Beating the odds: successful establishment of a phase II/III clinical research trial in resource-poor Liberia during the largest-ever Ebola outbreak. Contemp Clin Trials Commun. 2016;4:68–73. https://doi.org/10.1016/j.conctc.2016.06.008.

Fassassi A. Managing rumours and misinformation in West Africa. SciDevNet; 2015.

Feldmann H, Feldmann F, Marzi A. Ebola: lessons on vaccine development. Ann Rev Microbiol. 2018;72:423. https://doi.org/10.1146/annurev-micro-090817-062414.

Henao-Restrepo AM, Camacho A, Longini IM, Watson CH, Edmunds WJ, Egger M, et al. Efficacy and effectiveness of an rVSV-vectored vaccine in preventing Ebola virus disease: final results from the Guinea ring vaccination, open-label, cluster-randomised trial (Ebola Ca Suffit!). Lancet. 2017;389(10068):505–18. https://doi.org/10.1016/S0140-6736(16)32621-6.

Higgs ES, Dubey SA, Coller BAG, Simon JK, Bollinger L, Sorenson RA, et al. Accelerating vaccine development during the 2013-2016 west African Ebola virus disease outbreak. Curr Top Microbiol Immunol. 2017;411:229–61. https://doi.org/10.1007/82_2017_53.

Holmes EC, Dudas G, Rambaut A, Andersen KG. The evolution of Ebola virus: insights from the 2013-2016 epidemic. Nature. 2016;538(7624):193–200. https://doi.org/10.1038/nature19790.

Iserson KV. The next pandemic: prepare for "disease X". West J Emerg Med. 2020;21(4):756–8. https://doi.org/10.5811/westjem.2020.5.48215.

Kiiza P, Mullin S, Teo K, Adhikari NKJ, Fowler RA. Treatment of Ebola-related critical illness. Intensive Care Med. 2020;46(2):285–97. https://doi.org/10.1007/s00134-020-05949-z.

Kobayashi M, Beer KD, Bjork A, Chatham-Stephens K, Cherry CC, Arzoaquoi S, et al. Community knowledge, attitudes, and practices regarding Ebola virus disease—five counties, Liberia, September-October, 2014. Morb Mortal Wkly Rep. 2015;64(26):714–8.

Lakoff A. Unprepared: global health in a time of emergency. Oakland, CA: University of California Press; 2017.

Lane HC, Marston HD, Fauci AS. Conducting clinical trials in outbreak settings: points to consider. Clin Trials (London, England). 2016;13(1):92–5. https://doi.org/10.1177/1740774515618198.

London AJ, Omotade OO, Mello MM, Keusch GT. Ethics of randomized trials in a public health emergency. PLoS Negl Trop Dis. 2018;12(5):e0006313. https://doi.org/10.1371/journal.pntd.0006313.

Mathieu E, Spooner F, Dattani S, Ritchie H, Roser M. Mpox (monkeypox). Our World in Data. 2023. https://ourworldindata.org/monkeypox#citation. Accessed 8 June 2023.

McCartney M. Courage is treating patients with Ebola. BMJ. 2014;349:g4987. https://doi.org/10.1136/bmj.g4987.

Ministry of Health Liberia. National policy and strategic plan on health promotion, Liberia, 2016–2021. Monrovia, LR: Ministry of Health Liberia; 2016.

Morens DM, Folkers GK, Fauci AS. The challenge of emerging and re-emerging infectious diseases. Nature. 2004;430(6996):242–9. https://doi.org/10.1038/nature02759.

Mulangu S, Dodd LE, Davey RT Jr, Tshiani Mbaya O, Proschan M, Mukadi D, et al. A randomized, controlled trial of Ebola virus disease therapeutics. N Engl J Med. 2019;381(24):2293–303. https://doi.org/10.1056/NEJMoa1910993.

NASEM. Conducting clinical research during an epidemic. In: Busta ER, Mancher M, Cuff PA, McAdam K, Keusch G, editors. Integrating clinical research into epidemic response: the Ebola experience. Washington, DC: National Academies of Sciences Engineering and Medicine Publications, National Academices Press; 2017a. p. 37–82.

NASEM. Integrating clinical research into epidemic response: the Ebola experience. Washington, DC: National Academies of Sciences Engineering and Medicine Publications, The National Academies Press; 2017b.

National AIDS Control Program. Ministry of Health of the Republic of Liberia, Monrovia, LR. 2022. https://nacpliberia.org/. Accessed 25 July 2022.

National Malaria Control Program. Central Medical Stores, Monrovia, LR. 2021. https://nds-cms.gov.lr/national-malaria-control-program/. Accessed 25 July 2022.

Ollmann Saphire E. A vaccine against Ebola virus. Cell. 2020;181(1):6. https://doi.org/10.1016/j.cell.2020.03.011.

Onishi N. Back to the slums of his youth, to defuse the ebola time bomb. New York Times. 2014.

Osterholm MT, Olshanker M. Coronavirus: chronicle of a pandemic foretold. Foreign Aff. 2020;99(4).

Otu A, Ameh S, Osifo-Dawodu E, Alade E, Ekuri S, Idris J. An account of the Ebola virus disease outbreak in Nigeria: implications and lessons learnt. BMC Public Health. 2018;18(1):3. https://doi.org/10.1186/s12889-017-4535-x.

Prevail II Writing Group. A randomized, controlled trial of ZMapp for Ebola virus infection. N Engl J Med. 2016;375(15):1448–56. https://doi.org/10.1056/NEJMoa1604330.

Randolph DG, Refisch J, MacMillan S, Wright CY, Bett B, Robinson D et al. Preventing the next pandemic: zoonotic diseases and how to break the chain of transmission. UNEP Frontiers. Nairobi: United Nations Environmental Program International Livestock Research Institute; 2020.

Thielman NM, Cunningham CK, Woods C, Petzold E, Sprenz M, Russell J. Ebola clinical trials: five lessons learned and a way forward. Clin Trials (London, England). 2016;13(1):83–6. https://doi.org/10.1177/1740774515619897.

Towers S, Afzal S, Bernal G, Bliss N, Brown S, Espinoza B, et al. Mass media and the contagion of fear: the case of Ebola in America. PLoS One. 2015;10(6):e0129179. https://doi.org/10.1371/journal.pone.0129179.

Tucker JB. Updating the international health regulations. Biosecur Bioterror. 2005;3(4):338–47. https://doi.org/10.1089/bsp.2005.3.338.

Wells CR, Pandey A, Ndeffo Mbah ML, Gauzere BA, Malvy D, Singer BH, et al. The exacerbation of Ebola outbreaks by conflict in The Democratic Republic of the Congo. Proc Natl Acad Sci USA.

2019a;116(48):24366–72. https://doi.org/10.1073/pnas.1913980116.
Wells CR, Pandey A, Parpia AS, Fitzpatrick MC, Meyers LA, Singer BH, et al. Ebola vaccination in The Democratic Republic of the Congo. Proc Natl Acad Sci USA. 2019b;116(20):10178–83. https://doi.org/10.1073/pnas.1817329116.
Wenham C. What we have learnt about the World Health Organization from the Ebola outbreak. Philos Trans R Soc Lond Ser B Biol Sci. 2017;372(1721):20160307. https://doi.org/10.1098/rstb.2016.0307.
WHO. Ethical considerations for use of unregistered interventions for Ebola viral disease. Contract No.: WHO/HIS/KER/GHE/14.1. Geneva: World Health Organization. 2014a.
WHO. Meeting summary of the WHO consultation on potential Ebola therapies and vaccines. Geneva: World Health Organization; 2014b.
WHO. WHO meeting of the scientific and technical advisory committee on Ebola experimental interventions: briefing note. Geneva: World Health Organization; 2014c.
WHO. International Health Regulations (2005). 3rd ed. Geneva: World Health Organzation; 2016.
WHO. E-SPAR state party annual report. Geneva: World Health Organization; 2019a. https://extranet.who.int/e-spar. Accessed 3 Dec 2020.
WHO. WHO prequalifies Ebola vaccine, paving the way for its use in high-risk countries.pdf. Geneva: World Health Organizaion; 2019b.
WHO. Ending an Ebola outbreak in a conflict zone. Geneva: World Health Organization; 2020. https://storymaps.arcgis.com/stories/813561c780d44af38c57730418cd96cd. Accessed 7 Dec 2020.
WHO. WHO director-General's statement at the press conference following IHR emergency committee regarding the multi-country outbreak of monkeypox. Geneva: World Health Organization; 2022.
Yong E. How the pandemic defeated America. Atlantica. 2020.

17.1 In Practice: Integration of Clinical Research and Patient Care in the DRC PALM Ebola Therapeutics Trial

Richard Kojan

Contents

Learning Track Note: This chapter appears in Learning Tracks: Clinical Research; Research Ethics; Social Science Response Research

E. S. Higgs and R. A. Sorenson (eds.), *Principles and Practice of Emergency Research Response*, https://doi.org/10.1007/978-3-031-48408-7_24

Learning Objectives

This chapter will help readers understand and describe:

- How clinical research can be integrated with emergency medical treatment amid civil conflict in a low-resource setting
- Determination of whether an investigational drug worsens the clinical condition of an unstable patient
- Obtaining informed consent from a patient in critical condition
- Community engagement under the pressures of limited time and local conflict
- How providing quality patient care contributes to clinical trial success

1 Introduction and Background

Rigorous research to determine what treatments and supportive care demonstrably help patients is essential to improving their medical care. In the case of dangerous emerging diseases like SARS, Ebola, Nipah virus, or COVID-19, epidemics may be the only opportunity to move candidate medical interventions from preclinical development into Phase II and III clinical trials. Research done during the 2014–2016 West Africa Ebola outbreak and the 2018–2020 Democratic Republic of the Congo (DRC) Ebola virus disease (EVD) outbreaks has gone a long way toward putting to rest arguments that "Randomized clinical trials … were neither ethical nor feasible in an environment of limited health infrastructure and severe disease with a high fatality rate" (Ellenberg et al. 2018). The Ebola experience demonstrates that rigorous clinical research can

- Be conducted ethically during an emergency
- Provide a vital contribution to outbreak response
- Generate data for regulatory approval of medical countermeasures
- Enhance rather than detract from patient care (Jacob et al. 2020; Mulangu et al. 2019; NASEM 2017; Wolf et al. 2021)

The northeastern DRC at the time was coping with more than an Ebola outbreak. For many years armed groups had contended with each other and the DRC military for control over mining areas, where they "violently exploit civilians to retain access to valuable minerals" (Global Witness 2009). There was long-standing regional disaffection from a central government in Kinshasa that provided neither services nor security (Stearns 2012). Suspicion of incomers extended to both DRC Ministry of Health staff and foreign healthcare workers (Nguyen 2019). International humanitarian organizations nevertheless fielded staff with the courage and confidence to set up Ebola treatment centers (ETCs) to treat those infected and encourage the integration of Ebola isolation measures and other public health measures into regional health practice.

Even though armed attacks on ETCs took the lives of healthcare personnel, destroyed facilities (◘ Fig. 1), and disrupted the response, most ETCs continued to operate (Mueller and Rebmann 2019). They not only continued operating in the face of such dangers but were willing to accommodate a research program, which bespeaks both their courage and their ability to retain a perspective that looks beyond the immediate crisis to the longer term (Farrar 2018). For without the cooperation of the NGOs providing care for those infected with Ebola, the trial that led to two Ebola therapeutic agents being approved by the U.S. Food and Drug Administration (FDA) could not have occurred (FDA 2020a, b; Tshiani Mbaya et al. 2021).

High-quality clinical research must be carried out even in such circumstances because outbreaks are rare opportunities to counter dangerous diseases that, while episodic so far, can potentially spread and infect many more people over much wider areas. The clinical element of the response is urgent because a successful response will help end disease transmission overall, meaning there will then be too few potential research participants to allow for the collection of solid research data. Though doubts about whether high-quality clinical research and high-quality patient care can be conducted simultaneously persist, it is incumbent on both clinicians and researchers to ensure patients do not suffer because they consent to participate in a trial. They need to resolve important questions:

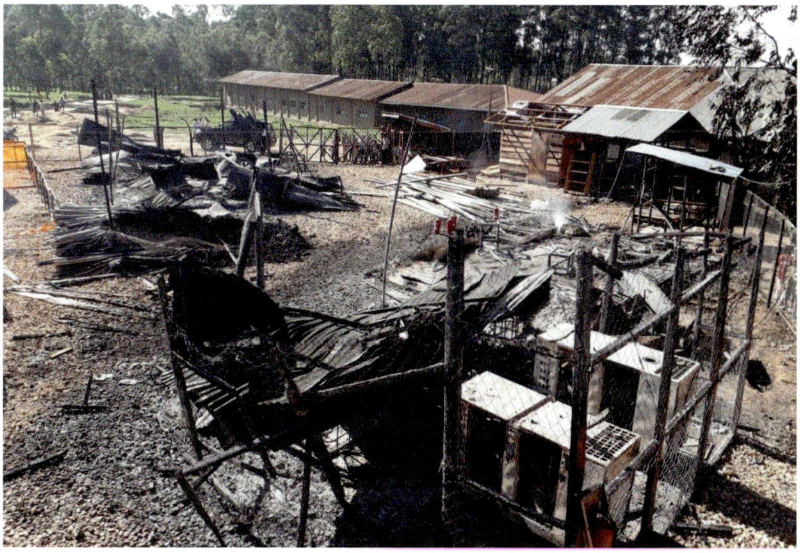

Fig. 1 Unidentified attackers set fire to an Ebola treatment center in Katwa, North Kivu, DRC in 2019. (Photo: Laurie Bonnaud/MSF)

- Could the drugs in a trial worsen the clinical condition of an unstable patient?
- How does one obtain informed consent from a patient in critical condition?
- How can one gain community support, especially when there is time pressure and the area is riven by conflict?

To address some of these questions and provide a concrete example of how clinical research can succeed amidst an infectious disease outbreak without compromising patient care, we describe here how diverse research and clinical care teams from several institutions worked together during the 2018–2020 EVD outbreak in the DRC to complete a clinical trial for Ebola therapeutics, while improving patient care and responding to community and population needs.

2 The PALM Trial

The *Pamoja Tulinde Maisha* (PALM) trial, "Together Save Lives" in Swahili, compared four investigational therapies for EVD to each other (meaning none of the participants received a placebo). The trial was a joint effort led by the DRC National Institute for Biomedical Research (*Institut National de la Recherche Biomédicale*, INRB) and the U.S. National Institutes of Health (NIH), in collaboration with the World Health Organization (WHO), the Alliance for International Medical Action, (ALIMA), Médecins Sans Frontières (MSF), International Mercy Corps and others; a complete list of partners can be found in Mulangu et al. (2019). The trial was urgently needed because there was then no licensed, effective therapy to reduce mortality for patients with EVD. A Phase I trial conducted by U.S. and Liberian partners during the 2014–2016 outbreak in West Africa had indicated that the monoclonal antibody ZMapp was safe for patients, but data were insufficient for a clear efficacy finding (Prevail II Writing Group 2016).

In the DRC study, consenting patients who tested positive for the Ebola virus were enrolled at Ebola treatment centers (ETCs) that agreed to support the study. All participants received standard medical care and were randomly assigned to receive one of the four therapies:

- ZMapp, which served as the control arm of the study
- The antiviral agent remdesivir
- The monoclonal antibody MAb114
- The antibody cocktail REGN-EB3

A total of 681 patients had enrolled by August 9, 2019, when the trial's data and safety monitoring board recommended stopping the remdesivir and Zmapp arms and that all patients be assigned either to the MAb114 or the REGN-EB3 groups for the remainder of the trial because interim analysis showed the clear superiority of Mab114 and REGN-EB3 over the other two agents with respect to mortality. Both MAb114 and REGN-EB3 were ultimately licensed by the FDA for the treatment of EVD based on the full trial results (FDA 2020a, b; Mulangu et al. 2019). Without the PALM trial, the world would not have approved Ebola therapeutics.

2.1 ALIMA in the Northeast DRC

ALIMA was a major contributor to the success of the PALM trial, and more than half the patients in the study were enrolled at ETCs run by ALIMA, the first organization to integrate the research into its treatment programs. Based in Dakar, Senegal, ALIMA provides humanitarian medical care and works to integrate research into clinical care in West and Central Africa along with a network of partners (ALIMA 2022). ALIMA previously provided care for Ebola patients in Guinea during the 2014–2016 West African outbreak. ALIMA has implemented health projects in the DRC since 2011 and provided treatment for EVD during the two 2018 outbreaks there (▶ In Practice 40.1). ALIMA had first undertaken Ebola response operations in the DRC in 2017. The ALIMA response to the outbreak that began in mid-2018, ultimately the largest seen in the DRC, began within days after the outbreak was declared on August 1, 2018, and continued until September 2019, when ALIMA operations were transitioned to MSF (Aruna et al. 2019).

For ALIMA, responding to the DRC outbreak was far more difficult than working in the West African countries affected by Ebola from 2014 to 2016. In both cases responders had to cope with minimal infrastructure and a barely functioning health care system. These troubles, along with a shortage of qualified personnel and the resulting heavy workload, required frequent rotations for the sake of staff members' physical and mental health, led to frequent resignations, and increased training needs for rotations and new hires. Despite such tribulations, the "trial showed that it is possible to conduct scientifically rigorous and ethically sound research during an outbreak, even in a conflict zone" (Mulangu et al. 2019).

2.2 Implementation of the PALM Trial in Beni and Katwa, DRC

ALIMA managed two of the ETCs (◘ Fig. 2) conducting the study in the cities of Beni and Katwa, North Kivu Province, where all the security and infrastructure problems described above were present. Nevertheless, while working with PALM trial organizers, ALIMA met the rigorous requirements of the study protocol approved by the DRC and the U.S. National Institute of Allergy and Infectious Diseases and their research ethics committees (Mulangu et al. 2019). Many obstacles had to be overcome to comply with trial protocol requirements, Good Clinical Practice, and Good Participatory Practice guidelines (ICH 2016; UNAIDS/AVAC 2011), and the DRC's and other regulators' regulatory requirements. Meeting those standards resulted in better patient care and a successful research study.

2.2.1 A Complex Implementing Partnership

Implementation of PALM at the research sites was carried out by the NIH and the DRC's National Institute of Biomedical Research (INRB) and teams from the DRC Ministry of Health (MoH) and ALIMA, with the Mitchell Group and Leidos, firms under contract with NIH, as administrative partners. Though it required considerable coordination, this approach worked well. Multiple partners bringing their respective strengths to the project not only accomplished the necessary tasks, but they also contributed to the

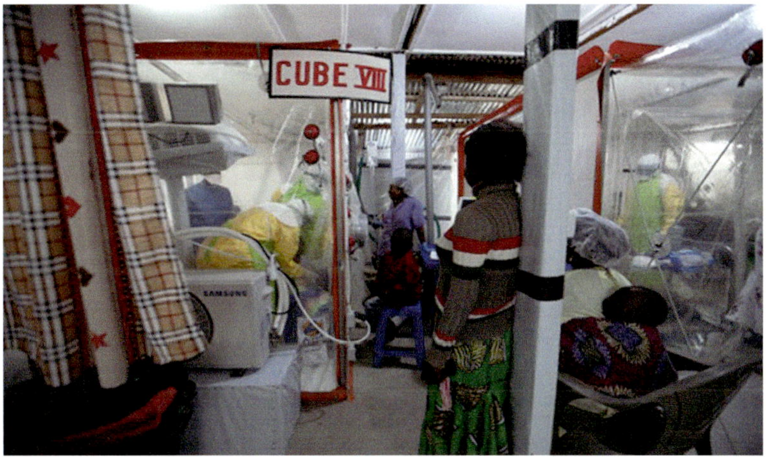

Fig. 2 A snapshot of the treatment environment where ALIMA implemented the PALM study. (Courtesy ALIMA)

training and education of each other's staff. Many of these staff members, building on career technical education training on implementing a standard clinical research protocol and their experience during the PALM Trial, can now perform higher-level tasks independently. The Beni ETC, inside Beni General Hospital, served as a model for patient care and research training.

2.2.2 Admission of Patients to the ETC

Upon arrival at the ETC, potential EVD patients were evaluated and had blood drawn for testing. Those testing positive for Ebola were admitted to an isolation ward or CUBE (▶ In Practice 40.1) at the ETC. Physicians then assessed their current medical status and undertook urgent measures to stabilize the patient's clinical condition if necessary. This was done in accordance with the prevailing ALIMA protocol, which had been reworked with help from WHO and approved by the DRC MoH. Then, in partnership with experts from Africa and around the world, WHO published guidelines to optimize supportive care for EVD before the end of the outbreak. In most cases the patient received standard care measures for stabilization, provided informed consent, and was immediately administered a candidate therapeutic drug within 24 h of admission; in a few cases, candidate drug administration was delayed until the hemodynamic instability of the patient could be addressed.

2.2.3 Informed Consent

During the patient's first day in the ETC, the investigator or another qualified member of the team reviewed the study with the patient and obtained informed consent; in cases where the patient was a minor or too ill to provide meaningful consent, a surrogate chosen in accordance with DRC law and local custom was asked to provide consent. This process included questions and answers. If necessary, a staff member explained the study in the local language, which is preferred by study participants or their representatives, rather than in Swahili. Each consent was witnessed, and the witness also signed the informed consent document.

2.2.4 Randomization of Participants

The gold standard of randomization is centralized, online randomization. In view of the low speeds and occasional outages of internet connections in Beni and Katwa, the PALM study team carried out "randomization by envelope": the centralized online randomization was carried out elsewhere, and the results were printed and sent to the sites as precise written procedures to be strictly followed, one of many adaptations but about as effective as a centralized, online system.

2.2.5 Participant Data Management

Because of security and resource constraints, participants' case report forms (CRFs) could not be well-protected in secure, controlled-access premises as is standard procedure. In anticipation of potential security incidents at the ETC, only the CRFs for currently hospitalized patients were on site, with the others being better secured in other locations in the city. Due to the poor quality of the internet network, participant data were not directly entered into the database by the field teams but manually entered on paper CRFs. These were scanned daily, and the copies were sent to the PALM electronic platform. The data were then extracted from the scans and entered into the trial database by a team of data managers in Kinshasa.

2.3 Contribution of Quality Standard Care to the Success of the Trial

The rapid implementation of the trial at the Beni ETC (beginning the day authorization from the ethics committee arrived) and the high quality of the trial at this site—replicated subsequently at other sites—were due to several factors:

- By the time the trial began, the Beni ETC was routinely providing the optimal standard of care to EVD patients within the limits imposed by resources and circumstances.
- The Beni ETC staff was familiar with the standard operating procedures for the preparation and administration of investigational products thanks to experience with the WHO Monitored Emergency Use of Unregistered and Investigational Interventions (MEURI) protocol, which had provided for the administration of investigational products on compassionate grounds for several months before the PALM RCT began (Fallah and Skrip 2019; WHO 2020).
- ALIMA also had previous experience in the implementation of clinical trials, meeting Good Clinical Practice and protocol requirements similar to those of PALM during PREVAC and PREVAIL IV studies in Guinea (NIAID 2019). This background in clinical research on EVD meant ALIMA could provide staff who were already experienced in clinical research, facilitating the prompt launch of the PALM trial.

2.4 Contribution of Research to Improving Patient Care

The implementation of research and the provision of standard care to patients by the same clinical teams at the same sites at the same time made it possible to pool resources and reduce costs. For example, the daily patient assessments for the trial also provided the information needed for clinical care. Having both clinical and research staff performing the assessments lightened the burden on both. Treatment administration, case analyses of deceased patients, death or discharge reporting, etc., used similar data and common patient input shared by research and clinical care staff. In addition, and concurrently, the implementation team's daily psychological assessment and supportive psychotherapy for the benefit of patients and their caregivers greatly contributed to patients' compliance with treatment regimens.

The research project contributed to an improved standard of care for patients in many ways. Since the patients with EVD at the sites where the study was implemented were participants in the PALM trial, there was better monitoring and management of standard care. One might call it dual monitoring: once for the PALM Trial and once for the clinician. Even though the data from a single assessment were used for both purposes, the regular updates required by the trial helped the clinical care teams to better adapt therapeutic measures to patients.

- The PALM safety team was directly involved in the real-time management of serious adverse events (SAE) in patients, and management of SAEs was integrated into overall patient management. Input from the PALM safety team was an added benefit for most of the patients concerned since most reported SAEs were attributed to the patients' disease and not to investigational products (▶ Chap. 36).

- The PALM coordination team included study coordinators, clinical research assistants, and a medical advisor at ALIMA headquarters, all of whom were clinicians experienced in the management of EVD. Their regular participation in medical meetings discussing how to adapt medical measures given to each patient contributed to better patient management.
- Each death of a participant was reported as soon as possible in the CRFs. Death reports were analyzed in detail by the PALM pharmacovigilance team research coordinators and the medical specialist working on the trial at ALIMA headquarters. Once again, this meant more input from qualified personnel with different perspectives, leading to better-informed recommendations for the management of patients to reduce morbidity and mortality.

Continuous training for better patient care. The PALM coordination team participated in the ongoing training of medical care staff through formative supervision (clinical research assistants, study coordinators, medical research advisors at ALIMA headquarters) and more formal training, with illustrated presentations, in various areas of quality and patient care (trial coordinators and director). Together with the daily discussions between research and care teams on specific patients, this has helped improve the technical skills and capacities of staff, thus providing a better standard of care for patients.

3 Recommendations and Conclusions

Proper assessment of surrounding conflict and the prevalence of mistrust in the community requires working with local partners and staff to establish the best possible collaboration between local health institutions and other local government units on the one hand, and local communities, traditional and religious leaders, youth, and other groups on the other. It is essential to convince people with possible EVD symptoms to seek treatment early; the earlier in the course of the infection they get care, the better their chances of survival. It is also essential to take an open, flexible approach to community and professional communications and partnerships. Allowing all stakeholders to be heard and to contribute as far as possible to patient care and research projects builds trust in the surrounding environment and can provide essential elements of patient support.

Whenever possible, integrate research management and standard patient care with the reciprocal sharing of workloads. The patient care team must have clinical research skills and researchers need culturally appropriate patient care skills. Establish an environment where each team learns from the other. Pool technical resources for patient care and research: establish joint teams working on the administration of standard care, meeting patients' needs, and ensuring proper implementation of clinical study protocols.

Support mutual and reciprocal capacity building between partners in both research and patient care response. Clinicians and researchers can learn much from each other, as can partners from developed and developing countries. Mutual respect and assistance are ethical imperatives that are also practical necessities for acceptance by communities to meet MoH training and education objectives, to ameliorate the frequent shortages of qualified medical personnel in acute health crises, and to assist developed-country researchers and clinicians in coping with the exigencies of resource-constrained environments.

Discussion Questions

1. Could the drugs in a trial worsen the clinical condition of an unstable patient?
2. How does one obtain informed consent from a patient in critical condition?

3. How can one gain community support, especially when there is time pressure and the area is riven by conflict?
4. How does research contribute to patient care improvement?
5. How does standard-of-care medical treatment contribute to the success of clinical trials?

References

ALIMA. Alliance for International Medical Action. Dakar, Senegal: Alliance for International Medical Action. 2022. https://alima.ngo/en/home/. Accessed 11 Aug 2022.

Aruna A, Mbala P, Minikulu L, Mukadi D, Bulemfu D, Edidi F, et al. Ebola virus disease outbreak—Democratic Republic of the Congo, August 2018-November 2019. MMWR Suppl. 2019;68(50):1162–5. https://doi.org/10.15585/mmwr.mm6850a3.

Ellenberg SS, Keusch GT, Babiker AG, Edwards KM, Lewis RJ, Lundgren JD, et al. Rigorous clinical trial design in public health emergencies is essential. Clin Infect Dis. 2018;66(9):1467–9. https://doi.org/10.1093/cid/cix1032.

Fallah MP, Skrip LA. Ebola therapies: an unconventionally calculated risk. Lancet. 2019;393(10174):850–2. https://doi.org/10.1016/s0140-6736(19)30160-6.

Farrar J. It isn't crazy to conduct an Ebola clinical trial in a war zone—it's necessary. Stat; 2018.

FDA. FDA approves first treatment for Ebola virus. Washington, DC: U.S. Food and Drug Administration; 2020a.

FDA. FDA approves treatment for Ebola virus. Washington, DC: U.S. Food and Drug Administration; 2020b.

Global Witness. "Faced with a gun, what can you do?" war and the militarisation of mining in eastern Congo. London: Global Witness; 2009.

ICH. Good clinical practice: ICH harmonised guideline. Integrated addendum to ICH E6(R1): guideline for good clinical practice ICH E6(R2) ICH consensus guideline. Geneva: International Council for Harmonisation of Technical Requirements for Pharmaceuticals for Human Use (ICH); 2016.

Jacob ST, Crozier I, Fischer WA 2nd, Hewlett A, Kraft CS, Vega MA, et al. Ebola virus disease. Nat Rev Dis Primers. 2020;6(1):13. https://doi.org/10.1038/s41572-020-0147-3.

Mueller ED, Rebmann T. Analyzing targeted violence against medical workers and EVD incidence in the 2018-19 Democratic Republic of the Congo outbreak using vector autoregression and granger causality. Health Security. 2019;17(6):477–84. https://doi.org/10.1089/hs.2019.0087.

Mulangu S, Dodd LE, Davey RT Jr, Tshiani Mbaya O, Proschan M, Mukadi D, et al. A randomized, controlled trial of Ebola virus disease therapeutics. N Engl J Med. 2019;381(24):2293–303. https://doi.org/10.1056/NEJMoa1910993.

NASEM. Integrating clinical research into epidemic response: the Ebola experience. National Academies of sciences engineering and medicine publications. Washington, DC: The National Academies Press; 2017.

Nguyen V-K. An epidemic of suspicion—Ebola and violence in the DRC. N Engl J Med. 2019;380:1298. https://doi.org/10.1056/NEJMp1902682.

NIAID. Researching Ebola in Africa: the Partnership for Research on Ebola virus in Liberia (PREVAIL). Bethesda, MD: National Institute of Allergy and Infecious Diseases; 2019. https://www.niaid.nih.gov/diseases-conditions/researching-ebola-africa. Accessed 26 Feb 2020.

Prevail II Writing Group. A randomized, controlled trial of ZMapp for Ebola virus infection. N Engl J Med. 2016;375(15):1448–56. https://doi.org/10.1056/NEJMoa1604330.

Stearns J. North Kivu: the background to conflict in north Kivu province of eastern Congo. Usalama Project. London: Rift Valley Institute; 2012.

Tshiani Mbaya O, Mukumbayi P, Mulangu S. Review: insights on current fda-approved monoclonal antibodies against ebola virus infection. Front Immunol. 2021;12:721328. https://doi.org/10.3389/fimmu.2021.721328.

UNAIDS/AVAC. Good participatory practice: guidelines for biomedical HIV prevention trials. Geneva: UNAIDS (Joint United Nations Programme on HIV/AIDS); 2011.

WHO. Ebola—African Region (AFRO), Democratic Republic of the Congo. Disease Outbreak News; 2020.

Wolf J, Jannat R, Dubey S, Troth S, Onorato MT, Coller B-A, et al. Development of pandemic vaccines: ERVEBO case study. Vaccines (Basel). 2021;9(3):190. https://doi.org/10.3390/vaccines9030190.

18 Good Participatory Practice: Social Mobilization, Communications, and Community Engagement

Robert A. Sorenson, Yvette Delph, Bartholomew Wilson, Mosoka P. Fallah, and Elizabeth S. Higgs

Contents

Learning Track Note: This chapter appears in Learning Tracks: Clinical Research; Emergency Research Response, Research Operations; Global Health; Preparedness; Public Health & Epidemiology; Research Ethics; Social Science, Response Research

E. S. Higgs and R. A. Sorenson (eds.), *Principles and Practice of Emergency Research Response*,
https://doi.org/10.1007/978-3-031-48408-7_25

Trust is crucial to the medical research enterprise. Absence of trust in research and researchers … can disrupt and delay the conduct of studies. Of greater consequence in a pandemic, it can have a negative effect on the public acceptability and, hence, the uptake of research results, including the new treatments and vaccines needed to respond effectively to novel pathogens. Lack of trust, in other words, risks undermining the fundamental rationale for undertaking research in the first place.
(Wilson et al. 2021)

Learning Objectives

Readers should understand and be able to discuss:

- Good participatory practice (GPP) or social mobilization, communication, and community engagement (SMC)
- Why active stakeholder engagement *must* be part of an emergency research response; possible consequences resulting from lack of trust in medical research
- Integration of GPP into the study life cycle
- How to identify research stakeholders and thereby help ensure that communities are adequately reached by GPP/SMC efforts
- Critical requirements for laying the groundwork for GPP during an emergency research response
- Fundamental elements of clinical research that partners in research and community members need to understand to be informed and participate in dialogue; the utility of a regularly updated list of frequently asked questions
- Development of a plan (roadmap) for ongoing engagement through the course of the trial as dialogue with stakeholders continues
- Successful implementation of GPP in Liberia during the 2014–2016 Ebola outbreak
- The principles that a research response program must implement during preparedness and emergencies

1 Introduction

The primary goals of clinical research during a health emergency are to advance medical countermeasures (MCMs) for use by physicians and communities to reduce morbidity and mortality and accelerate the end of an outbreak, epidemic, or pandemic. An underlying requirement for use of MCMs is doctor and patient confidence that they are safe and effective and that benefits outweigh risks for individual and community use. A broad view of research, as spanning the progress of medical countermeasures (MCMs) from the laboratory to use in the population or "lab to jab" for vaccines, elucidates why *public trust in the research process is indispensable*. Widespread vaccine hesitancy during the coronavirus disease 2019 (COVID-19) pandemic often reflected poor understanding or misinformation about the research that produced vaccines and therapeutics for the disease. Trust can be engendered by reaching out to all stakeholders, that is, those who are affected by the research or who can impact the research, and including them in the research program from beginning to end. This kind of engagement is known by different names in different places, but its core is respectful dialogue with stakeholders. In much of the world, the best-known term is good participatory practice (GPP), while in sub-Saharan Africa, it is often referred to as social mobilization, communication, and community engagement (SMC); another widely used term is risk communication and community engagement (RCCE).

Historically, community engagement has become a clinical research priority only recently, most clearly since the emergence of HIV/AIDS in the 1980s, with the first publication of GPP guidelines as such coming only in 2007. Paternalistic, "doctor knows best" attitudes in research date back much further, as does the colonial legacy of the metropole providing and the colonized passively receiving. It is hardly surprising, then, that clinical research may be perceived as exploitation and as contrary to local custom and ethical norms. Involving the community in the design and conduct of clinical research, as well as in the development of public health interventions and policies, reflects an understanding that such activities have inherent risks and benefits that affect more than just individuals. Individual liberty and survival in some situations, such as the 2014–2016 West Africa

Ebola outbreak, rely heavily on the interdependent and overlapping communities to which all humans belong.

While GPP/SMC should be part of all clinical research efforts, active engagement with stakeholders *must* be part of an emergency research response. When populations are under stress from an emerging infectious disease and its disruptive social consequences, their active participation and understanding of the research purpose, goals, and process and their confidence in research integrity, ethics, and oversight become pragmatic as well as normative requirements. Without community backing, a research program may not be feasible, and if the research identifies an MCM as safe and efficacious but it is not used for lack of confidence, it does little good.

Ideally, engagement with stakeholders precedes an emergency, but researchers do not choose the sites of infectious disease outbreaks and cannot prepare everywhere. Furthermore, GPP must be tailored to context. On one hand, this means the pathogen causing the outbreak, the dynamics of the outbreak, and the type of clinical study. On the other hand, it requires understanding the communities, languages, and cultures of trial participants, as well as the scientific and medical response practitioners in the area. It means understanding factors like income level, degree of access to healthcare, the security of the communities, and their attitudes toward their government. Effective GPP implementation strengthens communities and contributes to healthcare and research capacity. To illustrate these themes, this chapter explores some common patterns evident in different times and places, such as the public reactions to the 2014–2016 Ebola outbreak in West Africa and the COVID-19 epidemic.

GPP is both an ethical requirement and a pragmatic one. It must be a funded trial budget item from the start. Constructive stakeholder engagement is indispensable to ethical and scientific quality of research, acceptance of the data generated by rigorous research for decision making on MCMs, acceptability of the research to stakeholders, and ultimately public confidence in MCMs. Lack of trust in medical research can lead to:

- Reluctance to enroll in clinical trials
- Fertile ground for rumors and misinformation
- Physical violence directed against researchers, medical personnel, and treatment facilities
- Poor adherence to study protocols by participants
- Lack of confidence in vaccines and therapeutics
- Low compliance with public health measures
- Acceptance of ineffective "alternative" remedies
- Refusal to cooperate with health workers, e.g., in contact tracing
- Prolonging an epidemic due to noncompliance with public health measures and rejection of MCMs
- Greater morbidity and mortality

2 Integration of GPP into the Study Life Cycle

> *Communities of people affected by research should … play an active, informed role in all aspects of its planning and conduct, as well as the dissemination of results.* (UNAIDS and WHO 2012)

2.1 Before the Study

Ideally, there would be clinical research sites distributed around the world in proportion to need, conducting clinical research that would help communities where they operate and contribute to preparedness for potential pandemics. Ongoing clinical research would include GPP as a matter of course. In fact, clinical research tends to be concentrated in developed countries and investigates candidate medical countermeasures primarily intended for use in developed countries, and GPP or equivalent guidelines have yet to become a standard feature of all clinical trials (Wicks et al. 2018).

For emergency clinical research, GPP is indispensable and needs to be fully incorporated from beginning to end. GPP needs to be integrated into template or prototype research protocols drafted between emergencies, in readiness to be adapted when the need arises; requests for proposals and other grant funding mechanisms; preparedness planning and budgets drafted in advance for emergency response; and the mindset of every clinical research scientist.

2.2 Emergency Engagement

Assuming an outbreak requiring an emergency research response has occurred in a place without an existing research program, the steps outlined in ◘ Fig. 1 indicate the necessary sequence of actions. As soon as a research partnership with the affected country or jurisdiction is formed (▶ Chaps. 3, 17, and 32), partners from the locus of the outbreak need to bring their knowledge to the table to inform planning for GPP. Partners, in this case, must include not only scientists from the capital city of the affected country but medical practitioners and community leaders from the area of the outbreak.

Existing plans for emergency response in every country should include plans for GPP as part of preparedness. If not, the country's incident management system (IMS) or equivalent is often the best place to begin. Most African IMS systems include SMC (also known as risk communication and community engagement, or RCCE) pillars into the IMS plans. If community stakeholders have not already been consulted and identified, this needs to begin early in the outbreak response, so they can participate in the process and advise on immediate outreach to the community as study plans are taking shape. In a large, low-income country like the Democratic Republic of the Congo (DRC), where emergency clinical research has been conducted, the chances that previous clinical research efforts have been made in the outbreak area are low. Nevertheless, GPP should be treated as a clinical research requirement in such cases, one just as essential to clinical trial success as a sound study design. Review boards should ensure research proposals include a commitment to GPP and a description of how it will proceed and that GPP is incorporated into the trial protocol, manual of operations, and standard operating procedures (SOPs) (Baron et al. 2018). According to the widely accepted guidelines of the Council for International Organisations of Medical Sciences:

> The research protocol or other documents submitted to the research ethics committee should include a description of the plan for community engagement, and identify resources allocated for the proposed activities. This documentation must specify what has been and will be done, when and by whom, to ensure that the community is clearly defined and can be proactively engaged throughout the research to ensure that it is relevant to the community and is accepted. The community should participate, when feasible, in the actual discussion and preparation of the research protocol and documents. (CIOMS 2016)

Clinical research sites should be selected carefully in partnership with local experts and outreach to ensure the community will not oppose the research (▶ Chap. 40). Trials should also be harmonized with local response and research plans (Baron et al. 2018), and they may take place in treatment facilities run by local authorities or by humanitarian medical non-governmental organizations (NGOs) like Médecins Sans Frontières (MSF) or International Medical Corps (IMC) (▶ In Practice 17.1). As the research team begins the dialogue with the community in a new location, initial knowledge will need to be obtained on social and cultural dynamics through social science research (▶ Chap. 26), including social analytics to track community sentiment in near real time (▶ In Practice 18.2). As a site continues operating, a locally hired GPP team is essential for conveying information to the community about a disease emergency and the research program being planned and implemented in response, as well as for information on the climate of opinion in the community and providing feedback to the research team (WHO 2016) (▶ Chap. 42).

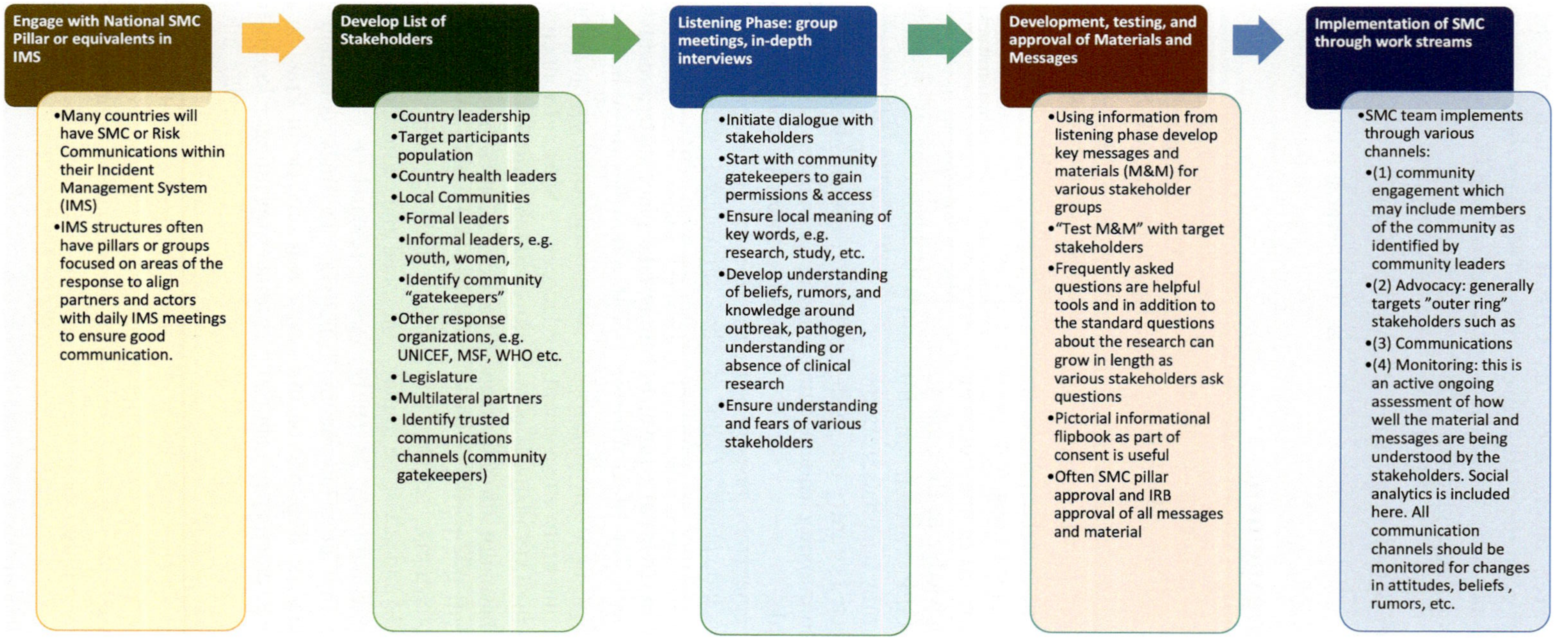

Fig. 1 A simplified road map for conducting social mobilization, communications, and community outreach, including many of the essential requirements for reaching and listening to communities. (Elizabeth S. Higgs)

3 Identifying Stakeholders

In the broadest sense, stakeholders include all individuals, groups, organizations, or governments at local, national, and international levels who are affected by or can influence the clinical research. SMC should include all the stakeholders, but the most important are the trial participants and their communities, as shown in Fig. 1 and as reflected in the CIOMS guidelines as well as more GPP specific guidance (AVAC 2012; CIOMS 2016; WHO 2016). This does not mean stakeholders more distal from the participants and their communities should be ignored (Fig. 2). Quite the contrary, all actors in the health emergency need to understand the need for GPP, corresponding implementation plans, and its potential impact on research. Therefore, when a SMC road map (Fig. 1) is developed, it must start with identifying all those with whom dialogue about the research is necessary.

There is a rich literature and many guideline documents on protecting human research participants and obligatory ethics reviews focused on *individual* protections for trial participants (▶ In Practice 4.2 and Chap. 33). But clinical trial protocols must also protect trial participants as people living in *communities*, and this has been a less central concern in Western (Northern) research ethics until recently (Brown et al. 2020; Folayan et al. 2021). "Communities" must be understood not only in the narrow sense of a neighborhood where people live but as all the social groups to which people belong and which shape their identities. This includes groups defined by gender, ethnicity, religion, profession, income, and other categories. Marginalized people may be least represented in community forums but most affected by disease. Women, usually the largest population group, are key stakeholders, in part because they are generally the primary caregivers in families and vital voices for themselves and for children, adolescents, and the elderly (WHO 2016); however, women are sometimes discouraged from participating in public life. In some communities, it may be difficult to hold direct, open discussions with those who are disempowered by the social structure, such as women or certain ethnic groups, and researchers must take special care to reach disempowered and vulnerable people for appropriate dialogue. Stakeholders thus include potential trial participants, their families, their communities, and others who could be affected or benefited by trial results; other stakeholders are health practitioners, service providers, political and informal leaders, and those whom the leaders may tend to ignore or dismiss.

Stakeholder identification may begin with reaching out to respected community members. Without support from community lead-

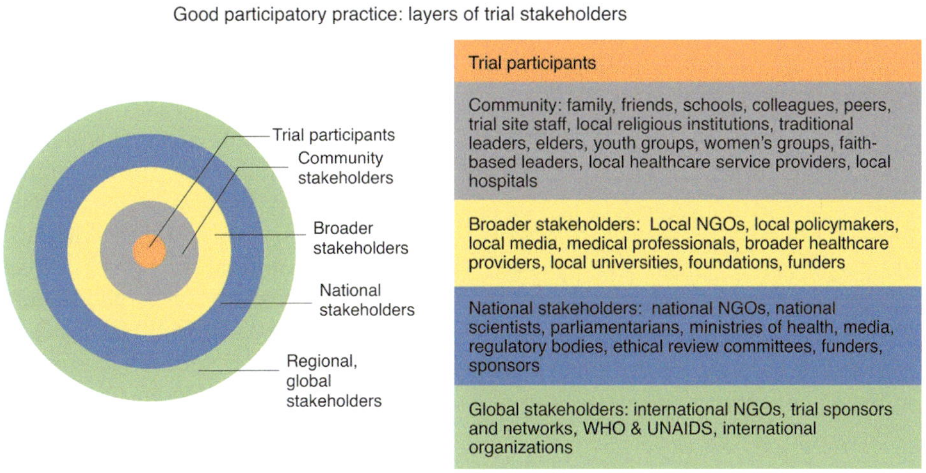

Fig. 2 GPP-EP stakeholders. (Wilson et al. 2021) (Bartholomew Wilson and Elizabeth S. Higgs)

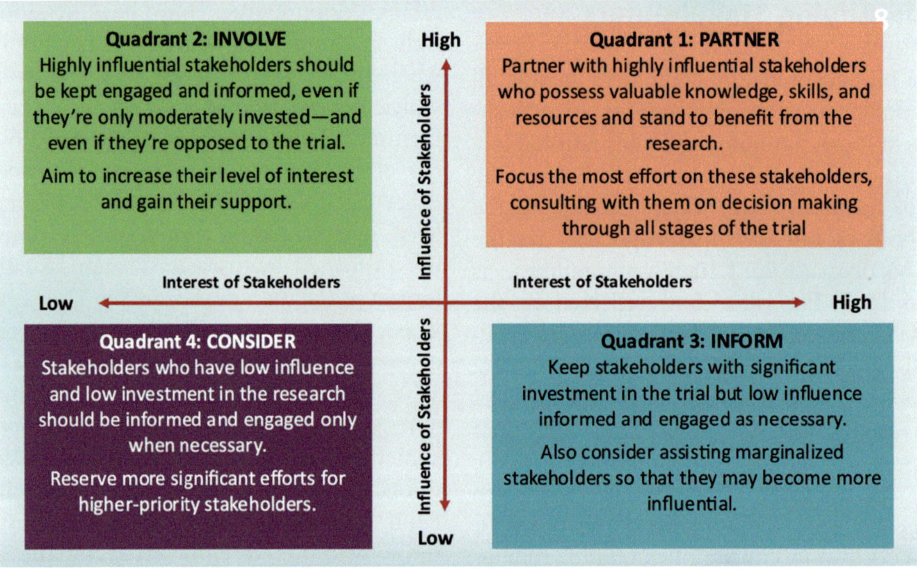

Fig. 3 Categorizing stakeholders by their levels of influence and engagement/interest in the research helps ensure that communities are adequately reached by GPP/SMC efforts. (AVAC 2014)

ers, the community engagement team is likely to encounter resistance (Chua et al. 2005; Cohen 2004, 2005; Ditmore 2005; Jintarkanon et al. 2005; Wilkinson et al. 2017). One of the major lessons from the 2014–2016 Ebola outbreak in West Africa was that the messenger sometimes mattered more than the message. People were more willing to follow advice and seek treatment if local leaders communicated recommendations (Svoboda 2022). By default, researchers may partner with the highest-ranking officials in a locality, but these may be the face of a mistrusted government rather than trusted leaders. As Lange noted in the aftermath of unimplemented human immunodeficiency virus (HIV) pre-exposure prophylaxis (PrEP) trials (Lange 2005) (Fig. 3):

> In clinical research, investigators may end up in situations in which they may have had an intense dialogue and come to an agreement with what they have identified to be the relevant community organizations, and yet a day later are put on the standby yet another activist group.

4 Laying the Groundwork

4.1 Outlines of Dialogue

Identifying and engaging with community members and other stakeholders is not a box to check but an ongoing, iterative process that continues as researchers learn about the community while members of the community, with trial participants at the forefront, learn to know the researchers and to understand the research. There is nothing inherently complex in this process, except in cases of severe local tensions in or among communities (Fig. 4).

A basic principle of GPP is bidirectional communication, mutual respect, and reciprocity. Reciprocity implies a partnership that ensures all partners work together to reach meaningful solutions to concerns that may hinder research or harm the community. Listening is a first step in the dialogue process. This may require additional training and ongoing conversation to ensure that all part-

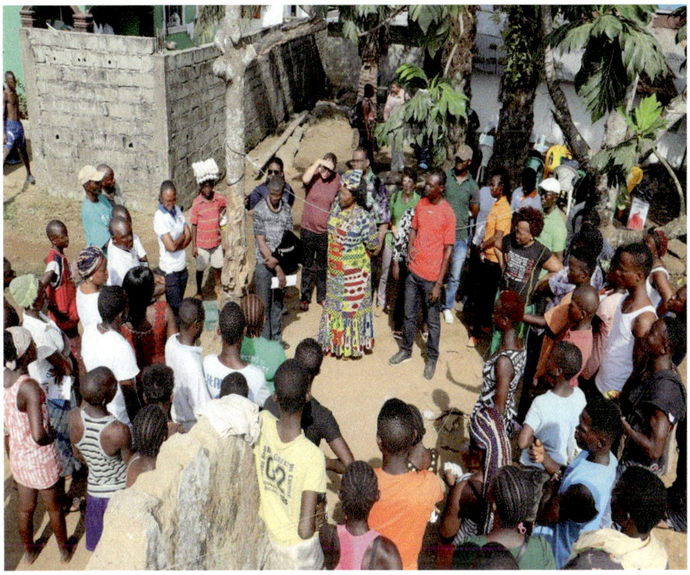

Fig. 4 Informal community gathering to discuss clinical trials in Liberia (faces blurred to protect privacy). (Photo: Laura McNay)

ners understand, to take one example, that a randomized trial cannot provide the most promising experimental intervention to all participants (▶ In Practice 4.1). Local partners, community leaders and members, and anthropologists can provide essential knowledge and methods to strengthen dialogue and improve emergency response (▶ Chap. 26). Effective partnerships recognize and integrate the expertise and experience of all partners, identifying roles and responsibilities for each partner throughout the research process and identifying opportunities for ongoing collaboration. Continued community engagement is critical for building the reputation of the research program as a trustworthy partner mindful of community needs; continued engagement signals long-term commitment to the health of the community (▶ Chap. 5).

Clinical research teams rely on partners to communicate honestly and authentically with each other, with communities and potential participants, and to judiciously work with people trusted by communities to answer questions about candidate MCM safety and side effects, equitable inclusion in clinical trials, product development, and post-trial access to any resulting MCMs. Community leaders who serve as guardians and gatekeepers must often be approached first to gain their cooperation in engaging the communities. In many places where community belonging has high social importance, it would be seen as morally unacceptable for an individual to participate in clinical research in which the community is not also a partner. Bringing organizations and community leaders together to co-coordinate and co-host educational sessions and other community activities strengthens partnerships.

4.2 Commitment to GPP

GPP staff cannot work effectively without involving principal investigators (PIs) and other senior research team members. PIs and clinicians should personally communicate with the community to debunk myths, clarify study procedures, and discuss concerns (Baron et al. 2018). They need to demonstrate that GPP is central to the research effort and join in pre-trial outreach to reduce misinformation, rather than react to rumors (Singh and Mills 2005). The whole research team, in other words, must work continually to build trust and share information with communities. They must listen to community concerns, input, and feedback, translate science into lay language, and disseminate science through appropriate community channels by working with community media and local community influencers. GPP is not something that can be put in the hands of community outreach (SMC) teams and forgotten. When they are heard by senior leadership, effective community engagement teams become advocates for both the study population and the goals of the research.

As they plan their outreach to the community, research teams need to tailor their approach to:

- The type of study being planned or implemented
- The characteristics of the outbreak emergency
- National and local societal and cultural norms
- Needs of impacted populations, especially marginalized groups
- National and local media landscapes
- Pertinent legislation

Since stakeholders' perspectives, the conduct of the trial (especially those with an adaptive design), and the course of the outbreak may all change, dialogue must be flexible and continual (WHO 2016). Adequate funding must be allocated to GPP from the start. GPP should not be limited to traditional recruitment, retention, community advisory board (CAB) meetings, and dissemination of study results. Social and other media campaigns, focus groups, town halls, and other outreach for broad community engagement are needed (Baron et al. 2018).

As research teams develop their research questions and concepts, they must work with other responders to ensure that the research is aligned with the emergency response (◘ Fig. 1) (WHO 2016) and that all the other responders understand the research. In cooperation with national health systems, healthcare NGOs often play a central response role, and their treatment centers may be the best sites for clinical trials (▶ In Practice 17.1). Health emergency NGOs increasingly accept the need for research response in infectious disease emergencies and may themselves conduct research (Nuffield Council on Bioethics 2020) (▶ In Focus 30.1).

4.3 Community Advisory Mechanisms

While the most important requirements for meaningful dialogue are commitment, mutual respect, and honesty, research teams can use formal organizational approaches to facilitate meaningful community involvement and partnership.

4.3.1 Expert Panels

Expert Panels review protocols, offer guidance, seek to reduce trial participant burdens, and improve dialogue between research teams and study populations of interest. Expert panels typically include 10–12 scientists and community leaders who either represent the study population or have biomedical, social, or behavioral science expertise. Productive relationships among expert panelists are vital for establishing clinical research sites and engaging community leaders in the research.

4.3.2 Inclusion of Community Members on Protocol Teams

As clinical trial concepts and protocols are developed, research teams should provide for community representatives, such as community advisory board (CAB) members and locally hired site staff, to express their perspectives. Their input helps ensure that participants' burdens are reasonable, that appropriate compensation or mitigation is provided, and that informed consent materials are appropriate for the intended audience. For example, in some places COVID-19 studies used electronic diaries for tracking post-vaccination reactions, and community members identified the need for paper alternatives or for provision of appropriate devices to some study participants.

4.3.3 Community Advisory Structures

Community Working Groups should include experienced community educator staff members and community advisory board representatives from participating clinical research sites. Whether new or experienced, working groups should ensure that community involvement is integral to the research endeavor. Organized and led by research team members tasked with overseeing GPP/SMC, these groups facilitate community participation throughout the course of a research trial or program. They advise study protocol teams and sponsors on aspects of protocol development, adapt consent forms for local use, advise on community education needs, develop messages and study-related materials, inform strategies for recruitment and retention, and assist in monitoring emerging issues. It may be helpful to hold some community working group meetings without research team leadership so members can freely express their concerns.

Community Advisory Boards. The Division of AIDS (DAIDS) of the National Institute of Allergy and Infectious Diseases (NIAID) defines a CAB as "an active group of individuals representing the local population(s) impacted by or at risk of acquiring HIV. The organization and composition of each CAB (or similar groups using different names) should reflect local community representation, promote community engagement, and provide local perspective(s) on the implementation of the NIAID clinical research plan(s)." DAIDS expects that every clinical research site (CRS) will have a minimum of one CAB, while multiple CABs may be required to "...enable effective representation of the populations involved, for example, to represent geographically, culturally, or other distinct populations" (HHS 2019). These groups should meet regularly with the principal investigator and other members of the research team to build trusting relationships.

The central function of CABs is to represent the community of potential and enrolled participants and provide insight into what works best in their local culture and geography. Members provide input into the research agenda, review protocols and informed consent materials, serve as a focus group for development of new materials and messages, and advise on outreach and recruitment strategies, events, and locations. They participate in community forums to provide research updates and in street and community outreach activities but do not recruit trial participants. A well-functioning CAB can go back to the communities it represents, discuss important scientific issues, convey up-to-date information on the research, bring community concerns back to the investigators, and build trust and transparency between the research site and the community. In successful CABs, about 40% of members represent the research population. Diversity in age, gender, race, ethnicity, and professional expertise should reflect the makeup of the community.

4.3.4 Early Warning Mechanisms

Resilient partnerships require flexibility to adapt to evolving outbreak dynamics and withstand crises (Donnelly et al. 2021). Establishing early warning mechanisms (e.g., a community liaison officer, social analytics) to monitor and quickly identify areas of misunderstanding and disagreement helps prevent crises.

5 Frequently Asked Questions

To be truly informed and able to participate in dialogue, partners in research and community members need to understand the key elements of clinical research. While not every study has all elements, these include (Singh and Mills 2005):

- Randomization
- Placebos and control groups
- Standard of care
- Informed consent
- Safety and side effects
- Protection of research participants
- Use of data and samples
- Compensation for participation and for study-related injuries
- Post-trial benefits

Public forums, community group meetings, and other venues can provide useful avenues for identifying interests and areas of concern and building community understanding. Such meetings must be safe spaces where community members feel comfortable expressing views that challenge the status quo and powerful persons (Sayani et al. 2021). Critically, research teams must respond to issues identified and not engage with communities as mere tokenism

(Sayani et al. 2021). Teams should track commitments made to communities and provide periodic updates on research progress. Concerns expressed by the community should be addressed and resolved when possible. Developing a list of frequently asked questions and adding to it as additional questions are asked is a functional tool for dialogue with communities and stakeholders. Various stakeholders will require different types of information. While the community cannot be permitted to insist on changes that could threaten the scientific validity of the research, the research team should be sensitive to concerns and cultural norms of communities (CIOMS 2016) (◘ Fig. 5).

6 Drawing a Roadmap

As dialogue with stakeholders becomes an ongoing process, the next useful step is to draw a roadmap (◘ Fig. 1) or plan for ongoing engagement through the course of the trial. As the course of a clinical trial can change unpredictably, the map must always be subject to revision. A roadmap or stakeholder engagement plan should cover the trial life cycle and include (AVAC 2014; WHO 2016):

- A budget including costs for dedicated GPP staff and planned activities
- How to identify stakeholders
- Goals and objectives for engagement with stakeholders
- Plans for stakeholder meetings—how, where, and when
- Draft roles and responsibilities of stakeholders and research teams, to be revised in dialogue
- Anticipated differences of opinion or conflicts with suggestions for resolution
- A communications plan harmonized with corresponding plans with local partners, healthcare providers, and national outbreak response authorities

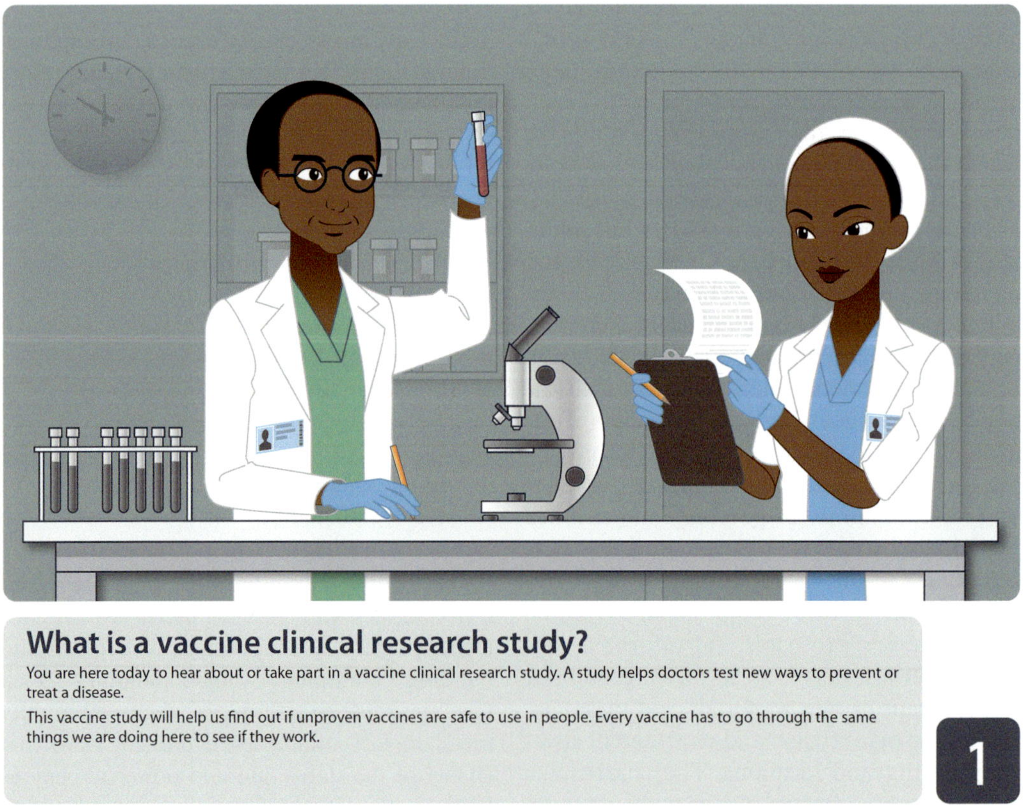

◘ **Fig. 5** Simplified but accurate illustrated information can be useful for community understanding, as well as for ensuring individual study participants can provide informed consent. (Credit: NIAID/NIH)

- Plans to track major issues and record discussions and resolution
- Methodology for strategy review and modification
- Monitoring and evaluation metrics

An SMC or GPP plan facilitates and organizes communications with stakeholders, describing
- Strategies to create supportive trial environments
- How to identify and resolve issues
- Strategies to convey accurate, understandable trial information to broad audiences
- How to coordinate communication between research teams and stakeholders
- How research teams intend to manage issues or adverse developments

Building community support depends on cultivation and maintenance of relationships and partnerships between research teams and the wider community. Pre-existing relationships between a community and a research program carrying out non-emergency research of value to the community provide opportunities to cement community relations (G7 2021; WHO 2022). In initial emergency response to an outbreak, however, researchers may not have had the chance to make such connections in advance. GPP is just as essential as ever—indeed more so. Work in partnership with trusted community organizations needs to begin immediately.

The research team and its public sector health and governance partners should forge relationships and partnerships with:
- Social service providers
- Advocacy organizations
- Community-based organizations
- Tribal leaders
- Community leaders
- Physician and medical professional associations
- Media and journalists
- Academic institutions
- Faith-based organizations
- Non-governmental organizations
- Organizations serving or representing marginalized communities

For example, outreach to essential worker organizations and corporations (such as nursing homes, assisted living facilities, and industry) was critical in COVID-19 prevention research efforts. Establishing partnerships opened important channels of communication and information dissemination, better enabling clinical trial sites to recruit study participants. Reaching beyond the health system to an array of community leaders and traditional structures in West Africa was essential to the research response during the 2014–2016 Ebola outbreak.

7 GPP in Liberia During the 2014–2016 Ebola Outbreak

The 2014–2016 outbreak in West Africa of Ebola, a disease not previously seen in that part of the world, disrupted the lives of West Africans for more than 18 months. Individual and community liberties were constrained by movement restrictions while the Ebola virus spread. Very little clinical research had been conducted in Liberia before the Ebola outbreak, and most people were "research naïve." As it began its work in October 2014, the Liberia-U.S. Partnership for Research on Ebola Vaccines in Liberia (PREVAIL) research team quickly identified community engagement as essential to the success of its planned Ebola vaccine trial, which was launched in February 2015 (Kennedy et al. 2016). The team developed and implemented a stakeholder engagement strategy for ongoing dialogue and information exchange. It built trust and a foundation for sustainable collaboration with community leaders and members who could influence or be affected by the study or its results. Instituting a genuine research partnership in accordance with GPP standards and SMC practice resulted in rapid enrollment and 98% compliance by trial participants with study requirements in the PREVAIL I Ebola Vaccine Trial (Doe-Anderson et al. 2016). Amid the fear and social disruption of a high-mortality public health emergency, rumors and misinformation seem to be much more transmissible among the human species than scientific knowledge with all its nuance and uncertainty.

In Liberia, the Ebola virus spread through the same networks that bind people most closely together. Liberian cultural norms stress hands-on, compassionate care for the ill and ceremonial care for their bodies if they die. The Ebola virus, generally transmitted through contact with bodily fluids, thus spread first within families and households via person-to-person transmission. Subsequently, transmission occurred among households (cluster transmission) and then from one cluster to another in community transmission (Skrip et al. 2017). These rapidly expanding rings of virus transmission stoked fear and many misconceptions among community dwellers. Fears escalated as misinformation spread through everyday conversations, promulgating disbelief in the epidemiology and myths about Ebola and exacerbating lack of trust in an already marginal healthcare system and political leaders. "Ebola" evoked horror movies in the minds of many Liberians. These beleaguering events resulted in social disruption, shuttered healthcare facilities, and the introduction of curfews and quarantine measures, among other consequences.

The Liberian government quickly became overwhelmed and recognized that it lacked the capacity to respond to a severe, sustained, and unprecedented public health crisis (WHO 2015). The government and its partners, including the World Health Organization (WHO), were overburdened with public health and medical demands complicated by cultural, geographic, and logistical challenges. These and other factors, including the behavior of the virus, created a volatile situation that evaded conventional control measures and constantly delivered surprises.

However, the courage, resilience, and commitment of communities in Liberia to combat this global health crisis gave birth to hope, the beginning of what turned out to be Liberia's success story. Communities became the bedrock of response. Community leaders set up response teams to conduct contact tracing, case investigation, and reporting. The community-based Ebola task force also instituted quarantine measures and provided food and water for those confined to their homes. The Ministry of Health, realizing the successes of these community-based efforts, decided to provide formal support to these informal response structures (Nyenswah et al. 2016). The Community-Based Initiative (CBI) program was established to support community volunteers. Today in Liberia, it is well documented that the success of the government and people in overcoming Ebola was not primarily a result of international support but of the resilience and commitment of community members to free their society from Ebola. As several experts have noted, when technical interventions cross purposes with entrenched cultural practices, control efforts must work within the culture, not against it (► Chap. 26).

The PREVAIL team developed and implemented a broad social mobilization and community engagement strategy comprising four distinct but integrated pillars: (1) advocacy, (2) community engagement, (3) communication, and (4) monitoring and evaluation. This strategy provided the platform to understand community concerns, culture, traditional values, and social norms and to gain community support for conducting research.

Advocacy. Advocacy engagements are held with local and national leaders, influencers, and gatekeepers to solicit political will and build trust and support for research among key decision makers. These engagements facilitate researchers' understanding of cultural diversity, social norms, and decision-making dynamics within communities. Advocacy engagements include informative interviews and focus group discussions with key influencers and meetings with leaders at all levels.

Community engagement includes outreach activities and meetings with study populations, community leaders, and members of the communities affected by the research. These activities support community awareness and understanding of clinical research and enlist community support for research participation. Community engagement activities address concerns about stigma, confidentiality, risk and benefit, and strengthen community ownership and sustainable partnerships.

Media engagement. Mass communication and engaging the media are very important for research, particularly in an emergency response, because of the ignorance and consequent gullibility that can characterize an unfamiliar situation. Media interactions allow researchers to build trust with local journalists, editors, on-air personnel, and commentators and to strengthen their knowledge of science and clinical research and their scientific reporting skills. Building research literacy among media institutions, journalists, and commentators is an effective way of preventing or countering rumors, negative propaganda, misconceptions, and conspiracy theories from inundating public perception.

Monitoring & evaluation (M&E) frameworks should be developed for the stakeholder engagement plan to document evolving beliefs; the impact of social mobilization on community awareness, rumors, and false beliefs; understanding of clinical research; community knowledge; attitudes and practices in epidemic response; and research participation. Stakeholders can use the monitoring and evaluation data to assess stakeholder engagement efforts and ensure GPP guidelines are in alignment with the goals of outbreak response. It is important to document the effectiveness of these engagement mechanism to better inform strategy for future programming and intervention.

Before Liberian communities were involved in PREVAIL, they tended to feel like objects of the research rather than partners in the process. This fueled distrust and misconceptions, which negatively impacted the process and, ultimately, the outcome of the research. Building trust with potential study participants, community members, leaders, and other stakeholders is not an event; it is a process that requires extensive dialogue, transparency, and bidirectional communication in a coordinated and involving manner. The PREVAIL SMC strategies employed during the 2014–2016 Ebola outbreak are a landmark example of successful implementation of GPP during a public health emergency. Continuing engagement with the communities where research participants live shows respect for them, their culture, the traditions and norms that bind them together as a people, and the ethical principle of treating people as means and not merely as ends to another goal (Kant 1785). Investigators and funders sometimes see GPP as taking time that cannot be spared in an emergency and can be tempted to make GPP a peripheral rather than foundational requirement. On the contrary, community engagement accelerated the conduct of the PREVAIL I Ebola Vaccine Trials in Liberia during the 2014–2016 Ebola outbreak. Although community engagement does take time and resources, clinical research without community engagement is more than likely to be hindered by unanticipated stumbling blocks. In Liberia, community engagement played a cardinal role, first in the acceptance of an accelerated clinical research program in the community and then in the recruitment, retention, and overall response rate of study participants.

As we have noted, the PREVAIL I Ebola vaccine trial was conducted amid an epidemic. With public fear, misconceptions, and lack of trust in public officials and the healthcare delivery system, obtaining community acceptance of an Ebola vaccine clinical trial would have been a challenge for any investigator. Rumors about the vaccine trials as a means of infecting the local population with the Ebola virus had spread widely. Resentment of well-equipped health responders and research scientists stoked suspicion about their motives. Media published and broadcast misleading stories about vaccine trials, aggravating public fear and resistance. Nevertheless, the PREVAIL I study team achieved excellent study participant recruitment and retention rates, thanks to its well-planned community engagement strategies and to the hard work of team members who understood the social and cultural context because they were from the communities involved. Such integration between research program and community is a prerequisite for willing cooperation; respect for communities, their members, and their social norms; and protection of individual autonomy and well-being. What is more, it greatly improves the odds of successful trial implementation, sound research conclusions, and ultimate benefit to the community.

Box 1: An Example of Community Skepticism of Official Leadership

An example of community skepticism of official leadership occurred early in the COVID-19 pandemic. By September 2020, the Navajo Nation, the largest tribal nation in the United States, had reported nearly 10,000 confirmed COVID-19 cases and 530 deaths. The Office of the Navajo Nation President and the Vice President's Facebook page notified the Nation of its participation in the Pfizer-BioNTech COVID-19 vaccine trial, which had received expedited approval from the Navajo Nation Human Research Review Board. In more than 250 comments, many asked, "Why do this?" While others said, "No, thanks" (Walker 2020). Ten days later, the Navajo Nation hosted a video town hall. In *Indian Country Today*, a nonprofit news organization, Dr. Christine Ami criticized the Navajo leadership and the town hall (Ami 2020):

Our own Navajo Nation government is now joining those calls to just get over the deep past of dirty research conducted on Native lands. … Their adamant endorsement of this trial without demonstrating official community input, their clear avoidance of any discussion about their failures to enforce the current CDC guidelines, their focus on proselytizing instead of consulting with traditional medicine people, and their unwillingness to present and discuss at length on local levels the very real side effects of this trial—both biologically and culturally—demonstrate their complete disregard for the health and safety of our Navajo people in the quest for a questionable solution. …

Many Native Americans live in rural areas with limited Internet availability, making online events a poor choice for community inclusiveness. In looking at the public reaction in the Navajo case, Alec Calac et al. (2021) found that many people expressed suspicion, skepticism, and concerns about safety. The virtual town hall event left many community members dissatisfied.

8 Benefits of GPP

8.1 More Relevant and Better Designed Research

Stakeholder involvement in research design ensures that research is relevant to communities, trial procedures are culturally appropriate, and greater equity exists in the eligibility criteria for study participation and level and duration of ancillary care. This promotes long-term sustainability of research capacity.

8.1.1 Better Understanding of How to Interact with Surrounding Cultures

Effective community engagement helps funders, sponsors, and research teams better understand and appreciate local cultures, norms, and values. This includes concerns of marginalized populations, local priorities, and community practices that may facilitate or prevent epidemic spread. Transparent, mutually respectful stakeholder engagement minimizes misunderstandings and reduces chances for unnecessary conflict or controversy. Community representatives can suggest study procedure modifications to reduce friction and increase acceptance of the research; assure that public notices, educational materials, and consent forms are culturally appropriate; and advocate study participation.

8.1.2 Amelioration of Power Imbalances

Power imbalances between research teams, funders, and sponsors and communities where clinical trial participants live are common, often along global North-South lines.

Moreover, marginalized groups (e.g., sex workers, infected individuals, and certain ethnic, cultural, social, or religious groups) are often disempowered. Meaningful engagement, strengthened by social science, identifies such imbalances, avoids reinforcing them, empowers the vulnerable, and increases awareness of marginalized populations' needs.

8.1.3 Community Empowerment

An essential component of stakeholder engagement is improving stakeholder understanding of research. When communities are educated and informed, their input is sought and respected, strengthening trust and overcoming suspicions and misconceptions.

8.1.4 Reduction of Stigma and Risks

Community engagement can identify risks resulting from fear of the disease being studied (e.g., Ebola) and strategies to counter unfounded fears, promote scientifically sound precautions against infection, and prevent social ostracism of trial participants. For example, pregnant Ebola survivors were often turned away from hospitals in Liberia when they arrived for childbirth. The research team helped set up care centers able to take care of Ebola survivors. Fears of Ebola virus being reactivated peripartum and transmission to the infant or medical personnel during delivery or via breast milk to newborns led the PREVAIL research team to undertake a birth cohort study (Fallah et al. 2023). The results of this and other studies of Ebola survivors were funneled back to communities and helped allay fears and superstitions.

8.1.5 Understanding Community Perspectives

Community perspectives can help inform important research questions as well as pragmatic operational issues, such as helping researchers determine:

- The compensation research participants should receive for their time and expenses
- Standard of care (the level of care provided for all patients enrolled in the study)
- Ancillary care (medical care for conditions unrelated to the study)
- A well-designed informed consent process to ensure participants understand essential elements of research and the risks and benefits of their participation

Early, in-depth interviews with community members and the target population can help researchers understand what is important to the participants. This early feedback helps in the design, implementation, and reporting of study results.

8.1.6 Enhanced Recruitment and Study Conduct

Community partnership helps stakeholders anticipate problems and agree on solutions. Incorporating local views into research planning, building community capacity to understand the research and raise concerns, and ensuring that trial procedures and study outreach materials are culturally appropriate are essential components of GPP. These contributions improve recruitment, informed consent, adherence to protocol, participant retention, and data quality.

8.1.7 Greater Uptake of Study Results and Likelihood of Future Research

When research teams and their studies are trusted, the credibility of researchers and research results increase. Participants and communities in partnership with researchers are more likely to understand and accept trial results and incorporate them into healthcare practice. Capacity building in conjunction with clinical trials paves the way for future research.

Box 2: Mistrust of Research, Reluctance to Use Medical Countermeasures

The accelerated development, authorization, and approval of multiple vaccines, therapeutics, and diagnostics for COVID-19 soon after the pandemic began was a demonstration of the capabilities of modern medical science and technology. For a large minority of the population in many countries, though, it intensified or engendered mistrust, especially about vaccines. *Vaccine hesitancy* was listed by WHO as one of ten major threats to world health even before the apparent deterioration of global *vaccine confidence* during the COVID-19 pandemic (Eagan et al. 2023; WHO 2019). Vaccines were the subject of prominent and often vehement public and private discussion. Misinformation and disinformation ran neck and neck with accurate information. Uptake of COVID-19 vaccines was lower than expected in many countries, despite their well-demonstrated safety and efficacy in most cases.

What do "vaccine hesitancy" and "vaccine confidence" mean? The definitions suggested by a WHO Strategic Advisory Group of Experts in 2014 are a good starting point:

- *Vaccine confidence* is "trust in (1) the effectiveness and safety of vaccines; (2) the system that delivers them, including the reliability and competence of the health services and health professionals and (3) the motivations of the policy-makers who decide on the needed vaccines."
- *Vaccine hesitancy* "refers to delay in acceptance or refusal of vaccines despite availability of vaccination services. Vaccine hesitancy is complex and context specific, varying across time, place, and vaccines. It is influenced by factors such as complacency, convenience and confidence" (WHO 2014).

Vaccine hesitancy may be motivated by worries about vaccine efficacy, safety, and side effects, as well as convenience and cost, though most governments undertook extraordinary efforts to make access to COVID-19 vaccine easy and cost-free. Fear about safety and efficacy were often cited by those reluctant to be vaccinated against COVID-19, along with a belief that the assessment of the vaccines was rushed because of the health emergency. Many other misconceptions lay behind suspicions about the vaccines—that the severity of COVID-19 was exaggerated for financial gain or other nefarious ends, lack of long-term safety follow-up, or that countermeasures were meant to control or harm the population, by causing sterility, for example (Cascini et al. 2021). Underlying such concerns in many countries is increasing mistrust in authorities, from government officials to academics and healthcare practitioners (Jennings et al. 2021).

Whatever terms one uses (Dudley et al. 2020), misconceptions that decrease uptake of safe and effective medical countermeasures defeat the purpose of emergency research response—to save lives, accelerate the end of the outbreak or pandemic, and develop measures to prevent and mitigate future outbreaks. The underlying causes of mistrust and unfounded beliefs are many and can be based on anything from individual disposition and subjective perceptions to economic and social insecurity. Skepticism about vaccines has led to outbreaks of measles in countries where it had been eliminated, hindered the eradication of polio, and led to many unnecessary deaths with COVID-19 around the world.

What does this have to do with clinical research and good participatory practice? As suggested above, concerns about safety, efficacy, and side effects of COVID-19 and other vaccines are often motivated by mistrust of the research that found them to be safe and effective. Was it hurried? Were corners cut? Were the researchers honest and motivated by people's best interests? Were they only interested in profits, or did they have other hidden motives?

Community outreach or GPP may seem a puny tool for influencing mass public opinion, but "retail" GPP has repeatedly proven effective with the communities involved and can provide a solid foundation for broader public understanding. Talking to people one knows who have direct experience as participants in clinical trials often carries more weight than secondhand reports. Public understanding would thus benefit from consistent implementation of GPP. In uncontroversial clinical trials in developed countries, GPP may be ignored or considered merely a recruitment tool. Public understanding of and appreciation for scientific research have dropped in recent years (Kennedy et al. 2022), and community outreach and other measures to promote a closer acquaintance between researchers and those who benefit every day from the work they do should help build trust between communities that otherwise seldom cross paths. GPP and similar outreach programs should help counter the mistrust that has led to countless preventable deaths from infectious diseases new and old.

9 Conclusion

GPP should be part of all clinical research, especially that conducted during epidemics and pandemics. Without community engagement, research teams jeopardize the successful completion of clinical trials. Without community support, there may be no trial participants, specimens, data, or acceptance of valid results. Response to public health emergencies will be inadequate without advance preparation. Clinical trials may still have to move rapidly in places where there has been no preparation. GPP is an indispensable element of emergency research response and can doom a trial to failure if neglected.

As global population and consumption grow, people increasingly encroach on wildlife habitats, climate change shifts the ranges of disease vectors and melts the permafrost to expose ancient pathogens, and intensifying meteorological disasters leave fertile environments for disease transmission in their wake, we cannot respond adequately to outbreaks without making the people affected partners in the research response (David et al. 2021; Lemieux et al. 2022; Morand and Walther 2020; Morens and Fauci 2020).

Discussion Questions

1. Define good participatory practice (GPP), also known as social mobilization, communication, and community engagement (SMC) and risk communication and community engagement (RCCE).
2. Discuss why active stakeholder engagement *must* be part of an emergency research response, and list possible consequences resulting from lack of trust in medical research.
3. Explain how GPP can be integrated into the study life cycle.
4. How are research stakeholders identified? Provide some examples of stakeholders.
5. When laying the groundwork for GPP during an emergency research response, the following factors are critical. Why?
   (a) Dialogue: bidirectional communication, mutual respect, and reciprocity
   (b) Genuine commitment to GPP
   (c) Community advisory mechanisms
6. What are the key elements of clinical research that research partners and community members need to understand for successful dialogue?
7. As dialogue with stakeholders is begun, a roadmap or plan for ongoing engagement through the course of the trial must follow. What needs to be included?
8. When planning for an emergency research response, a budget for GPP needs to be developed (as part of a funding plan/request). What needs to be included in the budget?
9. Summarize the implementation of GPP in Liberia during the 2014–2016 Ebola outbreak.

References

Ami C. Politics of distrust: the Navajo Nation's use of propaganda devices to recruit participants for COVID-19 trial vaccine. Indian Country Today. 2020.

AVAC. Presentation on good participatory practice (GPP) guidelines for biomedical HIV prevention trials 2011. 2nd ed. Geneva: AVAC, Global Advocacy for HIV Prevention; 2012.

AVAC. Good participatory practice tools: GPP blueprint for stakeholder engagement. New York: Global Advocacy for HIV Prevention (AVAC); 2014.

Baron D, Essien T, Pato S, Magongo M, Mbandazayo N, Scorgie F, et al. Collateral benefits: how the practical application of good participatory practice can strengthen HIV research in sub-Saharan Africa. J Int AIDS Soc. 2018;21(Suppl 7):e25175. https://doi.org/10.1002/jia2.25175.

Brown B, Taylor J, Dubé K, Kuzmanović D, Long Y, Marg L. Ethical reflections on the conduct of HIV research with community members: a case study. J Empir Res Hum Res Ethics. 2020;16(1–2):65–77. https://doi.org/10.1177/1556264620970802.

Calac AJ, Bardier C, Cai M, Mackey TK. Examining Facebook community reaction to a COVID-19 vaccine trial on the Navajo Nation. Am J Public Health. 2021;111(8):1428–30. https://doi.org/10.2105/AJPH.2021.306202.

Cascini F, Pantovic A, Al-Ajlouni Y, Failla G, Ricciardi W. Attitudes, acceptance and hesitancy among the general population worldwide to receive the COVID-19 vaccines and their contributing factors: a systematic review. EClinicalMedicine. 2021;40:101113. https://doi.org/10.1016/j.eclinm.2021.101113.

Chua A, Ford N, Wilson D, Cawthorne P. The tenofovir pre-exposure prophylaxis trial in Thailand: researchers should show more openness in their engagement with the community. PLoS Med. 2005;2(10):e346. https://doi.org/10.1371/journal.pmed.0020346.

CIOMS. International ethical guidelines for health-related research involving humans. Geneva: Council for International Organisations of Medical Sciences; 2016.

Cohen J. AIDS research. Cambodian leader throws novel prevention trial into limbo. Science. 2004;305(5687):1092. https://doi.org/10.1126/science.305.5687.1092a.

Cohen J. AIDS clinical trials. More woes for novel HIV prevention approach. Science. 2005;307(5716):1708. https://doi.org/10.1126/science.307.5716.1708a.

David PM, Le Dévédec N, Alary A. Pandemics in the age of the Anthropocene: is 'planetary health' the answer? Glob Public Health. 2021;16(8–9):1141–54. https://doi.org/10.1080/17441692.2021.1893372.

Ditmore M. Response to Joep M. A. Lange. PLoS Med. 2005;2(10):e347. https://doi.org/10.1371/journal.pmed.0020347.

Doe-Anderson J, Baseler B, Driscoll P, Johnson M, Lysander J, McNay L, et al. Beating the odds: successful establishment of a phase II/III clinical research trial in resource-poor Liberia during the largest-ever Ebola outbreak. Contemp Clin Trials Commun. 2016;4:68–73. https://doi.org/10.1016/j.conctc.2016.06.008.

Donnelly EK, Toof R, Silka L. Community based participatory research during the COVID-19 crisis: lessons for partnership resiliency. J High Educ Outreach Engagem. 2021;25(3).

Dudley MZ, Privor-Dumm L, Dube E, MacDonald NE. Words matter: vaccine hesitancy, vaccine demand, vaccine confidence, herd immunity and mandatory vaccination. Vaccine. 2020;38(4):709–11. https://doi.org/10.1016/j.vaccine.2019.11.056.

Eagan RL, Larson HJ, de Figueiredo A. Recent trends in vaccine coverage and confidence: a cause for concern. Hum Vaccin Immunother. 2023;19(2):2237374. https://doi.org/10.1080/21645515.2023.2237374.

Fallah MP, Reilly C, Van Ryn C, Badio M, Camanor SW, Kaler SG, et al. Pregnancy, pregnancy outcomes, and infant growth and development after recovery from Ebola virus disease in Liberia: an observational cohort study. Lancet Glob Health. 2023;11(7):e1053–e60. https://doi.org/10.1016/S2214-109X(23)00210-3.

Folayan MO, Brown B, Haire B, Babalola CP, Ndembi N. Considerations for stakeholder engagement and COVID-19 related clinical trials' conduct in sub-Saharan Africa. Dev World Bioeth. 2021;21(1):44–50. https://doi.org/10.1111/dewb.12283.

G7. In: HaS C, editor. G7 therapeutics and vaccines clinical trials charter. London: HMG Government (UK); 2021.

HHS. HIV:AIDS clinical trials units (UM1 clinical trial required). Washington, DC: HHS; 2019.

Jennings W, Stoker G, Bunting H, Valgarðsson VO, Gaskell J, Devine D, et al. Lack of trust, conspiracy beliefs, and social media use predict COVID-19 vaccine hesitancy. Vaccine. 2021;9(6):593. https://doi.org/10.3390/vaccines9060593.

Jintarkanon S, Nakapiew S, Tienudom N, Suwannawong P, Wilson D. Unethical clinical trials in Thailand: a community response. Lancet. 2005;365(9471):1617–8. https://doi.org/10.1016/s0140-6736(05)66501-4.

Kant I. Grundlegung zur Metaphysik der Sitten. 1st ed. Riga: Johann Friedrich Hartknoch; 1785.

Kennedy SB, Neaton JD, Lane HC, Kieh MWS, Massaquoi MBF, Touchette NA, et al. Implementation of an Ebola virus disease vaccine clinical trial during the Ebola epidemic in Liberia: design, procedures, and challenges. Clin Trials (London, England). 2016;13(1):49–56. https://doi.org/10.1177/1740774515621037.

Kennedy B, Tyson A, Funk C. Americans' trust in scientists, other groups declines. Pew Research Center; 2022.

Lange JM. We must not let protestors derail trials of pre-exposure prophylaxis for HIV. PLoS Med.

2005;2(9):e248. https://doi.org/10.1371/journal.pmed.0020248.
Lemieux A, Colby GA, Poulain AJ, Aris-Brosou S. Viral spillover risk increases with climate change in high Arctic lake sediments. Proc Biol Sci. 2022;289(1985):20221073. https://doi.org/10.1098/rspb.2022.1073.
Morand S, Walther BA. The accelerated infectious disease risk in the Anthropocene: more outbreaks and wider global spread. BioRxiv. 2020. https://doi.org/10.1101/2020.04.20.049866.
Morens DM, Fauci AS. Emerging pandemic diseases: how we got to COVID-19. Cell. 2020;182(5):1077–92. https://doi.org/10.1016/j.cell.2020.08.021.
Nuffield Council on Bioethics. Research in global health emergencies: ethical issues. Oxford, UK: Nuffield Council on Bioethics; 2020.
Nyenswah TG, Kateh F, Bawo L, Massaquoi M, Gbanyan M, Fallah M, et al. Ebola and its control in Liberia, 2014-2015. Emerg Infect Dis. 2016;22(2):169–77. https://doi.org/10.3201/eid2202.151456.
Sayani A, Maybee A, Manthorne J, Nicholson E, Bloch G, Parsons JA, et al. Building equitable patient partnerships during the COVID-19 pandemic: challenges and key considerations for research and policy. Healthcare Policy. 2021;17(1):17–24.
Singh JA, Mills EJ. The abandoned trials of pre-exposure prophylaxis for HIV: what went wrong? PLoS Med. 2005;2(9):e234. https://doi.org/10.1371/journal.pmed.0020234.
Skrip LA, Fallah MP, Gaffney SG, Yaari R, Yamin D, Huppert A, et al. Characterizing risk of Ebola transmission based on frequency and type of case–contact exposures. Philos Trans R Soc Lond Ser B Biol Sci. 2017;372(1721):20160301. https://doi.org/10.1098/rstb.2016.0301.
Svoboda E. Mastering the art of persuasion during a pandemic. Nature. 2022;610(7933):S34–s6. https://doi.org/10.1038/d41586-022-03354-8.
UNAIDS and WHO. Ethical considerations in biomedical HIV prevention trials: UNAIDS/WHO guidance document. Geneva: Joint United Nations Programme on HIV/AIDS (UNAIDS); 2012. p. 71.
Walker D. Navajo nation takes part in COVID vaccine study. Indian Country Today. 2020.
WHO. Report of the SAGE working group on vaccine hesitancy. Geneva: SAGE; 2014.
WHO. One year into the Ebola epidemic: a deadly, tenacious and unforgiving virus. Geneva: World Health Organization; 2015.
WHO. Good participatory practice guidelines for trials of emerging (and re-emerging) pathogens that are likely to cause severe outbreaks in the near future and for which few or no medical countermeasures exist (GPP-EP). Geneva: World Health Organization; 2016. p. 53.
WHO. Ten threats to global health in 2019. World Health Organization, Geneva. 2019. https://www.who.int/news-room/spotlight/ten-threats-to-global-health-in-2019. Accessed 18 Sept 2023.
WHO. Strengthening clinical trials to provide high-quality evidence on health interventions and to improve research quality and coordination. WHA 75.8. Geneva: World Health Organization; 2022.
Wicks P, Richards T, Denegri S, Godlee F. Patients' roles and rights in research. BMJ. 2018;362:k3193. https://doi.org/10.1136/bmj.k3193.
Wilkinson A, Parker M, Martineau F, Leach M. Engaging 'communities': anthropological insights from the west African Ebola epidemic. Philos Trans R Soc Lond Ser B Biol Sci. 2017;372(1721) https://doi.org/10.1098/rstb.2016.0305.
Wilson B, Wright K, Taylor R, Higgs E. Beyond recruitment: good participatory practice enhances the impact of research in a pandemic. Nat Med. 2021;27(3):369–71. https://doi.org/10.1038/s41591-021-01271-3.

18.1 In Practice: Building Community Engagement for Clinical Research Response

Michele Andrasik, Gail Broder, Linda Oseso, Patricia Segura, Kagisho Baepanye, Luciana Kamel, and Nelson Michael

Contents

Learning Track Note: This chapter appears in Learning Tracks: Clinical Research; Emergency Research Response, Research Operations; Preparedness; Public Health and Epidemiology; Research Ethics; Social Science Response Research

Supplementary Information The online version contains supplementary material available at https://doi.org/10.1007/978-3-031-48408-7_26.

E. S. Higgs and R. A. Sorenson (eds.), *Principles and Practice of Emergency Research Response*,
https://doi.org/10.1007/978-3-031-48408-7_26

Learning Objectives

This chapter will help readers understand and describe:

- How good participatory practice (GPP) provides a framework for community engagement by clinical research teams
- The process of building community support and some examples of working with devalued communities
- Approaches to community involvement and increasing scientific understanding in the community
- Avenues for conveying accurate knowledge and correcting misperceptions and misinformation
- Difficulties encountered when applying GPP in public health and the need for implementation science

1 Good Participatory Practice as a Framework

Community members are the heart of all clinical trials, particularly for prevention (including vaccine) research where healthy individuals will be enrolled. Community engagement is the process of respectfully and honestly sharing information and perspectives among community members, researchers, research sponsors, and other stakeholders to facilitate collaboration based on mutual trust with communities where clinical trials are implemented. Community engagement via good participatory practice (GPP) is a feature that continues throughout the lifecycle of a clinical trial, from concept generation through dissemination of results (▶ Chap. 18). It includes community education, study recruitment, and participant retention.

GPP guidelines were originally developed by UNAIDS and AVAC (Global Advocacy for HIV Prevention) (UNAIDS and AVAC 2011) to improve stakeholder engagement in biomedical HIV prevention trials, following community protests in several countries against planned trials about which they had not been well informed (Allman et al. 2014; Chua et al. 2005; Cohen 2005; Ditmore 2005; Duan 2005; Haire 2011; Lange 2005; Mills et al. 2005; Page-Shafer et al. 2005; Peterson and Folayan 2019; Singh and Mills 2005). "The GPP guidelines set global standard practices for stakeholder engagement. When applied during the entire lifecycle of a biomedical trial, they enhance both the quality and outcomes of research" (Broder et al. 2020). GPP guidelines have been foundational to developing global standards for engaging stakeholders in the design, conduct, and outcomes of clinical trials. Since their genesis, the concepts embodied in GPP have been further refined. Below are a few of many examples:

- *Good Participatory Practice Guidelines for Trials of Emerging (And Re-Emerging) Pathogens that Are Likely to Cause Severe Outbreaks in the Near Future and for which Few or No Medical Countermeasures Exist* (GPP-EP) (WHO 2016)
- *Good Participatory Practice for COVID-19 Clinical Trials: A Toolbox* (WHO 2020)
- *Research in Global Health Emergencies: Ethical Issues* (Nuffield Council on Bioethics 2020)
- *Good Participatory Practice Guidelines for TB Vaccine Research* (AERAS 2017)

2 Building and Maintaining Foundational Relationships

Building community support depends on the cultivation and maintenance of relationships and partnerships between the research team and the wider community, including, but not limited to:

- Social service providers
- Advocacy and community-based organizations
- Tribal leaders
- Medical professional associations and traditional healers
- Information media
- Academia
- Public sector health and governance partners
- Faith-based organizations
- Organizations that serve or represent communities that have been economically and socially marginalized
- Other non-governmental organizations (NGOs) and nontraditional partners

Working in partnership with community groups that have established relationships of trust with the community is invaluable, especially in communities with devalued identities, e.g., men who have sex with men, sex workers, racial and ethnic minorities, and transgender people. Partnerships must incorporate bidirectional communication and reciprocity, building capacity for all partners to work together. Anthropologists, local partners, and community leaders can provide essential knowledge, guidance, and direction to make partnerships work (▶ Chap. 26). Effective partnerships recognize and integrate the expertise and experience of all partners, identifying roles and responsibilities for each partner. Continued community engagement, even when a clinical trial site is not enrolling participants, helps build an institutional reputation of trustworthiness and concern for the needs of the communities being served. It also demonstrates that the research team is committed to the community's long-term health and is not merely engaged at times that benefit their own purposes.

Clinical research programs rely on such partnerships to communicate honestly and openly with communities and potential research participants. They can provide trusted individuals to answer questions and assuage concerns about safety and side effects, equitable inclusion in clinical trials, and product development. The principal investigator, along with the clinic staff, must work continually to build trust and share information, acting collaboratively with media and community leaders to do so. Listening to community concerns, input, and feedback, translating science into understandable and accurate terms, and disseminating information through appropriate community channels are all indispensable.

2.1 Real-World Examples

2.1.1 Rio de Janeiro, Brazil

In 2015, an art-focused program, known as *Transcrições* Art Project, was conceived to build bridges and foster relationships with transgender women (TGW) through art-related activities. The program was designed as a preparedness step for establishing a TGW referral center for healthcare and research at the Fiocruz clinical research site, a major public health research institution in Rio de Janeiro. The project supported art activities centered on the principles of self-respect, empowerment, and community building among transgender women. Activities included classes (e.g., Afro dance, acting, make-up), movie exhibitions, capacity building and advocacy workshops. A TGW leader and two highly skilled art educators who were paid members of the site's community engagement team conducted these activities. From its inception through 2019, over 700 TGW participated in workshops, museum tours, dramatic play attendance, and public presentations. During the COVID-19 pandemic, *Transcrições* moved to a virtual space, and weekly activities were organized through WhatsApp to maintain the connection between the TGW community and the research site. This was particularly important as the pandemic disproportionately impacted TGW across Brazil (◘ Fig. 1).

2.1.2 Buenos Aires, Argentina

For more than 20 years, the Balvanera clinical research site in Buenos Aires has focused on the care of people living with HIV. To enhance their community engagement, in October 2001 Balvanera established CePAD,[1] an HIV testing center providing confidential, anonymous, no-cost HIV testing, eliminating the need to go to a doctor's office for a test referral. CePAD helped cultivate a strong and enduring relationship with the local lesbian, gay, bisexual, transgender, queer, and/or questioning (LGBTQ+) community. In 2012, CEPAD expanded its services through a project focused on providing peer training to transgender community members. These efforts were further expanded in 2017 with the establishment of Clinsex, a sexual health clinic focused on preventing sexually trans-

1 Los Centros de Prevención, Asesoramiento y Diagnóstico (Centers for Prevention, Counseling, and Diagnosis). Website: ▶ https://buenosaires.gob.ar/salud/coordinacion-salud-sexual-vih-infecciones-de-transmision-sexual/test-de-vih-y-sifilis-y.

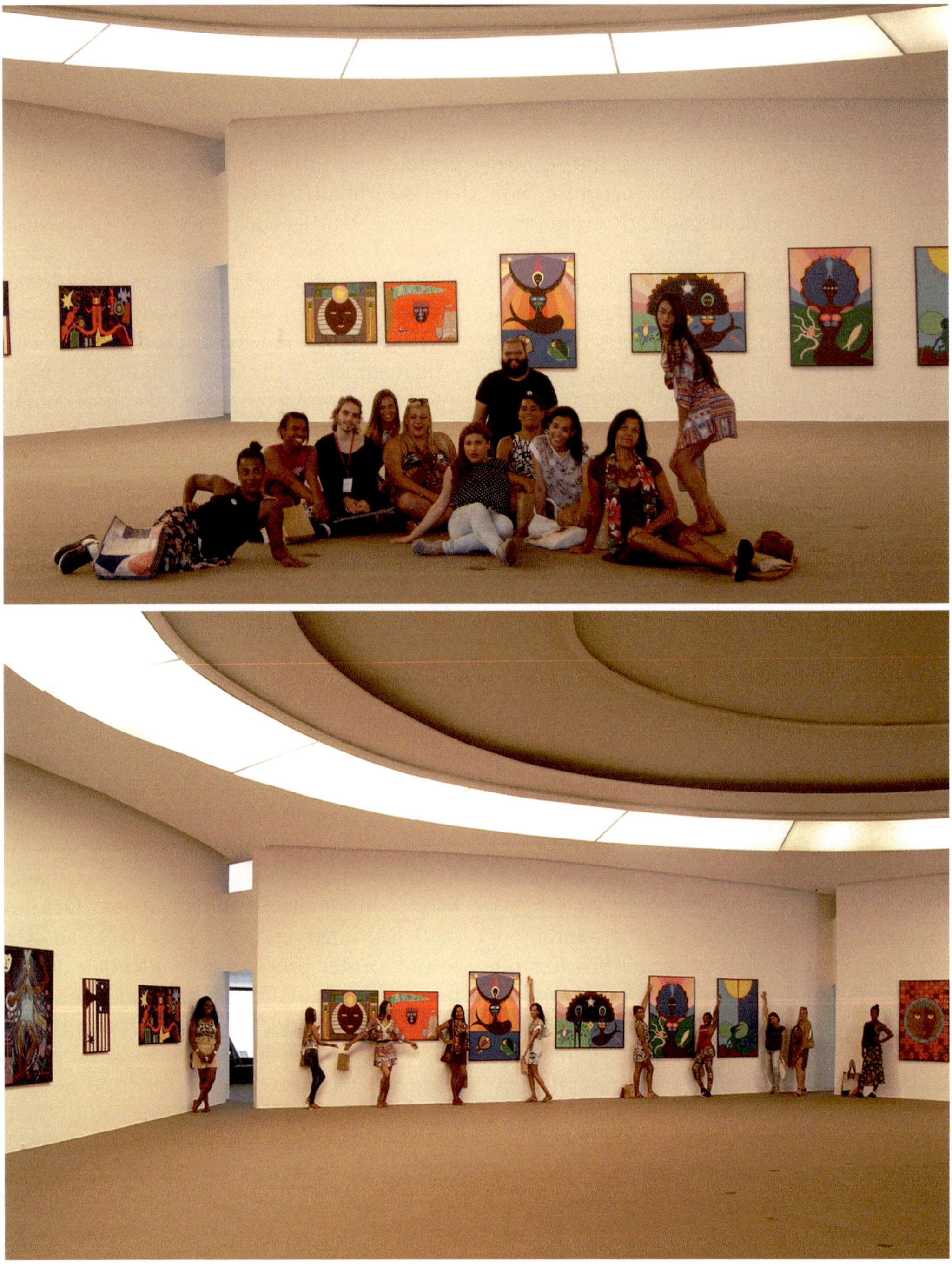

Fig. 1 Transcrições Art Project for fostering relationships with TGW in Rio de Janeiro, Brazil. (Courtesy Fred Hutch)

mitted infections by offering specialized, friendly, high-quality care. Clinsex facilitates access to safe sexual health services for people vulnerable to HIV, promoting the availability of preventive, diagnostic, and treatment tools. Clinsex has also conducted research aimed at responding to specific public health problems and facilitating training for health professionals to increase effective engagement with and care for vulnerable populations.

3 Meaningful Community Involvement Throughout the Research Process

> *Failure to properly and genuinely engage communities early in the stages of research planning may result in an inability to properly conduct and complete important trials. … Communities of people affected by research should … play an active, informed role in all aspects of its planning and conduct, as well as the dissemination of results.*
> (UNAIDS and WHO 2007)

Increasing community awareness and knowledge to address and correct misperceptions and misinformation requires using community-based participatory research (CBPR) approaches that involve the community meaningfully from the outset of any research program (Wallerstein et al. 2017). Communication with community members and leaders must use respectful language (e.g., older adult vs. elderly, priority vs. target populations, transgender vs. transgendered), inclusive identifiers (e.g., men who have sex with men *and* gay men), and materials that can be easily understood by priority populations (NIH 2023). Communities where various languages are spoken require special attention because preferred terms will vary, and some languages may not have words for specific scientific terms. Even among those fluent in Western languages like Portuguese, French, or English, speakers will have varying levels of scientific literacy, requiring additional efforts to ensure understanding of the biomedical product development process. Challenges can be addressed by developing appropriate outreach materials (◘ Fig. 2), creating meaningful and consistent metaphors for unfamiliar concepts, and using illustrated media.

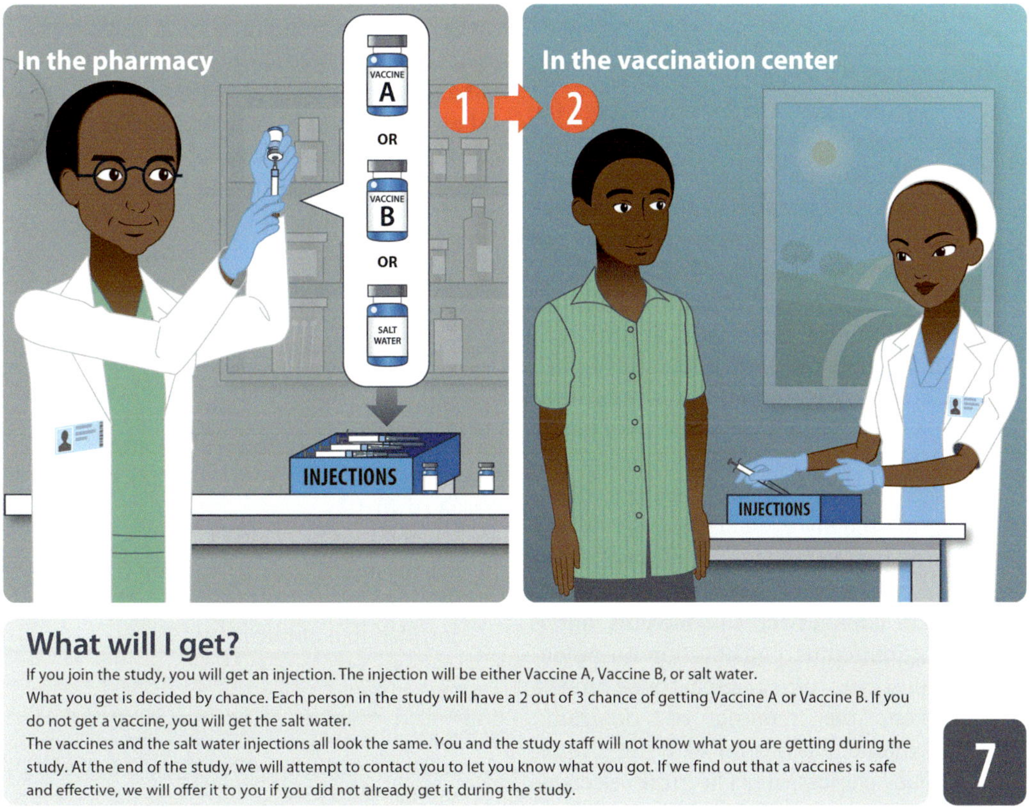

◘ **Fig. 2** First page of a "flipbook" produced by NIAID to explain a clinical trial to participants with little previous understanding of the topic. (NIAID)

The following approaches can help ensure meaningful community involvement:

1. *Establishing expert panels* composed of scientists and community leaders whose members represent priority communities. In addition to working with the communities, members review protocols and offer guidance and direction on considerations for their respective populations.
2. *Inclusion of community members on every protocol team* as specific clinical trial concepts are identified and developed.
3. *Establishing Community Advisory Structures, which may* include:
   (a) *Community working groups* composed of experienced community educator staff members and community advisory board (CAB) representatives from participating clinical research sites, who ensure adherence to community involvement principles in a form suitable for the community. CAB members advise on specific projects that their sites are involved in.
   (b) *Clinical Research Site community advisory boards (CABs)* represent the community of potential and enrolled participants. CABs are composed of community members who have insight into what works best in their local cultural and geographic context.
   (c) *Global CAB.* As each site is advised by a local CAB, these local groups each designate a representative to serve on a Global CAB that advises the broader network. The group meets virtually by webinar, with simultaneous interpretation provided by professionals, facilitating the involvement of those whose primary language differs from the primary language used in the clinical trial. This advice can include, but is not limited to, consultation on potential scopes of research to be undertaken, the naming of programs, recommendations for working groups, policy choices, etc. The group elects its chairpersons and designates members to serve on network governance committees.

3.1 Real-World Examples

3.1.1 USA, Peru, Brazil, South Africa

The COVID-19 Prevention Network (CoVPN) staff at clinical research sites across the world recognized the need to enhance community awareness and education and reduce misinformation and disinformation circulating in communities about COVID-19 and COVID-19 vaccines and broadly neutralizing antibody (bnAb) therapeutics.

To better understand how to convey accurate information to local communities and to train clinical research site staff in the importance of community understanding for successful study conduct, the CoVPN conducted virtual consultations in partnership with site staff and community stakeholders, identifying the need to develop educational videos. Site staff, community advisory board members, and other community stakeholders were engaged at each stage of video development—content solicitation, concept sheet development, script review, review of draft videos, review of translated scripts, review of finalized videos, and review of final videos in languages other than English. Videos were first developed in English and adapted into Spanish (for the USA and Peru) and Portuguese (for Brazil), resulting in 24 videos. In addition, videos were adapted into seven African languages for African clinical research sites. The videos[2] addressed the following themes:

- The importance of enrolling diverse participants in COVID-19 studies
- How can vaccine and antibody studies move so quickly and still be safe?
- Using antibodies for the prevention of COVID-19
- Vaccines do not cause COVID-19!
- What happens during vaccine study visits?
- What happens if I get COVID-19 while enrolled in a clinical study?

---

2 Playlist of animated videos: ▶ https://www.youtube.com/playlist?list=PLyV7_IecAhEqW6fWzXwaN1g0U7IoYjF4u.

Prevent Covid 19 YouTube page with playlists for English, Spanish, and Portuguese: ▶ https://www.youtube.com/@preventcovid19.

- Is one vaccine or antibody regimen against COVID-19 enough?
- Addressing nine COVID-19 myths and facts

4 Maintaining and Sustaining Engagement

Multiple NIAID funded clinical trial networks were repurposed as the CoVPN to address the COVID-19 pandemic in March 2020 (CoVPN 2021). CoVPN capitalized on existing HIV/AIDS research infrastructure and historic community engagement efforts. The effort was further supplemented by including other federally funded partners, such as other NIH institutes, the Veterans Administration, the Biomedical Advanced Research and Development Authority, and the Walter Reed Army Institute of Research (all in the United States). CoVPN successfully sustained community partnerships through continued support and focus on community engagement (Andrasik et al. 2021). At the CoVPN, particularly at clinical research sites, community engagement continued to be a collective responsibility shared by persons in all roles—investigators, community outreach, clinicians, and CAB members—and across the research lifecycle. Effective community engagement programs are characterized by the development of permanent teams of full-time staff (two to four staff members at each site) who lead and facilitate engagement efforts.

Each clinical research site must employ a minimum of one local, full-time community educator responsible for developing and implementing site-specific community engagement work plans that outline goals, objectives, and the scope of work. Community educators collaborate with the CAB to assess community education needs and identify appropriate educational strategies and materials. They also ensure that CAB representatives have input into study-specific issues, such as addressing community misconceptions, determining appropriate and non-coercive incentives for trial participation and retention, and determining the package of services that make up the local standard of prevention. An effective community educator develops and maintains collaborative community partnerships and ensures that all clinical research staff are involved in community engagement activities as appropriate.

CoVPN required its clinical research sites to develop annual work plans that outline their plans and objectives for community engagement. Work plans were reviewed and approved by the network's Community Engagement Unit and developed in partnership with site staff, including investigators, clinicians, CAB members, and community staff members. The work plans described community education, recruitment, and retention efforts, as well as how the CAB would be developed, educated, and utilized. CAB members provided input into the community engagement work plans developed by their respective sites and were required to co-sign the final plan.

4.1 Real-World Examples (Fig. 3)

4.1.1 South Africa

Even when they are not actively recruiting, clinical research sites across South Africa provide ongoing support for stakeholder programs through:

- Participation in activities planned by stakeholders.
  - Site staff often participate as unpaid speakers to address health issues without speaking about specific studies.
- Promoting and advertising activities taking place in the community.
- Site community educator participation in virtual and in-person community groups and dissemination of information regarding new developments and scientific advances.
- Site participation in local community radio station "healthy day" events, which reinforce the connection between the community and the research site.

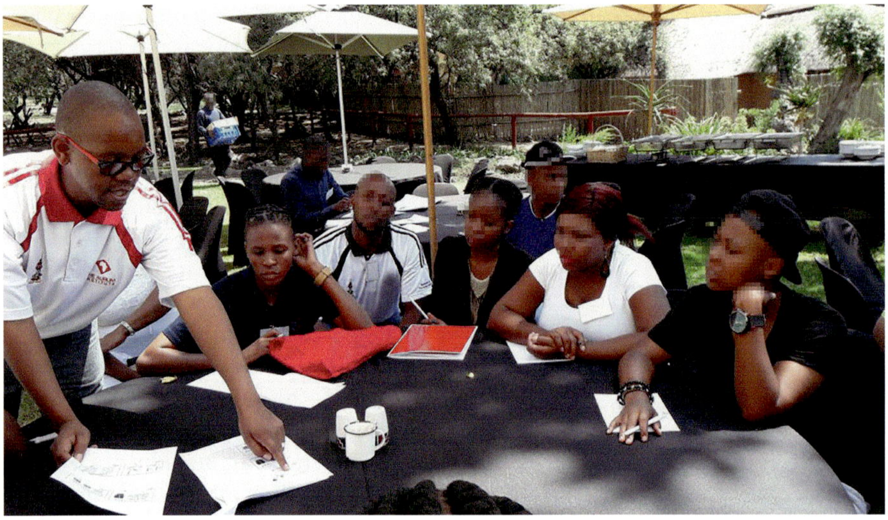

Fig. 3 Kagisho Baepanye conducting a community advisory board workshop on HIV at the Aurum Klerksdorp Clinical Research Site in Klerksdorp, South Africa. (Courtesy Fred Hutch)

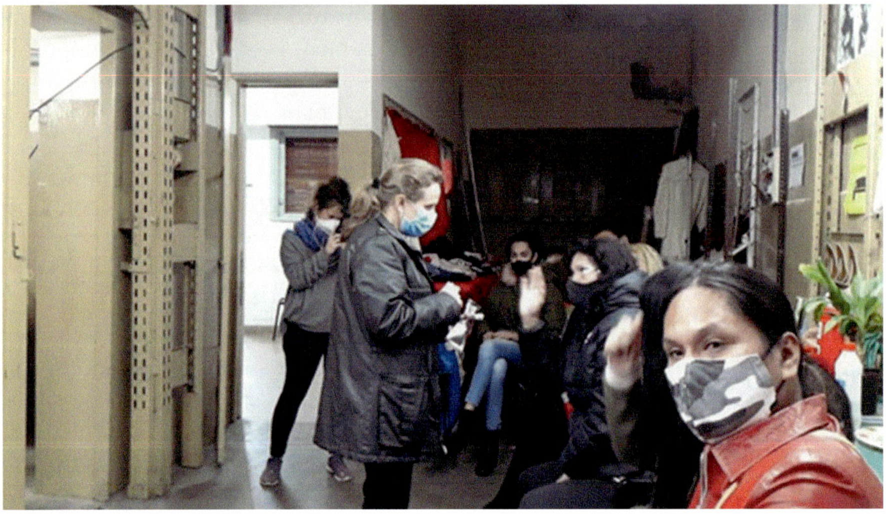

Fig. 4 The Fundación Huésped clinical research site in Buenos Aires. (Credit: Gastón Devisich/Huésped)

4.1.2 Buenos Aires, Argentina

The Fundación Huésped clinical research site in Buenos Aires has long worked to develop a presence and reputation for transparency and trust in their local community, particularly during the sanitary crisis that resulted from the COVID-19 pandemic. The site staff sought funding through Coalition Plus (of which Fundación Huésped is a member) and implemented several economic assistance projects for the local community, working in collaboration with partners like the Argentine LGBTQ + Federation (FALGBT) and Migrantes × Migrantes and La Garganta (Migrants × Migrants and the Powerful Throat) (Fig. 4).

Poderosa. Together they organized efforts to distribute basic food (e.g., milk, oil, rice) and disinfection (e.g., alcohol, facemasks, etc.) supplies for community members. They also successfully secured donations of kitchen and cleaning supplies for distribution through their partnerships with Hotel Gondolin (an institution where approximately 30 transgender people live) and Casa Trans. These institutions were critical in the design, planning, and implementation of a home-care project, through which an interdisciplinary team provided HIV and STI prevention, care, diagnosis, and treatment services; COVID-19 vaccination; training on active management of COVID-19 cases; and community mental health interventions. Additionally, the site offered its endocrinological clinic for hormone therapy for transgender women, services that were not provided at general health centers.

4.1.3 São Paulo, Brazil

Over the past few years, the Cerqueira Cesar clinical research site in São Paulo has achieved continuity of activity by using video and social media. Many social media posts have supported festive dates for the LGBTQ+ community and promoted information about health, human rights, and sexuality. The site also conducts live streams on its Instagram channel and through channels hosted by community partners. The site's community educator also participates in WhatsApp groups, maintaining direct, almost daily dialogue with community members. Additionally, site staff participate in city and municipal committees where health policy issues are discussed and strategies are developed. In 2019, as part of an advanced course for postgraduate students and health professionals on HIV pathogenesis at a local university, the community engagement team facilitated discussions about the lived experiences of transgender women, including bringing transgender women to engage in dialogue with the class (◘ Fig. 5).

4.1.4 Lima, Peru

The use of social networks became a strategic tool utilized by several Peruvian sites in response to COVID-19 restrictions to share information with participants and communities. Local teams were challenged to learn how to use various internet platforms to maintain contact with community-based organizations in such an expedited, short time. Clinical research sites in Lima and Iquitos have created successful communication channels (i.e., Facebook, Instagram, TikTok) to convey research achievements, ensure that the local community is included in research, and allow community leaders to share their experiences and perspectives. For clinical research sites in Lima, the primary communication channels are social network apps (e.g., Facebook, Instagram, TikTok). For the Asociacion Civil Selva Amazonica (ACSA), covering clinical research sites in the Peruvian jungle region, face-to-face approaches remain the most important channel.

As COVID persisted in Peru, it became common to watch news about vaccine development on TV, listen to discussions focusing on vaccines, and ask others what vaccines they had taken. As a result of this normative focus on vaccines, communities in Lima are more familiar with terms like vaccine, research, and protection. This is a window of opportunity to link this knowledge to benefit future HIV vaccine development and all the steps needed to achieve this goal (◘ Fig. 6).

4.1.5 Iquitos, Peru

The sanitary emergency caused by the COVID pandemic revealed the fragility of health systems, which in some cities became more evident than others. Iquitos, a city located in the northeastern part of Peru, was severely impacted early in the pandemic, challenging local community leaders to take extraordinary actions in the face of the overflow of cases and the limited response of the local health system. In view of the health system's limited ability to provide oxygen, for example, Raymond Portelli, a local priest and medical doctor, successfully led a national virtual fundraising campaign supporting two local oxygen centers, partially alleviating the crisis that the most vulnerable populations were experiencing. Dr. Portelli has cared for people with HIV for many years and works with the ACSA, a vaccine research center in Iquitos, Peru. Having an authentic community leader as an ally for the development of HIV research, and now for COVID research response, is the kind of strength that research centers must identify and maintain (◘ Fig. 7).

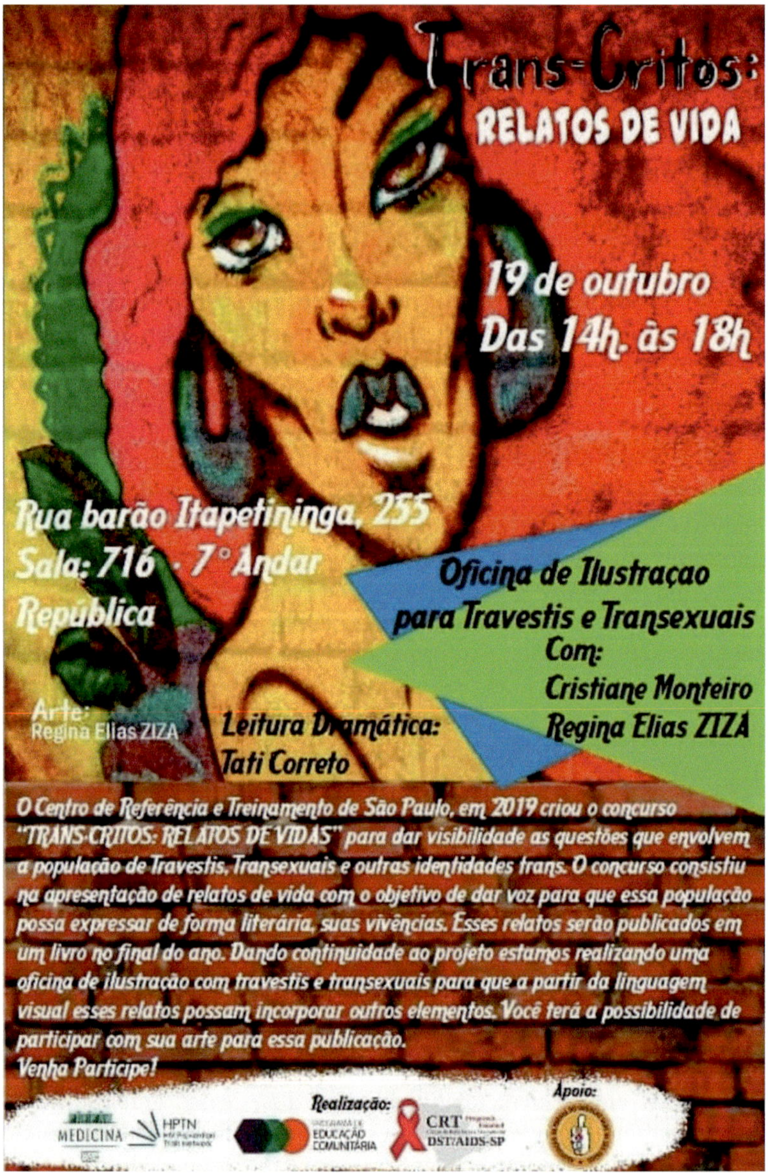

Fig. 5 Poster promoting a health information meeting for the transgender community in São Paulo. (Credit: Regina Elias da Costa)

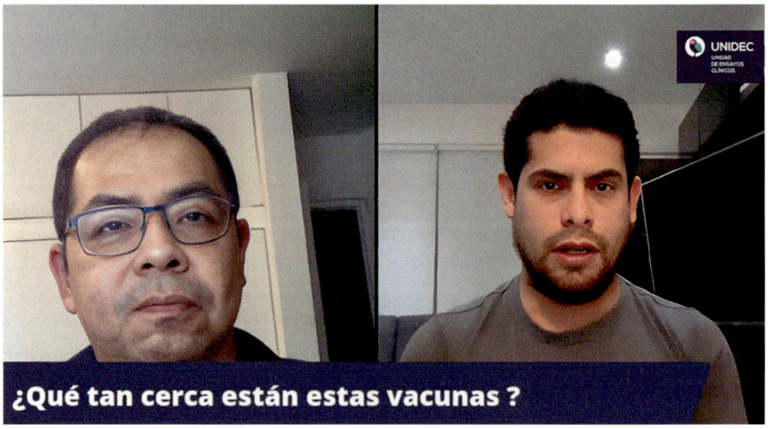

Fig. 6 A virtual community talk about COVID-19, Lima Peru

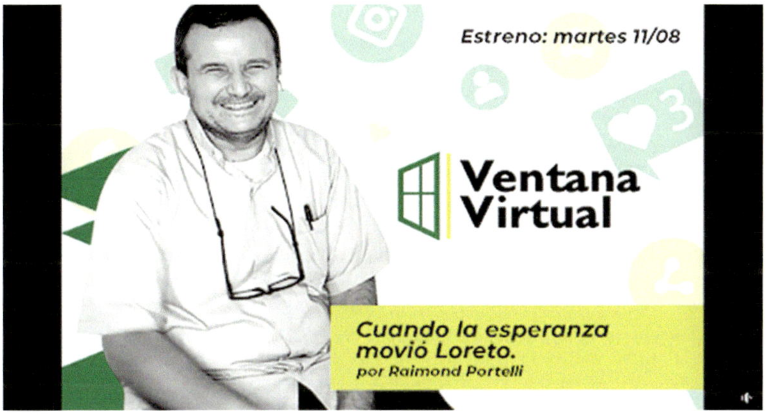

Fig. 7 Raymond Portelli participating in one of the TV shows broadcast locally with the support of Asociacion Civil Selva Amazonica (ACSA CRS) in Iquitos, Peru. (Courtesy ACSA CRS)

5 Implementation Science: A Call for Support

The conduct of biomedical prevention and treatment studies, especially in the context of a global pandemic, needs to be guided by research into the best ways to implement new public health tools. This concept is grounded in lessons learned from the clinical trials of new vaccines, monoclonal antibodies, drugs, and/or other products that have been proven to be safe and effective in clinical trials, and that have received initial approvals by appropriate regulatory authorities. Such rational development of ways to use new technologies for the good of communities has been termed implementation research. While critical to ultimately taking ideas from the bench to the bedside, funding for this type of research has historically been very limited compared with funding for basic, translational, and other clinical trials research. GPP will remain difficult to implement in public health in the absence of public and philanthropic research support of implementation science (Holtrop et al. 2021; Proctor et al. 2009).

Discussion Questions

1. How does good participatory practice (GPP) help build community engagement for clinical research?
2. Community support depends on relationships and partnerships of trust and mutual respect between the research team and various community groups.
   (a) List some of these community groups.
   (b) Provide one or two examples of building bridges and fostering relationships with devalued communities.
3. Meaningful community involvement must occur from the outset of the research process and be sustained throughout.
   (a) Describe approaches to meaningful community involvement.
   (b) How can the research team increase community awareness and correct misperceptions and misinformation?
   (c) Provide examples of efforts by CoVPN to enhance community awareness and reduce the impact of COVID-19 misinformation and disinformation.
4. What difficulties may be encountered when applying GPP to public health?
5. What is implementation science and why is it needed in this context?

References

AERAS. Good participatory practice guidelines for TB vaccine research. Rockville, MD. 2017.

Allman D, Ditmore MH, Kaplan K. Improving ethical and participatory practice for marginalized populations in biomedical HIV prevention trials: lessons from Thailand. PLoS One. 2014;9(6):e100058. https://doi.org/10.1371/journal.pone.0100058.

Andrasik MP, Broder GB, Wallace SE, Chaturvedi R, Michael NL, Bock S, et al. Increasing black, indigenous and people of color participation in clinical trials through community engagement and recruitment goal establishment. PLoS One. 2021;16(10):e0258858. https://doi.org/10.1371/journal.pone.0258858.

Broder GB, Lucas JP, Davis J, Wallace SE, Luthuli N, Baepanye K, et al. Standardized metrics can reveal region-specific opportunities in community engagement to aid recruitment in HIV prevention trials. PLoS One. 2020;15(9):e0239276. https://doi.org/10.1371/journal.pone.0239276.

Chua A, Ford N, Wilson D, Cawthorne P. The tenofovir pre-exposure prophylaxis trial in Thailand: researchers should show more openness in their engagement with the community. PLoS Med. 2005;2(10):e346. https://doi.org/10.1371/journal.pmed.0020346.

Cohen J. AIDS clinical trials. More woes for novel HIV prevention approach. Science. 2005; 307(5716):1708. https://doi.org/10.1126/science.307.5716.1708a.

CoVPN. COVID-19 prevention network. Washington, DC. 2021. https://www.coronaviruspreventionnetwork.org/. Accessed 11 July 2021.

Ditmore M. Response to Joep M. A. Lange. PLoS Med. 2005;2(10):e347. https://doi.org/10.1371/journal.pmed.0020347.

Duan N. Listening to consumers and HIV vaccine preparedness. Lancet. 2005;365(9465):1119–21. https://doi.org/10.1016/s0140-6736(05)71857-2.

Haire BG. Because we can: clashes of perspective over researcher obligation in the failed PrEP trials. Dev World Bioeth. 2011;11(2):63–74. https://doi.org/10.1111/j.1471-8847.2010.00292.x.

Holtrop JS, Estabrooks PA, Gaglio B, Harden SM, Kessler RS, King DK, et al. Understanding and applying the RE-AIM framework: clarifications and resources. J Clin Transl Sci. 2021;5:e126. https://doi.org/10.1017/cts.2021.789.

Lange JM. We must not let protestors derail trials of pre-exposure prophylaxis for HIV. PLoS Med. 2005;2(9):e248. https://doi.org/10.1371/journal.pmed.0020248.

Mills EJ, Singh S, Singh JA, Orbinski JJ, Warren M, Upshur RE. Designing research in vulnerable populations: lessons from HIV prevention trials that stopped early. BMJ. 2005;331(7529):1403–6. https://doi.org/10.1136/bmj.331.7529.1403.

NIH. Person-first and destigmatizing language. In: NIH style guide. Bethesda, MD: National Institutes of Health; 2023. https://www.nih.gov/nih-style-guide/person-first-destigmatizing-language. Accessed 7 Sept 2023.

Nuffield Council on Bioethics. Research in global health emergencies: ethical issues. Oxford, UK: Nuffield Council on Bioethics; 2020.

Page-Shafer K, Saphonn V, Sun LP, Vun MC, Cooper DA, Kaldor JM. HIV prevention research in a resource-limited setting: the experience of planning a trial in Cambodia. Lancet. 2005;366(9495):1499–503. https://doi.org/10.1016/s0140-6736(05)67146-2.

Peterson K, Folayan MO. Ethics and HIV prevention research: an analysis of the early tenofovir PrEP trial in Nigeria. Bioethics. 2019;33(1):35–42. https://doi.org/10.1111/bioe.12470.

Proctor EK, Landsverk J, Aarons G, Chambers D, Glisson C, Mittman B. Implementation research in mental health services: an emerging science with conceptual, methodological, and training challenges. Admin Pol Ment Health. 2009;36(1):24–34. https://doi.org/10.1007/s10488-008-0197-4.

Singh JA, Mills EJ. The abandoned trials of pre-exposure prophylaxis for HIV: what went wrong? PLoS Med. 2005;2(9):e234. https://doi.org/10.1371/journal.pmed.0020234.

UNAIDS and AVAC. Good participatory practice: guidelines for biomedical HIV prevention trials. Geneva: UNAIDS (Joint United Nations Programme on HIV/AIDS); 2011.

UNAIDS and WHO. Ethical considerations in biomedical HIV prevention trials. Geneva: Joint United Nations Programme on HIV/AIDS (UNAIDS); 2007.

Wallerstein N, Duran B, Oetzel JG, Minkler M. Community-based participatory research for health: advancing social and health equity. San Francisco: Wiley; 2017.

WHO. Good participatory practice guidelines for trials of emerging (and re-emerging) pathogens that are likely to cause severe outbreaks in the near future and for which few or no medical countermeasures exist (GPP-EP). Geneva: World Health Organization; 2016. p. 53.

WHO. Good participatory practice for COVID-19 clinical trials—a toolbox. Geneva: World Health Organization; 2020.

18.2 In Practice: Adapting Social Analytics for Research Response

Rhys O'Neill, David Cyprian, and Elizabeth S. Higgs

Contents

The two first authors provided social analytics support to NIH-supported EVD vaccine research trials while employed by Novetta, a data analytics firm.
Learning Track Note: This chapter appears in Learning Tracks: Clinical Research; Emergency Research Response, Research Operations; Public Health and Epidemiology; Research Ethics; Social Science Response Research

E. S. Higgs and R. A. Sorenson (eds.), *Principles and Practice of Emergency Research Response*,
https://doi.org/10.1007/978-3-031-48408-7_27

Learning Objectives

This chapter should enable readers to understand and discuss:

- Social analytics and its holistic approach to available data
- Key capabilities of social analytics systems
- The mechanics of effective social analytics
- The role of social media in monitoring beliefs and public opinion during health emergencies
- Why social media data should be interpreted cautiously
- What determines the success or failure of social analytics in practice
- Examples from Liberia and the Democratic Republic of Congo (DRC) where social analytics was successful and why
- Examples of misinformation and recurring behaviors of information flow

1 Introduction

Ensuring accurate, real-time understanding of individual, community, and societal beliefs, levels of trust, attitudes, and understanding of interventions during health emergencies is fundamental to effective response efforts. Social analytics is a powerful tool enabling governments, responders, and researchers to gauge real-time, geographically specific beliefs during health emergencies.

Epidemics occur in the real world. The disease appears and spreads in cities, remote villages, and nations that long predate the arrival of a pathogen. Health emergencies cause enhanced fear and anxiety among populations (Dragioti et al. 2022). Health emergencies often disrupt societal structures such as schools, hospitals, and businesses, including restrictions on individual and community liberties such as quarantines and curfews. Societal disruption aside, there are fears about the disease's threat to individuals and families. In many health emergencies, there is also a stigma associated with the disease (e.g., Ebola, mpox) that can result in social and employment ostracism. Moreover, in contrast to Western societies, which place relatively high emphasis on the individual, many cultures place greater emphasis on community or tribal identity. The ability to effectively respond to an infectious disease emergency requires individual, community, and population cooperation in the case of pandemics. Ending an outbreak may require non-pharmaceutical public health interventions such as masks, hand washing, and physical distancing or medical countermeasures (MCMs) like vaccines, therapeutics, and diagnostics—in most cases both sorts of response. Uptake and application of these interventions are obviously necessary for them to be effective. Clearly for research response—for acceptance of the interventions assessed to be safe and effective by research—support and participation by individuals and communities is critical to success.

Communities and populations are not monolithic. There are significant differences among individuals, communities, and groups that influence the acceptance of response interventions. Cultural practices, personal economies, politics, prejudices, education, religion, previous experiences, communal beliefs around who is trustworthy, and other factors intersect and can profoundly impact whether public health interventions, research responses, and response objectives are achieved. Marginalized and vulnerable groups may react differently than the dominant population.

An additional layer of complexity is that prevalent beliefs evolve over the course of health emergencies. In the beginning, disbelief or denial is common, e.g., Ebola is not real, COVID-19 is not that serious, etc. Over time, once the emergency is accepted as real, blame sets in, e.g., Ebola was created by industry, and the Chinese are responsible for SARS-CoV-2. With medical countermeasures (MCMs), false beliefs and rumors can undercut acceptance and uptake, as seen clearly with vaccine hesitancy, refusal to seek care, use of "alternative" treatments, etc. (◘ Fig. 1).

The ability to conduct a research response requires dialogue with stakeholders. The most important are the individuals and communities directly participating in research (► Chap. 18). It is essential that responders, governments, and researchers have real-time data specific to the beliefs, attitudes, knowledge,

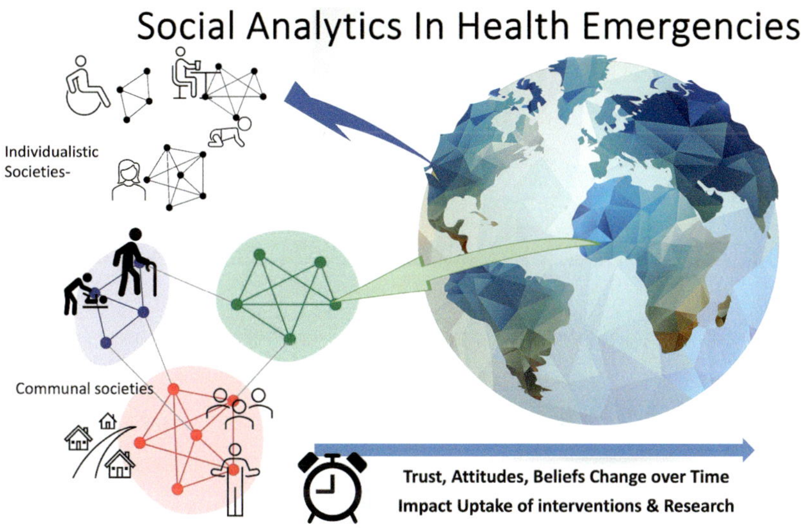

Fig. 1 Dynamics of belief systems may differ among societies that are more individualist as against those with a more communal orientation, but in all cases changing conceptions of medical research and the MCMs it produces has an impact on compliance with public health and medical advice. (Elizabeth S. Higgs)

and social mores of communities and populations where they are working so the responders can communicate as effectively as possible with target populations.

A new obstacle, or at least a greatly enlarged one, is intentional misinformation by individuals and entities trying to advance agendas other than that of the emergency response, with motives ranging from monetary gain to strategic calculation at the nation-state level (Toepfl et al. 2023). Social media increase the volume and speed of rampant disinformation, rumors, and misinformation,[1] increasing the risk posed by unscientific beliefs and disruptive social behaviors and further amplifying fear and mistrust.

While at the data analytics company Novetta, authors Rhys O'Neill and David Cyprian developed sophisticated methodologies and technology processes to parse and analyze social media in conflict zones like Syria and Iraq for clients in the national security domain. Innovative and pragmatic applications of modern technology, including machine learning (ML), natural language processing (NLP), computer vision, and data science tools, enable the processing of raw content at the scale required to discover, extract, measure, and analyze social data for narrative power and capacity to change behavior. During the 2014–2016 West Africa Ebola outbreak, the National Institute for Allergy and Infectious Diseases (NIAID) saw the potential to conduct real-time monitoring of beliefs, attitudes, and rumors to support social mobilization, communication, and community engagement (SMC) as part of its research response in Liberia.

Social Analytics became a valuable tool in the SMC efforts in Liberia and later in the eastern Democratic Republic of the Congo (DRC) during the large EVD outbreak between 2018 and 2020. The latter research response took place in near war-zone conditions, and social analytics information was particularly valuable for characterizing risk. The value of social analytics for health applications is expanding rapidly, and it has now been used in the recent Sudan virus outbreak in Uganda and several locations in response to the COVID-19 pandemic.

1 As Bernard et al. (2021) explain, "It is important to distinguish between disinformation and misinformation: misinformation is typically classified as 'accidental falsehood,' or wrong and misleading information shared without malice, while disinformation is 'deliberate falsehood,' or wrong or misleading information shared in full knowledge of its falsehood, often with malicious intent."

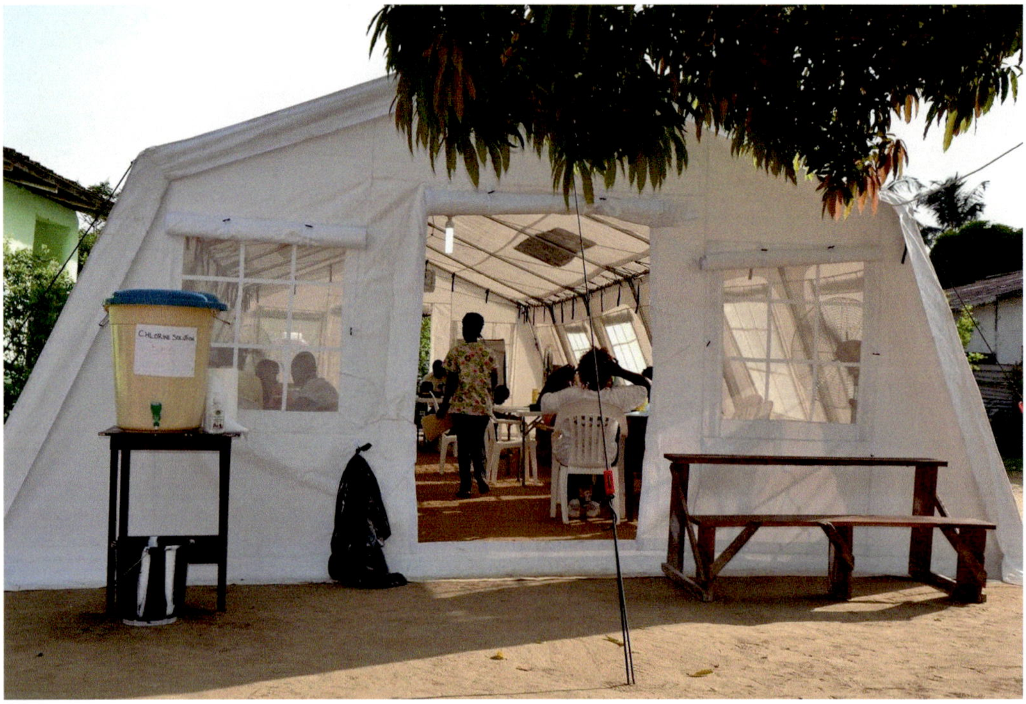

Fig. 2 Clinical trial site in Liberia. (Photo: Laura McNay)

Effective social analytics requires a holistic approach to available social data, including online content, news and broadcast content, and field research. It falls flat unless it includes data from the operational environment that can inform effective countermeasures and risk communications. The benefit and operational utility of the social mobilization, community engagement, and communications (SMC) structure that had already been established for the response and research in Liberia became the context for analysis.

Having the SMC in place allowed us to implement two adaptations from our conflict-zone work, which was more removed from in-country events because of security concerns. In the disease outbreak environment, especially in Libera, we could (1) include a rumor tracking process from in-country field research networks and (2) focus specifically on using the inputs from social analytics to inform SMC activities, including the determination of when to intervene with SMC messaging, followed by rapid assessment of the effectiveness of these interventions. A critical element of social mobilization, communication, and community engagement (or good participatory practice [GPP]) in support of research response is current information on community beliefs, rumors, and attitudes toward both the viral threats and the medical and non-medical interventions intended to mitigate the outbreak, and toward the health personnel leading the response (Fig. 2).

The two EVD environments were very different: In Liberia, we supported post-peak clinical research for treatments, vaccines, and survivor studies. In DRC, we supported the PALM[2] randomized clinical trial of Ebola therapeutics at the height of the epidemic, with ongoing violence, regional instability, and open warfare raging in the region (Mulangu et al. 2019; Nguyen 2019). Working with the SMC teams, we had the opportunity to field test, refine, and apply an approach to social analytics to support the research response. The weekly social analytics reports developed during the 2018 North Kivu, DRC

2 Pamoja Tulinde Maisha (PALM): "Together Save Lives" in Swahili.

Ebola outbreak were provided to WHO, the government of the DRC, response groups, and other responders. The reports provided geographically precise feedback on evolving community beliefs and sentiments. They also enabled critical alerts and operational recommendations for the epidemic response and clinical trial teams, as well as the social mobilization teams responsible for risk communications and community engagement (RCCE). The process of providing accurate monitoring required the synthesis of information from many sources, both online and offline. Critical threats had to be rapidly extracted from the noise of low-risk chatter, processed for veracity and threat level, and transmitted to those who could act to mitigate the threat of additional exposure to the Ebola virus or physical threats to clinical sites.

The global threat of coronavirus disease 2019 (COVID-19) remains, even after more than four years. While EVD was largely confined to distinct areas, with a few cases spreading to other continents from the West Africa outbreak, COVID-19 is truly global. Nevertheless, social analytics insight frameworks, observations, and tools apply in these very different situations in a great many respects. Social analytics collects real-time "fake news" and misinformation, localized economic, cultural, and political attitudes, and the influence of trusted voices on the population groups that trust them. The causes of counterproductive social behaviors, including refusal to comply with public health measures and vaccine hesitancy, can thus be better understood. The data sourcing, critical threat monitoring, and analytical frameworks refined for the EVD outbreak have also proven effective and relevant for COVID-19 management. However, the application and response channels for COVID-19's global reach require different messengers and mediums.

Effective social analytics for epidemic preparedness begins with understanding and accounting for the predictable elements within the social context of disease outbreaks. Rapid adaptation of data collection tools, data processing algorithms, and measurable indicators is possible within proven frameworks built on known factors that will occur, reoccur, and potentially disrupt global health response. What follows is a playbook for the resources and elements that should be included in social analytics cells to maximize the breadth and utility of support. We also include numerous examples from our work with EVD and COVID-19 to illustrate use cases where social analytics can make a positive difference in desired global health outcomes.

2 The Mechanics of Effective Social Analytics

Social analytics is a versatile and essential tool for epidemic response. As we learned, social analytics itself must be constructed from a broad array of sources that includes social media and other online content, but offline conversations and traditional news and broadcast media must not be neglected. In addition, it must be acknowledged at the outset that this type of social data is inherently messy, difficult to collect consistently, and requires significant interpretation to derive value. It requires both technology tools that can convert unstructured text and media snippets into structured data for pattern discovery and regional experts who can interpret the information in the local context.

The key capability of any social analytics system is to listen: to hear the motivations, the stories, the misinformation, and the fears that circulate and resonate among a target population regarding specific public health interventions, activities, and messaging. With this capability, a critical monitoring function is fulfilled. Early warnings of false beliefs, rumors, and the prevalence of narratives (harmful and helpful) are collected.

With the data in hand, the next step is the ability to extract, parse, and sort large streams of unstructured data to discover relevant or dangerous patterns. Categorizing circulating narratives to correlate with operational goals and adapting ML techniques to quickly classify content according to this taxonomy provide critical context to SMC to determine which rumors need a response and which can be ignored. This process allows the SMC team to craft appropriate social interventions. The monitoring capability then fulfills a spot evaluation role, indicating the degree of influence the intervention may have had in the narrative environment (◘ Figs. 3 and 4).

Typical technology would include social listening software (to extract social media conversations), a media monitoring service or software, and a data analysis system that allows for data manipulation and ML and

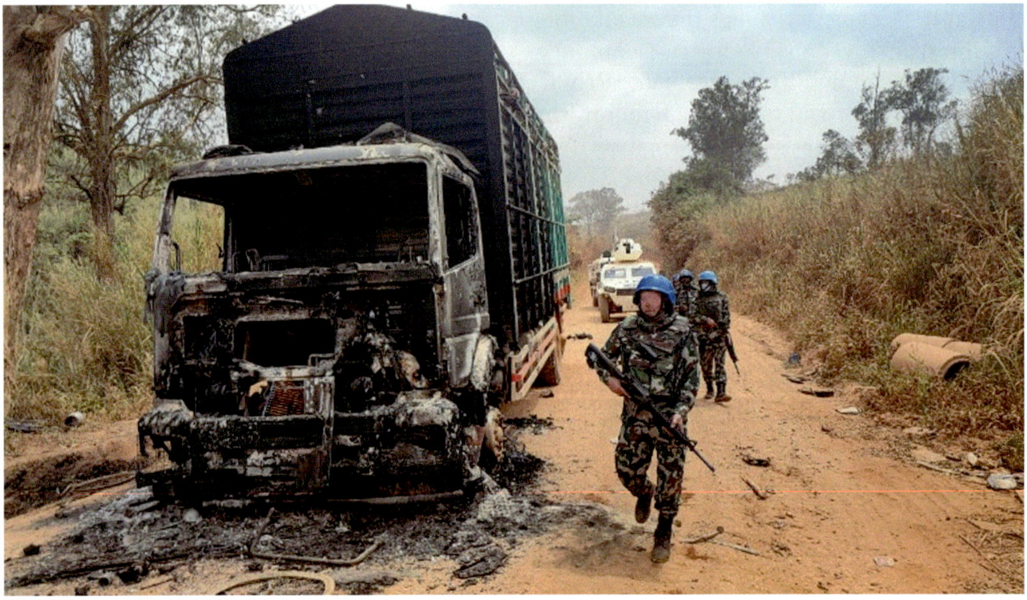

◘ **Fig. 3** Alerted about an attack by militiamen against a civilian vehicle on National Road Number 2y near the northeastern DRC city of Ituri, UN Stabilization Mission (MONUSCO) peacekeepers intervene in March 2022 to repel the assailants and protect the civilian population. (Photo: MONUSCO/Force)

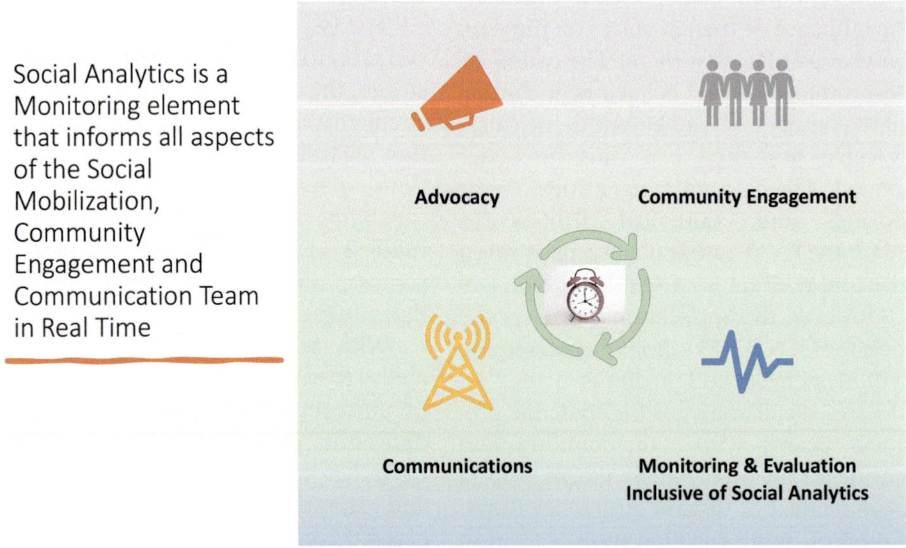

◘ **Fig. 4** Social analytics can become a vital part of the cycle of community engagement, allowing social communications teams to better understand the results of their efforts and refine their messaging to address the evolving concerns of communities near research sites. (Elizabeth S. Higgs)

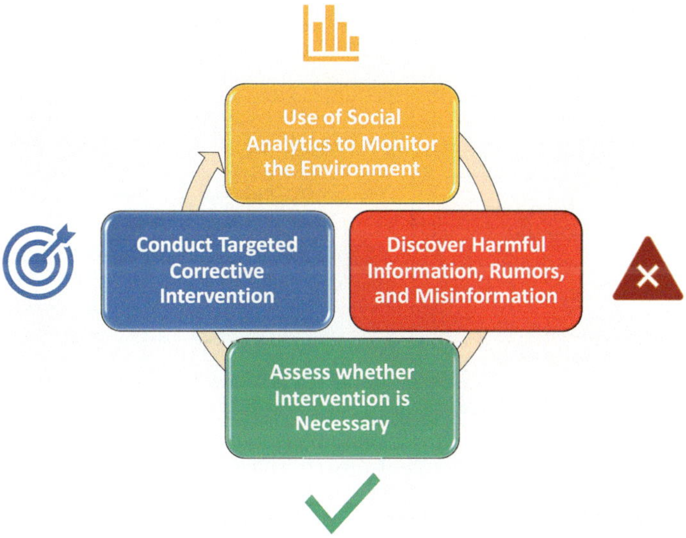

Fig. 5 This virtuous loop depicts the lifecycle of social analytics and interventions. The same process used to monitor the baseline environment becomes an assessment tool for the impact of interventions. (Authors)

NLP data analytics modules. Social media monitoring provides nearly immediate and cost-effective access to a vast array of issues and narratives. ML and NLP techniques (including geolocation, bot detection, topic modeling, named entity recognition, and object recognition) can help to formulate clusters of topics and clusters of users. Analysis techniques can also help determine whether social conversations are increasing in virality and intensity or waning (Fig. 5).

However, social media data must be interpreted cautiously for several reasons. The availability of social media data for researchers to collect is limited by the platforms themselves. Companies like Meta restrict the availability of Facebook and Instagram data. Overreliance on Twitter (now X), the one major social media platform with relatively open access, is common and can be a poor substitute in many regions, including Africa, where daily Twitter usage is minuscule compared to Facebook and WhatsApp. Another challenge is gathering an appropriate target audience sample, although diaspora populations and inorganic users (bots, troll farms, etc.) require that even the best analytic techniques accept some imprecision.

Therefore, regional expertise and additional data sources can significantly improve confidence in findings. These experts can conduct media landscape research to determine what sources have the most active reach into the target populations. These experts can also tap local field networks to validate or disprove whether online narratives and misinformation are reaching or influencing target populations. This validation can also help uncover patterns and motivations causing behavior of interest that may not be apparent from the initial data discovered in social media or news (Fig. 6).

Social analytics work for the Ebola response in DRC was a good example of complementary regional expertise and social listening technology providing crucial information and informing interventions. In 2019 in Beni and Butembo we identified influential public Facebook pages administered by youth groups (La Lucha, Veranda Mutsanga, etc.). Via social listening tools, we extracted and categorized hundreds of mischaracterizations of the Ebola response, e.g.: *Ebola is not real, Ebola is fabricated by the international public health response, Ebola is a tool to use against the Congolese people*. Due to the misinformation consistently found on these pages, Facebook removed the pages from its platform. However, our regional experts subsequently confirmed that removing these pages did not significantly curb misinformation spread online (as a social media monitoring analysis of public data would suggest). The influencers spreading this misinformation quickly migrated to private communication

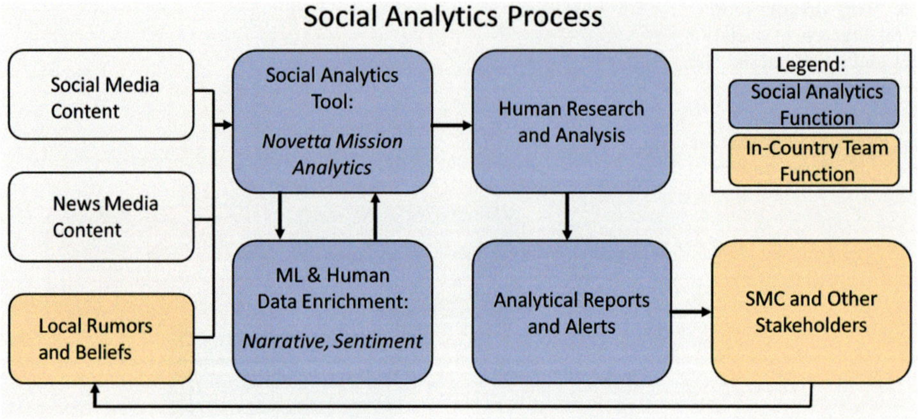

Fig. 6 Social analytics is most effective with a combination of human and machine analytic techniques and when the process is implemented with a field team capable of using the findings to target effective interventions. (Authors)

channels, principally WhatsApp. These private channels produced echo chambers that potentially drove deeper distrust of EVD response without an appropriate opportunity for public health voices to respond. Our awareness of the channels allowed us to advise the risk communications team that the beliefs were still being widely shared among the target population.

3 Applying Social Analytics During Epidemics

A social analytics system for epidemic preparedness and response should be organized to directly support key public health and health research objectives. Frequently, this includes building trust, respect, and communication pathways between the international community and local populations. Large international organizations operate more effectively in a country when the staff of these organizations is aware of local context and biases causing barriers to access and when local populations understand the organizations to be working on behalf of at-risk populations rather than to exploit, abuse, or harm their communities. Thus, social analytics can also inform pre-mission preparedness training for staff. The objective is to identify likely barriers to success that can be detected in social conversations.

Information from social analytics has a myriad of uses for response actors and governments. For SMC and GPP efforts, truly understanding societal attitudes, beliefs, and understandings enables course correction. It can sometimes detect and provide valuable insights into unintended consequences of response actions. The SMC teams in NIH research partnerships—PREVAIL in Liberia and PALM in the DRC—used social analytics to monitor the effectiveness of SMC and research response efforts and received real-time reports, enabling the SMC team to adjust their activities accordingly. The information provided a great deal of geographic community specificity, helping to inform actions on a hyperlocal scale.

Social analytics has value beyond the research response, extending to other elements of emergency response. For example, in the weekly social analytics report for March 9–15, 2019 from North Kivu, DRC, the team received the following information (Fig. 7):

One essential use of social analytics is to provide for the safety of health staff, healthcare workers, and patients. Political, military, paramilitary, economic, and other non-healthcare events can sometimes lead to rapid

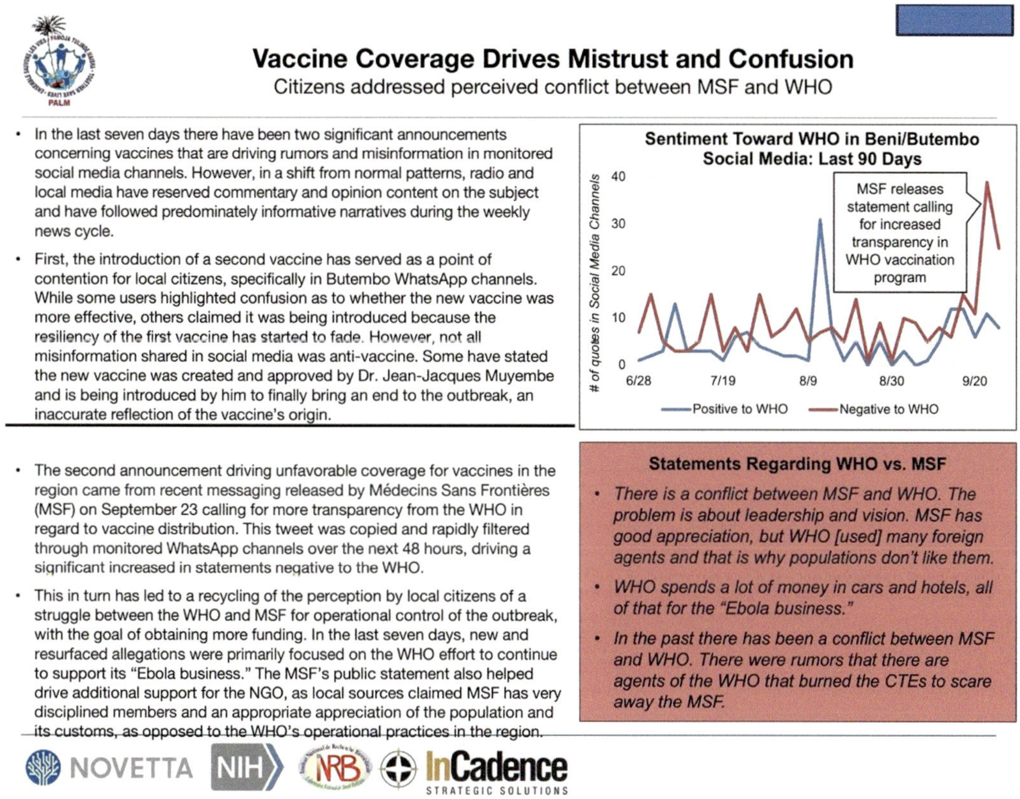

Fig. 7 A weekly social analytics report on events related to the Ebola response in the eastern DRC, September 2019. (NIAID)

destabilization. In our work for both EVD and COVID-19 responses, we have seen examples (see below) where social analytics discovered or validated indications of deteriorating safety conditions and provided this context rapidly to operations teams.

3.1 Liberia

We supported the clinical trial response to Liberia's West Africa Ebola outbreak from October 2014 to March 2019. We provided feedback on how the public viewed clinical trials in focus regions, helping to ensure there were enough willing participants in EVD studies based on more than 200,000 social data points from more than 50,000 unique sources online and through in-country field research. Our work supported the Partnership for Research on Vaccines and Infectious Diseases in Liberia (PREVAIL), described elsewhere in this book; specifically, we supported the risk communications and community engagement pillar (Higgs et al. 2017). Our assessment of the social landscape, the discovery of barriers to success, and recommendations for action were all conducted in close, near-daily coordination with the PREVAIL SMC. This allowed the findings from our social analytics work to translate directly into SMC activities to improve outcomes for trial enrollment.

One example was when a local disc jockey (DJ) on Radio Kintoma falsely alleged that a news story about the United States Agency for International Development (USAID)-supported research into the origin of Ebola in bats meant that a novel Ebola strain was returning to Liberia in August 2018. Because of the responsive and integrated framework we had built with social analytics and the PREVAIL SMC team (which had relationships with local government officials), the misinformation was quickly identified, and just three days later, Radio Kintoma hosted a Liberian health official from the national health ministry who corrected the record. This prevented a potentially damaging drop in enrollment in PREVAIL's ongoing local research trials.

Also in 2018, we discovered rumors on Facebook that the John F. Kennedy (JFK) Hospital in Monrovia was secretly harboring patients with new Ebola cases. Since PREVAIL was operating a clinic at JFK, this rumor had the potential to be extremely disruptive to clinical studies. We notified PREVAIL SMC within 24 hours of discovering the rumor, and PREVAIL immediately set to work correcting the misinformation in reputable local news sources and the community.

3.2 The Democratic Republic of the Congo

The 2018–2020 outbreak of EVD in the eastern DRC, designated the tenth DRC outbreak, claimed over 2000 lives. One of the primary obstacles to controlling it was longstanding, deeply rooted mistrust of authorities—including medical response personnel—on the part of the local communities most heavily affected (Stearns 2012; Wells et al. 2019; WHO 2020). While there was progress in combating stubborn resistance to EVD response teams, misinformation and damaging rumors continued throughout the response. Large-scale EVD information campaigns by the international community were undermined by misinformation in the media, which was accepted and amplified among trusted community members. Understanding where and how such rumors and misinformation originated was essential for community buy-in, especially at the fringes of an outbreak spreading into regions that did not have preparedness or support systems (Spinney 2019).

In an unstable and often dangerous region, social analytics enhances the security of operations through near real-time collection of threats of violence, often signaled on local social media. This also allows for rapid assessment of public opinion and media in regions that are either seeing their first EVD cases or are at risk of the disease in the immediate future.

Social analytics played a crucial role, for example, in understanding community members who carried out two separate raids on morgues in Beni. On June 24, 2019, several young men removed the body of an EVD victim from a Beni morgue. The body was that of the brother of one of the group members, who believed response team members would harvest organs from the cadaver. Multiple members of the group came into contact with the body with no protective gear. This message circulated on WhatsApp immediately following the event:

> We entered the morgue. There we had seen Florice. He was there. We transported him to the outside. We have seen it. It was already cut by the response agents [Author comment: this is likely false]. There were five dead in the morgue, but we managed to go out with Florice. But the forces of the police and the army came to us, and we had to throw the body and run away. There are many of our friends who are arrested. The innocents are arrested (since the morning,

including the young people who are suspected to be the authors of the fire of the responders' jeep). They fired live ammunition and tear gas. We were already in the street with the body, but we could not go so fast because we were only 5 people carrying the body. The other people had fled, and we had to disperse. I should have beaten this young responder who insisted that our friend be brought here to the morgue for the test. But he managed to escape and flee. Fools, they eat the money behind the dead. I know they have already cut off Florice's organs.

Have you ever seen a dead person bleeding as was the case with Florice's body? This proves that they had already cut off the private parts like the testicles. And his sex is gone. They cut him everything off I assure you because it was I who opened this place (the body bag). Florice should not be abandoned like this. (saved by authors)

On September 9, 2019 another body was removed from a morgue by members of two civil society groups in Beni. Though the individual had died in a skirmish, the body may have contained the Ebola virus, and those in contact with the body may have initiated a new close contact chain of Ebola infection. Moreover, civil society groups then called for a 2-day cessation of all business in Beni, including the Ebola response, to draw attention to inadequate government security measures—meaning the violence had direct and indirect impacts on preventing the spread of EVD. Local civic groups essential for securing support for the Ebola response instead became roadblocks to success, fueled by a potent mix of disaffection and misinformation.

Communities in the DRC were often unwilling to allow EVD response units into their neighborhoods based on a lack of trust, fearing community members would be wrongfully taken to a treatment center and not return, whether they had Ebola or not, and unwilling to let their family members be kept in a morgue rather than buried according to their own traditions. Fear and mistrust led to response teams being attacked as they entered these communities and turned Ebola treatment centers into symbolic, stationary targets for expressing local disapproval of the Ebola response's presence. Treatment centers were often attacked (shot at or burned), though these acts usually did not come without warning. Social analytics tools applied at the time highlighted offline written letters posted in the community (retrieved by field team networks) threatening violence, as well as online threats and warnings posted in more private social media channels. This allowed adequate threat assessment and warning to be provided to operational teams so they could be better prepared for potential violence.

Throughout the PALM study, the Social Analytics team provided weekly updates. Since the SMC team included the DRC Ministry of Health, the MOH representative could provide the information to the Incident Management Team. With permission from the DRC MOH the information was provided to the WHO (◘ Fig. 8).

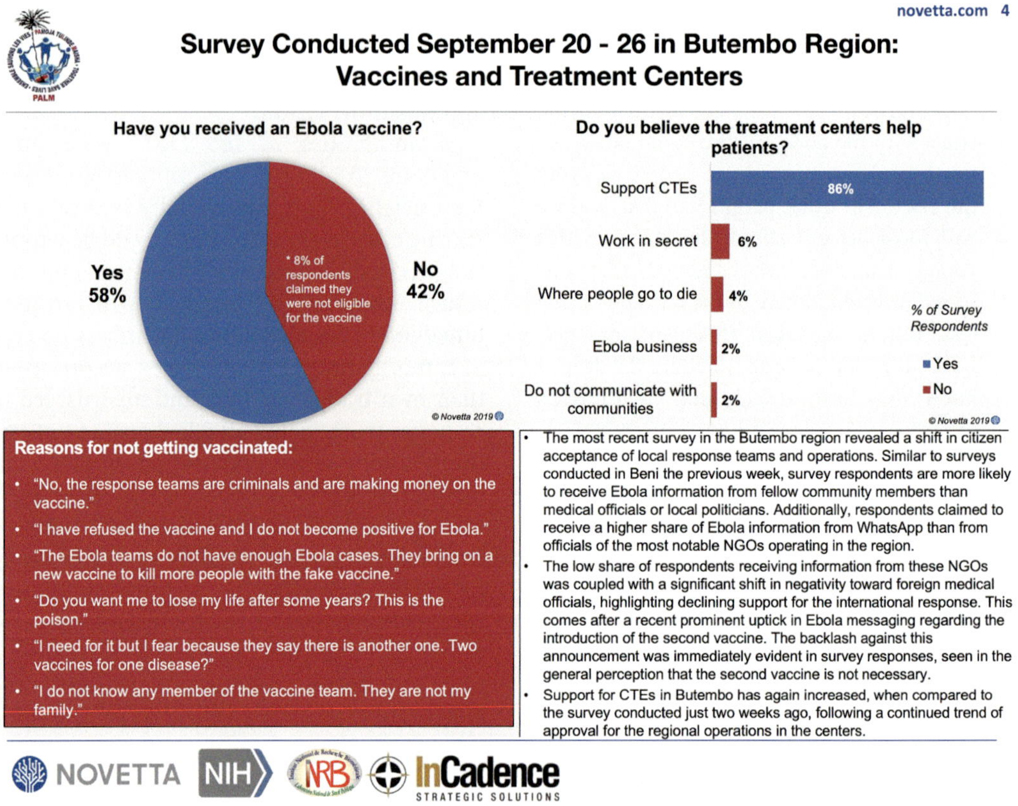

Fig. 8 Results of an opinion survey during the Ebola outbreak in eastern DRC. Public attitudes matter not only for vaccine uptake but also for assessment of the threat environment health care responders and researchers face. (NIAID)

4 Information and Misinformation Flow During Epidemics

4.1 COVID-19

As of 2023, the world appears to be slowly emerging from multiple waves of the COVID-19 pandemic. Sharp application of social analytics in this framework has been essential, especially considering the global scale of the at-risk population and the storm of misinformation, disinformation, and dangerous rumors that have characterized the pandemic. Obviously, hyper-local field teams for RCCE do not scale as well in this environment. Still, countless information campaigns operated locally benefit from social analytics tools for their own intake and analysis of public narratives in regional media and social media to measure their impact on local perceptions.

As we examine misinformation concerning COVID-19, we see significant patterns informed by our previous work on EVD. The intensity of feeling is very strong, specifically concerning the numerous COVID-19 vaccines that have become available since 2021. The vaccine question is, therefore, of particular interest since we expect cultural patterns that developed and hardened for COVID-19 to endure and repeat themselves when effective but novel and misunderstood vaccines are approved for future disease response. Vaccine skepticism, already classified as one of the top ten global health threats by WHO in 2019, seems to be growing in the wake of COVID-19 and may even be imperiling routine childhood vaccinations (Hotez 2022; WHO 2019). The next section will examine some of these high-level themes and detailed examples we have observed from misinformation concerning EVD and COVID-19.

4.2 The Velocity of Misinformation

"Falsehood flies, and the Truth comes limping after it" (Swift 1710). In a rapidly spreading outbreak, rumors and misinformation may be the only thing that outpaces the pathogen. The specifics of exactly what narratives are circulating among certain subgroups in a given week are extremely volatile. The WHO has introduced the term "infodemic," meaning "too much information, including false or misleading information in digital and physical environments during a disease outbreak" (WHO 2022). We have seen information echo chambers, splintered channels of communication, large and urgent information gaps, and other difficult situations (Briand et al. 2021). This is a key application for social analytics.

Patterns and themes in rumors and misinformation during disease outbreaks reoccur and mutate but are largely predictable in some form. This chapter focuses on disease misinformation in Africa, but it is reasonable to expect overlap with these patterns and themes anywhere an epidemic occurs, and experience confirms the assumption. As a hurricane picks up strength from warm water and winds, misinformation draws on novel facts and events that draw public and media attention but becomes much more dangerous when it feeds into preexisting stories, narratives, and attitudes that live within a culture. These include mistrust of authorities and experts, skepticism about public health measures and vaccines, and tales of vast conspiracies underlying apparent events. Social analytics helps us better understand how misinformation arises and spreads from small communities to runaway "viral" dissemination. And like a hurricane, while the lifecycle of the misinformation may have some predictability correlated to epidemiological and pharmacological lifecycles, the exact path is uncertain and can cause great damage in unexpected places.

From our work on EVD and COVID-19, we observe *two umbrella themes* of misinformation, each with multiple mature subthemes, which we expect to persist long past the COVID-19 pandemic. We also observe *two recurring behaviors of information flow* that can be but are not necessarily misinformation but should be expected to occur during epidemics and cause damage. We will examine all four in detail.

4.2.1 Global North to Global South Tensions

The first umbrella theme is framed by the Global North exploiting the Global South. This narrative framework is grounded in numerous historical paradigms with enduring economic and political consequences, including emotional overtones. It has its own vast literature (Young 2016), ranging from sober historical analysis and Nobel-prize-winning fiction to unhinged conspiracy theories. The misinformation gathering social currency within this theme frequently draws on subtexts like resisting corrupting influence from Europe, the United States, and multinational corporations or formerly colonized people asserting their power and value by rejecting patronage.

One example, from June 2020, is the U.S. National Institutes of Health (NIH) partnership with the University of Witwatersrand in South Africa to conduct a randomly controlled trial (RCT) for COVID-19 vaccine for patients with and without HIV (Madhi et al. 2021). Numerous voices on social media from central and southern Africa expressed outrage that such trials were not being conducted in the United States or Europe. The common tagline was that the West was treating Africans as guinea pigs for "their" new disease that was not harming Africans as significantly. Another example is the ubiquity of Microsoft founder Bill Gates in rumors and conspiracy theories about the disease, although such rumors are hardly confined to formerly colonized countries (Islam et al. 2021). A fixture of misinformation, in Africa and elsewhere, is that Bill Gates has worked with pharmaceutical companies to include computerized microchips in vaccines to monitor and control individuals who receive it (Ugwu 2021).

4.2.2 Traditional Beliefs and Cultural Stigma

The second umbrella theme arises when public health recommendations create tension with or are counter to traditional beliefs or cultural practices within a local community. Instances of resistance to health advice on such grounds (either by global health workers or local community health officials) can often be hyper-localized to small regions or villages and spread worldwide as well. Social analytics can be a very effective tool in deconstructing and addressing these issues because of its capability to monitor large-scale data from different media (social media, news, field research) and use analytic techniques to surface problematic developments.

Many of these traditional beliefs are rooted in religiosity. During the COVID-19 pandemic, one of the most consistent retorts to public health guidance shared online has been comments (e.g., from Facebook users) that elevate faith in religion above scientific medical advice. A sample of characteristic comments on Facebook in reaction to a factual video about the Omicron variant from December 2021 includes: (1) "GOD ALMIGHTY is in CONTROL…" (2) "COVID 19 pandemic is a created problem, let us wake-up and involve our Almighty God to make it disappear." (3) "We have God, who is bigger than your viruses, keep digging deep and finding names to scare us Our God is well able" (WHO AFRO 2021).

The "mark of the beast" is another consistent anti-vaccine epithet with Christian New Testament origins (NRSV Rev. 13:11–18), that has remained widespread in community conversations during both the Ebola epidemics and the COVID-19 pandemic. The mark of the beast, in the biblical text a visible brand signifying collaboration with evil, has been equated with having received a vaccine that is somehow satanic. This and related ideas have been prevalent for experimental EVD vaccines still in research trials and fully vetted COVID-19 vaccines that have completed clinical trials (Exline et al. 2022).

Another major category of misinformation on COVID-19 is the purported existence of effective herbal remedies, such as COVID Organics. This herbal product has been produced, marketed, and sold by the President of Madagascar and has become a very popular (unproven) therapeutic. Countries across Africa ordered and supplied the herbal treatment to such an extent that the Africa Centres for Disease Control and Prevention (AfCDC) ran clinical trials on its efficacy (Koigi 2021). Incidentally, the remedy contains artemisinin, which, when used improperly, could increase resistance by the malaria parasite to this widely used and proven malaria countermeasure (Nordling 2020). Moreover, when a head of state markets an ineffective medicine, trust in authorities is likely to suffer over the longer term. Misinformation can have many repercussions (◘ Fig. 9).

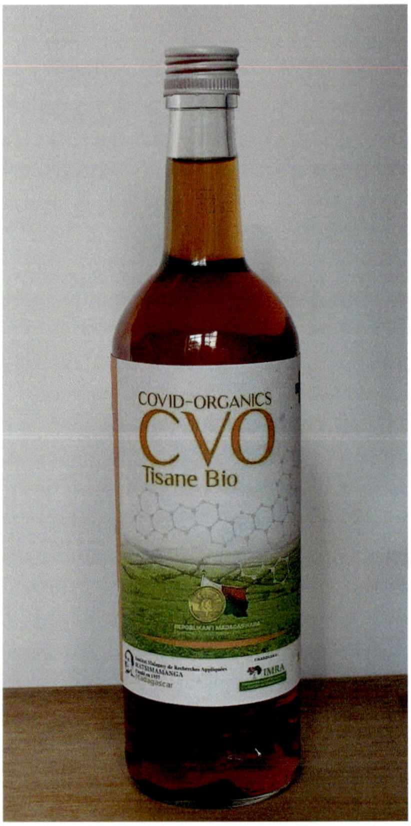

◘ **Fig. 9** Step right up, get your COVID oil! (Photo: Garreth Brown)

4.2.3 External Content Resonating Locally

A characteristic of viral misinformation resonating with local populations in Africa during the COVID-19 pandemic was the sharing of content generated elsewhere, particularly in the media-rich Global North. Social analytics can be extremely useful for anticipating this content as well. While global health operations are necessarily organized geographically for response, they can miss massive viral stories originating outside their area of responsibility. Social analytics can detect these stories, measure their global virality, and prepare epidemic response teams to prevent or respond to any local belief or behavior change the content may influence. This pattern was not as relevant during EVD outbreaks, as the disease had very little direct impact in most of the world and therefore did not generate as much misinformation outside of Africa. However, it was far from absent in the United States (Evans et al. 2016).

A recent example is the discussion of the therapeutic hydroxychloroquine. Several small clinical trials, in most cases not randomized, suggested that hydroxychloroquine had benefits for COVID-19 patients. Larger, better-designed trials found no significant efficacy. Several leaders in the Global North nevertheless promoted hydroxychloroquine, leading to widespread off-label use. The massive resources and media infrastructure of the Global North, combined with widespread mistrust of authorities by many in the population, make it fertile ground for popular rumors and misinformation that are subsequently spread by target populations globally, including in Africa (Equere 2020; Lee et al. 2021).

4.2.4 Lack of Information, Context, and Understanding

Another social behavioral pattern is how the lack of critical information and understanding damages relations between at-risk populations and health providers. One might assume social analytics is not well equipped to make these observations, which may be true in some cases. With good social analytics practice, though, it can sometimes be obvious when two groups of people who should have aligned incentives for epidemic management are talking about wildly different priorities, with each group making assumptions about the other that are simply not true.

A frequent example of this pattern is that global health workers, who are intently focused on mitigating a specific health risk in a community, such as Ebola, may overestimate the level of concern a local population has for that specific disease risk in comparison to other concerns (e.g., other diseases, poverty, physical safety, etc.). Social analytics can play a crucial role in eliciting such information via informed listening to local communities. Sometimes, this data can be misinterpreted to suggest that the target population is simply unaware of certain desirable health advice, but the strategic design of social data gathering can provide insight that the population does know key facts (e.g., COVID-19 vaccines are safe and effective) but have chosen to prioritize other needs.

In the previous section, we discussed how these mismatched perceptions manifested themselves in a chaotic, high-risk security situation in the DRC. There was a strong perception in the early stages that the response to the EVD outbreak in the DRC was disproportionate given the many other hardships in the region. Casualties at the hands of local rebel factions or DRC security forces in the northeastern DRC region where the 2018–2020 Ebola outbreak was centered were viewed as a matter for the DRC government and United Nations (UN) peacekeepers but largely ignored otherwise (MacLean 2017). Well-funded EVD response teams would test for new cases and hire security protection for treatment facilities while leaving citizens in harm's way, leading to quickly developed anger and resentment toward the Ebola response, a disease about which many in the region had little or no real understanding. In fact, a 2019 measles outbreak in the DRC killed more than twice as many people as died of Ebola, while international attention remained focused on the latter (Nachega et al. 2020).

5 Conclusion

How can we counter damaging misinformation and rumors during health emergencies, given they are constantly changing and vary among populations and communities? Real-time, community-specific, frequently updated information is invaluable for research response and overall emergency response. During the age of rapid misinformation and intentional disinformation, the value of social analytics in health is critical and expanding. Social analytics offers a versatile tool in places with little understanding or acceptance of measures to prevent and respond to disease. It can rapidly identify and assess misinformation, rumors, and obstacles to response.

Tailored analysis of current, high-resolution data helps responders tailor messaging and other interventions. Where unbiased reports are scarce, and misinformation is rampant, applying these lessons can make a real difference.

Discussion Questions

1. The benefits and operational utility of social analytics techniques to evaluate the social characteristics of communities at risk enabled the authors to support the NIAID EVD research response in Liberia and the eastern DRC. In this context,
   (a) Define social analytics in terms of its holistic approach to available social data.
   (b) Discuss the mechanics of effective social analytics.
   (c) What is the key capability of any social analytics system?
   (d) Why must social media data be interpreted cautiously?
   (e) Under what circumstances may social analytics fall flat?
2. One essential application of social analytics is to monitor potential threats to the safety of research staff, healthcare workers, and patients. When did social analytics discover, validate, and rapidly communicate signs of deteriorating safety conditions to operations teams in Liberia and the DRC?
3. Effective social analytics for outbreak preparedness begins with understanding and accounting for predictable elements within the social context of disease outbreaks. When using social analytics to compare the flow of information, misinformation, and disinformation during EVD epidemics and the COVID-19 pandemic, the authors observed the emergence of certain predictable, harmful patterns: *umbrella themes* of misinformation and *recurring behaviors of information flow.* Discuss an example of each.

References

Bernard R, Bowsher G, Sullivan R, Gibson-Fall F. Disinformation and epidemics: anticipating the next phase of biowarfare. Health Secur. 2021;19(1):3–12. https://doi.org/10.1089/hs.2020.0038.

Briand SC, Cinelli M, Nguyen T, Lewis R, Prybylski D, Valensise CM, et al. Infodemics: a new challenge for public health. Cell. 2021;184(25):6010–4. https://doi.org/10.1016/j.cell.2021.10.031.

Dragioti E, Li H, Tsitsas G, Lee KH, Choi J, Kim J, et al. A large-scale meta-analytic atlas of mental health problems prevalence during the COVID-19 early pandemic. J Med Virol. 2022;94(5):1935–49. https://doi.org/10.1002/jmv.27549.

Equere F. Dr Stella Immanuel Covid hydroxychloroquine video: Facebook remove viral post of doctor Wey say she use di drug to treat over 300 coronavirus patients for US. BBC News. 2020.

Evans NG, Smith TC, Majumder MS. Sections III, The politics of Ebola, and IV, Mainstream and social media response. In: Evans NG, Smith TC, Majumder MS, editors. Ebola's message: public health and medicine in the twenty-first century. Basic bioethics. MIT Press; 2016. p. 83–172.

Exline JJ, Pait KC, Wilt JA, Schutt WA. Demonic and divine attributions around COVID-19 vaccines: links with vaccine attitudes and behaviors, QAnon and conspiracy beliefs, anger, spiritual struggles, religious and political variables, and supernatural and apocalyptic beliefs. Religions. 2022;13(6):519.

Higgs ES, Dubey SA, Coller BAG, Simon JK, Bollinger L, Sorenson RA, et al. Accelerating vaccine development during the 2013-2016 west African Ebola virus disease outbreak. Curr Top Microbiol Immunol. 2017;411:229–61. https://doi.org/10.1007/82_2017_53.

Hotez PJ. Will anti-vaccine activism in the USA reverse global goals? Nat Rev Immunol. 2022;22(9):525–6. https://doi.org/10.1038/s41577-022-00770-9.
Islam MS, Kamal A-HM, Kabir A, Southern DL, Khan SH, Hasan SMM, et al. COVID-19 vaccine rumors and conspiracy theories: the need for cognitive inoculation against misinformation to improve vaccine adherence. PLoS One. 2021;16(5):e0251605. https://doi.org/10.1371/journal.pone.0251605.
Koigi R. Madagascar's controversial herbal remedy for COVID-19. Fair Planet. 2021.
Lee Z, Rayner CR, Forrest JI, Nachega JB, Senchaudhuri E, Mills EJ. The rise and fall of hydroxychloroquine for the treatment and prevention of COVID-19. Am J Trop Med Hyg. 2021;104(1):35–8. https://doi.org/10.4269/ajtmh.20-1320.
MacLean D. Impact of violence on medical and humanitarian services in North Kivu, DRC. Brussels: Médecins Sans Frontières. Analysis Department M, Brussels; 2017.
Madhi SA, Koen AL, Izu A, Fairlie L, Cutland CL, Baillie V, et al. Safety and immunogenicity of the ChAdOx1 nCoV-19 (AZD1222) vaccine against SARS-CoV-2 in people living with and without HIV in South Africa: an interim analysis of a randomised, double-blind, placebo-controlled, phase 1B/2A trial. Lancet HIV. 2021;8(9):e568–e80. https://doi.org/10.1016/s2352-3018(21)00157-0.
Mulangu S, Dodd LE, Davey RT Jr, Tshiani Mbaya O, Proschan M, Mukadi D, et al. A randomized, controlled trial of Ebola virus disease therapeutics. N Engl J Med. 2019;381(24):2293–303. https://doi.org/10.1056/NEJMoa1910993.
Nachega JB, Mbala-Kingebeni P, Otshudiema J, Zumla A, Tam-Fum JM. The colliding epidemics of COVID-19, Ebola, and measles in The Democratic Republic of the Congo. Lancet Glob Health. 2020;8(8):e991–e2. https://doi.org/10.1016/s2214-109x(20)30281-3.
Nguyen V-K. An epidemic of suspicion—Ebola and violence in the DRC. N Engl J Med. 2019;380:1298. https://doi.org/10.1056/NEJMp1902682.
Nordling L. Unproven herbal remedy against COVID-19 could fuel drug-resistant malaria, scientists warn. Science. 2020. https://doi.org/10.1126/science.abc6665.
Spinney L. Fighting Ebola is hard. In: Congo, fake news makes it harder. Science; 2019. https://doi.org/10.1126/science.aaw6657.
Stearns J. North Kivu: the background to conflict in north Kivu province of eastern Congo. Usalama Project. London: Rift Valley Institute; 2012.
Swift J. Essay upon the art of political lying. The Examiner. 1710;(15):2
Toepfl F, Kravets D, Ryzhova A, Beseler A. Who are the plotters behind the pandemic? Comparing Covid-19 conspiracy theories in Google search results across five key target countries of Russia's foreign communication. Inf Commun Soc. 2023;26(10):2033–51. https://doi.org/10.1080/1369118X.2022.2065213.
Ugwu K. There is silence. Facebook; 2021.
Wells CR, Pandey A, Ndeffo Mbah ML, Gauzere BA, Malvy D, Singer BH, et al. The exacerbation of Ebola outbreaks by conflict in The Democratic Republic of the Congo. Proc Natl Acad Sci USA. 2019;116(48):24366–72. https://doi.org/10.1073/pnas.1913980116.
WHO. Ten threats to global health in 2019. Spotlight; 2019.
WHO. Ending an Ebola outbreak in a conflict zone. Geneva: World Health Organization; 2020. https://storymaps.arcgis.com/stories/813561c780d44af38c57730418cd96cd. Accessed 7 Dec 2020.
WHO. Infodemic. Geneva: World Health Organization; 2022. https://www.who.int/health-topics/infodemic#tab=tab_1. Accessed 16 Feb 2022.
WHO AFRO. Here are the facts on the new #Omicron variant. Facebook; 2021.
Young RJC. Postcolonialism: a historical introduction. Chichester, UK: Wiley; 2016.

19 Understanding and Reporting the Natural History of an Infectious Disease

Ian Crozier

Contents

This project has been funded in whole or in part with federal funds from the National Cancer Institute, National Institutes of Health, under Contract No. 75N91019D00024. The content of this publication does not necessarily reflect the views or policies of the Department of Health and Human Services, nor does mention of trade names, commercial products, or organizations imply endorsement by the U.S. Government.
Learning Track Note: This chapter appears in Learning Tracks: Clinical Research

E. S. Higgs and R. A. Sorenson (eds.), *Principles and Practice of Emergency Research Response*,
https://doi.org/10.1007/978-3-031-48408-7_28

Learning Objectives

This chapter should enable readers to understand and discuss:

- The stages, outcomes, and potential modification of the natural history of an infectious disease in patients
- The importance of understanding the natural history
- The intrinsic determinants of the natural history
- Common obstacles to conducting natural history studies in outbreaks
- Strategies to improve the natural history research response in outbreaks

1 Introduction

When a novel or reemerging pathogen begins to infect large numbers of people in a short period, a concerted emergency research response is required. Preclinical and clinical research to characterize and understand the natural history of a disease and its determinants is critical for improving patient care and outcomes, including through the development of medical countermeasures (MCMs). For example, HIV/AIDS almost inevitably resulted in disability and death for many years after the first clinical descriptions (CDC 1981, 1982; Fauci and Lane 2020; Lundgren et al. 2023). After an inexcusably slow start in the eyes of many patients, HIV/AIDS ultimately motivated collaborative, well-resourced research attention to understand the natural history in a broad global effort (Fauci 2021) that led to effective therapeutics. Persons infected with HIV/AIDS now generally enjoy a high quality of life for a near-normal span, provided they receive timely diagnosis and standard treatment. This represents a remarkable redirection of the natural history of an infectious disease once correctly seen as a death sentence.

Four decades later, but far more rapidly, the natural history of COVID-19 after SARS-CoV-2 infection has arguably received more clinical, research, and public health attention than any infectious disease in history. Well-resourced research at unprecedented scale, pace, and high level of resolution has made it possible relatively quickly to provide better care and improve clinical outcomes. A detailed understanding of the natural history of the human-SARS-CoV-2 interaction has been essential to the accelerated development of preventive and therapeutic countermeasures.

Until the COVID-19 pandemic response made it plain, the need to integrate research into infectious disease emergency response was slow to win broad acceptance, even as the scientific tools facilitating an accelerated research response were becoming increasingly powerful and available. Similar efforts were not normative in the past; with few exceptions, understanding and reporting the natural history of clinical disease caused by novel or new-variant pathogens lagged behind public health response and other research efforts. An absent, incomplete, or at best low-resolution picture of the natural history of clinical disease in humans has historically been the rule for most emerging or reemerging infectious diseases. We focus in this chapter on general principles important to understanding and reporting natural history to improve patient outcomes, illustrating these using prototypic examples of infectious diseases that have posed historical and may pose future challenges.

2 Framework

2.1 Defining Terms: The Natural History of an Infectious Disease

As articulated by the U.S. Food and Drug Administration (FDA), *natural history* refers to the "course a disease takes in the absence of intervention in individuals with the disease, from the disease's onset until either the disease's resolution or the individual's death" (FDA/CDER 2019). Another description adds detail: the "natural course of a disease from the time immediately prior to its inception, progressing through its pre-symptomatic phase and different clinical stages to the point where it has ended and the patient is either cured, chronically disabled, or dead without external intervention" (de la Paz et al. 2010; Jewell 2016). Although typically emphasized in the study of cancer and rare genetic diseases, fundamental concepts of the natural history are crucial to consider in understanding and treating diseases caused by infectious pathogens.

A distinguishing feature of the natural history of an *infectious* disease is that it emerges from an evolving host–pathogen interaction, including an exposure that leads to an infection (acute or persistent); the onset of a disease syndrome (acute or chronic); and outcomes traditionally captured at either individual (as disability, dysfunction, or death); or population levels (as morbidity or mortality). We consider these stages in greater depth below, focusing on the clinical bedside and patient outcomes, the importance of understanding the natural history, factors determining the natural history, and how the natural history is optimally captured, understood, and reported to improve clinical outcomes.

2.2 Context: Infectious Disease Outbreaks

Effectively understanding and reporting disease natural history presents particular challenges for patients, clinicians, and researchers in infectious disease outbreaks.[1] This chapter focuses on understanding and reporting natural history in the context of historic, current, and future infectious disease outbreaks of epidemic and pandemic potential, i.e., the infectious diseases that have given rise to Public Health Emergencies of International Concern (PHEIC) since the International Health Regulations were revised in 2005 (WHO 2016) and those considered high risk for future emergencies. Past is prologue, and the research measures that have been most effective should carry forward into response to future outbreaks, with improvements made possible by scientific and technological advances and organizational refinements (Simpson et al. 2020; Van Kerkhove et al. 2021). For example, virus families of concern are included in the prototype pathogen approach (▶ Chap. 12) (Cassetti et al. 2022; Ford et al. 2023). A few selected examples—COVID-19, Ebola virus disease, Lassa fever, and mpox—will be explored here in more depth, with reference to other infectious diseases where relevant.

1 There is no bright line distinction between ongoing infectious disease burdens and outbreak emergencies, which can arise because of a new genetic variant rather than a new pathogen, particularly in the era of antimicrobial resistance. For example, the ancient global burden of tuberculosis (TB) has in recent years produced an extensively drug-resistant strain considered a global health emergency requiring urgent action (CDC 2007; Gandhi et al. 2006; Raviglione and Smith 2007). Outbreaks of artemisinin-resistant malaria in southeast Asia and Africa (Ashley et al. 2014; Balikagala et al. 2021; Dondorp et al. 2009; Raviglione and Smith 2007) or the threat of other antibiotic-resistant bacterial pathogens also elide the distinction (Laxminarayan 2022; Murray et al. 2022).

2.3 Target: Patient-Centered Care

The interplay between the natural history of the *individual's* health and *public or community* health cannot be disentangled, especially in infectious disease outbreaks. Though perspectives on the relative primacy of the individual or the community vary dramatically among cultures, we focus here primarily on how an infectious disease evolves in individual patients. In the clinical and clinical research setting, natural history may be best characterized at the level of resolution of the individual patient (or larger groups of individual patients) as disease manifests, evolves, and is modulated. There is much to be said about how an infectious disease outbreak evolves at population and community levels, but these themes are covered elsewhere (▶ Chaps. 21 and 26, In Focus 21.1).

2.4 Approach: Principles and Practice

In considering the importance of understanding and reporting the natural history of an infectious disease with the goal of improving care for patients, each section will first consider general principles broadly applicable across diseases and outbreaks, while recognizing that each infection, disease, and outbreak setting is unique. More concrete examples will follow, drawing predominantly from a few exemplary infectious diseases (COVID-19, Ebola virus disease [EVD], Lassa fever, and mpox). Practical examples may highlight disease-specific successes, but more often than not illustrate knowledge gaps, cautionary notes related to current uncertainty, research attention needed to remedy uncertainty, and suggested strategies to address these gaps in the future.

3 Stages of the Natural History and Outcomes in Outbreaks

3.1 Overview: Through the Lens of the Host–Pathogen–Care Interaction

The clinician working in emergency outbreak response usually interacts with patients presumed to be ill with the disease of concern, either presenting for care or having received some initial care. The provision of even the most basic clinical care is by definition an "intervention." Despite the natural history definitions above, observation absent any medical intervention would be unethical in human clinical care or research (unlike animal modeling). We will consider the natural history and its outcomes through the *host–pathogen–care* framework, focusing specifically on medical aspects of clinical care. Effective redirection of the natural history requires consideration of the features of the host–pathogen interaction that determine infection, disease, and the outcomes of that disease in an infected individual. General considerations applicable to most infectious diseases will be illuminated by pathogen- and disease-specific examples.

As seen in ◘ Fig. 1, the natural history can be considered in stages, beginning with an *exposure* (1A) of a human host to a virus that may lead to an *infection*. An infection may cause (1B) symptoms or signs of *disease* that vary across a spectrum of severity; those with significant disease are more likely to come to medical attention and receive clinical care (1C), eventually leading to immediate (acute) and longer-term *outcomes* (1D). Understanding the determinants of outcomes requires consideration of features intrinsic to the host, the virus, and the exposure. The interplay between these antecedents determines emergent features of the natural history. For example, peak viral load or viral load at admission, often among the strongest predictors of outcome, is not determined solely by the virus, the host, or the exposure, but emerges from their complex interaction, which in turn reflects increasingly complex interactions at multiple levels between a pathogen and human physiological systems, organs, tissues, cells, and so on. This host–pathogen–care heuristic will anchor much of the subsequent discussion which focuses on the clinical bedside and outcomes. Later sections consider how intrinsic host, virus, and exposure characteristics might determine the natural history.

3.1.1 Distinguishing Between Infection and Disease

As defined epidemiologically (as distinguished from a molecular virological definition), "pathogenicity" describes the proportion of infected persons who develop signs or symptoms, while "virulence" refers to the proportion who develop severe disease or death (CDC 2012). Characterization of the natural history is most important in hospitalized patients, who are at risk for the worst outcomes, and on whom we focus in ► Sect. 3.2. However, it is important to recognize the disease spectrum after most viral infections includes subclinical or mild disease in many if not most cases: failure to recognize this might impact the clinician or clinical researcher's analysis of risk-benefit in decision making and research study design. For most viral infections, the longer-term natural history in infected patients with asymptomatic or only mild disease is unclear, but might reasonably be assumed to be less consequential. Whether

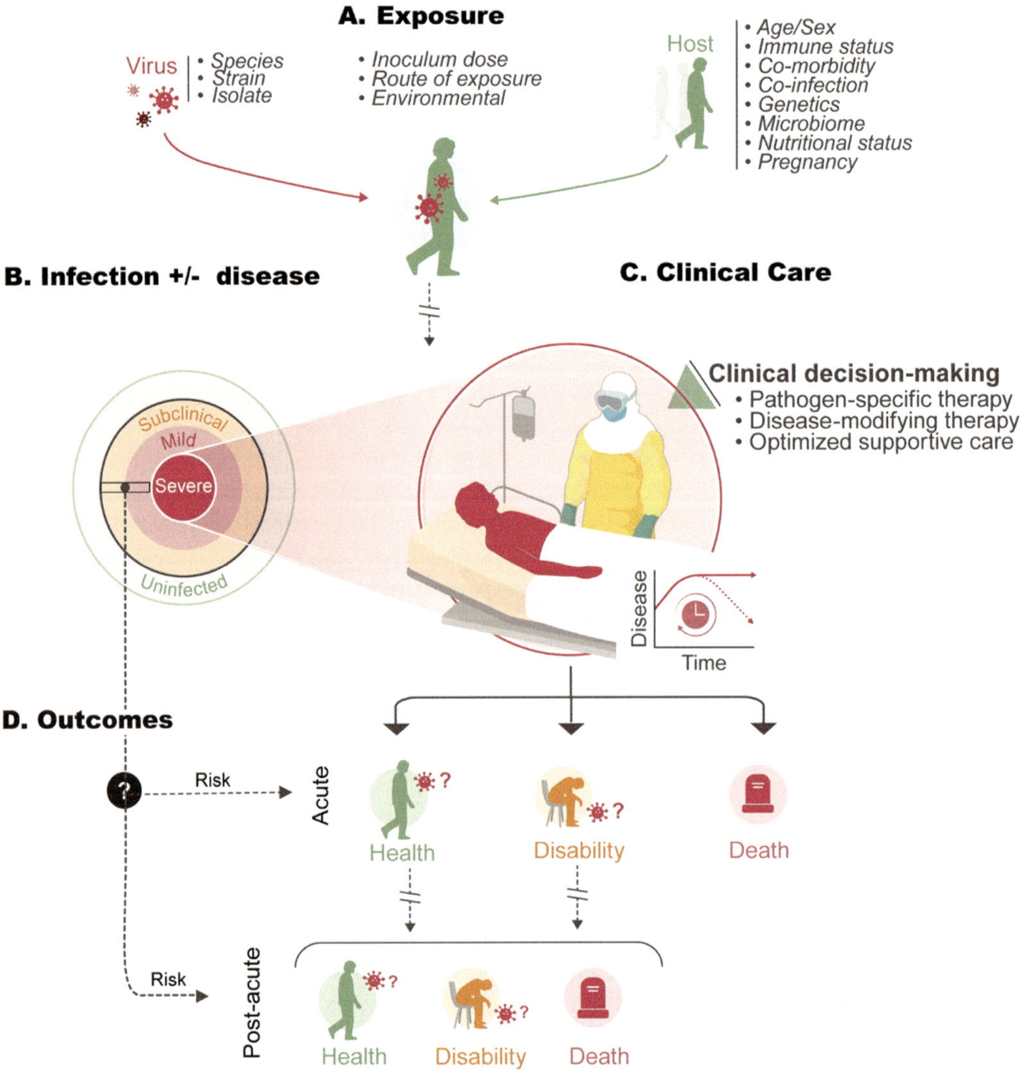

Fig. 1 Stages of the natural history and outcomes. (Author, artwork by Jiro Wada)

the same is true for the public-health risks associated with asymptomatic or subclinical infection, namely, viral persistence that could cause new outbreaks, most likely depends on the specific viral infection.

3.1.2 Practice: Distinction Between the Infection Fatality Rate (IFR) and the Case Fatality Rate (CFR)

The COVID-19 pandemic has demonstrated the importance of distinguishing between outcomes in all those infected vs. those who come to medical attention. With rare exceptions, this holds true for almost all viral pathogens. It has long been recognized, for example, that most serologically confirmed infections with Lassa virus (LASV) do not cause clinical disease, producing a very low IFR. Hospitalization with confirmed Lassa fever, by contrast, is associated with CFRs >20 to 50% (Buba et al. 2018; Grant et al. 2023; Okokhere et al. 2018). Some of these distinctions have only become apparent when large outbreaks prompted careful research into the infection vs. disease spectrum. For example, the CFR of Ebola virus disease

(EVD) was presumed for many years to be >70 to 80% and to approximate the IFR. Since the first identification of EVD in 1976, the CFRs from the few larger outbreaks (of >100 patients) corroborated this assumption (Jacob et al. 2020). More recent outcomes from much larger outbreaks in West Africa (2014–2016) suggest a lower overall CFR even in the absence of virus-specific therapeutics (Rojek et al. 2019), and a wider spectrum of disease that includes individuals who were exposed and infected but did not develop, recognize, or recall clinical symptoms (Gayedyu-Dennis et al. 2023; Glynn et al. 2017; Kelly et al. 2022; Timothy et al. 2019).

3.2 The Clinical Bedside and the Evolving Natural History

3.2.1 Overview

For obvious reasons, understanding the natural history of disease in the hospitalized patient is paramount: disease outcomes are typically modified here as the host–pathogen–care interaction evolves. In that regard, effective clinical management redirects the natural history of an infectious disease on three fronts (◘ Fig. 1c):

1. Safe and effective *pathogen-targeted* therapeutic intervention (e.g., antiviral therapeutics)
2. Safe and effective *disease-modifying* therapeutic intervention (e.g., immunomodulators)
3. Provision of appropriate *supportive care* (e.g., intravenous fluids, organ support) across a spectrum of disease severity

The importance of a clear understanding of the natural history to inform tactics on each front will be further explored after outlining key principles that include several cautions. Inadequate characterization of the natural history is the rule early in infectious disease outbreaks and is inescapable with a novel pathogen. Timely capture and reporting of early clinical signals are crucial to urgently informing patient care, optimizing standards of supportive care (▶ Chap. 20), and setting the stage for well-designed, well-conducted clinical trials to identify safe and effective medical countermeasures (MCMs). Accurate natural history begins to resolve key research questions to be answered in clinical trials:

- Is a specific intervention safe and effective?
- For which patient population?
- At what stage of infection or disease?
- At which dose and by which route?
- In which clinical setting?

3.2.2 Capturing Natural History Data at the Clinical Beside

After diagnosis, characterization of clinical disease should routinely capture:

- Host demographics
- Medical history (including clinical symptoms of presenting illness, antecedent treatment, and targeted review of systems; exposures; comorbid conditions; chronic medications; and vaccination history)
- Clinical signs (including vital signs; relevant physical examination, including the presence of intravenous access)
- Clinical laboratory features (especially of organ dysfunction or disease-related complications)
- Viral load (in blood and other relevant diagnostic samples)
- Clinical or postmortem pathology when available

Additional technical capacity, when available, captures more data, often at higher resolution. Electrocardiography and medical imaging, for example, can be very useful but have typically not been available during most outbreaks.

In addition to descriptive characterization of the presenting illness, investigation should also follow disease evolution over time and in response to intervention. Especially with the severe disease seen in outbreaks that become emergencies, a single snapshot at the clinical bedside cannot reliably predict disease course or outcomes. Indeed, accurately describing the natural history requires effectively mapping dynamic interactions between the pathogen (load, location) and the host (response, damage), with the goal of illuminating how the interactions determine outcomes and if, how, and when the disease trajectory may be redirected. As observations accrue, clinicians and researchers are increasingly able to delineate key phases of disease expression to inform therapeutic intervention.

3.2.3 Caution: Beware of Assumptions

Predictors of outcome may exist for diseases caused by some of these pathogens, but their reliability is often uncertain. Knowledge is often very limited; even in the rare cases when a relatively thorough understanding of the natural history is available, outcome predictors generated in under-resourced clinical settings may not be predictive in others. For example, the delivery of advanced supportive care, including extracorporeal support, to critically ill patients with Ebola virus disease had been considered by some clinicians to be futile prior to 2014. Albeit in a limited number of patients, the delivery of advanced care provided proof-of-principle that the natural history of EVD could be redirected even in patients with extremely high viral loads and multisystem organ failure (see ▶ Sect. 3.2.5) (Uyeki et al. 2016b).

3.2.4 Caution: Beware of Magic-Bullet Thinking

Clinical and research attention in outbreak settings has historically focused first on pathogen-specific interventions; more recent attention during the COVID-19 pandemic has also focused on host-directed disease-modifying therapies, e.g., immunomodulatory approaches. At times historically, supportive care efforts have lagged, and have often been under-emphasized during infectious disease outbreaks. Disease-specific therapeutics may be critical to success at the bedside, but are not "magic bullets" that can be uncoupled from effective supportive care as part of a complete bundle of optimized standard of care (SOC). With optimized SOC, all available strategies are deployed to prevent or mitigate clinical symptoms and signs, organ dysfunction and damage, severe disease and death, and clinical sequelae and pathogen persistence in survivors. Effective use of available treatment strategies depends on efficient understanding and reporting of the natural history and rapid dissemination of findings. Increasingly, "living" clinical care guidelines (▶ Chap. 20) that are regularly updated as the evidence base evolves provide clinicians in outbreak settings with near real-time access to the most current standard of care (SOC) recommendations.

3.2.5 Caution: Beware of Clinical Operational Gaps

Understanding the natural history and redirecting it effectively are resource-intensive endeavors, whether one relies on pathogen-directed interventions, disease-modifying interventions, or optimized SOC. Many clinical operational challenges arise in outbreak settings, including shortages of requisite medical staff, infrastructure, supplies, systems, and security. Renewed motivation and capacity improvements to provide more advanced clinical care and clinical research support in resource-limited outbreak settings have been increasingly evident in recent years, and further efforts are under active discussion at both national and international levels (GPMB 2023; WHO 2022a, b). Nevertheless, challenges intrinsic to under-resourced settings are likely to hinder optimal SOC and clinical research for years to come. Even in well-resourced settings, inadequate understanding of the natural history of a novel infectious disease, as in the early phase of the COVID-19 pandemic response, can lead to suboptimal clinical care, flawed research study design, and unintended harm to patients.

3.2.6 Practice: The Evolving Role of Optimized SOC in EVD

Over many decades after Ebola virus was first identified in 1976, typical clinical care provided in "Ebola isolation units" consisted only of the most basic case management. Patients received limited supportive care targeting the relief of symptoms (fever, pain), the prevention and treatment of dehydration (usually oral), and basic empiric treatment of possible bacterial or malarial coinfections. Delivery of even this minimal bundle of supportive care was constrained by lack of well-trained staff and supplies, suboptimal care environments, and uncertainty about protecting caregivers from infection; even the use of intravenous fluid replacement was considered controversial. Clinical laboratory testing was often unavailable near treatment units. Recognition of the need to improve care, especially in the face of consistently high case fatality, led to calls from the community to refocus on the clinical bedside and patient (Bausch et al. 2007).

Early in the historically largest West Africa EVD outbreak (2014–2016), calls to improve supportive care continued, but progress was limited by frequent resource-mission mismatches as unprepared healthcare facilities and rapidly erected treatment units were overwhelmed in a rapidly expanding outbreak. During the outbreak, a small number of EVD patients were cared for in well-resourced healthcare settings in the United States and Europe. Based on these few observations, the delivery of advanced supportive care that included extracorporeal organ support provided an important proof-of-principle that optimal SOC could be provided safely and effectively to critically ill EVD patients (Uyeki et al. 2016b). These observations also enabled the first high-resolution descriptions of multi-system organ dysfunction and "critical illness phenotypes" in EVD. The asymmetry in care provided and outcomes led to renewed emphasis on the need to develop the evidence base and improve delivery of optimal SOC in African settings (Lamontagne et al. 2018). Though efforts continued to be limited by resource constraints, exemplary fit-for-purpose EVD treatment units were able to provide advanced SOC to infected healthcare workers in West Africa by the end of the outbreak (Dickson et al. 2018).

Building on these initial steps, the delivery of optimal SOC took a major step forward during the 2018–2020 EVD outbreak in the eastern Democratic Republic of Congo. Significant advances during this outbreak that have become standard of care included key components:

- Novel care structures optimized to provide safe and effective patient-centered care and improve communications between providers, patients, and families (▶ In Practice 40.1)
- Near-treatment unit diagnostic clinical laboratories using standard testing platforms
- Specific guidelines for standardizing optimal SOC in EVD that were rapidly developed, distributed, and trained during the outbreak (WHO 2019)
- Provision of well-trained staff, including in key specialty areas
- Procurement of requisite supplies to operationalize optimal SOC

The commitment to provide this capacity and facilitate the standard delivery of improved SOC was evident throughout this outbreak (Fischer et al. 2019). Importantly, these advances also enabled optimal SOC as part of the PALM RCT that led to the first regulatory approval of two effective Ebola virus-specific therapeutics (▶ In Practice 17.1, 23.1, and 40.1) (Mulangu et al. 2019).

A continued commitment to maintain and improve these standards will be crucial to improve EVD outcomes in the future, particularly in patients with high viral loads and multi-system organ dysfunction, in whom case fatality remains high despite the receipt of effective, pathogen-specific therapeutics. For example, the presence of acute kidney injury (AKI) predicts poorer outcomes even in EVD patients receiving effective therapeutics (Mulangu et al. 2019). Efforts to optimize prevention and management will require a more detailed understanding of the clinical presentation, evolution, risk factors, and pathogenesis of AKI in EVD. Building on prior lessons learned from the care of severely ill patients in the United States and Europe, characterizing the natural history of differing critical illness phenotypes in African patients will be crucial to future success. As illustrated in ◘ Fig. 2, current SOC guidelines for EVD focus on a number of key features of illness and clinical management. Each of these areas

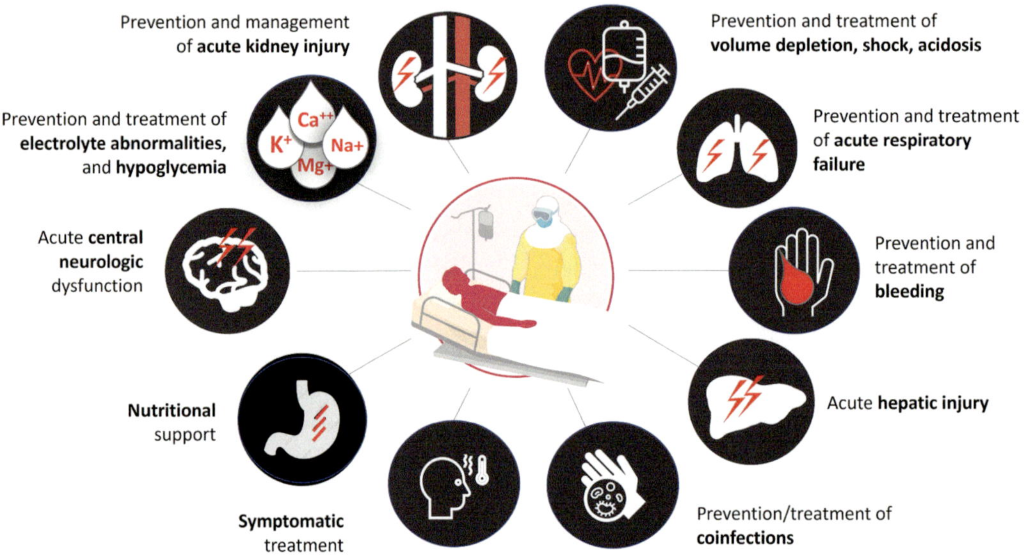

Fig. 2 Advancing optimized standard of care for Ebola virus disease: key focus areas. (Author)

reflects key focus areas for further clinical research to understand the natural history of EVD.

3.3 Outcomes of the Natural History

Accurately describing and reporting outcomes is crucial for clinicians and clinical researchers alike (Fig. 1, 1d). Indeed, the optimal design of clinical studies to identify safe and effective interventions requires defining appropriate candidate interventions with *clinical benefit*, namely improving how a patient *"feels, functions, or survives"* (FDA 2020). Clinical outcomes may be clinician-reported, patient-reported, non-clinician observer-reported, or based on a performance assessment. Assessing both acute and longer-term clinical outcomes is important, as is evaluating viral clearance or persistence.

3.3.1 Acute Clinical and Virologic Outcomes

Historically, the outcomes reported from the clinical bedside in outbreak emergencies have often been limited to death or survival. Caution is needed in extrapolation or comparison of historical or current outbreak case fatality ratios to individual outcomes. Each viral disease comes to be associated with an epidemiologically observed case fatality ratio (CFR); over time and multiple outbreaks, average CFRs are assumed to provide a good indicator for natural history. However, early in outbreaks, the proportion of poor outcomes may seem high, since severe or fatal cases are usually the first to bring a new or re-emerging viral pathogen to attention. These early signals thus tend to exaggerate the severity of the disease based on a subset of the most severe cases. Furthermore, overall outbreak CFRs include all outbreak cases, many of whom may have died in the community rather seeking care at a treatment center.

In addition, accurate understanding of natural history requires characterization of the entire spectrum of clinical outcomes, ranging from full health and well-being to long-term disability or death, along with observed and laboratory-measured indications. Even in patients who fully recover, the individual and public health risks of viral persistence argue for investigation and documentation of pathogen clearance.

3.3.2 Post-acute Clinical and Virologic Outcomes

The potential for acute severe viral infections to leave survivors with fixed (non-evolving) or ongoing (evolving) clinical sequelae has been long recognized, perhaps most famously in the *encephalitis lethargica* syndromes described after the 1918 influenza pandemic (Berger and Vilensky 2014). Given the emergency response required in infectious disease outbreaks, often in challenging and under-resourced settings, and the difficulty in following large numbers of survivors, it is perhaps not surprising that post-acute clinical sequelae of these diseases have not received a great deal of clinical or research attention until recently. Renewed interest was provoked by follow-up of survivors of the 2014–2016 West Africa EVD outbreak (see ▶ Sect. 3.3.3), and more recently by "long COVID," or post-acute sequelae of COVID-19 (PASC). Determining the causes of post-acute sequelae can be challenging. They may be a generic consequence of severe and prolonged critical illness, as in the increasingly recognized "post-intensive care syndrome" (Nakanishi et al. 2021; Quinn et al. 2023). They may be specific to the viral infection and disease of interest. Further considerations include defining whether sequelae are a fixed consequence of organ dysfunction/damage that occurred during acute illness or represent an evolving pathobiologic process—either ongoing infection and/or host immunopathology in the presence or absence of the pathogen. Understanding the natural history and longer-term outcomes accurately likely requires prospective, longitudinal, and well-controlled observational cohorts of survivors.

Recent decades have highlighted the potential for viruses, even those once presumed to cause only acute infections, to persist in tissues or bodily fluids considered to be "immune-privileged". It is heuristically useful to consider viral persistence in terms of consequences for individual and for public health. As illustrated below for EVD survivors, viral persistence poses risks for the individual patient, including recrudescent organ-specific inflammatory syndromes and potential "relapse" of systemic disease that may be clinically indistinguishable from the primary acute infection syndrome. Persistent virus or viral antigens may also contribute to nonspecific post-acute symptoms and signs (e.g., fatigue, arthralgia, and myalgia) or systemic inflammatory syndromes in survivors. Viral persistence may also pose a risk to public health, potentially reigniting human transmission months or even years after an outbreak has ended. For almost all the pathogens under discussion, the host–virus determinants of persistence and these individual or public health consequences remain underdetermined. Viral clearance from blood and other bodily fluids during and after acute infection has become an important virologic outcome, even in clinically recovered patients.

3.3.3 Practice: Clinical Sequelae and Viral Persistence in EVD Survivors

Though long-lasting effects of EVD had been infrequently described since 1976, usually from patient self-report, no controlled observational studies had been published prior to the West Africa outbreak. In its aftermath, case reports and series initially called attention to the need to understand the natural history in EVD survivors in order to address their urgent care needs, and potentially to protect public health. Rapidly assembled small observational cohorts of EVD survivors contributed to a growing understanding, but conclusions from these studies were often limited by the absence of physical examination and clinical laboratory findings. An array of clinical symptoms and signs have been noted in case reports, case series, and observational studies that (at minimum) included physical examination (see ◘ Fig. 2).

However, these data generally came from studies that *did not include closely matched control groups*, which are critical to determine whether particular sequelae are truly associated with EVD. Highlighted in ◘ Fig. 2 are the clinical features that were significantly different between EVD survivors and a group of close contact controls at 1 year of the 5-year PREVAIL III longitudinal natural history study of EVD survivors (Sneller et al. 2019).

Notably, only two of these post-acute clinical syndromes (red dots in ◘ Fig. 3) have been associated with Ebola virus (EBOV) persistence. This result highlights the need to consider both clinical and virologic outcomes and their rare but potential overlap.

Before the West Africa EVD outbreak, very limited data suggested that EBOV or EBOV RNA could persist in survivors, but individual or public health consequences had not been shown (Thorson et al. 2016). It became clear during and after that outbreak that EBOV persistence in immune-privileged tissues and/or bodily fluids had consequences for both the individual survivor and public health (◘ Fig. 4). Emerging data indicated the longer-term persistence of EBOV RNA and in some studies infectious EBOV in the semen of male EVD survivors (Barnes et al. 2017; Deen et al. 2017; Diallo et al. 2016; Fischer et al. 2017; Sissoko et al. 2017a; Sneller et al. 2019; Subtil et al. 2017; Thorson et al. 2021; Uyeki et al. 2016a) (◘ Fig. 4a). Viral persistence in semen was further associated with rare instances of sexual transmission that resulted in ongoing transmission (Diallo et al. 2016; Mate et al. 2015). Case reports of maternal-fetal transmission in pregnant EVD survivors, after resolution of acute EVD or absent previously recognized EBOV infection, signaled a similar public health risk, albeit a rare one (Bower et al. 2016) (◘ Fig. 4b). Finally, the relative risk of maternal-infant transmission of EBOV via breastmilk remains undetermined, but has been strongly suspected to lead to fatal EVD in at least one infant (◘ Fig. 4c) (Sissoko et al. 2017b). Notably, in several of these reports, the mother was not known to have been infected with EBOV, presumably having survived an unrecognized, mild, or subclinical infection.

Individual consequences for EVD survivors have included well-documented case reports of recrudescent organ-specific inflammatory syndromes (uveitis, meningoencephalitis) associated with infectious EBOV persistence (◘ Fig. 4d–e) (Jacobs et al. 2016; Varkey et al. 2015). Though only rarely reported, the actual prevalence of viral persistence and these inflammatory syndromes in the central nervous system (CNS) and eye is unknown. Uncertainty remains about whether such cases presented a public health risk: it had generally been assumed that survivors with viral persistence in the eye or CNS did not pose a threat outside of direct contact with intraocular fluid, cerebrospinal fluid, or associated tissues. During the 2018–2020 EVD outbreak in the Democratic Republic of the Congo (DRC), however, a previously vaccinated patient who was diagnosed with acute EVD subsequently cleared EBOV RNA in blood after treatment with a monoclonal antibody-based therapeutic and recovered. Six months later, the same patient developed severe systemic "EVD-like" illness with detectable EBOV RNA in blood, rapidly decompensated, and died with what was considered an EVD "relapse" after genetic sequencing confirmed relatedness to his initial infection. Given the setting and the severity of illness, cerebrospinal fluid could not be sampled, and relapse from a central nervous system or similar source could not be ruled out. This case led to ongoing human-to-human transmission and more than 90 subsequent EVD cases over a wide geographic area (Mbala-Kingebeni et al. 2021).

Many open questions remain about the risks posed by EBOV persistence in EVD survivors. Routine outbreak genetic sequencing has demonstrated several outbreaks in the DRC to be related to transmission from an EVD survivor (likely from semen) rather than a new zoonotic spillover (Mbala-Kingebeni 2022; Pratt 2021). In 2021, genetic sequencing suggested a new outbreak in Guinea was related to transmission from a survivor from the earlier West Africa EVD outbreak, though the epidemiology and mechanisms of transmission remain unclear (Keita et al. 2021). Open questions include:

- What are the determinants and risk factors for sexual (or other modes of) transmission from EVD survivors with viral persistence?
- Does persistence of virus or viral RNA in semen, which poses a rare but consequential public health risk for sexual transmission, have any health consequences for the individual male survivor?

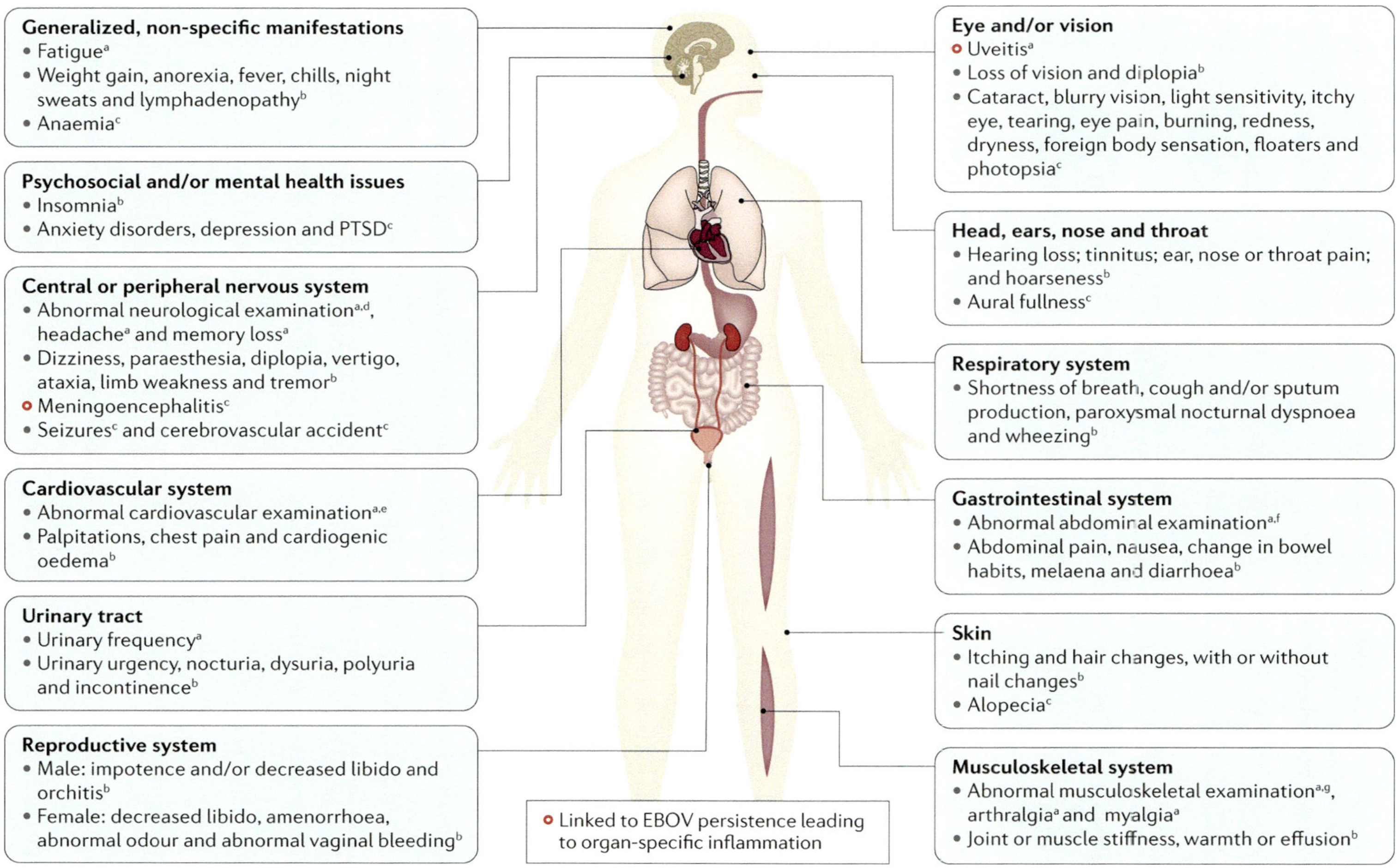

Fig. 3 Post-acute clinical sequelae in observational studies of EVD survivors that included physical examination. Items labeled [a] and [b] are symptoms or signs that were significantly different versus close contact controls in the PREVAIL III Natural History Study (Sneller et al. 2019). Data marked [c] are from uncontrolled cohorts, case series, or case reports. Details of abnormal exam findings ([d–f]) may be found in Jacob et al. (2020) from which figure 3 was reprinted by permission

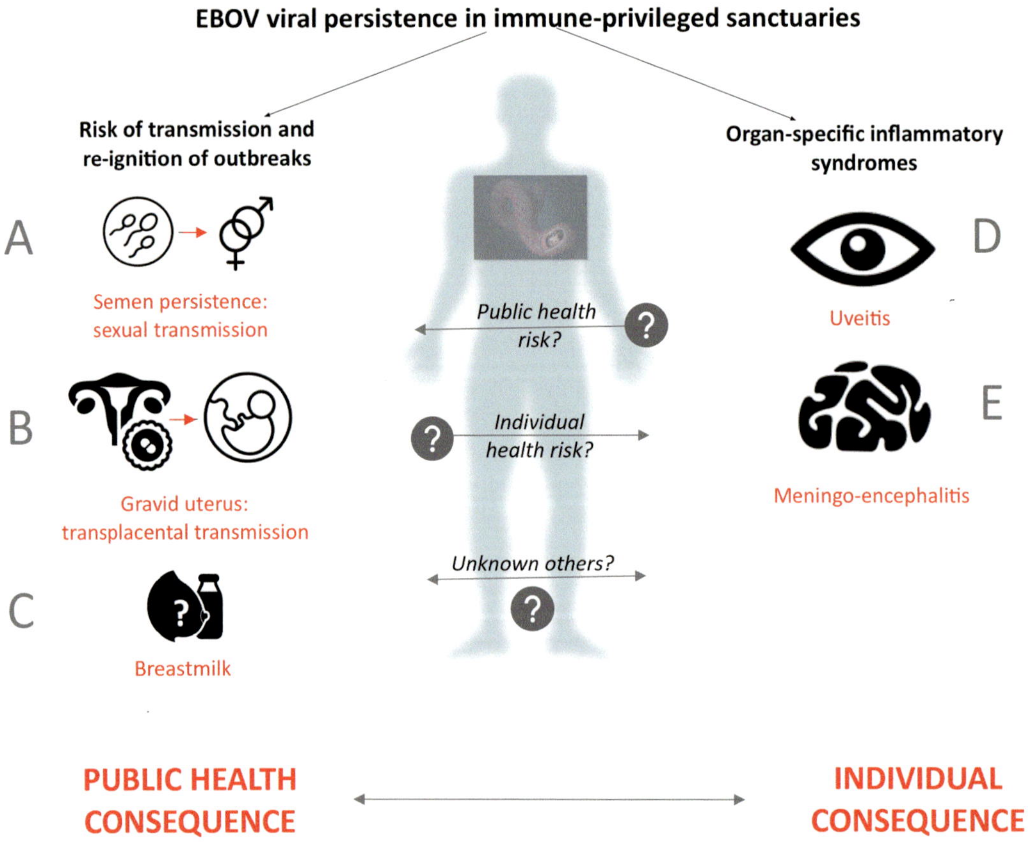

Fig. 4 Individual and public health implications of Ebola virus persistence in EVD survivors. (Author)

- Is EBOV or EBOV antigen persistence associated with very common generalized symptoms (e.g., fatigue, arthralgia/myalgia) seen in many survivors? (Thus far, other tissues or organs in which EBOV persists have not been identified.)
- Are EVD survivors of subclinical infection at risk for viral persistence?
- During acute EVD, what role could EVD-specific therapeutics play in preventing, mitigating, or treating EBOV persistence?
- In EVD survivors, what is the role of EBOV-specific antivirals to clear EBOV RNA (e.g. from the semen of male survivors as one signal suggests) (Higgs et al. 2021)?

Studies to date confirm the need to better understand the host-virus-therapeutic determinants of viral persistence and its recrudescent inflammatory or public health consequences at molecular, cellular, organ/tissue, individual, and population levels. Answering these questions will require well-designed natural history studies of EVD survivors that enable longitudinal long-term follow-up and comparison with well-matched controls.

3.3.4 Viral Persistence in Other Diseases of Interest

Lassa fever virus (LASV) and LASV RNA have recently been shown to persist in the semen of male Lassa fever survivors; thus far, any association with human transmission or any clinical sequelae have not been described (Thielebein et al. 2022). Longer-term viral persistence after acute infection has been documented with SARS-CoV-2, though not in immune-privileged sites in particular. Rather, prolonged detection of virus or viral antigen has been most commonly associated with immunodeficient hosts and with ongoing clinical signs and symptoms. The clinical significance of viral antigen in autopsy tissues from patients who died with COVID-19, even long after the resolution of acute illness, remains unclear (Stein et al. 2022). The relationship of SARS-CoV-2 viral or antigen persistence to post-acute sequelae of COVID-19 (PASC) is also unclear, but it is a hypothetical contributor (Davis et al. 2023; Proal et al. 2023). Similarly, prolonged, severe acute clinical disease associated with mpox (monkeypox) virus (MPXV) has been described in immunodeficient people living with HIV/AIDS, but has not so far been associated with typical immune-privileged sites (Fink et al. 2023; Govind et al. 2023).

4 Why Is Understanding and Reporting the Natural History Important?

4.1 Informing and Optimizing Patient Care and Care Guidelines

Rapid characterization of disease in extremely important to inform the urgent development of standards for clinical care in an outbreak, epidemic, or pandemic. It requires both the experience of clinicians directly caring for patients in the field who are qualified to characterize disease processes as well as expertise capable of gathering and considering evidence as it emerges to develop evidence-based consensus guidelines. In recent infectious disease outbreaks, curation of this development has been managed through globally supported outbreak response networks and rapidly established local, national, and global clinical discussions and guidelines panels. Early results should be published or otherwise disseminated as soon as possible. The widespread use of pre-print servers in medicine since the COVID-19 outbreak began has accelerated access to information before peer review is complete. This has contributed to the ability of emergency clinical guideline panels to gather needed evidence but has also made their expertise essential to weigh that evidence, determine any consensus, and identify outstanding questions. Such expert panels have become a key feature of recent large outbreaks (EVD, mpox, COVID-19) and have produced "living" clinical guidelines that can be updated frequently as new evidence emerges (▶ Chap. 20). These efforts are just the beginning of more careful research efforts to characterize the natural history. A subsequent section will consider how to best continue characterization in the research environment typical of ongoing outbreaks. Early clinical characterization not only informs SOC guidelines but also supports the design of interventional clinical trials to evaluate medical countermeasures (MCMs).

4.2 Informing Rational Design and Implementation of Clinical Trials

Accurate characterization of the natural history is crucial to the rational design of clinical trials to identify safe and effective interventions. Indeed, insufficient or inaccurate understanding of the natural history may lead to clinical trials that are poorly designed, poorly stratified, over- or under-powered, or cannot be generalized to meaningfully impact outcomes. Though clinical trial design and implementation is a focus elsewhere in this volume, a few rational design implications merit mention in this chapter (▶ Chaps. 12, 14, and 22).

4.2.1 Who: Selecting Study Populations

Accurate natural history information is important to identify, define, and select study populations most likely to benefit or at higher risk of harm from an intervention. In clinical trials of a candidate dengue virus vaccine, recognition that excess hospitalizations for dengue fever were observed among vaccine recipients 2–5 years of age who had not had prior dengue virus exposure/seropositivity was an instructive lesson (Sridhar et al. 2018). Prior understanding of the natural history may be valuable to risk stratification in designing randomization strategies. For example, previously described associations between EBOV load at admission (as proxied by the RT-PCR cycle threshold value) and survival informed rational allocation of randomization in the context of the PALM randomized trial of EVD therapeutics (Mulangu et al. 2019).

4.2.2 When: Timing Therapeutic Interventions

High-resolution characterization of the natural history can help distinguish key phases of an infectious disease that may have implications for the best timing of an intervention. For example, early recognition an early "virologic" phase of COVID-19 (driven by viral replication), and a later, "hyperinflammatory" phase (driven by host immunopathology) informed the design of therapeutic trials of antivirals and disease-modifying immunomodulation (Horby et al. 2021; RECOVERY Collaborative Group 2021, 2022).

4.2.3 How: Adequate Statistical Power for Meaningful Clinical Trial Results

The natural history informs selection of meaningful primary and secondary outcomes in clinical trial design. Outcomes of the natural history are discussed, but the identification of meaningful measures of how a patient "feels, functions, or survives" help determine the statistical power and generalizability of study findings (FDA 2020). Such information is especially valuable in clinical trials of emergency therapeutics with survival as the primary endpoint. Calculating statistical power is especially fraught early in outbreaks, when the typical disease course is not yet clear and CFRs may be biased toward the severe end of a disease spectrum.

4.2.4 How: Identifying Biomarkers of Disease

As defined by the FDA-NIH Biomarker Working Group, a biomarker is a "defined characteristic that is measured as an indicator of normal biological processes, pathologic processes, or biological responses to an exposure or therapeutic intervention" (FDA 2023; FDA-NIH Biomarker Working Group 2021). Well-designed natural history studies can identify key biomarkers that, when validated, serve as useful endpoints for clinical trials (as proxies for outcomes that may be more difficult to measure). Biomarkers can be categorized based on their utility for understanding and intervening in disease history, and include susceptibility/risk, diagnostic, monitoring, predictive, prognostic, response, and safety biomarkers. Clear criteria have been defined to determine when a biomarker might be a surrogate for clinical benefit (Institute of Medicine 2010).

4.2.5 Practice: The Kole Nat Hx of Mpox Study and Clinical Trials of Tecovirimat

After the first human case of mpox (then monkeypox) was described in the Democratic Republic of the Congo (Ladnyj et al. 1972), endemic disease was described over the next decades (Breman et al. 1980; Ježek et al. 1987) (Breman et al. 1980; Ježek et al. 1987). Two decades later, an increasing incidence of mpox was observed, thought in part to be related to waning cross-reactive immunity after the cessation of smallpox vaccination (Rimoin et al. 2010). Though smaller case series had been published, more detailed studies of the natural history of mpox were lacking. An important prospective observational natural history study conducted in Kole, DRC from 2007 to 2001 provided detailed clinical, virological, and pathologic characterization of the natural history of disease (Pittman et al. 2023). Findings from this pivotal natural history directly informed deliberations around rational design and selection of primary outcomes in an ongoing randomized, placebo-controlled evaluation of the safety and efficacy of tecovirimat in pediatric and adult patients with clade I mpox in DRC (The PALM007 trial; NCT05559099). Furthermore, after the global spread of clade II mpox was detected in 2022, the design of the PALM 007 DRC trial subsequently served as an important protocol template to inform the design of a number of international randomized clinical trials to evaluate tecovirimat in the treatment of clade IIb mpox (Rojek et al. 2023).[2]

4.2.6 Practice: The LASCOPE Study of Lassa Fever to Inform Clinical Trials

Much of the limited natural history data on Lassa Fever are retrospective and preceded the availability of reliable diagnostics and clinical laboratories. LASCOPE (NCT03655561) was a prospective observational cohort study to more fully characterize the natural history of Lassa Fever, standardize case management, and set the stage for clinical trials. In addition to characterizing disease and identifying risk factors for poor outcomes, the study helped define a reference mortality rate to inform future clinical trials; furthermore, results suggested that the need for dialysis should also be considered an important outcome in any evaluation of therapeutics. (Duvignaud et al. 2021).

4.3 Informing Preclinical Development of Novel and Repurposed Pathogen-Directed and Disease-Modifying Therapeutics

Especially in outbreaks of understudied infectious diseases, early description of the natural history in humans can rapidly inform the development of in vitro assays and animal models enabling studies of pathogenesis and the evaluation of novel or repurposed countermeasures. This needs to be considered for both pathogen-targeted therapeutics and host-targeted interventions. Early and accurate characterization of severe disease clinical phenotypes may also provide insight into specific sub-phenotypes within the larger clinical disease presentation.

4.3.1 Practice: Characterizing Pathophysiologic Stages in COVID-19

As the first natural history signals began to be reported early in the COVID-19 pandemic, poor patient outcomes were associated with hyperinflammation, including increased C-reactive protein and interleukin-6 (IL6) levels. Further understanding of the pathophysiologic signatures of this inflammation led to the study of broad (e.g., corticosteroids) and targeted (e.g., tocilizumab and baricitinib) immunomodulation to improve outcomes in particular subsets of COVID-19 patients (Horby et al. 2021; RECOVERY Collaborative Group 2021, 2022).

4.3.2 Practice: Characterizing Severe Illness Phenotypes in EVD

The care of severely ill EVD patients in well-resourced settings provided the first higher-resolution characterization of previously undescribed multi-organ dysfunction syndromes and critical illness phenotypes, including acute kidney injury, acute respiratory failure, circulatory shock, and central nervous system dysfunction (Uyeki et al. 2016b). Though based on a small number of observations, these case reports/series provided important insight into pathogenesis and the first proofs-of-principle that extracorporeal organ support could be safely and effectively provided to EVD patients. Deeper exploration of the mechanisms of organ dysfunction is needed to improve supportive care in the outbreak setting. Further study of severe EVD in some of these patients also suggested shared features between EVD and hyperinflammatory macrophage activation

---

2 These trials include:
STOMP (NCT05534984) (USA)
PLATINUM (NCT05534984) (UK)
PLATINUM-CAN (NCT05534165) (Canada)
EPOXI (EUCT 2022-501979-10-00) (Europe)
UNITY (NCT05597735) Brazil, Switzerland.

syndromes seen in other infectious diseases and autoimmune syndromes (McElroy et al. 2019), leading to further research in non-human primate models (Liu et al. 2023). Whether this shared "sub-phenotype" is truly a shared "endotype" reflecting common pathobiology and thus shared opportunities to modify disease is not yet clear (Reddy et al. 2020); nonetheless, higher-resolution characterization of the natural history of disease may generate hypotheses useful in the search for effective MCMs, including immunomodulatory approaches.

5 Determinants of the Natural History

As illustrated above (◘ Fig. 1, 1a), the true natural history of any infectious disease, absent intervention, is ultimately determined by intrinsic characteristics of the host, the virus, and the exposure that are antecedent to the development of infection and disease. Though we focus much of the prior discussion on the natural history of clinical disease (and its emergent features), these host, viral, and exposure factors merit consideration in understanding how the natural history is determined.

5.1 Host Determinants

5.1.1 General Principles

Several host factors have been identified or hypothesized to contribute to susceptibility or resistance to infection and disease and to short- and long-term outcomes. Host risk factors (◘ Fig. 1a) include, but are not limited to age; sex; immune status, including prior exposures (i.e., vaccinations, previous infections) and immunodeficiency states; nutritional status; pregnancy; co-morbidities; co-infections; host genetic factors; and host microbiome. Individual host factors may impact the risk and progression of infection and disease with similar effect, or they may influence each stage differently; therefore, a determinant of the risk for infection may or may not be a determinant of disease severity or outcomes. For many of the diseases under consideration, data on host contributory factors have been limited to what is easiest to capture (e.g., host demographics like age and sex, pregnancy, and basic nutritional status). Determining risk related to less easily measured host factors has been more challenging in outbreaks, especially in low-resource areas where more complex clinical or research laboratory capacity may be unavailable. Missing capabilities may include diagnostics for co-infections or comorbidities, the measurement of non-routine biomarkers, DNA characterization, and the absence of large data sets.

5.1.2 Practice: COVID-19

Recent experience with COVID-19 suggests that focused, well-resourced research on large datasets can expeditiously define the complex host determinants of a novel disease. Early in the COVID-19 pandemic, it became evident that age, sex, and certain comorbidities were associated with severe disease and death (Russell et al. 2023). Large, collaborative, multi-center international studies identified inborn errors in Type I interferon (IFN) responses (Zhang et al. 2020) or autoantibodies (Bastard et al. 2020; Reynolds et al. 2006b) against components of the Type I IFN immune response as major genetic or immunologic determinants of COVID-19 severity. As the pandemic progressed, these studies have continued to identify new genetic factors critical to understanding risk, elucidating pathophysiology, and informing immunomodulatory strategies for antiviral therapy (Covid-19 Host Genetics Initiative 2023; Kalil et al. 2021; Pairo-Castineira et al. 2023; Recovery Collaborative Group 2022; Reynolds et al. 2006a). More recently, genetic associations between human leukocyte antigen type and asymptomatic SARS-CoV-2 infection have emerged (Augusto et al. 2023). Finally, genome-wide association studies are beginning to describe host genetic variants in large cohorts of patients with PASC (Vilma et al. 2023). For almost all the other pathogens and diseases under discussion in this chapter, we still have a limited understanding of how host genetic factors influence the risk of infection and disease severity. In the future, similar efforts to define host genetic risks could inform clinical care and improve patient outcomes.

5.2 Viral Determinants of the Natural History

5.2.1 Viral Toolkits, Infection, and Disease

Each virus (as a member of a conceptual virus species) has its own molecular tools enabling infection, replication, local or systemic dissemination, and possible transmission to another host. Viral toolkits evolve to evade both innate and virus-specific adaptive immune responses in an ongoing host–pathogen evolutionary arms race (Crespo-Bellido and Duffy 2023; Ploquin et al. 2018). En route to replication and forward transmission, viral infection may cause dysfunction of or damage to cells, tissues, and organs or organ systems by direct (cytopathic) or indirect (noncytopathic) mechanisms and may provoke immunopathologic responses; clinical symptoms and signs of disease result. Detailed discussion of virus-specific molecular mechanisms of infection and disease is outside the scope of this chapter.

5.2.2 Within-Outbreak Viral Evolution and the Natural History

Sustained human-to-human transmission and replication enables viral evolutionary exploration of the human host. Theoretically, viral evolutionary trajectories should be oriented toward enhanced replication, transmission, and avoidance of host immune responses. The effects of ongoing evolution on pathogenicity are less clear, though they are generally thought to trend toward more transmissible and immune-evasive variants rather than variants that cause more severe disease. Sustained SARS-CoV-2 transmission over time has provided a clear example: early SARS-CoV variants (e.g., Alpha, Delta) appeared to cause more severe disease in humans and animal models than later variants (e.g., Omicron) (Nyberg et al. 2022); whether this trend will continue is unclear. The capacity for rapid genetic sequencing to provide near real-time molecular epidemiologic information during an outbreak is a recent phenomenon, having been deployed for the first time at scale during the 2014–2016 EVD outbreak in West Africa. During that relatively long period of human-to-human transmission, certain mutations became dominant in circulating EBOV, suggesting some fitness benefit to the virus. Efforts to determine any impact on the natural history, however, even in animal models, have not been revealing (Marzi et al. 2018). We do not have such detailed sequence data for most viral pathogens that infect and transmit among humans.

5.2.3 Intra-Species Viral Strains and the Natural History

In general, differentiation of virulence among viral variants (within a viral species) is limited to epidemiologically derived CFRs associated with different variants. Determining whether increased CFRs are caused by a more virulent virus strain (or isolate) typically requires in vitro and animal modeling studies that do not provide a complete picture of human infection and disease even when they can be conducted. For some viruses, animal models have not identified significant differences in virulence between specific outbreak strains; for example, EBOV-Mayinga, EBOV-Kikwit, and EBOV-Makona variants associated with different outbreaks do not appear to differ in severity in animal models (Yamaoka and Ebihara 2021). Subspecies differences in disease severity have been identified for other viral infections. Observations of higher CFR with mpox virus clade I (CFR 5–11%) versus clade II (CFR 1–3%), for example, suggest viral genomic variance contributes to an altered natural history of mpox. However, these observations may be confounded by other variables, including geographic origin, host genetic variation, and the availability and quality of care (Gessain et al. 2022). Comparisons in nonhuman primate models suggest differential lethality, viral loads, and organ-tropism between mpox virus clade I and clade II (Saijo et al. 2009). Similar observations have been made in Lassa fever caused by different clades of the Lassa virus in humans and in animal models (Grant et al. 2023; Stein et al. 2021).

5.3 Exposure Determinants of the Natural History

5.3.1 Dose, Route, Sample Matrix, Environment

Exposure to a larger quantity of infectious material is generally presumed to increase the likelihood of infection. A similar correlation with disease severity is likely, though simple exposure dose–response relationships (to either infection or disease severity) are challenging to demonstrate in either animal-to-human or human-to-human transmission and must rely instead on proxy animal modeling. In general, dose-ranging of viral exposure in animal models suggests that increased exposure increases either the disease severity or its progression. Determining the impact of the route of exposure generally must also rely on animal modeling. It is likely that infectivity and transmission also depends on the exposure matrix (e.g., blood versus bodily fluid versus semen) but this is not well understood beyond epidemiologic observations. It is also likely that the exposure environment affects infectivity and secondary attack rates given the differential stability of viruses in particular environments (e.g., relative humidity and air flow for viruses transmitted by aerosol particles or respiratory droplets) (Thornton et al. 2022).

5.3.2 Practice: Monkeypox Virus (MPXV) Exposure and the Natural History of Mpox

It has been long recognized that the route or site of initial exposure to orthopoxviruses directly impacts the clinical presentation. The cowpox pustules on the hands of infected milkmaids observed by Edward Jenner are perhaps the best-known example (Cowpox and paravaccinia 1967; Jenner 1798). In the context of endemic mpox (caused by Clade I MPXV infection) in the DRC, the route of exposure has been previously associated with more severe disease, though this may be confounded by a dose effect (Pittman et al. 2023; Reynolds et al. 2006b). During the global spread of mpox through human-to-human transmission in 2022–2023 (caused by Clade IIb MPXV infection), atypical clinical presentations were frequently described after high-risk sexual exposures, including localized skin lesions and regional lymphadenopathy, anogenital lesions, and proctitis. Clinical comparison to the disseminated skin lesions more typical of endemic mpox, and more often associated with animal-to-human or human-to-human transmission without high-risk sexual contact (clade I or II MPXV), suggests an important contribution of the exposure route to the natural history (Mitjà et al. 2023). Recently reported descriptions of mpox cases after likely heterosexual transmission of the virus (clade II MPXV) in Nigeria suggest a similar route dependence (Ogoina and James 2023).

5.3.3 Practice: Ebola Virus (EBOV) Exposure and the Natural History of EVD

Human-to-human transmission of EBOV is thought to occur predominantly from mucosal exposure to blood or body fluids from symptomatic or deceased patients (Vetter et al. 2016). Though an exposure dose response has not been confirmed in human studies, animal models suggest dose-dependent differences in the severity, character, or pace of illness after mucosal (oral or conjunctival) versus intramuscular inoculation (Cross et al. 2023; Johnson et al. 2023). However, dose-ranging studies have also demonstrated 100% lethality even after very small inocula after intramuscular or aerosol exposures. Limited observations after accidental laboratory exposures suggest that intravenous or intramuscular exposure (via a needlestick injury, for example) poses a high risk of infection and severe disease in humans (Vetter et al. 2016). Uncertainty remains around the effect of bodily fluid matrix on EBOV transmission, though its influence is very plausible. In comparison to human-to-human transmission of acute EVD, the paucity of cases associated with exposure to the semen of male EVD survivors (with high viral loads in semen, especially early in convalescence) suggests a matrix effect that lowers sexual transmission risk among other potential bottlenecks (Jacob et al. 2020).

6 Natural History Studies: Optimal Design and What Can Be Achieved in Outbreaks

6.1 Outbreak Realities: Challenges to Natural History Studies

Historically, the realities of outbreak settings have limited opportunities for well-designed natural history studies. Outbreaks occur unpredictably, often in remote, under-resourced settings. The immediate urgencies of outbreak response are not well suited to pre-planned, prospective studies, so understanding and reporting the natural history often proceeds as shown in ◘ Fig. 5. It is perhaps understandable that true natural history studies have typically only been established during prolonged outbreaks and are often focused on survivors rather than acute disease.

6.1.1 Rapid Communication via Existing Clinical Networks

As described above, the first signals of the natural history typically come from discussions of the clinical disease from providers caring for patients in the outbreak setting. In recent outbreaks (e.g., COVID-19, mpox, and filovirus disease outbreaks), connecting external subject matter experts to in-field clinicians has been invaluable to discuss emerging clinical challenges, begin to inform or update clinical guidelines, identify research questions, and rapidly inform preclinical and clinical research strategies.

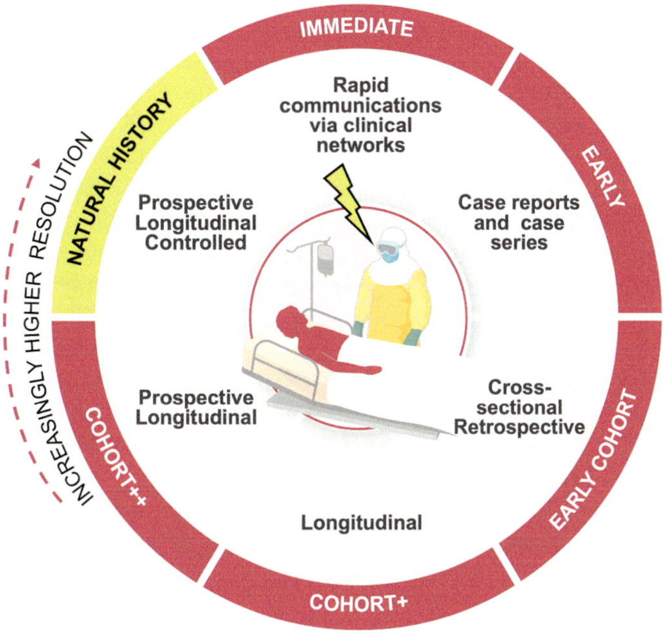

◘ **Fig. 5** Understanding the natural history in infectious disease outbreaks: typical progression. (Author)

6.1.2 Early Observational Studies of Natural History

During an outbreak, observational data is often first published as descriptive case reports, series, or small cohort studies. In these cases, data is derived retrospectively from already available clinical charts and medical records. Typically, these are also cross-sectional (collected during a specified limited time period). While this enables rapid design, analysis, and publication, these studies are susceptible to biases and limitations, including:

- Missing or inconsistent data or methods of data collection from existing records not designed to reliably capture all relevant data
- A bias toward a particular patient population may limit generalizability of findings. This is particularly true of case and series reports early in outbreaks, in which unusual or particularly severe clinical presentations may be more likely to be published
- Limited cross-sectional observation periods may not capture evolution of disease over time

Nonetheless, in most novel outbreaks, early descriptions of clinical disease play an important role in informing care and in shaping clinical research. For example, the first reports of clinical disease from China early in the COVID-19 pandemic critically set the stage to describe phases of disease, begin to identify risk factors for poor outcomes, and suggest strategic approaches for interventional redirection of the natural history (Guan et al. 2020).

6.1.3 Optimal Design of Natural History Studies: Prospective, Longitudinal, and Controlled Observations

Prospective studies evaluate events based on a prespecified study design. Longitudinal studies collect data from all patients in a pre-defined cohort over a defined period and are more likely to yield information about the onset and evolution of disease. Prospective, longitudinal observational cohorts with well-matched controls (where relevant) provide the most comprehensive, reliable, and generalizable information about the natural history of an emerging infectious disease. Optimally, over the outbreak period, these studies would provided an increasingly resolved picture of the natural history. However, the time, resources, and effort required to implement such studies during an emergency have limited their use in infectious disease outbreaks. Conducting effective natural history studies in infectious disease outbreaks likely requires alternative strategies.

6.2 Strategies to Improve Understanding of Natural History During Outbreaks

6.2.1 Early Identification of Research Gaps

The identification of key research gaps for any disease often requires systematic reviews—efforts that require considerable expertise, effort, and time, limiting their utility in emergency research response. For recognized priority pathogens with pandemic potential, formulation of a research agenda should emphasize understanding natural history to inform development of diagnostics and MCMs. A "rapid research needs appraisal" (RRNA) protocol aiming "to identify important gaps in evidence and knowledge in a robust, systematic, and replicable manner to rapidly inform clinical research prioritization" within five days is under development. It was recently piloted using a Lassa Fever outbreak scenario, with online rapid-review software, and evaluated in comparison with an expert Lassa fever panel (Sigfrid et al. 2019). This and analogous efforts to accelerate identification of key research gaps are needed.

6.2.2 Standardized Clinical Characterization Protocols (CCP) for Specific Diseases or Disease Syndromes

Another obstacle to urgently and widely collecting data for understanding natural history is the lack of standardized data collection protocols to enable harmonized collection from multiple sites and independent outbreaks of the same disease. "Prototype pathogen" approaches to help understand viral families should be paralleled by the development of "prototype protocols" that could be pre-positioned to understand the disease caused by those pathogens. Developing disease-specific or syndrome-specific clinical characterization protocols agreed upon by stakeholders in advance would help resolve this issue. Depending on the syndrome, these CCPs are easily adapted to novel diseases presenting with similar syndromes. For example, generic International Severe Acute Respiratory and Emerging Infection (ISARIC) CCPs have proven useful in understanding the natural history of COVID-19 from large international datasets, including in disease characterization (Drake et al. 2021; Millar et al. 2022; Sullivan et al. 2021; Swann et al. 2020), risk assessment (Knight et al. 2022), and evaluation of clinical care. In addition, proposed "perpetual observational studies" could become standard for characterization of the natural history of disease across outbreaks (Hassoun-Kheir et al. 2022).

6.2.3 Prepositioned Clinical Research Networks (and Researchers)

Establishing and strengthening clinical research networks (and researchers) across geographic areas susceptible to the same infectious diseases is a valuable strategy to improve understanding of novel diseases or endemic infectious diseases with significant knowledge gaps. These networks might be initiated in response to specific disease threats but maintained during inter-outbreak periods and able to pivot to new threats. For example, at the national level, the PREVAIL, PREGUI, and PALM collaborative efforts (in Liberia, Guinea, and the DRC, respectively) had origins in research responses to EVD outbreaks but have pivoted to other emergence research needs. Regional examples include The African Coalition for Epidemic Research, Response and Training (ALERRT), and the Pan-African Network for Rapid Research, Response, Relief and Preparedness for Infectious Disease Epidemics (Pandora-ID-Net) as well as focused training networks like the Clinical Research During Outbreaks (CREDO) initiative (ALERRT 2023; Kayem et al. 2019; PANDORA 2022).

6.2.4 Global Clinical Platforms

To enhance the understanding of the natural history in emerging infectious diseases, the WHO has proposed the use of "Global Clinical Platforms" (GCP) in which secure web-based databases could capture individual-level anonymized clinical data from patients around the world, providing large datasets for analysis. Platforms are to be disease or syndrome-adapted and focused on understanding natural history. For example, the aims of the WHO GCP for Viral Hemorrhagic Fever (WHO 2023) are to:

- Describe the disease course, its natural history, and severity.
- Identify the association of clinical characteristics of viral hemorrhagic fevers with outcomes.
- Inform strategies for use of clinical resources to provide high-quality supportive care.

6.2.5 Core Protocols: Integrating Natural History Studies into Clinical Trials of Medical Countermeasures

The challenges of conducting interventional clinical trials in unpredictable outbreak settings have led to calls to implement core (or master) protocols that could make it possible to continue a study across successive independent outbreaks (Dean et al. 2020). In addition to evaluating the safety and efficacy of a candidate therapeutic, the standardized clinical characterization collected during interventional studies could provide important insights into the natural history of disease. For example, platform adaptive randomized core trial protocols under discussion for the evaluation of new and repurposed treatments for filovirus diseases likely could also valuably improve our understanding of natural history.

7 Conclusion

Understanding and reporting the natural history of infectious diseases is an important but challenging component of emergency research response. A clear understanding of natural history not only informs clinical care but also sets the stage for better design of preclinical and clinical research to evaluate medical countermeasures. Recent experience in the COVID-19 pandemic suggests that unprecedented research goals can now be accomplished, albeit with exceptional collaborative effort and resources. Characterization of the evolving host–pathogen–care interaction has been much more limited for diseases caused by most priority pathogens. Any disease caused by a novel pathogen will require new characterization efforts to begin as soon as possible. As we plan for better preparedness for and response to future infectious disease emergencies, we must devise and incorporate strategies to rapidly and effectively characterize, understand, and redirect disease natural history.

Discussion Questions

1. Why is it important to develop an early, detailed understanding of the natural history of a novel disease in patients when there is a novel infectious disease outbreak?
2. What are the intrinsic determinants of the natural history of a disease in a human patient?
3. Name some obstacles to conducting natural history studies during outbreaks.
4. Suggest some ways of better preparing to conduct future natural history studies of novel infectious diseases.

References

ALERRT. African coaLition for Epidemic Research, Response and Training (ALERRT). 2023. https://www.alerrt.global. Accessed 10 Sept 2023.

Ashley EA, Dhorda M, Fairhurst RM, Amaratunga C, Lim P, Suon S, et al. Spread of artemisinin resistance in plasmodium falciparum malaria. N Engl J Med. 2014;371(5):411–23. https://doi.org/10.1056/NEJMoa1314981.

Augusto DG, Murdolo LD, Chatzileontiadou DSM, Sabatino JJ, Yusufali T, Peyser ND, et al. A common allele of HLA is associated with asymptomatic SARS-CoV-2 infection. Nature. 2023;620:128. https://doi.org/10.1038/s41586-023-06331-x.

Balikagala B, Fukuda N, Ikeda M, Katuro OT, Tachibana S-I, Yamauchi M, et al. Evidence of artemisinin-resistant malaria in Africa. N Engl J Med. 2021;385(13):1163–71. https://doi.org/10.1056/NEJMoa2101746.

Barnes KG, Kindrachuk J, Lin AE, Wohl S, Qu J, Tostenson SD, et al. Evidence of Ebola virus replication and high concentration in semen of a patient during recovery. Clin Infect Dis. 2017;65(8):1400–3. https://doi.org/10.1093/cid/cix518.

Bastard P, Rosen LB, Zhang Q, Michailidis E, Hoffmann HH, Zhang Y et al. Autoantibodies against type I IFNs in patients with life-threatening COVID-19. Science. 2020;370(6515). https://doi.org/10.1126/science.abd4585.

Bausch DG, Feldmann H, Geisbert TW, Bray M, Sprecher AG, Boumandouki P, et al. Outbreaks of filovirus hemorrhagic fever: time to refocus on the patient. J Infect Dis. 2007;196(Supplement_2):S136–S41. https://doi.org/10.1086/520542.

Berger JR, Vilensky JA. Encephalitis lethargica (von Economo's encephalitis). Handb Clin Neurol. 2014;123:745–61. https://doi.org/10.1016/b978-0-444-53488-0.00036-5.

Bower H, Grass JE, Veltus E, Brault A, Campbell S, Basile AJ, et al. Delivery of an Ebola virus-positive stillborn infant in a rural community health center, Sierra Leone, 2015. Am J Trop Med Hyg. 2016;94(2):417–9. https://doi.org/10.4269/ajtmh.15-0619.

Breman JG, Kalisa R, Steniowski MV, Zanotto E, Gromyko AI, Arita I. Human monkeypox, 1970-79. Bull World Health Organ. 1980;58(2):165–82.

Buba MI, Dalhat MM, Nguku PM, Waziri N, Mohammad JO, Bomoi IM, et al. Mortality among confirmed Lassa fever cases during the 2015-2016 outbreak in Nigeria. Am J Public Health. 2018;108(2):262–4. https://doi.org/10.2105/ajph.2017.304186.

Cassetti MC, Pierson TC, Patterson LJ, Bok K, DeRocco AJ, Deschamps AM, et al. Prototype pathogen approach for vaccine and monoclonal antibody development: a critical component of the NIAID plan for pandemic preparedness. J Infect Dis. 2022;227:1433. https://doi.org/10.1093/infdis/jiac296.

CDC. Pneumocystis pneumonia—Los Angeles. MMWR Morb Mortal Wkly Rep. 1981;45(34):729–33.

CDC. Update on acquired immune deficiency syndrome (AIDS)—United States. MMWR Morb Mortal Wkly Rep. 1982;31(37):507–8, 13–4.

CDC. Extensively drug-resistant tuberculosis—United States, 1993–2006. MMWR Morb Mortal Wkly Rep. 2007;56(11):250–3.

CDC. Principles of epidemiology in public health practice, third edition: an introduction to applied epidemiology and biostatistics. Atlanta: U.S. Centers for Disease Control and Prevention; 2012.

Covid-19 Host Genetics Initiative. A second update on mapping the human genetic architecture of COVID-19. Nature. 2023;621(7977):E7–E26. https://doi.org/10.1038/s41586-023-06355-3.

Cowpox and paravaccinia. Br Med J. 1967;4(5575):308–9.

Crespo-Bellido A, Duffy S. The how of counter-defense: viral evolution to combat host immunity. Curr Opin Microbiol. 2023;74:102320. https://doi.org/10.1016/j.mib.2023.102320.

Cross RW, Prasad AN, Woolsey CB, Agans KN, Borisevich V, Dobias NS, et al. Natural history of nonhuman primates after conjunctival exposure to Ebola virus. Sci Rep. 2023;13(1):4175. https://doi.org/10.1038/s41598-023-31027-7.

Davis HE, McCorkell L, Vogel JM, Topol EJ. Long COVID: major findings, mechanisms and recommendations. Nat Rev Microbiol. 2023;21(3):133–46. https://doi.org/10.1038/s41579-022-00846-2.

de la Paz MP, Villaverde-Hueso A, Alonso V, János S, Zurriaga Ó, Pollán M, et al. Rare diseases epidemiology research. In: de la Paz MP, Groft SC, editors. Rare diseases epidemiology. advances in experimental medicine and biology. Dordrecht: Springer Netherlands; 2010. p. 17–39.

Dean NE, Gsell P-S, Brookmeyer R, Crawford FW, Donnelly CA, Ellenberg SS, et al. Creating a framework for conducting randomized clinical trials during disease outbreaks. N Eng J M. 2020;382(14):1366–9. https://doi.org/10.1056/NEJMsb1905390.

Deen GF, Broutet N, Xu W, Knust B, Sesay FR, McDonald SLR, et al. Ebola RNA persistence in semen of Ebola virus disease survivors—final report. N Engl J Med. 2017;377(15):1428–37. https://doi.org/10.1056/NEJMoa1511410.

Diallo B, Sissoko D, Loman NJ, Bah HA, Bah H, Worrell MC, et al. Resurgence of Ebola virus disease in Guinea linked to a survivor with virus persistence in seminal fluid for more than 500 days. Clin Infect Dis. 2016;63(10):1353–6. https://doi.org/10.1093/cid/ciw601.

Dickson SJ, Clay KA, Adam M, Ardley C, Bailey MS, Burns DS, et al. Enhanced case management can be delivered for patients with EVD in Africa: experience from a UK military Ebola treatment Centre in Sierra Leone. J Infect. 2018;76(4):383–92. https://doi.org/10.1016/j.jinf.2017.12.006.

Dondorp AM, Nosten F, Yi P, Das D, Phyo AP, Tarning J, et al. Artemisinin resistance in Plasmodium falciparum malaria. N Engl J Med. 2009;361(5):455–67. https://doi.org/10.1056/NEJMoa0808859.

Drake TM, Riad AM, Fairfield CJ, Egan C, Knight SR, Pius R, et al. Characterisation of in-hospital complications associated with COVID-19 using the ISARIC WHO clinical characterisation protocol UK: a prospective, multicentre cohort study. Lancet. 2021;398(10296):223–37. https://doi.org/10.1016/S0140-6736(21)00799-6.

Duvignaud A, Jaspard M, Etafo IC, Gabillard D, Serra B, Abejegah C, et al. Lassa fever outcomes and prognostic factors in Nigeria (LASCOPE): a prospective cohort study. Lancet Glob Health. 2021;9(4):e469–e78. https://doi.org/10.1016/S2214--109X(20)30518-0.

Fauci A. Victories against AIDS have lessons for COVID-19. Nature. 2021;600(7887):9. https://doi.org/10.1038/d41586-021-03569-1.

Fauci AS, Lane HC. Four decades of HIV/AIDS—much accomplished, much to do. N Engl J Med. 2020;383(1):1–4. https://doi.org/10.1056/NEJMp1916753.

FDA. Clinical outcome assessment (COA): frequently asked questions. Silver Spring, MD: U.S. Food and Drug Administration; 2020. https://www.fda.gov/about-fda/clinical-outcome-assessment-coa-frequently-asked-questions. Accessed 16 Aug 2023.

FDA. Biomarker Qualification Program. Silver Spring, MD: U.S. Food and Drug Administration; 2023. https://www.fda.gov/drugs/drug-development-tool-ddt-qualification-programs/biomarker-qualification-program. Accessed 16 Aug 2023.

FDA/CDER. Rare diseases: natural history studies for drug development guidance for industry (draft). FDA; 2019.

FDA-NIH Biomarker Working Group. BEST (biomarkers, EndpointS, and other tools) resource. Silver Spring, MD: U.S. Food and Drug Administration, U.S. National Institutes of Health; 2021.

Fink DL, Callaby H, Luintel A, Beynon W, Bond H, Lim EY, et al. Clinical features and management of individuals admitted to hospital with monkeypox and associated complications across the UK: a retrospective cohort study. Lancet Infect Dis. 2023;23(5):589–97. https://doi.org/10.1016/S1473--3099(22)00806-4.

Fischer WA, Brown J, Wohl DA, Loftis AJ, Tozay S, Reeves E, et al. Ebola virus ribonucleic acid detection in semen more than two years after resolution of acute Ebola virus infection. Open Forum Infect Dis. 2017;4(3):ofx155. https://doi.org/10.1093/ofid/ofx155.

Fischer WA, Crozier I, Bausch DG, Muyembe J-J, Mulangu S, Diaz JV, et al. Shifting the paradigm—applying universal standards of care to Ebola virus disease. N Engl J Med. 2019;380(15):1389–91. https://doi.org/10.1056/NEJMp1817070.

Ford A, Hwang A, Mo AX, Baqar S, Touchette N, Deal C, et al. Meeting summary: global vaccine and immunization research forum, 2021. Vaccine. 2023;41(11):1799–807. https://doi.org/10.1016/j.vaccine.2023.02.028.

Gandhi NR, Moll A, Sturm AW, Pawinski R, Govender T, Lalloo U, et al. Extensively drug-resistant tuberculosis as a cause of death in patients co-infected with tuberculosis and HIV in a rural area of South

Africa. Lancet. 2006;368(9547):1575–80. https://doi.org/10.1016/s0140-6736(06)69573-1.

Gayedyu-Dennis D, Fallah MP, Drew C, Badio M, Moses JS, Fayiah T, et al. Identifying Paucisymptomatic or asymptomatic and unrecognized Ebola virus disease among close contacts based on exposure risk assessments and screening algorithms. J Infect Dis. 2023;227(7):878–87. https://doi.org/10.1093/infdis/jiac359.

Gessain A, Nakoune E, Yazdanpanah Y. Monkeypox. N Engl J Med. 2022;387(19):1783–93. https://doi.org/10.1056/NEJMra2208860.

Glynn JR, Bower H, Johnson S, Houlihan CF, Montesano C, Scott JT, et al. Asymptomatic infection and unrecognised Ebola virus disease in Ebola-affected households in Sierra Leone: a cross-sectional study using a new non-invasive assay for antibodies to Ebola virus. Lancet Infect Dis. 2017;17(6):645–53. https://doi.org/10.1016/s1473-3099(17)30111-1.

Govind A, Lazarte SM, Kitchell E, Chow JY, Estelle CD, Fixsen E, et al. Severe mpox infections in people with uncontrolled human immunodeficiency virus. Clin Infect Dis. 2023;76(10):1843–6. https://doi.org/10.1093/cid/ciad052.

GPMB. A manifesto for preparedness: three tests of global reforms. Geneva: Global Preparedenss and Monitoring Board; 2023.

Grant DS, Samuels RJ, Garry RF, Schieffelin JS. Lassa fever natural history and clinical management. Curr Top Microbiol Immunol. 2023;440:165. https://doi.org/10.1007/82_2023_263.

Guan W-j, Ni Z-y, Hu Y, Liang W-h, Ou C-q, He J-x, et al. Clinical characteristics of coronavirus disease 2019 in China. N Eng J Med. 2020;382(18):1708–20. https://doi.org/10.1056/NEJMoa2002032.

Hassoun-Kheir N, van Werkhoven CH, Dunning J, Jaenisch T, van Beek J, Bielicki J, et al. Perpetual observational studies: new strategies to support efficient implementation of observational studies and randomized trials in infectious diseases. Clin Microbiol Infect. 2022;28(12):1528–32. https://doi.org/10.1016/j.cmi.2022.07.024.

Higgs ES, Gayedyu-Dennis D, Fischer Ii WA, Nason M, Reilly C, Beavogui AH, et al. PREVAIL IV: a randomized, double-blind, 2-phase, phase 2 trial of Remdesivir vs placebo for reduction of Ebola virus RNA in the semen of male survivors. Clin Infect Dis. 2021;73(10):1849–56. https://doi.org/10.1093/cid/ciab215.

Horby P, Lim WS, Emberson JR, Mafham M, Bell JL, Linsell L, et al. Dexamethasone in hospitalized patients with Covid-19. N Engl J Med. 2021;384(8):693–704. https://doi.org/10.1056/NEJMoa2021436.

Institute of Medicine, editor. Transforming clinical research in the United States: challenges and opportunities: workshop summary. Transforming clinical research in the United States: challenges and opportunities. Washington, DC: National Academies Press; 2010.

Jacob ST, Crozier I, Fischer WA 2nd, Hewlett A, Kraft CS, Vega MA, et al. Ebola virus disease. Nat Rev Dis Primers. 2020;6(1):13. https://doi.org/10.1038/s41572-020-0147-3.

Jacobs M, Rodger A, Bell DJ, Bhagani S, Cropley I, Filipe A, et al. Late Ebola virus relapse causing meningoencephalitis: a case report. Lancet. 2016;388(10043):498–503. https://doi.org/10.1016/s0140-6736(16)30386-5.

Jenner E. An inquiry into the causes and effects of the variolac vaccinae; a disease discovered in some of the western counties of England, particularly Gloucestershire, and known by the name of the cow pox. London: Simon Low; 1798.

Jewell NP. Natural history of diseases: statistical designs and issues. Clin Pharm Therapeut. 2016;100(4):353–61. https://doi.org/10.1002/cpt.423.

Ježek Z, Szczeniowski M, Paluku KM, Mutombo M. Human monkeypox: clinical features of 282 patients. J Infect Dis. 1987;156(2):293–8. https://doi.org/10.1093/infdis/156.2.293.

Johnson DM, Brasel T, Massey S, Smith J, Garron T, Wallace S et al. Characterization of Ebola virus mucosal challenge routes in Cynomolgus macaques. J Virol. 2023:e0188822. https://doi.org/10.1128/jvi.01888-22.

Kalil AC, Patterson TF, Mehta AK, Tomashek KM, Wolfe CR, Ghazaryan V, et al. Baricitinib plus Remdesivir for hospitalized adults with Covid-19. N Engl J Med. 2021;384(9):795–807. https://doi.org/10.1056/NEJMoa2031994.

Kayem ND, Rojek A, Denis E, Salam A, Reis A, Olliaro P, et al. Clinical REsearch during outbreaks (CREDO) training for low- and middle-income countries. Emerg Infect Dis. 2019;25(11):2084–7. https://doi.org/10.3201/eid2511.180628.

Keita AK, Koundouno FR, Faye M, Düx A, Hinzmann J, Diallo H, et al. Resurgence of Ebola virus in 2021 in Guinea suggests a new paradigm for outbreaks. Nature. 2021;597(7877):539–43. https://doi.org/10.1038/s41586-021-03901-9.

Kelly JD, Van Ryn C, Badio M, Fayiah T, Johnson K, Gayedyu-Dennis D, et al. Clinical sequelae among individuals with pauci-symptomatic or asymptomatic Ebola virus infection and unrecognised Ebola virus disease in Liberia: a longitudinal cohort study. Lancet Infect Dis. 2022;22(8):1163–71. https://doi.org/10.1016/s1473-3099(22)00127-x.

Knight SR, Gupta RK, Ho A, Pius R, Buchan I, Carson G, et al. Prospective validation of the 4C prognostic models for adults hospitalised with COVID-19 using the ISARIC WHO clinical characterisation protocol. Thorax. 2022;77(6):606. https://doi.org/10.1136/thoraxjnl-2021-217629.

Ladnyj ID, Ziegler P, Kima E. A human infection caused by monkeypox virus in Basankusu territory, Democratic Republic of the Congo. Bull World Health Organ. 1972;46(5):593–7.

Lamontagne F, Fowler RA, Adhikari NK, Murthy S, Brett-Major DM, Jacobs M, et al. Evidence-based guidelines for supportive care of patients with Ebola

virus disease. Lancet. 2018;391(10121):700–8. https://doi.org/10.1016/s0140-6736(17)31795-6.
Laxminarayan R. The overlooked pandemic of antimicrobial resistance. Lancet. 2022;399(10325):606–7. https://doi.org/10.1016/S0140-6736(22)00087-3.
Liu DX, Pahar B, Cooper TK, Perry DL, Xu H, Huzella LM, et al. Ebola virus disease features Hemophagocytic lymphohistiocytosis/macrophage activation syndrome in the rhesus macaque model. J Infect Dis. 2023;228:371. https://doi.org/10.1093/infdis/jiad203.
Lundgren JD, Babiker AG, Sharma S, Grund B, Phillips AN, Matthews G et al. Long-term benefits from early antiretroviral therapy initiation in HIV infection. NEJM Evid. 2023;2(3). https://doi.org/10.1056/evidoa2200302.
Marzi A, Chadinah S, Haddock E, Feldmann F, Arndt N, Martellaro C, et al. Recently identified mutations in the Ebola virus-Makona genome do not Alter pathogenicity in animal models. Cell Rep. 2018;23(6).1806–16. https://doi.org/10.1016/j.celrep.2018.04.027.
Mate SE, Kugelman JR, Nyenswah TG, Ladner JT, Wiley MR, Cordier-Lassalle T, et al. Molecular evidence of sexual transmission of Ebola virus. N Engl J Med. 2015;373(25):2448–54. https://doi.org/10.1056/NEJMoa1509773.
Mbala-Kingebeni P. EVD case in DRC linked to 2018-2020 Nord Kivu EVD outbreak. Virological.org: Virological.org; 2022.
Mbala-Kingebeni P, Pratt C, Mutafali-Ruffin M, Pauthner MG, Bile F, Nkuba-Ndaye A, et al. Ebola virus transmission initiated by relapse of systemic Ebola virus disease. N Engl J Med. 2021;384(13):1240–7. https://doi.org/10.1056/NEJMoa2024670.
McElroy AK, Shrivastava-Ranjan P, Harmon JR, Martines RB, Silva-Flannery L, Flietstra TD, et al. Macrophage activation marker soluble CD163 associated with fatal and severe Ebola virus disease in humans. Emerg Infect Dis. 2019;25(2):290–8. https://doi.org/10.3201/eid2502.181326.
Millar JE, Neyton L, Seth S, Dunning J, Merson L, Murthy S, et al. Distinct clinical symptom patterns in patients hospitalised with COVID-19 in an analysis of 59,011 patients in the ISARIC-4C study. Sci Rep. 2022;12(1):6843. https://doi.org/10.1038/s41598-022-08032-3.
Mitjà O, Ogoina D, Titanji BK, Galvan C, Muyembe JJ, Marks M, et al. Monkeypox. Lancet. 2023;401(10370):60–74. https://doi.org/10.1016/s0140-6736(22)02075-x.
Mulangu S, Dodd LE, Davey RT Jr, Tshiani Mbaya O, Proschan M, Mukadi D, et al. A randomized, controlled trial of Ebola virus disease therapeutics. N Engl J Med. 2019;381(24):2293–303. https://doi.org/10.1056/NEJMoa1910993.
Murray CJ, Ikuta KS, Sharara F, Swetschinski L, Aguilar GR, Gray A, et al. Global burden of bacterial antimicrobial resistance in 2019: a systematic analysis. Lancet. 2022;399(10325):629–55. https://doi.org/10.1016/S0140-6736(21)02724-0.
Nakanishi N, Liu K, Kawakami D, Kawai Y, Morisawa T, Nishida T et al. Post-intensive care syndrome and its new challenges in coronavirus disease 2019 (COVID-19) pandemic: a review of recent advances and perspectives. J Clin Med. 2021;10(17). https://doi.org/10.3390/jcm10173870.
Nyberg T, Ferguson NM, Nash SG, Webster HH, Flaxman S, Andrews N, et al. Comparative analysis of the risks of hospitalisation and death associated with SARS-CoV-2 omicron (B.1.1.529) and delta (B.1.617.2) variants in England: a cohort study. Lancet. 2022;399(10332):1303–12. https://doi.org/10.1016/s0140-6736(22)00462-7.
Ogoina D, James HI. Mpox among linked heterosexual casual partners in Bayelsa, Nigeria. N Eng J Med. 2023;388:2101. https://doi.org/10.1056/NEJMc2300866.
Okokhere P, Colubri A, Azubike C, Iruolagbe C, Osazuwa O, Tabrizi S, et al. Clinical and laboratory predictors of Lassa fever outcome in a dedicated treatment facility in Nigeria: a retrospective, observational cohort study. Lancet Infect Dis. 2018;18(6):684–95. https://doi.org/10.1016/s1473-3099(18)30121-x.
Pairo-Castineira E, Rawlik K, Bretherick AD, Qi T, Wu Y, Nassiri I, et al. GWAS and meta-analysis identifies 49 genetic variants underlying critical COVID-19. Nature. 2023;617:764. https://doi.org/10.1038/s41586-023-06034-3.
PANDORA. Pan-African network for rapid research, response, relief and preparedness for infectious disease epidemics (Pandora-ID-Net). PANDORA; 2022.
Pittman PR, Martin JW, Kingebeni PM, Tamfum JM, Mwema G, Wan Q, et al. Clinical characterization and placental pathology of mpox infection in hospitalized patients in The Democratic Republic of the Congo. PLoS Negl Trop Dis. 2023;17(4):e0010384. https://doi.org/10.1371/journal.pntd.0010384.
Ploquin A, Zhou Y, Sullivan NJ. Ebola immunity: gaining a winning position in lightning chess. J Immunol. 2018;201(3):833–42. https://doi.org/10.4049/jimmunol.1700827.
Pratt C. EVD case in DRC linked to 2018-2020 Nord Kivu EVD outbreak. Virological.org: Virological.org; 2021.
Proal AD, VanElzakker MB, Aleman S, Bach K, Boribong BP, Buggert M, et al. SARS-CoV-2 reservoir in post-acute sequelae of COVID-19 (PASC). Nat Immunol. 2023;24:1616. https://doi.org/10.1038/s41590-023-01601-2.
Quinn KL, Stukel TA, Huang A, Abdel-Qadir H, Altaf A, Bell CM, et al. Comparison of medical and mental health sequelae following hospitalization for COVID-19, influenza, and sepsis. JAMA Intern Med. 2023;183:806. https://doi.org/10.1001/jamainternmed.2023.2228.

Raviglione MC, Smith IM. XDR tuberculosis—implications for global public health. N Engl J Med. 2007;356(7):656–9. https://doi.org/10.1056/NEJMp068273.

RECOVERY Collaborative Group. Tocilizumab in patients admitted to hospital with COVID-19 (RECOVERY): a randomised, controlled, open-label, platform trial. Lancet. 2021;397(10285):1637–45. https://doi.org/10.1016/s0140-6736(21)00676-0.

Recovery Collaborative Group. Baricitinib in patients admitted to hospital with COVID-19 (RECOVERY): a randomised, controlled, open-label, platform trial and updated meta-analysis. Lancet. 2022;400(10349):359–68. https://doi.org/10.1016/S0140-6736(22)01109-6.

Reddy K, Sinha P, O'Kane CM, Gordon AC, Calfee CS, McAuley DF. Subphenotypes in critical care: translation into clinical practice. Lancet Respir Med. 2020;8(6):631–43. https://doi.org/10.1016/s2213--2600(20)30124-7.

Reynolds MG, Anh BH, Thu VH, Montgomery JM, Bausch DG, Shah JJ, et al. Factors associated with nosocomial SARS-CoV transmission among healthcare workers in Hanoi, Vietnam, 2003. BMC Public Health. 2006a;6:207. https://doi.org/10.1186/1471-2458-6-207.

Reynolds MG, Yorita KL, Kuehnert MJ, Davidson WB, Huhn GD, Holman RC, et al. Clinical manifestations of human monkeypox influenced by route of infection. J Infect Dis. 2006b;194(6):773–80. https://doi.org/10.1086/505880.

Rimoin AW, Mulembakani PM, Johnston SC, Lloyd Smith JO, Kisalu NK, Kinkela TL, et al. Major increase in human monkeypox incidence 30 years after smallpox vaccination campaigns cease in the Democratic Republic of Congo. Proc Natl Acad Sci USA. 2010;107(37):16262–7. https://doi.org/10.1073/pnas.1005769107.

Rojek AM, Salam A, Ragotte RJ, Liddiard E, Elhussain A, Carlqvist A, et al. A systematic review and meta-analysis of patient data from the West Africa (2013-16) Ebola virus disease epidemic. Clin Microbiol Infect. 2019;25(11):1307–14. https://doi.org/10.1016/j.cmi.2019.06.032.

Rojek A, Dunning J, Haynes R, Horby P, Peto L. Randomised controlled trials for mpox in endemic countries. Lancet Infect Dis. 2023;23(3):281. https://doi.org/10.1016/S1473-3099(23)00045-2.

Russell CD, Lone NI, Baillie JK. Comorbidities, multimorbidity and COVID-19. Nat Med. 2023;29(2):334–43. https://doi.org/10.1038/s41591--022-02156-9.

Saijo M, Ami Y, Suzaki Y, Nagata N, Iwata N, Hasegawa H, et al. Virulence and pathophysiology of The Congo Basin and west African strains of monkeypox virus in non-human primates. J Gen Virol. 2009;90(Pt 9):2266–71. https://doi.org/10.1099/vir.0.010207-0.

Sigfrid L, Moore C, Salam AP, Maayan N, Hamel C, Garritty C, et al. A rapid research needs appraisal methodology to identify evidence gaps to inform clinical research priorities in response to outbreaks-results from the Lassa fever pilot. BMC Med. 2019;17(1):107. https://doi.org/10.1186/s12916-019-1338-1.

Simpson S, Kaufmann MC, Glozman V, Chakrabarti A. Disease X: accelerating the development of medical countermeasures for the next pandemic. Lancet Infect Dis. 2020;20(5):e108–e15. https://doi.org/10.1016/S1473-3099(20)30123-7.

Sissoko D, Duraffour S, Kerber R, Kolie JS, Beavogui AH, Camara AM, et al. Persistence and clearance of Ebola virus RNA from seminal fluid of Ebola virus disease survivors: a longitudinal analysis and modelling study. Lancet Glob Health. 2017a;5(1):e80–e8. https://doi.org/10.1016/s2214--109x(16)30243-1.

Sissoko D, Keïta M, Diallo B, Aliabadi N, Fitter DL, Dahl BA, et al. Ebola virus persistence in breast Milk after no reported illness: a likely source of virus transmission from mother to child. Clin Infect Dis. 2017b;64(4):513–6. https://doi.org/10.1093/cid/ciw793.

Sneller MC, Reilly C, Badio M, Bishop RJ, Eghrari AO, Moses SJ, et al. A longitudinal study of Ebola sequelae in Liberia. N Engl J Med. 2019;380(10):924–34. https://doi.org/10.1056/NEJMoa1805435.

Sridhar S, Luedtke A, Langevin E, Zhu M, Bonaparte M, Machabert T, et al. Effect of dengue serostatus on dengue vaccine safety and efficacy. N Engl J Med. 2018;379(4):327–40. https://doi.org/10.1056/NEJMoa1800820.

Stein DR, Warner BM, Audet J, Soule G, Siragam V, Sroga P, et al. Differential pathogenesis of closely related 2018 Nigerian outbreak clade III Lassa virus isolates. PLoS Pathog. 2021;17(10):e1009966. https://doi.org/10.1371/journal.ppat.1009966.

Stein SR, Ramelli SC, Grazioli A, Chung JY, Singh M, Yinda CK, et al. SARS-CoV-2 infection and persistence in the human body and brain at autopsy. Nature. 2022;612(7941):758–63. https://doi.org/10.1038/s41586-022-05542-y.

Subtil F, Delaunay C, Keita AK, Sow MS, Touré A, Leroy S, et al. Dynamics of Ebola RNA persistence in semen: a report from the Postebogui cohort in Guinea. Clin Infect Dis. 2017;64(12):1788–90. https://doi.org/10.1093/cid/cix210.

Sullivan MK, Lees JS, Drake TM, Docherty AB, Oates G, Hardwick HE, et al. Acute kidney injury in patients hospitalized with COVID-19 from the ISARIC WHO CCP-UK study: a prospective, multicentre cohort study. Nephrol Dial Transplant. 2021;37(2):271–84. https://doi.org/10.1093/ndt/gfab303.

Swann OV, Holden KA, Turtle L, Pollock L, Fairfield CJ, Drake TM, et al. Clinical characteristics of children and young people admitted to hospital with covid-19 in United Kingdom: prospective multicentre observational cohort study. BMJ.

2020;370:m3249. https://doi.org/10.1136/bmj.m3249.

Thielebein A, Ighodalo Y, Taju A, Olokor T, Omiunu R, Esumeh R, et al. Virus persistence after recovery from acute Lassa fever in Nigeria: a 2-year interim analysis of a prospective longitudinal cohort study. Lancet Microbe. 2022;3(1):e32–40. https://doi.org/10.1016/s2666-5247(21)00178-6.

Thornton GM, Fleck BA, Dandnayak D, Kroeker E, Zhong L, Hartling L. The impact of heating, ventilation and air conditioning (HVAC) design features on the transmission of viruses, including the 2019 novel coronavirus (COVID-19): a systematic review of humidity. PLoS One. 2022;17(10):e0275654. https://doi.org/10.1371/journal.pone.0275654.

Thorson A, Formenty P, Lofthouse C, Broutet N. Systematic review of the literature on viral persistence and sexual transmission from recovered Ebola survivors: evidence and recommendations. BMJ Open. 2016;6(1):e008859. https://doi.org/10.1136/bmjopen-2015-008859.

Thorson AE, Deen GF, Bernstein KT, Liu WJ, Yamba F, Habib N, et al. Persistence of Ebola virus in semen among Ebola virus disease survivors in Sierra Leone: a cohort study of frequency, duration, and risk factors. PLoS Med. 2021;18(2):e1003273. https://doi.org/10.1371/journal.pmed.1003273.

Timothy JWS, Hall Y, Akoi-Boré J, Diallo B, Tipton TRW, Bower H, et al. Early transmission and case fatality of Ebola virus at the index site of the 2013-16 west African Ebola outbreak: a cross-sectional seroprevalence survey. Lancet Infect Dis. 2019;19(4):429–38. https://doi.org/10.1016/s1473--3099(18)30791-6.

Uyeki TM, Erickson BR, Brown S, McElroy AK, Cannon D, Gibbons A, et al. Ebola virus persistence in semen of male survivors. Clin Infect Dis. 2016a;62(12):1552–5. https://doi.org/10.1093/cid/ciw202.

Uyeki TM, Mehta AK, Davey RT Jr, Liddell AM, Wolf T, Vetter P, et al. Clinical Management of Ebola Virus Disease in the United States and Europe. N Engl J Med. 2016b;374(7):636–46. https://doi.org/10.1056/NEJMoa1504874.

Van Kerkhove MD, Ryan MJ, Ghebreyesus TA. Preparing for "disease X". Science. 2021;374(6566):377. https://doi.org/10.1126/science.abm7796.

Varkey JB, Shantha JG, Crozier I, Kraft CS, Lyon GM, Mehta AK, et al. Persistence of Ebola virus in ocular fluid during convalescence. N Engl J Med. 2015;372(25):2423–7. https://doi.org/10.1056/NEJMoa1500306.

Vetter P, Fischer WA 2nd, Schibler M, Jacobs M, Bausch DG, Kaiser L. Ebola virus shedding and transmission: review of current evidence. J Infect Dis. 2016;214(suppl 3):S177–s84. https://doi.org/10.1093/infdis/jiw254.

Vilma L, Tomoko N, Samuel EJ, Shea JA, Juha K, Beatriz C et al. Genome-wide Association Study of Long COVID. medRxiv. 2023. https://doi.org/10.1101/2023.06.29.23292056.

WHO. International Health Regulations (2005). 3rd ed. Geneva: World Health Organzation; 2016.

WHO. Optimized supportive care for Ebola virus disease: clinical management standard operating procedures. Geneva: World Health Organization; 2019.

WHO. Strengthening clinical trials to provide high-quality evidence on health interventions and to improve research quality and coordination. WHA 75.8. Geneva: World Health Organization; 2022a.

WHO. WHO director-general's opening remarks at first meeting of the intergovernmental negotiating body to draft and negotiate a WHO convention, agreement or other international instrument on pandemic prevention, preparedness and response. Geneva: World Health Organization; 2022b.

WHO. The WHO global clinical platform forms to support the case management of viral haemorrhagic fever. Geneva: World Health Organization; 2023. https://www.who.int/tools/global-clinical-platform/viral-haemorrhagic-fever. Accessed 10 Sept 2023.

Yamaoka S, Ebihara H. Pathogenicity and virulence of ebolaviruses with species- and variant-specificity. Virulence. 2021;12(1):885–901. https://doi.org/10.1080/21505594.2021.1898169.

Zhang Q, Bastard P, Liu Z, Le Pen J, Moncada-Velez M, Chen J et al. Inborn errors of type I IFN immunity in patients with life-threatening COVID-19. Science. 2020;370(6515). https://doi.org/10.1126/science.abd4570.

20 Turning Research Results into Clinical Practice Guidelines in Public Health Emergencies

Donna M. Jacobsen, Henry Masur, Michael S. Saag, and Paul A. Volberding

Contents

Learning Track Note: This chapter appears in Learning Tracks: Clinical Research

E. S. Higgs and R. A. Sorenson (eds.), *Principles and Practice of Emergency Research Response*,
https://doi.org/10.1007/978-3-031-48408-7_29

Learning Objectives

This chapter will help readers and describe:

- The typical process for developing clinical practice guidelines (CPGs)
- How the CPG process has been modified during public health emergencies
- Conflicts of interest that may arise for panel members
- The kinds and reliability considerations of evidence used to formulate CPGs
- How clinical practice guidelines (CPGs) are conveyed to health care practitioners during an emergency when the providers are under stress and the guidelines may be subject to rapid changes

1 Overview and Role of Clinical Practice Guidelines

1.1 Clinical Practice Guidelines Background

Clinical practice guidelines (CPGs) are a vital tool to provide clinicians with recommendations for medical decision making for patient care, including diagnosis, prevention, and management of medical conditions. CPGs are generally designed specifically to provide clinical *guidance* but are not intended to be mandates or directives. They are written with health care practitioners as the intended audience but are frequently consulted by patients, payers (insurance companies or health systems), and public health authorities, among others; they may also be used in judicial proceedings like malpractice litigation (Ruhl and Siegal 2017). CPGs are not designed to set reimbursement policies or to replace a healthcare professional's clinical judgment about an individual patient's unique circumstances. Such distinctions are often lost on healthcare systems or insurance companies that see a benefit in measurable uniformity in practice by their clinicians. CPGs in well-established areas of medicine can usually rely on rich sources of definitive data, like reports of properly conducted randomized trials published in the peer-reviewed scientific literature, to comprise the evidence base from which the recommendations are made. Many, but not all, questions might be answered with available rigorous evidence.

This chapter addresses CPG development for emerging and urgent diseases for which evidence accumulates rapidly and may be of varying quality, particularly in a public health emergency. Examples with human immunodeficiency virus (HIV), hepatitis, and especially the National Institutes of Health (NIH) coronavirus disease 2019 (COVID-19) guidelines are described, and suggestions for creating a CPG are provided.

1.2 How CPGs in New and Emerging Diseases Are Different from more Established Diseases

When a new or emerging disease rises to the level of a public health emergency, such as Zika or COVID-19, clinicians often find themselves in unfamiliar clinical situations for which adequate published data and established treatments are lacking. As more information about the pathogenesis of the new disease is understood, patient risk factors for disease progression become clear, clinical trials provide results, and new clinical management strategies evolve, clinicians need a way to access information from a reliable, impartial source that balances the need to stay current with rapidly evolving knowledge with a careful critique of new studies for rigor, reliability, and generalizability. (A summary of elements of a CPG for emerging diseases is provided in ◘ Table 1).

1.3 CPGs for Public Health Emergencies Before COVID-19

1.3.1 HIV

The response to HIV is a prime example of how CPGs informed clinicians about best management practices for a new disease in the pre-internet era. HIV (CDC 1981, 1982) had a rapid evolution in terms of understanding

Table 1 Sample steps for developing clinical practice guidelines (CPGs) in public health emergencies (authors)

Sample steps for developing a CPG	
Establish trust	Ensure the sponsoring organization(s) is well-respected
	Appoint panel leadership and members with strong scientific reputations, leadership skills, and experience in developing CPGs
	Establish a transparent recruitment process
Empanel a CPG committee	Appoint panel members with expertise in the subject area, from an array of scientific disciplines based on the condition being addressed, who are committed to investing the necessary time needed
	Consider including members from affected communities and regulatory agencies
	Include members with sex/gender, racial, ethnic, institutional, and geographic diversity
	Educate members on the processes and requirements, including evidence to be considered, decision-making process, rating the recommendations, confidentiality, and dissemination
	Ensure disclosure and management of any financial or scientific conflicts of interest
	Bring in some prior experience in managing CPGs
Establish an administrative support team	Generate and manage ongoing literature reviews and other information sources
	Manage communications among panel and with stakeholders
	Provide operational support for leadership and members
	Prepare minutes, agendas, and working materials
	Manage the CPG document
	Generate and manage timelines and assignments to optimize workflow and deadlines
	Organize panel into teams as needed with designation of team leadership
Generate recommendations and create the "document"	Review all relevant data with systematic and regular information searches
	Develop recommendations that are concise, clear, unambiguous
	Rate each recommendation (e.g., for strength of the *recommendation* and quality of *evidence*), with clear definition of rating system (see Fig. 4)
	Generate text that supports the recommendations
	Include key citations that support the recommendation, rather than an exhaustive listing of all supporting evidence or a review of the literature
	Design length to be appropriate for a CPG (vs. a review article or book chapter)
	Create tables, figures, and boxes to communicate recommendations in a clear, concise, and readily accessible fashion
	Update the document as dictated by the emergence of new data and availability of new diagnostic technologies or therapeutic interventions
	Consider the best format for the presentation of a "living document" that can be updated as needed and is widely available and accessible
	Review the content regularly for currency, accuracy, readability
	Terminate online CPG when the need for immediately updated recommendations has diminished and the information is available from other sources such as print and online textbooks and journals

pathogenesis, and in terms of recognizing evolving diagnostics, preventive strategies, and therapeutics for the primary viral disease and for the HIV-associated comorbidities. In the early 1980s, HIV was recognized as a public health emergency. Information about natural history, diagnosis, and therapy evolved rapidly. There was much controversy in the lay press and medical literature about best practices for management. Clinicians needed help understanding the new data, new claims in the mass media, and actions supported by advocacy groups.

From 1982 to 1987, as the type and nature of HIV-related opportunistic diseases were recognized, data about diagnosing, preventing, and managing these complications were beginning to become available. Given how rapidly information emerged, the number of journals that were publishing important information, and the delay in getting information to clinicians, NIH initiated a CPG for managing individual opportunistic infections (e.g., *Pneumocystis carinii* [now *P. jirovici*] pneumonia and *Mycobacterium avium* complex infections) in 1989 and 1993. This guidance was expanded to a CPG for all HIV-related opportunistic infections in 1995 (CDC 1989; Kaplan et al. 1995). The initial CPGs were published in *Morbidity and Mortality Weekly Report* as an attempt to reduce the time from completion of the CPG to publication of the recommendations, compared with publication in print journals and reviews in books. Clinical trials were being conducted that required experience and expertise to interpret. Book chapters and journal review articles lagged the release of emerging data about therapies that patients were desperate to access. Online resources like UpToDate® and the online version of the Sanford Guide did not exist at that time.

The U.S. Department of Health and Human Services (HHS) published recommendations on the use of azidothymidine (AZT, zidovudine) from a state-of-the-art conference of experts in 1990, nine years after the first patients with acquired immunodeficiency syndrome (AIDS) were described (NIH 1990). This document was updated three years later as clinical trial data were emerging about single agents and combination regimens (Sande et al. 1993); however, any further updates would need to await new clinical endpoint (e.g., survival) data.

In December 1995, as data on more combination antiretroviral therapy emerged based on studies with viral load endpoints rather than survival or progression to AIDS, the International AIDS Society-USA (IAS-USA, now the International Antiviral Society-USA) assembled an expert panel of physician scientists and developed a CPG that was published in a high-impact journal within 8 months of the panel being appointed. Subsequent revisions initially were published annually and later biannually, based on the emergence of new evidence (Carpenter et al. 1996; Saag et al. 2020). By the mid-2000s, the pace of new, practice-changing developments had slowed, and country-specific, HIV CPGs were becoming available. IAS-USA continues to publish its CPG in the mainstream literature because of the credibility associated with publication in the peer-reviewed literature and the journal's ability to publish the CPG within 3–4 months of submission. The impact of the worldwide dissemination via publication in a respected, multi-specialty journal is clear; the IAS-USA CPGs have consistently reached Web of Science's highly cited status (meaning that they are in the top 1% of papers cited in the field of clinical medicine overall for the publication year). However, CPGs published in the literature will be quickly outdated if new major developments emerge.

In 2003, HHS began reissuing its CPG as a web-based resource, which improved its timeliness and accessibility. This transition to a web-based document required an increased budgetary commitment to support additional staff. The supporting team was expanded to include individuals with experience creating and maintaining a website, and editorial support was expanded. Furthermore, the panel leadership and members shifted their process to ongoing attention to new data and more frequent updates of the CPG.

1.3.2 Hepatitis C

After the discovery of the hepatitis C virus (HCV) in the late 1980s, newly available diagnostic testing began to reveal the unexpectedly high prevalence of hepatitis C in the United States and worldwide. As the link between hepatitis C and morbidity and mortality became more evident, clinicians and patients were eager to learn how to treat the infection and prevent or halt the progression of associated liver disease. A new generation of drugs entered clinical trials around 2012 and showed dramatic rates of "cure"—elimination of virus from the body—that were more than twice that observed with the previous, more toxic alfa interferon-based regimens, reaching success rates of more than 95%. The new drugs escalated the demand for treatment even more (Wang et al. 2016). However, most clinicians were unfamiliar with hepatitis C and needed guidance about host factors and viral factors that would influence therapeutic choices. Clinicians also needed to learn how to monitor treatment. Between 2012 and 2016, more than a dozen individual direct-acting antivirals (DAAs) were approved by the U.S. Food and Drug Administration (FDA) for use in the treatment of hepatitis C (FDA 2017). Clinical trial results were published frequently in various journals.

Clinicians clearly needed guidance about using the new, highly effective drugs for HCV. Historically, hepatitis C was diagnosed mostly by liver specialists, who also managed the limited treatments available to patients. With the new treatments, an expanded cadre of practitioners was required to ensure treatment was available to the many patients with HCV infection. The Infectious Diseases Society of America (IDSA), the American Association for the Study of Liver Diseases (AASLD), and the IAS-USA cosponsored a web-based HCV CPG targeted to liver specialists, infectious disease physicians, and general practitioners. The IAS-USA had the necessary expertise in developing CPGs, operational infrastructure, and website development, as well as special experience effectively managing a panel of experts and creating a web-based document quickly, one that was accessible, appropriately focused, credible, and nimble enough to be frequently updated as new clinical trial data emerged. The HCV CPG was initially updated 6–12 times a year as new DAA drugs and combinations were released. In some instances, the AASLD/IDSA/IAS-USA CPG was updated within a week of formal FDA approval of a new DAA, regimen, or indication. Such updates required an extensive volunteer effort and a substantial administrative support organization.

The HCV Guidance is an example of three professional organizations working together to cosponsor a CPG format that was enthusiastically received by its target audience of internet-familiar clinicians and was a marked advance from how CPGs for HIV-related opportunistic infections and antiretroviral therapy were initially developed and deployed.

2 CPG for COVID-19

At the end of January 2020, a month after China reported a cluster of unusual pneumonia cases in the city of Wuhan, the WHO declared a Public Health Emergency of International Concern (WHO 2020). The novel coronavirus, subsequently named severe acute respiratory syndrome coronavirus-2 (SARS-CoV-2), had been identified as the cause of the disease now called coronavirus disease 2019 (COVID-19). The disease quickly became a public health emergency and spread to virtually every corner of the world. As with HIV/AIDS, SARS-CoV-1, hepatitis C virus (HVC), and other emerging or re-emerging infectious diseases, clinicians urgently needed to understand the natural history, transmission, diagnosis, treatment, and prevention of this often lethal virus, which caused nearly two million deaths worldwide in the first year (Masur 1993; Ravelo and Jerving 2021). As of January 2023, the global death toll is estimated at more than 6.7 million. As so often with a new disease, or with an established but intractable one, untested, poorly investigated, unproven, and sometimes harmful and fraudulent therapies and preventives were soon being touted in social media by celebrities and politicians and, in some cases, by physicians (Grimes 2021). Internet sites, social media, and the 24-hour news cycle bombarded healthcare practitioners with unverified, often inaccurate, information and opinions. Volumes of preliminary clinical trial results and anecdotal observations were reported on websites, many of which were picked up and often exaggerated or distorted in mass media. Even the number of peer-reviewed articles published in conventional medical journals soon rose well beyond the capacity of any one physician or practice team to follow (CROI 2021; Stevenson 2021) (see Figs. 1 and 2).

With the rapid spread of COVID-19 worldwide and the lack of reliable, evidence-based guidance for clinicians, NIH began to assemble the information needed for a panel of experts to prepare a CPG that would be universally available online and updated as often as deemed necessary.

The COVID-19 CPG Panel published its first set of recommendations on April 21, 2020, 30 days after its first meeting (NIH 2020). As of August 2022, it continues to meet as a full panel every week and in subgroups at least four more times each week to update the guidelines, publishing changes 25 times in its first year to ensure that recommendations reflected careful review of rapidly accumulating knowledge about SARS-CoV-2 and were based on the most recent evidence.

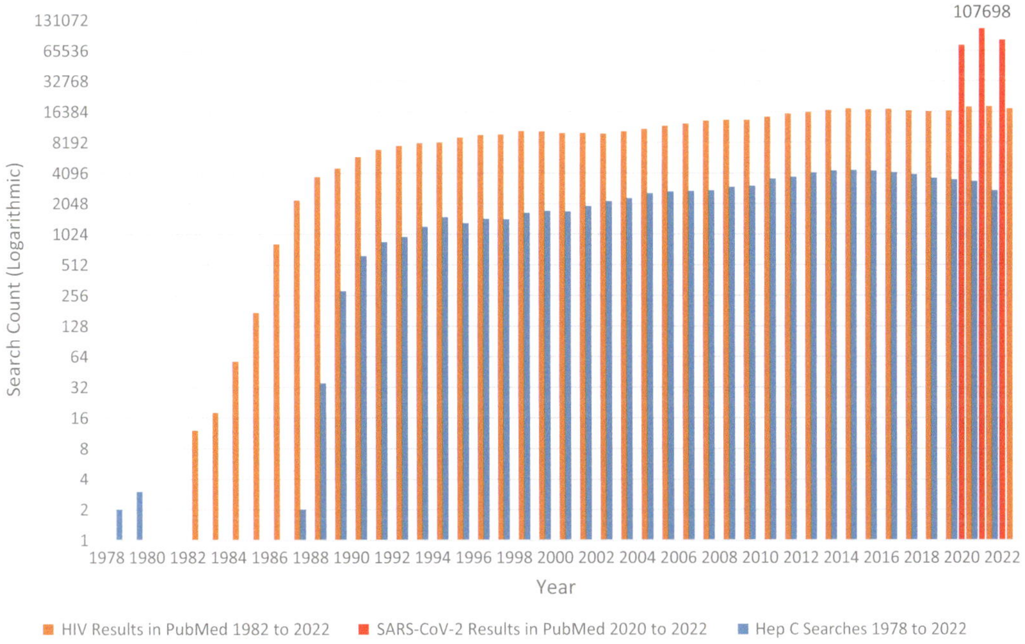

Fig. 1 Publications in PubMed for HIV, HCV, and COVID-19 from the first recognition of the disease entities through December 31, 2022, illustrating the relative volume and rate of new information for clinicians to consider around COVID-19. (Authors' work)

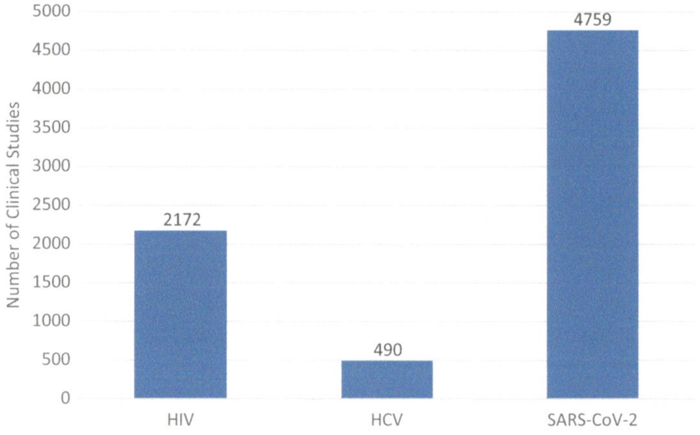

Fig. 2 Ongoing clinical studies listed in ▶ ClinicalTrials.gov for HIV, hepatitis C virus, and SARS-CoV-2 as of December 31, 2022. (Authors' work)

3 Creating a Credible CPG

3.1 Getting Started: Sponsoring Organization(s) and Leadership

A CPG will have little impact if stakeholders do not have confidence in its accuracy, objectivity, and timeliness. Trust in a CPG is essential and depends on many factors, including the reputation(s) of the sponsoring organization(s), the expertise of the individuals comprising the CPG panel and its leadership, and the usefulness of its recommendations. Government health agencies may often be able to quickly deploy the resources, expertise, and relative freedom from commercial conflicts of interest necessary to produce a credible CPG. Healthcare practitioners often relate best to members of their specialty or subspecialty and medical societies typically have leadership and expertise within their organization to sponsor CPGs that engender trust of their members. Other organizations with a reputation for high-quality information or continuing medical education that also have broad resources and trust may have the scientific expertise, operational experience, and administrative resources necessary to produce a CPG rapidly.

Once the decision is made to develop a CPG in response to a public health emergency, a panel and operational plan need to be developed. Use of an existing CPG infrastructure will expedite the process. The obvious challenge of redeploying an existing administrative team or individual employees is that such staff are often already consumed with their existing responsibilities and commitments to their other CPG activities. Leadership may have to make a well communicated and strategic decision to have targeted staff defer some of their ongoing obligations and focus on responding to the public health emergency.

Ideally, the CPG leader(s) will have prior CPG experience, management capabilities, a vision for the CPG, and broad professional recognition in pertinent areas of expertise. The leader(s) must have the commitment to devote sufficient time to the project to make it successful, the objectivity to determine whether they will have the time to follow through, and if such a commitment is realistic. Some degree of flexibility in the time commitment is required with the understanding that the initial assessment of time required likely is underestimated. Experience with HIV, hepatitis C, and COVID-19 CPGs indicates that many busy professionals will respond to volunteer roles for CPG leadership and membership if they see a national or global need, a high likelihood of having a major impact, and adequate infrastructure support. Confidence in the sponsoring organization and the named leaders is important to recruiting appropriate expertise.

Candidates for CPG leadership include well-respected subject-matter experts; government health ministry or research institute leaders; professional society or association leaders; and persons with CPG experience.

Each public health emergency is likely to require a different skill set. The initial IAS-USA CPG for HIV treatment benefitted from choosing well-known and well-respected academic leaders with experience in HIV CPG development (Carpenter et al. 1996). Panel members were national and international leaders in HIV research and active HIV practitioners. Members were recruited from outside the United States as well as domestically because, unlike some other CPGs, the document was intended for an international (developed world) audience.

For the HIV-related CPG sponsored by NIH, leaders largely came from NIH but with major contributions from academic leaders, the FDA, and the U.S. Centers for Disease Control and Prevention (CDC). All members were recruited from the United States because the target audience was intended to be domestic rather than international. For the IDSA/AASLD/IAS-USA HCV Guidance, academic authorities chosen by the collaborating CPG organizations provided leadership. For the NIH COVID-19 CPG, a mix of government and academic leaders, all of whom had worked together on other CPGs, accelerated the development of the CPG to respond to an urgent public health emergency that had disrupted virtually every aspect of day-to-day life. The resulting acute need for credible, science-based guidelines was complicated by political, social, and economic factors.

3.2 Assembling the Panel

Assembling the panel requires a strategy for identifying potential members from a variety of scientific and medical disciplines: research scientists, clinicians, clinical trialists, pathogen and disease experts, pharmacists, biostatisticians, regulatory scientists, and others. In the case of COVID-19, nursing and respiratory therapy expertise was essential. Panel membership should be diverse to be credible to all stakeholders, especially groups disproportionately affected by the emergency. Leadership needs to determine what scientific or financial biases would make resolving any conflicts of interest unmanageable and apply those criteria consistently (see below). Sex/gender identity, race/ethnicity, geographic location, specialty, institutional affiliation, and prior history of scientific advocacy are important considerations.

Representatives of patient advocacy groups and communities at risk can provide important perspectives. For the HHS/NIH HIV CPGs, there were well-developed advocacy groups with members who were eager to join the panel and who made important contributions. For the NIH COVID-19 CPG initially, the lack of well-defined advocacy groups made the identification of candidate community members difficult.

In a rapidly evolving public health emergency, there may not be time for an initial public request for applications, a methodical search for panel members, or careful vetting of applicants. Relying on experts identified by panel leadership from their professional contacts may be the most practical approach to launching the CPG quickly. Accepting nominations from other relevant organizations allows other groups to add their credibility to the process and to provide outside perspectives to the selection of panel members.

The selection process for CPG membership should be transparent and the criteria used for inclusion should be described in the methods section of the CPG. For the panel to operate effectively, panel member selection must consider personal and professional behavior and conduct. Panel members must have a history of reliability in expectations of participation, commitment to attending the majority of meetings, diligence in studying the relevant materials, and must contribute to panel work products. They must comply with expectations for confidentiality and timely disclosure of potential conflicts of interest and recuse themselves from discussions that are deemed to represent a conflict.

Importantly, members must have a record of working collegially in groups. Although candid discussions and differences of opinion

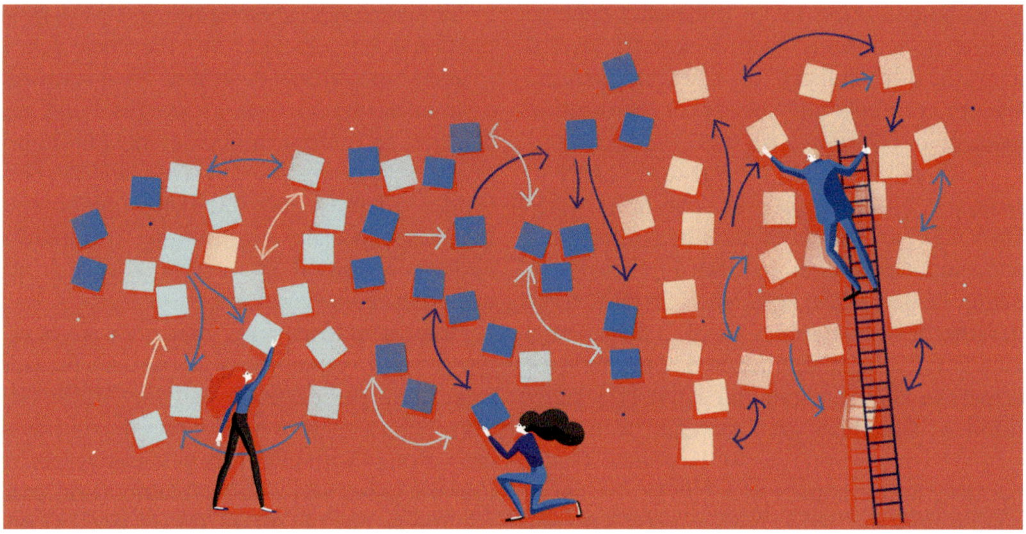

Fig. 3 When getting a CPG panel up and running, there are a lot of disparate inputs to place in some sort of rational order. (Giovanna Giuliano)

are expected and necessary aspects of the CPG process, members must be able to listen as well as speak, accept group decisions or votes without perseverating, consider differences as professional rather than personal issues, and publicly support the panel consensus recommendations.

Once the initial CPG is empaneled, additional expertise may be identified and new members added as necessary. CPG membership should be a flexible process with members added or retired as expertise needs change and as member performance may suggest that some choices were not a good match for the panel.

3.3 Administrative Support Team

Most CPG panels have administrative professionals who support the panel in a variety of ways, including organizing meetings, setting deadlines, holding members accountable for assignments, producing cogent summaries of meeting minutes and panel decisions, and ensuring that that the decisions of the panel discussions are accurately reflected in the revisions of the CPG in progress. The administrative team also includes members who support technical aspects of preparing the versions of the document, such as proper referencing, preparation of visually appealing tables and figures, and for online CPGs, website posting that includes initial document linking from text to graphics and vice-versa. Skills they need include medical editing, medical or health-related experience, and strong project management experience. Prior experience in managing a team of volunteer members and holding them to deadlines, scheduling panel and subcommittee meetings, overseeing the budget, and managing contractors is useful (Saag et al. 2018, 2020) (Fig. 3).

4 Sources of Information

In CPG development for well-established diseases, evidence is generally drawn from data published in well-regarded peer-reviewed journals selected by the panel. Abstracts from scientific conferences and expert opinions are often considered too preliminary, brief, and variable to be acceptable, and such information may change after submission and review by academic journals.

In public health emergencies, healthcare practitioners and patients need to have access as quickly as possible to information that is as reliable as possible given the early state of knowledge. In addition to published articles, then, CPG panels may seek access to conference abstracts, unpublished manuscripts, safety reports, and government communications, and in some cases, they will consider press releases, news stories, blogs, and social media posts. The latter sources, of course, must be used carefully. CPGs need to develop a systematic method to collect information from credible sources, starting with conventional literature searches in databases like PubMed or Embase (Institute of Medicine 2011). Finding a way to monitor and review all other sources of information, particularly those that are not usually peer reviewed, like preprints, is a challenge without an easy answer. Some new pathogenetic, epidemiologic, or clinical trial data are so striking that a responsible CPG should not wait for a journal to publish the data, or even until the data are published online. Some panels perform their own peer review of unpublished manuscripts and other evidence, especially when the research team is willing to present the data, answer questions, or both. These CPGs need a well-defined, comprehensive process for obtaining and analyzing data, but they may also be flexible when information comes to them in various formats, if the panel is able to satisfy itself that the data are reliable and relevant (Canadian Task Force on the Periodic Health Examination 1979).

4.1 Decision-Making Process

The CPG sponsor(s) and leadership needs to determine how decisions for recommendations will be made. Recommendations are best made by consensus of the full panel, based on initial recommendations from subcommittees if applicable. Some CPGs have a formal voting process, with or without publication of the actual voting tally. How decisions are made should be described in the methods, but the discussions among members leading up to the recommendation should be confidential to allow frank discussions and encourage members to be open minded about changing their minds in the face of convincing arguments or evidence.

4.2 Rating the Recommendations

An important part of developing a CPG is determining a rating scale for the recommendations. All recommendations are based on some sort of evidence, which can range in assumed rigor from numerous, well-conducted RCTs down to biologic plausibility or the panel's analysis of accumulated experience (expert opinion).

Various systems for rating recommendations have been used, from the relatively restrictive GRADE (Grading of Recommendations, Assessment, Development, and Evaluations) system (Guyatt et al. 2008) to those unique to specific CPGs that provide ratings for the *strength of the recommendation* and separately for the *quality of the evidence* supporting that recommendation (see ◘ Fig. 4). Rating the *quality of the evidence* is relatively straightforward from the data used to support the recommendation and cited in the document. Rating the *strength of the recommendation,* however, is not so simple. Some of the most robust discussion at CPG meetings involves how to rate the strength of a recommendation, often related to the difficulty of distinguishing between the strength of the recommendation and strength of the evidence. A recommendation may have high-quality evidence (e.g., from numerous well-designed RCTs) but still have a weak recommendation from the panel. Likewise, the evidence may be based on biologic plausibility or expert opinion (low quality) but have a strong recommendation from the panel, such as a strong recommendation for the use of a parachute for jumping from an aircraft with only weak supporting evidence (Yeh et al. 2018). Panel leadership and members need to apply the designated recommendation rating system consistently.

In an emerging public health crisis, a CPG panel may need to adapt previous rating systems to address the unique circumstances of the disease and the available evidence used to formulate the recommendations. Regardless of which system is used, it should be described in the methods section and summarized in a table or box.

Category, Rating	Definition
Strength of recommendation	
A	Strong panel support for the recommendation
B	Moderate panel support for the recommendation
C	Limited or weak panel support for the recommendation
Quality of evidence	
Ia	Evidence from one or more randomized clinical trials published in the peer-reviewed literature
Ib	Evidence from one or more randomized clinical trials presented in abstract form at peer-reviewed scientific meetings
IIa	Evidence from nonrandomized clinical trials or cohort or case-control studies published in the peer-reviewed literature
IIb	Evidence from nonrandomized clinical trials or cohort or case-control studies presented in abstract form at peer-reviewed scientific meetings
III	Recommendation based on biologic plausibility or the panel's analysis of the accumulated available evidence (i.e., "expert opinion."

Fig. 4 Examples of a strength of recommendation and quality of evidence rating scale. (Adapted from ▶ https://www.covid19treatmentguidelines.nih.gov/about-the-guidelines/guidelines-development/) (USG public domain)

4.3 Mitigating Financial and Scientific Biases

Panel members must be able to make decisions that are not biased by their individual financial or professional commitments. Organizations should determine in advance what financial relationships will be permitted and how potential conflicts will be managed (e.g., abstain from certain discussions or recommendations vs. exclusion from the panel), and maintain full transparency regarding the panel members' and the sponsoring organization's relevant financial relationships. The panel leadership and members' relevant financial relationships should be reviewed frequently and updated in the CPG as necessary.

Scientific bias of members must also be considered. Principal investigators of studies and funded investigators might be perceived as having a conflict of interest in terms of interpreting their own trial data or the data of competing studies when formulating a treatment recommendation. Although there are no absolute rules on when panel members with such potential conflicts should recuse themselves or be excluded, potential commitments to specific scientific approaches need to be considered to ensure a balanced and rational decision process about recommendations.

Decisions to exclude individuals with certain potential conflicts from panel membership, or to recuse them from certain discussions, often involve detailed consideration of the exact nature of the financial or scientific conflict. Such decisions are often based on qualitative assessments that not all adjudicators will necessarily agree on. There should be clear standards on what kind of relationships and over what period (e.g., in the past 3 years) are permitted or require abstention from panel deliberations to help with managing potential conflicts.

4.4 Sources of Evidence

In the earlier era of CPG development and still with some CPGs for well-established diseases, data usually had to be published in a peer-reviewed journal to be considered as acceptable evidence for developing CPG recommendations. In some of these cases, data from abstracts presented at scientific conferences are considered too preliminary and too brief to be acceptable.

Especially during public health emergencies, healthcare practitioners and patients need to be aware of new information and all pertinent evidence as quickly as possible. As a result, CPG members may want to review abstracts, preprints, government communications, safety reports, unpublished manuscripts, press releases, news stories, and social media posts, as well as published medical literature. A crucial source of trial result information before it is publicly available may be the trial team itself.

CPGs need to develop systematic methods to collect information from credible sources that start with conventional literature searches from databases such as PubMed or Embase. Finding a way to monitor all the other releases of information in a comprehensive way is a challenge without an easy solution. Some new clinical trial data are so striking that a responsible CPG should not wait for a journal to publish the trial, even online. Many panels feel that they can provide their own peer review of unpublished manuscripts, especially if amplified by presentations of the data with opportunities to question the research team. CPGs need a well-defined process for obtaining and analyzing data, a process that is flexible enough to accommodate circumstances in which information comes in various formats if in fact the panel is confident in the reliability and validity of such data (Institute of Medicine 2011) (see ◘ Fig. 4).

Box 1: Elements to Describe in the Methods Section of Clinical Practice Guidelines

- Type of evidence to be considered (or excluded)
- Evidence identification
- Literature search
- Other sources that are considered, such as abstracts presented at peer-reviewed scientific conferences, unpublished manuscripts, safety reports, personal communications, press releases, social media
- Selection process for the panel members, including
- Subject matter experts
- Representation of the biologic systems affected
- Representation of the communities affected
- Representation of other stakeholders
- Expertise
- Management of potential conflicts of interest
- Decision-making process: consensus, voting, etc.
- Process for rating the recommendations
- Strength of the recommendations and quality of the supporting data
- Other rating system relevant to the condition or disease

4.5 Readability: Format, Text, and Supplemental Materials

It is imperative that the CPG be user-friendly. For web-based material, because of the perception of unlimited space, there is a temptation to provide extensive details. This can make the writers' tasks a bit easier but not necessarily so for the CPG users. Excessively long documents are unlikely to be read thoroughly by most of the intended audience. Readers are usually most interested in the recommendations and the details primarily for the studies that were pivotal to make the recommendations. In some cases, discussion of the subtleties that are not apparent from reading the literature may be included if they had a major impact on a particular recommendation. Some other relevant studies can be included in references, but a CPG should not attempt to be a comprehensive review article or compendium of references that are simply confirmatory or are not relevant to specific recommendations.

The discussion for each recommended approach or treatment needs to describe the benefits and any risks and include discussion of any circumstances that require particular attention (e.g., the presence of comorbidities, age- sex/gender- or race-related differences, pregnancy, and socioeconomic factors). Recommendations should be clearly articulated, using the term "recommended," even if panel members assume the recommendation should be implicit to the reader. Use of language that suggests the user "consider" a specific intervention is generally not helpful and should be avoided. It is more useful for the statement to clarify under what circumstances a modified recommendation would not apply or to recommend an alternative. For example, "XYX is recommended in adults with HIV (rating AIa). However, XYZ is not recommended for adults with HIV who are receiving treatment for active tuberculosis infection (rating BIIa)."

As to editorial style, the CPG sponsor may have its own in-house style or use one of the established style manuals such as the *Chicago Manual of Style* or the *AMA Style Guide*. The panel members charged with drafting sections and recommendations should have a general overview of the style and format so there is some consistency across the document. In terms of terminology, each sponsor usually has preferred terminology, although some general suggestions are as follows.

1. Use "people first" language such as "people with HIV" rather than "HIV-infected people."
2. Similarly, avoid characterizing people by their conditions. "People with diabetes" is preferred over "diabetics"; "patients with cirrhosis" rather than "cirrhotics"; "people who inject drugs" rather than "drug abusers."
3. Out of respect and gratitude to the individuals who agree to participate in scientific studies that advance knowledge in the field, the individuals should be referred to as study "participants" or "volunteers" and not "subjects."

Tables, boxes, and figures, especially those that summarize the recommendations (with ratings) are particularly useful to the reader, recognizing that many readers have neither the time nor the focus to read detailed analyses. Over time, as the online CPG becomes more detailed and complex, it is increasingly important to harmonize and update recommendations across all relevant sections, including tables, figures, and references. Similarly, as the document evolves, the outdated and less useful sections and graphics need to be retired. Drugs that were widely considered and discussed at one time may be completely irrelevant a short time later (Henderson 2021). Summarizing the most recent updates in a table and at the beginning of the CPG, prominently showing the date of the update, and in some cases highlighting updates (with the date) are extremely helpful for the user to rapidly locate any new recommendations or ratings. Some CPGs maintain a separate table of all updates over time, by date.

4.6 Publication and Dissemination of CPG

Publication of a CPG in a respected peer-review journal has been the traditional approach to CPG dissemination and still has considerable value for the reader, the field overall, and the sponsoring organization. However, for public health emergencies, there is a need for a CPG that is accessible to a wide audience beyond one journal's audience, in a format that can be updated quickly and regularly, as needed.

In urgent diseases, publishing a CPG in a traditional journal runs the risk of providing outdated information as soon as the CPG is published. Several organizations created online platforms for their CPGs with specific web addresses that can be easily searched for and accessed. Examples include Clinical Info HIV Clinical Guidelines (▶ https://clinicalinfo.hiv.gov/en/guidelines), the NIH COVID-19 CPG (▶ https://www.covid19treatmentCPGs.nih.gov/), and the IDSA/AASLD/IAS-USA-HCV (▶ https://www.hcvguidelines.org/). These web addresses can also be publicized by media outreach via journals, press releases, Twitter (now X), and Facebook, as well as on organizational websites.

4.7 Managing a Web-Based Living Document

For web-based CPGs in urgent and rapidly evolving areas, updates need to be done as often as required to maintain currency of the CPG. The CPG needs ongoing surveillance to ensure that the organization of the CPG site is logical and easy to access and use.

Sections of the web-based CPG can quickly become out of date. In addition, panel membership may change, new potential conflicts of interest may arise, references may need updating, and tables, boxes, and figures may need harmonization with updated text. Harmonization is particularly important as the CPG grows in complexity overtime. A simple change may well require updates in several parts of the document as well as in tables, figures, boxes, and supplementary material. It is essential to ensure that all materials and statements in the CPG are consistent. Maintaining the CPG so that it is accurate, consistent, and current requires dedicated support and attention to detail.

4.8 Lifespan of a CPG

The goal of all CPGs is to serve their target audience to improve patient outcomes. Success, therefore, is best measured by utilization data and user feedback. For a web-based CPG utilization data typically includes the number and type of users who access the CPGs. Beyond simply recording the number of "hits" or downloads from the website, metrics such as length of time on the webpage, visitation to linked sites, table viewing, and number of pages viewed per visit can be useful. User feedback can be solicited formally on the live website or can be sought via surveys. Letters to the editors or other forms of direct communication from the end users serve as an effective quality assurance service. Feedback from other stakeholders is another way to measure success. Federal agencies and funders, such as insurance companies, along with the public, all have an interest in the effectiveness, accuracy, and efficiency of CPGs.

Based on feedback from the CPG leadership and panel members as well as these other sources, the CPGs can be kept updated and relevant. The feedback also can indicate when the CPG may not be needed any longer. In certain instances, the clinical disease state is either no longer a problem or has become straightforward in approach to management, making the web-based, frequently updated CPG and urgent attention of the volunteers panel no longer necessary. In such instances, the CPG should be "sun-setted" and put out to pasture, or, if appropriate, published only as needed in the more traditional literature. If the website is left online for historical purposes, notice that the CPG is not being actively updated and the date of last update should be displayed prominently on the website.

5 Conclusion

CPGs are especially important in improving care outcomes in the setting of new and rapidly evolving medical conditions and require innovative approaches in development and distribution. The lack of an existing base of knowledge of effective treatment, along with rapid explosion of new information, much of which is conveyed before the peer-reviewed standard of medical literature takes place, makes it difficult to ensure care is optimal. CPGs in this setting can be developed by taking lessons from prior instances of creating CPGs during other emerging diseases. CPGs for HIV, HCV, and COVID-19 can be used as current exemplars; future CPGs can adopt approaches used in prior public health emergencies to develop, update, and communicate effective recommendations to healthcare practitioners.

Appointing leaders and representative panel members with expertise in the field and prior CPG development experience who are able to collaborate under the pressure of rapid change, along with experienced staff, are key to this effort. Transparency in the process and instituting standards for mitigating any potential conflicts of interest are essential as well. Finally, defining methods of collating and reviewing all relevant evidence, which may include abstracts, preprints, and other early data, along with a process of rapid dissemination such as that afforded by internet-based platforms, can enable successful implementation of this crucial activity. At the time of this writing, dissemination of recommendations via a web-based platform—something not imagined possible even 30 years ago—allows immediate updates with free and widespread access to all users worldwide. With the rapid advances in new technologies, however, GPG sponsors need to continue to evaluate the best ways to disseminate their CPGs.

As we can anticipate continued rapid change in the current COVID-19 pandemic and in future ones, applying the lessons learned and implementing new strategies as necessary is vital to our field.

Discussion Questions

1. *Conflicts of interest*: Financial relationships between commercial entities and panel members and leaders may include research support, consultancy, stock options or ownership, payment for speeches, employment, and payments for work on data and safety monitoring boards (DSMBs), among other possibilities.
   (a) How should such relationships and possible financial conflicts of interest be managed for a CPG panel: Is disclosure enough? Are any financial relationships acceptable? Are there some relationships that are more allowable than others are? Should there be a dollar amount threshold? Should panel leadership be held to a different standard than members?
   (b) How might conflicts of interest unduly influence CPG discussions? (Same discussion points as above.)
2. *Evidence used in creating CPGs*: In urgent public health crises, new information emerges quickly but not always reliably.
   (a) What types of review and validation might be important for including data that are not peer reviewed? Create a rating scale for the strength of the recommendations, quality of the evidence, and other parameters that can be used in this setting.
3. *Delivering CPG Content in Urgent Public Health Crises*: Although the World Wide Web was only launched in the early 1990s, it did not begin to be the everyday tool we know today until about 2000. The internet has made instant access to information available to almost anyone with access to a computer, which as discussed in this chapter, has been essential for CPGs in urgent public health crises.
   (a) *Discussion*: Look forward to 20 years from now. In what ways might technology have evolved to deliver credible CPGs that are widely accessible and user friendly to their various audiences?

References

Canadian Task Force on the Periodic Health Examination. The periodic health examination. Can Med Assoc J. 1979;121(9):1193–254.

Carpenter CCJ, Fischl MA, Hammer SM, Hirsch MS, Jacobsen DM, Katzenstein DA, et al. Antiretroviral therapy for HIV infection in 1996: recommendations of an international panel. JAMA. 1996;276(2):146–54. https://doi.org/10.1001/jama.1996.03540020068031.

CDC. Pneumocystis pneumonia—Los Angeles. MMWR Morb Mortal Wkly Rep. 1981;45(34):729–33.

CDC. Update on acquired immune deficiency syndrome (AIDS)—United States. MMWR Morb Mortal Wkly Rep. 1982;31(37):507–8, 13–4.

CDC. Guidelines for prophylaxis against *pneumocystis carinii* pneumonia for persons infected with human immunodeficiency virus. MMWR Morb Mortal Wkly Rep. 1989;38(S5):1–9.

CROI. Program committee workshop for new investigators and trainees. Conference on retroviruses and opportunistic infections (CROI) San Francisco. 2021.

http://www.croiwebcasts.org/s/2021croi/Workshop-1;jsessionid=A9EBBA8EC3684AD683C424869A9781BF. Accessed 27 Oct 2021.

FDA. Chronic hepatitis C virus infection: developing direct-acting antiviral drugs for treatment: guidance for industry. Silver Spring, MD: U.S. Food and Drug Administration; 2017.

Grimes DR. Medical disinformation and the unviable nature of COVID-19 conspiracy theories. PLoS One. 2021;16(3):e0245900. https://doi.org/10.1371/journal.pone.0245900.

Guyatt GH, Oxman AD, Vist GE, Kunz R, Falck-Ytter Y, Alonso-Coello P, et al. GRADE: an emerging consensus on rating quality of evidence and strength of recommendations. BMJ. 2008;336(7650):924–6. https://doi.org/10.1136/bmj.39489.470347.AD.

Henderson J. More hospitals sued over right to try ivermectin. MedPage Today; 2021.

Institute of Medicine. Clinical practice guideline we can trust. Washington, DC: National Academies Press; 2011.

Kaplan JE, Masur H, Holmes KK, McNeil MM, Schonberger LB, Navin TR, et al. USPHS/IDSA guidelines for the prevention of opportunistic infections in persons infected with human immunodeficiency virus: introduction. Clin Infect Dis. 1995;21(Supplement_1):S1–S11. https://doi.org/10.1093/clinids/21.Supplement_1.S1.

Masur H. Recommendations on prophylaxis and therapy for disseminated *Mycobacterium avium* complex disease in patients infected with the human immunodeficiency virus. Public health service task force on prophylaxis and therapy for *Mycobacterium avium* complex. N Engl J Med. 1993;329(12):898–904. https://doi.org/10.1056/nejm199309163291228.

NIH. State-of-the-art conference on azidothymidine therapy for early HIV infection. Am J Med. 1990;89(3):335–44. https://doi.org/10.1016/0002-9343(90)90347-g.

NIH. Coronavirus disease 2019 (COVID-19) treatment guidelines. Bethesda, MD: National Institutes of Health; 2020.

Ravelo JL, Jerving S. COVID-19 in 2020—a timeline of the coronavirus outbreak. Dev Dent. 2021. https://www.devex.com/news/covid-19-in-2020-a-timeline-of-the-coronavirus-outbreak-99634. Accessed 27 Oct 2021.

Ruhl DS, Siegal G. Medical malpractice implications of clinical practice guidelines. Otolaryngol Head Neck Surg. 2017;157(2):175–7. https://doi.org/10.1177/0194599817707943.

Saag MS, Benson CA, Gandhi RT, Hoy JF, Landovitz RJ, Mugavero MJ, et al. Antiretroviral drugs for treatment and prevention of HIV infection in adults: 2018 recommendations of the international antiviral society–USA panel. JAMA. 2018;320(4):379–96. https://doi.org/10.1001/jama.2018.8431.

Saag MS, Gandhi RT, Hoy JF, Landovitz RJ, Thompson MA, Sax PE, et al. Antiretroviral drugs for treatment and prevention of HIV infection in adults: 2020 recommendations of the international antiviral society–USA panel. JAMA. 2020;324(16):1651–69. https://doi.org/10.1001/jama.2020.17025.

Sande MA, Carpenter CCJ, Cobbs CG, Holmes KK, Sanford JP, Coombs RW, et al. Antiretroviral therapy for adult HIV-Infected patients: recommendations from a state-of-the-art conference. JAMA. 1993;270(21):2583–9. https://doi.org/10.1001/jama.1993.03510210069030.

Stevenson M. CROI 2021: summary of basic science research in HIV and SARS-CoV-2. Top Antivir Med. 2021;29(3):355–60.

Wang LS, D'Souza LS, Jacobson IM. Hepatitis C—a clinical review. J Med Virol. 2016;88(11):1844–55. https://doi.org/10.1002/jmv.24554.

WHO. 2019 novel coronavirus (2019-nCoV): strategic preparedness and response plan. Geneva: World Health Organization; 2020.

Yeh RW, Valsdottir LR, Yeh MW, Shen C, Kramer DB, Strom JB, et al. Parachute use to prevent death and major trauma when jumping from aircraft: randomized controlled trial. BMJ. 2018;363:k5094. https://doi.org/10.1136/bmj.k5094.

Methodology for Research Response

Peter G. Smith

Overview of Book Section V: The major methodologies applicable in research response to an infectious disease outbreak are described, illustrating that effective response is by necessity an interdisciplinary endeavor.

Arthur Reingold (▶ Chap. 21) emphasizes the crucial role of the rapid implementation of observational epidemiologic studies, often done in conjunction with laboratory, environmental and behavioral investigations. Well-designed epidemiologic studies are crucial, particularly, but not only, in the early stages of an out-break or epidemic, and may guide the development and implementation of both non-pharmaceutical interventions and medical counter measures (MCMs) that can ameliorate or put a stop to the outbreak.

Bjarke Frost Nielsen et al. (▶ In Focus 21.1) emphasize the importance of very early studies to estimate the percentage of infected individuals responsible for most (80%) of transmissions. The so-called "super-shedders" are a characteristic of many infectious diseases, including SARS-CoV-2, for which about 10% of those infected were responsible for 80% of transmissions. Knowledge of their role is important, not only in designing control strategies but in modeling the likely development of an epidemic.

Rebecca Kahn et al. (▶ Chap. 22) outline design considerations for trials of vaccines as part of epidemic response, including classic randomized controlled trials and adaptive and other designs tailored to the nature of the epidemic. In this regard, Natalie Dean and Ira Longini (▶ In Focus 22.1) discuss the advantages and disadvantages of the "ring trial" design, illustrated through the first use of the design for the "Ebola Ça Suffit" ring trial successfully implemented in Guinea to evaluate the first vaccine against Ebola disease.

Michael Proschan and Birgit Grund (▶ Chap. 23) review the very important role that Data Safety and Monitoring Boards (DSMBs) have in trials of interventions, including vaccines and therapeutics, especially with respect to early identification of efficacious, non-efficacious or unsafe interventions, so that further research and/or rapid deployment of the intervention can be considered. Proschan and David DeMets (▶ In Practice 23.1) illustrate the demanding, complex task of the DSMB for the PALM trial of four potential therapeutics in the DRC, which was conducted despite minimal basic infrastructure, widespread popular suspicion and hostility, and outbreaks of violence.

Mathematical modeling has increasingly become an essential component of planning for and responding to infectious disease outbreaks. Bradford Greening and Martin Meltzer (▶ Chap. 24) introduce the principal types of mathematical models used to inform infectious disease response, along with best practices for communicating conclusions to decision makers. Modeling, though limited in the early stages of an epidemic by fragmentary data, can provide early insight into possible futures, including best- and worst-case scenarios, which may inform intervention strategies and can provide increasingly reliable guidance on likely outcomes as more data become available. With respect to mathematical modeling of the COVID-19 pandemic, Natsuko Imai et al. (▶ Chap. 25) summarize some of the advanced analytics and mathematical modeling used, focusing on key retrospective analyses and prospective modeling approaches. Joseph Wu and Corey Peak (▶ Case Study 25.1) describe how mathematical modeling was used to rapidly assess a proposed yellow fever vaccination campaign with reduced vaccine dosage to ameliorate supply shortages—correctly predicting the strategy would prevent more infections than using the available vaccine at standard dosage.

Finally, Nina Gobat and colleagues (Chap. ▶ 26) note that infectious disease outbreaks are social events as much as biomedical ones and review principles and practices for rapidly generating evidence about social and behavioral dynamics in health emergencies. Credible and robust social and behavioral studies contribute to a holistic understanding of the social complexities involved in disease transmission, prevention, and control. Their rapid initiation and analysis is likely to be relevant to both policy and response, including providing guidance for messaging and avoiding potential missteps with stakeholder communities.

Contents

21 Epidemiologic Research in the Setting of Outbreak Response

Arthur Reingold

Contents

You can observe a lot by just watching.
—Yogi Berra, New York Yankees (1925–2015)

Learning Track Note: This chapter appears in Learning Tracks: Biostatistics; One Health; Preparedness; Public Health & Epidemiology

E. S. Higgs and R. A. Sorenson (eds.), *Principles and Practice of Emergency Research Response*,
https://doi.org/10.1007/978-3-031-48408-7_30

Learning Objectives

This chapter will help readers understand and describe:

- What observational epidemiological study designs can be employed to quickly assess the effectiveness of public health, clinical, or medical countermeasure intervention modalities in reducing disease transmission and the need for hospitalization
- How well-designed and efficiently executed observational studies guide the development and implementation of effective interventions
- Major threats to the validity of such studies and how to minimize these threats
- The prerequisites for carrying out studies that evaluate the impact (or lack thereof) of policies and what study designs can be employed

1 Introduction

The subject of this chapter is observational epidemiology in the context of investigating and responding to an outbreak, epidemic, or pandemic. Laboratory and environmental studies (▶ Chap. 9); behavioral, anthropological, and other social science studies (▶ Chap. 26); mathematical modeling (▶ Chap. 24); and experimental studies (i.e., randomized trials of therapies and vaccines) (▶ Chap. 22) may also be critically important components of the research carried out in the context of an outbreak or epidemic/pandemic. Because those topics are all addressed in other chapters, they will not be covered here, although the observational epidemiological studies discussed here are almost invariably conducted in conjunction with, benefit from, or provide benefit to such studies.

Modern-day epidemiological investigations of outbreaks of infectious diseases typically involve the collection and testing of specimens from patients, the environment, or both, as well as the application of sophisticated laboratory methods for pathogen discovery, identification, or subtyping, in an earlier era, epidemiological studies alone often provided important insights into the epidemiological features of infectious diseases and informed prevention efforts. Thus, John Snow's well-known nineteenth-century research on cholera in London (◘ Fig. 1) identified water as the source of illness and helped lay the foundations for epidemiology as a discipline (Snow 1854).

Perhaps less well known to many is the work of Peter Panum, who investigated an epidemic of measles on the Faroe Islands in 1846 and showed that the incubation period was 10–14 days; patients are infectious during the prodromal stage (after the first symptoms appear but before the diagnostic features of the disease appear) and early in the course of their illness but not at the time of desquamation (i.e., subsequent peeling of the skin); the immunity produced by measles is lifelong; and there is little or no transmission by fomites (Panum 2018). Similarly, in 1846, Ignaz Semmelweis observed that puerperal sepsis, an almost universally fatal postpartum group A streptococcal infection, occurred at a much higher rate among women delivered by medical students and doctors, who often came to the delivery suite straight from the autopsy suite, than among women delivered by midwives (Carter and Carter 2019). He then showed that having medical students and doctors wash their hands with chlorinated lime between the autopsy theater and the delivery room reduced the mortality rate from puerperal sepsis by 90%, to a rate comparable to that among women delivered by midwives.

Thus, while modern investigation of outbreaks and epidemics of infectious diseases almost invariably benefits from close collaboration with the laboratory and often benefits from the results of a parallel environmental investigation, observational epidemiological

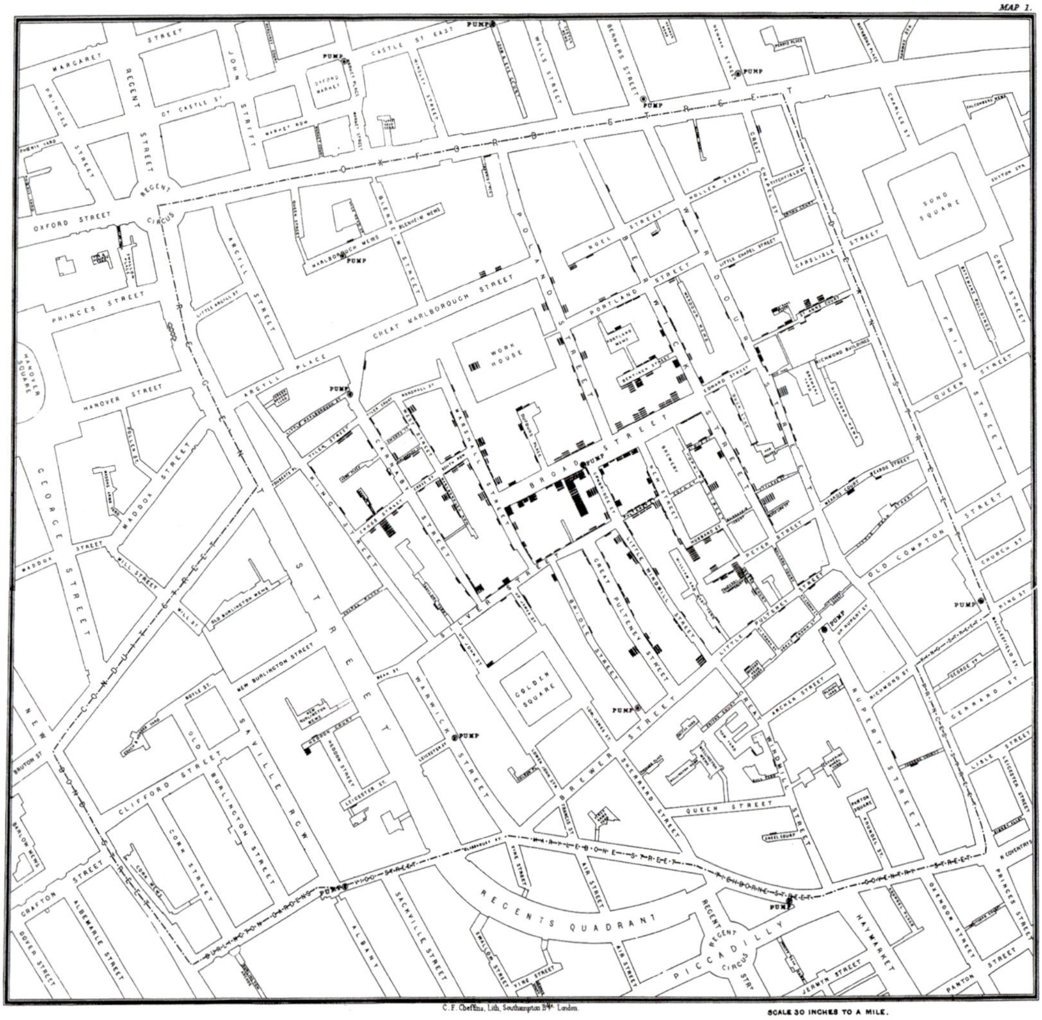

Fig. 1 John Snow's famous map, centered on the Broad Street pump in London and displaying recorded cholera cases as black bars. (Snow 1854) (Public domain)

studies, when well-designed, conducted, and analyzed, can guide control and prevention efforts. A somewhat more recent example, that of Brainerd diarrhea, reinforces this point (Mintz 2003). Despite multiple attempts by modern laboratories to identify the etiologic agent that causes this severe, often chronic watery diarrhea, the etiologic agent has never been identified. Nevertheless, in multiple outbreaks, a common source (e.g., untreated water or raw milk) has been identified by an observational epidemiological study and appropriate interventions developed and implemented.

Box 1: Confounding

Confounding provides an alternative explanation for an observed association between an exposure (X) and an outcome. It occurs when the observed association is distorted because the exposure is also correlated with another risk factor (Y). This risk factor Y is also associated with the outcome, but independently of X, the exposure under investigation. As a consequence, the estimated association is not the same as the true effect of exposure X on the outcome.

Because of the ever-present threat of various forms of bias, especially confounding, observational epidemiological studies are seen as inferior to and to produce a lower quality of evidence than randomized trials. Everyone who has taken an introductory epidemiology course or read an epidemiology textbook will be familiar with the axiom "correlation does not prove causation" or a variation of that phrase. While the concept is valid, it remains the case that many important epidemiological questions about a disease can never be subjected to a randomized trial, for either practical or ethical reasons. Fortunately, well-designed and carefully implemented observational studies can often provide useful and reliable answers to such questions, particularly in the context of an outbreak or epidemic.

2 Types and Sequence of Observational Epidemiological Studies

2.1 Types of Observational Epidemiological Studies

Epidemiological studies that do not involve randomly assigning individuals or groups to one or more treatment groups can be classified into six broad types in terms of their design, although these types comprise important subtypes and hybrids. While it is beyond the scope of this chapter to provide the detail concerning various study designs that are found in standard epidemiology textbooks (e.g., *Essentials of Epidemiology in Public Health*; Aschengrau and Seage III, Third Edition and *Modern Epidemiology*, and Rothman, Greenland, and Lash, Third Edition), the key attributes of the various types of observational epidemiological studies are summarized in ◘ Table 1. With the exception of descriptive epidemiological studies, all of these study designs are used to test hypotheses concerning the relationship between one or more exposures and one or more outcomes of interest, as well as to quantify such relationships. In the context of an outbreak, epidemic, or pandemic, the outcome(s) of interest might include transmission of the infectious agent; infection, whether symptomatic or asymptomatic; illness; and severity of illness, as measured by signs and systems, the need for hospitalization or intensive care, or death. The choice of an appropriate study design may be influenced by many factors, including the time needed to complete the study, the resources available, and ethical considerations, among others.

2.2 Sequence of Observational Epidemiological Studies

Several factors are likely to influence the sequence and timing of various epidemiological studies in the context of an outbreak or emerging epidemic, particularly the state of knowledge about the etiologic agent—unknown, suspected, newly identified, a new variant (especially germane to influenza and SARS-CoV-2), or relatively well understood. However, the relative priority for some types of information (e.g., response to various treatment regimens) and the timeframe in which needed data will be available will often dictate when various studies can and should be conducted. Other types of studies, including laboratory investigation to identify the causative agent, randomized trials of therapeutic modalities and of vaccine candidates, and modeling studies, will inevitably proceed along their own timelines (these topics are covered elsewhere in this volume), but expedited information sharing among investigators pursuing different disciplinary approaches to an emergency is an oft-noted area of weakness in emergency response (Degeling et al. 2015; International Vaccines Task Force 2018; Lees et al. 2020).

Table 1 Observational epidemiological study designs (author)

Study type	Common application(s)	Design elements	Key advantages	Key disadvantages
1. Descriptive	Describe the person, place, and time characteristics of cases	Tabulate cases by personal characteristics, geographic location, and time period	• Inexpensive • Can generate hypotheses concerning etiology and risk factors	• Not hypothesis testing • Susceptible to diagnostic and reporting biases
2. Ecological	Examine the relationship between aggregate, environmental, or global measures and the risk or rate of an infection, disease, or transmission	Assess relationship between group level measures of exposures and group level outcomes (e.g. incidence)	• Inexpensive • Rapid • Can examine effects of group level exposures and policies	• Susceptible to various biases, including confounding and the "ecologic fallacy"
3. Cohort	Compare the risk or rate of infection or disease or death by level of exposure	Follow individuals in various exposure groups over time; detect incidence of infections or cases; and calculate risks or rates, as well as risk/rate differences or ratios	• Less bias in measurements of exposure • Can establish temporal relationship between exposure and outcome • Can assess multiple outcomes	• Can be expensive and take a long time • Loss to follow up • Confounding by unmeasured factors • Exposure status may change over time
4. Cross sectional	Measure the prevalence of infection, disease, or risk/behavioral factors in a population at a given time	Recruit a population and collect information and specimens to measure current or past exposure and outcome information	• Inexpensive • Rapid • Can examine multiple exposures and outcomes	• Inefficient for studying rare exposures or outcomes • Cannot always establish temporal sequence of exposure and outcome • May not be representative of the population
5. Case control	Assess the association between suspected causal or protective factors and infection, illness, or death	Identify and enroll individuals with and without the condition under study and collect data regarding prior exposure and possible confounding factors	• Inexpensive • Rapid • Can examine multiple exposures	• Can study only one outcome • Confounding by unmeasured factors • Selection and information biases (e.g. recall bias)
6. Case only	Assess the relationship between an exposure that varies over time (e.g. recent vaccination) and the risk or odds of an adverse health event within a relatively short time window	Identify cases and compare the distributions of exposure status in those individuals immediately prior to the adverse health event to the distributions of exposure status in other (e.g. outlier) time intervals	• Controls for or eliminates time invariant confounding • No need for control subjects	• Not suitable for many outcomes • Only useful for adverse events with a short induction period

All epidemiological studies depend on having one or more case definitions, whether laboratory confirmed or based on clinical or epidemiological criteria. Similarly, such studies depend upon some form of case detection or reporting. Given one or more case definitions and a means of identifying cases, case reports, and case series can be quickly assembled, often within a few weeks, starting with the first steps below and continuing with further research.

- Development of case definition(s) and case finding/case reporting mechanisms
- Case reports and case series
- Descriptive epidemiologic and clinical studies
- Studies of risk factors and protective factors for infection or illness, hospitalization, or death, including treatment effectiveness and route(s) of transmission/sources of infection
- Studies of the impact of prevention measures and policies
- Studies of vaccine safety and efficacy (clinical trials)
- Studies of vaccine effectiveness, duration of vaccine-induced protection, and factors influencing them

The collation of cases, particularly if a standard, unbiased case definition can be employed, can quickly (within a few weeks or months) enable implementation of descriptive epidemiological studies describing the personal, temporal, and geographic features of the cases, as well as clinical information, such as signs, symptoms, laboratory test results, and outcomes. Concurrently or soon thereafter, analytic studies of the factors that increase or reduce the risk of infection, illness, hospitalization, and death are of high priority to help guide prevention, control, and treatment efforts; the study designs most often employed are case-control studies and either retrospective or prospective cohort studies. These studies also are critical to determining the route(s) and source(s) of infection; secondary attack rates; and the reproductive number, R_0 (i.e., the expected number of new infections directly generated by one infected individual in a population where all individuals are susceptible to infection), among other epidemiological features of the disease.

As prevention and control measures targeting individuals and communities are implemented and revised, their impact and effectiveness can be assessed, using either case-control or cohort studies to measure interventions targeting individuals, and using ecologic and modeling studies to assess the impact of community-level interventions. Finally, once a vaccine against the responsible etiologic agent has been deployed, many dimensions of vaccine effectiveness can be examined: effectiveness in various subgroups; effectiveness of varying schedules or numbers of doses of the vaccine; and effectiveness over time or against diverse strains of the etiologic agent. Again, the most common study designs employed are case-control and cohort studies of different types. At the same time, vaccine safety, as reflected in adverse events following immunization, can be monitored and investigated, again, using case-control or cohort studies or one of the case-only study designs. These studies, even under the best of circumstances, have rarely been feasible until at least 12–18 months after the onset of an outbreak or epidemic caused by a novel agent has begun, although they can be undertaken more rapidly if a vaccine against the causative agent is already in existence at the time the outbreak begins, or if the ambitious preparedness plans currently being considered come to fruition (Pandemic Preparedness Partnership 2021).

In any event, it is clear that there will be considerable investment, at least in the short term, in accelerating outbreak response research, including its epidemiological dimensions. Assuring that such research is thoughtfully designed and carefully implemented is of high priority.

3 Case Reports, Case Series, and Descriptive Studies

3.1 Case Definitions and Case Finding or Reporting

Early in the course of studying any outbreak or epidemic (or, for that matter, any illness or disease), it is essential to develop one or more case definitions that can be employed to classify individuals as having or not having the disease under study, so that cases can be tabulated and described. Case definitions may or may not include laboratory confirmation of the role of a specific etiologic agent. In many instances, it may be useful to develop and deploy multiple case definitions, including definitions for laboratory- or culture-confirmed cases; clinical cases; suspect or probable cases; epidemiologically linked cases; etc. Standardization and publication of these definitions allow for meaningful comparisons of data collected by diverse investigators in equally diverse settings and time intervals. See ► Box 2 for an example of an epidemiological case definition formulated for a newly recognized disease that was developed for toxic shock syndrome (TSS) caused by *Staphylococcus aureus*.

Box 2: Criteria for Staphylococcal Toxic Shock Syndrome (TSS)

Clinical Criteria

An illness with the following clinical manifestations:

- Fever: temperature greater than or equal to 102.0 °F (38.9 °C)
- Rash: diffuse macular erythroderma
- Desquamation: 1–2 weeks after onset of rash
- Hypotension: systolic blood pressure less than or equal to 90 mmHg for adults or less than fifth percentile by age for children aged less than 16 years
- Multisystem involvement (three or more of the following organ systems):
  - Gastrointestinal: vomiting or diarrhea at onset of illness
  - Muscular: severe myalgia or creatine phosphokinase level at least twice the upper limit of normal
  - Mucous membrane: vaginal, oropharyngeal, or conjunctival hyperemia
  - Renal: blood urea nitrogen or creatinine at least twice the upper limit of normal for laboratory or urinary sediment with pyuria (greater than or equal to 5 leukocytes per high-power field) in the absence of urinary tract infection
  - Hepatic: total bilirubin, alanine aminotransferase enzyme, or asparate aminotransferase enzyme levels at least twice the upper limit of normal for laboratory
  - Hematologic: platelets less than 100,000/mm^3
  - Central nervous system: disorientation or alterations in consciousness without focal neurologic signs when fever and hypotension are absent

Laboratory Criteria for Diagnosis

Negative results on the following tests, if obtained:

- Blood or cerebrospinal fluid cultures (blood culture may be positive for *Staphylococcus aureus*)
- Negative serologies for Rocky Mountain spotted fever, leptospirosis, or measles

Case Classification

Probable

A case which meets the laboratory criteria and in which four of the five clinical criteria described above are present.

Confirmed

A case which meets the laboratory criteria and in which all five of the clinical criteria described above are present, including desquamation, unless the patient dies before desquamation occurs.

At the same time, feasible approaches to identifying and reporting possible cases of the disease in question are essential prerequisites for conducting surveillance for that disease, including either passive or active surveillance systems. Passive reporting systems tend to be faster and less expensive to establish and maintain but often lead to incomplete, variable, and biased identification and reporting of cases. Active surveillance systems are typically more expensive to establish and maintain, but produce more complete and unbiased data. Surveillance systems, whether active or passive, may be laboratory-based or clinically based (or both) and may or may not be legally mandated—that is, there are certain diseases that must be reported to public health authorities by law in a given jurisdiction. Development of a standardized case report or case investigation form is also essential to the data-gathering process.

3.2 Case Reports and Case Series

In the earliest phase of an outbreak or epidemic, case reports and case series can be invaluable sources of information about the clinical manifestations of and laboratory findings in individuals with the disease. Such case reports and case series, which typically are generated by those involved in the diagnosis and management of the illness in a clinical setting, can be used in the development and refinement of one or more case definitions. They can also be very useful in the generation of hypotheses about risk factors and the etiology of the disease. As an example, the fact that the earliest cases of AIDS occurred in sexually active men-who-have-sex-with-men and in injection drugs users and hemophiliacs led to the development of hypotheses related to sexual practices, drug use practices, and exposure to blood as possible risk factors for the disease (De Cock et al. 2012). At the same time, case reports and case series typically cannot be used to test such hypotheses, unless the risk factor exposure distribution among the cases can be meaningfully distinguished from the exposure distribution in the population from which the cases originated, for example by using data from a recent, representative population survey. Case series are often used to assess the correlation of underlying co-morbid conditions or other factors (e.g., age, sex, and race/ethnicity) with the severity of illness (as measured by the need for mechanical ventilation, admission to the intensive care unit, or case fatality proportion). In addition, the beneficial or harmful effect of a given treatment (e.g., a medication) on such outcomes among those with the disease can sometimes be estimated (see below).

3.3 Descriptive Epidemiological Studies

Descriptive epidemiological studies, which typically have less clinical information but more epidemiological information than case series, generally provide details about the personal (e.g., age, sex, race/ethnicity, occupation, and socio-economic status), geographic (distribution of cases by location of residence), and temporal (distribution of cases over time) characteristics of the cases. Such early descriptive studies have been central to the early (and subsequent) investigations of SARS, Ebola in West Africa, and COVID-19, among other epidemic diseases (Aylward et al. 2014; Novel Coronavirus Pneumonia Emergency Response Epidemiology Team 2020; Zhong et al. 2003). Beyond providing information about the "who, where, and when" characteristics of the disease, descriptive studies can help generate hypotheses about risk factors for the disease (e.g., if a disproportionate share of the cases are in healthcare workers). In addition, they may provide information about the incubation period (the time period between infection and the onset of symptoms), the mean serial interval (the time period between the onsets of symptoms in successive cases in a chain of transmission), and other parameters. Descriptive studies can also provide vital information for modeling the likely future course of the outbreak (Aylward et al. 2014).

4 Analytic Epidemiological Study Designs

While epidemiologists have at their disposal a limited number of analytic observational study designs, as summarized in ◘ Table 1, all of them have been and can be used successfully in the context of an outbreak or epidemic to answer important questions concerning individual-level risk factors for infection, illness, hospitalization, and death; the effectiveness and safety of various treatment regimens; the effectiveness at the individual level of interventions, including diverse non-pharmaceutical interventions and vaccines; and the effectiveness or impact of group level policies.

4.1 Risk or Protective Factors for Infection, Disease, Hospitalization, or Death

Early in the course of an outbreak or epidemic, analytic epidemiological studies are almost invariably used to examine the role of various factors in determining the risk of infection, illness, hospitalization, or death; such studies can also be useful subsequently. Cohort, case-control, and cross-sectional study designs are all used, depending on the circumstances. Case-control studies are often deployed first. Because of the speed with which they can be designed and carried out, the results can be used to inform early development and subsequent refinement of prevention and control measures, as well as to assess their effectiveness. For example, case-control studies of the factors related to development of SARS in the community setting in 2003 in China, Hong Kong, and Vietnam found that exposures associated with an increased risk of SARS included having visited a fever clinic; eating outside the home; taking taxis frequently; and providing care for a symptomatic individual with laboratory-confirmed SARS (Lau et al. 2004; Tuan et al. 2007; Wu et al. 2004). Factors associated with a decreased risk of SARS included frequent mask use in public, frequent handwashing, and disinfecting living quarters (Anderson et al. 2004). In the COVID-19 pandemic, case-control studies in diverse countries found that factors such as recent close contact with someone with confirmed COVID-19, eating or drinking at a restaurant or bar, carpooling, and having a child in daycare were associated with increased odds of contracting COVID-19, while teleworking, wearing a mask at all times, and physical distancing of 1 m or more were associated with decreased odds of COVID-19 (Chu et al. 2020; Doung-Ngern et al. 2020; Fisher et al. 2020; Galmiche et al. 2021).

Cohort studies of various designs (i.e., retrospective, prospective, and ambi-directional) have also been used to study the factors associated with the risk of transmission or acquisition of the etiologic agents responsible for epidemic diseases. For example, studies of hemorrhagic fever viruses, such as Ebola, have demonstrated that an increased risk of infection is related to direct physical contact with patients or the cadavers of those who had died of Ebola, with exposure to body fluids conferring additional risk (Aylward et al. 2014; Brainard et al. 2016; Dowell et al. 1999; Robert et al. 2019; Tiffany et al. 2017). An exceptionally large cohort study (12 million adults) in England assessing risk factors for acquisition of SARS-CoV-2 infection and the development of COVID-19 has, interestingly, found that among adults ≤65 years of age, living in the same household with children was associated with a small but statistically significant increased risk of reported SARS-CoV-2 infection and COVID-19 outcomes during the second wave of the epidemic there, but not during the first wave (Forbes et al. 2021).

Cross-sectional studies have been used in the context of a pandemic to measure the prevalence of current infection, serologic evidence of past infection, and risk factors for infection with SARS-CoV-2. One such study, in San Francisco, California, found an estimated prevalence of current infection of 2.3% and an estimated cumulative incidence of

6.1% (Routledge et al. 2021). Risk factors for infection included Latinx ethnicity, inability to shelter in place and maintain income, frontline service work, unemployment, and household income <$50,000/year (Rubio et al. 2021). Similarly, a multistate study in the U.S. demonstrated that the prevalence of SARS-CoV-2 infection was higher in adolescents (10–19 years of age) and youth (15–24 years of age) than in older adults (≥60 or ≥65 years of age) during a surge in cases (Rumain et al. 2021).

4.2 Case Contact Investigations

Case contact investigations, which are a form of cohort study, can be invaluable in defining a number of features of an epidemic or pandemic disease, providing essential inputs into mathematical models and projections. A good example of such studies was an assessment in Taiwan of transmission of SARS-CoV-2 infection by laboratory-confirmed index cases to their close contacts. Through follow-up and testing of 2761 contacts of 100 individuals with COVID-19, investigators were able to measure the overall secondary attack rate (0.7%), show that only exposures to the index case within 5 days of symptom onset led to transmission of SARS-CoV-2, and estimate the median incubation period (4.1 days) and the median serial interval (4.1 days) (Cheng et al. 2020). They were also able to demonstrate transmission to contacts whose exposure to the index case was exclusively before the onset of symptoms in that individual.

For infections that can be transmitted from patients to healthcare workers providing care to them or working in a healthcare setting, analytic epidemiological studies are often employed to assess what factors are associated with either an increased or decreased risk of acquisition of infection in healthcare workers. Case-control studies have been employed to examine factors associated with acquisition of Ebola, SARS, and COVID-19 by healthcare workers (Barakzaie 2021; Doshi et al. 2020; Lau et al. 2004; Lentz et al. 2021; Reynolds et al. 2006). Factors such as inconsistent use or availability of personal protective equipment (e.g., gloves, masks, eye protection, and gowns) and fewer hours of infection control training have been associated with an increased risk of infection among healthcare workers for one or more of these diseases, while respirator use during aerosol-generating procedures has been associated with a decreased risk. Interestingly, and perhaps not surprisingly, some studies of healthcare workers have found substantial evidence that extra-occupational (i.e., community) exposure may account for many SARS-CoV-2 infections and COVID-19 cases in healthcare workers, rather than occupational exposures (Lentz et al. 2021).

4.3 Effects of Treatment Modalities

As noted above, observational analytic studies are often used not only to summarize the clinical and descriptive epidemiological features of a disease when it first appears but also to assess the impact of one or more treatment modalities (e.g., antimicrobial or antiviral drugs and corticosteroids) on outcomes (e.g., mortality). While it is widely recognized that in the absence of randomization, such analyses are subject to various sources of bias, particularly confounding by severity of illness, they can nevertheless be informative, especially before randomized trials can be designed and carried out. To take one example, a retrospective cohort analysis of mortality among recipients of various antimicrobial agents showed that individuals who acquired Legionnaires' disease in the first recognized outbreak in Philadelphia in 1976 were far less likely to die if they were treated with erythromycin rather than a penicillin or a cephalosporin (Fraser et al. 1977; Tsai et al. 1979). These results were available to guide treatment of future cases before microbiologists were able to cultivate the causative bacterium and demonstrate that in vitro sensitivities matched the epidemiologic findings.

On the other hand, such retrospective cohort studies may find no benefit from a particular treatment or even evidence of harm. For example, retrospective cohort studies of patients with SARS, for which randomized trials were not conducted, suggested that the anti-viral drug ribavirin and corticosteroids were each associated with possible harm (Stockman et al. 2006). Similarly, observational cohort studies of patients with COVID-19 suggested that the drug hydroxychloroquine was not beneficial, a result subsequently confirmed in randomized trials (Rosenthal et al. 2020). On the other hand, many observational cohort studies of the effect of corticosteroids on outcomes in patients with COVID-19 failed to find the beneficial effect demonstrated in subsequent randomized trials, perhaps because the observational studies included COVID-19 patients with diverse levels of severity, while the benefit demonstrated in the randomized trials was limited to patients with severe COVID-19 (Figliozzi et al. 2020; RECOVERY Collaborative Group 2020; Sahilu et al. 2021).

4.4 Localized Outbreaks within Defined Populations

Within a widespread epidemic or pandemic, cases and clusters of cases often occur in settings with a defined population or a limited time of exposure. When carefully investigated, such cases or clusters can provide valuable epidemiologic information about the infection and its transmission that can otherwise be difficult to obtain. For example, studies of the transmission (or not) of the etiologic agents of SARS and COVID-19 when an infected individual had flown on a commercial flight have been able to assess the extent to which transmission by asymptomatic vs. symptomatic individuals occurs, as well as the likelihood of transmission, depending on proximity of one's seat to that of the infected individual (Blomquist et al. 2021; Olsen et al. 2003). Similarly, studies of secondary attack rates among household contacts of index cases of COVID-19 have quantified the extent to which transmission of SARS-CoV-2 occurs in this setting, as well as differences in the risk of transmission, depending on the age (i.e., children vs. adults) of the index case, the SARS-CoV-2 variant, and the COVID-19 vaccination status of the index case (Madewell et al. 2021; Peng et al. 2021; Telle et al. 2021). Investigations of clusters of cases, such as a cluster of SARS cases in the Amoy Gardens housing complex in Hong Kong in 2003 or a cluster of cases of COVID-19 at a call center in South Korea in 2020, have provided strong evidence that SARS-CoV-1 and SARS-CoV-2 can be transmitted by small, airborne particles over distances exceeding 2 m (Park et al. 2020a; Yu et al. 2004).

4.5 Sequelae of Acute Infection

While the investigation of most outbreaks and epidemics focuses on the immediate, short-term health outcomes (e.g., illnesses, hospitalizations, and deaths) caused by the etiologic agent, there can be a need for studies of the longer-term impacts on health or other types of sequelae of acute infection. For example, there are numerous reports of persistent ill health among COVID-19 survivors (so-called COVID-long haulers) with diverse clinical manifestations. Longer-term follow-up of such individuals, most likely in the form of cohort studies, will be needed to characterize and quantify the long-term impacts of COVID-19 among survivors. Similarly, while the Zika virus epidemic of 2015–2016 caused large numbers of acute febrile illnesses, it was the effects of exposure to the virus in utero that led to a World Health Organization (WHO) declaration of a Public Health Emergency of International Concern (McCloskey and Endericks 2017). As a result, diverse analytic epidemiologic studies, including cohort, case-control, and cross-sectional studies, were conducted to assess the relationship between in utero exposure to the virus and various developmental and other outcomes in the fetus or newborn, such as microcephaly, prematurity, low birth weight, and fetal death (Brady et al. 2019). These studies found a strong association between microcephaly and in utero Zika virus infection, particularly during the first trimester (Aguilar Ticona et al. 2021; de Araújo et al. 2016; Souza et al. 2021).

4.6 Vaccine Effectiveness and Safety

Measuring the "real world" effectiveness and safety of vaccines deployed is almost invariably of interest, whether or not there is an outbreak or epidemic (▶ Chap. 36). While the randomized, placebo-controlled trial(s) demonstrating the efficacy and safety of a vaccine that support approval or licensure of that vaccine provide critical information about efficacy and safety, they are inherently limited by their size, duration of follow-up, and composition of the study population, among other factors. With regard to efficacy, trials leading to licensure or approval of a vaccine typically have short follow-up, meaning that the duration of clinical protection afforded by the vaccine can rarely be determined. In addition, the efficacy of the vaccine in preventing relatively rare outcomes (e.g., death from the disease) often cannot be calculated with precision, due to the small number of such events. Efficacy of a vaccine in various subgroups of the population (e.g., by age, underlying illness, and race/ethnicity) may similarly be not well characterized in the trial(s) because of the relatively small numbers of such individuals included. Moreover, if new strains or variants of the etiologic agent have arisen or become more prevalent since the trial was conducted, such as the Delta or Omicron variants of SARS-CoV-2, the trial results will shed little or no light on the efficacy of the vaccine against such new strains or variants.

Laboratory studies characterizing the immune response (e.g. neutralizing antibody levels and in vitro T cell responses) can be helpful in answering such questions, especially if data and samples from a vaccine trial allow for the determination of immune correlates of clinical protection, but they are not a substitute for direct estimates of vaccine-induced protection. Furthermore, the efficacy of a vaccine in the "ideal world" of a trial may not be identical to the effectiveness of that vaccine in the "real world" for diverse reasons.

While estimating the real-world effectiveness of influenza vaccines, including those developed and deployed in the context of the 2009 influenza A (H1N1) pandemic, provides an example of the utility of observational studies of vaccine effectiveness, the SARS-CoV-2 pandemic is even more noteworthy for demonstrating the utility of such studies. The reporting of "breakthrough" SARS-CoV-2 infections and cases of COVID-19 in fully vaccinated individuals, while expected, has raised concerns about the effectiveness of the various COVID-19 vaccines being deployed in countries around the world—concerns that have been exploited in many instances by those opposing vaccination against SARS-CoV-2 (Bergwerk et al. 2021; Wu 2021). It is important to note that the existence of breakthrough infections and cases, while proving that a given vaccine is not 100% effective (which is not surprising, as no vaccine is 100% effective), cannot by itself allow the estimation of a vaccine's effectiveness, nor can the proportion of cases occurring in fully vaccinated individuals, at least not without additional data, such as the proportions of fully and partially vaccinated people in the populations being studied. In a population with 100% coverage with a vaccine that is 99.9% effective, 100% of cases will be in fully vaccinated individuals.

There is currently enormous interest in measuring the real-world effectiveness of the various COVID-19 vaccines that are being used globally. As of the end of June 2021, ~70 such studies had been completed or initiated in the United Stats, Canada, Brazil, Israel, multiple European countries, and elsewhere. Study designs being employed include the screening method (in which the proportion of cases of the disease in previously vaccinated individuals is compared to the coverage with the vaccine in the source population), retrospective and prospective cohort studies, and case-control studies, including test-negative case-control studies (i.e., case-control studies in which the controls have been selected from among those tested for the disease/infection and found to be negative). Outcomes being studied include documented SARS-CoV-2 infection, transmission of SARS-CoV-2, symptomatic SARS-CoV-2 infection, COVID-19 hospitalization, and COVID-19-

related death. Study populations include healthcare workers, residents of long-term care and skilled nursing facilities, adults in the community, and immunosuppressed individuals (Haas et al. 2021; Harris et al. 2021; Moustsen-Helms et al. 2021; Zacay et al. 2021).

The advantage of such observational studies of vaccine effectiveness is that they can answer questions that the randomized trials of COVID-19 vaccine(s) were in many cases not designed to and could not answer, beyond the real-world performance of a given vaccine. Among the questions such studies can potentially answer are the duration of vaccine-induced clinical protection, the effectiveness of the vaccines in distinct sub-populations; the effectiveness of regimens and dosing schedules not examined in the trials (e.g., the effectiveness of regimens in which the number or spacing of doses differ and the effectiveness of regimens comprised of doses of different types or manufacturers of vaccines); and the effectiveness against variants of SARS-CoV-2 that were not circulating at the time the trial was conducted. These studies, while susceptible to various forms of bias, particularly confounding, will provide information critical to informing COVID-19 vaccination policies, such as whether, when, and to whom booster doses of COVID-19 vaccine should be given, as well as the composition of any such booster doses. They may also show that one or more COVID-19 vaccines or vaccination schedules currently being used have an effectiveness that is sufficiently low as to lead to re-consideration of its use and its replacement by vaccines or schedules with higher levels of effectiveness.

Because vaccines are typically designed and intended to be given to large numbers of individuals, many or most of whom are healthy, their safety is of paramount importance. Given that even a single report of an adverse event following receipt of a vaccine can, when publicized on social media platforms and in other types of media, markedly decrease confidence in the vaccine, provide talking points for anti-vaccination propaganda, and decrease vaccine uptake, it is critically important to monitor vaccine safety; investigate reports of adverse events; conduct appropriate observational epidemiologic studies to test the hypotheses generated by such reports; and explain their significance to the public.

With very few exceptions, the size of a randomized placebo-controlled trial of a candidate new vaccine is determined based on the expected incidence rate(s) of the outcome(s) the vaccine is intended to prevent, as well as the minimum efficacy considered important to establish and the desired precision of the estimate of the efficacy. Such trials, which rarely exceed several tens of thousands of individuals (only a subset of whom receive the candidate vaccine), have more than adequate power to measure with precision the frequency of common short-term side effects, such as injection site pain and swelling, fever, malaise, and headache. However, they are not large enough to measure or detect rare but potentially serious adverse events associated with receipt of the vaccine, which may not become apparent until the vaccine is given to much larger numbers (e.g., millions to tens of millions) of persons.

Rare, but potentially important adverse events associated with receipt of a vaccine can, therefore, typically only be studied using observational epidemiological study designs. The need to monitor adverse events following administration of vaccines is widely recognized, and wealthy countries like the United States have well-established systems for doing so, including both passive and active systems. The Vaccine Adverse Events Reporting System (VAERS), which is co-administered by the U.S. Food and Drug Administration (FDA) and Centers for Disease Control and Prevention (CDC), is an example of a passive reporting system: vaccine recipients, family members, and health care providers are all encouraged to report any adverse health event following receipt of any vaccine (HHS 2022). The Vaccine Safety Datalink (VSD), which is a joint activity of the CDC and nine healthcare provider organizations, is an example of an active adverse event reporting system, which uses electronic medical records to identify events in the days, weeks, and months following administration of a vaccine (CDC 2020). In the context of the COVID-19 pandemic, these systems have been augmented to enhance their ability to detect "safety signals" and conduct epidemiologic studies to test hypotheses generated by reports of adverse events following receipt of a vaccine. While the importance of having such systems in place in low- and middle-income countries has been widely recognized and discussed, progress in implementing such systems in most such countries has been slow, impeded by lack of funding and other obstacles (Amarasinghe et al. 2013).

Given a hypothesis that receipt of a particular vaccine is associated with an increased risk of an adverse health event, whether generated by analogy to another vaccine or by a report from a patient, family member, or health care provider, the observational epidemiological study designs employed to test such hypotheses and estimate the magnitude of the risk include cohort studies, case-control studies, and case-only studies. Examples of these different approaches can be seen in the investigation of the hypothesis that receipt of the influenza A (H1N1) 2009 monovalent vaccine was associated with an increased risk of Guillain–Barré Syndrome or of narcolepsy, and the hypothesis that receipt of a COVID-19 vaccine was associated with an increased risk of venous thromboembolism, thrombocytopenia, and bleeding.

The hypothesis that receipt of influenza A (H1N1) 2009 monovalent vaccine might be associated with an increased risk of Guillain–Barré Syndrome was predicated on earlier findings, suggesting that influenza vaccine, particularly the 1976 swine influenza vaccine, was associated with an increased risk of developing this syndrome. Both case-control and self-control risk-interval (a form of case only study in which only vaccinated individuals with the adverse event are included) studies have been performed for various influenza vaccines, leading to estimates of the incidence rate ratio or odds ratio and the number of excess cases of Guillain–Barré Syndrome per million people vaccinated (Vellozzi et al. 2014).

When case reports and an increase in the incidence of narcolepsy following widespread use of pandemic influenza A (H1N1) vaccine in 2009–2010 generated the hypothesis of an association between receipt of one or more of the vaccines being used and narcolepsy, similar study designs were used to test this hypothesis. Observational epidemiological study designs employed included retrospective cohort studies, case-control studies, and self-controlled case series, again producing estimates of the incidence rate ratio, the odds ratio, and the number of cases of narcolepsy per million vaccine recipients attributable to the vaccine. Only one formulation of an adjuvanted vaccine was associated with a significantly increased risk of narcolepsy (Hallberg et al. 2019; Miller et al. 2013; Montplaisir et al. 2014; O'Flanagan et al. 2014).

More recently, following the rapid development, testing, and deployment of multiple types of COVID-19 vaccine, reports of venous thromboembolism accompanied by thrombocytopenia and bleeding in recipients of viral vectored COVID-19 vaccines and reports of myocarditis in recipients of mRNA COVID-19 vaccines were received in Europe and the United States. In each instance, the earliest attempts to assess the relationship between receipt of the vaccine in question and the outcome of interest have included population-based cohort studies comparing rates of the respective outcomes among those who have and have not received the vaccine of interest or comparing the incidence rate among those who have been recently vaccinated with an expected incidence rate, based on studies of similar populations (Pottegård et al. 2021). There has been particular interest in making these assessments for vaccine recipients of different ages and sexes, and, when appropriate, by dose of vaccine administered (i.e., first vs. second), so as to possibly guide recommendations concerning use of the vaccines in various subpopulations. As more safety signals related to the use of various COVID-19 vaccines arise, these and the other types of observational study designs alluded to above will undoubtedly be deployed to assess the relationship, if any, between receipt of a vaccine and diverse adverse events.

5 Policies and Structural Factors

Many of the most important policies and interventions deployed to prevent or contain outbreaks or epidemics do not act at the individual level, and thus their effectiveness or impact cannot be assessed using analytic epidemiologic studies with individuals as the unit of observation, such as cohort studies and case-control studies. Mathematical modeling (▶ Chap. 24) can help estimate the plausible effects of such policies and interventions under various sets of assumptions; ecologic studies can be used to detect and directly estimate such effects in certain circumstances. While various biases, particularly confounding and the "ecologic fallacy" (when an association between an exposure and an outcome at the ecologic/group level is not an accurate measure of the association at the individual level), are known limitations of ecologic studies, they do not render such studies useless.

One illustration of how an ecologic study can inform efforts to prevent spread of an epidemic infectious disease within hospitals was conducted in Guangzhou and Hong Kong during the SARS epidemic. The investigators compared environmental and administrative characteristics of two groups of hospital wards—those where a "superspreader event" occurred following admission of a patient with SARS and those on which no transmission of the SARS virus (SARS-CoV-1) occurred, despite the admission of a patient with SARS (Yu et al. 2007). Altogether, 124 wards in 26 hospitals were included in the study. Among the ward-level factors associated with an increased odds of transmission of SARS-CoV-1 on the ward were a minimum distance between beds of ≤ 1 m; administration on the ward of positive airway pressure ventilation; whether resuscitation was ever performed on the ward; and whether staff members worked while having symptoms, while the availability of washing or changing facilities for staff was associated with reduced odds transmission.

Ecologic studies have also been used in the context of the more recent COVID-19 pandemic to investigate the effects of various policies imposed at the community level to reduce transmission of the SARS-CoV-2 virus, policies that had measurable adverse social, economic, educational, and other types of impacts. Policies examined using one or another form of ecologic study, such as time series and difference-in-differences analyses, have included school closures, stay-at-home orders, mask mandates, international travel restrictions, and continuation of on-premises restaurant dining, among others. Outcomes examined have included both the incidence of COVID-19 cases and of COVID-19 mortality during various time intervals following implementation of the policy. As shown in individual studies and as summarized in a recent systematic review of such studies, the policies associated with a reduced incidence of COVID-19 cases or deaths in a population include quarantine and isolation; mask mandates; stay at home orders; closures of schools, workplaces, and businesses; limiting social gatherings; and bans on public events and on international travel (Auger et al. 2020; Fowler et al. 2021; Guy Jr. et al. 2021; Mendez-Brito et al. 2021). On the other hand, allowing indoor dining has been associated with an increased rate of growth in the incidence of COVID-19 cases and deaths (Zweig et al. 2021).

Other strategies deployed in the context of a pandemic include temperature and symptom screening of various groups or in various settings, such as travelers, students, and employees, in order to identify and exclude or isolate those who are infected and could transmit the infection to others, with results typically reported in terms of sensitivity and specificity of such screening. To date, studies of exit and entry screening, whether for fever or for reported symptoms, have shown that such screening typically has had very low (often zero) sensitivity and very low specificity when applied in the context of SARS, Ebola, pandemic influenza A (H1N1), and dengue (Khaksari et al. 2021; Mitra et al. 2020; Mouchtouri et al. 2019; St. John et al. 2005). Other studies have shown that a policy of initial quarantine accompanied by laboratory testing for SARS-CoV-2 infection will detect a high proportion (68–92%) of international travelers who are infected (Burns et al. 2021).

Identification and tracing of contacts of an individual with an infectious disease (contact tracing) is a venerable component of efforts to control tuberculosis; syphilis, HIV, and other sexually transmitted infections; and diverse other endemic infections (e.g., hepatitis B and leprosy), for some of which effective treatment can be administered to contacts, preventing disease, onward transmission, or both. Contact tracing has also been deployed in the context of outbreaks and epidemics, such as Ebola and COVID-19. The assessments of the impact of contact tracing for Ebola during the 2014–2015 West Africa epidemic generally have reported on the proportions of cases for which contact tracing was initiated and of cases identified as a result (Swanson et al. 2018). Contact tracing has been seen as an integral and an essential component of the public health response to the COVID-19 pandemic, with substantial resources devoted to this set of activities in many countries. Assessments of contact tracing (or a testing–tracing–treatment) strategy have often focused on calculating the proportions of cases successfully interviewed or interviewed within 24 h of reporting; the number of contacts identified per case and the proportion of those contacts successfully traced and interviewed; and the proportion of contacts interviewed who were tested for SARS-CoV-2, positive for SARS-CoV-2, monitored, etc. (Bi et al. 2020; Spencer et al. 2021). Authors have sometimes inferred from these data that contact tracing was having a "suboptimal impact on SARS-CoV-2 transmission, largely because 2 of 3 cases were either not reached for interview or named no contacts when interviewed" (Lash et al. 2021).

Other studies have reported on the proportion of SARS-CoV-2 positive individuals who were asymptomatic at the time of diagnosis; the time from symptom onset to quarantine/isolation; the proportion of cases with an unknown source of infection; the mean number of contacts of infected individuals; and the time-varying reproductive number, showing improvements in some or all of these metrics (Liu et al. 2021; Park et al. 2020b). A retrospective cohort study in Portugal found no differences in the number of secondary cases per index case or the proportion of cases with one or more subsequent secondary cases, based on whether or not cases were subject to contact tracing and quarantine measures before laboratory confirmation of the COVID-9 case (Malheiro et al. 2020). An ecologic study examining the association between national contact tracing policies and COVID-19 case fatality proportions in 138 countries reported that countries that implemented comprehensive contact tracing had significantly lower case fatality proportions (Yalaman et al. 2021); however, the methods section of the paper did not provide a case definition of COVID-19. Increasing the number of asymptomatic individuals who undergo testing for SARS-CoV-2 as a result of contact tracing would invariably lower the case fatality proportion—if a case is defined as anyone with a positive test for SARS-CoV-2—but without necessarily reducing transmission of the virus or improving health outcomes in those who are infected. Thus, it is difficult to assess whether this association is indicative of a beneficial effect.

6 Summary and Conclusion

While Yogi Berra was right that you can "observe a lot by just watching," you can learn even more by taking a thoughtful approach to identifying important questions that need to be answered in the context of an outbreak or epidemic to improve knowledge and guide treatment and prevention efforts. Outbreaks and epidemics represent "natural experiments" and often present unique learning opportunities. While some questions concerning treatment and prevention can and should be answered using experimental study designs, many other equally important questions can only be answered using well-designed and conducted observational studies, acknowledging their limitations and possible biases. The results of such studies can not only inform medical and public health practices and policies but can also provide "real world" estimates of parameters used in epidemiological modeling and projections. Textbooks and "off-the-shelf" protocols, while important resources, are not a substitute for having well-trained, experienced epidemiologists available to formulate important research questions; select appropriate observational study designs for answering those questions; and implement, analyze, and interpret the results of those studies.

Discussion Questions

1. *Assessing the effectiveness of treatment modalities during a pandemic.* A pandemic involving a novel pathogen is producing substantial morbidity and mortality worldwide. While well-designed randomized trials of one or more treatment regimens are being planned and initiated, there is enormous pressure to assess the effectiveness of various treatment modalities being employed in clinical settings.

   Question: What observational epidemiological study designs can be employed to quickly assess the effectiveness of one or more treatment modalities in reducing the need for hospitalization; the need for care in an intensive care unit; and death? What are the major threats to the validity of such studies, and can those threats be minimized?
2. *Assessing the impact of population-level policies and restrictions put into place during a pandemic.* In response to pandemic spread of an infectious agent globally, countries, states, and localities often enact policies and restrictions (e.g., mask mandates, school closures, and travel bans) in an effort to reduce transmission of the infectious agent and resultant illness.

   Question: What are the prerequisites for carrying out studies to evaluate the impact (or lack thereof) of such policies, and what study designs can be employed?

References

Aguilar Ticona JP, Nery N Jr, Ladines-Lim JB, Gambrah C, Sacramento G, de Paula Freitas B, et al. Developmental outcomes in children exposed to Zika virus in utero from a Brazilian urban slum cohort study. PLoS Negl Trop Dis. 2021;15(2):e0009162. https://doi.org/10.1371/journal.pntd.0009162.

Amarasinghe A, Black S, Bonhoeffer J, Carvalho SM, Dodoo A, Eskola J, et al. Effective vaccine safety systems in all countries: a challenge for more equitable access to immunization. Vaccine. 2013;31(Suppl 2):B108–14. https://doi.org/10.1016/j.vaccine.2012.10.119.

Anderson RM, Fraser C, Ghani AC, Donnelly CA, Riley S, Ferguson NM, et al. Epidemiology, transmission dynamics and control of SARS: the 2002-2003 epidemic. Philos Trans R Soc Lond Ser B Biol Sci. 2004;359(1447):1091–105. https://doi.org/10.1098/rstb.2004.1490.

Auger KA, Shah SS, Richardson T, Hartley D, Hall M, Warniment A, et al. Association between statewide school closure and COVID-19 incidence and mortality in the US. JAMA. 2020;324(9):859–70. https://doi.org/10.1001/jama.2020.14348.

Aylward B, Barboza P, Bawo L, Bertherat E, Bilivogui P, Blake I, et al. Ebola virus disease in West Africa—the first 9 months of the epidemic and forward projections. N Engl J Med. 2014;371(16):1481–95. https://doi.org/10.1056/NEJMoa1411100.

Barakzaie B. A case-control study of risk factors for corona virus (COVID-19) among health care workers. J Bacteriol Parasitol. 2021;12(2):392.

Bergwerk M, Gonen T, Lustig Y, Amit S, Lipsitch M, Cohen C, et al. Covid-19 breakthrough infections in vaccinated health care workers. N Engl J Med. 2021;385:1474. https://doi.org/10.1056/NEJMoa2109072.

Bi Q, Wu Y, Mei S, Ye C, Zou X, Zhang Z, et al. Epidemiology and transmission of COVID-19 in 391 cases and 1286 of their close contacts in Shenzhen, China: a retrospective cohort study. Lancet Infect Dis. 2020;20(8):911–9. https://doi.org/10.1016/s1473-3099(20)30287-5.

Blomquist PB, Bolt H, Packer S, Schaefer U, Platt S, Dabrera G, et al. Risk of symptomatic COVID-19 due to aircraft transmission: a retrospective cohort study of contact-traced flights during England's containment phase. Influenza Other Respir Viruses. 2021;15(3):336–44. https://doi.org/10.1111/irv.12846.

Brady OJ, Osgood-Zimmerman A, Kassebaum NJ, Ray SE, de Araújo VEM, da Nóbrega AA, et al. The association between Zika virus infection and microcephaly in Brazil 2015-2017: an observational analysis of over 4 million births. PLoS Med. 2019;16(3):e1002755. https://doi.org/10.1371/journal.pmed.1002755.

Brainard J, Hooper L, Pond K, Edmunds K, Hunter PR. Risk factors for transmission of Ebola or Marburg virus disease: a systematic review and meta-analysis. Int J Epidemiol. 2016;45(1):102–16. https://doi.org/10.1093/ije/dyv307.

Burns J, Movsisyan A, Stratil JM, Biallas RL, Coenen M, Emmert-Fees KM, et al. International travel-related control measures to contain the COVID-19 pandemic: a rapid review. Cochrane Database Syst Rev. 2021;3(3):Cd013717. https://doi.org/10.1002/14651858.CD013717.pub2.

Carter KC, Carter BR. Childbed fever: a scientific biography of Ignaz Semmelweis. 3rd ed. New Brunswick, NJ: Transaction Publishers; 2019.

CDC. Vaccine Safety Datalink (VSD). U.S. Centers for Disease Control and Prevention; 2020. https://www.cdc.gov/vaccinesafety/ensuringsafety/monitoring/vsd/index.html. Accessed 27 Feb 2022.

Cheng HY, Jian SW, Liu DP, Ng TC, Huang WT, Lin HH. Contact tracing assessment of COVID-19 transmission dynamics in Taiwan and risk at different exposure periods before and after symptom onset. JAMA Intern Med. 2020;180(9):1156–63. https://doi.org/10.1001/jamainternmed.2020.2020.

Chu DK, Akl EA, Duda S, Solo K, Yaacoub S, Schünemann HJ. Physical distancing, face masks, and eye protection to prevent person-to-person transmission of SARS-CoV-2 and COVID-19: a systematic review and meta-analysis. Lancet. 2020;395(10242):1973–87. https://doi.org/10.1016/s0140-6736(20)31142-9.

de Araújo TVB, Rodrigues LC, de Alencar Ximenes RA, de Barros Miranda-Filho D, Montarroyos UR, de Melo APL, et al. Association between Zika virus infection and microcephaly in Brazil, January to May, 2016: preliminary report of a case-control study. Lancet Infect Dis. 2016;16(12):1356–63. https://doi.org/10.1016/s1473-3099(16)30318-8.

De Cock KM, Jaffe HW, Curran JW. The evolving epidemiology of HIV/AIDS. AIDS. 2012; 26(10):1205–13. https://doi.org/10.1097/QAD.0b013e328354622a.

Degeling C, Johnson J, Kerridge I, Wilson A, Ward M, Stewart C, et al. Implementing a one health approach to emerging infectious disease: reflections on the socio-political, ethical and legal dimensions. BMC Public Health. 2015;15(1):1307. https://doi.org/10.1186/s12889-015-2617-1.

Doshi RH, Hoff NA, Bratcher A, Mukadi P, Gadoth A, Nicholson BP, et al. Risk factors for Ebola exposure in healthcare workers in Boende, Tshuapa Province, Democratic Republic of the Congo. J Infect Dis. 2020;226:608. https://doi.org/10.1093/infdis/jiaa747.

Doung-Ngern P, Suphanchaimat R, Panjangampatthana A, Janekrongtham C, Ruampoom D, Daochaeng N, et al. Case-control study of use of personal protective measures and risk for SARS-CoV 2 infection, Thailand. Emerg Infect Dis. 2020;26(11):2607–16. https://doi.org/10.3201/eid2611.203003.

Dowell SF, Mukunu R, Ksiazek TG, Khan AS, Rollin PE, Peters CJ. Transmission of Ebola hemorrhagic fever: a study of risk factors in family members, Kikwit, Democratic Republic of the Congo, 1995. Commission de Lutte contre les Epidémies à Kikwit. J Infect Dis. 1999;179(Suppl 1):S87–91. https://doi.org/10.1086/514284.

Figliozzi S, Masci PG, Ahmadi N, Tondi L, Koutli E, Aimo A, et al. Predictors of adverse prognosis in COVID-19: a systematic review and meta-analysis. Eur J Clin Investig. 2020;50(10):e13362. https://doi.org/10.1111/eci.13362.

Fisher KA, Tenforde MW, Feldstein LR, Lindsell CJ, Shapiro NI, Files DC, et al. Community and close contact exposures associated with COVID-19 among symptomatic adults ≥18 years in 11 outpatient health care facilities—United States, July 2020. MMWR Morb Mortal Wkly Rep. 2020;69(36):1258–64. https://doi.org/10.15585/mmwr.mm6936a5.

Forbes H, Morton CE, Bacon S, McDonald HI, Minassian C, Brown JP, et al. Association between living with children and outcomes from covid-19: open SAFELY cohort study of 12 million adults in England. BMJ. 2021;372:n628. https://doi.org/10.1136/bmj.n628.

Fowler JH, Hill SJ, Levin R, Obradovich N. Stay-at-home orders associate with subsequent decreases in COVID-19 cases and fatalities in the United States. PLoS One. 2021;16(6):e0248849. https://doi.org/10.1371/journal.pone.0248849.

Fraser DW, Tsai TR, Orenstein W, Parkin WE, Beecham HJ, Sharrar RG, et al. Legionnaires' disease: description of an epidemic of pneumonia. N Engl J Med. 1977;297(22):1189–97. https://doi.org/10.1056/nejm197712012972201.

Galmiche S, Charmet T, Schaeffer L, Paireau J, Grant R, Chény O, et al. Exposures associated with SARS-CoV-2 infection in France: a nationwide online case-control study. Lancet Reg Health Eur. 2021;7:100148. https://doi.org/10.1016/j.lanepe.2021.100148.

Guy GP Jr, Lee FC, Sunshine G, McCord R, Howard-Williams M, Kompaniyets L, et al. Association of state-issued mask mandates and allowing on-premises restaurant dining with county-level COVID-19 case and death growth rates—United States, march 1-December 31, 2020. MMWR Morb Mortal Wkly Rep. 2021;70(10):350–4. https://doi.org/10.15585/mmwr.mm7010e3.

Haas EJ, Angulo FJ, McLaughlin JM, Anis E, Singer SR, Khan F, et al. Impact and effectiveness of mRNA BNT162b2 vaccine against SARS-CoV-2 infections and COVID-19 cases, hospitalisations, and deaths following a nationwide vaccination campaign in Israel: an observational study using national surveillance data. Lancet. 2021;397 (10287):1819–29. https://doi.org/10.1016/s0140-6736(21)00947-8.

Hallberg P, Smedje H, Eriksson N, Kohnke H, Daniilidou M, Öhman I, et al. Pandemrix-induced narcolepsy is associated with genes related to immunity and neuronal survival. EBioMedicine. 2019;40:595–604. https://doi.org/10.1016/j.ebiom.2019.01.041.

Harris RJ, Hall JA, Zaidi A, Andrews NJ, Dunbar JK, Dabrera G. Effect of vaccination on household transmission of SARS-CoV-2 in England. N Engl J Med. 2021;385(8):759–60. https://doi.org/10.1056/NEJMc2107717.

HHS. VAERS: Vaccine Adverse Events Reporting System. Washington, DC: U.S. Deptartment of Health and Human Services; 2022. https://vaers.hhs.gov/index.html. Accessed 27 Feb 2022.

International Vaccines Task Force. Money and microbes: strengthening clinical research capacity to prevent epidemics. Washington, DC: World Bank; 2018.

Khaksari K, Nguyen T, Hill B, Quang T, Perreault J, Gorti V, et al. Review of the efficacy of infrared thermography for screening infectious diseases with applications to COVID-19. J Med Imaging (Bellingham). 2021;8(Suppl 1):010901. https://doi.org/10.1117/1.JMI.8.S1.010901.

Lash RR, Moonan PK, Byers BL, Bonacci RA, Bonner KE, Donahue M, et al. COVID-19 case investigation and contact tracing in the US, 2020. JAMA Netw Open. 2021;4(6):e2115850. https://doi.org/10.1001/jamanetworkopen.2021.15850.

Lau JTF, Tsui H, Lau M, Yang X. SARS transmission, risk factors, and prevention in Hong Kong. Emerg Infect Dis. 2004;10(4):587–92. https://doi.org/10.3201/eid1004.030628.

Lees S, Palmer J, Procureur F, Blanchet K. Contested legitimacy for anthropologists involved in medical humanitarian action: experiences from the 2014-2016 West Africa Ebola epidemic. Anthropol Med. 2020;27(2):125–43. https://doi.org/10.1080/13648470.2020.1742576.

Lentz RJ, Colt H, Chen H, Cordovilla R, Popevic S, Tahura S, et al. Assessing coronavirus disease 2019 (COVID-19) transmission to healthcare personnel: the global ACT-HCP case-control study. Infect Control Hosp Epidemiol. 2021;42(4):381–7. https://doi.org/10.1017/ice.2020.455.

Liu H, Ye C, Wang Y, Zhu W, Shen Y, Xue C, et al. The effectiveness of active surveillance measures for COVID-19 cases in Pudong new area Shanghai, China, 2020. J Med Virol. 2021;93(5):2918–24. https://doi.org/10.1002/jmv.26805.

Madewell ZJ, Piontti APY, Zhang Q, Burton N, Yang Y, Longini IM et al. Using simulated infectious disease outbreaks to guide the design of individually randomized vaccine trials. medRxiv. 2021. https://doi.org/10.1101/2021.01.29.21250703.

Malheiro R, Figueiredo AL, Magalhaes JP, Teixeira P, Moita I, Moutinho MC, et al. Effectiveness of contact tracing and quarantine on reducing COVID-19 transmission: a retrospective cohort study. Public Health. 2020;189:54–9. https://doi.org/10.1016/j.puhe.2020.09.012.

McCloskey B, Endericks T. The rise of Zika infection and microcephaly: what can we learn from a public health emergency? Public Health. 2017;150:87–92. https://doi.org/10.1016/j.puhe.2017.05.008.

Mendez-Brito A, El Bcheraoui C, Pozo-Martin F. Systematic review of empirical studies comparing the effectiveness of non-pharmaceutical interventions against COVID-19. J Infect. 2021;83(3):281–93. https://doi.org/10.1016/j.jinf.2021.06.018.

Miller E, Andrews N, Stellitano L, Stowe J, Winstone AM, Shneerson J, et al. Risk of narcolepsy in children and young people receiving AS03 adjuvanted pandemic A/H1N1 2009 influenza vaccine: retrospective analysis. BMJ. 2013;346:f794. https://doi.org/10.1136/bmj.f794.

Mintz E. A riddle wrapped in a mystery inside an enigma: Brainerd diarrhoea turns 20. Lancet. 2003;362(9401):2037–8. https://doi.org/10.1016/s0140-6736(03)15148-3.

Mitra B, Luckhoff C, Mitchell RD, O'Reilly GM, Smit V, Cameron PA. Temperature screening has negligible value for control of COVID-19. Emerg Med Australas. 2020;32(5):867–9. https://doi.org/10.1111/1742-6723.13578.

Montplaisir J, Petit D, Quinn MJ, Ouakki M, Deceuninck G, Desautels A, et al. Risk of narcolepsy associated with inactivated adjuvanted (AS03) A/H1N1 (2009) pandemic influenza vaccine in Quebec. PLoS One. 2014;9(9):e108489. https://doi.org/10.1371/journal.pone.0108489.

Mouchtouri VA, Christoforidou EP, An der Heiden M, Menel Lemos C, Fanos M, Rexroth U, et al. Exit and entry screening practices for infectious diseases among travelers at points of entry: looking for evidence on public health impact. Int J Environ Res Public Health. 2019;16(23):4638. https://doi.org/10.3390/ijerph16234638.

Moustsen-Helms IR, Emborg H-D, Nielsen J, Nielsen KF, Krause TG, Mølbak K et al. Vaccine effectiveness after 1st and 2nd dose of the BNT162b2 mRNA Covid-19 vaccine in long-term care facility residents and healthcare workers—a Danish cohort study. medRxiv. 2021. https://doi.org/10.1101/2021.03.08.21252200.

Novel Coronavirus Pneumonia Emergency Response Epidemiology Team. The epidemiological characteristics of an outbreak of 2019 novel coronavirus diseases (COVID-19)—China, 2020. China CDC Wkly. 2020;2(8):113–22.

O'Flanagan D, Barret A, Foley M, Cotter S, Bonner C, Crowe C, et al. Investigation of an association between onset of narcolepsy and vaccination with pandemic influenza vaccine, Ireland April 2009-December 2010. Euro Surveill. 2014;19(17):15–25.

Olsen SJ, Chang H-L, Cheung TY-Y, Tang AF-Y, Fisk TL, Ooi SP-L, et al. Transmission of the severe acute respiratory syndrome on aircraft. N Engl J Med. 2003;349(25):2416–22. https://doi.org/10.1056/NEJMoa031349.

Pandemic Preparedness Partnership. 100 days mission to respond to future pandemic threats: reducing the impact of future pandemics by making diagnostics, therapeutics and vaccines available within 100 days: a report to the G7. London: G7 United Kingdom 2021; 2021.

Panum PL. Observations made during the epidemic of measles on The Faroe Islands in the year 1846. Creative Media Partners, LLC; 2018.

Park SY, Kim YM, Yi S, Lee S, Na BJ, Kim CB, et al. Coronavirus disease outbreak in call center, South Korea. Emerg Infect Dis. 2020a;26(8):1666–70. https://doi.org/10.3201/eid2608.201274.

Park Y, Huh IS, Lee J, Kang CR, Cho SI, Ham HJ, et al. Application of testing-tracing-treatment strategy in response to the COVID-19 outbreak in Seoul, Korea. J Korean Med Sci. 2020b;35(45):e396. https://doi.org/10.3346/jkms.2020.35.e396.

Peng J, Liu J, Mann SA, Mitchell AM, Laurie MT, Sunshine S, et al. Estimation of secondary household attack rates for emergent spike L452R SARS-CoV-2 variants detected by genomic surveillance at a community-based testing site in San Francisco. Clin Infect Dis. 2021;74:32. https://doi.org/10.1093/cid/ciab283.

Pottegård A, Lund LC, Karlstad O, Dahl J, Andersen M, Hallas J, et al. Arterial events, venous thromboembolism, thrombocytopenia, and bleeding after vaccination with Oxford-AstraZeneca ChAdOx1-S in Denmark and Norway: population based cohort study. BMJ. 2021;373:n1114. https://doi.org/10.1136/bmj.n1114.

RECOVERY Collaborative Group. Dexamethasone in hospitalized patients with Covid-19. N Engl J Med. 2020;384(8):693–704. https://doi.org/10.1056/NEJMoa2021436.

Reynolds MG, Anh BH, Thu VH, Montgomery JM, Bausch DG, Shah JJ, et al. Factors associated with nosocomial SARS-CoV transmission among healthcare workers in Hanoi, Vietnam, 2003. BMC Public Health. 2006;6:207. https://doi.org/10.1186/1471-2458-6-207.

Robert A, Edmunds WJ, Watson CH, Henao-Restrepo AM, Gsell PS, Williamson E, et al. Determinants of transmission risk during the late stage of the west African Ebola epidemic. Am J Epidemiol. 2019;188(7):1319–27. https://doi.org/10.1093/aje/kwz090.

Rosenthal N, Cao Z, Gundrum J, Sianis J, Safo S. Risk factors associated with in-hospital mortality in a US National Sample of patients with COVID-19. JAMA Netw Open. 2020;3(12):e2029058. https://doi.org/10.1001/jamanetworkopen.2020.29058.

Routledge I, Epstein A, Takahashi S, Janson O, Hakim J, Duarte E, et al. Citywide serosurveillance of the initial SARS-CoV-2 outbreak in San Francisco using electronic health records. Nat Commun. 2021;12(1):3566. https://doi.org/10.1038/s41467--021-23651-6.

Rubio LA, Peng J, Rojas S, Rojas S, Crawford E, Black D, et al. The COVID-19 symptom to isolation cascade in a Latinx community: a call to action. Open Forum Infect Dis. 2021;8(2):ofab023. https://doi.org/10.1093/ofid/ofab023.

Rumain B, Schneiderman M, Geliebter A. Prevalence of COVID-19 in adolescents and youth compared with older adults in states experiencing surges. PLoS One. 2021;16(3):e0242587. https://doi.org/10.1371/journal.pone.0242587.

Sahilu T, Sheleme T, Melaku T. Severity and mortality associated with steroid use among patients with COVID-19: a systematic review and meta-analysis. Interdiscip Perspect Infect Dis. 2021;2021:6650469. https://doi.org/10.1155/2021/6650469.

Snow J. On the mode of communication of cholera. 2nd ed. London: John Churchill; 1854.

Souza JP, Meio M, de Andrade LM, Figueiredo MR, Gomes Junior SC, Pereira Junior JP, et al. Adverse fetal and neonatal outcomes in pregnancies with confirmed Zika virus infection in Rio de Janeiro, Brazil: a cohort study. PLoS Negl Trop Dis. 2021;15(1):e0008893. https://doi.org/10.1371/journal.pntd.0008893.

Spencer K, Chung C, Stargel A. COVID-19 case investigation and contact tracing efforts from health departments—United States, June 25–July 24, 2020. MMWR Morb Mortal Wkly Rep. 2021; 70:83–7. https://doi.org/10.15585/mmwr.mm7003a3external.

St. John R, King A, de Jong D, Bodie-Collins M, Squires SG, Tam S. Border screening for SARS. Emerg Infect Dis. 2005;11(1):6–10. https://doi.org/10.3201/eid1101.040835.

Stockman LJ, Bellamy R, Garner P. SARS: systematic review of treatment effects. PLoS Med. 2006;3(9):e343. https://doi.org/10.1371/journal.pmed.0030343.

Swanson KC, Altare C, Wesseh CS, Nyenswah T, Ahmed T, Eyal N, et al. Contact tracing performance during the Ebola epidemic in Liberia, 2014-2015. PLoS Negl Trop Dis. 2018;12(9):e0006762. https://doi.org/10.1371/journal.pntd.0006762.

Telle K, Jorgensen SB, Hart R, Greve-Isdahl M, Kacelnik O. Secondary attack rates of COVID-19 in Norwegian families: a nation-wide register-based study. Eur J Epidemiol. 2021;36(7):741–8. https://doi.org/10.1007/s10654-021-00760-6.

Tiffany A, Dalziel BD, Kagume Njenge H, Johnson G, Nugba Ballah R, James D, et al. Estimating the number of secondary Ebola cases resulting from an unsafe burial and risk factors for transmission during the West Africa Ebola epidemic. PLoS Negl Trop Dis. 2017;11(6):e0005491. https://doi.org/10.1371/journal.pntd.0005491.

Tsai TF, Finn DR, Plikaytis BD, McCauley W, Martin SM, Fraser DW. Legionnaires' disease: clinical features of the epidemic in Philadelphia. Ann Intern Med. 1979;90(4):509–17. https://doi.org/10.7326/0003-4819-90-4-509.

Tuan PA, Horby P, Dinh PN, Mai LT, Zambon M, Shah J, et al. SARS transmission in Vietnam outside of the health-care setting. Epidemiol Infect.

2007;135(3):392–401. https://doi.org/10.1017/S0950268806006996.

Vellozzi C, Iqbal S, Broder K. Guillain-Barre syndrome, influenza, and influenza vaccination: the epidemiologic evidence. Clin Infect Dis. 2014;58(8):1149–55. https://doi.org/10.1093/cid/ciu005.

Wu KJ. Post-vaccination infections come in 2 different flavors. Atlantica. 2021.

Wu J, Xu F, Zhou W, Feikin DR, Lin C-Y, He X, et al. Risk factors for SARS among persons without known contact with SARS patients, Beijing, China. Emerg Infect Dis. 2004;10(2):210–6. https://doi.org/10.3201/eid1002.030730.

Yalaman A, Basbug G, Elgin C, Galvani AP. Cross-country evidence on the association between contact tracing and COVID-19 case fatality rates. Sci Rep. 2021;11(1):2145. https://doi.org/10.1038/s41598-020-78760-x.

Yu ITS, Li Y, Wong TW, Tam W, Chan AT, Lee JHW, et al. Evidence of airborne transmission of the severe acute respiratory syndrome virus. N Engl J Med. 2004;350(17):1731–9. https://doi.org/10.1056/NEJMoa032867.

Yu IT, Xie ZH, Tsoi KK, Chiu YL, Lok SW, Tang XP, et al. Why did outbreaks of severe acute respiratory syndrome occur in some hospital wards but not in others? Clin Infect Dis. 2007;44(8):1017–25. https://doi.org/10.1086/512819.

Zacay G, Shasha D, Bareket R, Kadim I, Hershkowitz Sikron F, Tsamir J, et al. BNT162b2 vaccine effectiveness in preventing asymptomatic infection with SARS-CoV-2 virus: a nationwide historical cohort study. Open Forum Infect Dis. 2021;8(6):ofab262. https://doi.org/10.1093/ofid/ofab262.

Zhong NS, Zheng BJ, Li YM, Poon LLM, Xie ZH, Chan KH, et al. Epidemiology and cause of severe acute respiratory syndrome (SARS) in Guangdong, People's Republic of China, in February, 2003. Lancet. 2003;362(9393):1353–8. https://doi.org/10.1016/s0140-6736(03)14630-2.

Zweig SA, Zapf AJ, Xu H, Li Q, Agarwal S, Labrique AB, et al. Impact of public health and social measures on the COVID-19 pandemic in the United States and other countries: descriptive analysis. JMIR Public Health Surveill. 2021;7(6):e27917. https://doi.org/10.2196/27917.

21.1 In Focus: The Impact and Mechanisms of Superspreading

Bjarke Frost Nielsen, Kim Sneppen, and Lone Simonsen

Contents

Learning Track Note: This chapter appears in Learning Tracks: Biostatistics; One Health; Preparedness; Public Health and Epidemiology

E. S. Higgs and R. A. Sorenson (eds.), *Principles and Practice of Emergency Research Response*, https://doi.org/10.1007/978-3-031-48408-7_31

Learning Objectives

This chapter will help readers understand and describe:

- Potential mechanisms underlying the phenomenon of superspreading
- Superspreading mitigation strategies, including those developed through mathematical modeling
- The *k* value of COVID-19 and other infectious diseases
- How early determination of the *k* value of a novel pathogen, along with R_0, can inform outbreak response
- Examples of how superspreading varies among diseases

1 Introduction

In the spring of 2020, nations around the globe responded to the emerging coronavirus disease 2019 (COVID-19) pandemic with lockdowns of varying stringency. All in all, more than half the world's population had been asked to stay at home by the beginning of April (Sandford 2020). As a mitigation strategy, lockdowns turned out to be very effective, far more so than mathematical models and experience from past pandemics would have predicted (Hatchett et al. 2007; Sneppen et al. 2021; Fraser et al. 2011). The explanation behind the unexpected success of lockdowns turns out to involve a particular feature of the transmission pattern of the SARS-CoV-2 virus known as superspreading. It refers to the finding that most individuals who contract COVID-19 do not transmit the disease, while a small fraction of them infect large numbers of people (Bi et al. 2020; Kirkegaard and Sneppen 2021; Lau et al. 2020; Miller et al. 2020; Pozderac and Skinner 2021; Endo et al. 2020).

In this special focus text, we review the role that superspreading plays in determining the effects of interventions. This understanding is critical because early detection of superspreading patterns in a future pandemic is in fact feasible and translates into possibilities for more effective mitigation of transmission or even elimination of an emerging pathogen.

The superspreading concept has received growing attention in recent decades, especially following the severe acute respiratory syndrome (SARS) outbreak in 2003 where superspreading was described as an important mechanism of spread (Leo et al. 2003; Lipsitch et al. 2003; Shen et al. 2004). Now, in the COVID-19 pandemic, superspreading is understood to be a key feature that must be included in models guiding the rapid response to the emerging virus.

During the SARS outbreak, superspreading was quickly noted as a defining feature; outbreaks were observed to occur in clusters. A Singapore study identified more than 100 secondary cases from only six patients (Leo et al. 2003). This was discussed at the time, and several researchers noted the need for more detailed models of transmission that could realistically incorporate the effects of heterogeneities (Dye and Gay 2003; Lipsitch et al. 2003). However, the outbreak ended the same year, and models able to capture the interactions between superspreading and mitigation strategies were not developed.

Since 2012, another highly lethal coronavirus has emerged and caused outbreaks, primarily in the Middle East. The "hospital superspreading" phenomenon noted with SARS was also seen with Middle East respiratory syndrome coronavirus, MERS-CoV. In one MERS-CoV outbreak in South Korea, one patient caused 23 secondary cases, leading to major outbreaks in two hospitals. The effective transmission may have been associated with intensive treatment that aerosolized the virus (Park et al. 2016).

The phenomenon of superspreading is not limited to coronaviruses; one of the very early studies of superspreading—preceding the terminology itself—was an ingenious experiment involving tuberculosis patients and guinea pigs (Riley et al. 1962). The researchers were able to show that out of the 77 patients, just 3 accounted for 73% of the infectious burden

(Frieden and Lee 2020; Riley et al. 1962). Furthermore, the experiment conclusively showed that this was a result of high biological infectiousness since the experimental setup ruled out any differences in behavior or environmental factors. Many of the patients, although smear-positive (i.e., with at least one positive respiratory sample prior to the initiation of anti-tuberculosis therapy), were simply not very infectious, whereas a minority was highly infectious. In modern parlance, these would be called super-shedders. In general, the term superspreading covers a spectrum from individuals who are super-shedders to circumstantial superspreading events; it almost always refers to a combination of behavioral, environmental, and biological contributing factors. However, some infectious diseases have been shown to be more prone to superspreading than others, even among respiratory diseases with similar routes of transmission (Chen et al. 2021a, b; Fraser et al. 2011; Goyal et al. 2021; Lloyd-Smith et al. 2005). It is thus important to recognize, and is widely accepted, that heterogeneous transmission is inherent to certain diseases.

2 Early Detection of a Superspreading Signature

On March 11, 2020, the World Health Organization (WHO) declared COVID-19 a pandemic. Even before this date, data had been obtained that allowed estimation of the overdispersion of transmission, a measure of the superspreading tendency of the emerging virus (Bi et al. 2020; Endo et al. 2020). In practice, this is determined by computing the relative standard deviation in the number of new infections that each infected person gives rise to (Lloyd-Smith et al. 2005; Woolhouse et al. 1997). Bi et al. (2020) used contact tracing data recorded in January and February of 2020 by the Shenzhen Center for Disease Control and Prevention and found that just 9% of infected persons accounted for 80% of new infections. Outside China, aggregated data from a WHO situation report published in late February formed the basis for one of the early estimates of the *k* value (the superspreading parameter) of COVID-19 (Endo et al. 2020; WHO 2020). It was calculated to be around 0.1, a figure which corresponds to approximately 10% of infected persons accounting for 80% of new infections.

This substantial level of superspreading was later corroborated by other studies using multiple independent methods from phylodynamics to analysis of aggregated time series (Kirkegaard and Sneppen 2021; Miller et al. 2020). Clearly, early detection of the level of superspreading is possible. With the increased attention given to the phenomenon and the advances in quantification seen during the COVID-19 pandemic, it is likely that such epidemiological investigations (▶ Chap. 21) into superspreading will be even more timely for future pandemic threats.

The significance of the basic reproductive number, R_0, has been recognized for close to a century. This is the average number of infections that each infected person gives rise to in a susceptible population. From an epidemiological perspective, there is no other single numerical quantity that better characterizes the spread of an infectious disease. However, in light of our increasing appreciation of the importance of variability in transmission, we argue that the *k* value should be adopted as a similarly central metric characterizing transmission. A low *k* value (e.g., approximately 0.1, as in COVID-19) indicates a high superspreading potential, while a higher *k* value (around 1 or greater, as in pandemic influenza) signals fairly homogeneous transmission. In ◘ Fig. 1, we show characteristic chains of transmission arising from a superspreading and a non-superspreading disease, respectively. The central panel gives examples of *k* values for some respiratory infectious diseases, along with the closely associated metric, "Which fraction of infected individuals accounts for 80% of next-generation infections?" If this number is low, it follows that transmission is highly heterogeneous.

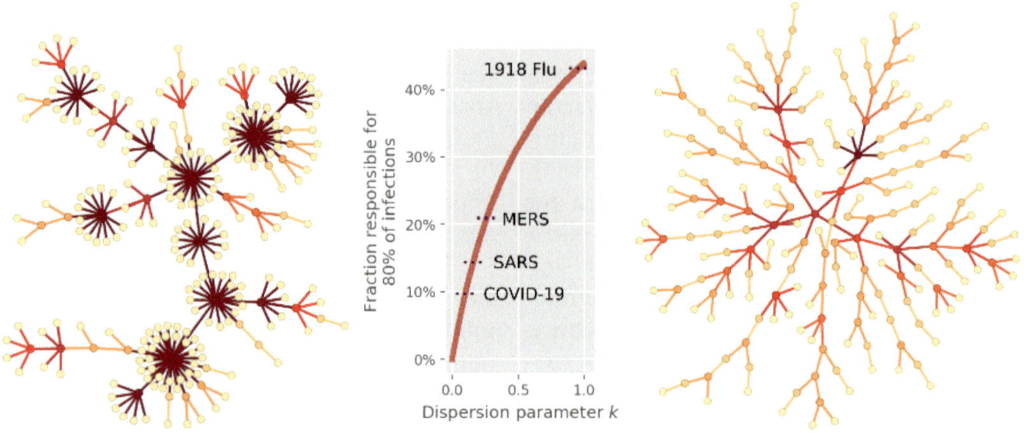

Fig. 1 The level of superspreading varies between respiratory infectious diseases. This affects the structure of infection networks, which in turn has implications for the effects of mitigation strategies used to control an outbreak. The left and right panels show simulated infection networks at different levels of superspreading. In the left panel is a superspreading disease with $k = 0.1$, similar to SARS-CoV-2. In the right panel is a homogeneously spreading disease, more akin to pandemic influenza. Both diseases were assumed to have an R_0 value of 3. The central panel shows the superspreading degree of three recent coronavirus threats and the 1918 pandemic influenza. Lower k values indicate a more pronounced tendency toward superspreading. (Nielsen et al. 2021)

3 The Mechanism of Superspreading in COVID-19

As we have seen, superspreading has an enormous impact on transmission patterns. This, in turn, greatly affects the choice of suitable mitigation and containment strategies. In some cases, the knowledge that transmission is highly heterogeneous is sufficient, and further information on the type of superspreading is not necessary. In other cases, the "etiology" is important. In general, the mechanisms underlying the phenomenon of superspreading can be categorized into three principal components (Althouse et al. 2020):

- Biological, owing to highly infectious individuals (super-shedders).
- Social, owing to high numbers of susceptible contacts for some infected individuals.
- Environmental: high-risk settings and activities. This may include environments where aerosol transmission becomes more likely due to environmental factors such as humidity. High-risk activities may include behaviors such as singing and certain aerosol-generating medical procedures, such as bronchoscopy and intubation (Davies et al. 2009; Judson and Munster 2019; Yu et al. 2007).

For any given respiratory infectious disease outbreak, the transmission pattern will result from a combination of the above factors. However, for COVID-19, there are by now several indications that the observed superspreading tendency has a strong biological component (i.e., that a subset of infected persons become super-shedders). Perhaps the most direct piece of evidence for this is the very large variation in respiratory viral loads seen in SARS-CoV-2-positive individuals. In Fig. 2, we show a viral load distribution obtained by Kidd et al. (2021) showing that just 10% of positive individuals accounted for 90% of the total viral particles. Similarly, Jones et al. (2021) reported that "viral load was highly variable" and wrote that "of the 25,381 positive subjects, about 8% showed very high viral loads." Yang et al. (2021) used the term "supercarriers" after finding that only 2% of infected students on a Colorado university campus accounted for 90% of the

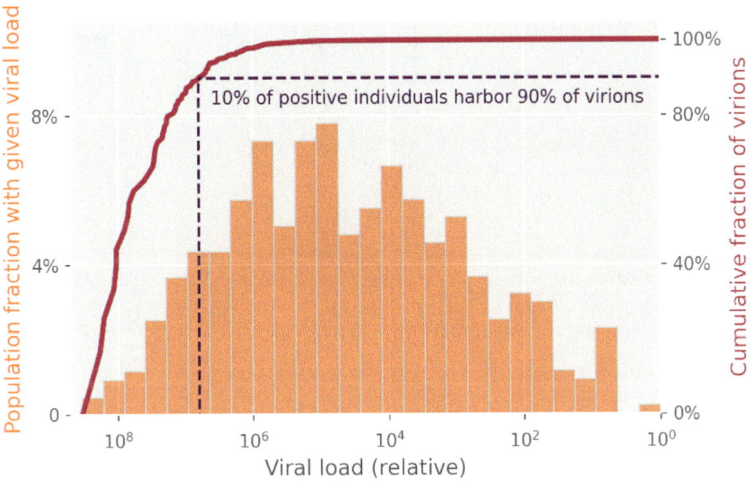

Fig. 2 Distribution of SARS-CoV-2 respiratory viral loads obtained by reverse-transcriptase quantitative polymerase chain reaction (RT-qPCR) testing analyzed with respect to the N (nucleocapsid) gene. Note that the horizontal viral load scale is logarithmic and varies over eight orders of magnitude. Just 10% of the population were found to harbor 90% of the virions, exemplifying the large variability in SARS-CoV-2 respiratory viral loads. (Original figure design inspired by Yang et al. (2021) (CC BY 4.0), data from Kidd et al. (2021))

circulating virus. These individuals were all asymptomatic or pre-symptomatic, but the authors went on to show that the viral load distribution among symptomatic patients was similar.

In a recent controlled-environment study, it was shown that the respiratory viral load of a SARS-CoV-2-positive individual is highly correlated with the concentration of virions in the immediate environment (Parhizkar et al. 2021). In other words, high variation in viral load between infected individuals is expected to coincide with a highly variable number of expelled virions. Chen et al. (2021b) ask why superspreading drives the COVID-19 pandemic but not the influenza A/H1N1pdm09 pandemic of 2009, and write, "inherently, most COVID-19 cases are minimally infectious, but highly infectious individuals are estimated to expel hundreds to thousands of virions per minute while talking, singing, or coughing. Meanwhile, a greater proportion of people infected with A/H1N1pdm09 are inherently infectious but expel virions at low rates."

4 Superspreading as a Key Factor Determining the Effects of Mitigation Strategies

Instances of superspreading are inherently concerning and it is natural to think that the stochasticity conferred by superspreading is always bad news. However, recent research has shown that a heterogeneous transmission pattern actually renders some mitigation strategies drastically more effective, while it is detrimental to other strategies (Endo et al. 2021; Lewis 2021; Nielsen et al. 2021; Sneppen et al. 2021).

For a disease characterized by super-shedding, the obvious strategy to control it should naturally be to prevent highly infectious individuals from causing large outbreaks—in other words, to prevent them from infecting others to their full potential. Some authors have therefore suggested concentrating on finding and isolating super-shedders or otherwise taking them out of the equation (Althouse et al. 2020; Kain et al. 2020; Lloyd-Smith et al. 2005). However, this seemingly

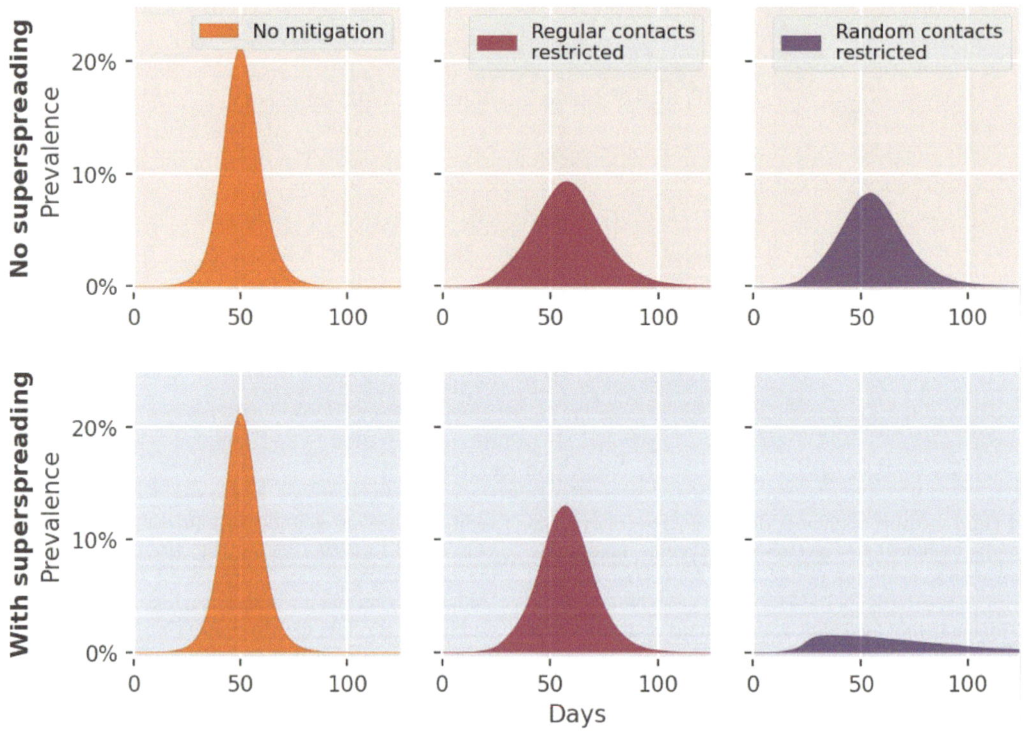

Fig. 3 Superspreading renders certain mitigation strategies much more powerful while it impedes others. In a homogeneously spreading disease, mitigation strategies such as lockdowns, which rely on population-wide reductions in contacts, are only expected to "flatten the curve." In a highly heterogeneous (superspreading) disease, however, such mitigation strategies can be highly effective, as long as they target venues where people are likely to have many random contacts with persons they do not regularly meet. Examples include restrictions imposed on bars, restaurants, and public transportation. The three upper panels show the course of a homogeneously spreading disease in three scenarios: unmitigated, subject to mitigation of regular contacts (workplace, school classes, etc.), and subject to mitigation of random contacts (as described above). The three lower panels show the effects of the same mitigation strategies in a superspreading disease, where restriction of random contacts evidently has an outsized effect. (Data from Sneppen et al. (2021))

obvious strategy relies on preemptively recognizing or identifying super-shedders before they get out and about—something which is not usually possible. Thus, a different approach is needed.

First, we will review how an outbreak of a superspreading disease is affected by reductions in contact numbers. It is this key aspect which explains the high efficacy of lockdowns in the COVID-19 pandemic. Using an agent-based modeling approach that can capture the heterogeneity, we have recently demonstrated that reducing activity in those areas of society where many random encounters occur has an enormous effect on a superspreading disease (Sneppen et al. 2021). In contrast, such restrictions are much less effective as means to control a more homogeneously spreading disease. This means that restrictions on large gatherings, closure of bars and nightclubs, and interventions to reduce crowding in public transport are more effective at curbing a superspreading disease than a homogeneous one.

In Fig. 3, we demonstrate how two classes of contact-restricting, population-wide mitigation strategies fare for a superspreading and non-superspreading disease, respectively. One mitigation strategy is as described above: based on minimizing "random" encounters. The other is based on restricting contact only among more regular contacts (e.g., workplaces and school classes). While the strategy based on just restricting regular contacts has a moderate effect (and actually fares worse in a superspreading disease outbreak), the strategy based on restricting random contacts is highly effective in a superspreading scenario.

The mechanism, which we explored further in a subsequent paper (Nielsen et al. 2021), is that superspreading diseases are highly sensitive to what one could call contact diversity (i.e., the number of distinct persons each infected individual comes into contact with) rather than the total contact time. Interestingly, for a homogeneous disease such as influenza, the reverse is true. The finding is determined by the very high infectiousness of super-shedders, which gives them the potential to cause many infections, given enough susceptible contacts. In a homogeneously spreading disease, most infected individuals become infectious but generally only expel virions at a lower rate, meaning that the exposure time is the more determinative factor.

Contact tracing is another type of mitigation strategy that exhibits increased effectiveness for superspreading diseases. However, this is only true if a suitable contact tracing scheme is chosen. Here, it is important to distinguish between forward and backward and retrospective contact tracing. When an infected person (the index case) is identified, forward contact tracing tries to answer the question, "Who may the index case have infected?" Backward or retrospective tracing, on the other hand, tries to identify the person who infected the index case and then, by tracing forward from that person asks, "Who may that source person also have infected?" The strength of this latter approach relies on an analog of the so-called friendship paradox of network theory. The friendship paradox is the counterintuitive statement that "on average, your friends have more friends than you do," which holds true as soon as there is some variability in the number of friends that people have (Feld 1991). Going back to the infection networks in Fig. 1, an analogous statement can be clearly made for the superspreading infection network: the person who infected you is likely to infect many more people than you are likely to infect. In the non-superspreading infection network, this is of course much less true. Endo et al. (2021) studied the implications of superspreading for retrospective contact tracing in a mathematical model and found that it was a drastically superior mode of contact tracing when transmission was heterogeneous, and cases occurred in clusters.

More broadly, these theoretical studies of the implications of superspreading for mitigation emphasize the role that mathematical modeling can play in the rapid response to an emerging pathogen (▶ Chaps. 24 and 25). The mechanisms revealed by mathematical models in the SARS-CoV-2 pandemic are likely to help further shorten the time delay between identification of key signature features of an emerging disease and the implementation of suitable countermeasures.

In light of our increasing understanding of the implications that heterogeneous transmission has for outbreak control, we call for including early determination of superspreading potential as an integral part of the assessment work for a future "Disease X" (WHO 2018). From a quantitative perspective, this entails including the dispersion parameter k as a key variable characterizing transmission alongside the well-known basic reproduction number R_0.

While the mechanisms of superspreading in the case of COVID-19 are becoming clearer, the within-host dynamics that lead to high variability in shedding are still not well understood, and further research in this direction will be crucial. An improved understanding of the mechanisms behind this variability is likely to increase our chances during future outbreaks of identifying individuals at risk of becoming super-shedders. In the meantime, we can take solace in the fact that it is possible to design population-wide mitigation strategies that work effectively for superspreading diseases.

Discussion Questions

1. Identify potential risks for a scenario of superspreading of COVID-19 at an international scientific meeting with social events planned:
   (a) Describe potential mechanisms underlying the phenomenon of superspreading.
   (b) What mitigation strategies could be implemented?
   (c) Could mathematical models be used to guide mitigation strategies at the event? How?
2. What is the significance of the *k* value of COVID-19 and other infectious diseases?
   (a) Why is the *k* value a key statistical property of SARS-CoV-2 transmission?
   (b) What do low and high *k* values indicate?
   (c) How does the *k* value for COVID-19, in relation to the basic reproductive number R_0, affect the options for non-pharmaceutical interventions to minimize the pandemic?
   (d) How can early determination of the *k* value of a novel pathogen, along with R_0, inform outbreak response?
2. Superspreading can have very different origins across diseases.
   (a) What are some examples?
   (b) How are the examples explained by the properties of each disease (mode of transmission, duration, symptoms, immunology, etc.)?

Acknowledgements The authors acknowledge financial support from the Danish National Research Foundation (grant DNRF170) and from the Carlsberg Foundation under its Semper Ardens programme (grant CF20-0046). BFN also acknowledges separate financial support from the Carlsberg Foundation (grant CF23-0173). The authors would like to thank Robert J. Taylor, who is sadly no longer with us, for his contributions to research into the superspreading phenomenon.

References

Althouse BM, Wenger EA, Miller JC, Scarpino SV, Allard A, Hébert-Dufresne L, Hu H. Superspreading events in the transmission dynamics of SARS-CoV-2: opportunities for interventions and control. PLoS Biol. 2020;18(11):e3000897. https://doi.org/10.1371/journal.pbio.3000897.

Bi Q, Wu Y, Mei S, Ye C, Zou X, Zhang Z, et al. Epidemiology and transmission of COVID-19 in 391 cases and 1286 of their close contacts in Shenzhen, China: a retrospective cohort study. Lancet Infect Dis. 2020;20(8):911–9. https://doi.org/10.1016/s1473-3099(20)30287-5.

Chen PZ, Bobrovitz N, Premji Z, Koopmans M, Fisman DN, Gu FX. Heterogeneity in transmissibility and shedding SARS-CoV-2 via droplets and aerosols. elife. 2021a;10:e65774. https://doi.org/10.7554/eLife.65774.

Chen PZ, Koopmans M, Fisman DN, Gu FX. Understanding why superspreading drives the COVID-19 pandemic but not the H1N1 pandemic. Lancet Infect Dis. 2021b;21(9):1203–4. https://doi.org/10.1016/S1473-3099(21)00406-0.

Davies A, Thomson G, Walker J, Bennett A. A review of the risks and disease transmission associated with aerosol generating medical procedures. J Infect Prev. 2009;10(4):122. https://doi.org/10.1177/1757177409106456.

Dye C, Gay N. Modeling the SARS epidemic. Science. 2003;300(5627):1884–5. https://doi.org/10.1126/science.1086925.

Endo A, Centre for the Mathematical Modelling of Infectious Diseases COVID-19 Working Group, Abbott S, Kucharski AJ, Funk S. Estimating the overdispersion in COVID-19 transmission using outbreak sizes outside China. Wellcome Open Res. 2020;5:67. https://doi.org/10.12688/wellcomeopenres.15842.3.

Endo A, Centre for the Mathematical Modelling of Infectious Diseases COVID-19 Working Group, Leclerc QJ, Knight GM, Medley GF, Atkins KE, et al. Implication of backward contact tracing in the presence of overdispersed transmission in COVID-19 outbreaks. Wellcome Open Res. 2021;5:239. https://doi.org/10.12688/wellcomeopenres.16344.3.

Feld SL. Why your friends have more friends than you do. Am J Sociol. 1991;96(6):1464–77.

Fraser C, Cummings DAT, Klinkenberg D, Burke DS, Ferguson NM. Influenza transmission in households during the 1918 pandemic. Am J Epidemiol. 2011;174(5):505–14. https://doi.org/10.1093/aje/kwr122.

Frieden TR, Lee CT. Identifying and interrupting superspreading events-implications for control of severe acute respiratory syndrome coronavirus 2. Emerg Infect Dis. 2020;26(6):1059–66. https://doi.org/10.3201/eid2606.200495.

Goyal A, Reeves DB, Cardozo-Ojeda EF, Schiffer JT, Mayer BT. Viral load and contact heterogeneity predict SARS-CoV-2 transmission and super-spreading events. elife. 2021;10:e63537. https://doi.org/10.7554/eLife.63537.

Hatchett RJ, Mecher CE, Lipsitch M. Public health interventions and epidemic intensity during the 1918 influenza pandemic. Proc Natl Acad Sci USA. 2007;104(18):7582–7. https://doi.org/10.1073/pnas.0610941104.

Jones TC, Biele G, Mühlemann B, Veith T, Schneider J, Beheim-Schwarzbach J, et al. Estimating infectiousness throughout SARS-CoV-2 infection course. Science. 2021;373(6551):eabi5273. https://doi.org/10.1126/science.abi5273.

Judson SD, Munster VJ. Nosocomial transmission of emerging viruses via aerosol-generating medical procedures. Viruses. 2019;11(10):940. https://doi.org/10.3390/v11100940.

Kain MP, Childs ML, Becker AD, Mordecai EA. Chopping the tail: how preventing superspreading can help to maintain COVID-19 control. medRxiv. 2020. https://doi.org/10.1101/2020.06.30.20143115.

Kidd M, Richter A, Best A, Cumley N, Mirza J, Percival B, et al. S-variant SARS-CoV-2 lineage B1.1.7 is associated with significantly higher viral load in samples tested by TaqPath polymerase chain reaction. J Infect Dis. 2021;223(10):1666–70. https://doi.org/10.1093/infdis/jiab082.

Kirkegaard JB, Sneppen K. Variability of individual infectiousness derived from aggregate statistics of COVID-19. medRxiv. 2021. https://doi.org/10.1101/2021.01.15.21249870.

Lau MSY, Grenfell B, Thomas M, Bryan M, Nelson K, Lopman B. Characterizing superspreading events and age-specific infectiousness of SARS-CoV-2 transmission in Georgia, USA. Proc Natl Acad Sci. 2020;117(36):22430–5. https://doi.org/10.1073/pnas.2011802117.

Leo Y, Chen M, Heng B, Lee C, Paton N, Ang B, et al. Severe acute respiratory syndrome—Singapore, 2003. MMWR Morb Mortal Wkly Rep. 2003;52(18):405–11.

Lewis D. Superspreading drives the COVID pandemic—and could help to tame it.pdf. Nature. 2021;590:544. https://www.nature.com/articles/d41586-021-00460-x.

Lipsitch M, Cohen T, Cooper B, Robins JM, Ma S, James L, et al. Transmission dynamics and control of severe acute respiratory syndrome. Science. 2003;300(5627):1966–70. https://doi.org/10.1126/science.1086616.

Lloyd-Smith JO, Schreiber SJ, Kopp PE, Getz WM. Superspreading and the effect of individual variation on disease emergence. Nature. 2005;438(7066):355–9. https://doi.org/10.1038/nature04153.

Miller D, Martin MA, Harel N, Tirosh O, Kustin T, Meir M, et al. Full genome viral sequences inform patterns of SARS-CoV-2 spread into and within Israel. Nat Commun. 2020;11(1):5518. https://doi.org/10.1038/s41467-020-19248-0.

Nielsen BF, Simonsen L, Sneppen K. COVID-19 superspreading suggests mitigation by social network modulation. Phys Rev Lett. 2021;126(11):118301. https://doi.org/10.1103/PhysRevLett.126.118301.

Parhizkar H, Dietz L, Olsen-Martinez A, Horve P, Barnatan L, Northcutt D, Wymelenberg KVD. Quantifying human and environmental viral load relationships amidst mitigation strategies in a controlled chamber with participants having COVID-19. ResearchSquare. 2021. https://doi.org/10.21203/rs.3.rs-940891/v1.

Park SH, Kim Y-S, Jung Y, Choi SY, Cho N-H, Jeong HW, et al. Outbreaks of Middle East respiratory syndrome in two hospitals initiated by a single patient in Daejeon, South Korea. Infect Chemother. 2016;48(2):99–107. https://doi.org/10.3947/ic.2016.48.2.99.

Pozderac C, Skinner B. Superspreading of SARS-CoV-2 in the USA. PLOS-One. 2021;16(3):e0248808. https://doi.org/10.1371/journal.pone.0248808.

Riley RL, Mills CC, O'Grady F, Sultan LU, Wittstadt F, Shivpuri DN. Infectiousness of air from a tuberculosis ward. Am Rev Respir Dis. 1962;85(4):511–25. https://doi.org/10.1164/arrd.1962.85.4.511.

Sandford A. Half of humanity on lockdown in 90 countries. Eur Secur. 2020. https://www.euronews.com/2020/04/02/coronavirus-in-europe-spain-s-death-toll-hits-10-000-after-record-950-new-deaths-in-24-hou.

Shen Z, Ning F, Zhou W, He X, Lin C, Chin DP, et al. Superspreading SARS events, Beijing, 2003. Emerg Infect Dis. 2004;10(2):256–60. https://doi.org/10.3201/eid1002.030732.

Sneppen K, Nielsen BF, Taylor RJ, Simonsen L. Overdispersion in COVID-19 increases the effectiveness of limiting nonrepetitive contacts for transmission control. Proc Natl Acad Sci. 2021;118(14):e2016623118. https://doi.org/10.1073/pnas.2016623118.

WHO. 2018 Annual review of diseases prioritized under the Research and Development Blueprint. 2018. https://www.who.int/docs/default-source/blueprint/2018-annual-review-of-diseases-prioritized-under-the-research-and-development-blueprint.pdf?sfvrsn=4c22e36_2.

WHO. Coronavirus disease 2019 (COVID-19) situation report—38. Geneva: World Health Organization; 2020. https://apps.who.int/iris/handle/10665/331226.

Woolhouse ME, Dye C, Etard JF, Smith T, Charlwood JD, Garnett GP, et al. Heterogeneities in the transmission of infectious agents: implications for the design of control programs. Proc Natl Acad Sci USA. 1997;94(1):338–42. https://doi.org/10.1073/pnas.94.1.338.

Yang Q, Saldi TK, Lasda E, Decker CJ, Paige CL, Muhlrad D, et al. Just 2% of SARS-CoV-2-positive individuals carry 90% of the virus circulating in communities. medRxiv. 2021. https://doi.org/10.1101/2021.03.01.21252250.

Yu IT, Xie ZH, Tsoi KK, Chiu YL, Lok SW, Tang XP, et al. Why did outbreaks of severe acute respiratory syndrome occur in some hospital wards but not in others? Clin Infect Dis. 2007;44(8):1017–25. https://doi.org/10.1086/512819.

22 Vaccine Trial Designs

Rebecca Kahn, Sofia S. Villar, Natalie E. Dean, and Marc Lipsitch

Contents

Learning Track Note: This chapter appears in Learning Tracks: Biostatistics; Clinical Research; Global Health; Preparedness; Public Health and Epidemiology

E. S. Higgs and R. A. Sorenson (eds.), *Principles and Practice of Emergency Research Response*, https://doi.org/10.1007/978-3-031-48408-7_32

Learning Objectives

This chapter will help readers understand and describe:

- The three main objectives of vaccine efficacy trials conducted during infectious disease emergencies: testing the null hypothesis, estimating efficacy, and maximizing public health impact.
- Five key choices of trial design: randomization, comparators, trial population, implementation, and primary endpoint.
- Opportunities, challenges, and trade-offs of employing adaptive designs and placebo controls for vaccine trials.
- Vaccine trial designs that have been successful.

1 Introduction

In vaccine efficacy trials conducted during epidemics of emerging infectious diseases, there are three major objectives, in addition to evaluating safety.

1. *Test the null hypothesis* (of no efficacy or efficacy below a minimally acceptable threshold) of the vaccine candidate in a rigorous fashion.
2. *Estimate the efficacy of the vaccine candidate*.
3. *Maximize the public health impact* of the vaccine trial for both trial participants and the broader community, which we could roughly characterize as
   (a) The net benefit (protection from infection or disease minus adverse events) to trial participants.
   (b) The benefit to the broader community if the vaccine is shown to be safe and efficacious by the trial.

All of these objectives create urgency for planning vaccine trials. For hypothesis testing and effect estimation, it is important to start a trial quickly so that enough people at risk of infection can be enrolled in the trial, in order to obtain sufficient power for the trial and so that early efficacy estimates can be obtained as soon as possible. If the vaccine candidate is effective, these early estimates can be used to apply for emergency use authorization and/or licensure, which will help enable widespread use and maximize the public health benefit.

The aims of a trial should lead to a design that best delivers those aims. This can be difficult, as sometimes all aims of the trial favor the same design choices but at other times there may conflicting considerations and no clear superior design option. Several studies have quantified the tradeoffs of different design decisions in clinical trials in terms of possible aims (Robertson et al. 2021; Villar et al. 2015; Williamson et al. 2017) and specifically in the context of vaccine trials (Halloran et al. 2017; Johnson et al. 2021).

During the 2014–2016 West African Ebola virus disease epidemic, many vaccine efficacy trial designs were proposed (NASEM 2017). Only one design—the cluster-randomized ring vaccination design, which enrolled contacts and contacts of contacts of individuals with Ebola—was used successfully (Henao-Restrepo et al. 2017). However, the debates surrounding efficacy trial design during this outbreak underscored the need for planning and discussion of trial design choices prior to future outbreaks. During the COVID-19 pandemic, dozens of vaccine efficacy trials were conducted, and several vaccines received emergency use authorization within record time, drastically altering the course of the pandemic. Balancing speed of result (objective 3) with scientific value (objectives 1 and 2) created tradeoffs in the design of these trials. The scientific and public health communities continue to learn lessons about trial design and about the properties of these vaccines as rollout continues.

Ideally, a preferred design, based on the anticipated aims of a trial, should be chosen as early as possible, as all three trial objectives become more challenging to attain if and when an epidemic declines (Camacho et al. 2015). In the context of the Zika virus PHEIC, the World Health Organization (WHO) released a document and online tool to aid in choosing among existing trial designs (WHO 2019). A sample decision tree (Fig. 1) prepared with the tool by Bellan et al. (2019)

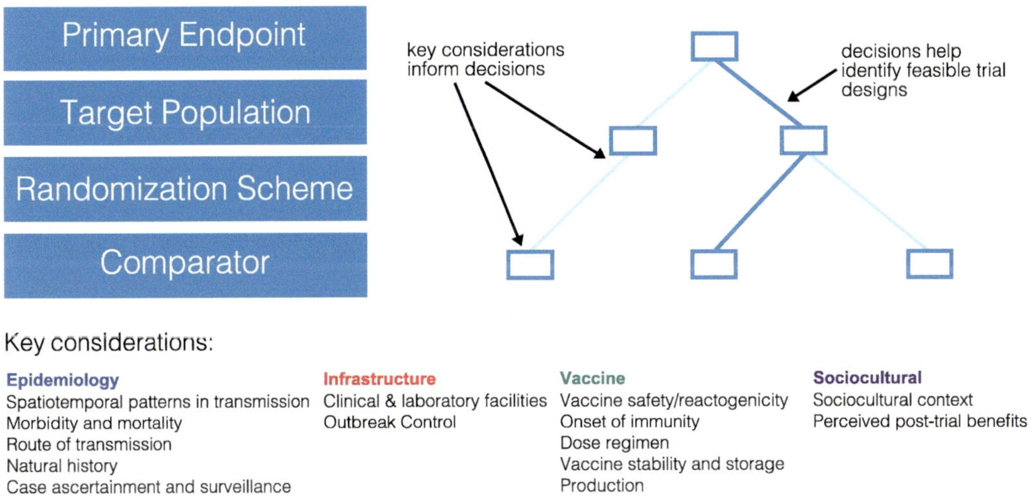

Fig. 1 Example of a decision tree: Schematic of InterVax-Tool's decision process. Within each of four decision tree branches (solid blue bars at left), users navigate a set of hierarchical decisions following guidance on how each of 14 key considerations affects the decision to pick one choice (open blue boxes at right) over another. During this process, users take notes on the scenario under consideration as well as on their justifications for the decisions chosen through the four decision trees. (Bellan et al. 2019)

helps illustrate a few of the factors and steps involved.

In this chapter, we highlight five main choices in conventional vaccine efficacy trial designs. We also describe the opportunities and challenges of employing adaptive designs for vaccine trials, though these have primarily been used in therapeutics and non-vaccine prophylactics trials in recent experience ► www.protect-trial.net (PROTECT-CH 2021; RECOVERY trial 2022). Drawing on examples from the West African Ebola outbreak and the COVID-19 pandemic, we show how different pathogen characteristics and outbreak contexts can influence decisions on vaccine trial design. Where possible, simple, familiar designs should be chosen to make the trial easier to conduct, results easier to interpret, and authorization or approval easier to obtain. SARS-CoV-2 vaccine efficacy trials have largely followed this principle, and the speed with which emergency use authorization was achieved reinforces its value. However, in some circumstances, innovative designs may be called for, and having preapproved protocols with adaptive elements incorporated can help expedite such trials during an outbreak.

2 Choices in Vaccine Trial Design

Trialists and sponsors must make many choices in the design and analysis of vaccine trials (Dean et al. 2018; Kahn et al. 2018). Here, we discuss five key choices (Fig. 2) in relation to the three desired objectives described above (Kahn et al. 2018):

1. randomization unit
2. comparator intervention
3. trial population
4. trial implementation
5. primary endpoint

These are separate choices that must be made in trial design; they may be combined in multiple ways. Some combinations, such as individually randomized, placebo-controlled trials, are well established, commonly used, and often preferred in many regulatory frameworks; others, such as the innovative cluster-randomized ring vaccination compared against delayed vaccination used in the "Ebola Ça Suffit!" trial conducted in Guinea (► In Focus 22.1) (Henao-Restrepo et al. 2017), have been used only once. Still other combinations of choices (e.g., ring vaccination with an active or placebo comparator) have never

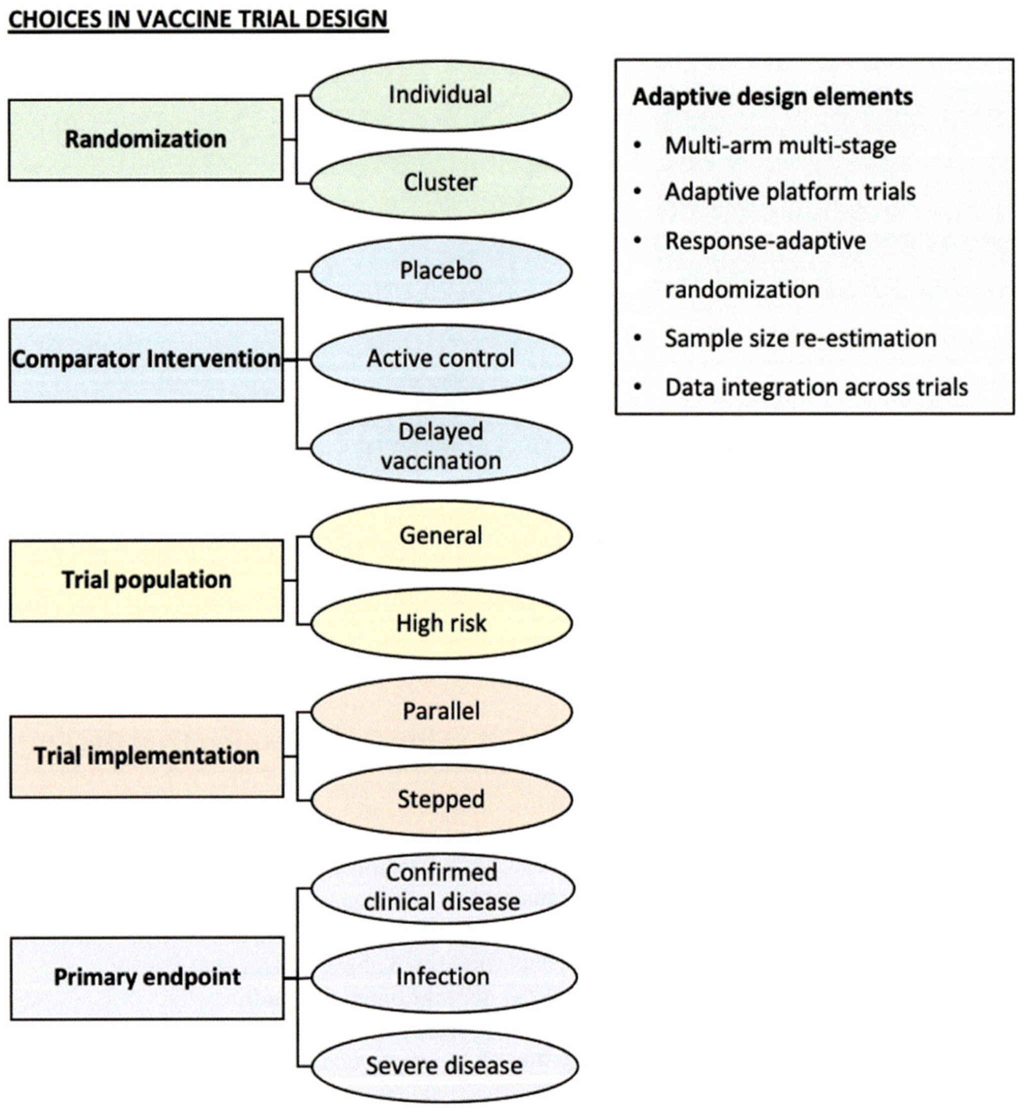

Fig. 2 Schematic of major clinical trial design choices discussed below. (Authors)

been used. Examples of choices that have been made to date are shown in Table 1.

2.1 Randomization

Randomized efficacy trials are considered the gold standard and are typically required for vaccine licensure (Lipsitch et al. 2016), and for good reasons (Lipsitch and Eyal 2017). Therefore, this section will focus on the choice between individual and cluster randomization rather than the choice between randomization and complete roll-out without a randomized trial, which has been proposed for extreme emergencies (WHO 2014) and did in fact occur with some SARS-CoV-2 vaccines (Burki 2020; Mahase 2020).

The choice between individual and cluster randomization depends on both scientific and feasibility considerations. Individual randomization simply means that individuals are randomized, independently and one at a time, to be offered the candidate vaccine or control

Table 1 Comparison of selected trial designs: Individually randomized trials are statistically more efficient than cluster randomized trials, meaning they require a smaller sample size for detecting a given effect and conclude (or reach interim analysis points) faster. The sample size of the cluster randomized trial must be increased to account for correlation between people in the same cluster (Donner et al. 1981). If the vaccine proves effective, a more rapid conclusion (usually available from an individually randomized trial) permits more rapid rollout to those at greatest risk, and presumably a greater benefit to that population. If this at-risk population is much larger than the trial population, as is most often the case, this will be the dominant effect (Kahn et al. 2018)

No	Trial design type, with examples[a]	Comparison	Population	Implementation
I. Individually randomized				
1	"Classic" individually randomized controlled trial[b] Ex: Pneumococcal vaccine, California (Black et al. 2000) Rotavirus vaccine, Niger (Isanaka et al. 2017) PREVAIL Ebola vaccine, Liberia (Kennedy et al. 2016)	Placebo or other vaccine ("active control")	General or high-risk	Parallel
2	Serodiscordant couples[c] Ex: Herpes simplex virus, type 2 (Stanberry et al. 2002)	Placebo	High-risk	Parallel
3	Individually randomized, comparison to delayed vaccination Ex: STRIVE Ebola vaccine, Sierra Leone, as performed (Widdowson et al. 2016)	Delay (without a placebo)	High-risk	Parallel
4	Individually randomized controlled trial with deliberately stepped rollout Ex. Proposed for Ebola vaccine (Lipsitch et al. 2015b)	Placebo	General or high-risk	Stepped
II. Cluster randomized				
5	"Classic" parallel, cluster-randomized controlled trial Ex: Pneumococcal vaccine, Navajo Nation (O'Brien et al. 2003)	Placebo or other vaccine ("active control")	General	Parallel
6	Stepped-wedge design Ex: Hepatitis B vaccine, the Gambia (Gambia hepatitis intervention study 1987) STRIVE Ebola vaccine, as proposed (Bellan et al. 2015)	Delay (without a placebo)	High-risk	Stepped
7	Ring-vaccination trial versus delayed vaccination[d] Ex: Ebola Ça Suffit Ebola vaccine, Guinea (Henao-Restrepo et al. 2017)	Delay (without a placebo)	High-risk	Ring (stepped)

[a] Abbreviations: For example; *PREVAIL* Partnership for Research on Ebola Virus in Liberia; *STRIVE* Sierra Leone Trial to Introduce a Vaccine Against Ebola

[b] Most common design used for vaccine efficacy trials. (A search on ▶ clinicaltrials.gov with filters "Interventional (or Clinical Trial)" for study type, "Phase III" for study phase, and search term "vaccine" for intervention found 1251 trials, of which 989 were randomized. Out of a randomly selected 50 of these trials, all were individually randomized and 44 specified a parallel rollout

[c] Seronegative partner of a seropositive person is at high risk for exposure to infection and is randomized to vaccine or placebo

[d] Choice of delayed vaccination comparison due to perceived challenges to the use of placebo in this setting

(see ▶ Sect. 2.2). In cluster randomization, whole groups of individuals, defined for example by geography (e.g., the villages they live in) or social contacts (e.g., the contacts of a particular person) are randomized as a group to one of these two arms. This design choice has several consequences (Kahn et al. 2018). First, individual randomization compares the risk of disease or infection between those who receive the vaccine and those who receive the control, yielding estimates of the direct effect of the vaccine, defined as how much the vaccine reduces an individual's risk of disease or infection (Halloran et al. 2010). Cluster randomization compares the risk between persons in the vaccine candidate clusters and persons in the control clusters, providing a combined estimate of the direct and indirect (herd) effects of the vaccine candidate, which may be quantified as the total effect or the overall effect (Halloran et al. 2010). These combined effects are more challenging to extrapolate to other settings than the direct effect because the magnitude of the combined effects depends not only on the direct effect, but also on factors including the intensity of transmission, the contact network structure, and the phase of the epidemic at which a vaccine is deployed (Hitchings et al. 2018; Staples et al. 2015). Additionally, licensure decisions are based primarily on the product's ability to prevent a defined health condition in individuals (i.e., the direct effect), favoring individual randomization.

In general, because of the shorter time required for a trial, statistical efficiency, estimation of the more generalizable direct effect, and precedent as the standard for authorization and licensure, individual randomization should be considered the default (Kahn et al. 2018). However, there may be certain situations in which cluster randomization is preferred. For example, the combined effects from cluster randomization may be of interest to policy makers, as they more closely approximate the effect of a mass vaccination campaign. Additionally, there may be situations where a cluster-randomized trial is more feasible than individual randomization (e.g., due to simplified procedures as all participants in an area receive either the vaccine or control), meaning a cluster-randomized trial could start considerably earlier, and perhaps even recruit and randomize individuals faster than in an individually randomized trial.

2.2 Comparator Intervention

In randomized trials, the comparator arm may receive a placebo, another vaccine (i.e., active control), or delayed administration of the vaccine candidate. A placebo-controlled trial is considered preferable to a delayed-administration control, as it permits use of a double-blind design in which neither the investigators nor participants know who is in which arm of the trial, preventing changes in behavior based on knowledge of trial arm assignment. Delayed administration of the vaccine candidate during the trial, such as in a stepped-wedge design (described below), provides access to the vaccine candidate to all trial participants during the trial but has several limitations. Participants will be aware of their vaccine status, which might lead to changes in behavior that could bias assessment of the vaccine candidate's true efficacy. In addition, while long-term follow-up is challenging after any trial in which efficacy has been demonstrated, delayed vaccination for the comparator arm further limits long-term follow-up as there is no longer a control arm to which the investigational arm may be compared even during the trial.

Methodologically, placebo control is "cleaner" than active control because while the latter may provide some benefit to participants in the control arm against another disease, it may complicate the assessment of safety and efficacy as compared to trials with a placebo. For example, it may be hard to distinguish whether an adverse event that occurs more often in the experimental arm than in the active control arm is a harm caused by the experimental vaccine or an unanticipated protective effect of the active control (Gessner et al. 2017).

Because they permit double-blinding, allow a straightforward comparison between arms, and typically have higher power than delayed administration (Dean et al. 2018), placebo-controlled trials are more likely to provide the most accurate and efficient estimates of a vaccine's efficacy and safety. Thus, placebo-controlled trials are favored when considering the scientific objectives of the trial. If the vaccine candidate is highly likely to be effective, delayed vaccination can provide clear advantages over its alternatives for the third desired objective of maximizing public health benefit during the trial, as more vaccinated people will be protected. Offering the vaccine to all control participants as soon as efficacy is demonstrated can reduce this difference substantially (Eyal and Lipsitch 2017) but may compromise the scientific and social value of the trial and have other disadvantages (Rid et al. 2021) (► In Practice 4.1); a blinded crossover design, which was used in the Novavax SARS-CoV-2 trial (Follmann et al. 2021), can help address some of these limitations. The ethics of the use of placebo in clinical trials in epidemics is a topic of much discussion (Eyal and Lipsitch 2021; Kahn et al. 2018; Millum and Grady 2013; Millum and Wendler 2018; Rid et al. 2014), and some ethics committees may not sanction a placebo arm (Ebola Ça Suffit Ring Vaccination Trial Consortium 2015). This choice of comparator arm highlights the potential tension between the three desired objectives of vaccine trials, as well as the possibility of relieving this tension by, for example, providing vaccine to all participants at the end of follow-up or analysis or conducting an adaptive trial designed to vaccinate as many participants as possible while collecting efficacy and safety data.

2.3 Trial Population

A vaccine trial may enroll participants from the general population or from a population at high risk of infection or severe disease, such as healthcare workers or contacts of confirmed cases in an Ebola outbreak. Conducting a trial in the general population can increase the generalizability of the trial's results and provide important estimates regarding safety and efficacy for the population in which the vaccine would be used if proven efficacious. However, given the urgency created by an epidemic and the short window of opportunity epidemics create for trials to be completed before transmission declines, especially for rarer diseases, all desired objectives can provide justification for conducting the trial in a population at high risk for the trial endpoints. This is one reason why a ring vaccination strategy is particularly useful in a declining epidemic when there is limited time remaining to conduct a trial, as it enrolls only those at the highest risk of infection. This strategy requires identifying, locating, and randomizing individuals at high risk, which may be easier to accomplish as the epidemic is waning and conditions are returning to normal than during an epidemic's peak. Indeed, the ring vaccination trial design (► In Focus 22.1) is perhaps the most innovative trial design for vaccines that has been implemented in recent years.

Because high-risk populations have a higher rate of events, and these events are likely to be observed earlier, efficacy estimates from a trial conducted in a high-risk population may not be generalizable to the general population but at the same time may be more statistically efficient, requiring both a smaller sample size and shorter follow-up period to reach a correct conclusion (Johnson et al. 2021). There is some theoretical justification to expect that vaccine efficacy may differ according to the risk experienced by a population, and in particular that efficacy will be lower in populations with more exposures or typically exposed to a higher dose (Gomes et al. 2014). Limited empirical evidence from animal and human studies supports this expectation (Langwig et al. 2019). In this respect, one could envisage a situation where efficacy is lower in a trial in a high-risk population than it would be in the general population, and even where this fact leads to lower power to test the hypothesis of no effect, but these concerns have not been widely explored.

Not all vaccines are intended for use in the general population (e.g., Ebola), so a further consideration is to match the trial population to that in which the vaccine is intended for use once approved. In regard to the third objective of maximizing public health benefit, if the vaccine candidate proves highly effective, and given a limited supply of vaccines, vaccinating high-risk populations could have a larger impact on incidence and transmission than a trial conducted in the general population.

The choice of trial population becomes more complicated when there are safety concerns with conducting the trial in the ideal target population for a vaccine, as was the case for pregnant women who would have been an ideal trial group for Zika vaccine trials because of the devastating consequences of congenital Zika syndrome. However, these concerns should not result in the default exclusion of pregnant women and other populations, and efforts should be made to include at-risk populations in trials whenever possible (Ethics Working Group on ZIKV Research and Pregnancy 2017; PREVENT Working Group 2018). Additional complications arise when restricting the trial population to those who have not been previously infected. In addition to the expense and logistics required to test all potential participants for previous infection prior to enrollment in the trial, this restriction may limit the generalizability of the trial, as participants who are both at high risk for infection and have avoided infection in the past may be less likely to get infected (Kahn et al. 2018; Tuite and Fisman 2011). A compromise may be to collect sera from all participants at baseline and the end of follow-up and test some or all of these at the conclusion of the trial to stratify efficacy analyses by prior infection (Lipsitch et al. 2020). SARS-CoV-2 trials showed that this approach also enables estimation of additional endpoints (serologically confirmed infection); see ▶ Sect. 2.5 (Kahn et al. 2019; Sadoff et al. 2021).

2.4 Trial Implementation

Participants may be enrolled into the trial as quickly as possible in a "parallel" rollout, or enrollment may be intentionally phased in over time in a "stepped" rollout, for example, to facilitate comparisons based on geography or to follow an outbreak. In some cases, such as a stepped-wedge trial (Bellan et al. 2015; Gambia hepatitis intervention study 1987), clusters receive the vaccine at randomly assigned, staggered calendar times, and incidence is compared between clusters that have received the vaccine candidate and clusters that have not, using statistical techniques that continue to be refined and expanded (Kennedy-Shaffer and Lipsitch 2020; Thompson et al. 2018). Ring vaccination of cases' contacts and contacts of contacts by design (Henao-Restrepo et al. 2017) is stepped, as enrollment in the trial occurs based on when and where cases arise; in addition, during the Ebola Ça Suffit! trial, the control clusters received the vaccine candidate 21 days after enrollment, which could be seen as a delayed comparator and/or as another form of stepped rollout.

If there are sufficient resources and logistics in place (▶ Chap. 37) and the geographic area of the trial is clearly identified, a parallel rollout (i.e., enrollment, informed consent, randomization, and vaccination occurring essentially simultaneously) can result in a shorter trial than a stepped rollout and therefore obtain an efficacy estimate sooner. Additionally, if the vaccine candidate is effective, more people will receive this beneficial intervention earlier during the trial in a parallel rollout than in a stepped rollout. Thus, under these assumptions, for a vaccine candidate that works, all objectives lend support to a parallel rollout. However, when incidence is very patchy in space and time, and it is practical to implement the trial over time in areas (or among contact networks) of high transmission, stepped rollout may be favored, as in the case of Ebola Ça Suffit! (Henao-Restrepo et al. 2017). Moreover, a very fast rollout could prevent potentially useful adaptations of the trial (discussed more below). For example, if the trial concludes futility of the vaccine at its end, the same trial participants cannot be re-enrolled to test a different vaccine, which could delay testing of the second vaccine.

The choice of rollout and its impact is an area of active research. For example, a novel variant of the stepped-wedge design has been proposed that allows areas at the highest risk to be prioritized for the earliest rollout in order to maximize public health benefit while preserving randomization (Harling et al. 2017). Likewise, individual randomization with stepped rollout can prioritize areas of predicted high incidence for earlier trial starts, similarly increasing public health benefit as well as trial power (Lipsitch et al. 2015a).

2.5 Primary Endpoints

Another important decision for a trial design is the choice of the primary endpoint. This choice is a balance between selecting an endpoint of the greatest public health relevance and ensuring the feasibility of the trial. Often vaccine trials use clinical disease, typically combined with a confirmatory diagnostic test, as the primary endpoint. Vaccine efficacy against confirmed clinical disease was the primary endpoint for many SARS-CoV-2 vaccine trials (Baden et al. 2021; Logunov et al. 2021; Polack et al. 2020; Sadoff et al. 2021; Shapiro et al. 2021; Voysey et al. 2021a). This endpoint is clinically relevant and easier logistically than other endpoints, such as infection, which may require testing of all or a large sample of trial participants on a regular basis. Efficacy against severe disease may be of greater public health interest, but the endpoint may occur too infrequently to be feasible. There are several additional endpoints of interest, which were often secondary endpoints of these trials, such as vaccine efficacy against severe disease, asymptomatic infection, hospitalization, or death, as well as vaccine efficacy among high-risk groups, such as the elderly (Lipsitch and Dean 2020).

Vaccine efficacy against all infections, not only symptomatic infections, is important for certain kinds of pathogens. A vaccine's efficacy in preventing infection (even asymptomatic) is important if asymptomatic infection plays a role in onward transmission, as with Nipah, MERS, and SARS-CoV-2 for example (Clayton et al. 2012; Johansson et al. 2021; Kahn et al. 2019; Omrani et al. 2013; Rodriguez-Barraquer et al. 2013) or can result in long-term sequelae, such as congenital Zika syndrome (CDC 2019). While still requiring testing of some participants, approaches exist for accurately estimating this endpoint by testing only a fraction of trial participants (Kahn et al. 2019). This requires a laboratory assay that can distinguish between natural infection and vaccine-induced immunity (Sadoff et al. 2021). Some studies of SARS-CoV-2 vaccines included secondary endpoints of asymptomatic virus infection or serologically detected infection (Baden et al. 2021; Voysey et al. 2021a). Measures of viral positivity and viral load may also provide additional information about the vaccines' effects on the potential for onward transmission (Kennedy-Shaffer et al. 2021; Lipsitch and Kahn 2021). A complication that has been recently recognized is that vaccination itself may prevent seroconversion in some vaccinated persons who do become infected, leading to a risk that the use of serologic endpoints may overestimate vaccine efficacy against infection (Follmann et al. 2022). Finally, vaccine efficacy against progression to symptoms is another potential endpoint of trials (Halloran et al. 2010; Kahn et al. 2019; WHO 2013).

If trials are stopped based on aggregate numbers of clinical disease cases, they may not have sufficient power to detect efficacy against rarer outcomes, such as severe disease, or efficacy in different subgroups (e.g., age, comorbidities) (Lipsitch and Dean 2020). Generalizability of the results may therefore be limited if, for example, a population of interest has a different age structure than that of the trial population. To ensure that SARS-CoV-2 vaccines were well evaluated in highest-risk populations, the U.S. FDA specified that trials "should include adequate representation of elderly individuals and individuals with medical comorbidities" (FDA 2020). Moderna's COVID-19 vaccine trial set minimum enrollment targets for adults over 65 and adults under 65 who were categorized as being at increased risk upon screening (Moderna 2020). They also adjusted site selection and enrollment processes during the conduct of the trial to increase the numbers of participants from racial and ethnic minorities (Baden et al. 2021). Other potential solutions include (1) setting minimum thresholds for the number of cases in each subgroup that must be met before interim analyses are performed, (2) continuing placebo-controlled follow-up for longer (though this has other implications as discussed above), or (3) obtaining estimates in post-approval observational studies (discussed below).

In vaccine trials, the usual endpoint is a time-to-event one. This requires being able to know robustly the time at which an individual acquires the disease, which is not always possible or easy. An alternative primary endpoint is disease or infection status at the end of the study or at a follow up, a "binary" endpoint. Here there are competing considerations for satisfying the first two scientific objectives of the trial. While a trial with a binary endpoint may require fewer resources and enable the trial to start (and finish) earlier, all else equal; a time-to-event analysis has higher power to detect an effect because it uses more information (George et al. 2014; Syed et al. 2016); however, given that events are rare, the results are typically very similar. Though often unknown, the nature of the vaccine mechanism (i.e., leaky vs. all-or-nothing) also impacts the choice of analysis (Smith et al. 1984).

3 Adaptive Vaccine Trial Design

3.1 Adaptive Designs: Basic Concepts

A traditional, non-adaptive trial (Fig. 3) is implemented in three steps: a trial design and study size are chosen, then the trial is conducted, and finally the data are analyzed at the end of the trial according to a pre-defined analysis plan. Adaptive designs (Fig. 3) make clinical trials flexible (Shih 2006) by allowing the use of data accumulating in the trial to modify the trial's course according to pre-specified rules while maintaining the validity and integrity of the trial. Crucially, such a priori planned adaptations are fundamentally different from unplanned ad hoc modifications, which are common in traditional trials (e.g., alterations to the eligibility criteria). A second defining feature of an adaptive design is that, because data will be examined during the course of the trial, ensur-

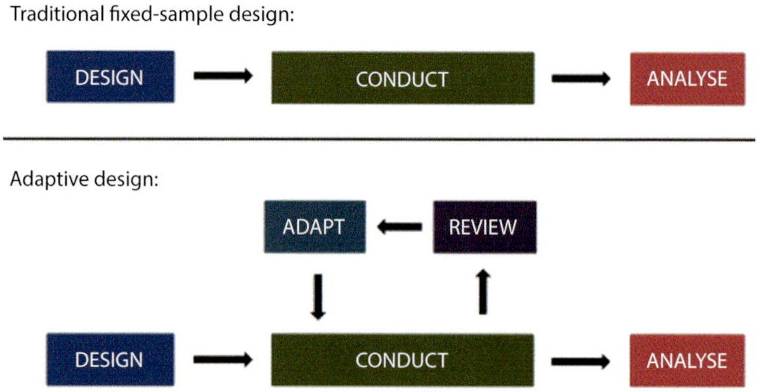

Fig. 3 Schematic of a traditional clinical trial design with fixed sample size (top), and an adaptive design with pre-specified review(s) and adaptation(s). Adaptive designs are useful for addressing analysis challenges, such as some of those that arose during the COVID-19 pandemic. (Pallmann et al. 2018) (Creative Commons Attribution 4.0)

ing the integrity and validity of results as part of the design is crucial. Integrity of the trial requires ensuring that trial data and processes are not compromised, e.g., minimizing information leakage at the interim analyses that could introduce biases in the rest of the study (Fleming et al. 2008). To ensure the validity of an adaptive design one must ensure that the trial answers the original research questions adequately, e.g., by ensuring type I error (rejection of a true null hypothesis or false positive) is controlled at a target level despite the multiple looks at the data (Graf et al. 2014) and by producing accurate estimates of treatment effects and correct p-values (Bauer et al. 2009).

Well-recognized adaptations that these designs permit include: stopping the trial at an early stage to declare success or lack of efficacy (futility) by sequential monitoring, changing the randomization ratio of patients to trial arms during the trial interim analysis, re-estimating the sample size needed to detect a certain treatment effect, changing the doses or arms examined during the trial (i.e., abandoning existing arms/doses or adding new ones), and identifying patients most likely to benefit from a treatment in order to focus the study and recruitment efforts on them. Whenever feasible, adaptive designs may allow for clinical trials that are more efficient, informative, and/or ethical than trials with a fixed design (Graf et al. 2014). Early stopping for success or futility is common in vaccine efficacy trials, particularly in the emerging infectious disease setting where urgency is heightened. Most COVID-19 trials included one or more interim looks, timed according to the number of primary endpoints observed. In a Phase I/II/III trial of Pfizer-BioNTech's BNT 162b2 vaccine, a first analysis was planned after 32 cases. After discussion with the FDA, the company revised their first interim analysis to 62 cases. Because of high incidence rates during the conduct of the trial, the evaluable case count reached 94 cases when the data monitoring committee reviewed the first analysis (Pfizer and BioNTech 2020). The vaccine met its pre-specified efficacy success criteria at that time.

Adaptive trial designs have been used in therapeutic trials across early and late stages for more than 25 years now (Bauer et al. 2009). Despite their obvious benefits in many situations, there still remain some important practical barriers for a more widespread use of these designs, such as lack of expertise or experience. Before the COVID-19 pandemic started, concerns of how funders and regulators would perceive adaptive designs were an important reason why they were still far from an established practice (Pallmann et al. 2018). Despite that, they had been increasingly used over the decade preceding COVID-19 (Bothwell et al. 2018).

The COVID-19 pandemic and the unprecedented response in terms of clinical research activity that came with it dramatically changed the picture for adaptive designs. This research needed to be conducted as rapidly as possible and under considerably large uncertainty (e.g., over the natural history of the disease, the number and population of patients affected, and the emergence of new potential therapies/vaccines). These challenges made the use of adaptive designs for clinical trials a particularly attractive option in the context of a novel infectious disease such as COVID-19 (Stallard et al. 2020). Additionally, adaptive design methods were also found useful to address the consequences the pandemic had on ongoing clinical trials begun in non-COVID-19 conditions (many clinical trials answering important questions were stopped, or temporarily paused to possibly restart later, some with important modifications) (Kunz et al. 2020). Adaptive trial design analytical methodology proved useful for getting interpretable results from trials that had to be stopped before their original endpoints or were stopped and later restarted.

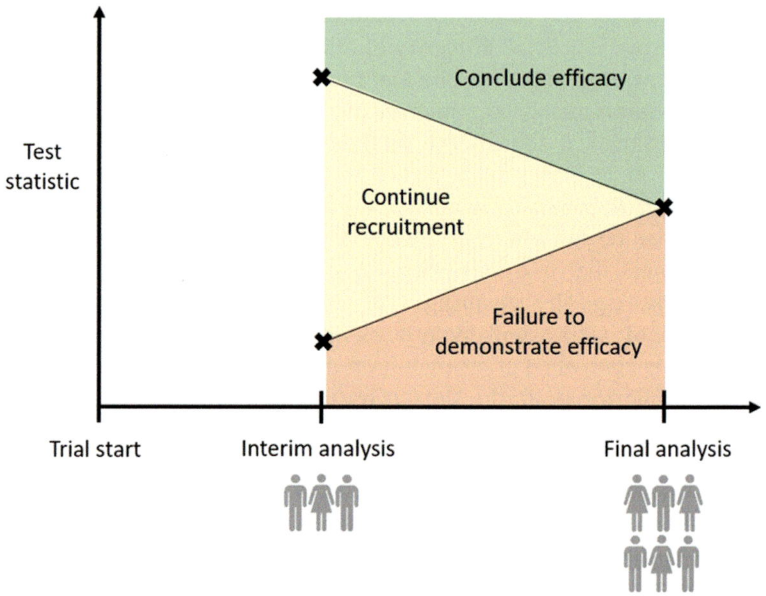

Fig. 4 Demonstration of stopping boundaries in a two-stage group sequential design. (Burnett et al. 2020) (CC BY 4.0)

3.2 Possible Adaptations for Innovative Vaccine Trials

In this section, we will consider some popular forms of adaptations that have been proposed and used in therapeutic trials (including for COVID-19 treatments). To the best of the authors' knowledge, most of these adaptations have not yet been implemented in vaccine trials. Some have been proposed or used within the context of an emerging epidemic for therapeutic trials (e.g., changes to the randomization). Here, we discuss the potential for specific benefits and challenges of the different adaptations in a vaccine trial context.

3.2.1 Multi-arm Multistage Trials

In general, a sequential monitoring approach can be applied to two-armed or multi-arm trials (also known as multi-armed, multi-stage trials). In the latter case, a trial may start with a number of experimental treatment arms (or vaccine candidates) and a common control arm to which all arms are compared. These designs include interim decision points at which data will be analyzed and a decision for each arm compared to control will be made: either an arm is dropped for futility or its superiority is declared (in both cases early stopping of the arm is decided); or the trial continues to the next stage (if the final recruitment target has not been reached yet). The trial as a whole can also stop early if all arms are dropped because of futility, and at the final stage of the trial, a decision (either efficacy or futility) must be made.

Possible adaptations in a multi-arm setting include early stopping boundaries to either select arms during the trial or to early stop the complete trial (that preserves power and type I error (Fig. 4) (Jennison and Turnbull 1999)). These boundaries can be defined using a frequentist approach, e.g., based on Magirr et al. (2012), using traditional statistics (Ghosh et al. 2017), or based on a Bayesian approach, using posterior probabilities of the treatments being efficacious. Brueckner et al. (2018) compare different approaches to boundary definition for evaluating treatment options in the context of emerging epidemics.

Testing several vaccine candidates at the same time (those with promising efficacy and safety data from Phases I and II) allows for a faster speed of development (compared to parallel trials that may start at different time points and require multiple study set ups) and for readily concentrating resources on promising vaccine candidates. An additional advantage of these designs comes from extra efficiency gains from a common control group (Parmar et al. 2008). In terms of a vaccine trial, a common control arm would reduce the number of unvaccinated participants when the control arm is a placebo arm, which could enhance the public health benefit of the trial if the vaccines are effective (objective 3). Specific statistical considerations for vaccine trials with multiple candidates may need consideration. Some of particular importance from the Ebola virus disease (EVD) crisis centered around the appropriateness of multiplicity adjustment when doing hypothesis testing and type I error control (which impacts on the required size of the study), the optimal size for a placebo control group in a multi-arm setting (i.e., optimal in terms of efficiency), and the timing of interim analysis in terms of overall or pairwise comparisons (Nason 2016).

A potential disadvantage of adaptive designs that allow for early stopping is that even if their expected sample size is smaller than that for a fixed trial design, their maximum sample size could indeed be larger than that (Lai and Shih 2004). These families of adaptive designs may potentially impact all objectives in a vaccine trial; for example, when early stopping is triggered there are efficiency gains (objective 1), negative impact on precision of the estimate (objective 2), and possibly earlier roll-out (objective 3).

3.2.2 Adaptive Platform Trials

Adaptive Platform Trials provide a recent example of the ideas described above. These trials "study multiple interventions in a single disease (or condition) in a perpetual manner, with interventions allowed to enter or leave the platform on the basis of a decision algorithm" (Adaptive Platform Trials Coalition 2019). A specific adaptation that is possible in a platform trial is to add new experimental treatments as the trial progresses. Platform trials provide considerable operational efficiency (Schiavone et al. 2019). This approach enabled the Randomized, Embedded, Multifactorial Adaptive Platform trial for Community Acquired Pneumonia (REMAP-CAP, NCT0273570) trial to be rapidly adapted to study COVID-19 patients. An FDA (2021) guidance cites platform trials as a potential approach for evaluating drugs intended to treat or prevent COVID-19. There are several other recent examples of platform trials, such as the Solidarity and RECOVERY trials (▶ In Practice 14.1) (RECOVERY trial 2022; WHO 2022a, b).

3.2.3 Response-Adaptive Randomization

Response-Adaptive Randomization uses accumulating outcome data to change the randomization probabilities within a trial to meet a predefined objective. These objectives include efficiency (e.g., maximizing power for a given sample size), ethical advantages (e.g., allocating more participants to the superior arm if it exists), or a combination of both (e.g., minimizing treatment failures subject to a power constraint) (Hu and Rosenberger 2006). While the most popular randomization method aims for a balanced allocation of treatments, most commonly 1:1 in two-arm trials, this may be suboptimal where multiple experimental objectives compete against each other. The use of response-adaptive randomization during a vaccine trial could, for example, try to attain a minimum power level for the trial (objective 1) while maximizing the number of participants that receive an active vaccine (objective 3). An additional advantage, particularly in multi-arm platform trials, is to identify groups of patients in which a vaccine works (or works better). The use of response adaptive randomization for treatments in an emerging epidemic was considered by Berry et al. (2016) and has been used in REMAP-CAP. More recently, Johnson et al. (2021) discuss the use of this adaptation in simulated COVID-19 two-armed vaccine trials.

Response-adaptive randomization has generated controversy over its use in practice since it was first proposed. For a review on the practical and statistical issues discussed see Robertson et al. (2023). For a debate on its use in the context of the COVID-19 pandemic see Proschan and Evans (2020) and Villar et al.

(2020). Of course, changes in the randomization ratio during the trial require specific analysis at the end to protect the study from bias and preserve inferential validity of the results (Brueckner et al. 2018).

3.2.4 Sample Size Re-estimation

Sample size calculations are performed prior to the start of a trial and require assumptions about both the hypothesized treatment effect and its variability. Sample size re-estimation uses data accumulated during the trial to update the estimated sample size. If information on the estimated treatment effect is used to re-estimate sample size, the analysis must be adjusted to preserve validity of the inference (Proschan 2009), but there are forms of sample size re-estimation—based on nuisance parameters such as the estimated variability of the treatment effect—that permit the trial to be analyzed in the same manner as if the sample size had been decided upon in advance.

Vaccine trials, especially those designed rapidly, may make their sample size calculations based on highly uncertain assumptions about both incidence in the control arm and the magnitude of vaccine effect. A planned sample size re-estimation could involve an interim look at the data after some number of events have been observed in the trial to decide whether to prolong follow-up, add participants, or both in the event that the interim look suggests the planned follow-up will be inconclusive. During the COVID-19 pandemic, the sample size of a large Phase III trial of the single dose Ad26.COV2.S vaccine from Janssen was reduced from 60,000 to approximately 40,000 (Sadoff et al. 2021). This change reflected the higher than anticipated incidence of COVID-19 during the trial.

3.2.5 Integrating Data Across Trials

Ideally, a single vaccine trial will be sufficiently large to reliably assess the efficacy and safety of a vaccine. For COVID-19 vaccine trials, this was achieved by running trials with very large numbers of participants (>30,000) and, in some cases, over 100 distinct participating sites across multiple global regions. For example, the randomized, double-blind, placebo-controlled, individually randomized Phase III ENSEMBLE trial of the single-dose Janssen Ad26.COV2.S vaccine had sites in Argentina, Brazil, Chile, Colombia, Mexico, Peru, South Africa, and the United States (Sadoff et al. 2021). By including sites in distinct geographic regions, this multi-site design is considered more robust to uncertainty in COVID-19 epidemiology, as the trial can continue to accrue endpoints even if incidence wanes in one region (Dean et al. 2020a). As new SARS-CoV-2 variants emerged in these regions, the ENSEMBLE trial was fortuitously one of the first to provide randomized estimates of vaccine efficacy against these novel strains.

A multi-country trial with a shared master or core protocol is ideal, as it ensures consistency of the study procedures (Dean et al. 2020a). Nonetheless, situations can occur where there are multiple, independently run trials evaluating the same vaccine. In that case, it may be advantageous to combine information across these trials to create a stronger evidence base. An interim report on the Oxford-AstraZeneca ChAdOx1 nCoV-19 vaccine published in the *Lancet* included data from four distinct blinded, randomized, controlled trials in three countries (Voysey et al. 2021b). These studies had a variety of differences in their design, including study populations and control arm (i.e., placebo, or meningococcal conjugate vaccine), yet they were deemed sufficiently similar to be pooled into a combined analysis. This required extensive discussion with regulators to ensure that the results were of acceptable quality.

3.3 Opportunities and Challenges for Adaptive Designs in Vaccine Trials

Adaptive designs, in their many different forms, can offer efficiency gains (understood as a higher power to detect a certain vaccine efficacy level), the possibility of gathering conclusive evidence sooner or with fewer subjects than a traditional trial, or even the chance of vaccinating more participants during the trial and afterward. Each adaptation considered can produce one of these effects or a combination of them.

In some cases, the adaptations considered can alleviate trade-offs between the objectives, while in other cases they can create new trade-offs. As mentioned before, allowing for early stopping for efficacy can reduce the number of trial participants needed to achieve a certain statistical power level while simultaneously allowing for more participants to receive the vaccine due to earlier roll-out (positively impacting both objectives 1 and 3). However, as shown in Johnson et al. (2021), certain types of response adaptive randomization considerably increase the number of participants vaccinated during a 2-arm trial compared to a traditional fixed randomized design, but they also require a larger sample size, creating a conflict between objectives 2 and 3.

In general, adaptive designs also present practical challenges for implementation, some of which will perhaps be more relevant in a vaccine context than in a treatment one. First, most adaptive designs require a quickly observable endpoint that needs to also be clinically meaningful. For long-term observable endpoints, as in vaccine trials, early predictors of final outcome can be considered as endpoints for adaptation purposes, and the long-term outcome can be used for the final analysis of the trial (Krams et al. 2009). The utility of adaptive designs also depends on recruitment pace. If most or all patients are recruited and treated at the same time, adaptations are harder or impossible to implement. This creates a tension between the desire to complete recruitment as fast as possible (objectives 1 and 2) and the recruitment pace that would be ideal for an adaptive design with different objectives (objectives 1 and 3).

Methodological papers proposing adaptive designs usually do not consider the pace of recruitment versus the length of follow-up of the endpoint when quantifying the efficiency advantages of adaptive designs (Wason et al. 2019). Establishing the optimal recruitment pace for a given endpoint and a given adaptive design can be done by running simulations that resemble potential scenarios and exploring the impact that these can have on different operating characteristics of the designs.

An additional issue to consider is that adaptive designs require interim analyses to be conducted quickly and to a high standard. This requires an effective infrastructure that will, for example, return data for the interim analysis promptly and completely; data queries and cleaning also have to be dealt with fairly quickly (Wason et al. 2019). Adaptive designs naturally imply staggered randomization and treatment of participants so that data can be partially observed and used to inform future decisions. If the pace of the adaptation matches that of practical recruitment constraints (given, for example, by vaccine availability), then the design will not artificially slow down the trial's progress. If an adaptive design is to be considered in situations in which the trial's duration might have to be extended in order to adapt, then the effects of the epidemic's dynamics should be factored into reporting the operating characteristics and resulting trade-offs of such a design (Pallmann et al. 2018).

A final point to consider is that communicating the adaptive design to stakeholders or trial participants may be more challenging than for traditional trials. Specifically, this could create a challenge at the time of obtaining regulatory approval for the study. Adaptive designs can raise more questions than traditional trials as to how the integrity and validity of conclusions are ensured by the more complex design (a priori planned *adaptations* are fundamentally different from unplanned ad hoc modifications and require pre-planned analysis methods that avoid introducing bias into the trial). Explaining simulation results to stakeholders usually helps to increase their understanding of the benefits and risks of any particular design. When possible, seeking regulatory approval of more complex designs as early as possible can help prevent delays (Berry et al. 2016; Multiple treatments for Ebola virus disease (EVD) 2015; REMAP-CAP response to COVID-19 pandemic 2021).

With respect to this last point, it is worth noting that the major regulatory agencies for Europe and the United States have issued detailed guidelines on the use of adaptive designs (EMA 2007; FDA 2016, 2019), which suggest that the agencies are generally well-disposed toward adaptive trials, especially when the design is properly justified and concerns about its validity are addressed.

3.4 Further Considerations for Adaptive Designs for Vaccine Trials

The adaptive designs described in the previous sections have been proposed and used in the context of clinical trials for treatments and/or vaccines. Further innovative adaptive approaches could be developed specifically for a vaccine trial designed to be run during an emerging epidemic. For example, an adaptive design could use accumulated data on the primary endpoints or an available surrogate endpoint to inform the decision on when and where to start the trial (which locations and at which moment of time) in order to meet a desired objective or combination of multiple objectives. This would require a complex (and novel) trial design that would closely integrate practical realities of outbreak epidemiology and predictions of the epidemic's trajectory to support decision making. It would also require careful consideration of the type of epidemics and how this may influence the different weights objectives 1, 2, and 3 of a vaccine trial may receive. For example, in the context of EVD, a vaccine trial could have had a much larger role as a control strategy than in a pandemic like COVID-19, in which the population at risk—essentially every human on earth—cannot be included in the trial. A similar consideration has been made for the relative benefits of adaptive designs and the proportion of patients included in a clinical trial (Berry and Eick 1995).

Laber et al. (2018) propose an approach for a trial meant to serve as part of an optimal disease control strategy in the context of an emerging epidemic. Harling et al. (2017) have used simulations to study designs that adaptively incorporate information about cluster connectivity in the design of cluster randomized trials. Their results show that this can increase the public health impact of trials, especially in acute outbreak settings, but they also highlight the computational and modeling challenges of developing such an adaptive design and the key role of simulations for designing and implementing them in practice.

The use of adaptive designs has implications for the five decisions discussed in ► Sect. 3. The choices of randomization unit (individual or cluster) and primary endpoint (binary or continuous time to event) directly affect the portfolio of adaptive methods available for the final design. Some adaptive designs may have been more developed methodologically for individual randomization and/or for binary endpoints rather than for cluster randomized trials and/or continuous (time to event) endpoints. For example, the adaptive multi-armed multistage approach offers no clear advantages in terms of requiring smaller expected sample sizes if the primary endpoint is a time to event one and trial participants can and will be followed indefinitely until the event of interest occurs (Emerson et al. 2011); response-adaptive randomization methods have been extensively developed for binary outcomes and individual randomization, and less work has been done for continuous endpoints or cluster trials (Williamson and Villar 2019). Similarly, methodological work in adaptive designs has mostly considered the control arm to be placebo or active standard of care rather than a delayed administration of the same treatment.

Finally, the choice of trial population (general versus high risk) may be revisited during the trial rather than being fixed in advance. An adaptive design could aim to dynamically identify groups of patients that benefit more from a specific treatment, similar to the way biomarker-led adaptive trials use accumulated data on efficacy endpoints to determine which population (if any) maximizes power of a trial by being included in it (Harling et al. 2017; Wason et al. 2015).

4 Additional Considerations

4.1 Seamless Designs

Traditional drug and vaccine development consists of a sequence of independent experiments in different phases. In vaccine trials,

Phase I experiments that study safety profiles of vaccine candidates and Phase II immunogenicity studies are conducted before a study focusing on efficacy of the vaccine takes place. Usually, not only is there a considerable time interval between the phases, but also late phase trials are evaluated as stand-alone trials, ignoring data from previous phases.

Seamless designs formally link trials of different phases by combining them into one single trial implemented in two or more stages (Bretz et al. 2006; Kennedy et al. 2017). In the first example mentioned above, one or more treatments are selected after the first stage based on the available data, and carried on for further study in the second stage. Seamless designs can offer different advantages and may be classified as operationally or inferentially seamless (Cuffe et al. 2014; Mahajan and Gupta 2010). This design was used in evaluation of some SARS-CoV-2 vaccines (NIH 2021b).

An *operationally* seamless design—an early trial followed by a confirmatory one wherein the data of each stage is analyzed separately—has a common protocol, allowing for time savings on logistics, approvals, etc., and therefore positively impacting objectives 1 and 3. An *inferentially* seamless design combines data from both phases to make the final inference, which may provide further advantages in terms of power and the resulting estimation, potentially impacting objectives 1 and 2 of a vaccine trial. Furthermore, inferential seamless designs may also be adaptive (Maca et al. 2006) if there is a treatment of subgroup selection based on the first-stage data that will determine the hypothesis to be studied in the second stage of the trial.

4.2 Observational Study Designs

Randomization ensures that under a null hypothesis of no vaccine effect, the distribution of the outcome (e.g., time of infection) will be closely similar on average between the arms of the trial, with variability that can be predicted statistically. This strengthens inference compared to a situation where access to the vaccine is not assigned randomly but depends on factors about the individual participant, such as belonging to a cluster or a vulnerable group; the latter case raises the possibility that those who do and do not get the vaccine have systematically different distributions of the outcome, even apart from any effect of the vaccine, which could result in incorrectly observed vaccine efficacy under the null hypothesis (Senn 2012). However, as discussed above, not all measures of interest regarding vaccine efficacy will be obtainable in most trials (e.g., subgroup efficacy). Observational studies, while limited by the potential for confounding and selection bias, provide an opportunity to gain additional information about vaccines' effectiveness. A wealth of additional questions can be answered post authorization or approval, as has been seen with the COVID-19 pandemic, including information about effectiveness in different subgroups; after a single dose in a two-dose regimen; in populations different from the trial population; against genetic variants not common at the time of trials; and against transmission, asymptomatic infection, and viral load (CDC 2021; Lipsitch and Dean 2020; Richterman et al. 2021). Ongoing work to enhance the robustness of observational studies is important both for their routine use in areas like influenza (Lipsitch et al. 2016; Sullivan et al. 2016), and for their potential use in emergencies (WHO 2021a).

4.3 Incorporating Pathogen Sequence Data into Vaccine Evaluation

As evidenced during the West African Ebola epidemic (Emmett et al. 2015; Gire et al. 2014; Park et al. 2015) and the COVID-19 pandemic, advances in pathogen sequencing technology are making sequencing during an epidemic more of a reality (Martin et al. 2021). The ability to reconstruct transmission networks using a combination of sequence and epidemiologic data could enhance the estimates obtained from vaccine trials. For example, it could permit estimation of vaccine efficacy against infectiousness, that is, the reduction in transmission by an infected vaccinated individual compared to an infected unvaccinated individual (Kahn et al. 2021). This would provide a more complete understanding of the public health and cost-effectiveness of future vaccination campaigns. Sequencing can also help provide estimates of vaccine efficacy or effectiveness against genetic variants, a critical question for SARS-CoV-2 as more variants continue to emerge.

4.4 Simulations

Computer simulations are useful tools for better understanding stochastic disease transmission dynamics and for assessing the impact different interventions could have on the course of outbreaks (▶ Chap. 24). For vaccine trial design and analysis, simulations can provide important insights (Halloran et al. 2017; Martin et al. 2021). They can be used to compare and contrast the different choices described above, such as the implications of randomization unit on power and sample size (Hitchings et al. 2017, 2018); to identify efficient methods for estimating vaccine efficacy against all infection (Kahn et al. 2019); to make area-specific predictions, aid in trial site selection, and assess feasibility (Dean et al. 2020b; Madewell et al. 2021); or to quantify ethical tradeoffs in design choices (Bellan et al. 2017), including impact on operating characteristics of different types of adaptive designs for a therapeutic trial in the context of an epidemic (Brueckner et al. 2018; Johnson et al. 2021).

Advance preparation of principles and protocols for vaccine trials before epidemics emerge is critical for ensuring vaccine trials can start as early as possible in the course of an epidemic, as has been recognized in pandemic planning for some time (HHS 2016; Pandemic Preparedness Partnership 2021). Simulations can be very valuable for illustrating a design choice to stakeholders and for assessing the robustness of design to different assumptions, for example, studying the effect of different recruitment and participation rates on key operating characteristics. Simulations also provide a fast and efficient way to narrow down the range of possible trial designs and to identify innovative solutions both before an epidemic emerges and in the early days of an outbreak (▶ Chap. 25).

4.5 Comparing Ebola and SARS-CoV-2 Vaccine Trial Experiences

Experiences during the West African Ebola epidemic led to insightful and innovative research on improving vaccine trials in these urgent settings. The distinct experience of the COVID-19 pandemic has further challenged us but has also yielded new growth and insights. The contrast between vaccine trial conditions and choices in these two episodes is a reminder of the unique challenges arising in each infectious disease emergency and the importance of these conditions in guiding vaccine and treatment trial design. Future epidemics are likely to challenge us in new ways and may call for the use of more innovative designs.

Broadly speaking, among the major practical challenges facing Ebola vaccine trials were patchy, episodic outbreaks that were beginning to decline as trials were being rolled out, while intense debates about the ethics of placebo control were ongoing. This led to numerous proposals and eventually to an innovative, cluster-randomized, stepped-rollout delayed-vaccination-controlled, ring vaccine trial in Guinea that followed cases and vaccinated rings of contacts and contacts-of-contacts (Henao-Restrepo et al. 2017).

In contrast, the COVID-19 pandemic was global with high attack rates in the general population. Large, uncontrolled epidemics in multiple countries with experience and infrastructure for vaccine trials (e.g., the United States, United Kingdom, Brazil, and South Africa) created the conditions for rapid results to be obtained from trials of multiple vaccines with very traditional designs: individually randomized, placebo-controlled, parallel-rollout, in the general population, with laboratory-confirmed symptomatic infection as primary endpoints. At the other extreme, some vaccines (e.g., Sputnik V, EpiVacCorona, and Convidecia) were rolled out before formal efficacy trials were completed (Corona Virus Vaccine Tracker: Russia 2021). Likely due in part to the different disease severity profiles between SARS-CoV-2 and Ebola and the intended use case to vaccinate billions globally, debates about the ethics of placebo (at least for trials of first-generation vaccines) were remarkably absent for COVID-19 vaccine trials (Eyal and Lipsitch 2021).

5 Conclusion

Multiple factors will influence the choices made in the design and analysis of vaccine trials conducted during an outbreak of an emerging or re-emerging infectious disease. Many of the decisions made will depend on the setting and epidemiologic characteristics of the outbreak and will likely be influenced by factors beyond researchers' control, such as the impact of conflict on outbreak response strategies (Maxmen 2019). To recapitulate, we have discussed five key choices that must be made in all trials:

1. individual vs. cluster randomization
2. placebo vs. active control vs. delayed administration
3. general vs. high-risk trial population
4. parallel vs. stepped implementation
5. clinical and statistical end points

These choices must be made in the context of the three main objectives noted at the beginning:

1. Test the null hypothesis of no or minimum effect of the vaccine candidate in a rigorous fashion.
2. Estimate the efficacy of the vaccine candidate.
3. Maximize the public health impact of the vaccine trial, for both trial participants and the broader community, which we could roughly characterize as
   (a) The net benefit (protection from infection minus adverse events) to trial participants.
   (b) The benefit to the broader community if the vaccine is shown to be safe and efficacious by the trial.

When these three objectives conflict, innovative designs can help balance competing objectives. We have highlighted potential ways adaptive designs can aid in this, as well as the need for simulations to enhance the robustness of trial design and analysis. We also advocate careful consideration of the importance of the different aims of a vaccine trial up front, before the trial starts, in order to find and select a design (adaptive or not) that is optimal with respect to those aims and practically feasible. Whenever possible, harmonization and standardization of trial protocols should be considered to help ensure consistent evaluation of vaccine candidates (NIH 2021a; WHO 2021b).

Discussion Questions

Short Questions

1. What are the three main objectives of vaccine efficacy trials conducted during epidemics of emerging infectious diseases?
2. List the five key choices that must be made in trial design.
3. What is the historical default vaccine trial design?
4. Provide four examples of factors and steps involved in the selection of trial design.
5. List the guiding principles of vaccine trial design.
6. Explain the differences between individual and cluster randomization and give an example where each may be used.
7. Discuss the advantages and disadvantages of placebo-controlled trials.
8. Give examples of target vaccine trial populations.
9. Describe two examples of primary endpoints in vaccine trials and how these might be measured.
10. Explain the basic concepts of adaptive design.

Long Questions

1. Describe the opportunities and challenges of employing adaptive designs for vaccine trials.
2. Discuss how different pathogen characteristics and outbreak contexts can influence decisions on vaccine trial design.

Fig. 5 Contrasting trials. (Authors)

Contrasting and similar features	Ebola Ça Suffit!	Most COVID-19 vaccine efficacy RCTs
Randomization unit	Cluster (ring)	Individual
Comparator intervention	Delayed vaccination	Placebo or active control
Trial population	High risk (contacts and contacts of contacts)	General population
Trial implementation	Stepped (ring)	Parallel
Primary endpoint	Laboratory confirmed symptomatic disease	Laboratory confirmed symptomatic disease
Adaptivity	Interim analyses and early stopping	Interim analyses and early stopping

Application of Knowledge to Scenario

Vaccine trials in response to Ebola virus and SARs-CoV-2 have followed different paths, as illustrated in Fig. 5.

Apply the lessons learned from prior vaccine trials to a scenario of a future unknown pathogen (Pathogen X) or a current pathogen of concern (e.g., Nipah virus) requiring a vaccine trial:

1. Describe a planning and implementation process for a vaccine trial (identify different aims up front before trial starts that is practically feasible).
2. Identify the potential trial types you would consider.
    (a) What interventions could mitigate potential conflicts among the three main objectives of efficacy trials?
    (b) What simulation tools could be utilized to enhance the robustness of trial design and analysis?
    (c) What examples of harmonization and standardization of trial protocols should be considered, when possible, to help ensure consistent evaluation of vaccine candidates?

References

Adaptive Platform Trials Coalition. Adaptive platform trials: definition, design, conduct and reporting considerations. Nat Rev Drug Discov. 2019;18(10):797–807. https://doi.org/10.1038/s41573-019-0034-3.

Baden LR, El Sahly HM, Essink B, Kotloff K, Frey S, Novak R, et al. Efficacy and safety of the mRNA-1273 SARS-CoV-2 vaccine. N Engl J Med. 2021;384(5):403–16. https://doi.org/10.1056/NEJMoa2035389.

Bauer P, Koenig F, Brannath W, Posch M. Selection and bias: two hostile brothers. Stat Med. 2009;29:1. https://doi.org/10.1002/sim.3716.

Bellan S, Pulliam J, Pearson C, Champredon D, Fox S, Skrip L, et al. Statistical power and validity of Ebola vaccine trials in Sierra Leone: a simulation study of trial design and analysis. Lancet Infect Dis. 2015;15(6):703–10. https://doi.org/10.1016/S1473-3099(15)70139-8.

Bellan S, Pulliam J, van der Graaf R, Fox S, Dushoff J, Meyers L. Quantifying ethical tradeoffs for vaccine efficacy trials during severe epidemics. bioRxiv. 2017:193649. https://doi.org/10.1101/193649.

Bellan S, Eggo R, Gsell P-S, Kucharski A, Dean N, Donohue R, et al. An online decision tree for vaccine efficacy trial design during infectious disease epidemics: the InterVax-tool. Vaccine. 2019;37(31):4376–81. https://doi.org/10.1016/j.vaccine.2019.06.019.

Berry DA, Eick SG. Adaptive assignment versus balanced randomization in clinical trials: a decision analysis. Stat Med. 1995;14(3):231–46. https://doi.org/10.1002/sim.4780140302.

Berry S, Petzold E, Dull P, Thielman N, Cunningham C, Corey G, et al. A response adaptive randomization platform trial for efficient evaluation of Ebola virus treatments: a model for pandemic response. Clin Trials (London, England). 2016;13(1):22–30. https://doi.org/10.1177/1740774515621721.

Black S, Shinefield H, Fireman B, Lewis E, Ray P, Hansen JR, et al. Efficacy, safety and immunogenicity of heptavalent pneumococcal conjugate vaccine in children. Northern California Kaiser Permanente Vaccine Study Center Group. Pediatr Infect Dis J. 2000;19(3):187–95. https://doi.org/10.1097/00006454-200003000-00003.

Bothwell L, Avorn J, Khan N, Kesselheim A. Adaptive design clinical trials: a review of the literature and ClinicalTrials.gov. BMJ Open. 2018;8(2):e018320. https://doi.org/10.1136/bmjopen-2017-018320.

Bretz F, Schmidli H, König F, Racine A, Maurer W. Confirmatory seamless phase II/III clinical trials with hypotheses selection at interim: general concepts. Biom J. 2006;48(4):623–34. https://doi.org/10.1002/bimj.200510232.

Brueckner M, Titman A, Jaki T, Rojek A, Horby P. Performance of different clinical trial designs to evaluate treatments during an epidemic. PLoS One. 2018;13(9):e0203387. https://doi.org/10.1371/journal.pone.0203387.

Burki TK. The Russian vaccine for COVID-19. Lancet Respir Med. 2020;8(11):e85–e6. https://doi.org/10.1016/S2213-2600(20)30402-1.

Burnett T, Mozgunov P, Pallmann P, Villar SS, Wheeler GM, Jaki T. Adding flexibility to clinical trial designs: an example-based guide to the practical use of adaptive designs. BMC Med. 2020;18(1):352. https://doi.org/10.1186/s12916-020-01808-2.

Camacho A, Eggo R, Funk S, Watson C, Kucharski A, Edmunds W. Estimating the probability of demonstrating vaccine efficacy in the declining Ebola epidemic: a Bayesian modelling approach. BMJ Open. 2015;5(12):e009346. https://doi.org/10.1136/bmjopen-2015-009346.

CDC. Zika virus. Atlanta, GA: Centers for Disease Control and Prevention, National Center for Emerging and Zoonotic Infectious Diseases (NCEZID), Division of Vector-Borne Diseases (DVBD); 2019. https://www.cdc.gov/zika/index.html. Accessed 28 Jan 2020.

CDC. Science brief: background rationale and evidence for public health recommendations for fully vaccinated people. 2021. https://www.cdc.gov/coronavirus/2019-ncov/science/science-briefs/fully-vaccinated-people.html#print. Accessed 16 July 2021.

Clayton B, Middleton D, Bergfeld J, Haining J, Arkinstall R, Wang L, et al. Transmission routes for Nipah virus from Malaysia and Bangladesh. Emerg Infect Dis. 2012;18(12):1983–93. https://doi.org/10.3201/eid1812.120875.

Corona Virus Vaccine Tracker: Russia. New York Times, New York. 2021. https://www.nytimes.com/interactive/2020/science/coronavirus-vaccine-tracker.html#gamaleya. Accessed 14 July 2021.

Cuffe R, Lawrence D, Stone A, Vandemeulebroecke M. When is a seamless study desirable? Case studies from different pharmaceutical sponsors. Pharm Stat. 2014;13(4):229–37. https://doi.org/10.1002/pst.1622.

Dean N, Halloran M, Longini I. Design of vaccine trials during outbreaks with and without a delayed vaccination comparator. Ann Appl Stat. 2018;12(1):330–47. https://doi.org/10.1214/17-AOAS1095.

Dean NE, Gsell P-S, Brookmeyer R, Crawford FW, Donnelly CA, Ellenberg SS, et al. Creating a framework for conducting randomized clinical trials during disease outbreaks. N Eng J M. 2020a;382(14):1366–9. https://doi.org/10.1056/NEJMsb1905390.

Dean NE, Pastore YPA, Madewell ZJ, Cummings DAT, Hitchings MDT, Joshi K, et al. Ensemble forecast modeling for the design of COVID-19 vaccine efficacy trials. Vaccine. 2020b;38(46):7213–6. https://doi.org/10.1016/j.vaccine.2020.09.031.

Donner A, Birkett N, Buck C. Randomization by cluster. Am J Epidemiol. 1981;114(6):906–14. https://doi.org/10.1093/oxfordjournals.aje.a113261.

Ebola ça Suffit Ring Vaccination Trial Consortium. The ring vaccination trial: a novel cluster randomised controlled trial design to evaluate vaccine efficacy and effectiveness during outbreaks, with special reference to Ebola. BMJ. 2015;351:h3740. https://doi.org/10.1136/bmj.h3740.

EMA. Reflection paper on methodological issues in confirmatory clinical trials planned with an adaptive design. Contract No.: Doc. Ref. CHMP/EWP/2459/02. London: European Medicines Agency. (CHMP) CfMPfHU. 2007.

Emerson S, Rudser K, Emerson S. Exploring the benefits of adaptive sequential designs in time-to-event endpoint settings. Stat Med. 2011;30(11):1199–217. https://doi.org/10.1002/sim.4156.

Emmett K, Lee A, Khiabanian H, Rabadan R. High-resolution genomic surveillance of 2014 ebolavirus using shared subclonal variants. PLoS Currents. 2015;7:ecurrents.outbreaks.c7fd7946ba606c982668a96bcba43c90. https://doi.org/10.1371/currents.outbreaks.c7fd7946ba606c982668a96bcba43c90.

Ethics Working Group on ZIKV Research & Pregancy. Pregnant women & the Zika virus vaccine research agenda: ethics guidance on priorities, inclusion, and evidence generation. Baltimore. 2017.

Eyal N, Lipsitch M. Vaccine testing for emerging infections: the case for individual randomisation. J Med Ethics. 2017;43(9):625–31. https://doi.org/10.1136/medethics-2015-103220.

Eyal N, Lipsitch M. How to test SARS-CoV-2 vaccines ethically even after one is available. Clin Infect Dis. 2021;73:2332. https://doi.org/10.1093/cid/ciab182.
FDA. Adaptive designs for medical device clinical studies. Washington, DC: US Food and Drug Administration; 2016. p. 49.
FDA. Adaptive design clinical trials for drugs and biologics guidance for industry. Washington, DC: US Food and Drug Administration; 2019. p. 37.
FDA. Development and licensure of vaccines to prevent-COVID-19: guidance for industry. 2020.
FDA. COVID-19: master protocols evaulating drugs and biological products. 2021.
Fleming T, Sharples K, McCall J, Moore A, Rodgers A, Stewart R. Maintaining confidentiality of interim data to enhance trial integrity and credibility. Clin Trials (London, England). 2008;5(2):157–67. https://doi.org/10.1177/1740774508089459.
Follmann D, Fintzi J, Fay MP, Janes HE, Baden LR, El Sahly HM, et al. A deferred-vaccination design to assess durability of COVID-19 vaccine effect after the placebo group is vaccinated. Ann Intern Med. 2021;174:1118. https://doi.org/10.7326/M20-8149.
Follmann D, Janes HE, Buhule OD, Zhou H, Girard B, Marks K et al. Anti-nucleocapsid antibodies following SARS-CoV-2 infection in the blinded phase of the mRNA-1273 Covid-19 vaccine efficacy clinical trial. medRxiv. 2022. https://doi.org/10.1101/2022.04.18.22271936.
Gambia hepatitis intervention study. Cancer Res. 1987;47(21):5782.
George B, Seals S, Aban I. Survival analysis and regression models. J Nucl Cardiol. 2014;21(4):686–94. https://doi.org/10.1007/s12350-014-9908-2.
Gessner B, Knobel D, Conan A, Finn A. Could the RTS,S/AS01 meningitis safety signal really be a protective effect of rabies vaccine? Vaccine. 2017;35(5):716–21. https://doi.org/10.1016/j.vaccine.2016.12.067.
Ghosh P, Liu L, Senchaudhuri P, Gao P, Mehta C. Design and monitoring of multi-arm multi-stage clinical trials. Biometrics. 2017;73(4):1289–99. https://doi.org/10.1111/biom.12687.
Gire S, Goba A, Andersen K, Sealfon R, Park D, Kanneh L, et al. Genomic surveillance elucidates Ebola virus origin and transmission during the 2014 outbreak. Science. 2014;345(6202):1369–72. https://doi.org/10.1126/science.1259657.
Gomes MG, Lipsitch M, Wargo AR, Kurath G, Rebelo C, Medley GF, et al. A missing dimension in measures of vaccination impacts. PLoS Pathog. 2014;10(3):e1003849. https://doi.org/10.1371/journal.ppat.1003849.
Graf AC, Bauer P, Glimm E, Koenig F. Maximum type 1 error rate inflation in multiarmed clinical trials with adaptive interim sample size modifications. Biom J. 2014;56(4):614–30. https://doi.org/10.1002/bimj.201300153.
Halloran ME, Longini IM, Struchiner CJ. Design and analysis of vaccine studies. Statistics for biology and health. New York: Springer; 2010.
Halloran ME, Auranen K, Baird S, Basta NE, Bellan SE, Brookmeyer R, et al. Simulations for designing and interpreting intervention trials in infectious diseases. BMC Med. 2017;15(1):223. https://doi.org/10.1186/s12916-017-0985-3.
Harling G, Wang R, Onnela J-P, De Gruttola V. Leveraging contact network structure in the design of cluster randomized trials. Clin Trials (London, England). 2017;14(1):37–47. https://doi.org/10.1177/1740774516673355.
Henao-Restrepo AM, Camacho A, Longini IM, Watson CH, Edmunds WJ, Egger M, et al. Efficacy and effectiveness of an rVSV-vectored vaccine in preventing Ebola virus disease: final results from the Guinea ring vaccination, open-label, cluster-randomised trial (Ebola Ca Suffit!). Lancet. 2017;389(10068):505–18. https://doi.org/10.1016/S0140-6736(16)32621-6.
HHS. Ebola response improvement plan 2016. 2016.
Hitchings MDT, Grais RF, Lipsitch M. Using simulation to aid trial design: ring-vaccination trials. PLoS Negl Trop Dis. 2017;11(3):e0005470. https://doi.org/10.1371/journal.pntd.0005470.
Hitchings M, Lipsitch M, Wang R, Bellan S. Competing effects of indirect protection and clustering on the power of cluster-randomized controlled vaccine trials. Am J Epidemiol. 2018;187(8):1763–71. https://doi.org/10.1093/aje/kwy047.
Hu F, Rosenberger W. The theory of response-adaptive randomization in clinical trials. In: Wiley series in probability and statistics. Hoboken, NJ: Wiley; 2006.
Isanaka S, Guindo O, Langendorf C, Matar Seck A, Plikaytis BD, Sayinzoga-Makombe N, et al. Efficacy of a low-cost, heat-stable Oral rotavirus vaccine in Niger. N Engl J Med. 2017;376(12):1121–30. https://doi.org/10.1056/NEJMoa1609462.
Jennison C, Turnbull B. Group sequential methods with applications to clinical trials, Chapman & Hall/CRC interdisciplinary statistics series. 1st ed. New York: Chapman & Hall; 1999.
Johansson MA, Quandelacy TM, Kada S, Prasad PV, Steele M, Brooks JT, et al. SARS-CoV-2 transmission from people without COVID-19 symptoms. JAMA Netw Open. 2021;4(1):e2035057. https://doi.org/10.1001/jamanetworkopen.2020.35057.
Johnson R, Jackson C, Presanis A, Villar SS, De Angelis D. Quantifying efficiency gains of innovative designs of two-arm vaccine trials for COVID-19 using an epidemic simulation model. Stat Biopharm Res. 2021;14:33–41. https://doi.org/10.1080/19466315.2021.1939774.
Kahn R, Rid A, Smith P, Eyal N, Lipsitch M. Choices in vaccine trial design in epidemics of emerging infections. PLoS Med. 2018;15(8):e1002632. https://doi.org/10.1371/journal.pmed.1002632.
Kahn R, Hitchings M, Wang R, Bellan S, Lipsitch M. Analyzing vaccine trials in epidemics with mild and asymptomatic infection. Am J Epidemiol. 2019;188(2):467–74. https://doi.org/10.1093/aje/kwy239.

Kahn R, Wang R, Leavitt SV, Hanage WP, Lipsitch M. Leveraging pathogen sequence and contact tracing data to enhance vaccine trials in emerging epidemics. Epidemiology. 2021;32:698. https://doi.org/10.1097/ede.0000000000001367.

Kennedy SB, Neaton JD, Lane HC, Kieh MWS, Massaquoi MBF, Touchette NA, et al. Implementation of an Ebola virus disease vaccine clinical trial during the Ebola epidemic in Liberia: design, procedures, and challenges. Clin Trials (London, England). 2016;13(1):49–56. https://doi.org/10.1177/1740774515621037.

Kennedy SB, Bolay F, Kieh M, Grandits G, Badio M, Ballou R, et al. Phase 2 placebo-controlled trial of two vaccines to prevent Ebola in Liberia. N Engl J Med. 2017;377(15):1438–47. https://doi.org/10.1056/NEJMoa1614067.

Kennedy-Shaffer L, Lipsitch M. Statistical properties of stepped wedge cluster-randomized trials in infectious disease outbreaks. Am J Epidemiol. 2020;189(11):1324–32. https://doi.org/10.1093/aje/kwaa141.

Kennedy-Shaffer L, Kahn R, Lipsitch M. Estimating vaccine efficacy against transmission via effect on viral load. medRxiv. 2021. https://doi.org/10.1101/2021.05.03.21256556.

Krams M, Sharma A, Dragalin V, Burns D, Fardipour P, Padmanabhani S, et al. Adaptive approaches in clinical drug development. Pharm Med. 2009;23(3):139–48. https://doi.org/10.1007/bf03256762.

Kunz CU, Jorgens S, Bretz F, Stallard N, Van Lancker K, Xi D, et al. Clinical trials impacted by the COVID-19 pandemic: adaptive designs to the rescue? Stat Biopharm Res. 2020;12(4):461–77. https://doi.org/10.1080/19466315.2020.1799857.

Laber EB, Meyer NJ, Reich BJ, Pacifici K, Collazo JA, Drake JM. Optimal treatment allocations in space and time for on-line control of an emerging infectious disease. J R Stat Soc Ser C Appl Stat. 2018;67(4):743–70.

Lai TL, Shih MC. Power, sample size and adaptation considerations in the design of group sequential clinical trials. Biometrika. 2004;91(3):507–28. https://doi.org/10.1093/biomet/91.3.507.

Langwig KE, Gomes MGM, Clark MD, Kwitny M, Yamada S, Wargo AR, et al. Limited available evidence supports theoretical predictions of reduced vaccine efficacy at higher exposure dose. Sci Rep. 2019;9(1):3203. https://doi.org/10.1038/s41598-019-39698-x.

Lipsitch M, Dean NE. Understanding COVID-19 vaccine efficacy. Science. 2020;370:763. https://doi.org/10.1126/science.abe5938.

Lipsitch M, Eyal N. Improving vaccine trials in infectious disease emergencies. Science. 2017;357(6347):153–6. https://doi.org/10.1126/science.aam8334.

Lipsitch M, Kahn R. Interpreting vaccine efficacy trial results for infection and transmission. Vaccine. 2021;39(30):4082–8. https://doi.org/10.1016/j.vaccine.2021.06.011.

Lipsitch M, Eyal N, Halloran ME, Hernán MA, Longini IM, Perencevich EN, et al. Obtaining efficacy data in an environment of variable and uncertain incidence: Ebola and beyond. Science. 2015a;348(6230):46–8. https://doi.org/10.1126/science.aaa3178.

Lipsitch M, Eyal N, Halloran ME, Hernán MA, Longini IM, Perencevich EN, et al. Vaccine testing. Ebola and beyond. Science. 2015b;348(6230):46–8. https://doi.org/10.1126/science.aaa3178.

Lipsitch M, Jha A, Simonsen L. Observational studies and the difficult quest for causality: lessons from vaccine effectiveness and impact studies. Int J Epidemiol. 2016;45(6):2060–74. https://doi.org/10.1093/ije/dyw124.

Lipsitch M, Kahn R, Mina MJ. Antibody testing will enhance the power and accuracy of COVID-19-prevention trials. Nat Med. 2020;26(6):818–9. https://doi.org/10.1038/s41591-020-0887-3.

Logunov DY, Dolzhikova IV, Shcheblyakov DV, Tukhvatulin AI, Zubkova OV, Dzharullaeva AS, et al. Safety and efficacy of an rAd26 and rAd5 vector-based heterologous prime-boost COVID-19 vaccine: an interim analysis of a randomised controlled phase 3 trial in Russia. Lancet. 2021;397(10275):671–81. https://doi.org/10.1016/s0140-6736(21)00234-8.

Maca J, Bhattacharya S, Dragalin V, Gallo P, Krams M. Adaptive seamless phase II/III designs—background, operational aspects, and examples. Drug Inf J. 2006;40(4):463–73. https://doi.org/10.1177/216847900604000412.

Madewell ZJ, Piontti APY, Zhang Q, Burton N, Yang Y, Longini IM et al. Using simulated infectious disease outbreaks to guide the design of individually randomized vaccine trials. medRxiv. 2021. https://doi.org/10.1101/2021.01.29.21250703.

Magirr D, Jaki T, Whitehead J. A generalized Dunnett test for multi-arm multi-stage clinical studies with treatment selection. Biometrika. 2012;99(2):494–501. https://doi.org/10.1093/biomet/ass002.

Mahajan R, Gupta K. Adaptive design clinical trials: methodology, challenges and prospect. Indian J Pharmacol. 2010;42(4):201–7. https://doi.org/10.4103/0253-7613.68417.

Mahase E. Covid-19: Russia approves vaccine without large scale testing or published results. BMJ. 2020;370:m3205. https://doi.org/10.1136/bmj.m3205.

Martin MA, VanInsberghe D, Koelle K. Insights from SARS-CoV-2 sequences. Science. 2021;371(6528):466–7. https://doi.org/10.1126/science.abf3995.

Maxmen A. Science under fire: Ebola researchers fight to test drugs and vaccines in a war zone. Nature. 2019;572(7767):16–7. https://doi.org/10.1038/d41586-019-02258-4.

Millum J, Grady C. The ethics of placebo-controlled trials: methodological justifications. Contemp Clin Trials. 2013;36(2):510–4. https://doi.org/10.1016/j.cct.2013.09.003.

Millum J, Wendler D. The duty to rescue and randomized controlled trials involving serious diseases. J Moral Philos. 2018;15(3):298–323. https://doi.org/10.1163/17455243-20170012.

Moderna. Final mRNA-1273-P301 protocol amendment 6. 2020.

Multiple treatments for Ebola virus disease (EVD). 2015. https://clinicaltrials.gov/ct2/show/NCT02380625. Accessed 15 July 2021.

NASEM. Integrating clinical research into epidemic response: the Ebola experience. National Academies of sciences engineering and medicine publications. Washington, DC: The National Academies Press; 2017.

Nason M. Statistics and logistics: design of Ebola vaccine trials in West Africa. Clin Trials (London, England). 2016;13(1):87–91. https://doi.org/10.1177/1740774515620612.

NIH. Accelerating COVID-19 therapeutic interventions and vaccines (ACTIV). 2021a. https://www.nih.gov/research-training/medical-research-initiatives/activ. Accessed 20 Feb 2023.

NIH. Study to evaluate the safety, tolerability, and immunogenicity of an RNA vaccine candidate against COVID-19 in healthy children <12 years of age. 2021b. https://clinicaltrials.gov/ct2/show/NCT04816643. Accessed 15 July 2021.

O'Brien KL, Moulton LH, Reid R, Weatherholtz R, Oski J, Brown L, et al. Efficacy and safety of seven-valent conjugate pneumococcal vaccine in American Indian children: group randomised trial. Lancet. 2003;362(9381):355–61. https://doi.org/10.1016/s0140-6736(03)14022-6.

Omrani AS, Matin MA, Haddad Q, Al-Nakhli D, Memish ZA, Albarrak AM. A family cluster of Middle East respiratory syndrome coronavirus infections related to a likely unrecognized asymptomatic or mild case. Int J Infect Dis. 2013;17(9):e668–e72. https://doi.org/10.1016/j.ijid.2013.07.001.

Pallmann P, Bedding AW, Choodari-Oskooei B, Dimairo M, Flight L, Hampson LV, et al. Adaptive designs in clinical trials: why use them, and how to run and report them. BMC Med. 2018;16(1):29. https://doi.org/10.1186/s12916-018-1017-7.

Pandemic Preparedness Partnership. 100 days mission to respond to future pandemic threats: reducing the impact of future pandemics by making diagnostics, therapeutics and vaccines available within 100 days: a report to the G7. London: G7 United Kingdom; 2021.

Park D, Dudas G, Wohl S, Goba A, Whitmer S, Andersen K, et al. Ebola virus epidemiology, transmission, and evolution during seven months in Sierra Leone. Cell. 2015;161(7):1516–26. https://doi.org/10.1016/j.cell.2015.06.007.

Parmar MKB, Barthel FMS, Sydes M, Langley R, Kaplan R, Eisenhauer E, et al. Speeding up the evaluation of new agents in cancer. J Natl Cancer Inst. 2008;100(17):1204–14. https://doi.org/10.1093/jnci/djn267.

Pfizer and BioNTech. Pfizer and BioNTech announce vaccine candidate against COVID-19 achieved success in first interim analysis from phase 3 study. 2020.

Polack FP, Thomas SJ, Kitchin N, Absalon J, Gurtman A, Lockhart S, et al. Safety and efficacy of the BNT162b2 mRNA Covid-19 vaccine. N Engl J Med. 2020;383(27):2603–15. https://doi.org/10.1056/NEJMoa2034577.

PREVENT Working Group. Pregnant women and vaccines against emerging epidemic threats: ethics guidance for preparedness, research, and response. Baltimore: Johns Hopkins Berman Institute of Bioethics; 2018.

Proschan MA. Sample size re-estimation in clinical trials. Biom J. 2009;51(2):348–57. https://doi.org/10.1002/bimj.200800266.

Proschan M, Evans S. Resist the temptation of response-adaptive randomization. Clin Infect Dis. 2020;71(11):3002–4. https://doi.org/10.1093/cid/ciaa334.

PROTECT-CH. 2021. https://www.protect-trial.net/. Accessed 15 July 2021.

RECOVERY trial. University of Oxford, Oxford. 2022. https://www.recoverytrial.net/. Accessed 15 Apr 2022.

REMAP-CAP response to COVID-19 pandemic. 2021. https://www.remapcap.org/coronavirus. Accessed 27 June 2022.

Richterman A, Meyerowitz EA, Cevik M. Indirect protection by reducing transmission: ending the pandemic with SARS-CoV-2 vaccination. Open Forum Infect Dis. 2021;9 https://doi.org/10.1093/ofid/ofab259.

Rid A, Saxena A, Baqui AH, Bhan A, Bines J, Bouesseau MC, et al. Placebo use in vaccine trials: recommendations of a WHO expert panel. Vaccine. 2014;32(37):4708–12. https://doi.org/10.1016/j.vaccine.2014.04.022.

Rid A, Lipsitch M, Miller FG. The ethics of continuing placebo in SARS-CoV-2 vaccine trials. JAMA. 2021;325(3):219–20. https://doi.org/10.1001/jama.2020.25053.

Robertson JFR, Sewell HF, Stewart M. Delayed second dose of the BNT162b2 vaccine: innovation or misguided conjecture? Lancet. 2021;397:879–80. https://doi.org/10.1016/s0140-6736(21)00455-4.

Robertson DS, Lee KM, Lopez-Kolkovska BC, Villar SS. Response-adaptive randomization in clinical trials: from myths to practical considerations. Stat Sci. 2023;38(2):185–208.

Rodriguez-Barraquer I, Mier-y-Teran-Romero L, Burke DS, Cummings DAT. Challenges in the interpretation of dengue vaccine trial results. PLoS Negl Trop

Dis. 2013;7(8):e2126. https://doi.org/10.1371/journal.pntd.0002126.

Sadoff J, Gray G, Vandebosch A, Cardenas V, Shukarev G, Grinsztejn B, et al. Safety and efficacy of single-dose Ad26.COV2.S vaccine against Covid-19. N Engl J Med. 2021;384(23):2187–201. https://doi.org/10.1056/NEJMoa2101544.

Schiavone F, Bathia R, Letchemanan K, Masters L, Amos C, Bara A, et al. This is a platform alteration: a trial management perspective on the operational aspects of adaptive and platform and umbrella protocols. Trials. 2019;20(1):264. https://doi.org/10.1186/s13063-019-3216-8.

Senn S. Seven myths of randomisation in clinical trials. Stat Med. 2012;32(9):1439–50. https://doi.org/10.1002/sim.5713.

Shapiro J, Dean NE, Madewell ZJ, Yang Y, Halloran ME, Longini I. Efficacy estimates for various COVID-19 vaccines: what we know from the literature and reports. medRxiv. 2021. https://doi.org/10.1101/2021.05.20.21257461.

Shih W. Plan to be flexible: a commentary on adaptive designs. Biom J. 2006;48(4):656–9. https://doi.org/10.1002/bimj.200610241.

Smith PG, Rodrigues LC, Fine PEM. Assessment of the protective efficacy of vaccines against common diseases using case-control and cohort studies. Int J Epidemiol. 1984;13(1):87–93. https://doi.org/10.1093/ije/13.1.87.

Stallard N, Hampson L, Benda N, Brannath W, Burnett T, Friede T, et al. Efficient adaptive designs for clinical trials of interventions for COVID-19. Stat Biopharm Res. 2020;12(4):483–97. https://doi.org/10.1080/19466315.2020.1790415.

Stanberry LR, Spruance SL, Cunningham AL, Bernstein DI, Mindel A, Sacks S, et al. Glycoprotein-D-adjuvant vaccine to prevent genital herpes. N Engl J Med. 2002;347(21):1652–61. https://doi.org/10.1056/NEJMoa011915.

Staples PC, Ogburn EL, Onnela J-P. Incorporating contact network structure in cluster randomized trials. Sci Rep. 2015;5:17581. https://doi.org/10.1038/srep17581.

Sullivan SG, Tchetgen Tchetgen EJ, Cowling BJ. Theoretical basis of the test-negative study design for assessment of influenza vaccine effectiveness. Am J Epidemiol. 2016;184(5):345–53. https://doi.org/10.1093/aje/kww064.

Syed H, Jorgensen AL, Morris AP. Evaluation of methodology for the analysis of 'time-to-event' data in pharmacogenomic genome-wide association studies. Pharmacogenomics. 2016;17(8):907–15. https://doi.org/10.2217/pgs.16.19.

Thompson JA, Davey C, Fielding K, Hargreaves JR, Hayes RJ. Robust analysis of stepped wedge trials using cluster-level summaries within periods. Stat Med. 2018;37(16):2487–500. https://doi.org/10.1002/sim.7668.

Tuite AR, Fisman DN. Spectrum bias and loss of statistical power in discordant couple studies of sexually transmitted infections. Sex Transm Dis. 2011;38(1):50–6. https://doi.org/10.1097/olq.0b013e3181ec19f1.

Villar SS, Bowden J, Wason J. Multi-armed bandit models for the optimal design of clinical trials: benefits and challenges. Stat Sci. 2015;30(2):199–215. https://doi.org/10.1214/14-STS504.

Villar SS, Robertson DS, Rosenberger WF. The temptation of overgeneralizing response-adaptive randomization. Clin Infect Dis. 2020;73:e842. https://doi.org/10.1093/cid/ciaa1027.

Voysey M, Clemens SAC, Madhi SA, Weckx LY, Folegatti PM, Aley PK, et al. Safety and efficacy of the ChAdOx1 nCoV-19 vaccine (AZD1222) against SARS-CoV-2: an interim analysis of four randomised controlled trials in Brazil, South Africa, and the UK. Lancet. 2021a;397:99. https://doi.org/10.1016/S0140-6736(20)32661-1.

Voysey M, Costa Clemens SA, Madhi SA, Weckx LY, Folegatti PM, Aley PK, et al. Single-dose administration and the influence of the timing of the booster dose on immunogenicity and efficacy of ChAdOx1 nCoV-19 (AZD1222) vaccine: a pooled analysis of four randomised trials. Lancet. 2021b;397(10277):881–91. https://doi.org/10.1016/s0140-6736(21)00432-3.

Wason JMS, Abraham JE, Baird RD, Gournaris I, Vallier A-L, Brenton JD, et al. A Bayesian adaptive design for biomarker trials with linked treatments. Br J Cancer. 2015;113(5):699–705. https://doi.org/10.1038/bjc.2015.278.

Wason JMS, Brocklehurst P, Yap C. When to keep it simple—adaptive designs are not always useful. BMC Med. 2019;17(1):152. https://doi.org/10.1186/s12916-019-1391-9.

WHO. Correlates of vaccine-induced protection: methods and implications. Contract No.: WHO reference number: WHO/IVB/13.01. Geneva: World Health Organization. Immunization VaB; 2013.

WHO. Ethical considerations for use of unregistered interventions for Ebola viral disease. Contract No.: WHO/HIS/KER/GHE/14.1. Geneva: World Health Organization; 2014.

WHO. InterVax tool: decision support for vaccine efficacy trial design during an emerging outbreak. Geneva: World Health Organization; 2019. http://vaxeval.com/. Accessed 10 Aug 2021.

WHO. Evaluation of COVID-19 vaccine effectiveness interim guidance. Contract No.: WHO reference number: WHO/2019-nCoV/vaccine_effectiveness/measurement/2021.1. 2021a.

WHO. Standardization of vaccines for coronavirus disease (COVID-19). 2021b.

WHO. WHO COVID-19 solidarity therapeutics trial. Geneva: World Health Organization; 2022a. https://www.who.int/emergencies/diseases/novel-coronavirus-2019/global-research-on-novel-coronavirus-2019-ncov/solidarity-clinical-trial-for-covid-19-treatments. Accessed 7 Sept 2022.

WHO. WHO COVID-19 solidarity trial vaccines. Geneva: World Health Organization; 2022b. https://www.who.int/emergencies/diseases/novel-coronavirus-2019/

global-research-on-novel-coronavirus-2019-ncov/solidarity-trial-of-covid-19-vaccines. Accessed 7 Sept 2022.

Widdowson MA, Schrag SJ, Carter RJ, Carr W, Legardy-Williams J, Gibson L, et al. Implementing an Ebola vaccine study—Sierra Leone. MMWR Suppl. 2016;65(3):98–106. https://doi.org/10.15585/mmwr.su6503a14.

Williamson S, Villar S. A response-adaptive randomization procedure for multi-armed clinical trials with normally distributed outcomes. Biometrics. 2019;76:197. https://doi.org/10.1111/biom.13119.

Williamson S, Jacko P, Villar S, Jaki T. A Bayesian adaptive design for clinical trials in rare diseases. Comput Stat Data Anal. 2017;113:136–53. https://doi.org/10.1016/j.csda.2016.09.006.

22.1 In Focus: Ring Trial Design

Natalie E. Dean and Ira M. Longini Jr

Contents

Learning Track Note: This chapter appears in Learning Tracks: Biostatistics; Clinical Research

E. S. Higgs and R. A. Sorenson (eds.), *Principles and Practice of Emergency Research Response*,
https://doi.org/10.1007/978-3-031-48408-7_33

Learning Objectives

This chapter should enable readers to understand and discuss:

- Basic design features of a ring trial for a candidate medical intervention and its origins
- Rings and how they are identified
- Key advantages and disadvantages of a ring trial approach
- Settings in which a ring trial design would be most valuable or not feasible
- Modifications that could make the ring trial approach useful for other settings
- The Ebola vaccine ring trial conducted in Guinea and the validity of its results
- A hypothetical infectious disease emergency that lends itself to a ring trial of medical countermeasures

1 Introduction

A *ring trial* is a flexible trial design where recruited participants are directly or indirectly linked to a newly diagnosed infectious disease case (▶ Chap. 22). Participants linked to the same index case form a ring that can then be randomized as a cluster to an intervention or control, or individually randomized within the ring. The design thus targets a population at increased risk of disease, reducing sample size requirements relative to designs that enroll populations without this epidemiological link (Ebola Ça Suffit Ring Vaccination Trial Consortium 2015). This has the potential to accelerate the acquisition of evidence which is critical in a health emergency. Ring trials are also designed to be more responsive than other trial protocols to the evolving epidemiology of an epidemic. Mobile trial teams can move into new hotspots as they emerge and out of areas where incidence has waned. The ring design is well-suited to evaluate fast-acting interventions intended to interrupt transmission in an outbreak setting, such as single-dose vaccines and targeted antiviral prophylaxis (Halloran et al. 2007). The design will be valuable in settings where spatial and temporal trends in disease incidence are highly unpredictable, so trials with pre-selected sites risk being underpowered. In this section, we discuss the origins of the ring trial design and its use in the West Africa Ebola epidemic, summarize its advantages and disadvantages, and lay out considerations for generalizing the design to other contexts.

2 Origins of Ring Vaccination

Ring trials are closely modeled after the surveillance and containment strategy of *ring vaccination*. In this targeted strategy, vaccine is provided to individuals who are socially or geographically connected to an index case. This may include household contacts, neighbors, and contacts who visited the symptomatic patient (see ◘ Fig. 1). With an efficacious vaccine, ring vaccination creates a buffer of immune people around each new case in order to prevent further spread of infection. Importantly, secondary cases may not be preventable by vaccination as these individuals may already be infected at the time of vaccination (unless the vaccine has postexposure prophylactic effects), but an effective vaccine could prevent future spread within a ring. This strategy was central to the public health achievement of smallpox eradication in the 1970s (Foege et al. 1975).

Ring vaccination as a containment strategy is most effective when cases primarily occur within known transmission chains (Kucharski et al. 2016), requiring a sensitive contact tracing system. It is suited to diseases that are transmitted through person-to-person contacts and most transmission occurs after the onset of symptoms and asymptomatic infections either do not occur or are responsible for little onward transmission. The strategy is also most effective for controlling disease when the pathogen's reproduction number is not too high (Merler et al. 2016), so other concurrent control measures may be needed to bring down levels of transmission. The effectiveness of the approach depends upon how quickly the intervention can be deployed. It is most effective when response times are rapid and the vaccine is fast-acting (Merler et al. 2016).

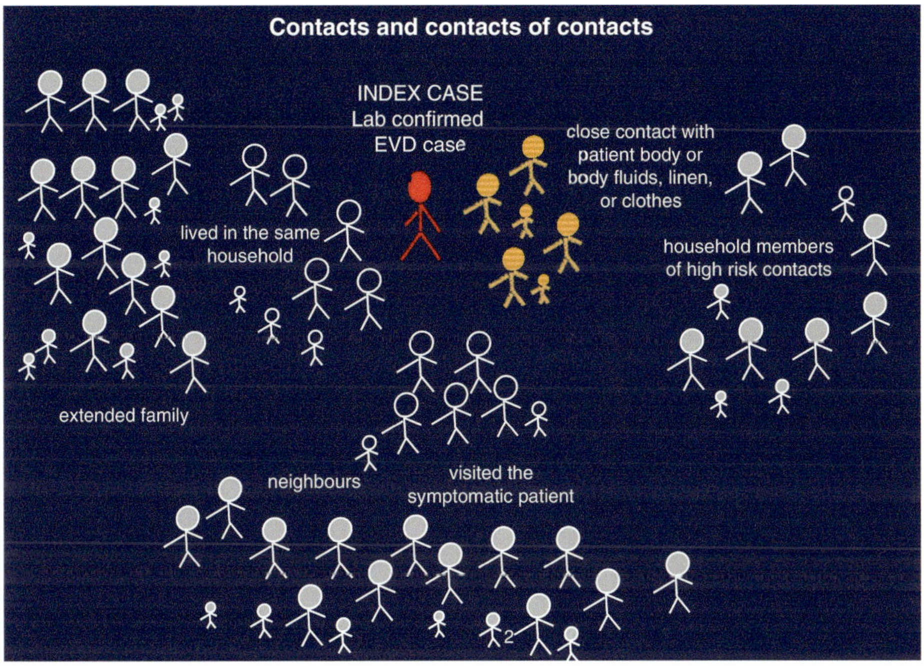

Fig. 1 What is a vaccination ring? Example from Ebola virus disease. (Figure from Henao-Restrepo et al. (2016))

3 Design of the Original Ring Trial

Though ring vaccination dates back to smallpox, the concept of a randomized ring trial was first described in 2015 (Ebola ça Suffit Ring Vaccination Trial Consortium 2015), and the first randomized ring trial was conducted in Guinea during the 2014–2016 West African Ebola epidemic to evaluate the efficacy and effectiveness of the candidate rVSV-ZEBOV vaccine (Foege et al. 1975; Henao-Restrepo et al. 2015). The Ebola ring vaccination trial design worked as follows (see also Fig. 2). Laboratory-confirmed cases of Ebola virus disease were detected by active or passive surveillance, and then served as potential index cases for the formation of new rings. As Ebola primarily spreads through person-to-person exposure to bodily fluids, the rings were comprised of contacts and contacts of contacts of the index Ebola virus disease (EVD) case (see Fig. 1). Contacts were individuals who lived in the same household, visited or were visited by the index case after the onset of symptoms, provided him or her with unprotected care, or prepared the body for the traditional funeral ceremony; contacts of contacts were neighbors of the index case plus the household members of any high-risk contacts living away from the index cases' residence (Henao-Restrepo et al. 2015). Importantly, rings were not contiguous geographic areas but reflected individuals' social networks, which could include contacts further afield.

Once an index case was identified, local social mobilization teams were deployed to visit the index patient's residence. With community consent for the trial (▶ Chaps. 18 and 30), a second team enumerated and listed contacts and contacts of contacts. Preliminary eligibility criteria (e.g., age) were applied to generate a list of ring members to be contacted for informed consent. On the basis of this preliminary list, an independent statistician randomly allocated rings to either immediate or delayed (21 days later) vaccination in a 1:1 ratio using a block randomization procedure stratified by location (urban vs. rural) and size of rings (≤20 vs. >20 eligible individ-

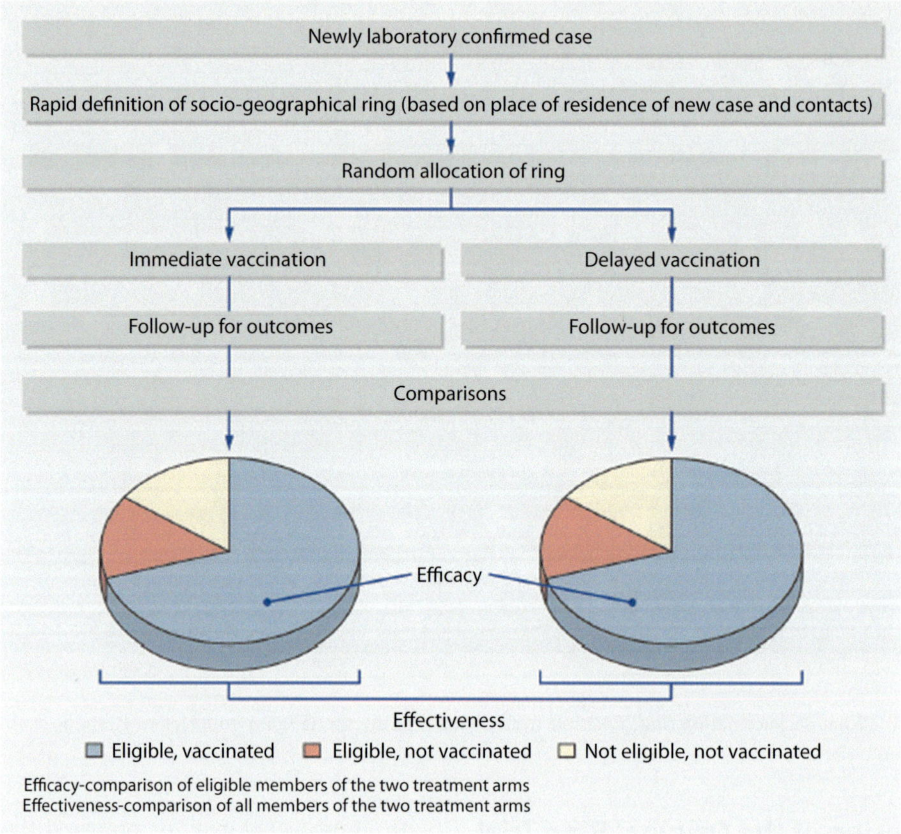

Fig. 2 Schematic presentation of the design of a ring vaccination trial during an outbreak of an infectious disease. (Ebola ça Suffit Ring Vaccination Trial Consortium 2015)

uals). Study teams obtained individual informed consent from eligible ring members, while reasons for non-enrolment were recorded. Study allocation was revealed after informed consent, at which time vaccine was administered per randomized schedule.

Participants were visited on days 3, 14, 21, 42, 63, and 84 to assess safety. Contacts were followed up in accordance with usual surveillance practices to identify new cases of EVD in enrolled and non-enrolled ring members. The primary outcome was laboratory-confirmed EVD 10 or more days after randomization; the analysis period was shifted to allow time for vaccinated individuals to develop protective immunity or for disease incubation, as symptom onset times were observed rather than infection times (Dean et al. 2018). Confirmed cases arising in non-enrolled ring members contributed to secondary analyses of vaccine effectiveness, including overall and indirect vaccine effectiveness (Halloran et al. 2010).

4 Results of the Original Ring Trial

The original ring trial started with a short pilot phase in which three clusters were allocated to immediate vaccination. Afterward, new confirmed cases were assessed for eligibility as index cases. Reasons for a case not becoming a ring index case included delayed case reporting, inadequate capacity, negative attitude toward the trial in the community, security issues, negative Ebola tests at the reference laboratory, or the case already having been included in an existing ring.

At a planned interim analysis, 90 clusters with a total of 7651 people had been randomized, of which 4394 contributed to the primary analysis. In the pre-specified primary analysis, no immediately vaccinated individuals developed symptoms 10 or more days after randomization, as compared to 16 individuals in seven clusters in the delayed vaccination arm. Estimated vaccine efficacy was 100% (95% confidence interval 74.7–100%). Following the interim analysis, the data safety monitoring board advised discontinuing the delayed vaccination arm. Subsequent clusters were allocated to immediate vaccination only, and a summary of 117 randomized and non-randomized clusters was published as a final analysis after the end of the epidemic (Henao-Restrepo et al. 2017). In 2016, during an EVD flare-up in Guinea, the then unlicensed rVSV-ZEBOV vaccine was deployed via a simplified version of the ring vaccination trial protocol without randomization, under an expanded access mechanism (Gsell et al. 2017).

5 Advantages of the Ring Trial Approach

The ring trial approach has several key features that make it well-suited for emergency response research (see ◘ Fig. 3). Its greatest advantage is that it enrolls a high-risk population expected to have comparatively high attack rates, reducing the total sample size requirements for the trial (see *Ring vaccination—by the numbers*). This is critically important during outbreaks, as low overall incidence and waning transmission are obstacles to assessing efficacy. Though the Ebola ring vaccination trial was launched after the peak of the epidemic in Guinea (see ◘ Figs. 3 and 4), the trial captured a sizable fraction of cases from the tail of the epidemic curve as new index cases, primary endpoints, or secondary endpoints in ring members not eligible for vaccination. The design is flexible, responsively following the epidemic as it progresses. As outbreaks are highly unpredictable, a standard design that pre-selects trial sites runs the risk of being conducted in locations where no transmission occurs, further contributing to low power.

The ring trial approach has practical advantages, including a naturally phased roll-out, which can be valuable where resources are limited (Kahn et al. 2018; Lipsitch et al. 2015). Another advantage is that mobile teams can efficiently vaccinate and conduct

Advantages	Disadvantages
Targets exposed individuals with a higher attack rate. Requires fewer overall participants than a trial in a more general population.	Exposed contacts may not be satisfactorily representative of the desired population. For example, there could be under-representation of age or risk groups.
Flexible design can quickly adapt to an evolving outbreak by focusing on where cases are spreading. Does not require exact pre-specification of trial populations.	Requires a flexible trial infrastructure that can be quickly activated to approve, enroll, and vaccinate at a new location when an index case is identified.
Phased roll-out, where participants are recruited over time, is useful when resources are limited.	More challenging to conduct the trial, including administering the vaccine and collecting laboratory samples, in the field than at health centers.
Aligns naturally with and can support the ongoing efforts of contact tracing teams.	Because the period of highest risk is concentrated around the time of vaccination, the results may be sensitive to the definition of the per protocol analysis period. May not be suitable for evaluating long-term vaccine effectiveness.
Based on the public health strategy of ring vaccination, the trial itself may aid in the overall reduction of disease spread.	Best for a vaccine that rapidly induces immunity. May not be appropriate for a vaccine that requires multiple doses.
The trial design can generate insights on the effectiveness of ring vaccination, indirect effects of the vaccine, and detailed data on transmission within rings.	The recruitment rate may be unpredictable, with uncertain periods between defining new rings.

◘ **Fig. 3** Summary of advantages and disadvantages of the ring trial design. (Author)

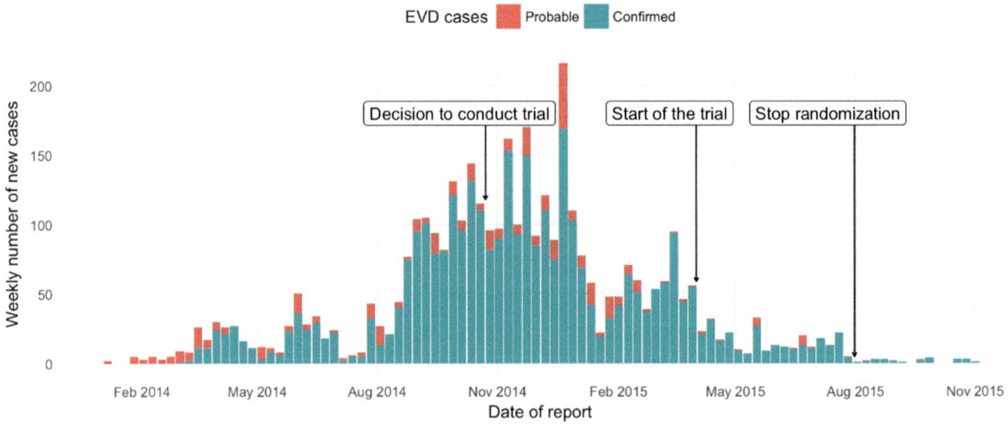

Fig. 4 Weekly incidence of Ebola in Guinea 2014–2015, and key dates in the ring vaccination trial. (Figure courtesy of Anton Camacho)

follow-up visits around the same time in the same location, at participants' places of residence. Trial teams can work in conjunction with outbreak response teams. The pragmatism of the design is evidenced by the success of the Guinea trial, which was conducted in a resource-poor setting and in a crisis.

Finally, the ring trial can yield several different useful estimates of intervention effectiveness. Though vaccine trials are typically analyzed per protocol, counting only cases that occur after a sufficient lag period, one can analyze the data without this lag using an intention-to-treat approach. This yields an estimate of the effectiveness of the ring strategy in that population. For fast-moving diseases, slow-acting vaccines, or if there are excessive delays in reaching communities, early cases would reduce the effectiveness of the strategy as measured by the intention-to-treat approach. It is possible for a vaccine to be efficacious when provided well in advance of exposure but for a ring trial to return a negative result, indicating that it would not be well-suited for ring vaccination (Yung 2015). Finally, because the design enrolls clusters of participants in common networks, cluster randomized ring trials can also be used to estimate indirect and overall effects of vaccines (Halloran et al. 2010).

Box 1: Ring Vaccination—By the Numbers

Although the largest recorded Ebola outbreak, Ebola virus disease was still a rare event in the general population during the West African epidemic. Over the entire epidemic, 28,616 cases were reported in the three highly affected countries of Guinea, Liberia, and Sierra Leone (WHO Ebola Response Team 2016); with a combined population size of 22 million, the overall attack rate was approximately 0.13%. Note that this attack rate includes the early peak of the epidemic before trials were launched, but we use this attack rate for the purposes of this example. Assuming 70% vaccine efficacy, an individually randomized controlled trial with a cumulative incidence of 0.13% would require sample sizes exceeding 20,000 people per arm to achieve power of 90% (two-sided log-rank test with $\alpha = 0.05$ to rule out a null hypothesis of 0% efficacy).

In contrast, for a ring trial, a cumulative incidence of Ebola virus disease of 2% within rings is possible. Even after inflating the sample size to account for an assumed intracluster correlation coefficient of 0.05, approximately 5000 people per arm (95 rings per arm) are required to achieve a power of 90% (vaccine efficacy = 70%, two-sided test with $\alpha = 0.05$ to rule out a null hypothesis of 0% efficacy). Thus, even though cluster-randomized trials are traditionally less statistically efficient, the planned sample size was one-quarter of that required for an individually randomized trial because of the increased event rate. An individually randomized trial within rings, which would not need to be inflated for intracluster correlation, would have an even smaller sample size requirement.

6 Limitations of the Ring Trial Approach

The ring trial approach also has several limitations (see Fig. 3). Primarily, the design must be weighed against a more traditional trial where eligibility is not defined by exposure. Unless the pathogen is especially slow moving, the ring trial approach is not well-suited to evaluate multi-dose vaccines. Because vaccination and exposure occur within the same narrow time window in a ring trial, the primary analysis is particularly sensitive to the definition of the per-protocol period (Dean and Longini 2022). To reduce bias, a conservative choice is to select a long time lag, yet this could result in reduced power if transmission rapidly wanes within rings due to other interventions (Dean et al. 2018). Relatedly, unless there are frequent reintroductions to the population, the design is not well-suited for evaluating long-term vaccine efficacy. Mathematical simulations are valuable for exploring the properties of a proposed design incorporating context-specific features and can guide the selection of this period (Hitchings et al. 2017).

As a practical limitation, the ring trial design requires a flexible trial infrastructure that can be activated quickly to approve, enroll, and vaccinate at a new location. This may not be logistically feasible in all settings. It may also be more challenging to conduct the trial procedures in the field than at health centers. Cold-chain technology to deliver the vaccine to remote locations may be needed. Where existing clinical research infrastructure exists within a region, it is advantageous to leverage this. Hybrid designs that use both clinical sites and mobile teams may be a compromise.

As recruitment into the trial is directly linked to incidence in the region, the rate of recruitment can be unpredictable, with uncertain periods between defining new rings. For zoonotic diseases with infrequent spillovers, like Nipah virus disease in Bangladesh, modeling suggests that even a targeted design like a ring trial may be infeasible because of low incidence (Nikolay et al. 2021). If new rings are relatively rare, so that only one or a few rings are defined during a time period or in a location, a cluster-randomized design is especially prone to chance imbalances across the trial arms. Individual randomization within rings is then preferred, as it is not prone to this problem. Finally, enrolling only exposed contacts could lead to under-representation of certain age or risk groups that are important to include for regulatory decision-making.

7 Applying the Ring Trial Approach to New Settings

The ring trial approach can be generalized in several ways to make it useful for other settings. As noted earlier, the unit of randomization could be individuals within rings instead of the entire rings (individual vs. cluster randomization), where the former is operationally feasible and acceptable to the community. Such a design would be expected to have a lower overall sample size requirement than the cluster-randomized equivalent (Hitchings et al. 2017). While participants of the original ring trial were not blinded to their allocation, a blinded control is recommended to reduce the potential for bias (Nason 2016). A wide array of control arms could be used, including placebo control, a product targeting an unrelated but geographically relevant disease, delayed intervention, or a product with previously demonstrated efficacy against the same target disease (in the form of a non-inferiority trial).

While the original conception of the ring trial was contact-based, it is clear that other definitions of "rings" could be utilized and might be preferred, depending on the nature of the disease (Dean et al. 2019). Rings could be geographically defined, as might be suitable for vector-borne diseases. Rings could be households or clusters of households. In the case of nosocomial transmission, rings could be hospitals. General guiding principles require a mechanism to maintain clear separation between rings and limit contamination, and that rings should be large enough to capture third (or beyond) generations of cases.

Finally, the trial design has a natural relationship with trials of targeted prophylaxis, including post-exposure prophylaxis. A ring trial approach has been proposed for evaluating post-exposure prophylaxis with lopinavir/ritonavir for the prevention of COVID-19 disease in adults exposed to SARS-CoV-2 (Smit et al. 2020). Single households are randomized as a cluster to the proposed regimen or no treatment, and the analysis follows an intention-to-treat approach.

8 Summary

The innovative ring trial approach is a prime example of how research activities can be an important part of emergency response. In Guinea, the ring vaccination trial was both a randomized clinical trial, generating valuable data on vaccine efficacy and effectiveness to support regulatory decision-making and a strategy for deploying a new technology likely to fight the spread of disease. The trial established that ring vaccination with rVSV was a feasible and useful intervention for Ebola (Gsell et al. 2017), supporting policymakers such as the WHO Strategic Advisory Group of Experts on Immunization. Overall, the ring trial was successful because it was flexible, feasible, and highly targeted. It has great potential for future applications in emergency response research to evaluate fast-acting interventions in settings where outbreaks are very localized and where infected individuals and exposed contacts can be readily identified. Individual randomization within rings is more statistically powerful than cluster randomization, and blinding is highly recommended to reduce the potential for bias. Alternative definitions of "rings" may be used to suit different pathogen and outbreak contexts, including geographically defined rings. Ring trials are expected to be most valuable when more traditional trial approaches are underpowered because of low or unpredictable future incidence.

Discussion Questions

Short Questions

1. Describe the design of a ring trial.
2. Describe the origins and design of the original ring trial in Guinea.
3. Outline the key advantages of a ring trial approach.
4. Outline the key disadvantages of a ring trial approach.
5. In what settings would a ring trial design be most valuable?
6. Describe at least one setting in which a ring trial approach may not be feasible.
7. Give examples of modifications that could be made to the ring trial approach to tailor it to different disease settings (Dean and Longini 2022).

Long Questions

1. Discuss the characteristics of a hypothetical emergency that would lend itself to a ring trial of medical countermeasures.
2. Describe how mathematical modeling can be used to explore the design and feasibility of a ring trial.

References

Dean NE, Longini IM. The ring vaccination trial design for the estimation of vaccine efficacy and effectiveness during infectious disease outbreaks. Clin Trials. 2022;19(4):402–6. https://doi.org/10.1177/17407745211073594.

Dean N, Halloran M, Longini I. Design of vaccine trials during outbreaks with and without a delayed vaccination comparator. Ann Appl Stat. 2018;12(1):330–47. https://doi.org/10.1214/17-AOAS1095.

Dean N, Gsell P-S, Brookmeyer R, De Gruttola V, Donnelly C, Halloran M, et al. Design of vaccine efficacy trials during public health emergencies. Sci Transl Med. 2019;11(499):eaat0360. https://doi.org/10.1126/scitranslmed.aat0360.

Ebola ça Suffit Ring Vaccination Trial Consortium. The ring vaccination trial: a novel cluster randomised controlled trial design to evaluate vaccine efficacy and effectiveness during outbreaks, with special reference to Ebola. BMJ. 2015;351:h3740. https://doi.org/10.1136/bmj.h3740.

Foege WH, Millar JD, Henderson DA. Smallpox eradication in west and Central Africa. Bull World Health Organ. 1975;52(2):209–22.

Gsell PS, Camacho A, Kucharski AJ, Watson CH, Bagayoko A, Nadlaou SD, et al. Ring vaccination with rVSV-ZEBOV under expanded access in response to an outbreak of Ebola virus disease in Guinea, 2016: an operational and vaccine safety report. Lancet Infect Dis. 2017;17(12):1276–84. https://doi.org/10.1016/s1473-3099(17)30541-8.

Halloran ME, Hayden FG, Yang Y, Longini IM Jr, Monto AS. Antiviral effects on influenza viral transmission and pathogenicity: observations from household-based trials. Am J Epidemiol. 2007;165(2):212–21. https://doi.org/10.1093/aje/kwj362.

Halloran ME, Longini IM, Struchiner CJ. Design and analysis of vaccine studies. Statistics for biology and health. New York: Springer; 2010.

Henao-Restrepo AM, Longini IM, Egger M, Dean NE, Edmunds WJ, Camacho A, et al. Efficacy and effectiveness of an rVSV-vectored vaccine expressing Ebola surface glycoprotein: interim results from the Guinea ring vaccination cluster-randomised trial. Lancet. 2015;386(9996):857–66. https://doi.org/10.1016/s0140-6736(15)61117-5.

Henao-Restrepo AM, Preziosi M-P, Wood D, Moorthy V, Kieny MP. On a path to accelerate access to Ebola vaccines: the WHO's research and development efforts during the 2014–2016 Ebola epidemic in West Africa. Curr Opin Virol. 2016;17:138–44. https://doi.org/10.1016/j.coviro.2016.03.008.

Henao-Restrepo AM, Camacho A, Longini IM, Watson CH, Edmunds WJ, Egger M, et al. Efficacy and effectiveness of an rVSV-vectored vaccine in preventing Ebola virus disease: final results from the Guinea ring vaccination, open-label, cluster-randomised trial (Ebola Ca Suffit!). Lancet. 2017;389(10068):505–18. https://doi.org/10.1016/S0140-6736(16)32621-6.

Hitchings MD, Grais RF, Lipsitch M. Using simulation to aid trial design: ring-vaccination trials. PLoS Negl Trop Dis. 2017;11(3):e0005470. https://doi.org/10.1371/journal.pntd.0005470.

Kahn R, Rid A, Smith P, Eyal N, Lipsitch M. Choices in vaccine trial design in epidemics of emerging infections. PLoS Med. 2018;15(8):e1002632. https://doi.org/10.1371/journal.pmed.1002632.

Kucharski AJ, Eggo RM, Watson CH, Camacho A, Funk S, Edmunds WJ. Effectiveness of ring vaccination as control strategy for Ebola virus disease. Emerg Infect Dis. 2016;22(1):105–8. https://doi.org/10.3201/eid2201.151410.

Lipsitch M, Eyal N, Halloran ME, Hernán MA, Longini IM, Perencevich EN, et al. Vaccine testing. Ebola and beyond. Science. 2015;348(6230):46–8. https://doi.org/10.1126/science.aaa3178.

Merler S, Ajelli M, Fumanelli L, Parlamento S, et al. Containing Ebola at the source with ring vaccination. PLoS Negl Trop Dis. 2016;10(11):e0005093. https://doi.org/10.1371/journal.pntd.0005093.

Nason M. Statistics and logistics: design of Ebola vaccine trials in West Africa. Clin Trials (London, England). 2016;13(1):87–91. https://doi.org/10.1177/1740774515620612.

Nikolay B, Ribeiro Dos Santos G, Lipsitch M, Rahman M, Luby SP, Salje H, et al. Assessing the feasibility of Nipah vaccine efficacy trials based on previous outbreaks in Bangladesh. Vaccine. 2021;39(39):5600–6. https://doi.org/10.1016/j.vaccine.2021.08.027.

Smit M, Marinosci A, Nicoletti GJ, Perneger T, Ragozzino S, Andrey DO, et al. Efficacy of pragmatic same-day ring prophylaxis for adult individuals exposed to SARS-CoV-2 in Switzerland (COPEP): protocol of an open-label cluster randomised trial. BMJ Open. 2020;10(11):e040110. https://doi.org/10.1136/bmjopen-2020-040110.

WHO Ebola Response Team. After Ebola in West Africa - unpredictable risks, preventable risks. NEJM 2016;375:587–96. https://doi.org/10.1056/NEJMsr1513109.

Yung CF. Ebola: evaluating vaccines during epidemics. BMJ. 2015;351:h3861. https://doi.org/10.1136/bmj.h3861.

23 Data and Safety Monitoring of Clinical Trials During Public Health Emergencies

Michael A. Proschan and Birgit Grund

Contents

Learning Track Note: This chapter appears in Learning Tracks: Biostatistics; Clinical Research; Public Health and Epidemiology

E. S. Higgs and R. A. Sorenson (eds.), *Principles and Practice of Emergency Research Response*, https://doi.org/10.1007/978-3-031-48408-7_34

Learning Objectives

This chapter will help readers understand and describe:

- The (data and safety monitoring board) DSMB role in clinical trials
- Why the DSMB should review protocols and monitoring plans before participant enrollment
- How DSMB responsibilities may change for trials conducted in response to public health emergencies. How this difference may influence DSMB composition
- Monitoring boundaries for interim review and the importance of specifying them beforehand
- Why a DSMB might stop a clinical trial at an interim review during a public health emergency
- The DSMB role in the PREVAIL I Ebola vaccine trial and what differed from that of a DSMB monitoring a non-emergency trial
- How the integrity of trial results could be damaged by unblinding interim data while the trial is ongoing
- When unblinding data from an ongoing clinical trial is acceptable

1 Introduction

Clinical trials are essential for the development of evidence-based treatments and vaccines. During infectious disease outbreaks, there is substantial pressure to implement and conclude trials very quickly to meet three strategic goals: (1) save lives and avert suffering; (2) accelerate the end of the outbreak; and (3) develop nonpharmaceutical and medical countermeasures (MCMs) to prevent and mitigate future outbreaks (▶ Chap. 22). In this chapter, we describe the monitoring of clinical trials in general, with special emphasis on trials of infectious disease MCMs during public health emergencies. We present issues arising from COVID-19 treatment trials and a case study of the Partnership for Research on Ebola Vaccines in Liberia (PREVAIL) first trial comparing two candidate Ebola vaccines versus placebo during and after the 2014–2015 Ebola outbreak in West Africa (▶ In Practice 23.1) (Kennedy et al. 2017).

Clinical trials are monitored by a group of outside experts not affiliated with the trial called the *Data and Safety Monitoring Board (DSMB)*, also called *Data Monitoring Committee (DMC)*, among other names. An excellent reference on the workings of DSMBs and practical aspects of monitoring clinical trials is Ellenberg et al. (2019). Useful guidelines for DSMBs may be found in Calis et al. (2017) and Fleming et al. (2017). A DSMB usually consists of three to nine experts including physicians, statisticians, and an ethicist. Their role is to (1) ensure the safety of participants; (2) monitor outcome data to determine whether the data conclusively support superiority of one arm over another at an interim analysis; (3) monitor the integrity of the trial, including trial participant accrual, timeliness in submitting forms, loss to follow-up, and so on; and (4) stop the trial for futility if enough evidence has accrued to indicate the trial will not be able to answer its intended question, or the treatment under study has no chance of being shown superior.

It is critical that DSMB members are not affiliated with the trial and have no major conflicts of interest, as this could jeopardize their impartiality or the perception of impartiality. For example, if they have a consulting arrangement with a company that has a competing product, their objectivity may be questioned. Consequently, before each DSMB meeting, members must sign conflict of interest forms disclosing any conflicts or certifying that there are none.

The first DSMB meeting usually occurs before the trial begins enrolling. The board reviews the protocol for the trial, including the design, statistical analysis, and monitoring plans for safety, efficacy, and futility. The study team often presents mock tables and graphs with made-up data to illustrate the format in which data will be presented to the DSMB throughout the trial. The board may express concerns or require modifications to these. This initial DSMB meeting is vital to ensure that the study team and DSMB agree on and understand their roles and responsibilities and the plan for monitoring, particularly with respect to the ongoing provision of information of adverse safety events as the trial progresses and on the frequency of any interim analyses of efficacy. Disagreements or confusion should be clarified before any real data from the trial are presented.

After the trial has begun, the DSMB meets periodically to review data and make recommendations to the trial sponsor about whether to continue as is, make changes such as dropping a poorly performing arm, or pausing or stopping the entire trial. The trial could be paused or stopped because of concerns about safety or study integrity or stopped because one arm is clearly superior to the other or the trial is very unlikely to show benefit of the treatment. Recommendations are expressed in a written summary provided by the DSMB after each meeting. Generally, no data by treatment group or information about the interim estimates of efficacy is given in such reports for ongoing trials.

A DSMB sometimes recommends discontinuation of the trial in a subgroup of participants. For example, in the Adaptive COVID-19 Treatment Trial 3 (ACTT-3) (▶ Chap. 15) comparing interferon beta 1-a plus remdesivir to remdesivir alone for the treatment of patients with COVID-19, an excess of serious adverse events on interferon 1-a among participants requiring high-flow oxygen or non-invasive ventilation caused the DSMB to recommend stopping enrollment of such patients to the trial, while continuing enrollment of participants requiring less oxygen (NIAID 2020). The DSMB further recommended against opening enrollment to patients on invasive mechanical ventilation or extra-corporeal membrane oxygenation (ECMO). The trial sponsor implemented these changes. It is important to note that recommendations from the DSMB are advisory to the trial sponsor and the sponsor makes the final decision about what action to take, but it would be very unusual for the sponsor not to implement the recommendations of the DSMB.

In many trials, a DSMB might meet once or twice per year, but in emerging infectious disease trials in the context of a public health emergency they may meet more frequently, especially early in the trial. This is because the safety profile of experimental agents may not be well understood, there is pressure to find vaccines and treatments quickly, and enrollment and the occurrence of outcome events can be very fast. The DSMB monitoring the Adaptive COVID-19 Treatment Trial 1 (ACTT-1) of remdesivir plus standard care versus placebo plus standard care received weekly safety data electronically (Beigel et al. 2020).

2 Monitoring for Efficacy

One key role of a DSMB is monitoring for efficacy of the investigational treatment. Consider a two-arm trial where patients are assigned at random to the experimental treatment or the control group. During interim monitoring, comparisons of the treatment versus control groups are repeatedly reviewed. In a single comparison, the treatment would be considered effective if it is superior to control with respect to the pre-defined primary outcome (e.g., if mortality is lower in the treatment group compared to control) and the probability of such a strong result if there was no true difference, called *p*-value, is below a pre-specified limit. Small *p*-values suggest that chance alone is unlikely to explain observed results if there really is no difference between treatment arms: formally, a *p*-value is the probability of a difference in outcomes as large or larger than that observed, computed under the assumption that the treatment has no effect. While *p*-values of 0.05 or less are often considered sufficient evidence for superiority in a single comparison, when a trial is monitored many times, otherwise unlikely results might eventually occur by chance even if the treatment has no real effect. This phenomenon may be illustrated by considering the chance that an unskilled dart thrower throws a dart and hits the bull's eye. The chance of this may be very low in a single throw, but if allowed enough tries, even an unskilled dart thrower will eventually hit the bull's eye. The standard way to account for multiple tries (interim analyses) in clinical trials is to require stronger evidence at each look than would be needed if there were only a single look. This is accomplished through *monitoring boundaries,* on which a very brief introduction is given below. More statistical detail may be found in Jennison and Turnbull (2000) or Proschan et al. (2006).

A monitoring boundary may be expressed in terms of values for test statistics or in terms of *p*-values for the treatment difference. For example, DSMB guidelines may recommend stopping a trial for efficacy at an interim review if the *p*-value for the treatment difference is smaller than the *p*-value boundary for this review, i.e., when the interim data provide high confidence that the experimental treatment is superior. Examples of monitoring boundaries are given in ◘ Fig. 1.

An intuitive approach for constructing monitoring boundaries would be to divide the acceptable limit of false positives (called the "Type I error rate," e.g., 5%) by the number of interim looks, which is called the Bonferroni method for multiple comparisons (i.e., if two looks are planned, the Type 1 error rate would be set at 2.5% for each look). That would result in equal cut-offs for the tests at each interim look, but it would also require a very small *p*-value for the final comparison when the trial is complete and, thus, a large sample size. Therefore, monitoring boundaries are often constructed by distributing the total acceptable Type I error unequally, requiring overwhelming evidence for a treatment difference early in the trial and relaxing the Type I error to closer to 5% when the trial nears completion. This corresponds to very high boundaries for the z-statistics and very small *p*-values to end the trial at an early interim analysis. In the early stages of a trial, unusual things can happen that might not occur once investigators are more familiar with the trial procedures. The last thing we want is to stop an important, expensive trial and then realize that the observed difference between arms could be explained by things like misunderstandings or incorrect measurements. Furthermore, patients admitted early in a trial may differ from later patients.

Analysis	Haybittle-Peto	O'Brien-Fleming
1	0.001	0.00005
2	0.001	0.004
3	0.001	0.019
4	0.047	0.043

◘ **Fig. 1** *P*-value boundaries for Haybittle–Peto and O'Brien–Fleming procedures with four equally spaced looks. (Authors)

A recent trial of the antiviral molnupiravir against Covid-19 illustrates this point (Bernal et al. 2022). In an interim analysis, the antiviral was shown to reduce risk of hospitalization or death by 50% (28/385 vs. 53/377), and emergency approval of the treatment was sought with these results. However, in analysis of the full data, the risk reduction was only 30% (48/709 vs. 68/699 for hospitalization or death). Temporal differences in infectious disease trials can result from changing standard of care, introduction of vaccines, different variants, and other factors. Using very high early z-score boundaries also allows the level of evidence required to declare a statistically significant result at the planned end of the trial to be close to what it would be with no monitoring.

A counterargument to having very high early boundaries in an epidemic setting is that there is an imperative to quickly find effective vaccines and treatments, but also to quickly discard ineffective vaccines and treatments, so that limited resources can be redirected. Therefore, some have argued for more lenient early monitoring boundaries such as those provided by the *triangular test* (Whitehead 1997). There is a tradeoff: for a fixed sample size, power is greater using traditional, high early boundaries and lower late boundaries, but the trial is more likely to stop early for either efficacy or futility with lower early boundaries. As a result, the expected duration of a trial is shorter with lower early boundaries, but the results are more robust with high early boundaries. We eschew this debate and focus on traditional, higher early boundaries and lower later boundaries.

The *Haybittle-Peto* and *O'Brien-Fleming boundaries* (Haybittle 1971; O'Brien and Fleming 1979) are high early and low at the end. Expressed in terms of the *p*-value required to declare statistical significance, these boundaries require very small *p*-values to stop early, but the *p*-value required at the end of the trial is close to 0.05. For a trial with four equally spaced analyses, the p-value thresholds at each analysis using the Haybittle–Peto or O'Brien–Fleming methods are shown in ◘ Fig. 1. The first three analyses would be planned to be conducted when 25, 50, and 75% of data have accrued, and the fourth ("final") analysis would be conducted when the trial is completed.

The Haybittle–Peto boundary is crossed at any interim analysis if the p-value is 0.001 or less, and at the final analysis if the p-value is $0.05–3 \times (0.001) = 0.047$ or less. One appealing feature of the Haybittle–Peto boundary is its simplicity. Regardless of the number of interim looks, each uses the same p-value cutoff 0.001, and the p-value cutoff at the final analyses is 0.05 minus the product of the number of interim analyses and 0.001. The O'Brien–Fleming boundary is much more difficult to cross than the Haybittle–Peto boundary at the first interim analysis; the p-value must be 0.00005 or less. By the halfway point, the O'Brien–Fleming boundary becomes less conservative than the Haybittle–Peto boundary. ◘ Figure 1 shows that the required p-values are 0.004 for O'Brien–Fleming versus 0.001 for Haybittle–Peto at the second interim analysis. Because the tiny p-value required by O'Brien–Fleming at the first analysis virtually precludes an early stop at the first analysis, some protocols truncate the O'Brien–Fleming early boundaries at, say, 0.001, and then fix later boundaries to ensure an overall error rate of 0.05.

Boundaries depend on the amount of data accrued at the time of review, expressed as "information time"; the boundaries in ◘ Fig. 1 were calculated for interim reviews conducted at equally spaced information times (25, 50, 75, and 100%). In a trial with a binary outcome like 28-day mortality, this corresponds to the first review conducted when 25% of participants reach 28 days of follow-up, the second review after 50% of participants reach 28 days, and so on. When the outcome is time to an event rather than occurrence of an event by a fixed, prespecified time, the relevant information is the proportion, among all events expected by the end of the trial, that has been observed by the time of the interim analysis. For example, in a trial that continues until 100 deaths have occurred, the amount of information after 46 deaths is 46%. Given that the DSMB may not be able to convene at the exact time required by an equal spacing of interim looks, Lan and DeMets (1983) proposed an alternative method whereby a pre-specified *spending function* dictates how much error probability to "spend" by different points in the trial, depending on the amount of information accrued. Whenever the DSMB meets, a boundary is constructed that spends the allotted error probability at that time. The best spending functions spend the error probability slowly at first and more quickly toward the end of the trial. This results in conservative early boundaries that are very similar to those of O'Brien–Fleming. Most trials today use the Lan-DeMets spending function approach for efficacy monitoring.

3 Monitoring for Futility

A DSMB sometimes recommends stopping a trial for *futility*. This could be *operational futility*, meaning that there are serious threats to the integrity of the trial that prevent meaningful conclusions. For example, accrual of trial participants may be so slow that the trial could not be completed within a reasonable time, or participants may be dropping out or changing treatments at a much higher rate than expected. Our focus is not on operational futility, but on futility in the sense that accumulating data show no effect, or even harmful effect, of treatment compared to control. In an extreme case, the final result might be completely determined at an interim analysis. For example, it is theoretically possible for the observed treatment effect to be so disappointing that even if planned enrollment were to be completed and all newly enrolled treatment patients were to have a good outcome and control patients a bad outcome, the result would not be statistically significant. In that case, there is little reason to continue. Stopping because the outcome is *guaranteed* to be null is known as *curtailment*. A much more common scenario is stopping when the final outcome is *very likely* to be null. We assess this through *conditional power*, the conditional

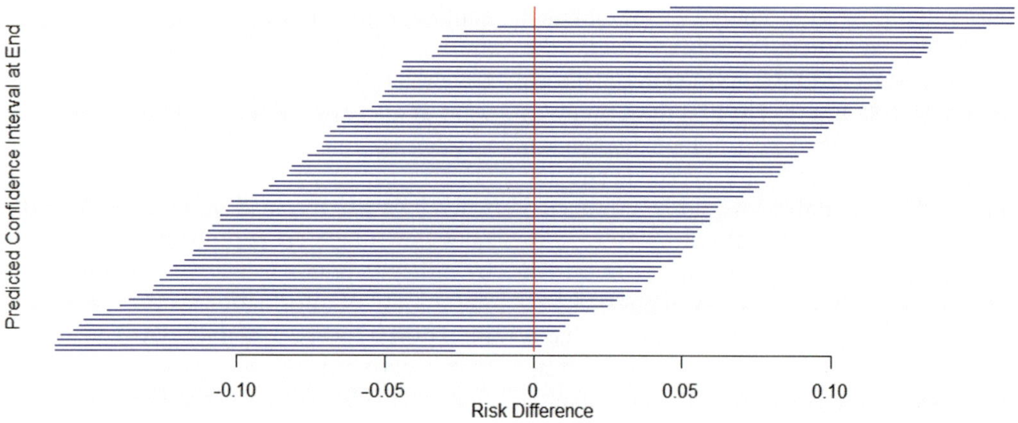

Fig. 2 Predicted interval plot based on observed data augmented with simulated future data. (Authors)

probability of reaching a statistically significant benefit at the end of the trial, given results observed so far (Lan et al. 1982; Lan and Wittes 1988). If conditional power is very low, we may want to stop for futility. This might be formalized by a rule such as: stop if conditional power drops below 20%. Such a rule is known as *stochastic curtailment* because it is a probabilistic variant of curtailment. (Be aware, though, that some authors use "stochastic curtailment" as a synonym for conditional power.)

Conditional power requires assumptions about future data. The primary conditional power calculation should use the pre-specified treatment effect for which the trial was powered. This is usually an assumption about treatment effect that has turned out to be overly optimistic, if stopping for futility is a current consideration. Another option is to compute conditional power assuming the treatment effect observed thus far will continue, the so-called *current trend.* That feels like it would result in a more accurate forecast, but there is a lot of variability in the current trend estimate of treatment effect. As a result, conditional power computed under the current trend has poor properties, especially if computed before approximately one-third of the trial has been completed. The probability of erroneously stopping for futility can be unacceptably high when conditional power is computed under the current trend. DSMBs often ask for conditional power to be computed in several different ways to get a full picture about whether continuation of the trial is futile.

A useful graphical display to accompany conditional power calculations is the *predicted interval plot* (Evans et al. 2007; Li et al. 2009). Projected confidence intervals at the end of the trial are computed using the current data, augmented with simulated future data. This gives a quick pictorial representation of conditional power; if most of the confidence intervals include the null value, conditional power is low. For example, Fig. 2 shows a predicted interval plot in which approximately 90% of the predicted confidence intervals for the risk difference between treatment and control include the null value of 0; each line represents an interval calculated with current data augmented with simulated data assuming the hypothesized treatment effect for future enrollments. Phrased differently, Fig. 1 illustrates a case where only about 10% of predicted confidence intervals at the end of the trial would indicate statistical significance (i.e., the lower bound of the interval exceeds zero), corresponding to a conditional power of 10%. Here, stopping for futility due to low conditional power would be a consideration.

4 Practical Aspects of Monitoring

The protocol-specified interim monitoring boundaries are typically considered guidelines, not mandates, for DSMB recommendations. Efficacy decisions are almost never driven solely by crossing a boundary but follow a comprehensive evaluation of all available data. In some circumstances, the DSMB might recommend continuation of a trial even though the interim monitoring boundary for efficacy has been crossed. For example, there may be safety signals in the interim data that, if confirmed, could potentially offset the benefit observed for the primary (efficacy) endpoint. In this case, the trial might continue until the benefit/risk profile is more firmly established. In the PROMISE trial of mother-to-child transmission of HIV, one regimen better prevented transmission of HIV but resulted in a higher proportion of birth complications (Fowler et al. 2016). In some cases, perceptions of the medical community may influence the level of evidence required to stop a clinical trial. A good example is the Cardiac Arrhythmia Suppression Trial (CAST), undertaken to determine whether suppression of cardiac arrhythmias in patients with a prior heart attack reduces the probability of sudden death/cardiac arrest (CAST II Investigators 1992; CAST Investigators 1989). DSMB deliberations included a concern that, because of the prevailing medical opinion that arrhythmia suppression was beneficial, only very convincing evidence to the contrary would be able to dispel this myth. CAST I and II did demonstrate convincing evidence that suppression of arrythmias with the medications used was harmful to patients. Because a DSMB must weigh all circumstances when making recommendations, efficacy boundaries are sometimes regarded as advisory rather than binding.

Futility boundaries are often considered even less binding than efficacy boundaries. For instance, suppose that a futility boundary is crossed after all participants have been recruited, but not all have completed their follow-up period. Unless participants might be harmed by ongoing use of the investigational treatment, or the incremental cost of following patients to completion is large, follow-up might be continued to better estimate the treatment effect or to obtain useful data on secondary outcomes. Alternatively, a trial might be stopped for futility before crossing a futility boundary if, in addition to the primary outcome, important secondary outcomes also show no benefit of treatment.

When stopping a trial for efficacy, DSMBs often want to see consistency of results across different endpoints, methods of analysis, and subgroups of participants. In the ACTT-1 trial alluded to earlier, the benefit seen for the primary endpoint of time to recovery was also observed for the secondary endpoint of clinical status at Day 15, which was based on an eight-point ordinal scale of assessment (Beigel et al. 2020). There was a suggestion of benefit on mortality, but those results were not statistically significant. Consequently, no claim of benefit was made for mortality.

The ACTT-1 trial illustrates the challenge of interpreting multiple subgroup analyses. One particularly tantalizing finding was that mortality for patients on low-flow oxygen at baseline seemed substantially lower on Remdesivir than on placebo. ◘ Figure 3 of Beigel et al. (2020) shows that at Day 29, there were 25 deaths on placebo and only 9 on Remdesivir in this subgroup, corresponding to a hazard ratio for mortality of 0.30, with 95% confidence interval (0.14, 0.64). Is this a real finding or could it be the play of chance?

After all, there were many subgroups, so the probability of at least one of them showing an apparent benefit is not small, even if remdesivir truly has no mortality benefit for anyone. Yusuf et al. (1985) warned of the dangers of over-interpreting subgroup results in the ISIS-2 trial of cardiovascular disease by illustrating that there was a very striking benefit of aspirin on mortality in patients whose astrological sign was other than Gemini or Libra, but results in those two signs showed a non-significant increase in mortality on aspirin. The point is that if one is allowed to rummage through enough subgroups, some subgroups will show significant differences by chance alone. A much larger trial testing remdesivir, the Solidarity trial, showed no benefit on mortality (Pan et al. 2021; WHO Solidarity Trial Consortium 2022) in its initial results, but updated results showed a statistically significant mortality benefit in non-intubated patients. Unfortunately, the Solidarity publication used a slightly different categorization

Table 2. Outcomes Overall and According to Score on the Ordinal Scale in the Intention-to-Treat Population.*

	Overall		Ordinal Score at Baseline							
			4		5		6		7	
	Remdesivir (N=541)	Placebo (N=521)	Remdesivir (N=75)	Placebo (N=63)	Remdesivir (N=232)	Placebo (N=203)	Remdesivir (N=95)	Placebo (N=98)	Remdesivir (N=131)	Placebo (N=154)
Recovery										
No. of recoveries	399	352	73	58	206	156	57	61	63	77
Median time to recovery (95% CI) — days	10 (9–11)	15 (13–18)	5 (4–6)	6 (4–7)	7 (6–8)	9 (7–10)	15 (10– 27)	20 (14– 26)	29 (24–NE)	28 (24–NE)
Rate ratio (95% CI)†	1.29 (1.12–1.49 [P<0.001])		1.29 (0.91–1.83)		1.45 (1.18–1.79)		1.09 (0.76–1.57)		0.98 (0.70–1.36)	
Mortality through day 14‡										
Hazard ratio for data through day 15 (95% CI)	0.55 (0.36–0.83)		0.42 (0.04–4.67)		0.28 (0.12–0.66)		0.82 (0.40–1.69)		0.76 (0.39–1.50)	
No. of deaths by day 15	35	61	1	2	7	21	13	17	14	21
Kaplan–Meier estimate of mortality by day 15 — % (95% CI)	6.7 (4.8–9.2)	11.9 (9.4–15.0)	1.3 (0.2–9.1)	3.2 (0.8–12.1)	3.1 (1.5–6.4)	10.5 (7.0–15.7)	14.2 (8.5–23.2)	17.3 (11.2–26.4)	10.9 (6.6–17.6)	13.8 (9.2–20.4)
Mortality over entire study period‡										
Hazard ratio (95% CI)	0.73 (0.52–1.03)		0.82 (0.17–4.07)		0.30 (0.14–0.64)		1.02 (0.54–1.91)		1.13 (0.67–1.89)	
No. of deaths by day 29	59	77	3	3	9	25	19	20	28	29
Kaplan–Meier estimate of mortality by day 29 — % (95% CI)	11.4 (9.0–14.5)	15.2 (12.3–18.6)	4.1 (1.3– 12.1)	4.8 (1.6–14.3)	4.0 (2.1–7.5)	12.7 (8.8–18.3)	21.2 (14.0–31.2)	20.4 (13.7–29.8)	21.9 (15.7–30.1)	19.3 (13.8–26.5)
Ordinal score at day 15 (±2 days) — no. (%)§										
1	157 (29.0)	115 (22.1)	38 (50.7)	28 (44.4)	90 (38.8)	62 (30.5)	18 (18.9)	14 (14.3)	11 (8.4)	11 (7.1)
2	117 (21.6)	102 (19.6)	20 (26.7)	15 (23.8)	70 (30.2)	58 (28.6)	22 (23.2)	19 (19.4)	5 (3.8)	10 (6.5)
3	14 (2.6)	8 (1.5)	8 (10.7)	4 (6.3)	6 (2.6)	4 (2.0)	0	0	0	0
4	38 (7.0)	33 (6.3)	3 (4.0)	7 (11.1)	17 (7.3)	13 (6.4)	12 (12.6)	4 (4.1)	6 (4.6)	9 (5.8)
5	58 (10.7)	60 (11.5)	3 (4.0)	5 (7.9)	25 (10.8)	18 (8.9)	2 (2.1)	14 (14.3)	28 (21.4)	23 (14.9)
6	28 (5.2)	24 (4.6)	1 (1.3)	0	5 (2.2)	7 (3.4)	12 (12.6)	11 (11.2)	10 (7.6)	6 (3.9)
7	95 (17.6)	121 (23.2)	1 (1.3)	3 (4.8)	13 (5.6)	21 (10.3)	16 (16.8)	20 (20.4)	57 (43.5)	74 (48.1)
8	34 (6.3)	58 (11.1)	1 (1.3)	1 (1.6)	6 (2.6)	20 (9.9)	13 (13.7)	16 (16.3)	14 (10.7)	21 (13.6)
Odds ratio (95% CI)	1.5 (1.2–1.9)		1.5 (0.8–2.7)		1.6 (1.2–2.3)		1.4 (0.9–2.3)		1.2 (0.8–1.9)	

* P values and confidence intervals have not been adjusted for multiple comparisons. NE denotes not possible to estimate.

† Recovery rate ratios and hazard ratios were calculated from the stratified Cox model; the P value for this ratio was calculated with the stratified log-rank test (overall model stratified by actual disease severity). Recovery rate ratios greater than 1 indicate a benefit with remdesivir; hazard ratios less than 1 indicate a benefit with remdesivir.

‡ Mortality over the first 14 days includes data from all patients who were still alive through 14 days postenrollment, with data censored on day 15, as if 14 days was the maximum follow-up time. Mortality over the entire study period uses the totality of the study data and censors data from patients who completed follow-up alive at 28 days postenrollment.

§ The ordinal score at day 15 is the patient's worst score on the ordinal scale during the previous day. Four patients died 15 days after randomization and are recorded as having died for the ordinal score at the day 15 outcome but not for the mortality day 15 outcome. Scores on the ordinal scale are as follows: 1, not hospitalized, no limitations of activities; 2, not hospitalized, limitation of activities, home oxygen requirement, or both; 3, hospitalized, not requiring supplemental oxygen and no longer requiring ongoing medical care (used if hospitalization was extended for infection-control reasons); 4, hospitalized, not requiring supplemental oxygen but requiring ongoing medical care (Covid-19–related or other medical conditions); 5, hospitalized, requiring any supplemental oxygen; 6, hospitalized, requiring noninvasive ventilation or use of high-flow oxygen devices; 7, hospitalized, receiving invasive mechanical ventilation or extracorporeal membrane oxygenation (ECMO); and 8, death. Odds ratios and P values were calculated with the use of a proportional odds model (overall model adjusted for actual disease severity). Odds ratio values greater than 1 indicate a benefit with remdesivir.

Fig. 3 Outcomes of ACCT-1 trial. (Beigel et al. 2020)

of patients, so it is not possible to compare mortality in ACTT-1 and Solidarity in patients on low-flow oxygen at baseline.

5 Case Study: Monitoring a Trial in a Public Health Emergency—The PREVAIL I Vaccine Trial

When the 2014–2016 Ebola virus disease outbreak in West Africa started, preclinical data were available for two candidate vaccines, a chimpanzee adenovirus 3-based vaccine (CHAd3-EBO-Z) and a recombinant vesicular stomatitis virus-based vaccine (rVSV-ZEBOV). To evaluate the efficacy and safety of the vaccine candidates, the National Institutes of Health (NIH) and the Liberian Ministry of Health jointly planned a randomized, placebo-controlled Phase II/III trial, the Partnership for Research in Ebola Virus in Liberia (PREVAIL) study (Kennedy et al. 2016, 2017). Volunteers aged 18 years or older were randomized 2:1:2:1 to receive the CHAd3-EBO-Z (2 mL) vaccine candidate or a matched 2 mL saline placebo, or the rVSV-ZEBOV (1 mL) vaccine candidate or a matched 1 mL placebo. The primary objective was to determine the efficacy of a single intramuscular dose of active vaccine versus the pooled placebo group, separately for each of the two vaccines. The primary efficacy outcome for the Phase III study was confirmed Ebola infection occurring 21 days or more after vaccination, and enrollment of 28,170 participants was planned. The primary safety outcome was the rate of serious adverse events (SAEs) experienced within 30 days of vaccination.

Because safety data for the dose to be studied were limited, expanded safety and immunogenicity data were to be collected for the first 600 participants in a Phase II substudy, later expanded to 1500 participants.

Follow-up visits occurred at week 1, month 1, month 2, and every 2 months through month 12. In addition to the primary safety endpoint (SAEs within 30 days of vaccination and through month 12), targeted symptoms and injection site reactions were collected within 30 min after vaccination, after 1 week and after 1 month. The targeted symptoms included, for example, fever, headache, nausea, and joint and muscle pain, which had been observed in preliminary studies. Other safety data included changes in blood plasma chemistries from baseline to week 1, such as blood cell counts and liver-related measures. To assess immunogenicity, antibody response was to be determined from stored plasma at a central lab, from specimens collected at baseline, week 1, and month 1; later, months 6 and 12 were added.

For the full Phase III vaccine trial, participants were to be contacted every 2 months to assess Ebola status, until a common closing date. Trial development started in October 2014, at the height of the outbreak, and 1500 participants were enrolled at the vaccination center at Redemption Hospital in Monrovia, Liberia for the Phase II sub-study between February 2 and April 30, 2015 (Kennedy et al. 2016).

An independent Data and Safety Monitoring Board (DSMB) was convened by the National Institute of Allergy and Infectious Diseases (NIAID) to oversee the study and review interim analyses. The eight DSMB members included internal medicine and infectious disease clinicians/researchers, a pharmacist, a bioethicist, and two biostatisticians. At least two of the DSMB members, including the chair, had deep knowledge of local healthcare delivery and cultural factors in Liberia, where the trial was conducted. The interim data reports were prepared by a team of three unblinded statisticians at the School of Public Health, University of Minnesota.

The main responsibilities of the DSMB were (1) to identify developing safety concerns, (2) based on the interim closed data, to advise whether and when the initial Phase II safety study of 600 participants should be expanded to the full Phase III trial, and (3) to monitor the full vaccine trial for safety and efficacy in preventing Ebola disease. For the latter, the Lan-DeMets error spending function analog of the O'Brien–Fleming boundary was to be used for vaccine efficacy, to preserve a one-sided significance level of 0.0125 for comparing each of the two vaccines versus placebo; because the trial tested two vaccine candidates versus placebo simultaneously, each of the two vaccines versus placebo comparisons was allocated one-half of the usual allowance of a one-sided Type I error (significance level) of 0.025. Interim monitoring boundaries for harm also were defined based on the primary efficacy endpoint (time to confirmed Ebola virus disease occurring 21 days or more after vaccination) but used the narrower Haybittle–Peto boundaries, at 2.5 standard deviations of the test statistic early in the trial (one-sided $p < 0.006$), and 2.0 standard deviations (one-sided $p < 0.023$) after 25% or more of the primary events had accrued. In addition, the protocol specified that the DSMB would monitor safety closely and could halt enrolment in the event of vaccine-related deaths or SAEs. At each interim review, extensive summaries of safety data were provided. These included comparisons of the vaccine versus placebo groups for the primary safety endpoint (rate of SAEs within 30 days of vaccination) as well as summaries and treatment comparisons for targeted symptoms and injection site reactions within 30 min of injection, after 1 week, and after 1 month.

Early, intense monitoring was important because available safety data were sparse and no safety data were available in the West African population where the study was taking place and the vaccine would be needed. It was expected that possible adverse effects would manifest themselves within days after vaccination, and certainly within the first month. The first participant enrolled on February 2, 2015, when Ebola was still epidemic in Liberia, and 276 participants were enrolled by February 18, the cut-date for the first DSMB report. Due to the fast enrollment, interim safety data accrued very quickly.

A short summary of the DSMB reviews is given below and in ◘ Fig. 4. At each meeting, the DSMB reviewed the accrued safety data

Date	Enrollment	No. of pts with Week 1 safety data	No. of pts with Month 1 follow-up	No. of pts with SAEs[*]	Main topics and recommendations[†]
01/26/2015	0	0	0	0	Review of protocol and DSMB charter
02/24/2015	276	155	0	2	First interim safety data review, plans for study expansion
03/10/2015	492	394	59	6	Interim safety data review, plans for Phase III expansion
03/20/2015	660	560	203	9	Update on study progress and protocol amendment: expand enrollment to 1,500 and add week 2 visit with data collection on joint pain
04/21/2015	1,194	1,058	647	21	Interim data review; support for the team's plan to add site in Guinea where Ebola was still active; discussed the sharing of blinded data with regulatory agencies while protecting the integrity of the trial
05/12/2015	1,500[‡]	1,441	995	28	Interim data review, request for additional safety analyses by subgroups; support for unblinding one-month safety data to selected stakeholders
06/09/2015	1,500[¶]	1,487	1,477	34	Interim data review; support for sharing one-month safety data but not immunogenicity data until trial was completed
08/18/2015	1,500[¶]	1,487	1,477	102	Unblinding report for the completed study, review of antibody response data

Fig. 4 Interim DSMB reviews for the PREVAIL I Ebola trial: Enrollment, number of participants with primary safety endpoint data (at month 1), and main topics. (Authors)

comparing the two active vaccines versus placebo. For both vaccines, adverse effects subsided within a few days after vaccination and tended to be low-grade, symptoms were consistent with preliminary data, and there were no safety concerns that would warrant stopping or modifying the trial. Visit attendance and data quality were excellent throughout the trial. Soon after the trial started enrolling, the Ebola outbreak waned in Liberia, and the study team worked on expanding the trial to areas where the Ebola epidemic was ongoing. Due to the pressing need for a vaccine, there was intense interest in the accruing safety data, and the DSMB repeatedly discussed requests for sharing confidential data from the ongoing trial.

At its first meeting on January 26, 2015, the DSMB discussed the study protocol, interim monitoring guidelines, DSMB responsibilities, and the frequency of DSMB reviews with the study team. The team had planned to enroll 600 participants within 4 weeks and asked the DSMB to meet as frequently as once a week during this phase to review safety and efficacy data. Beyond the initial phase, interim data were to be reviewed every 2–4 weeks, depending on safety and Ebola infection rates.

February 24, 2015: The team described efforts to develop infrastructure to add clinical sites in Liberia and expand the study to Sierra Leone. The DSMB supported the addition of sites and recommended that the study team should consider adding a simple but formal process to assess participants' understanding of the trial to the informed consent process. Also, the assay to measure antibody responses was complex, and the team described efforts to set up the infrastructure to rapidly determine antibody responses.

March 10, 2015: The study team asked the DSMB whether the accrued safety data permitted expansion of the study to the planned Phase III trial, in which large numbers of participants would be enrolled. The DSMB recommendation would have to be based on the accrued safety data for 394 participants with 1 week of follow-up (about 130 per treatment group), 59 participants with month 1 data, and immunogenicity antibody data for 35 participants. At this time, the Ebola outbreak was waning in Liberia; there had been no new Ebola cases since February 19, 2015. The study team described efforts to expand enrollment to countries where the Ebola outbreak remained active. The DSMB supported expansion of enrollment to the Phase III trial and the inclusion of new sites. Given the low Ebola incidence in Liberia, the DSMB recommended expanding the collection of immunogenicity data (in addition to Ebola status) beyond the originally planned 600 participants. The Board also recommended collecting immunogenicity data at months 6 and 12, to assess the durability of antibody responses. The DSMB deferred additional guidance regarding sample size for a planned Phase III study, requesting updated information of Ebola incidence in the proposed expansion area. The DSMB recommended including more women into the study; at this point, 18% of participants were women.

March 20, 2015: The team was in negotiations to add clinical sites in Guinea where Ebola cases were still occurring, and the DSMB recommended moving forward with enrolling the Phase III part at other clinical sites with Ebola outbreaks. The team noted receiving requests to share safety data with outside stakeholders. The DSMB recommended that only the study team leadership should have access to pooled outcome data at this time.

April 21, 2015: Version 2 of the protocol, with expanded sample size and added week 2 safety data collection, was approved by the Liberian and U.S. research ethics committees (RECs, aka institutional review boards or IRBs) on April 13–14. Requests by a regulatory agency to review closed safety data to determine whether the trial could be safely expanded were discussed. The DSMB stated that it was very closely monitoring the study and was interested in addressing regulatory concerns while minimizing dissemination of data summaries to protect the overall integrity of the trial.

May 12, 2015: Enrollment of 1500 participants into the Phase II safety trial was completed, and 995 participants had month 1 follow-up. The DSMB agreed that interim month 1 safety data could be shared with outside stakeholders, such as vaccine manufacturers, the U.S. Food and Drug Administration (FDA), and future study participants, to inform research and provide reassurance. Expansion of enrollment to Guinea for the Phase III vaccine efficacy study was again supported. At this point, the Ebola epidemic was waning, and the low incidence of new Ebola cases required a substantially larger sample size to assess efficacy of the two vaccines with respect to preventing new Ebola cases.

June 9, 2015: The team continued efforts to implement the study in Guinea. However, the incidence of Ebola had decreased substantially, and now a sample size of 200,000 would have to be enrolled to adequately power the Phase III trial unless incidence increased again. The DSMB recommended against sharing interim immunogenicity analyses before the DSMB could review more complete data. An unblinding report of the month 1 safety data was distributed to the study team leadership, the FDA, and industry partners on June 24, 2015.

August 18, 2015: A ring trial of the rVSV vaccine had shown efficacy in preventing Ebola disease; results had been published on July 31, 2015 (Henao-Restrepo et al. 2015) (► In Focus 22.1). The availability of an effective vaccine now ruled out placebo-controlled trials during an active Ebola outbreak. Therefore, plans to implement the Phase III part of the PREVAIL study were stopped. However, open research questions remained, including the durability of protection, efficacy of the CHAd3-EBO-Z vaccine and other vaccine candidates, the risk profile of the vaccines in children, and the risk-benefit profile of preventive, population-based vaccination as opposed to ring vaccination of persons who had come in contact with Ebola cases.

Designed at the height of the Ebola outbreak 2014–2015, PREVAIL I had the primary goal of evaluating the safety and efficacy of two candidate vaccines in preventing Ebola in a placebo-controlled trial. The outbreak was over shortly after the trial started, and none of the participants contracted Ebola. Therefore, there were no clinical endpoints to evaluate the efficacy of the vaccine. The trial was continued beyond the end of the outbreak to establish prolonged safety of the vaccine, and to evaluate durability of immunogenicity based on antibody responses. Final results of the PREVAIL I study were published in 2017 (Kennedy et al. 2017).

Based on the preliminary data gained from PREVAIL I and other studies, a new strategy vaccine trial was designed to investigate the risk/benefit profile of the rVSV vaccine with and without a second dose, and the J&J Ad26. ZEBOV and MVA-FN-Filo two-dose vaccine regimen. One of the main objectives of the follow-up trial was to establish safety and immunogenicity profiles among children aged 1–17 years, in addition to adults, and the duration of the antibody response with and without a boost. The Partnership for Research on Ebola Vaccination (PREVAC) trial enrolled adults and children in Liberia, Mali, and Guinea between 2017 and 2018 when Ebola was not endemic (Badio et al. 2021).

6 Lessons Learned

During an outbreak, clinical trials need to be developed in a short time frame, and enrollment can be very fast. There is substantial pressure to conclude the trials very quickly, so that desperately needed treatments or vaccines become available to the at-risk population. Nevertheless, it is essential to minimize the risk for trial participants and safeguard the scientific integrity of the trial. In this, independent DSMBs play an important role. Below, we list considerations for clinical trials during an epidemic that are relevant for the work of the DSMB, ranging from the design of the study to the composition of the DSMB and the conduct of interim monitoring reviews.

6.1 Study Design and Conduct

- During an epidemic, any health care system will be under stress. Consequently, intensive data collection may not be possible. Nevertheless, sufficient data need to be collected to ensure trial integrity, safety of the participants, and generalizability of results. For example, relevant demographic and clinical baseline characteristics are needed to identify subgroup differences in the effect of treatments. Clinically relevant endpoints are needed that can be reliably ascertained during the outbreak. In PREVAIL I, the primary efficacy endpoint was confirmed Ebola virus disease. In a vaccine trial, ascertaining immune correlates of protection can bolster results and greatly advance the field.
- Vaccines that are to be given to a large portion of the population in case of a future outbreak need to have an excellent safety profile, with very few side effects. While clinical vaccine efficacy can be established only while the disease is active, well-designed vaccine trials may be continued after the outbreak has ended to establish safety and allow the vaccine to be used to fight the next outbreak.

6.2 Composition of the DSMB

- DSMB members may need to be found at short notice. DSMB members should be experienced and must know what is expected of them. Finding specialists with the needed experience may be challenging and is necessarily so in the context of a novel disease such as COVID-19. Therefore, having the same DSMB review more than one trial in the given disease has great appeal. For example, a single DSMB reviewed multiple ACTT COVID-19 treatment trials.
- Because there may be requests by outside stakeholders (e.g., the WHO, FDA, investigators, and pharmaceutical companies planning other trials) to release interim data, the DSMB needs to have confident leadership and experience to evaluate the reliability of interim results, the consequences to the integrity of the trial of releasing those results, and how to respond

to justified requests for data sharing without jeopardizing the trial.

- Due to the compressed time frame for conducting the trial, frequent reviews are needed, requiring substantial time commitment from DSMB members. For example, the PREVAIL I trial was reviewed every 2–4 weeks, and the ACTT-1 trial of remdesivir for COVID-19 had weekly safety reviews.
- It is advisable to duplicate crucial expertise, so that the DSMB can meet at short notice even if one or two members cannot attend. Thus the DSMBs for the ACTT and PREVAIL trials included at least two experienced biostatisticians.
- In international trials, DSMBs must include representatives from the countries in which the study is conducted. When local investigators with prior DSMB expertise cannot be found at short notice, clinicians who have conducted clinical trials in the corresponding countries should be sought.

6.3 Preparing Interim Reports for the DSMB

- Requests to the DSMB by the study team should be clearly laid out in the open report, as well as responses of the team to previous DSMB recommendations.
- The unblinded statisticians who prepare the interim monitoring reports should anticipate the needs of the DSMB and write summaries that address the important points and can be easily digested. While this applies to any trial, the accelerated timetable during an outbreak does not leave time to "learn while doing"; an experienced team of statisticians is needed to produce the frequent reports.
- Given the short time to develop reports, statisticians need to work proactively to develop code allowing tables to be run automatically for the core of the report. Additional specific data reports may be requested by the DSMB as questions emerge, and statisticians need to be able to respond quickly.
- Interim reports for clinical trials are usually based on data that are "cut" about 2–4 weeks prior to the data lock date, to allow for delays in submission of data to the statistical center, and for resolving inconsistencies. Given the time pressure during an epidemic, reports may be prepared without any such lag time for data cleaning to provide up-to-date data.

6.4 Interim Reviews by the DSMB

- DSMB meetings typically contain both open and confidential closed sessions. In the open session, the study team presents updates on enrollment and participant characteristics and discusses study conduct and future plans with the DSMB. In the closed session, the DSMB evaluates safety and efficacy based on the confidential data summaries by treatment group. The closed session is also used to find consensus on recommendations to the study team.
- The fast-paced nature of the trials requires frequent meetings at short notice, which usually requires teleconferences rather than face-to-face meetings. In addition to the full DSMB reviews, abbreviated reports focused on safety outcomes may be provided at higher frequency so the DSMB can react quickly to emerging safety signals. The DSMB may choose to review such reports without meeting, for example by communicating via email.
- DSMB members have only a short time to review reports and thus need to plan carefully. Hundreds of pages of data summaries may be provided just 4 or 5 days before the review meeting. This also poses a challenge to the statisticians who prepare the reports, as reports need to be concise while still presenting the needed information to comprehensively evaluate safety and efficacy.

- DSMB members need to work closely as a team, as their joint expertise is needed. It is beneficial to have some face-to-face meetings to build trust for an efficient working relationship among DSMB members, as well as between the DSMB and the study team and other stakeholders. In particular, when the DSMB recommends closing or modifying a trial, the study leadership and investigators need to trust the DSMB to draw correct conclusions from interim data.

7 Conclusion

Clinical trials conducted during an outbreak are essential to provide evidence-based decisions on which treatments or vaccines are safe and efficacious. DSMBs overseeing such trials have a huge responsibility and dedicate an immense amount of time and effort.

DSMB members are under tremendous pressures: both to maintain the highest scientific standards before concluding that a treatment or vaccine works and to make decisions very quickly to discard ineffective interventions and implement effective ones. Decisions can be very difficult. Statistical tools like monitoring boundaries and conditional power can help guide decisions, but ultimately the most important tools are experience, good judgment, and the combined wisdom of DSMB members with diverse expertise. Each member may be an expert in one area: statistics, infectious disease, or ethics. One member can offer a perspective that may never have occurred to a member with a different background. That is why good communication skills and patience are essential.

Discussion Questions

1. What is the role of a DSMB for a clinical trial?
2. Why is it important that the DSMB review the protocol and monitoring plans before any participants are enrolled?
3. How do DSMB responsibilities differ for trials conducted in a public health emergency compared to other times? How would this influence the composition of the DSMB?
4. What are monitoring boundaries for interim reviews?
5. Why is it important to specify monitoring boundaries for efficacy and safety prior to the first interim review? Who is responsible for specifying such boundaries?
6. Usually, DSMBs will stop clinical trials for efficacy at an interim review only when there is clear and convincing evidence that the experimental treatment is superior to the control. Should this guideline be relaxed when there is a public health emergency?
7. Usually, DSMBs will stop clinical trials for futility at an interim review only when conditional power is very low, i.e., when there is no evidence for a beneficial effect of the experimental treatment and there remains little chance that the trial will show superiority of the experimental treatment even when the trial is fully enrolled and completed. Should experimental treatments be abandoned earlier when there is a public health emergency? What are arguments for and against?
8. In the ACTT-1 trial comparing remdesivir to placebo for the treatment of COVID-19 in hospitalized patients, 59 (11%) of 521 participants in the remdesivir group died by day 29, compared with 77 (15%) of 352 in the placebo group. The difference was not statistically significant. However, the observed difference in the subgroup of participants who needed low-flow supplemental oxygen was 9 (4%) of 232 versus 25 (13%) of 203, and the p-value was <0.05. Is this convincing evidence that remdesivir decreases mortality among hospitalized patients who need low-flow supplemental oxygen?
9. Did the PREVAIL I trial succeed in establishing safety and efficacy of vaccines against Ebola virus disease?
10. The PREVAIL I trial was developed during the 2014–2016 Ebola virus disease outbreak in West Africa to test the

clinical efficacy of vaccines, and the outbreak waned before the Phase III trial was fully enrolled. How did the role of the DSMB differ from monitoring a vaccine trial for an endemic disease that was not a current public health emergency?

11. How could the integrity of the final trial results be damaged by unblinding interim data while the trial is still ongoing?
12. Is unblinding data from an ongoing clinical trial ever acceptable? Why did the PREVAIL I investigators ask their DSMB for advice concerning unblinding requests?

References

Badio M, Lhomme E, Kieh M, Beavogui AH, Kennedy SB, Doumbia S, et al. Partnership for Research on Ebola VACcination (PREVAC): protocol of a randomized, double-blind, placebo-controlled phase 2 clinical trial evaluating three vaccine strategies against Ebola in healthy volunteers in four west African countries. Trials. 2021;22(1):86. https://doi.org/10.1186/s13063-021-05035-9.

Beigel JH, Tomashek KM, Dodd LE, Mehta AK, Zingman BS, Kalil AC, et al. Remdesivir for the treatment of Covid-19—final report. N Engl J Med. 2020;383(19):1813–26. https://doi.org/10.1056/NEJMoa2007764.

Bernal AJ, Gomes da Silva MM, Musungaie DB, Kovalchuk E, Gonzalez A, Reyes VD, Martín-Quirós A, Caraco Y, Williams-Diaz A, Brown ML, Du J, Pedley A, et al. Molnupiravir for oral treatment of covid-19 in nonhospitalized patients. N Engl J Med. 2022;386:509–20. https://doi.org/10.1056/NEJMoa2116044.

Calis KA, Archdeacon P, Bain R, DeMets D, Donohue M, Elzarrad MK, et al. Recommendations for data monitoring committees from the clinical trials transformation initiative. Clin Trials (London, England). 2017;14(4):342–8. https://doi.org/10.1177/1740774517707743.

CAST II Investigators. Effect of the antiarrhythmic agent moricizine on survival after myocardial infarction. N Engl J Med. 1992;327(4):227–33. https://doi.org/10.1056/nejm199207233270403.

CAST Investigators. Preliminary report: effect of encainide and flecainide on mortality in a randomized trial of arrhythmia suppression after myocardial infarction. N Engl J Med. 1989;321(6):406–12. https://doi.org/10.1056/nejm198908103210629.

Ellenberg SS, Fleming TR, Demets DL. Data monitoring committees in clinical trials: a practical perspective, Statistics in practice. 2nd ed. Hoboken, NJ: Wiley; 2019.

Evans SR, Li L, Wei LJ. Data monitoring in clinical trials using prediction. Drug Inf J. 2007;41(6):733–42. https://doi.org/10.1177/009286150704100606.

Fleming TR, DeMets DL, Roe MT, Wittes J, Calis KA, Vora AN, et al. Data monitoring committees: promoting best practices to address emerging challenges. Clin Trials (London, England). 2017;14(2):115–23. https://doi.org/10.1177/1740774516688915.

Fowler MG, Qin M, Fiscus SA, Currier JS, Flynn PM, Chipato T, et al. Benefits and risks of antiretroviral therapy for perinatal HIV prevention. N Engl J Med. 2016;375(18):1726–37. https://doi.org/10.1056/NEJMoa1511691.

Haybittle JL. Repeated assessment of results in clinical trials of cancer treatment. Br J Radiol. 1971;44(526):793–7 https://doi.org/10.1259/0007-1285-44-526-793.

Henao-Restrepo AM, Longini IM, Egger M, Dean NE, Edmunds WJ, Camacho A, et al. Efficacy and effectiveness of an rVSV-vectored vaccine expressing Ebola surface glycoprotein: interim results from the Guinea ring vaccination cluster-randomised trial. Lancet. 2015;386(9996):857–66. https://doi.org/10.1016/s0140-6736(15)61117-5.

Jennison C, Turnbull BW. Group sequential methods with applications to clinical trials. Boca Raton, FL: Chapman & Hall/CRC; 2000.

Kennedy SB, Neaton JD, Lane HC, Kieh MWS, Massaquoi MBF, Touchette NA, et al. Implementation of an Ebola virus disease vaccine clinical trial during the Ebola epidemic in Liberia: design, procedures, and challenges. Clin Trials (London, England). 2016;13(1):49–56. https://doi.org/10.1177/1740774515621037.

Kennedy SB, Bolay F, Kieh M, Grandits G, Badio M, Ballou R, et al. Phase 2 placebo-controlled trial of two vaccines to prevent Ebola in Liberia. N Engl J Med. 2017;377(15):1438–47. https://doi.org/10.1056/NEJMoa1614067.

Lan KK, DeMets DL. Discrete sequential boundaries for clinical trials. Biometrika. 1983;70(3):659–63. https://doi.org/10.1093/biomet/70.3.659.

Lan KK, Wittes J. The B-value: a tool for monitoring data. Biometrics. 1988;44(2):579–85.

Lan KK, Simon R, Halperin M. Stochastically curtailed tests in long–term clinical trials. Commun Stat C Seq Anal. 1982;1(3):207–19. https://doi.org/10.1080/07474948208836014.

Li L, Evans SR, Uno H, Wei LJ. Predicted interval plots (PIPS): a graphical tool for data monitoring of clinical trials. Stat Biopharm Res. 2009;1(4):348–55. https://doi.org/10.1198/sbr.2009.0041.

NIAID. NIAID stops enrollment of severely ill COVID-19 participants in clinical trial of investigational treatments. Bethesda, MD: National

Institute of Allergy and Infectious Diseases (NIAID); 2020.
O'Brien PC, Fleming TR. A multiple testing procedure for clinical trials. Biometrics. 1979;35(3):549–56.
Pan H, Peto R, Henao-Restrepo AM, Preziosi MP, Sathiyamoorthy V, Abdool Karim Q, et al. Repurposed antiviral drugs for Covid-19—interim WHO solidarity trial results. N Engl J Med. 2021;384(6):497–511. https://doi.org/10.1056/NEJMoa2023184.
Proschan MA, Lan KKG, Wittes JT. Statistical monitoring of clinical trials: a unified approach. Statistics for biology and health. New York: Springer; 2006.
Whitehead J. The design and analysis of sequential clinical trials (revised). 2nd ed. Chichester, UK: Wiley; 1997.
WHO Solidarity Trial Consortium. Remdesivir and three other drugs for hospitalised patients with COVID-19: final results of the WHO solidarity randomised trial and updated meta-analyses. Lancet. 2022;399:1941–53. https://doi.org/10.1016/S0140-6736(22)00519-0.
Yusuf S, Peto R, Lewis J, Collins R, Sleight P. Beta blockade during and after myocardial infarction: an overview of the randomized trials. Prog Cardiovasc Dis. 1985;27(5):335–71. https://doi.org/10.1016/s0033-0620(85)80003-7.

23.1 In Practice: Monitoring the PALM Ebola Therapeutics Study in the Democratic Republic of the Congo

Michael A. Proschan and David L. DeMets

Contents

Learning Track Note: This chapter appears in Learning Tracks: Biostatistics

E. S. Higgs and R. A. Sorenson (eds.), *Principles and Practice of Emergency Research Response*,
https://doi.org/10.1007/978-3-031-48408-7_35

Learning Objectives

This chapter should enable readers to understand and discuss:

- How to overcome some of the challenges of monitoring clinical trials in difficult circumstances
- Overview of the PALM trial
- Mitigation strategies for a DSMB to cope with delayed information
- The downsides of unblinded trials
- How the DSMB responded to the increase in the PALM sample size due to rapid recruitment
- The DSMB's calculation of mortality rates

1 Monitoring a Clinical Trial in an Epidemic Setting

The urgency and often the remoteness of an outbreak or epidemic can make the complex endeavor of a clinical trial exceptionally demanding. That includes the integral task of monitoring the trials, as described by DeMets et al. (2021) and DeMets and Fleming (2020). Here we briefly summarize some of these challenges. Recruitment of trial participants and accumulation of events can occur rapidly, in sharp contrast with traditional trials, which often take longer than anticipated to complete enrollment. To keep up with the frantic pace, the data and safety monitoring board (DSMB) must meet frequently and virtually instead of in person. This requires reliable and secure communication using a format such as Zoom, Webex, or Microsoft Teams. The fact that many trials evaluating similar interventions may take place at nearly the same time makes attractive the idea of sharing a DSMB across separate trials or across multiple treatments in the same platform trial. This is especially important for detecting safety signals in new interventions or interventions used in a new disease. Another important issue is that an epidemic emergency setting where both resources and medical personnel are at their limits makes it more difficult than would be desirable to collect and verify all the data. Therefore, streamlining the collection of data and focusing on the most critical outcomes for safety and efficacy monitoring is paramount.

2 Monitoring the PALM Trial of Ebola Therapeutics in the DRC

2.1 Overview of PALM Trial

The *Pamoja Tulinde Maishe* (PALM, Swahili for "together save lives") trial took place in the Democratic Republic of the Congo (DRC) in exceptionally difficult circumstances

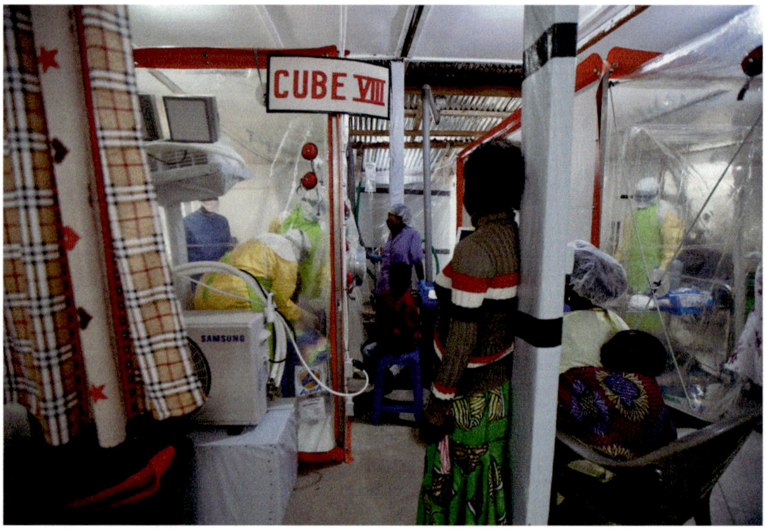

Fig. 1 Inside one of the improved Ebola treatment centers where the PALM trial was implemented. The facilities had to be set up rapidly in a resource-poor environment, under threat from various armed groups operating in the area. (Credit: Richard Kojan, ALIMA)

(◼ Fig. 1), which included minimal basic infrastructure, widespread suspicion and hostility among the population, and armed groups in more or less open rebellion against the central government (Nguyen 2019) (▸ In Practice 17.1). The trial, which began enrolling patients on November 20, 2019, randomized participants with Ebola virus disease who had been admitted to Ebola treatment centers to one of four treatments: (1) ZMapp, a triple monoclonal antibody product; (2) remdesivir, a direct-acting antiviral; (3) MAb114, a monoclonal antibody derived from an Ebola survivor; or (4) REGN-EB3, a mixture of three monoclonal antibodies (Mulangu et al. 2019). Based on promising, but not statistically significant, results from the PREVAIL II trial in Western Africa, which compared ZMapp to the then current standard of care, ZMapp was chosen in PALM as the control arm to which the other three arms were compared (Mulangu et al. 2019; Prevail II Writing Group 2016). The primary outcome in PALM was mortality within 28 days following randomization. REGN-EB3 was added after the other three arms had begun. To protect against the possibility of temporal trends in outcomes affecting trial findings, patients receiving REGN-EB3 were compared only to control arm participants randomized after REGN-EB3 was added. The planned sample size was 140 in each of the first three arms and 125 participants in the REGN-EB3 arm (545 total), which would ensure more than 85% power to detect a 50% relative reduction in mortality of an investigational arm compared to the ZMapp control.

Efficacy monitoring in the PALM trial used the Lan-DeMets spending function approach (Lan and DeMets 1983). The spending function is a method for adjusting the levels of evidence to control the error rate from multiple tests of statistical significance. Briefly, spending functions allow flexible monitoring concerning the number and timing of interim analyses by specifying the rate at which we "spend" the error probability rather than a specific boundary (▸ Chap. 23). The spending function selected mimics the O'Brien and Fleming (1979) boundary but truncated at a one-tailed p-value of 0.001. The reason for truncating the boundary is that, as pointed out in ▸ Sect. 2 of ▸ Chap. 23, the O'Brien-Fleming boundary is extremely conservative early. For example, even if the first 15 people in one arm survived and the first 15 in the comparator arm died, the O'Brien-Fleming boundary would not be crossed. Given the high mortality rate of Ebola virus disease and the need to identify effective treatments quickly, we decided to diminish the level of conservatism by truncating early boundaries.

Some people argued that ZMapp had not met the usual level of evidence in the PREVAIL II trial to be used as a control arm in PALM. They believed that it was preferable to simultaneously compare all arms rather than compare each to ZMAPP as the control arm. The downside of that proposal is that a simultaneous comparison of all arms would only indicate whether the hypothesis that all arms are equally effective should be rejected. Additional pairwise comparisons would be needed to decide which treatments differed. It is possible for the simultaneous comparison of more than two arms to be statistically significant while no pair on its own is statistically significantly different. There is another problem with the simultaneous comparison proposal. With four treatments, there are six pairwise comparisons. The prevailing opinion is that when many comparisons are made in a clinical trial, a multiple comparison adjustment must be made that requires stronger evidence for each one. Comparing each arm to the ZMapp control results in half the number of comparisons. We argued that because there were three comparisons rather than six, it was reasonable not to use a multiple comparison adjustment.

2.2 Monitoring Comparisons with Control

The decision to use ZMapp as a control raises an interesting possibility: what if no arm is shown different from ZMapp, but other differences in arms become apparent? One arm might appear clearly inferior to at least one other arm, but not to ZMapp. If a clear separation existed, it would be very difficult to continue randomizing participants to the inferior arm. In PALM, although the primary comparisons were of each arm to the ZMapp control, a chi-squared test comparing all arms was also conducted to check consistency of results. DSMBs are reluctant to make important decisions based on just a single way of analyzing data.

2.3 Lag Problem

One important issue for monitoring clinical trials of infectious diseases is that the epidemic can wax and wane. Periods of frantic enrollment can lead to a lag in information presented to the DSMB, as we explain next. To plan for the PALM DSMB meeting, unblinded statisticians specified an enrollment cutoff date such that all patients randomized by that date would have had 28 days of follow-up. This required the allowance of additional time to capture all deaths, write the DSMB report, and give the DSMB time to review it. The resulting enrollment cutoff date for the August 9, 2019, DSMB meeting of the PALM trial was June 26. A drawback to this approach is that by the time of the DSMB meeting, many more patients had been randomized but not included. Indeed, 369 patients were included in the primary analysis, but 671 patients had been enrolled as of August 6! Deaths other than those in the 369 patients were not included in the primary analysis. There was a serious potential risk that results of the primary analysis might be obsolete by the time of the meeting.

One idea to combat the data lag problem was to include all deaths in the DSMB report, regardless of whether patients had 28 days of follow-up. After all, patients who die by day 6, for example, will remain dead by the time they have had 28 days of follow-up. The problem with this method is that a patient with less than 28 days of follow-up is included in the analysis *only* if she/he dies. This leads to an overestimate of the probability of death. There is no problem from a testing perspective because, under the null hypothesis, the degree of overestimation should be the same in different arms. Still, we felt that the option described in the next paragraph was preferable.

In Ebola virus disease, the overwhelming majority of patients who die do so early after being randomized. Consequently, early mortality is an excellent surrogate for later mortality. For example, approximately 97% of the patients who died in PALM did so by 10 days after randomization. An updated analysis was presented to the DSMB that included deaths at any time up to 28 days in all patients with at least 10 days of follow-up. The updated analysis included all 499 participants with at least 10 days of follow-up, as opposed to the 369 patients in the primary analysis.

2.4 External Influences

PALM was not a blinded trial. The treatments under study required different numbers of infusions, so blinding would have required sham infusions that might endanger the health of very sick participants and expose staff to additional transmission risk. One problem with unblinded trials is that staff form opinions about which treatments work better than others, and that is exactly what happened in PALM. The prevailing opinion was that remdesivir was inferior to the other therapeutics in the trial. A nonrandomized, unblinded study in the DRC at the same time and using the same interventions as PALM, a World Health Organization (WHO) Monitored Emergency Use of Unregistered and Investigational Interventions (MEURI), reinforced that opinion by issuing a statement calling for deprioritizing the use of remdesivir in MEURI. The chosen wording was intended to have minimal effect on the successful completion of PALM, which was recognized as a more rigorous comparison by virtue of being a randomized trial. Unfortunately, there was already some concern in the community about outsiders conducting medical research in the DRC. If people came to believe that an inferior arm was continuing too long, the entire trial could be in jeopardy.

However, there was no statistically significant difference between remdesivir and ZMapp in PALM. An unblinded statistician attempted to reassure principal investigators that PALM had an extraordinary DSMB who were carefully monitoring safety and efficacy; if they believed that one treatment was inferior to another, they would not let that treatment continue. But this could only be expressed in vague terms. No specific information could be communicated to the study team about preliminary results. The question was whether the DSMB should be made aware of the mounting external pressure against remdesivir. On the one hand, the DSMB should not feel pressured. On the other hand, they needed to be aware of any serious threats to the successful completion of the trial. What if staff became so convinced that remdesivir was harmful that they refused to continue administering it? Alternatively, what if they spent more time caring for those on remdesivir in the belief that they were at greater risk of death? Either way, the integrity of PALM would be compromised. In the end, the DSMB was notified about the negative impression medical caregivers had about remdesivir.

2.5 Sample Size Increase

PALM was designed to detect a large treatment effect to keep the sample size manageable. It was believed that recruiting a much larger number of participants would take many years to complete, and results might be obsolete by the time the trial ended. However, recruitment was progressing much faster than anticipated. This prompted the study team to submit a protocol amendment to increase the sample size to enable detection of a mortality reduction of less than 50%. It would be very tempting for unblinded statisticians to opine about whether such an increase was necessary, but that would convey information to the study team about treatment effects. A crucial tenet of clinical trials is that the study team should not have knowledge of comparative efficacy data during the trial; that is restricted to the DSMB only. The amendment was implemented, increasing the sample size to 185/arm in the ZMapp, remdesivir, and MAb114 arms and 170 in the REGN-EB3 arm (725 total).

3 August 9, 2019: The DSMB Decision

Mortality rates in the MAb114 and REGN-EB3 arms had been lower than those of ZMapp and REGN-EB3 throughout the trial, although the boundary for the primary analysis of 28-day mortality had not been crossed. As mentioned in ► Sect. 2.3, only 369 of 671 patients randomized were included in the primary analysis at the August 9 meeting. The DSMB had requested updated data, so mortality in all participants with at least 10 days of follow-up was presented and treated as another official interim analysis. Based on that analysis, the DSMB recommended discontinuation of randomization to ZMapp and remdesivir. They further recommended that the final analysis of PALM data should be performed when all patients randomized by August 9, 2019, reached 28 days of follow-up. These recommendations were accepted by trial sponsors. Randomization to MAb114 and REGN-EB3 continued in an extension phase of PALM.

Whenever there are pending data at the time of a DSMB decision, there is always concern that once those pending data are resolved, the evidence will reverse itself. That is, a boundary that was crossed might not be crossed when data are updated. One very useful tool in such a circumstance is conditional power (Lan et al. 1982), the calculated probability that the full data result, namely, that produced by the interim data plus the pending cases, will remain over the boundary, given the interim data observed so far. Under reasonable assumptions about the pending cases, that conditional power was very high. Thus, even though there was a theoretical possibility that the final data could be below a boundary, we were very confident that would not happen. That confidence turned out to be well justified; the final results (◘ Fig. 2) showed that both MAb114 and REGN-EB3 were superior to ZMapp (Mulangu et al. 2019).

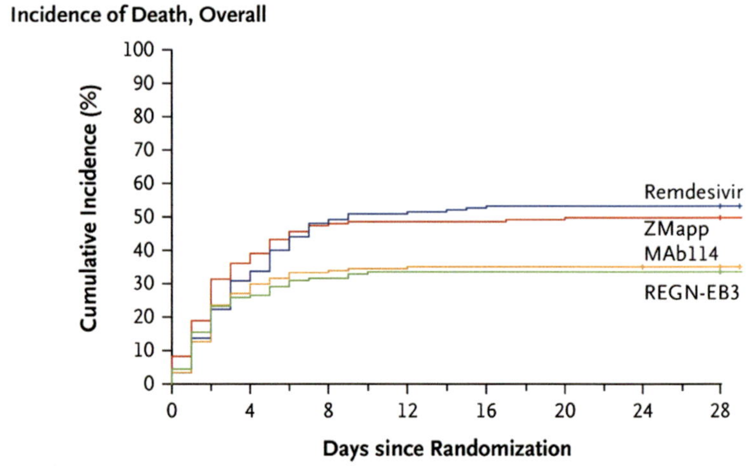

No. at Risk

ZMapp	169	137	108	96	89	87	87	87	87	86	86	85	85	85	85
Remdesivir	175	151	121	105	91	86	86	85	83	82	82	82	82	82	82
MAb114	174	152	127	119	116	114	114	113	113	113	113	113	113	112	112
REGN-EB3	155	131	115	110	106	104	103	103	103	103	103	103	103	103	103

Fig. 2 Cumulative incidence of death in the overall population in the PALM trial. (Kaplan-Meier estimates) (Mulangu et al. 2019)

Discussion Questions

1. Review some challenges of monitoring clinical trials in demanding epidemic settings.
2. What measures are available to redress the data lag in information presented to the DSMB that can result from uneven enrollment?
3. PALM was not blinded since that would have required sham infusions that posed health risks to trial participants and additional transmission risk to staff. What are the downsides of an unblinded trial?
4. To keep the sample size manageable, PALM was designed to detect a large treatment effect, but recruitment progressed faster than anticipated and increased the sample size. How did the study team respond?
5. How did the DSMB accommodate the evidence that that mortality rates in the MAb114 and REGN-EB3 arms were lower than those of ZMapp and REGN-EB3, even though the boundary for primary analysis of 28-day mortality had not been crossed?

References

DeMets DL, Fleming TR. Achieving effective informed oversight by DMCs in COVID clinical trials. J Clin Epidemiol. 2020;126:167–71. https://doi.org/10.1016/j.jclinepi.2020.07.001.

DeMets DL, Fleming TR, Ellenberg SS. Monitoring clinical trials in infectious diseases. J Allergy Infect Dis. 2021;2(1):29–32. https://doi.org/10.46439/allergy.2.019.

Lan KKG, DeMets DL. Discrete sequential boundaries for clinical trials. Biometrika. 1983;70(3):659–63. https://doi.org/10.1093/biomet/70.3.659.

Lan KKG, Simon R, Halperin M. Stochastically curtailed tests in long-term clinical trials. Commun Stat C Seq Anal. 1982;1(3):207–19. https://doi.org/10.1080/07474948208836014.

Mulangu S, Dodd LE, Davey RT Jr, Tshiani Mbaya O, Proschan M, Mukadi D, et al. A randomized, controlled trial of Ebola virus disease therapeutics. N Engl J Med. 2019;381(24):2293–303. https://doi.org/10.1056/NEJMoa1910993.

Nguyen V-K. An epidemic of suspicion—Ebola and violence in the DRC. N Engl J Med. 2019;380:1298. https://doi.org/10.1056/NEJMp1902682.

O'Brien PC, Fleming TR. A multiple testing procedure for clinical trials. Biometrics. 1979;35(3):549–56.

Prevail II Writing Group. A randomized, controlled trial of ZMapp for Ebola virus infection. N Engl J Med. 2016;375(15):1448–56. https://doi.org/10.1056/NEJMoa1604330.

24 Mathematical Modeling for Emergency Response: Using Models to Inform and Direct Response Priorities and Shape the Research Agenda

Bradford Greening Jr and Martin I. Meltzer

Contents

Learning Track Note: This chapter appears in Learning Tracks: Biostatistics; Clinical Research

E. S. Higgs and R. A. Sorenson (eds.), *Principles and Practice of Emergency Research Response*, https://doi.org/10.1007/978-3-031-48408-7_36

Learning Objectives

This chapter should enable readers to understand and discuss:

- Four key questions that decision-makers should ask about an outbreak
- The salient information decision-makers need early in a response to gauge the resources required and to explain the unfolding situation to the public
- The differences between statistical and mathematical modelling, and their usefulness and limitations in a real-world setting for emergency response decision-making
- The features of compartmental, decision-tree, patient flow and throughput, and individual or agent-based models
- Why methods of sensitivity analysis are important in dealing with uncertainty
- Five common types of sensitivity analyses
- Examples of how response leadership can use modeling results and communicate them effectively

1 Introduction: Decision-Making in an Emergency Response

Mathematical modeling has become an essential component of planning for and responding to dangers like infectious disease outbreaks and bioterrorism. The reason such modeling is now so widely used is that it can provide insights into possible scenarios when there are insufficient data for statistical analysis to produce a more definitive basis for decision-making. Even when historical data are available on outbreaks involving a specific pathogen, they must be used with caution, since context can change dramatically over time, rendering historical data less useful for predicting current risks. In a little over a century, for example, there have been four recognized influenza pandemics (1918, 1957, 1968, and 2009). These differed widely in the numbers infected and the severity of symptoms, with the greatest differences in impact being between 1918 and 2009 (Crosby 2003; Shrestha et al. 2010).

Given the obvious uncertainty about future infectious disease events, response planning can benefit from a set of scenarios generated by mathematical modeling. While there has never been a large-scale bioterrorist attack using anthrax, for example, providing planners with numbers illustrating both the unmitigated burden and the potential impact of various interventions can be done through modeling, e.g., CDC's Anthrax Assist model (Rainisch et al. 2017).

Mathematical modeling can encompass a wide array of techniques, varying in complexity and the type of mathematics used, which can be confusing to a non-modeling audience of planners and decision-makers. How are they to select the best model to use for planning and response? We present in this chapter some guidelines and recommendations for both modelers and public health emergency response managers about how to design and use mathematical models for planning and decision-making during emergency responses.

2 Common Modeling Questions in an Emergency Response

Despite the lack of reliable data from the field in the early stages of many outbreak responses, leadership needs data to inform response actions, especially during the initial stages of the response, when there is often pressure to take immediate action. In such scenarios, there are four categories of questions that emergency response leaders generally ask modelers (► Chap. 25). These categories, described in more detail below, can elicit fundamental information for informing the response. When answering such questions, it is important to clearly convey when fluctuations in input values may cause these predictions to change dramatically over time—e.g., due to rapidly changing circumstances early in an outbreak (see ► Sects. 6 and 7.4).

2.1 How Bad Could It Get?

One of the most salient pieces of information that decision-makers need early in a response is an estimate of how bad things could get (how many cases, hospitalizations, and deaths) in the absence of any effective interventions. Such estimates help leaders gauge the resources needed to mount a suitable response. They also help political, scientific, and community leaders to explain the unfolding situation to the public. Regular reassessment and updates are essential to keep both response management and public messaging on track. In addition to case numbers, hospitalizations, and deaths, managers will often request estimates of peak severity and impact on vulnerable populations, like the elderly, healthcare workers, children, and pregnant women. Planning for the maximum expected stress on healthcare systems and focusing response on those who need it most depends on such estimates.

2.2 When Will It End?

Leaders will also ask when the outbreak will end with an effective response. This estimate helps determine initial allocation of resources, such as personnel needs for staffing the myriad response activities. Further, letting decision-makers know when they can realistically expect the outbreak to end helps them better advise lower-level managers and the public.

2.3 How Much Stuff Will We Need?

Decision-makers also need sound information to request appropriate levels of medical countermeasures like therapeutic drugs and vaccines, trained staff, and facilities (e.g., places to screen patients, specialized hospital wards, or high-containment care facilities), along with the needed funding. Too little and the response could be inadequate, or leaders will have to go back to funders hat in hand; too much and accusations of waste and even malfeasance are likely to follow.

2.4 What Is the Impact of a Particular Decision or Intervention?

Response leaders, funders, and politicians need realistic estimates of the potential impact of interventions intended to slow and ultimately stop disease transmission. Potential interventions may include encouraging or mandating social distancing, physical isolation of suspected and fulminant cases, vaccination of those at risk of exposure, or post-exposure prophylaxis for those who may have been exposed but are not symptomatic. Impact estimates may also illuminate interventions underway, gauging the success of ongoing response efforts and guiding decision-making about new strategies.

3 Models

3.1 What Is a Model?

A common misperception is that a mathematical model is a crystal ball which modeling wizards use to predict the future with uncanny accuracy. The reality is not so mysterious. A mathematical model can be described as nothing more than a simplified, imperfect representation of a real-world entity, system, or phenomenon. The best mathematical models approximate the essential aspects of a system (e.g., how a disease spreads during an outbreak), allowing the modelers to rapidly answer questions that data currently available from the field cannot resolve. For example, models can be used to answer questions such as “What might happen if we vaccinate X% of Y population?” It is the ability to answer these what-if questions that make mathematical models such powerful tools to inform decision-making.

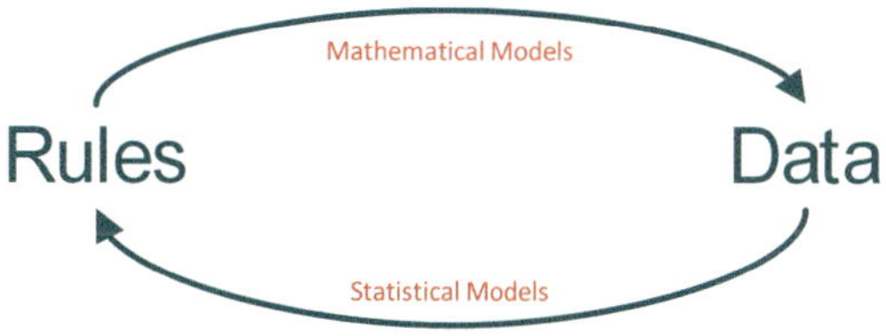

Fig. 1 A simple relationship between statistical models and mathematical models. (Authors)

3.2 Statistical Models Versus Mathematical Models

Most models used in public health can be broadly categorized as either statistical models or mathematical models (▶ Chap. 25). Generally, we can distinguish them by understanding how data are being used in each type of model (see Fig. 1). In terms of building either a statistical or mathematical model, we can think of the system being modeled as being split into two key parts:

1. A set of rules by which the system operates
2. A set of observable outcomes (i.e., data) produced by the system

3.2.1 Statistical Models

When creating statistical models, we use data gathered from studies of a system to generate a set of rules or equations that describe that system. For example, a statistical model could provide an equation describing how the risk of salmonella infection changes based on the consumption of a specified group of food products.

3.2.2 Mathematical Models

When creating a mathematical model, we start by creating a set of rules capturing the relevant features of how the system works to the best of our current knowledge. These rules are typically a set of mathematical equations that describes how interactions between inputs produce particular outputs (data). For example, a modeler may estimate how many new clinical cases of a disease might be generated per week during an outbreak by using the following inputs:

- Number of infectious persons at the start of the week
- Duration of infectivity
- Average number of cases infected per infectious person per day
- Average length of incubation
- Effectiveness of any interventions currently deployed (cf. ▶ Sect. 2.4).

For practical purposes, response leadership can view a mathematical model as a dashboard containing a set of dials, one dial for each input. These inputs are connected by a set of rules (equations). The modeler, in response to questions from the leadership (cf. ▶ Sect. 2), can "turn the dials" (change the input values) to see the impact of input changes on the output values. For example, a modeler can readily alter the presumed percentage of persons vaccinated in the next four weeks of an outbreak to estimate the resulting reduction in future cases. Similar approaches are familiar in mortgage payment or credit score calculators, where users can modify various inputs to see how they affect the output.

Manipulating input values allows us to understand better which inputs are primarily driving the results. For example, a modeler may estimate the number of future cases in an outbreak using a set of input values that a group of experts finds reasonable. Another plausible set of input values may produce a very different result. Such a difference would indicate that either (1) we lack a good understanding of what constitutes a reasonable estimate, relative to what is actually happening, of one or more of the inputs in the model or (2) the set of rules (equations) that we are using fails to capture some fundamental aspect of the system.

3.2.3 Critical Differences Between Statistical and Mathematical Models

The capability that mathematical models give the modeler to change the input values and rewrite the rules/equations accordingly is *the* critical difference between statistical and mathematical models. The mathematical model allows the modeler to answer almost innumerable what-if questions that arise as leaders seek the optimal set of responses to the outbreak. The remainder of this chapter will use the terms "models" and "modeling" to refer only to mathematical models.

4 Why Use Modeling? Contributions to Emergency Response

To better understand why modeling is useful for emergency response decision-making, let us examine more closely what modeling can and cannot do. Models cannot reliably predict the future. The most common misconception, as mentioned above, is that mathematical models can predict exactly what will occur. This is unrealistic, of course, but often the presence of uncertainty in model outputs makes response managers uneasy. To reiterate, models are simplified, imperfect representations of real-world systems. To maximize the operational value of estimates produced by models, the modeler must ensure that response leadership clearly understands the potential sources and implications of imperfections (e.g., flawed input data, faulty model assumptions, randomness, uncaptured processes).

If models cannot accurately predict the future, then why use them? The following set of short hypothetical examples illustrates ways in which response leadership can use modeling results and why they are useful. In addition, ▶ Sect. 7 contains a more detailed Worked Example.

You are the incident manager: To illustrate how models can help during an emergency response, assume for the remainder of ▶ Sect. 4 that you are the incident manager in charge of organizing the response to an infectious disease outbreak.

4.1 Provide Insights into Decision Thresholds

In an emergency response to almost any infectious disease, you, as the incident manager, might ask, "How many cases will there be by the time this is over?" We know we cannot give a precise number. However, estimating a plausible range for the likely number of cases helps you choose the type of response activities to set in motion. For example, if there is an efficacious vaccine against the agent, understanding the potential size of the outbreak, both at its peak(s) and in total, could help you decide between deploying a targeted vaccination strategy (such as ring vaccination) or undertaking a mass vaccination campaign in specific geographic areas. Some proposed activities have the potential to go beyond your vaccination capacity by exceeding either vaccine supply or availability of personnel to administer vaccines.

To help you decide among options, a mathematical model can help decision-makers determine thresholds at which one option becomes preferable to another. For example, a model could assess how varying levels of inaccuracy in daily case reports might affect estimates of future case counts, and the consequent effect on the estimated impact of different vaccination strategies (e.g., ring vaccination vs. targeted mass vaccination). The results would inform a conversation about which option to choose, given the probable inaccuracies. Note that approaching the problem in this way may also help you better understand what is known about the accuracy of case reporting.

4.2 Identify Key Mechanisms, Metrics, and Policy Levers

One of the most useful features of models during a response is that they can provide a sense of the critical resources needed as the outbreak progresses. These resources and how best to deploy them are the policy levers with which you, the incident manager, can potentially alter the trajectory of the outbreak (▶ Chap. 26) (i.e., shorten outbreak duration, reduce the number of cases, mitigate morbidity and mortality).

For example, laboratory testing of samples from suspected patients provides critical information on the size of the outbreak, as well as confirmation of whether particular patients are infected, to guide their treatment and infection control. As case counts grow, demand for laboratory tests can increase drastically. Mathematical models can help you estimate the potential number of samples that will need testing. A separate model may help you gauge whether laboratory capacity is sufficient to process projected samples expeditiously, or if additional laboratory capacity will be needed. Models assessing laboratory capacity can also highlight other possible bottlenecks in sample processing.

4.3 Simplify Complex Systems

As the number of factors that affect a system increases, it becomes intuitively less clear how changes in inputs affect outcomes. Models can help responders navigate the complexity and resultant uncertainty. For example, assume that you, as incident manager, need to know whether deploying a new point-of-care test will affect the time required, from initial presentation to test result, to screen patients for exposure to nuclear radiation. The new device will purportedly tell you more rapidly than previous methods whether a patient received more than a specified dose of radiation. You would like to know whether this improvement in the delivery of critical information will help route patients to proper care more rapidly and utilize limited human resources and medical countermeasures (MCMs) more efficiently.

The construction of a simple model (the queueing model, ▶ Sect. 5.3, that combines available data on the accuracy of the testing device, the time and number of trained staff needed for each step, and information on how patients will move through the system, may illustrate that deploying the new test will require a large increase in staffing needs. Such an increase in staff requirements could combine with an increased probability of false negatives or positives to tilt the balance against the new test. Increased patient throughput and better targeting of MCMs may not outweigh the downsides. In other words, the model can help you identify scenarios in which the new test could be useful and provide information to help improve the existing testing system.

4.4 Clarify the Question

During an influenza pandemic, an incident manager will need to know if there will be enough mechanical ventilators available for patients likely to experience acute respiratory failure. The modeler can illustrate that the supply of mechanical ventilators is not a standalone question, but that adequate hospital space and trained staff to use those ventilators are also essential components of mitigating serious outcomes (Ajao et al. 2015; Meltzer and Patel 2017). Mathematical models, such as CDC's FluSurge (Zhang et al. 2006) and COVID-19 Surge models (CDC 2016), can assist with predicting increases in demand for hospital services and associated staffing needs. Such models can help you re-assess your original question by focusing on the impact of actions and including other appropriate factors that may be critical to ensuring the success of a proposed intervention.

5 A Brief Technical Introduction to Mathematical Models

Models are simplifications of real-world systems that may, for example, be used to predict the spread of an infectious disease. Creating simplified (modeled) versions of the real world can help us test, explore, and understand how systems function and how changes to key inputs can affect them, helping us answer questions like, "What should we do to end an infectious disease outbreak?" Models can provide information when it is impractical, infeasible, or in some cases unethical to take measurements and perform tests. For example, amid an outbreak, we may not be able to conduct a carefully controlled trial to measure the impact of vaccination in a previously unvaccinated population or to wait for the results of an ongoing trial. In this section, we will discuss some standard types of mathematical models and provide some insights into how they can inform decision-making during public health emergency responses. For each type of model discussed below, a specific structure (set of equations) is built to track individuals or sections of a community. In practice, model design may blur the lines by incorporating or blending features from more than one category. A brief overview of some more complex model structures is given in ► Box 1.

5.1 Compartmental Models

Compartmental models are constructed using two major components—states and flows.

1. States, aka compartments: a set of characteristics used to group individuals within a population (e.g., susceptible-to-disease, infectious, or recovered with immunity). In compartmental models we must define these states so that all individuals will be in exactly one state at any point in time. Note that since these states are typically defined with respect to differences in disease transmission (such as differences in probability of transmission, for example), the states in our model may not directly align with traditional clinical or epidemiological disease states. To illustrate, for some pathogens, an infected individual may be both incubating (pre-symptomatic) and infectious to others. In our model then, we would define a compartment (state) as "incubating and infectious," since this differs in its risk of transmission relative to "incubating and not infectious" as well as "symptomatic and infectious."
2. Flows, aka transitions: process definitions (equations) that describe how individuals move between the compartments. First, for individuals in a given state, we describe which other states they could move into (e.g., an individual who is susceptible to disease cannot immediately move into the infectious state). Then, for each permitted transition, we describe the rate, or likelihood, of an individual making that transition. Note that many compartmental models do not, in practice, track specific individuals but rather percentages of a community (e.g., X% of a community are susceptible to infection, and they move into the infected state at a rate of Y% per day).

The SI model in ◘ Fig. 2 is a simple example of a compartmental model. The model is so named because of its states: individuals in the population can either be Susceptible to disease (S) or Infected/Infectious (I). In this very simple system, individuals can only flow from Susceptible to Infected/Infectious, where they will remain. There is no differentiation between becoming infected and becoming infectious. The rate of transition or movement between the two states is governed by the factor (an input) labeled β, which simultaneously accounts for the probability of individuals from I coming into contact with individuals from S and the probability of becoming infected during that contact. Note that this transition rate contains an implicit assumption that individuals in S are all equally likely to come into contact with individuals in I (an assumption known as homogeneous mixing).

In practice, additional states will often be needed, along with knowledge, or our best estimates, about how individuals move between all of the states included. For example, ◘ Fig. 3 shows CDC's simple model of the spread of Ebola Virus Disease through a

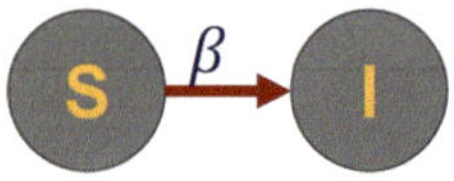

◘ **Fig. 2** S-I model of infectious disease transmission. (Authors)

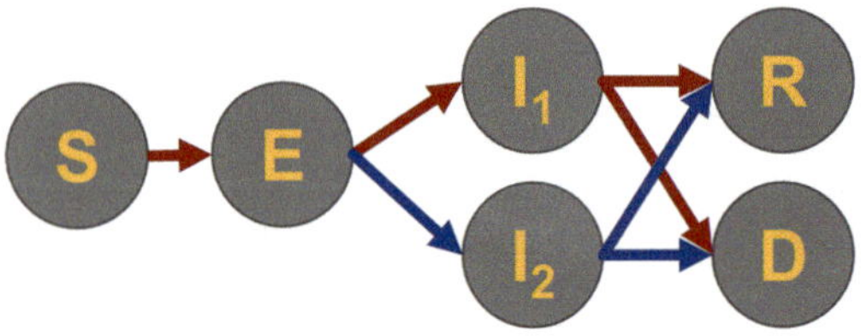

◘ **Fig. 3** Sample model structure for Ebola virus disease. (Authors)

population, an expanded SI model including the following states (Meltzer et al. 2014):

- E: individuals who have been exposed to (and infected with) the virus but who have not yet become infectious.
- I1: individuals who have become infectious but are properly isolated so that the risk they will infect others is drastically lower.
- I2: individuals who have become infectious but are not properly isolated.
- R: individuals who have recovered and are no longer infectious. These individuals do not return to the Susceptible category due to naturally acquired immunity (thought to be lifelong).
- D: individuals who died as a result of their infection.

5.2 Decision Tree Models

Decision tree models examine the possible outcomes that could occur as a result of a particular decision (e. g., to vaccinate or not to vaccinate). We construct a set of pathways, or branches, that begin with the choice being examined. Individuals or segments of a community are then modeled as passing through a set of probable intermediate states, terminating in one of several possible final outcomes (e.g., death, survival with lifelong sequelae, not infected). For each intermediate and final state, we give a probability of arriving in that state, as well as detail any costs that may be incurred by existing in that state.

Decision tree models are useful for assessing the potential costs and benefits of choosing one option over another. In an emergency response, these are choices of interventions to be implemented by the response (▶ Chap. 22). For example, during the 2014–2016 West Africa Ebola epidemic, Carias et al. (2016) examined the cost-effectiveness of prophylactically giving antimalarial drugs to people who had come into contact with suspected Ebola patients. The desired goal of this public health strategy was to reduce the number of persons arriving at Ebola treatment units (ETUs) who had early-stage malaria symptoms (e.g., sweating, fever) that are very similar to those of Ebola virus disease (EVD). The decision tree in Fig. 4 provides a straightforward, visual representation of the response process for possible contacts of suspected Ebola patients, beginning with the decision on whether to administer antimalarials.

When constructing a decision tree model, it is important to remember that individuals can only move through the model left-to-right (i.e., cannot reverse course). Therefore, individuals at each state are a subset of the group of individuals in the immediately preceding state. At each state, there is a defined probability that an individual will transition into a subsequent state. The sum of these probabilities at each branching point must add up to 1 (i.e., the options facing a patient are complete, and all patients at the branching point will move into *exactly* one of the subsequent states).

To illustrate these points, in Fig. 4 we would read a possible path from the beginning of the decision tree, stepwise, as follows:

1. Assume no malaria treatment is provided to contacts of suspect Ebola patients (the decision).
2. Then, X% of all contacts of suspect Ebola patients will develop fever due to malaria, Y% will develop fever due to EVD, while the remaining Z% will not develop a fever at all (where $X + Y + Z = 1$).
3. Then, of those who develop fever due to malaria, some portion will be mistakenly isolated in an ETU, while the rest will not.

5.3 Patient Flow/Throughput/Queuing Models

Throughput models are useful when we want to understand more about the *maximum capacity of a particular system* (a COVID-19 treatment ward, for example), or to determine bottlenecks that might be remedied to increase throughput. These models may also be referred to in the literature as patient flow models, queueing models, or capacity planning models. Their common thread is that they aim to answer the question, "How much can be accomplished with a given set of resources and constraints?"

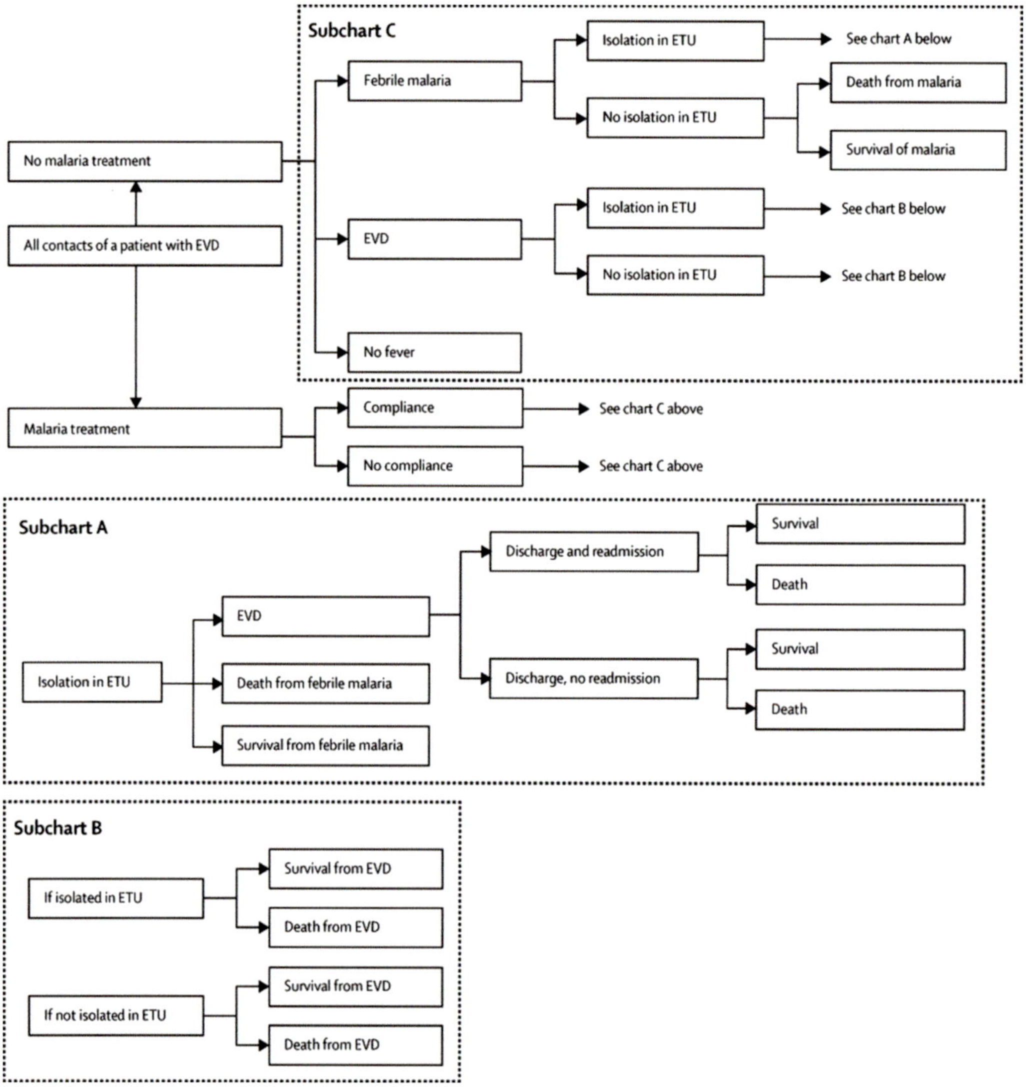

Fig. 4 Decision tree to assess cost-effectiveness of providing antimalarial drugs to suspected Ebola patients. (Carias et al. 2016)

Throughput models are often best visualized as a flow chart (Fig. 5), where patients move from one station to the next (e.g., initial screening or triage, taking biological specimens, placement in a treatment ward (▶ Chap. 40). Each station has specified resource and time requirements. Such models can also include patient waiting time as they move from station to station. The model is then programmed to add up all the resource and time requirements, providing estimates of total resources required and how fast patients may be processed.

Box 1: More Complex Model Types

Many models contain more detailed rules than those described in the main text. The expanded number of rules increases complexity as well as the amount of data or assumptions needed to define input values. The increased complexity (and resultant uncertainty) can cause these models to be used less frequently by emergency response leadership.

Network models: In public health, network models often represent individuals as points or "nodes," with nodes being connected by "edges." These edges are where interactions like disease transmission can occur. Defining rules for such interactions can provide insight into mechanisms of disease transmission that are not possible with compartmental models (e.g., highlighting the role of so-called superspreaders). These models require data measuring contact patterns between individuals that are almost universally unavailable during the timeframe of an emergency response, making their application in real time difficult at best.

Individual or agent-based models: These models contain rules that govern the behavior of specific individuals (agents). This class of models allows us to gain insights into how the behavior of individuals, when combined, produces outcomes at the community level, for example how X% of infectious individuals effectively self-isolating will affect the extent and duration of an outbreak. The most data-intensive requirement for these models is the set of probabilities describing who infects whom, which also requires an understanding of who contacts whom. Such contact data are usually not available during outbreaks, and modelers mostly have to use contact data collected from other communities, often measured during non-outbreak situations. CDC's Community Flu 2.0 is an example. Even though it is limited to modeling a representative 1000-household community, it requires approximately 300 data points (CDC 2016).

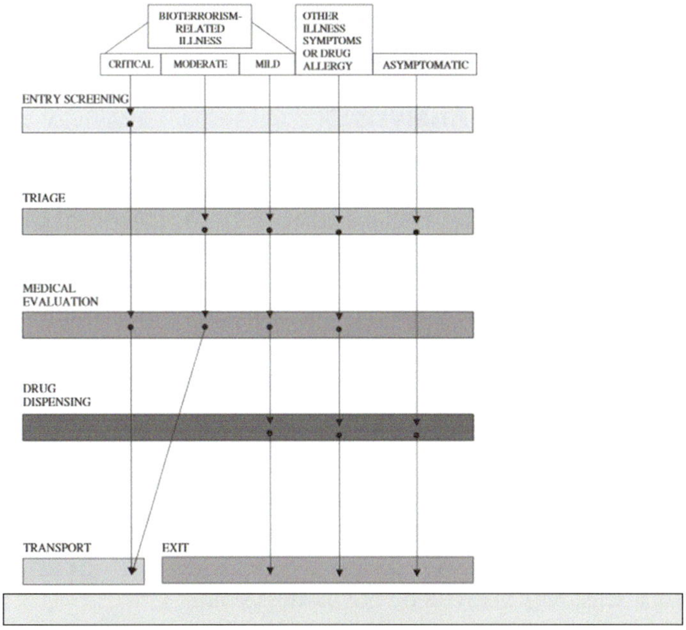

Fig. 5 Flowchart diagram from a published patient throughput model. (Hupert et al. 2002)

6 Dealing with Uncertainty: Methods of Sensitivity Analysis

Choosing the model structure is only the first step for providing useful modeling estimates in an emergency response. As noted, models are imperfect representations of reality, both in their structure and in the data used to populate them. When presenting modeling estimates to response leadership, it is therefore critical to convey the uncertainty of your estimates by conducting sensitivity analyses. A useful, disciplined contextualization of uncertainty through sensitivity analysis should accomplish at least one of the following goals:

1. Clearly illustrate the impact of uncertain input values upon the outputs.
2. Identify potential policy levers—inputs that represent options available to response leadership (e.g., number of persons who can be vaccinated in x time with y resources), and the changes likely to occur based on the options chosen.

We provide below a brief description of five common types of sensitivity analysis used to illustrate the consequences of uncertainty.

6.1 Univariate Analysis

The simplest form of sensitivity analysis is called univariate sensitivity analysis, in which the modeler assesses the impact on final outputs by changing the value of one input at a time. This method is good for illustrating the magnitude of impact that each input has on model outputs individually. Figure 6 illustrates the impact of changing model inputs (disease rates, intervention duration, vaccine efficacy, and vaccine uptake) within specified ranges on the number of estimated outpatient visits (one of the model outputs), relative to the baseline estimate. Of course, the fact that such sensitivity analyses do not address simultaneous changes in more than one input, or interconnections between inputs, places limits on their utility.

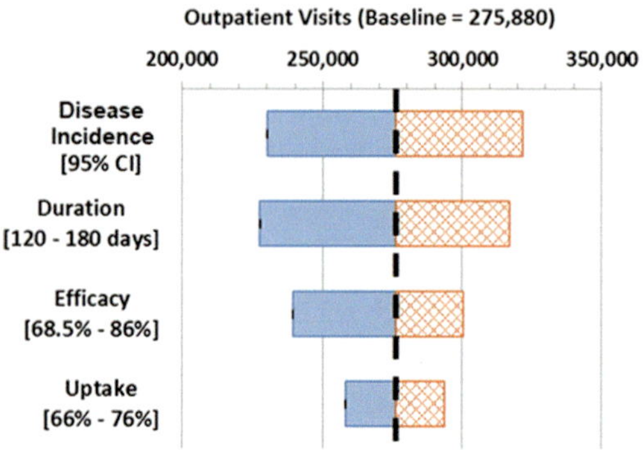

Fig. 6 A published example of univariate sensitivity analysis visualized using a tornado graph. (Adapted from Rainisch et al. (2020))

6.2 Multivariate Analysis

In a multivariate analysis, the modeler makes simultaneous changes to two or more input values, providing an illustration of the impact of uncertainty due to connections (correlations) between inputs. The greatest challenge in using this method, which can produce a large number of estimates, is finding the best way to explain the results, since response leaders do not typically have much time to spend understanding a complex model or examining its results. Figure 7 is a published visual representation of a multivariable sensitivity analysis. It shows how the cost-effectiveness of a proposed intervention changes when some key input variables are modified (namely age of contact, prevalence of malaria, and seasonality). This graphic allows modelers to visually explain that the intervention becomes more cost-effective (and perhaps even cost-saving) among older contacts as parasite prevalence increases, but that similar effects may not occur in contacts under age 14, and that this effect holds regardless of seasonality.

6.3 Scenario-Based Analysis

Another straightforward method to account for uncertainty is to construct several scenarios, each containing a different set of values

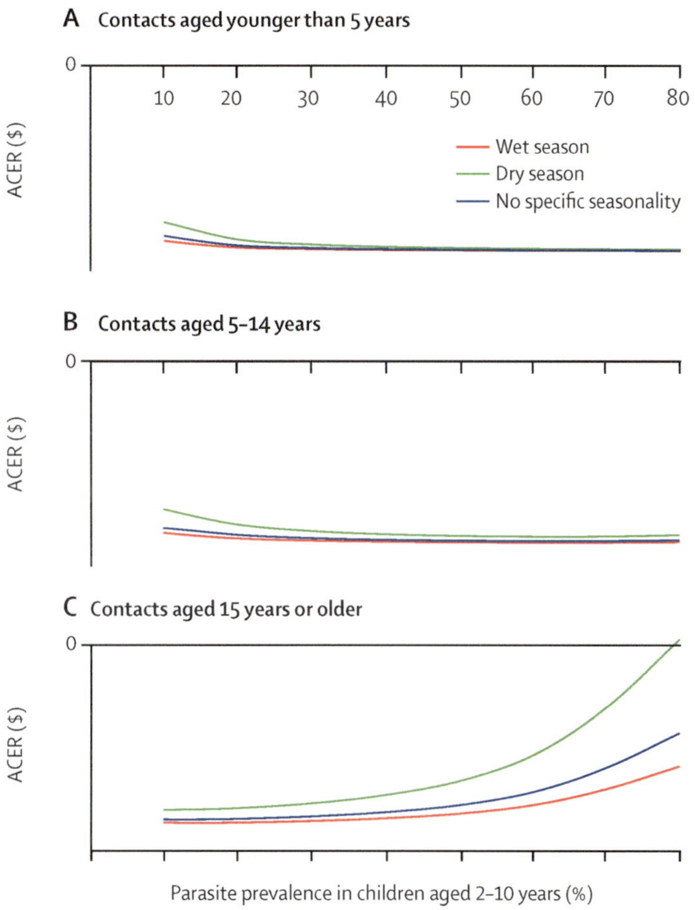

Fig. 7 Published example of multivariate sensitivity analysis (Carias et al. 2016). ACER is average cost-effectiveness ratio

and assumptions for the inputs—a what-if approach. The modeler and response leadership can then choose input values and assumptions to assess based on what they believe to be reasonable. Moreover, conveying results from this method is often easier than with other methods. The downside is that there is no inherent indication of the real-life probability with which a chosen scenario could occur.

6.4 Using Probabilities (Monte Carlo Simulation)

One of the more sophisticated methods of accounting for uncertainty is for the modeler to assign a probability distribution for each value (e.g., a distribution of the probability of an infectious person infecting others), instead of a single value. A specific value from the probability distribution is then randomly chosen and used to calculate an output (e.g., estimated total cases). This process is repeated numerous—often thousands—of times (iterations), producing a set of estimates illustrating the range, mean, median, and other measures of variability in the outcome. The biggest obstacle to using this method in emergency response scenarios is selecting the right probability distribution for each input value. Lack of data from the field for probability distributions forces the modeler to either use data from another source like a previous outbreak, or more often to make assumptions about the shape and dimensions of the probability distribution. An incorrect probability distribution could have a drastic impact on the conclusions drawn from the analysis, since sampling input values from an incorrect distribution over many iterations compounds the error(s). This method of accounting for uncertainty can also be hard to explain to a nontechnical audience.

6.5 Threshold Analysis

Response leaders typically understand that model estimates are uncertain due to inaccuracy or lack of data, especially in an outbreak. Leadership needs a clear illustration of what changes in estimated outputs (e.g., estimated rate of disease spread) would justify a change in response strategy. A modeler can generate information to guide decision-making by analyzing sets of input values to determine thresholds that warrant a change in policy or strategy. For example, response leaders would be well served by a model elucidating the set of conditions under which it would be prudent to stop building new Ebola treatment units (ETUs) and adopt a community-based isolate-and-treat strategy, which is less efficient at preventing disease transmission but quicker and cheaper to implement. Threshold analyses are often done in conjunction with other methods of sensitivity analysis, particularly multivariate sensitivity analyses (cf. ▶ Sect. 6.2). The key to making such threshold analyses useful is to avoid confining the analytical exploration of when to change response strategies to an overly limited range of input values.

7 Successful Modeling Is Not Just About the Model

A technically sound model is only one piece of a successful, model-based process to inform decision-making during a response. Given the high stakes of an emergency response and intense pressure to make consequential decisions quickly, effective communication between the response leadership and the modelers is crucial. Here we outline some effective communication strategies we have found beneficial for conveying modeling results that response leadership has used to make critical decisions (Meltzer et al. 2016).

7.1 Well-Defined Questions

Clearly defining the specific question that the modeler will seek to answer should be the very first step in any modeling project, regardless of setting. This becomes even more critical in an emergency because of the urgent need for results that can inform life-and-death decisions. Understanding what response leadership needs, and how the information will feed into decision-making, helps ensure that the analysis provides the most useful data possible. Keep in mind that there are many scenarios in which the question first proposed may not be the one that will provide the most useful information (see ▶ Sect. 4.4).

While there is no formula for creating a well-defined question, there are several well-tested criteria. A well-formed question should:

- be specific and lead to an informative, quantitative answer
- contain brief details of the problem being investigated, the interventions or strategies being assessed, and the outcome of interest
- contain some information about the intended audience, the analytic perspective, and the time horizon

Each analysis should focus on answering a single, well-formed question or a small, closely related set of questions. Attempting to answer multiple questions simultaneously invariably leads to an over-complicated, unfocused model and analysis. Large sets of questions should be broken down into several analyses, each focusing on a particular question. Defining specific, well-focused questions is frequently an iterative process, involving several rounds of discussion between the modelers and the response team. ▶ Box 2 contains an example of the iterative development of a focused question addressed by modeling during the 2014–2016 West Africa Ebola epidemic (Carias et al. 2016).

Box 2: Examples of Poor, Better, and Best Questions to Pose to Modelers

Poor: What is the value of providing antimalarial treatment to all contacts of suspected Ebola patients?

Better: How many cases of Ebola Virus Disease might be averted by providing anti-malarial treatment prophylactically to all contacts of suspected Ebola cases?

Best: Because of the similarity of symptoms for malaria and early-stage EVD, people with malaria may be referred to ETUs under the misimpression that they have EVD. Aside from burdening the ETUs, malaria patients awaiting screening results in an ETU may contract EVD. How many malaria patients could be prevented from presenting at an ETU if all those exposed to known Ebola patients received anti-malarial prophylaxis, and what would it cost the response per case averted?

7.2 Simple Approaches and Tools

When designing mathematical modeling methods and tools for emergency response one should take care to keep things as simple as possible while still effectively answering the question at hand. While complex models (cf. ► Box 1) are often useful in non-emergency research, there are many reasons to keep methods and tools simple during an emergency response.

7.2.1 Minimize the Likelihood of Error

The first reason to adopt simple models is that it reduces the errors and uncertainty associated with the larger numbers of inputs needed for more complex models. As noted, data from the field during an emergency response are usually limited and of uncertain reliability. Every existing input parameter based on uncertain data introduces more uncertainty into our results. Simplifying the model design where possible, without detracting from the model's ability to answer the question, allows the modeler to more directly interpret the outputs and relationships between inputs.

7.2.2 Enhance Usability and Dissemination

A simple model increases the chances of response leadership rapidly understanding and accepting the model and its results. Public health emergency response leaders often have diverse backgrounds, education, and experience. Few have formal training in modeling. A simple model is easier to explain to a diverse audience.

Producing a model that is successfully disseminated and used by response leaders depends upon the modeler keeping in mind the question (cf. ► Sect. 4.4), the intended audience (the response leadership team may include politicians, military officers, police chiefs, budget and public affairs professionals, and health care administrators as well as medical scientists), and their perspectives and needs. Emergency models should not be designed for research, nor should publication be the top concern.

7.3 Spreadsheet-Based Models

To enhance the likelihood that model results will aid decision-making, we have found it to be extraordinarily useful to provide copies of our models to the response leadership, typically in computer-based spreadsheet formats (Meltzer and Patel 2017). Disseminating spreadsheet-based models allows the leadership to explore the ramifications of changing particular inputs or assumptions at their own pace. This opportunity to "drive" the models themselves increases leaders' understanding of the results, the impact of uncertainty, and where decision thresholds may occur. Furthermore, professionals in many fields are familiar with spreadsheet programs like Excel, which can provide a level of accessibility and comfort that enhances user trust and uptake. ▶ Box 3 provides a few best practices, based on many years of emergency response modeling experience, that we have found useful in producing models suited for response leadership.

Box 3: Best Practices to Produce Simple Models for Emergency Response Decision-Making

Inputs and Input Values

- Use clear and direct names for each input, with additional notation as needed, so the user knows what each input represents, and the metric used to represent that unit.
- Divide long lists of inputs and group them by topic (e.g., epidemiological, logistical, and demographic parameters).
- Program the model so that users can immediately see the effect of changes in inputs.

Programming and Implementation

- Produce the model in a format that is widely used around the world and does not require a constant internet connection. Computer-based spreadsheet programs often meet this criterion.
- For greater transparency, break complex calculations down into intermediate steps.
- Produce a user-friendly interface that allows a user without modeling experience to easily enter or alter input data and readily interpret results.
- Provide non-technical documentation and notations, in the form of a manual if time permits.
- Improve user navigation through the model with color-coding of inputs and results.
- Minimize dependence on external computer programming technical package add-ins. For example, when using spreadsheet programs to produce a model, avoid programming macros, Visual Basic code, and other technical linkages that may introduce problems for the non-technical user who is making critical decisions.

7.4 Clearly Conveying Model Limitations

Again, models are simplifications. The simplifications and assumptions contained in models naturally lead to limitations in interpreting their outputs. Modelers should carefully note such limitations in their reports to encourage response leadership to think less about the precision of the results and more about the interaction of inputs and outputs, and the implications for choosing response actions. For example, even if model estimates of actual cases over time have been within 15% of actual reported cases, that is less important for decision-making than model results suggesting that increasing rates of vaccination by 10% might end an outbreak within 3 months. As the prominent statistician George Box (1979) said, "All models are wrong but some are useful."

7.5 Communicating with Response Leadership

Effective communication at all stages of the modeling process is vital to ensuring that modeling work will help response leadership make critical decisions. Clarifying the question at the outset (▶ Sect. 7.1) is essential to ensure all parties have common expectations for what the model will produce. Communication must continue during model development so that modelers and leaders agree on parameter choices and assumptions and on any changes to interventions and intermediate goals. Communication of results is pivotal, and modelers should ensure that the leadership fully understands how the results can be interpreted as well as the degree of uncertainty and limitations surrounding them (cf. ▶ Sect. 6). It frequently happens that providing a set of results raises a secondary set of questions that the response leadership will find useful, illustrating the iterative nature of modeling support for decision-making.

Particular sets of results may warrant dissemination beyond the immediate requestor. In such cases, the modeler should report the results in a form that allows diverse readers to understand the question analyzed by the model, as well as the most essential results. The modeler should also provide details—a brief description of methods, an explanation of limitations and caveats, some expanded results (including any sensitivity analyses), as well as a detailed technical appendix. This presentation style is quite different from writing for a peer-reviewed journal: the essential messages should be in the first paragraph ("bottom line up front"), with supporting details following, allowing a decision-maker with little time to get the gist quickly. ▶ Box 4 contains a guide to a memo format that has proven very successful at the CDC in effectively communicating model results to a diverse array of decision makers.

Box 4: Example Format of a Memo to Effectively Communicate Model Results to Response Leadership

Length: The Background, Question, Bottom Line Results, and one Key Fig. or Table should be presented in the first 2–3 pages. Higher-level authorities like cabinet ministers and heads of government may ask for even shorter memos. Additional sections, such the Brief Methods, Expanded Results, and Technical Appendix, can take several pages. Note that such sections will not be read as carefully as the first 2–3 pages, if at all.

Title: Should provide as much information as possible in non-technical language, so a reader will immediately have an idea of what they should expect to gain from reading the memo.

Date: When the memo was written and when the analysis was done; allows reader to assess whether the memo is the most recent and whether results may still apply.

Background: Brief information as to why the question addressed in the memo is important in the context of the current response.

Question: Tells the reader what the analysis was designed to answer. This should be written so the question and bottom-line results explain to the reader how the analysis informs the decision at hand.

Bottom-Line Results: Provides the reader with the most important set of results applicable to decision-making.

Key Fig. and/or Key Table illustrating bottom-line results.

Brief Methods: A brief, non-technical description of how the analysis was performed. More complete descriptions of methodology can be provided in a Technical Appendix.

Expanded Results: Additional results that may be relevant, but are not of immediate, critical importance to the decision at hand. This may include sensitivity analyses.

Limitations and Caveats: A clear statement of model limitations that impact the interpretation of the results.

Technical Appendices: Detailed information describing how the model was built, data sources, limitations, assessments of accuracy, etc. Ideally, this material will enable those with suitable skills and interest to independently replicate the model and results.

Version Control: Indicates sequentially produced memos and reduces confusion as to which set of results is being discussed. This may be up front or in a repeated heading but is mainly for the use of those producing rather than those reading the memo.

Change Log: Records changes between the memo versions (may be highlighted in text portions or placed in the Appendix).

8 Worked Example

8.1 Scenario

8.1.1 Situation

Assume an outbreak of hypothetical infectious disease ABV19 occurring on a large island (meaning a fixed population size). To date, there have been 1025 confirmed cases of ABV19 and 75,000 persons vaccinated in a population of approximately three million.

8.1.2 Epidemiology

Human-to-human transmission of ABV19 occurs with some probability through contact with the bodily fluids of an infected person. Risk of transmission is hypothesized to increase as an infected (and infectious) person's symptoms progress. The rate and degree of increased risk is unknown. Most cases (>95%) will begin to show recognizable symptoms within 15 days of contact with an infectious person (i.e., incubation period of up to 15 days). It is believed that a patient is infectious for approximately 7 days. Once patients infected with ABV19 have recovered they have lifelong immunity.

8.1.3 Public Health Interventions

Several public health interventions are underway:

1. *Case finding and isolation*: Reports of symptomatic persons are investigated, and the person is taken to a specialized treatment center and isolated to prevent the further spread of infection while receiving medical care.
2. *Contact tracing*: Persons who have been in contact with an infectious case are listed and then visited once a day for 30 days to check for the occurrence of any symptoms of the disease. If symptoms arise, they will be isolated temporarily and tested for infection. If the test returns positive, they are admitted to a specialized treatment center. If no symptoms have presented after 30 days, they are considered disease-free.
3. *Vaccination*: Persons listed as contacts are given the option of vaccination against the disease, as are those determined to have been in contact with these contacts (contacts-of-contacts). Previous studies have indicated that the vaccine requires 15 days to become fully protective. The ring vaccination strategy (▶ In Focus 22.1) is designed to produce a ring of protection around known transmission chains so that disease transmission will be contained within the ring and not "leak" into the general population.

8.1.4 Supply and Logistics

Supplies of vaccine are limited 75,000 doses of an existing 500,000 have already been expended, and response leadership fears supplies will run out. To conserve vaccine supplies, they are considering a fractional-dose strategy using either twofold or fourfold reduction of the standard vaccine dose, that is, half or one-quarter of the standard dose (▶ Case Study 25.1).

8.2 Clarifying the Question

The incident manager asks you, as the response modeler, to estimate the potential impact of using fractional doses of the vaccine. You discover that although using the fractional doses would indeed extend vaccine supplies, it would also, according to several available studies, prolong the interval before a vaccinated person acquires immunity. You immediately realize that there are realistic scenarios in which this extended period of susceptibility could increase the number of people infected. This would in turn raise the number of people requiring vaccination (contacts and contacts-of-contacts of these new cases) and potentially increase rather than reduce demand for vaccine and diminish outbreak control. (Case Study 25.1 discusses a use of mathematical modeling in which fractional dosing was found to be effective.)

You reframe the analytic question (▶ Sect. 4.4) to emphasize that the goal of the vaccination program is to prevent future cases, not to vaccinate as many people as possible. The question that you will now analyze is reformulated as follows:

- *Old question*: How many more people could be vaccinated using each proposed fractional vaccine dose (twofold and fourfold reduction)?
- *New question*: How will using the proposed fractional vaccine doses affect the number and timing of ABV19 cases averted and consequent vaccination requirements?

Discussion Question 1

How did rephrasing the analytic question improve your ability to convey actionable results to response leadership? (For example, it may have allowed you to identify thresholds or scenarios in which a fractional dosing strategy would be counterproductive (► Sects. 4.2 and 4.4).

8.3 Designing the Model

As you design the model, you realize that there are several inputs for which you do not have adequate data, including:

- The probability of acquiring the virus upon contact with an infectious case
- How transmission risk changes with progressing symptoms
- An understanding of the nature and frequency of contacts between persons in the population

8.3.1 Model Structure

To simplify the model's representation of the complex real-world system while accounting for missing data, you decide to produce a compartmental model (Sect. 5.1.1), which distributes and moves the population among the following compartments:

1. Susceptible (*S*): individuals who have neither been vaccinated against nor infected with ABV19.
2. Vaccinated within past 15 days (V<15): individuals vaccinated within the last 15 days and not infected.
3. Vaccinated more than 15 days ago (V15+): individuals vaccinated more than 15 days ago and not infected.
4. Infected (I): individuals who have been infected with ABV19.

8.3.2 Model Dynamics

You decide that disease transmission and vaccination will be modeled as follows in each 15-day timestep:

- We begin with a user-defined number of infectious cases.
- Each infectious case will be assigned a fixed number of contacts, and each contact will have a separate but also fixed number of contacts (i.e., contacts-of-contacts).
- Vaccination: eligible contacts and contacts-of-contacts (i.e., those not previously vaccinated or infected) will be offered vaccination. A percentage of them will accept the vaccine.
- Numbers vaccinated per day: Each day, eligible persons will be vaccinated as needed, up to a daily logistical limit defined by vaccination capacity.
- Order of vaccination: all contacts will be vaccinated before contacts-of-contacts.
- Disease transmission risks: You will compute the number of cases that will occur in the next time step by calculating the percentage of contacts that fall into each of the model's categories. Each category has a separate risk of infection:
  - Susceptible: not vaccinated, therefore no reduction in transmission risk.
  - Vaccinated within the last 15 days: vaccinated but do not have full immunity. Some proportion of these individuals may still become infected.
  - Vaccinated more than 15 days ago: vaccinated and have had time to build full immunity. A small risk of infection remains since the vaccine is not 100% effective.
  - Infected: these contacts have been infected and are either ill or have recovered; therefore, no risk of re-infection exists.

- Calculating the number of new cases: The number of new cases in the next time step is calculated by multiplying the number in each category by the category-specific risk of infection and then taking the sum across all four categories.

8.3.3 Data, Assumptions, and Simplifications

You will need to provide values or estimates for the following inputs for your model:

- *Number of contacts per case/Number of contacts per contact*

  Use the average number of contacts and contacts-of-contacts listed on contact tracing records available through the response operations center.
- *Vaccine acceptance rate*

  The number of persons offered vaccination and vaccinated to date should be available from response records, or you will have to make an educated guess based on discussions with experts involved in the response field activities.
- *Logistical limit on number of persons who can be vaccinated per day*

  You may be able to calculate the number of persons who can be vaccinated per day from reports available through the response operations center, which may also be able to help you calculate the extent to which they can increase the number with available resources.
- *Transmission risk (number infected per infectious person absent intervention)*

  Precise data is often unavailable. You will need to use the average number of new infections per case during the current outbreak to date as a proxy.
- *Vaccine effectiveness and days needed to build full vaccine-based immunity for full, half, and quarter doses*

  For this scenario, we will assume that the vaccine has undergone extensive clinical trials and field testing, at least for the full-strength dose. As for fractional doses, the experts believe that the twofold and fourfold reductions of the full vaccine dose will provide protection, but it will take three and five days longer, respectively, for vaccine-induced immunity to develop.

8.3.4 Other Assumptions

In addition to assumptions about parameter values, you have made some implicit assumptions as a result of your model design. For example, you have assumed that all contacts will receive vaccination before any contacts-of-contacts, which is unlikely to be true in practice. You have also simplified disease progression; even though there is a latent period when an individual is infected but has not yet become infectious, you have chosen not to include an "infected but not yet infectious" category in the model. Ensure that both you and your intended audience are aware of significant assumptions and simplifications (▶ Sect. 7.4).

Discussion Question 2

Identify some additional assumptions (either explicit or implicit) in the described ABV19 model and discuss how these assumptions may affect your presentation of model results to response leadership.

8.4 Presenting Useful Results

Once you have built your model and produced some estimates, you will need to present your results to response leadership as clearly and directly as possible. You decide to provide a written set of results in the memo format described in ▶ Sect. 7.5. Using that memo, you will likely want to request time at the next Incident Management meeting for a brief oral presentation of results. You should also plan to have an Excel version of your model available to help you answer leadership's questions (often of the what-if variety) through direct demonstration.

Your results indicate two main points that will inform a useful discussion about optimal vaccine dosing: first, because of the three and five extra days needed for full immunity for the half and quarter vaccine doses, respectively, the fractional dosing strategy will be unlikely to slow the rate of onward transmission as rapidly as the full-dose ring strategy and may end up requiring more vaccine (see ◘ Fig. 8). Second, your sensitivity analyses show how the uncertainty of the input values can affect the estimates. For example, in ◘ Fig. 9, you illustrate to leadership that uncertainty about the average number of new infections associated with each case of ABV19 could have a large impact on whether the outbreak can be successfully controlled and ended by public health interventions, or whether it could progress to an uncontrolled endpoint where the outbreak overwhelms the interventions and only ends for "natural" reasons. Regardless of the actual number of new infections per case, the impact of the extended susceptibility to infection increases as the vaccine dose decreases.

Policy implications: Extending the supply of vaccine will not itself help control and end the outbreak of ABV19. Further, there is a great deal of uncertainty regarding the potential impact of a fractional dosing strategy.

While you will touch on each of these conclusions and its policy implications, you intend to use the oral presentation to primarily highlight the first point: switching to fractional dosing may not be useful for maintaining vaccine supplies, since the additional doses gained from fractional dosing could be more than offset by the increase in persons requiring vaccination. To end the outbreak sooner, concurrent improvements in other aspects of the response are essential, such as increasing the proportion of cases discovered and isolated early on through improved surveillance

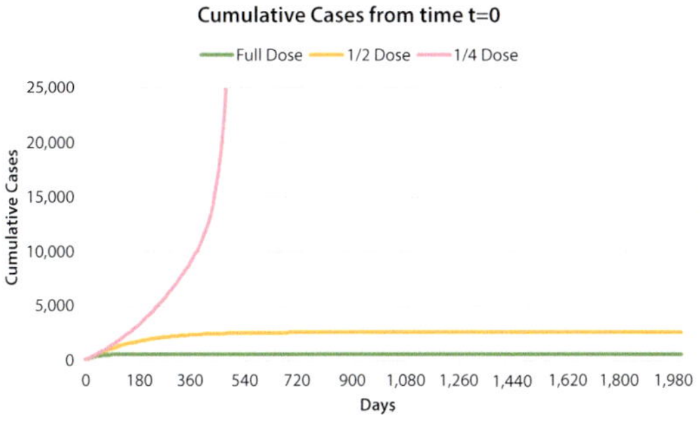

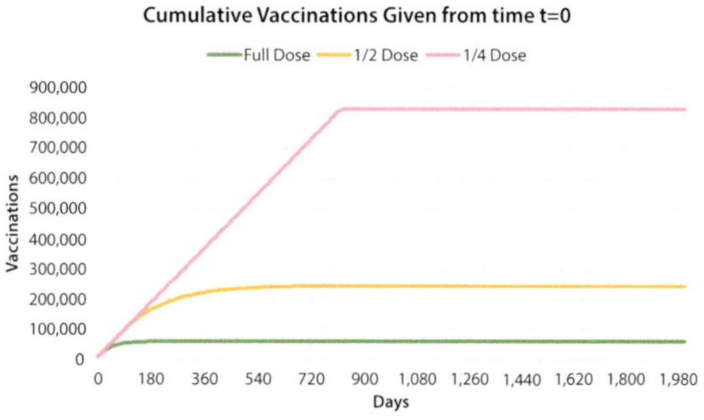

	Outbreak Controlled?	Days to End of Outbreak	Future Cases	Vaccinations Administered	mL of Vaccine Administered
Full Dose	✓	250	635	61,546	61,546 mL
1/2 Dose	✓	890	2,600	245,851	122,926 mL
1/4 Dose	✗				

◘ **Fig. 8** Example of policy-oriented visualization of model results. (Authors)

Univariate Threshold Analysis: # of New Infections per Case

# of New Infections per Case	# of Cases at End of Outbreak			# of Vaccinations Administered at End of Outbreak		
	Full	1/2 Dose	1/4 Dose	Full	1/2 Dose	1/4 Dose
1.20	242	433	572	20,326	37,372	50,012
1.47	348	1,392	*Uncontrolled*	29,793	118,852	*Uncontrolled*
1.58	421	*Uncontrolled*	*Uncontrolled*	36,476	*Uncontrolled*	*Uncontrolled*
1.80	725	*Uncontrolled*	*Uncontrolled*	63,351	*Uncontrolled*	*Uncontrolled*
2.10	*Uncontrolled*	*Uncontrolled*	*Uncontrolled*	*Uncontrolled*	*Uncontrolled*	*Uncontrolled*

◘ **Fig. 9** Example of a univariate threshold/sensitivity analysis on a key input parameter of your model. (Authors)

or contact tracing. Focusing on these key implications provides response leadership with a more comprehensive understanding of how using fractional vaccine doses could affect the trajectory of the outbreak.

You will provide a fuller exploration of results and sensitivity analyses in the written memo (▶ Sect. 7.5, ▶ Box 4). The memo will allow response leadership to learn the details at their own pace. You can also further highlight threshold input values at which policy decisions might change (▶ Sect. 6.5).

8.5 Avoiding a Data-First Approach

Note the order in which you approached the problem. The first step was to define the question so it would be most likely to yield an answer useful to the response leadership. Then you designed the model, concentrating on the structure needed to yield the answer to the question. Then, and only then, did you concentrate on the available data. It is a common mistake to look at the available data first and try to answer the question based on the data you have. If data are lacking in an emergency, that is (a) to be expected, (b) something the model is designed to help you cope with, and (c) itself something response leadership needs to know. Research efforts during an emergency to produce such data are possible, and a judgment on whether they are likely to be cost- and resource-effective will be within the purview of the response leadership.

9 Summary and Conclusion

Mathematical models are increasingly used to inform public health emergency response, particularly infectious disease response, as seen in the plethora of mathematical models devised to elucidate the spread of COVID-19 (Becker et al. 2021; James et al. 2021). The ability to take even minimal knowledge about a pathogen causing an outbreak and use a mathematical model to combine it with data from the current outbreak often provides a level of insight that is not available by any other means. Because mathematical models provide estimates for critical decision-making even when data are sparse, the use of such modeling during emergency responses will likely increase in the coming years. At the same time, the increasing viability of research during an outbreak into improving patient care, testing medical countermeasures, and conducting needed social science research (e.g., the nature and number of contacts between people in a particular culture with and without intervention) should provide modelers with better data faster to refine their models. It will remain essential for emergency response leadership to have a basic understanding of what modeling can and cannot do to improve the scope and effectiveness of response activities.

Discussion Questions

1. Leadership needs data to inform response actions during an outbreak, especially during the initial stages of the response when there is pressure to take immediate action. Discuss the four categories of questions that emergency response leaders generally ask modelers in such scenarios.
2. Discuss the salient pieces of information decision-makers need early in a response to gauge the resources required for a suitable response and to explain the unfolding situation to the public.
3. Define a model.
4. Explain critical differences between statistical and mathematical modelling, and their usefulness and limitations in a real-world setting for emergency response decision making.
5. Discuss what modeling can and cannot do and why modeling is useful for emergency response decision making.
6. Discuss compartmental, decision-tree, patient flow and throughput, and individual- or agent-based models.
7. Explain why methods of sensitivity analysis are important in dealing with uncertainty.
8. Describe the four common types of sensitivity analyses: univariate, multivariate, scenario-based, threshold.

9. Outline some effective communications strategies that are beneficial for conveying modeling results that response leadership can use for making critical decisions.

References

Ajao A, Nystrom SV, Koonin LM, Patel A, Howell DR, Baccam P, et al. Assessing the capacity of the US health care system to use additional mechanical ventilators during a large-scale public health emergency. Disaster Med Public Health Prep. 2015;9(6):634–41. https://doi.org/10.1017/dmp.2015.105.

Becker AD, Grantz KH, Hegde ST, Bérubé S, Cummings DAT, Wesolowski A. Development and dissemination of infectious disease dynamic transmission models during the COVID-19 pandemic: what can we learn from other pathogens and how can we move forward? Lancet Digit Health. 2021;3(1):e41–50. https://doi.org/10.1016/s2589-7500(20)30268-5.

Box G. Robustness in the strategy of scientific model building. Robustness in statistics. New York and London: Academic Press; 1979. p. 201–36.

Carias C, Greening B Jr, Campbell CG, Meltzer MI, Hamel MJ. Preventive malaria treatment for contacts of patients with Ebola virus disease in the context of the West Africa 2014-15 Ebola virus disease response: an economic analysis. Lancet Infect Dis. 2016;16(4):449–58. https://doi.org/10.1016/S1473-3099(15)00465-X.

CDC. Commuity flu 2.0. Atlanta, GA: U.S. Centers for Disease Control and Prevention; 2016. https://www.cdc.gov/flu/pandemic-resources/tools/communityflu.htm. Accessed 13 Mar 2020.

Crosby AW. America's forgotten pandemic: the influenza of 1918. Cambridge, UK: Cambridge University Press; 2003.

Hupert N, Mushlin AI, Callahan MA. Modeling the public health response to bioterrorism: using discrete event simulation to design antibiotic distribution centers. Med Decis Mak. 2002;22(1_suppl):17–25. https://doi.org/10.1177/027298902237709.

James LP, Salomon JA, Buckee CO, Menzies NA. The use and misuse of mathematical modeling for infectious disease policymaking: lessons for the COVID-19 pandemic. Med Decis Mak. 2021;41(4):379–85. https://doi.org/10.1177/0272989x21990391.

Meltzer MI, Patel A. Stockpiling ventilators for influenza pandemics. Emerg Infect Dis. 2017;23(6):1021–2. https://doi.org/10.3201/eid2306.170434.

Meltzer MI, Atkins CY, Santibanez S, Knust B, Petersen BW, Ervin ED, et al. Estimating the future number of cases in the Ebola epidemic—Liberia and Sierra Leone, 2014-2015. MMWR Suppl. 2014;63(3):1–14.

Meltzer MI, Santibanez S, Fischer LS, Merlin TL, Adhikari BB, Atkins CY, et al. Modeling in real time during the Ebola response. MMWR Suppl. 2016;65(3):85–9. https://doi.org/10.15585/mmwr.su6503a12.

Rainisch G, Meltzer MI, Shadomy S, Bower WA, Hupert N. Modeling tool for decision support during early days of an anthrax event. Emerg Infect Dis. 2017;23(1):46–55. https://doi.org/10.3201/eid2301.151787.

Rainisch G, Adhikari B, Meltzer MI, Langley G. Estimating the impact of multiple immunization products on medically-attended respiratory syncytial virus (RSV) infections in infants. Vaccine. 2020;38(2):251–7. https://doi.org/10.1016/j.vaccine.2019.10.023.

Shrestha SS, Swerdlow DL, Borse RH, Prabhu VS, Finelli L, Atkins CY, et al. Estimating the burden of 2009 pandemic influenza a (H1N1) in the United States (April 2009-April 2010). Clin Infect Dis. 2010;52(Supplement 1):S75–82. https://doi.org/10.1093/cid/ciq012.

Zhang X, Meltzer M, Wortley P. FluSurge—a tool to estimate demand for hospital services during the next pandemic influenza. Med Decis Mak. 2006;26(6):617–23. https://doi.org/10.1177/0272989X06295359.

25 Models in the COVID-19 Pandemic

Natsuko Imai, Marc Baguelin, and Neil M. Ferguson

Contents

Learning Track Note: This chapter appears in Learning Tracks: Biostatistics; Clinical Research

E. S. Higgs and R. A. Sorenson (eds.), *Principles and Practice of Emergency Research Response*, https://doi.org/10.1007/978-3-031-48408-7_37

Learning Objectives

This chapter should enable readers to understand and discuss

- The role of epidemiological analysis and mathematical modeling in providing insights for policymakers deciding on infectious disease emergency response options
- Basic features of the advanced analytics and mathematical modeling used during the COVID-19 pandemic, including key retrospective and prospective analyses and modeling
- How estimates of the SARS-CoV-2 reproduction number (R_0) from the start of the COVID-19 pandemic were important to decision-making
- What sort of investigations or data are needed to inform the optimal duration of case isolation or quarantine measures
- Why "nowcasts" are useful for improving situational awareness in addition to reported numbers of cases, hospitalizations, and deaths
- Why modeling of possible futures is useful for policymakers even if real-life outcomes can differ from model outputs

1 Introduction

The unprecedented scale and impact of the COVID-19 pandemic have challenged policymakers globally. Decisions on implementing socially and economically disruptive control measures have often had to be made on limited quantitative evidence. Epidemiological analysis and mathematical modeling are powerful tools for systematically synthesizing the knowns and unknowns, to highlight key knowledge gaps, and to provide quantitative insights into potential policy options. The pandemic has reinforced how modeling or advanced analytics can play an important role in informing policy responses.

For any emerging pathogen, rapid assessment and continuous monitoring of key metrics are crucial for response activities (◘ Table 1). Together, these help to address questions such as: What is the true scale of the epidemic? How fast is it spreading? How much of a threat does it pose? How bad will it get? And what can we do?

"Modeling" (▶ Chap. 24) is often used as a catch-all phrase that spans a wide range of interconnected quantitative analyses, including classical epidemiological studies; statistical models; mechanistic transmission models; and phylogenetic models. Modeling in the ongoing COVID-19 pandemic can be broadly split into three categories:

1. *Retrospective analysis* uses available data from the past to understand epidemic trends, estimate key parameters such as transmissibility and incubation period, and assess the impact of past interventions (e.g., estimating vaccine effectiveness).
2. *Prospective short-term forecasts* estimate how many new cases, hospitalizations, or deaths we might see in the next 3–6 weeks if current trends continue.
3. *Prospective scenario modeling and counterfactual analyses* explore what might happen in the future over the coming months under certain scenarios. The potential impact of different policy options can be quantitatively assessed, and the key uncertainties explored.

This chapter explores the advanced analytics and mathematical modeling used for planning and decision-making during the COVID-19 pandemic. ◘ Figure 1 shows the timeline of key analyses conducted during the pandemic up to December 31, 2021.

Table 1 Summary of key metrics required to address key public health questions (authors)

Public health question	Metric	Definition
How quickly will it spread?	Basic reproduction number (R_0)	The average number of secondary cases generated by a single case in a large entirely susceptible population
How many people will die?	Case fatality ratio (CFR) Infection fatality ratio (IFR)	The proportion of cases (CFR) or infections (IFR) that will eventually die from the disease
How many people will require healthcare?	Case hospitalization ratio (CHR) Infection hospitalization ratio (IHR)	The proportion of cases (CHR) or infections (IHR) that will be hospitalized
How easy will it be or how quickly will control measures need to be implemented?	Serial interval (SI) Generation time (T_g)	The time between symptom onset (SI) or infection (T_g) of the infector and infected in a successive transmission chain
How long should a case or contact be quarantined for? Or how long should they self-isolate?	Incubation period	The time between infection and symptom onset
	Duration of infectiousness	The time period that a symptomatic or asymptomatic case sheds infectious virus
Should close contacts of confirmed cases self-isolate? Or should routine testing of asymptomatic persons be introduced in certain settings?	Asymptomatic and infectious proportion	The proportion of infections that never develop symptoms but can transmit the virus
In what settings is the risk of transmission the highest?	Secondary attack rate	The proportion of known contacts that develop the disease
What are the drivers of transmission?	Overdispersion (k)	Heterogeneity in transmission
What is the potential healthcare capacity required?	Delay distributions	Duration of hospitalization or delay between symptom onset and death or recovery

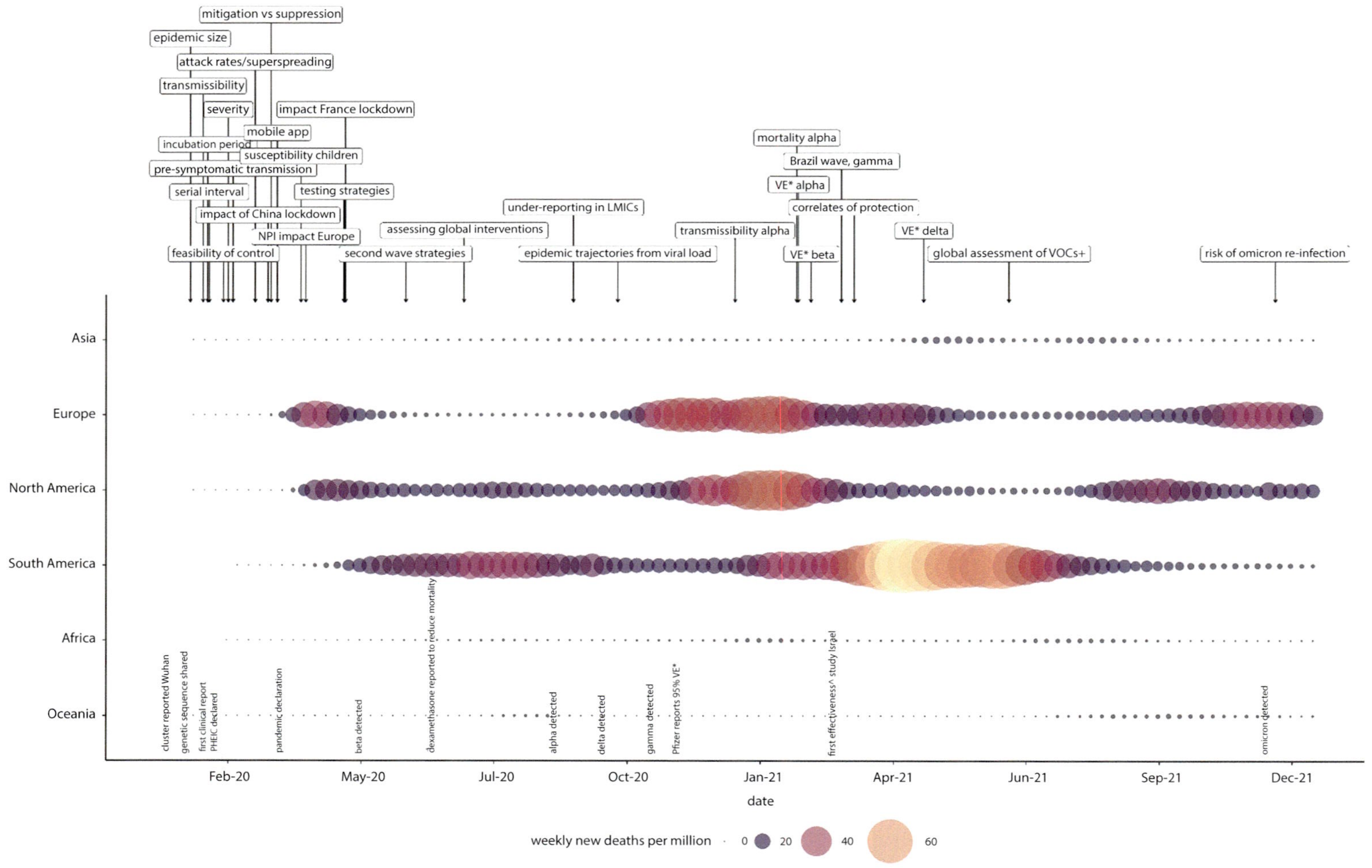

Fig. 1 New confirmed COVID-19 deaths per million population by continent over time (up to December 31, 2021). Labels along the top indicate key analyses and text along the bottom indicate key dates during the pandemic. Data as reported by Johns Hopkins University (Dong et al. 2020). *VE = vaccine efficacy, +VOC = variant(s) of concern. (Authors)

2 Retrospective Analysis

2.1 Assessment of Transmissibility

The basic reproduction number, R_0, defined as the average number of secondary cases generated by a single case in a large susceptible population, is a key metric that quantifies whether an epidemic is likely to take off. The epidemic will grow when $R_0 > 1$ and will shrink if $R_0 < 1$. Thus, the reproduction number helps to define the intensity of interventions required to bring the epidemic under control.

The earliest estimate of R_0 for COVID-19 was based on calibrating the proportion of simulations (generated using a branching process model and a range of R_0 values) that were statistically compatible with the estimated true size of the epidemic in Wuhan City (Imai et al. 2020a, b; Wu et al. 2020b). Estimates of R_0, growth rate and doubling times were also made directly from the initial epidemic curve of 425 patients (Li et al. 2020). When data are sparse, mathematical models can help to synthesize multiple data sets into a single quantitative framework. For example, the potential for sustained human-to-human transmission outside China was estimated by fitting a stochastic transmission model (a model that captures the randomness inherent in real infectious disease transmission and demographic processes) simultaneously to case data in Wuhan, in all of China, and internationally, and to the prevalence of SARS-CoV-2 infections in repatriation flights (Kucharski et al. 2020b). Alternatively, the outbreak aboard the *Diamond Princess* cruise ship in January–February 2020 provided an early opportunity to understand the transmission dynamics of SARS-CoV-2 within a closed setting. Using the daily incidence of new confirmed infections and a next-generation matrix approach, the effective reproduction number could be tracked in distinct populations (crew vs. passengers) over the course of the outbreak (Mizumoto and Chowell 2020). Furthermore, as cases were increasingly reported from provinces across China, using data on travel volumes and dates of travel, early transmissibility could be estimated by assuming or estimating the incubation period and serial interval distributions (Sanche et al. 2020). These early estimates of R_0, ranging between 1.5 and 3.5, established SARS-CoV-2 as a novel pathogen with pandemic potential and helped to define the level of interventions required to bring the epidemic(s) under control.

After the widespread implementation of nonpharmaceutical interventions (NPIs) such as school or workplace closures, the real-time estimation of SARS-CoV-2 transmissibility using branching processes (and extensions to this) (Cori et al. 2013; Thompson et al. 2019) became critical to understand the impact of measures and to assess by how much they could be lifted (Cowling et al. 2020; Leung et al. 2020).

2.2 Estimating Severity

The case and infection fatality ratios (CFR and IFR)—the proportion of cases or individuals infected who eventually die from the disease, respectively—are among the most important variables to quantify during an outbreak of a novel pathogen. However, the delay between the onset of symptoms and the eventual recovery or death of an individual and the bias in surveillance toward clinically severe cases may bias crude estimates of the severity of disease (Ghani et al. 2005).

The first clinical reports identified a high mortality associated with hospitalized patients, with risk of death increasing with age (Huang et al. 2020; CDC COVID-19 Response Team 2020; Zhou et al. 2020). However, estimating the denominator population (all cases or all infections) is challenging when diagnostic capacity is low and/or healthcare systems are overwhelmed. Thus, detailed data on outbreaks in closed populations such as onboard the *Diamond Princess* cruise ship can be beneficial for estimating CFR and IFRs (Russell et al. 2020).

Alternatively, synthesis of multiple data sources can help to provide robust estimates of severity by accounting for censoring (incomplete information about an individual due to the event of interest not occurring during the study period) and ascertainment biases (where some subgroups of the target population are less likely to be captured due to, for example, differences in clinical symptoms). By fitting to age-specific confirmed cases and deaths in Wuhan City, across mainland China, confirmed cases departing Wuhan international airport to destinations outside of China, and the prevalence of PCR-confirmed SARS-CoV-2 infection among repatriated individuals, a range of severity estimates could be generated (Verity et al. 2020; Wu et al. 2020a). The higher severity and rapidly increasing risk of death with age were informative for preparedness plans and exploration of potential policy options such as "shielding" the most vulnerable.

As data on SARS-CoV-2 seroprevalence became available, providing robust estimates of the number of infections within a population, this was combined with the age-specific number of cases and deaths within the same population to refine estimates of the IFR. A range of sophisticated analyses accounted for the delays between infection and seroconversion and infection and death, as well as uncertainty in seroprevalence estimates (Brazeau et al. 2020; O'Driscoll et al. 2021; Perez-Saez et al. 2021). These studies allowed more rigorous comparison of disease burden across different settings.

2.3 Incubation Period and Serial Interval

The incubation period (time between infection and onset of symptoms) and the serial interval (time between dates of onset of symptoms in consecutive cases in a chain of transmission) are important variables for interpreting trends in disease incidence. Closely related to the serial interval, the generation time is the time between the date of infection of an index case and that of a secondary case generated by that index. The incubation period and its variation require information on date of exposure and symptom onset and can help define the optimal duration of quarantine for contacts of cases. The serial interval requires contact-tracing data to identify potential chains of transmission and the dates of symptom onset within this chain. It indicates the controllability of an epidemic by determining the relationship between growth rate and R_0, the potential for pre-symptomatic transmission (Tindale et al. 2020), and how delays to case isolation may hinder control.

These key intervals were initially estimated empirically from clinical records (Guan et al. 2020; Xu et al. 2020) or by using data from international travelers with travel history to Wuhan. Fitting parametric probability distributions to these data allowed a probabilistic assessment of these intervals, for example, 95% of individuals developed symptoms within 12.5 days from infection (Backer et al. 2020; Li et al. 2020). Further analyses accounted for censoring, coarse data, or the sensitivity to the onset of specific symptoms, for example, cough vs. fever (Lauer et al. 2020; Linton et al. 2020).

Typically, contact-tracing or outbreak investigation data are needed to reconstruct transmission chains and estimate the serial interval from pairs of infector–infectees (Pung et al. 2020). Once interventions are implemented, it is important to account for the effect of isolation on truncating the serial interval (Bi et al. 2020). NPIs, and their implementation or relaxation, can affect the serial interval distribution over the course of an epidemic; this variation should be accounted for when assessing changes in the reproduction number (Ali et al. 2020). As SARS-CoV-2 has evolved over the course of the epidemic, the serial interval and generation time have changed, requiring estimates to be updated regularly (Hart et al. 2022).

2.4 Over-Dispersion and Attack Rates

The secondary attack rate (the proportion of known contacts who develop disease) and the degree of over-dispersion (heterogeneity in transmission) provide insights into the risk of transmission in different settings. By stratifying by the type of contact, such as household or workplace or by the age of the index case and/or contact, high-risk transmission settings or activities can be identified and targeted for interventions (Bi et al. 2020; Cheng et al. 2020; Jing et al. 2020; Laxminarayan et al. 2020). Systematic reviews and meta-analyses of attack rates pooling and stratifying estimates from multiple studies identified households and exposure in settings with close contacts, such as spouses, as high risk and an increased risk of transmission from symptomatic compared to asymptomatic index cases (Madewell et al. 2020; Thompson et al. 2021a).

At the start of the pandemic, some countries observed far fewer sustained chains of SARS-CoV-2 transmission than others. This suggested a high degree of variation in the number of secondary transmissions (often characterized by superspreading events—▶ In Focus 21.1). Early comparisons of imported and locally acquired cases identified a highly over-dispersed offspring distribution with approximately 10–20% of cases responsible for 80% of onward transmission (Endo et al. 2020). This finding was later validated by detailed contact-tracing studies and phylogenetic studies (Adam et al. 2020; Bi et al. 2020; Wang et al. 2020). Furthermore, the increasing transmissibility of the Alpha, Delta, and Omicron SARS-CoV-2 variants is associated with higher secondary attack rates—1.31 and 2 times higher for Alpha and Delta index cases, respectively, compared to non-VOC index cases (Buchan et al. 2022; Ng et al. 2021).

The combined findings of high-risk settings and evidence of superspreading events driving transmission helped to inform the World Health Organization's recommendation "avoid the 3 Cs": crowded places, close-contact settings, and confined and enclosed spaces (WHO 2020).

2.5 Assessing the Impact of Nonpharmaceutical Interventions

Assessing the impact of specific NPIs on transmission of a novel pathogen is critical for planning pandemic response measures—especially before, in the absence of, or where there is a shortage of vaccines or therapeutics. Early on, most countries implemented blunt "lockdown" measures in response to the exponentially growing pandemic.

The impact of restrictions imposed on movement between Wuhan and other cities across mainland China was estimated by combining detailed information on real-time mobility, the number of new cases outside Wuhan, and their travel histories, and showed that strict mobility measures could successfully reduce the growth rate (Kraemer et al. 2020). As restrictions were introduced in rapid succession across Europe, under fixed assumptions about parameters like the fatality rate and the delay between infection and death, information could be pooled across countries to estimate the time-varying reproduction number, R_t, and whether and how lockdown measures successfully drove this below the critical threshold of one (Flaxman et al. 2020). Gatto et al. (2020) used spatially explicit transmission models to estimate the effects of emergency containment measures as they were introduced in specific provinces before being implemented nationally in Italy and found that such measures reduced transmission by 45% (95% CI: 42–49). As surveillance for COVID-19 was established, transmission models could be fitted to detailed hospital data such as ICU admissions, hospital admissions, and bed occupancy to estimate changes in the reproduction number due to lockdown measures (Salje et al. 2020).

While studies agree that lockdowns were highly effective, quantifying which measures within the suite of social distancing measures were most impactful was vital as countries considered lockdown "exit strategies." In settings such as Hong Kong, where a package of interventions short of a total lockdown was implemented, comparisons of influenza R_t to previous years showed that the interventions additional to school closures (schools had been closed in previous influenza seasons) had a substantial effect on influenza transmission, which shares characteristics with SARS-CoV-2 (Cowling et al. 2020). Similarly, where different combinations or "tiers" of restrictions were implemented in specific regions in England, evidence synthesis approaches combining COVID-19 data with mobility and social contact data were used to quantify the impact of specific tiers on transmission (Davies et al. 2021b). Social mixing patterns have changed radically in response to behavioral changes and control measures. Comparisons of contact patterns collected through surveys before and after or during control measures can be used to estimate the change in the reproduction number and thus the impact of NPIs (Jarvis et al. 2020; Quaife et al. 2020; Zhang et al. 2020). Mathematical models can therefore be used to inform exit strategies but also to evaluate their success. In England, a stepwise lifting of interventions was planned alongside the rapid roll-out of vaccinations. By extending transmission models to account for vaccinations, the impact of increased transmission due to higher social mixing as interventions are lifted and the protective effects of vaccines can be disentangled (Sonabend et al. 2021).

2.6 Vaccine Effectiveness

Randomized controlled trials (RCTs) (► Chap. 22) have demonstrated high efficacy of multiple vaccines against COVID-19 (Baden et al. 2021; Polack et al. 2020; Sadoff et al. 2021; Voysey et al. 2021). However, the efficacies measured in tightly controlled RCTs are not always observed under real-world conditions. Robust estimates of vaccine effectiveness (VE), combined with age-specific estimates of severity and insights from modeling, can help to inform optimal vaccination strategies.

Following rollout of vaccines, a large number of vaccine effectiveness studies have been undertaken in multiple countries (Feikin et al. 2022). Large-scale cohorts (possible in settings where vaccination data can be linked to viral testing and outcome data) have been used to estimate interim single dose VE and VE against specific end-points, such as hospitalizations or death (Sheikh et al. 2021; Thompson et al. 2021b; Vasileiou et al. 2021). Analysis of these cohorts typically uses Poisson or negative binomial regression statistical models. Other observational studies have used matched cohort designs (Dagan et al. 2021) or test-negative case–control designs (Haas et al. 2021; Lopez Bernal et al. 2021a, b). The pandemic has also seen the development of novel approaches to assess VE against infection using large-scale asymptomatic testing, with commensurately more complex statistical analysis to account for potential biases (Pouwels et al. 2021).

2.7 Variants

The emergence and detection of new "variants of concern" (VOCs) of SARS-CoV-2, notably the lineages B.1.1.7 (Alpha), B.1.351 (Beta), P.1 (Gamma), B.1.617.2 (Delta), and B.1.1.529 (Omicron), have posed challenges for global pandemic control efforts. When a new variant emerges, rapid assessments of potential changes in severity and transmissibility must be made to inform policy responses. Genetic surveillance and the availability and timeliness of sequence data have been critical for these efforts.

Mathematical models can be fitted to data on the increase in frequency of a variant over time to quantify the relative growth rates of new variants (Davies et al. 2021a; Volz et al. 2021). Phylodynamic models can also estimate epidemic growth rates from the rates of genetic diversification over time (Volz et al. 2021). Mechanistic mathematical models can then be used to explore specific hypotheses for increased transmission such as variation in susceptibility by age, immune-escape properties, increased infectiousness, or longer durations of infectiousness (Davies et al. 2021a; Faria et al. 2021). Typically, new variants emerge and spread from a hotspot. Phylogeographic approaches integrating mobile phone mobility data were used to explore the spatial invasion dynamics of Alpha in England and the potential implications of the timing of NPIs and the levels of social mixing (Kraemer et al. 2021).

Where data on genetic testing and patient outcomes can be linked, survival models can quantify changes in disease severity associated with new variants (Davies et al. 2021c; Nyberg et al. 2022).

3 Prospective Modeling

3.1 Short-Term Forecasting

Real-time models, with parameters calibrated to an ongoing epidemic, can be used to provide insights into potential future trajectories and help with policy planning. Predictions about the course of an epidemic are often referred to as probabilistic forecasts (Cramer et al. 2022). A forecast is a set of time-bound outcomes associated with a probability distribution, for example, the number of beds occupied by COVID-19 patients at a certain date, with associated uncertainty (Gneiting and Katzfuss 2014). They are obtained by fitting a model to an ongoing epidemic and simulating outcomes based on the likely evolution of the parameters of the model. They are closely related to projections, where the model is fitted to ongoing epidemics and the outcome is based on assuming the parameters remain the same; and scenarios, where the outcome is based on parameters varied with predefined assumptions.

Short-term forecasts (less than 6 weeks) aid situational awareness and allow policymakers to plan for healthcare demand and allocate resources. A specific set of forecasts known as "nowcasts" can also provide a set of outcomes describing the current situation associated with a probability distribution. Due to reporting delays or lags to outcomes such as deaths associated with COVID-19, which can occur several weeks after the onset of symptoms, often, real-time data on cases or deaths may not be an accurate reflection of the true epidemic. This was true for COVID-19 when the rapid doubling time and exponential growth of the early epidemic meant that delaying control measures for a short period had a disproportionate impact on the final burden. For example, a 1-week delay in implementing lockdown in the first pandemic wave in England resulted in an estimated 20,000 additional deaths (Knock et al. 2021).

COVID-19 forecasting has benefited from existing forecasting consortiums for seasonal influenza (CDC 2019) or emerging outbreaks, such as Ebola (Viboud et al. 2018), led, for example, by the U.S. Centers for Disease Control and Prevention (CDC) (COVID-19 forecast hub 2022; Cramer et al. 2022). Many groups have made forecasting tools publicly available (Epiforecasts. 2022; Sheldon et al. 2020), and many countries reference forecasts or projections as part of their COVID-19 dashboards; for example, Australia (Australian Government 2020a, b, c), Hong Kong (Leung et al. 2021), Japan (National Institute of Infectious Diseases 2022), the Philippines (Philippines Dept of Health 2022), South Africa (National Institute for Communicable Diseases 2021), and the United Kingdom (Scientific Advisory Group for Emergencies 2022).

3.2 Scenario Modeling and Counterfactual Analysis

Policymakers have faced unprecedented situations during the multiple SARS-CoV-2 waves. In the initial absence of epidemiological studies quantifying the potential impact of the different intervention options, decision-makers often had to rely on and base their decisions on outputs of scenario modeling.

Scenario modeling shares many features of projections and forecasts obtained using models fitted to the current outbreak, often using a Bayesian methodology to integrate multiple data sources and reflect uncertainty. While forecasts and short-term projections can rely on simpler models, the modeling and exploration of policy scenarios require the inclusion of more complex mechanisms, such as explicitly modeling mass action transmission as a function of contacts in an age-stratified population.

These scenarios are usually built around a central scenario, commonly the *status quo* or else what is judged the most likely course of action, with alternative (counterfactual) scenarios. Each scenario provides outputs using a number of metrics, for example, the cumulative number of deaths or hospitalizations over time, or number of general or intensive care beds occupied at the peak of the predicted wave. This information allows decision-makers to balance the societal and economic cost of interventions with the potential scale of mortality or the risk of healthcare capacity being overwhelmed. Note that this type of modeling is primarily an aid to policy thinking, rather than scientific research per se.

Early in the pandemic, counterfactual analyses focused on the impact of potential restrictions to mitigate deaths and avoid health systems being overwhelmed by a sudden increase in hospitalizations. These analyses assumed an ability to impose restrictions that reduced R_0 below 1 and compared the feasibility of implementing strict "COVID-zero," a range of NPI measures, or a "laissez faire" strategy (Australian Government 2020a; Habib 2020; Imperial College COVID-19 Response Team 2020; Ministry of Health Manatu Hauora 2021).

Following the initial lockdowns, models then focused on modeling resurgence of transmission (second wave) based on seasonal factors and the degree of return to pre-pandemic social mixing (Monod et al. 2021; Panovska-Griffiths et al. 2020). The main public health question was the potential level of resurgence following the partial lifting of NPIs given the absence of widespread population immunity and no vaccine. In the United Kingdom, the potential for resurgence in the autumn and winter of 2020 was framed in terms of a "reasonable worst-case scenario." This uses a set of assumptions defined as "pessimistic" as assessed by expert opinion (or based on past data if available) but regarded as still plausible (Academy of Medical Sciences 2020; Spectator 2020). Such models provide policymakers with a useable benchmark for resourcing and planning.

"Novel" interventions, less stringent than lockdowns but still with potential to mitigate an increase in infections, were also explored in the second half of 2020. These included face coverings (IHME COVID-19 Forecasting Team 2021), contact-tracing and isolation to control COVID-19 transmission (Hellewell et al. 2020), various molecular testing strategies (Grassly et al. 2020), or a combination of multiple measures (Kucharski et al. 2020a). Other studies explored the feasibility of digital automated contact-tracing through dedicated mobile phone applications (Abueg et al. 2021; Cencetti et al. 2021; Ferretti et al. 2020).

The emergence of VOCs highlighted the importance of using scenario analyses to revise plans if necessary. A good example of this is the modeling informing "the roadmap out of lockdown" in England (Scientific Pandemic Influenza Group on Modelling 2021c, d; UK Government 2021). Analyses following the emergence of the Delta variant informed and led to the government delaying the final "step 4" lifting of COVID-19 restrictions by 1 month (Scientific Pandemic Influenza Group on Modelling 2021a, b).

The availability of effective vaccines starting at the end of 2020 led to modeling studies looking at their potential impact, examining a variety of allocation strategies and rollout scenarios (Bubar et al. 2021; Hogan et al. 2021). The initial vaccine prioritization from National Immunization Technical Advisory Groups[1] worldwide was largely driven by the age of vaccine recipients, given the marked age-specific severity profile (Verity et al. 2020) and the uncertainty around how effectively vaccines could protect against infections or onward transmission from breakthrough infections. This age-based prioritization was supported by early modeling studies (Foy et al. 2021) suggesting that strategies prioritizing younger age groups in order to reduce transmission, rather than to reduce hospitalizations and deaths, would only be practical with a large supply of transmission-blocking vaccines (Hogan et al. 2021). Regardless of strategy, economic modeling demonstrated the favorable cost–benefit of vaccines compared to NPIs (Sandmann et al. 2021).

1 National Immunization Technical Advisory Groups (NITAGs) are multidisciplinary groups of national experts responsible for providing independent, evidence-informed advice to policymakers and program managers on policy issues related to immunization and vaccines. The Global Vaccine Action Plan called for all countries to establish or have access to a NITAG by 2020. As of 2019, 120 countries reported the existence of a group meeting the criteria of a well-established NITAG (WHO 2021).

In early 2021, despite the emergence of the more severe and transmissible Alpha variant (Davies et al. 2021a; Volz et al. 2021), the wide availability of vaccines in some countries led to the potential of reaching high vaccine coverage in the most vulnerable groups. In this context, models have been used to define the pace at which NPIs could be lifted as a function of the vaccine roll-out plan, to avoid a substantial "exit wave." Such modeling informed England's "roadmap out of lockdown," which defined the lifting of restrictions in successive steps (Moore et al. 2021). While initial models did not consider new variants, the emergence and global spread of the Delta variant, which was even more transmissible and severe than the Alpha variant, forced a rethink of existing models. New models had to incorporate multiple variants (mechanism of replacement), impact of policy on behavior and transmission, a reduction in vaccine effectiveness (relative to Alpha), and increasing vaccine-induced immunity (Sonabend et al. 2021).

In October 2021, a new variant, Omicron, was first reported in South Africa. Modeling quickly estimated the potential for substantial immune escape, reflected in the high level of reinfections observed (Pulliam et al. 2022). Projections for other settings demonstrated how this new variant was likely to sustain and prolong the circulation of SARS-CoV-2 (Barnard et al. 2021).

Throughout the pandemic, its trajectory has depended not only on current epidemiological parameters but also on viral evolution, human behavior, and policy decisions. Additionally, longer term model-based projections can impact behavior or policies, subsequently making the initial projection "wrong" if the control measures in place are changed, for example. Counterfactual modeling scenarios have in some cases been misinterpreted by the public and media as predictions, with media often highlighting the most pessimistic of the many scenarios generated. Models rely on surveillance data to be calibrated, but new analyses are most needed when something new arises, for example, the emergence of a new variant, availability of a new vaccine, or a change in policy. In these situations, the key data to assess the impact of potential scenarios are often missing—such as the transmissibility or severity of the new variant, the effectiveness of the new vaccine, or the impact of the change in policy on transmission. Thus, analyses conducted early in the emergence of new variant carry large uncertainties. While such modeling is still valuable for policymakers, rigorous representation and characterization of such uncertainty are essential, as is assessment of the data needs and timescale required to reduce that uncertainty.

4 Conclusion

Epidemiological analyses and mathematical modeling have been vital tools in informing the COVID-19 response globally. As with any emerging pathogen, key policy questions need answers—"How quickly is it spreading?" "How severe will it be?" "What can we do?"—and the data necessary to address these questions have remained unchanged (Cori et al. 2017). While the speed and scale of the scientific response have been immense, the sheer volume of peer-reviewed and pre-print research produced has at times made it difficult to identify and robustly assess the emerging scientific evidence. Efforts to collate relevant information via evidence synthesis and systematic reviews have therefore been valuable in providing a wider overview of the pandemic, which has differed substantially by country. Furthermore, heterogeneity in data availability, particularly in low- and middle-income countries where testing capacity may be limited, has led to methodological developments using novel indicators including death certificates and changes in burial practices (Djaafara et al. 2021; Watson et al. 2021). Other advances include the development of guidelines for the standardized reporting of epidemic forecasts, which will improve the consistency and comparability of forecasts across settings (Pollett et al. 2021). However, there are substantial regional disparities in the technical capacity required to undertake rapid analysis and modeling to support the COVID-19 response, highlighting the need for in-country capacity strengthening, especially in low- and middle-income settings. Finally, as countries look toward lessons learned and future preparedness and response efforts, it will be vital to retain and build on the wide-ranging analytical capacity created and the strong international collaborative efforts taken in response to the pandemic.

Discussion Questions

1. Why is it important for decision-making to have estimates of the reproduction number (R_0) at the beginning of and throughout a pandemic, as well as in response to the emergence of new pathogen variants?
2. What sort of investigations (or data) are needed to inform the optimal duration of case isolation or quarantine measures?
3. How are "nowcasts" useful for improving situational awareness in addition to reported numbers of cases, hospitalizations, and deaths?
4. Why is modeling of future possible scenarios useful for policymakers even if we expect real-life outcomes to differ from model outputs?

References

Abueg M, Hinch R, Wu N, Liu L, Probert W, Wu A, et al. Modeling the effect of exposure notification and non-pharmaceutical interventions on COVID-19 transmission in Washington state. NPJ Digit Med. 2021;4(1):49. https://doi.org/10.1038/s41746-021-00422-7.

Academy of Medical Sciences. Coronavirus: preparing for challenges this winter. London: The Academy of Medical Sciences; 2020. https://acmedsci.ac.uk/policy/policy-projects/coronavirus-preparing-for-challenges-this-winter. Accessed 7 Apr 2022.

Adam DC, Wu P, Wong JY, Lau EHY, Tsang TK, Cauchemez S, et al. Clustering and superspreading potential of SARS-CoV-2 infections in Hong Kong. Nat Med. 2020;26(11):1714–9. https://doi.org/10.1038/s41591-020-1092-0.

Ali ST, Wang L, Lau EHY, Xu XK, Du Z, Wu Y, et al. Serial interval of SARS-CoV-2 was shortened over time by nonpharmaceutical interventions. Science. 2020;369(6507):1106–9. https://doi.org/10.1126/science.abc9004.

Australian Government. Impact of COVID-19 theoretical modelling of how the health system can respond. Canberra. 2020a. https://www.pm.gov.au/sites/default/files/files/covid19-icu-modelling-summary.pdf.

Australian Government. Modelling the current impact of COVID-19 in Australia. 2020b. https://www.health.gov.au/resources/publications/modelling-the-current-impact-of-covid-19-in-australia.

Australian Government. Update: modelling the current impact of COVID-19 in Australia. 2020c. https://www.health.gov.au/resources/publications/update-modelling-the-current-impact-of-covid-19-in-australia.

Backer JA, Klinkenberg D, Wallinga J. Incubation period of 2019 novel coronavirus (2019-nCoV) infections among travellers from Wuhan, China, 20–28 January 2020. Euro Surveill. 2020;25(5):2000062. https://doi.org/10.2807/1560-7917.Es.2020.25.5.2000062.

Baden LR, El Sahly HM, Essink B, Kotloff K, Frey S, Novak R, et al. Efficacy and safety of the mRNA-1273 SARS-CoV-2 vaccine. N Engl J Med. 2021;384(5):403–16. https://doi.org/10.1056/NEJMoa2035389.

Barnard RC, Davies NG, Pearson CAB, Jit M, Edmunds WJ. Projected epidemiological consequences of the Omicron SARS-CoV-2 variant in England, December 2021 to April 2022. medRxiv. 2021. https://doi.org/10.1101/2021.12.15.21267858.

Bi Q, Wu Y, Mei S, Ye C, Zou X, Zhang Z, et al. Epidemiology and transmission of COVID-19 in 391 cases and 1286 of their close contacts in Shenzhen, China: a retrospective cohort study. Lancet Infect Dis. 2020;20(8):911–9. https://doi.org/10.1016/s1473-3099(20)30287-5.

Brazeau NF, Verity R, Jenks S, Fu H, Whittaker C, Winskill P et al. Infection fatality ratio: estimates from seroprevalence. London: Imperial College COVID-19 response team, Imperial College London; 2020.

Bubar KM, Reinholt K, Kissler SM, Lipsitch M, Cobey S, Grad YH, et al. Model-informed COVID-19 vaccine prioritization strategies by age and serostatus. Science. 2021;371(6532):916–21. https://doi.org/10.1126/science.abe6959.

Buchan SA, Tibebu S, Daneman N, Whelan M, Vanniyasingam T, Murti M, et al. Increased household secondary attacks rates with variant of concern severe acute respiratory syndrome coronavirus 2 index cases. Clin Infect Dis. 2022;74(4):703–6. https://doi.org/10.1093/cid/ciab496.

CDC. About CDC's flu forecasting efforts. Atlanta: Centers for Disease Control and Prevention; 2019. https://www.cdc.gov/flu/weekly/flusight/about-flu-forecasting.htm. Accessed 6 Apr 2022.

CDC COVID-19 Response Team. Severe outcomes among patients with coronavirus disease 2019 (COVID-19)—United States, February 12–March 16, 2020. MMWR Morb Mortal Wkly Rep.

2020;69:343–6. https://doi.org/10.15585/mmwr.mm6912e2.
Cencetti G, Santin G, Longa A, Pigani E, Barrat A, Cattuto C, et al. Digital proximity tracing on empirical contact networks for pandemic control. Nat Commun. 2021;12(1):1655. https://doi.org/10.1038/s41467-021-21809-w.
Cheng HY, Jian SW, Liu DP, Ng TC, Huang WT, Lin HH. Contact tracing assessment of COVID-19 transmission dynamics in Taiwan and risk at different exposure periods before and after symptom onset. JAMA Intern Med. 2020;180(9):1156–63. https://doi.org/10.1001/jamainternmed.2020.2020.
Cori A, Ferguson NM, Fraser C, Cauchemez S. A new framework and software to estimate time-varying reproduction numbers during epidemics. Am J Epidemiol. 2013;178:1505–12.
Cori A, Donnelly CA, Dorigatti I, Ferguson NM, Fraser C, Garske T, et al. Key data for outbreak evaluation: building on the Ebola experience. Philos Trans R Soc Lond Ser B Biol Sci. 2017;372(1721):20160371. https://doi.org/10.1098/rstb.2016.0371.
COVID-19 forecast hub. The COVID-19 forecast hub, Amherst, MA. 2022. https://covid19forecasthub.org/. Accessed 6 Apr 2022.
Cowling BJ, Ali ST, Ng TWY, Tsang TK, Li JCM, Fong MW et al. Impact assessment of non-pharmaceutical interventions against Impact assessment of non-pharmaceutical interventions against coronavirus disease 2019 and influenza in Hong Kong: an observational study. Lancet Public Health 2020. 5:e279-ee88.
Cramer EY, et al. Evaluation of individual and ensemble probabilistic forecasts of COVID-19 mortality in the United States. Proceedings of the National Academy of Sciences. 2022;119(15):e2113561119.
Dagan N, Barda N, Kepten E, Miron O, Perchik S, Katz MA, et al. BNT162b2 mRNA Covid-19 vaccine in a nationwide mass vaccination setting. N Engl J Med. 2021;384:1412–23. https://doi.org/10.1056/NEJMoa2101765.
Davies NG, Abbott S, Barnard RC, Jarvis CI, Kucharski AJ, Munday JD, et al. Estimated transmissibility and impact of SARS-CoV-2 lineage B.1.1.7 in England. Science. 2021a;372(6538):eabg3055. https://doi.org/10.1126/science.abg3055.
Davies NG, Barnard RC, Jarvis CI, Russell TW, Semple MG, Jit M, et al. Association of tiered restrictions and a second lockdown with COVID-19 deaths and hospital admissions in England: a modelling study. Lancet Infect Dis. 2021b;21:482–92. https://doi.org/10.1016/S1473-3099(20)30984-1.
Davies NG, Jarvis CI, Edmunds WJ, Jewell NP, Diaz-Ordaz K, Keogh RH. Increased mortality in community-tested cases of SARS-CoV-2 lineage B.1.1.7. Nature. 2021c;593(7858):270–4. https://doi.org/10.1038/s41586-021-03426-1.
Djaafara BA, Whittaker C, Watson OJ, Verity R, Brazeau NF, et al. Using syndromic measures of mortality to capture the dynamics of COVID-19 in Java, Indonesia, in the context of vaccination rollout. BMC Med. 2021;19(1):146. https://doi.org/10.1186/s12916-021-02016-2.
Dong E, Du H, Gardner L. An interactive web-based dashboard to track COVID-19 in real time. Lancet Infect Dis. 2020;20(5):533–4. https://doi.org/10.1016/s1473-3099(20)30120-1.
Endo A, Centre for the Mathematical Modelling of Infectious Diseases COVID-19 Working Group, Abbott S, Kucharski AJ, Funk S. Estimating the overdispersion in COVID-19 transmission using outbreak sizes outside China. Wellcome Open Res. 2020;5:67. https://doi.org/10.12688/wellcomeopenres.15842.3.
Epiforecasts. London school of hygiene and tropical medicine, London. 2022. https://github.com/epiforecasts. Accessed 6 Apr 2022 2022.
Faria NR, Mellan TA, Whittaker C, Claro IM, Candido DDS, Mishra S, et al. Genomics and epidemiology of the P.1 SARS-CoV-2 lineage in Manaus, Brazil. Science. 2021;372(6544):815–21. https://doi.org/10.1126/science.abh2644.
Feikin DR, Higdon MM, Abu-Raddad LJ, Andrews N, Araos R, Goldberg Y, et al. Duration of effectiveness of vaccines against SARS-CoV-2 infection and COVID-19 disease: results of a systematic review and meta-regression. Lancet. 2022;399(10328):924–44. https://doi.org/10.1016/s0140-6736(22)00152-0.
Ferretti L, Wymant C, Kendall M, Zhao L, Nurtay A, Abeler-Dörner L, et al. Quantifying SARS-CoV-2 transmission suggests epidemic control with digital contact tracing. Science. 2020;368(6491):eabb6936. https://doi.org/10.1126/science.abb6936.
Flaxman S, Mishra S, Gandy A, Unwin HJT, Mellan TA, Coupland H, et al. Estimating the effects of non-pharmaceutical interventions on COVID-19 in Europe. Nature. 2020;584(7820):257–61. https://doi.org/10.1038/s41586-020-2405-7.
Foy BH, Wahl B, Mehta K, Shet A, Menon GI, Britto C. Comparing COVID-19 vaccine allocation strategies in India: a mathematical modelling study. Int J Infect Dis. 2021;103:431–8. https://doi.org/10.1016/j.ijid.2020.12.075.
Gatto M, Bertuzzo E, Mari L, Miccoli S, Carraro L, Casagrandi R, et al. Spread and dynamics of the COVID-19 epidemic in Italy: effects of emergency containment measures. Proc Natl Acad Sci USA. 2020;117(19):10484–91. https://doi.org/10.1073/pnas.2004978117.
Ghani AC, Donnelly CA, Cox DR, Griffin JT, Fraser C, Lam TH, et al. Methods for estimating the case fatality ratio for a novel, emerging infectious disease. Am J Epidemiol. 2005;162:479–86. https://doi.org/10.1093/aje/kwi230.
Gneiting T, Katzfuss M. Probabilistic forecasting. Annu Rev Stat Appl. 2014;1:125–51. https://doi.org/10.1146/ANNUREV-STATISTICS-062713-085831.
Grassly NC, Pons-Salort M, Parker EPK, White PJ, Ferguson NM. Comparison of molecular testing strategies for COVID-19 control: a mathematical

modelling study. Lancet Infect Dis. 2020;20(12):1381–9. https://doi.org/10.1016/s1473-3099(20)30630-7.

Guan W-j, Ni Z-y, Hu Y, Liang W-h, Ou C-q, He J-x, et al. Clinical characteristics of coronavirus disease 2019 in China. N Eng J Med. 2020;382(18):1708–20. https://doi.org/10.1056/NEJMoa2002032.

Haas EJ, Angulo FJ, McLaughlin JM, Anis E, Singer SR, Khan F, et al. Impact and effectiveness of mRNA BNT162b2 vaccine against SARS-CoV-2 infections and COVID-19 cases, hospitalisations, and deaths following a nationwide vaccination campaign in Israel: an observational study using national surveillance data. Lancet. 2021;397(10287):1819–29. https://doi.org/10.1016/s0140-6736(21)00947-8.

Habib H. Has Sweden's controversial covid-19 strategy been successful? BMJ. 2020;369:m2376. https://doi.org/10.1136/bmj.m2376.

Hart WS, Miller E, Andrews NJ, Waight P, Maini PK, Funk S, et al. Generation time of the alpha and delta SARS-CoV-2 variants: an epidemiological analysis. Lancet Infect Dis. 2022;22:603. https://doi.org/10.1016/s1473-3099(22)00001-9.

Hellewell J, Abbott S, Gimma A, Bosse NI, Jarvis CI, Russell TW, et al. Feasibility of controlling COVID-19 outbreaks by isolation of cases and contacts. Lancet Glob Health. 2020;8(4):e488–e96. https://doi.org/10.1016/s2214-109x(20)30074-7.

Hogan AB, Winskill P, Watson OJ, Walker PGT, Whittaker C, Baguelin M, et al. Within-country age-based prioritisation, global allocation, and public health impact of a vaccine against SARS-CoV-2: a mathematical modelling analysis. Vaccine. 2021;39(22):2995–3006. https://doi.org/10.1016/j.vaccine.2021.04.002.

Huang C, Wang Y, Li X, Ren L, Zhao J, Hu Y, et al. Clinical features of patients infected with 2019 Novel coronavirus in Wuhan, China. Lancet. 2020;395(10223):497–506. https://doi.org/10.1016/S0140-6736(20)30183-5.

IHME COVID-19 Forecasting Team. Modeling COVID-19 scenarios for the United States. Nat Med. 2021;27(1):94–105. https://doi.org/10.1038/s41591-020-1132-9.

Imai N, Cori A, Dorigatti I, Baguelin M, Donnelly CA, Riley S, et al. Report 3: transmissibility of 2019-nCoV. London: Imperial College London; 2020a.

Imai N, Dorigatti I, Cori A, Riley S, Ferguson NM. Report 1: estimating the potential total number of novel coronavirus cases in Wuhan City, China. 2020b.

Imperial College COVID-19 Response Team. Report 9—Impact of non-pharmaceutical interventions (NPIs) to reduce COVID-19 mortality and healthcare demand. Imperial College London; 2020.

Jarvis CI, Van Zandvoort K, Gimma A, Prem K, Klepac P, Rubin GJ, et al. Quantifying the impact of physical distance measures on the transmission of COVID-19 in the UK. BMC Med. 2020;18(1):124. https://doi.org/10.1186/s12916-020-01597-8.

Jing QL, Liu MJ, Zhang ZB, Fang LQ, Yuan J, Zhang AR, et al. Household secondary attack rate of COVID-19 and associated determinants in Guangzhou, China: a retrospective cohort study. Lancet Infect Dis. 2020;20(10):1141–50. https://doi.org/10.1016/s1473-3099(20)30471-0.

Knock ES, Whittles LK, Lees JA, Perez-Guzman PN, Verity R, FitzJohn RG, et al. Key epidemiological drivers and impact of interventions in the 2020 SARS-CoV-2 epidemic in England. Sci Transl Med. 2021;13(602):eabg4262. https://doi.org/10.1126/scitranslmed.abg4262.

Kraemer MUG, Yang CH, Gutierrez B, Wu CH, Klein B, Pigott DM, et al. The effect of human mobility and control measures on the COVID-19 epidemic in China. Science. 2020;368(6490):493–7. https://doi.org/10.1126/science.abb4218.

Kraemer MUG, Hill V, Ruis C, Dellicour S, Bajaj S, McCrone JT, et al. Spatiotemporal invasion dynamics of SARS-CoV-2 lineage B.1.1.7 emergence. Science (New York, N.Y.). 2021;373:889–95.

Kucharski AJ, Klepac P, Conlan AJK, Kissler SM, Tang ML, Fry H, et al. Effectiveness of isolation, testing, contact tracing, and physical distancing on reducing transmission of SARS-CoV-2 in different settings: a mathematical modelling study. Lancet Infect Dis. 2020a;20(10):1151–60. https://doi.org/10.1016/s1473-3099(20)30457-6.

Kucharski AJ, Russell TW, Diamond C, Liu Y, Edmunds J, Funk S, et al. Early dynamics of transmission and control of COVID-19: a mathematical modelling study. Lancet Infect Dis. 2020b;20:553–8. https://doi.org/10.1016/S1473-3099(20)30144-4.

Lauer SA, Grantz KH, Bi Q, Jones FK, Zheng Q, Meredith HR, et al. The incubation period of coronavirus disease 2019 (COVI-19) from publicly reported confirmed cases: estimation and application. Ann Intern Med. 2020;172(9):577–82. https://doi.org/10.7326/m20-0504.

Laxminarayan R, Wahl B, Dudala SR, Gopal K, Mohan BC, Neelima S, et al. Epidemiology and transmission dynamics of COVID-19 in two Indian states. Science. 2020;370(6517):691–7. https://doi.org/10.1126/science.abd7672.

Leung K, Wu JT, Liu D, Leung GM. First-wave COVID-19 transmissibility and severity in China outside Hubei after control measures, and second-wave scenario planning: a modelling impact assessment. Lancet. 2020;395:1382–93. https://doi.org/10.1016/S0140-6736(20)30746-7.

Leung K, Wu JT, Leung GM. Real-time tracking and prediction of COVID-19 infection using digital proxies of population mobility and mixing. Nat Commun. 2021;12(1):1501. https://doi.org/10.1038/s41467-021-21776-2.

Li Q, Guan X, Wu P, Wang X, Zhou L, Tong Y, et al. Early transmission dynamics in Wuhan, China, of novel coronavirus-infected pneumonia. N Engl J Med. 2020;382:1199–207. https://doi.org/10.1056/NEJMoa2001316.

Linton NM, Kobayashi T, Yang Y, Hayashi K, Akhmetzhanov AR, Jung SM, et al. Incubation period and other epidemiological characteristics of 2019 novel coronavirus infections with right truncation: a statistical analysis of publicly available case data. J Clin Med. 2020;9(2):538. https://doi.org/10.3390/jcm9020538.
Lopez Bernal J, Andrews N, Gower C, Gallagher E, Simmons R, Thelwall S, et al. Effectiveness of Covid-19 vaccines against the B.1.617.2 (Delta) variant. N Engl J Med. 2021a;385(7):585–94. https://doi.org/10.1056/NEJMoa2108891.
Lopez Bernal J, Andrews N, Gower C, Robertson C, Stowe J, Tessier E, et al. Effectiveness of the Pfizer-BioNTech and Oxford-AstraZeneca vaccines on covid-19 related symptoms, hospital admissions, and mortality in older adults in England: test negative case-control study. BMJ. 2021b;373:n1088. https://doi.org/10.1136/bmj.n1088.
Madewell ZJ, Yang Y, Longini IM Jr, Halloran ME, Dean NE. Household transmission of SARS-CoV-2: a systematic review and meta-analysis. JAMA Netw Open. 2020;3(12):e2031756. https://doi.org/10.1001/jamanetworkopen.2020.31756.
Ministry of Health Manatu Hauora. COVID-19 elimination strategy for Aotearoa New Zealand. Aotearoa New Zealand: Ministry of Health Manatu Hauora; 2021.
Mizumoto K, Chowell G. Transmission potential of the novel coronavirus (COVID-19) onboard the Diamond princess cruise ship, 2020. Infect Dis Model. 2020;5:264–70. https://doi.org/10.1016/j.idm.2020.02.003.
Monod M, Blenkinsop A, Xi X, Hebert D, Bershan S, Tietze S, et al. Age groups that sustain resurging COVID-19 epidemics in the United States. Science. 2021;371(6536):eabe8372. https://doi.org/10.1126/science.abe8372.
Moore S, Hill EM, Tildesley MJ, Dyson L, Keeling MJ. Vaccination and non-pharmaceutical interventions for COVID-19: a mathematical modelling study. Lancet Infect Dis. 2021;21(6):793–802. https://doi.org/10.1016/s1473-3099(21)00143-2.
National Institute for Communicable Diseases. Modelling consortium (projections). Johannesburg: National Institute for Communicable Diseases, Division of the National Health Laboratory Service; 2021. https://www.nicd.ac.za/diseases-a-z-index/disease-index-covid-19/surveillance-reports/modelling-consortium-projections/. Accessed 4 Dec 2022.
National Institute of Infectious Diseases. Coronavirus disease (COVID-19). Tokyo: National Institue of Infectious Diseases (Japan); 2022. https://www.niid.go.jp/niid/en/. Accessed 4 Dec 2022.
Ng OT, Marimuthu K, Koh V, Pang J, Linn KZ, Sun J, et al. SARS-CoV-2 seroprevalence and transmission risk factors among high-risk close contacts: a retrospective cohort study. Lancet Infect Dis. 2021;21(3):333–43. https://doi.org/10.1016/s1473--3099(20)30833-1.
Nyberg T, Ferguson NM, Nash SG, Webster HH, Flaxman S, Andrews N, et al. Comparative analysis of the risks of hospitalisation and death associated with SARS-CoV-2 omicron (B.1.1.529) and delta (B.1.617.2) variants in England: a cohort study. Lancet. 2022;399(10332):1303–12. https://doi.org/10.1016/s0140-6736(22)00462-7.
O'Driscoll M, Ribeiro Dos Santos G, Wang L, Cummings DAT, Azman AS, Paireau J, et al. Age-specific mortality and immunity patterns of SARS-CoV-2. Nature. 2021;590(7844):140–5. https://doi.org/10.1038/s41586-020-2918-0.
Panovska-Griffiths J, Kerr CC, Stuart RM, Mistry D, Klein DJ, Viner RM, et al. Determining the optimal strategy for reopening schools, the impact of test and trace interventions, and the risk of occurrence of a second COVID-19 epidemic wave in the UK: a modelling study. Lancet Child Adolesc Health. 2020;4(11):817–27. https://doi.org/10.1016/s2352--4642(20)30250-9.
Perez-Saez J, Lauer SA, Kaiser L, Regard S, Delaporte E, Guessous I, et al. Serology-informed estimates of SARS-CoV-2 infection fatality risk in Geneva, Switzerland. Lancet Infect Dis. 2021;21(4):e69–70. https://doi.org/10.1016/s1473-3099(20)30584-3.
Philippines Dept of Health. Updates on novel coronavirus disease (COVID-19). Manila: Republic of the Philippines Department of Health; 2022. https://doh.gov.ph/2019-ncov. Accessed 6 Apr 2022.
Polack FP, Thomas SJ, Kitchin N, Absalon J, Gurtman A, Lockhart S, et al. Safety and efficacy of the BNT162b2 mRNA Covid-19 vaccine. N Engl J Med. 2020;383:2603–15. https://doi.org/10.1056/NEJMoa2034577.
Pollett S, Johansson MA, Reich NG, Brett-Major D, Del Valle SY, Venkatramanan S, et al. Recommended reporting items for epidemic forecasting and prediction research: the EPIFORGE 2020 guidelines. PLoS Med. 2021;18(10):e1003793. https://doi.org/10.1371/journal.pmed.1003793.
Pouwels KB, Pritchard E, Matthews PC, Stoesser N, Eyre DW, Vihta KD, et al. Effect of Delta variant on viral burden and vaccine effectiveness against new SARS-CoV-2 infections in the UK. Nat Med. 2021;27(12):2127–35. https://doi.org/10.1038/s41591-021-01548-7.
Pulliam JRC, van Schalkwyk C, Govender N, von Gottberg A, Cohen C, Groome MJ, et al. Increased risk of SARS-CoV-2 reinfection associated with emergence of omicron in South Africa. Science. 2022;376:eabn4947. https://doi.org/10.1126/science.abn4947.
Pung R, Chiew CJ, Young BE, Chin S, Chen MI, Clapham HE, et al. Investigation of three clusters of COVID-19 in Singapore: implications for surveillance and response measures. Lancet. 2020;395(10229):1039–46. https://doi.org/10.1016/s0140-6736(20)30528-6.
Quaife M, van Zandvoort K, Gimma A, Shah K, McCreesh N, Prem K, et al. The impact of

COVID-19 control measures on social contacts and transmission in Kenyan informal settlements. BMC Med. 2020;18(1):316. https://doi.org/10.1186/s12916-020-01779-4.

Russell TW, Hellewell J, Jarvis CI, van Zandvoort K, Abbott S, Ratnayake R, et al. Estimating the infection and case fatality ratio for coronavirus disease (COVID-19) using age-adjusted data from the outbreak on the Diamond princess cruise ship, February 2020. Euro Surveill. 2020;25(12):2000256. https://doi.org/10.2807/1560-7917.Es.2020.25.12.2000256.

Sadoff J, Gray G, Vandebosch A, Cardenas V, Shukarev G, Grinsztejn B, et al. Safety and efficacy of single-dose Ad26.COV2.S vaccine against Covid-19. N Engl J Med. 2021;384(23):2187–201. https://doi.org/10.1056/NEJMoa2101544.

Sanche S, Lin YT, Xu C, Romero-Severson E, Hengartner N, Ke R. High contagiousness and rapid spread of severe acute respiratory syndrome coronavirus 2. Emerg Infect Dis. 2020;26:1470–7. https://doi.org/10.3201/eid2607.200282.

Sandmann FG, Davies NG, Vassall A, Edmunds WJ, Jit M. The potential health and economic value of SARS-CoV-2 vaccination alongside physical distancing in the UK: a transmission model-based future scenario analysis and economic evaluation. Lancet Infect Dis. 2021;21(7):962–74. https://doi.org/10.1016/s1473-3099(21)00079-7.

Scientific Advisory Group for Emergencies. UK Government, London. 2022. https://www.gov.uk/government/organisations/scientific-advisory-group-for-emergencies. Accessed 7 Apr 2022.

Scientific Pandemic Influenza Group on Modelling. Summary of further modelling of easing restrictions (7 July). Coventry, UK. 2021a.

Scientific Pandemic Influenza Group on Modelling. Summary of further modelling of easing restrictions (9 June). Coventry, UK. 2021b.

Scientific Pandemic Influenza Group on Modelling. Summary of modelling on easing restrictions. Coventry, UK: University of Warwick & Imperial University London. 2021c.

Scientific Pandemic Influenza Group on Modelling. Summary of modelling on scenario for easing restrictions. Coventry, UK. 2021d.

Sheikh A, McMenamin J, Taylor B, Robertson C. SARS-CoV-2 Delta VOC in Scotland: demographics, risk of hospital admission, and vaccine effectiveness. Lancet. 2021;397(10293):2461–2. https://doi.org/10.1016/s0140-6736(21)01358-1.

Sheldon D, Gibson C, Reich N. Bayesian compartmental models for COVID-19. Amherst, MA: University of Massachusetts Amherst; 2020. https://github.com/dsheldon/covid. Accessed 6 Apr 2022 2022.

Salje H, Tran Kiem C, Lefrancq N, et al. Estimating the burden of SARS-CoV-2 in France. Science (New York, NY). 2020. p. 208–11.

Sonabend R, Whittles LK, Imai N, Perez-Guzman PN, Knock ES, Rawson T, et al. Non-pharmaceutical interventions, vaccination, and the SARS-CoV-2 delta variant in England: a mathematical modelling study. Lancet. 2021;398(10313):1825–35. https://doi.org/10.1016/s0140-6736(21)02276-5.

Spectator. Covid in winter 2020, a worst-case scenario. The Spectator; 2020.

Thompson RN, Stockwin JE, van Gaalen RD, Polonsky JA, Kamvar ZN, Demarsh PA, et al. Improved inference of time-varying reproduction numbers during infectious disease outbreaks. Epidemics. 2019;29:100356. https://doi.org/10.1016/j.epidem.2019.100356.

Thompson HA, Mousa A, Dighe A, Fu H, Arnedo-Pena A, Barrett P, et al. Severe acute respiratory syndrome coronavirus 2 (SARS-CoV-2) setting-specific transmission rates: a systematic review and meta-analysis. Clin Infect Dis. 2021a;73(3):e754–e64. https://doi.org/10.1093/cid/ciab100.

Thompson MG, Burgess JL, Naleway AL, Tyner HL, Yoon SK, Meece J, et al. Interim estimates of vaccine effectiveness of BNT162b2 and mRNA-1273 COVID-19 vaccines in preventing SARS-CoV-2 infection among health care personnel, first responders, and other essential and frontline workers—eight U.S. locations, December 2020–March 2021. MMWR Morb Mortal Wkly Rep. 2021b;70(13):495–500. https://doi.org/10.15585/mmwr.mm7013e3.

Tindale LC, Stockdale JE, Coombe M, Garlock ES, Lau WYV, Saraswat M, et al. Evidence for transmission of COVID-19 prior to symptom onset. elife. 2020;9:9. https://doi.org/10.7554/eLife.57149.

UK Government. COVID-19 response—spring 2021. London: UK Government; 2021.

Vasileiou E, Simpson CR, Shi T, Kerr S, Agrawal U, Akbari A, et al. Interim findings from first-dose mass COVID-19 vaccination roll-out and COVID-19 hospital admissions in Scotland: a national prospective cohort study. Lancet. 2021;397(10285):1646–57. https://doi.org/10.1016/s0140-6736(21)00677-2.

Verity R, Okell LC, Dorigatti I, Winskill P, Whittaker C, Imai N, et al. Estimates of the severity of coronavirus disease 2019: a model-based analysis. Lancet Infect Dis. 2020;20(6):669–77. https://doi.org/10.1016/s1473-3099(20)30243-7.

Viboud C, Sun K, Gaffey R, Ajelli M, Fumanelli L, Merler S, et al. The RAPIDD ebola forecasting challenge: synthesis and lessons learnt. Epidemics. 2018;22:13–21. https://doi.org/10.1016/j.epidem.2017.08.002.

Volz E, Mishra S, Chand M, Barrett JC, Johnson R, Geidelberg L, et al. Assessing transmissibility of SARS-CoV-2 lineage B.1.1.7 in England. Nature. 2021;593(7858):266–9. https://doi.org/10.1038/s41586-021-03470-x.

Voysey M, Clemens SAC, Madhi SA, Weckx LY, Folegatti PM, Aley PK, et al. Safety and efficacy of the ChAdOx1 nCoV-19 vaccine (AZD1222) against SARS-CoV-2: an interim analysis of four randomised controlled trials in Brazil, South Africa,

and the UK. Lancet. 2021;397:99. https://doi.org/10.1016/S0140-6736(20)32661-1.
Wang L, Didelot X, Yang J, Wong G, Shi Y, Liu W, et al. Inference of person-to-person transmission of COVID-19 reveals hidden super-spreading events during the early outbreak phase. Nat Commun. 2020;11(1):5006. https://doi.org/10.1038/s41467--020-18836-4.
Watson OJ, Alhaffar M, Mehchy Z, Whittaker C, Akil Z, Brazeau NF, et al. Leveraging community mortality indicators to infer COVID-19 mortality and transmission dynamics in Damascus, Syria. Nat Commun. 2021;12(1):2394. https://doi.org/10.1038/s41467-021-22474-9.
WHO. Avoid the three Cs. World Health Organization; 2020.
WHO. National Immunization Technical Advisory Groups (NITAGs). Geneva: World Health Organization; 2021. https://www.who.int/teams/immunization-vaccines-and-biologicals/policies/national-advisory-committees-on-immunization. Accessed 8 Apr 2022 2022.
Wu JT, Leung K, Bushman M, Kishore N, Niehus R, de Salazar PM, et al. Estimating clinical severity of COVID-19 from the transmission dynamics in Wuhan, China. Nat Med. 2020a;26(4):506–10. https://doi.org/10.1038/s41591-020-0822-7.
Wu JT, Leung K, Leung GM. Nowcasting and forecasting the potential domestic and international spread of the 2019-nCoV outbreak originating in Wuhan, China: a modelling study. Lancet. 2020b;395:689–97. https://doi.org/10.1016/S0140-6736(20)30260-9.
Xu XW, Wu XX, Jiang XG, Xu KJ, Ying LJ, Ma CL, et al. Clinical findings in a group of patients infected with the 2019 novel coronavirus (SARS-Cov-2) outside of Wuhan, China: retrospective case series. BMJ. 2020;368:m606. https://doi.org/10.1136/bmj.m606.
Zhang J, Litvinova M, Liang Y, Wang Y, Wang W, Zhao S, et al. Changes in contact patterns shape the dynamics of the COVID-19 outbreak in China. Science. 2020;368(6498):1481–6. https://doi.org/10.1126/science.abb8001.
Zhou F, Yu T, Du R, Fan G, Liu Y, Liu Z, et al. Clinical course and risk factors for mortality of adult inpatients with COVID-19 in Wuhan, China: a retrospective cohort study. Lancet. 2020;395:1054–62. https://doi.org/10.1016/S0140-6736(20)30566-3.

25.1 Case Study: Modeling Fractional-Dose Emergency Vaccination Campaigns for Yellow Fever

Joseph T. Wu and Corey M. Peak

Contents

Learning Track Note: This chapter appears in Learning Tracks: Biostatistics

E. S. Higgs and R. A. Sorenson (eds.), *Principles and Practice of Emergency Research Response*, https://doi.org/10.1007/978-3-031-48408-7_38

Learning Objectives

This chapter should enable readers to understand and discuss:

- Why WHO warned against cutting mosquito control programs when the incidence of yellow fever (YF) dropped around the world.
- The basis of the proposal to provide one-fifth of the normally recommended YF vaccine dose in response to a 2016 YF outbreak in Central Africa.
- How a dose-sparing immunization regimen could reduce the infection rate even if the smaller dose is less effective in preventing infection and disease.
- The mathematical modeling used by the authors to assess the impact of potentially reduced vaccine efficacy with fractional dosing on the YF infection attack rate.
- How the conclusions of the modeling study were applied in urban Kinshasa.
- Conference recommendations for further research on the efficacy of fractional doses in outbreaks.

1 Modeling Fractional-Dose Emergency Vaccination Campaigns for Yellow Fever

Yellow fever (YF) is a mosquito-borne disease with no specific treatment (WHO 2019b). During the 1950s, mass vaccination and intensive mosquito-control programs largely eliminated YF, except in sub-Saharan Africa and sporadic hotspots in South America. However, as the burden of YF subsided, many mosquito control programs were dismantled. The World Health Organization (WHO) has been warning for decades that such policy failure, together with changes in demography, land use patterns, and international air travel, would set the stage for explosive outbreaks of urban YF.

This premonition was realized when YF resurged and spread widely in urban Angola in late 2015 (Chan 2016). By May 2016, more than 2500 suspected cases, including 301 deaths, had been reported from all 18 provinces of Angola. Cases had been exported to Kenya, China, and the Democratic Republic of the Congo (DRC), and the risk of further international spread was escalating. Although WHO maintained a YF vaccine stockpile of about six million doses for emergency use in reactive campaigns, the stockpile was intended for responding to sylvatic spillovers and was therefore insufficient in size for controlling sustained urban outbreaks. Facing severe shortages of YF vaccines, WHO proposed dose fractionation for an emergency YF vaccination campaign in August 2016 to vaccinate eight million people in Kinshasa, three million in anterior Angola, and 4.3 million along the DRC-Angola corridor (Schnirring 2016).

Although empirical evidence suggested that a fivefold fractional dose was not inferior to a standard dose in terms of safety and immunogenicity (largely due to the excess of infectious viral particles in routine YF vaccine batches) (Visser 2019), it was not known whether equal immunogenicity implies equal vaccine efficacy (VE) for YF vaccines. To strengthen the evidence base for the public health benefit of dose fractionation of YF vaccines, we used mathematical modeling to assess the impact of reduced VE in fractional dose vaccines on the infection attack rate (IAR), defined as the proportion of the population infected over the course of an epidemic (Wu et al. 2016). Such an assessment would be particularly useful if the pathogen was not highly transmissible (e.g., the basic reproductive number R_0 of influenza is below 2 (Riley et al. 2007)) because even if dose fractionation reduced VE, the resulting higher vaccine coverage (VC) might confer higher herd immunity, in which case the number of infections could be significantly reduced by the indirect effect of large-scale vaccination. However, the transmissibility of YF in urban settings had never been adequately characterized before due to limited data, and hence the importance of herd immunity for YF vaccination was unknown. As such, the first step of our study was to estimate the R_0 of YF in urban settings by analyzing the epidemic curve of YF in Luanda, Angola. We found that in the absence of interventions, the R_0 of YF was around 5–7, which suggested that the intrinsic transmissibility of YF was not low. Therefore, the herd effect would not likely be substantial unless the immunization coverage (VC x VE) was close to the control threshold $1-\frac{1}{R_0}$.

Let VE(n) and IAR(n) be the VE and IAR under n-fold dose fractionation. We assumed that vaccine action was all-or-nothing, i.e., vaccines provided 100% protection against infection in a proportion VE(n) of vaccinees and no protection in the remainder. Under this assumption,

$$\mathrm{IAR}(n) = S_0\left(1-\mathrm{VE}(n)\mathrm{nV}\right)\left[1-\exp\left(-R_0\cdot\left(I_0+\mathrm{IAR}(n)\right)\right)\right]$$

where V was the vaccine coverage achievable with standard-dose vaccines, and S_0 and I_0 were the initial proportion of population that were susceptible and infectious. This simple model indicated that n-fold dose fractionation reduced IAR if and only if $\mathrm{VE}(n) > \frac{\mathrm{VE}(1)}{n}$ regardless of the transmissibility of the pathogen and pre-existing population immunity.

Having established the minimum requirement on VE(n) for n-fold dose fractionation to be non-inferior, we then considered VE(5) = 1, 0.9, 0.6 and 0.3 and compared the IAR when vaccines were administered in standard dose only versus according to the fivefold dose-fractionation proposed by the WHO for its vaccination campaign in Kinshasa. We parameterized the population demographics and pre-campaign vaccine coverage in the model using (1) the age distribution of Angola and Kinshasa from the World Factbook (CIA 2020); (2) the annual routine immunization coverage among children aged 12–23 months between 1997 and 2015 from WHO/United Nations Children's Fund (UNICEF) immunization estimates (WHO 2019a); and (3) vaccine coverage conferred by the emergency vaccination of around one million people in Kinshasa during May–June 2016. We estimated that the dose-sparing strategy would avert 7.1, 7.1, 5.4, and 1.3 million infections if R_0 = 4, and around 7.9, 7.9, 4.0 and 1.0 million infections if R_0 = 8–12. These figures were based on the assumption of a sustained epidemic, such that transmission declined when the population of susceptible hosts was depleted.

In conclusion, our rapid risk assessment model, shared via preprint in May 2016, showed that the proposed WHO dose-sparing strategy for the YF vaccination campaign in Kinshasa, DRC, would be a robust and effective strategy for reducing infection attack rate; it would prevent many more infections than using the vaccine at standard dosage, even with a large margin for error in case fivefold fractional-dose vaccine efficacy turned out to be lower than expected. WHO formally recommended the dose-fractionation strategy in July 2016 (WHO 2016a), and it was implemented in August 2016 (Fig. 1), during which nearly 7.5 million residents of urban Kinshasa received fivefold fractional dose vaccines and nearly 0.5 million children under two and pregnant women received standard dose vaccines, achieving an estimated 98% coverage of the target population (WHO 2016b). In June 2017, WHO published an addendum to its 2013 position paper on YF vaccine stating, "As a dose-sparing strategy, a fractional YF vaccine dose meeting the WHO minimum requirement for potency is expected to be equivalent to a standard YF vaccine dose with respect to safety, immunogenicity, and effectiveness" (WHO 2013, 2017c). Research conferences in 2017 and 2019 drew on several clinical studies that supported the efficacy of fractional doses in outbreak circumstances, while recommending further research on the duration of immunity and potential need for booster doses (WHO 2017a, 2020; Casey et al. 2019).

Here, mathematical modeling (▶ Chaps. 24 and 25) provided insights into the tradeoffs between individual-level vaccine efficacy and population-level herd immunity conferred by dose-sparing strategies. This approach bears relevance for questions of dose-sparing for other vaccines, e.g., inactivated polio vaccine

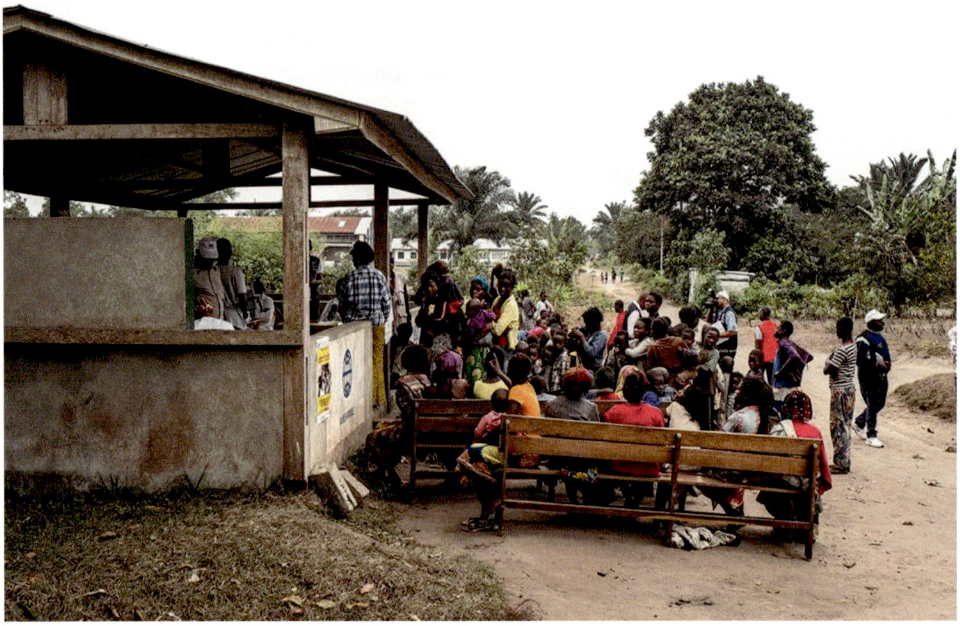

Fig. 1 Dose-sparing yellow fever vaccination campaign underway near Kinshasa. (Courtesy of WHO/E. Photo: Soteras Jalil)

(WHO 2017b), as well as dose-spacing approaches, for example with coronavirus disease 2019 (COVID-19) vaccines (Kadire et al. 2021; Tuite et al. 2021). With respect to the latter, delaying the administration of the second dose of a two-dose vaccine regimen has been implemented in some countries as a means to accelerate population coverage with the first dose, at the potential, uncertain cost of lower and/or waning efficacy during the time between when the second dose would be administered under the standard regimen and the second injection under the dose-spacing regimen. In principle, if during this period the average vaccine efficacy of the first dose remains above one-half of the vaccine efficacy following the second dose, then a dose-spacing regimen may reduce the infection attack rate.

Discussion Questions

1. During the 1950s, mass vaccination and intensive mosquito-control programs largely eliminated YF except in sub-Saharan Africa and sporadic hotspots in South America. As the burden of YF subsided, WHO warned against dismantling many mosquito control programs. Why?
2. Following YF's resurgence and spread in urban Angola in late 2015, cases were exported to Kenya, China, and the DRC, escalating the risk of further international spread. What prompted WHO to consider a fivefold fractional vaccine dose for an emergency YF vaccination campaign in August 2016?
3. The transmissibility of YF in urban settings had never been adequately characterized, so the importance of herd immunity in YF was also largely unknown. Briefly summarize the mathematical modeling used by the authors to assess the potential impact of vaccine efficacy being reduced by an uncertain amount by fractional dosing.
4. Briefly state the conclusions of this study and their application in urban Kinshasa.
5. Research conferences in 2017 and 2019 drew on several clinical studies that supported the efficacy of fractional doses in outbreak circumstances. What were

some recommendations for further research?

6. The mathematical modeling of this study provided insights into the tradeoffs between individual-level vaccine efficacy and population-level herd immunity conferred by dose-sparing strategies. Beside YF, this approach also bears relevance for questions of dose-sparing for inactivated polio vaccine and dose-spacing for COVID-19 vaccines. How could a dose-spacing regimen reduce the infection attack rate?

References

Casey R, Harris J, Ahuka-Mundeke S, Dixon M, Kizito G, Nsele P, et al. Immunogenicity of fractional-dose vaccine during a yellow fever outbreak—final report. N Engl J Med. 2019;381(5):444–54. https://doi.org/10.1056/NEJMoa1710430.

Chan M. Yellow fever: the resurgence of a forgotten disease. Lancet. 2016;387(10034):2165–6. https://doi.org/10.1016/S0140-6736(16)30620-1.

CIA. World factbook. Washington, DC: Central Intelligence Agency; 2020. https://www.cia.gov/library/publications/the-world-factbook. Accessed 2 Feb 2020.

Kadire SR, Wachter RM, Lurie N. Delayed second dose versus standard regimen for Covid-19 vaccination. N Engl J Med. 2021;384(9):e28. https://doi.org/10.1056/NEJMclde2101987.

Riley S, Wu JT, Leung GM. Optimizing the dose of pre-pandemic influenza vaccines to reduce the infection attack rate. PLoS Med. 2007;4(6):e218. https://doi.org/10.1371/journal.pmed.0040218.

Schnirring L. WHO plans to stretch vaccine as yellow fever persists in Africa. CIDRAP News. 2016.

Tuite AR, Fisman DN, Zhu L, Salomon JA. Alternative dose allocation strategies to increase benefits from constrained COVID-19 vaccine supply. Ann Intern Med. 2021;174(4):570–2. https://doi.org/10.7326/M20-8137.

Visser LG. Fractional-dose yellow fever vaccination: how much more can we do with less? Curr Opin Infect Dis. 2019;32(5):390–3. https://doi.org/10.1097/qco.0000000000000576.

WHO. Yellow fever vaccines position paper. Wkly Epidemiol Rec. 2013;88(27):269–84.

WHO. Fractional dose yellow fever vaccine as a dose-sparing option for outbreak response. WHO Secretariat information paper. Contract No.: WHO/YF/SAGE/16.1. Geneva: World Health Organization. Department of Immunization VaB; 2016a.

WHO. Yellow fever vaccination campaign in Kinshasa: More than 7 million vaccinated in 2 weeks. Geneva: World Health Organization; 2016b. https://www.who.int/news-room/feature-stories/detail/yellow-fever-vaccination-campaign-in-kinshasa-more-than-7-million-vaccinated-in-2-weeks. Accessed 23 Jan 2020.

WHO. Consultation on the research agenda for fractional yellow fever vaccination. Consultation on the research agenda for fractional yellow fever vaccination. Baltimore, MD/Geneva: World Health Organization; 2017a.

WHO. Use of fractional dose IPV in routine immunization programmes—considerations for decision-making.pdf. Geneva: World Health Organization. Initiative GPE; 2017b.

WHO. Yellow fever vaccine: WHO position on the use of fractional doses. Wkly Epidemiol Rec. 2017c;92(25):345–56.

WHO. WHO vaccine-preventable diseases: monitoring system. 2019 global summary. Geneva: World Health Organization; 2019a. http://apps.who.int/immunization_monitoring/globalsummary. Accessed 23 Jan 2020.

WHO. Yellow fever. Geneva: World Health Organization; 2019b. https://www.who.int/news-room/fact-sheets/detail/yellow-fever. Accessed 23 Jan 2020.

WHO. Consultation on the research agenda for fractional yellow fever vaccination. Washington, DC/Geneva: World Health Organization; 2020.

Wu J, Peak C, Leung G, Lipsitch M. Fractional dosing of yellow fever vaccine to extend supply: a modelling study. Lancet. 2016;388(10062):2904–11. https://doi.org/10.1016/S0140-6736(16)31838-4.

26 Social Science Evidence for Outbreak and Pandemic Response: Rapid Research and Analytics for Public Health Emergencies

Nina Gobat, Simone Carter, Ruth Kutalek, Sabina Faiz Rashid, Shelley Lees, and Julienne Ngoundoung Anoko

Contents

Learning Track Note: This chapter appears in Learning Tracks: Clinical Research; Preparedness; Research Ethics; Social Science Response Research

E. S. Higgs and R. A. Sorenson (eds.), *Principles and Practice of Emergency Research Response*,
https://doi.org/10.1007/978-3-031-48408-7_39

Learning Objectives

This chapter should enable readers to understand and discuss:

- Key considerations, practices, obstacles, and possible solutions for rapidly generating social and behavioral evidence in health emergencies
- How social-science data can help elucidate outbreak dynamics and how, when integrated with biomedical approaches, such data contribute to a holistic understanding of disease transmission, prevention, and control
- Ideal credentials for a social scientist who can be helpful in an emergency response
- Examples of practical questions social science scientists might ask at the start of an emergency infectious disease outbreak and how the resulting information can contribute to overcoming operational obstacles
- The concept of reflexivity
- How assessments of cultural, social, economic, and structural circumstances contribute to emergency response

1 Introduction

Outbreaks of new and re-emerging infectious diseases present an ongoing threat to global health security (WHO 2022c; Gostin et al. 2016). Human behavior and the underlying social, political, and economic structures of societies directly influence how disease outbreaks emerge and evolve (Farmer 1996; Lindahl and Grace 2015). Climate change, migration, deforestation, and urbanization are among the trends reshaping the social geography of the world, disrupting environments in ways that can favor the emergence or re-emergence of novel pathogens (Saker et al. 2004). Globalization and the ease of long-distance travel mean that once novel pathogens emerge, they can more easily and rapidly travel around the world and increase the spread of disease. In the absence of known medical interventions to prevent and treat infection, non-pharmaceutical measures to break chains of transmission are the first line of defense. Once novel medical countermeasures (MCM), such as vaccines, therapies, and diagnostics, have been developed, their potential to shift the trajectory of a health emergency depends on uptake and use. Moreover, health emergencies and the measures aimed at containing them disproportionately affect resource-poor settings, where many people live with fractured infrastructure, weak governance, fragile health systems, food insecurity, congested environments, or lack safe access to clean water. Evidence that draws attention to these social and behavioral dimensions of health emergencies is a key factor to inform inclusive, equitable and effective emergency response (Bedford et al. 2019; Carter et al. 2021; Afifi et al. 2020; Bedson et al. 2021).

The coronavirus disease 2019 (COVID-19) pandemic witnessed a step change in the use of evidence to guide policy and practice. Research was integrated into mainstream response. This was evident at local, national, and global levels. The breadth of social science research contributions became more visible during the pandemic and key areas of contribution were highlighted (Carter et al. 2020; Bedson et al. 2021; WHO 2020b; Bavel et al. 2020). Evidence from the social and behavioral sciences yielded data on the many social and cultural factors influencing uptake of response measures designed to slow the spread of the pandemic (Seale et al. 2020; van der Westhuizen et al. 2020; Martindale et al. 2021; Ryan et al. 2021; Voo et al. 2021). It provided explanations and insights into human behaviors that may seem counterintuitive, such as the zero-sum thinking that saw people in high income countries hoarding toilet paper, the politically aligned opposition to wearing of face masks, and rejection of safe and effective COVID-19 vaccines that brought promise of the end of the pandemic (Albrecht 2022; Mello et al. 2022; Andreas et al. 2022; van der Westhuizen et al. 2020). Social science also brought sharp focus to the immediate and longer-term impacts of the pandemic, highlighting biomedical and social vulnerability and the differential impacts of the pandemic on disadvantaged social groups. Understanding these dynamics is essential to shaping effective responses that account for social inequalities and seek to redress rather than perpetuate them (Rashid et al. 2020).

Research priorities

Objective 1

Generate high-quality evidence to achieving the goals of the strategic public health response plan.

- Promote the prioritization of knowledge needs according to epidemic dynamics
- Promote the production of knowledge according to local, national and regional needs
- Promote that knowledge outputs and methodological limitations are easily understood by non-social scientists

Objective 2

To develop and employ strong methodologies and theoretical frameworks to tackle current epidemic challenges

- Develop innovative interdisciplinary science
- Develop guidelines and Standard Operating Procedures (SOPs) to operationalized epidemic mitigation mechanisms
- Develop and connect global research networks with response partners
- Engage with communities to bring their voices to decision-making processes

Objective 3

To understand non-intended consequences of epidemic-control decisions

- Understand contextual vulnerability
- Understand how decisions in the field may inadvertently undermine response goals
- Understand how social and economic impacts need to be mitigated

Fig. 1 Summary of social science research objectives from the World Health Organization (WHO) Coordinated Global Research Map. (WHO 2020b)

Evidence from social science research drew attention to the impacts and adaptations of health services in community and hospital settings (Wanat et al. 2021; Hrynick et al. 2021; Chan et al. 2020), and to policy dynamics and the limitations of evidence informed practice (Vickery et al. 2022; Atkinson et al. 2020). Donors made important investments in social science research and the research community delivered an ambitious research program that impacted the way COVID-19 was managed around the world (Norton et al. 2021). Alongside these advances there were important innovations in how research was conceived and delivered, including research on infrastructure and the development of tools and novel rapid research methods (▶ Chap. 22) (WHO 2021, 2022a). For example, innovative data platforms enabled longitudinal data to be collected on public attitudes and practices related to public health and social measures (Collis et al. 2022; Betsch et al. 2020) (▶ In Practice 18.2). These socio-behavioral data were used at policy level to inform public health and social measures policy decisions, risk communications, and community engagement. The breadth and scale of COVID-19 expanded the scope and demand for social and behavioral evidence. However, as with other disciplinary approaches, a tremendous amount of social and behavioral evidence was produced and not all of it was used or useful (Fig. 1).

Drawing on lessons from COVID-19 and beyond, this chapter focuses on social science research to inform and strengthen emergency response. Social science is a broad academic field that includes behavioral science, psychology, anthropology, sociology, social epidemiology, economics, political science, bioethics, history, geography, health communications, and law, as well as other disciplines. These disciplines are united in their focus on societies, human behavior, and human relationships. The social sciences apply theories and scientific methodologies to the social, behavioral, historic, political, economic, and ecological processes that influence the emergence and evolution of disease outbreaks. To inform policy and operational decision-making during an emergency, different kinds of research are needed. Evidence aimed at impacting the trajectory of an outbreak during the acute phases needs to be rapidly produced. Longer term research, for example, research evaluating the wider impacts of an outbreak, is also valuable, particularly for recovery and for future outbreaks. By "research" we mean the systematic collection and analysis of data using appropriate and replicable methods to address a clearly articulated and well rationalized research question. Here we focus on the response phase of the health emergency cycle and address rapid production of data and evidence to highlight social and behavioral dynamics during an active outbreak. Without data, these dynamics often go unseen and unaccounted for. We include research to inform development or evaluation of interventions to tackle the acute phase of an outbreak. We do not include specific focus on monitoring and evaluation of programs. Our examples illustrate research conducted by social scientists as well as by others working in multidisciplinary emergency response teams.

Rapidly generated evidence provides timely data to inform decision-makers and make emergency response interventions better adapted, appropriate, and effective; helping slow disease transmission, reduce morbidity and mortality, and ultimately end an outbreak—the goals of all response research described in this volume. Understanding the lived experiences and needs of affected groups can help responders partner with affected communities to deliver disease prevention and control measures that are contextually appropriate, safe, and acceptable, and therefore more effective. These needs and realities are often highly dynamic and localized: what worked last year may not be successful now, and what is effective in one community will not necessarily work in the next one. Societies also vary greatly between rural and urban environments as well as within and across countries. Intersectional and large-scale factors such as power, class, gender, ethnicity, age, sex, religion, poverty, and politics also keep some groups more vulnerable than others. Awareness of these dynamics will influence the kinds of questions that are asked during a public health emergency, the types of data collected, and the ways in which those data are then used to inform community-centered response actions. ▶ Case Studies 1–5 provide examples of how evidence from the social sciences can help tackle operational challenges and inform response.

Case Study 1

Social Science Research to Inform Prevention of Nipah Virus Transmission in Bangladesh, 2009

Operational challenge: Preventing emergence of new zoonotic viruses depends on understanding the determinants of human risk. Nipah virus is a lethal zoonotic pathogen that has spilled over from bats into human populations, with limited person-to-person transmission. Human behavior patterns shaped by culture, social environment, poverty, etc. must be taken into account to understand transmission and to inform messages for transmission prevention. Social norms in affected communities in Bangladesh required that caregivers take close care of patients, often sharing the same bowls, cleaning up patients' bodily fluids, administering medicines, and often carelessly disposing of fluids, waste, etc.

Research: A collaborative team of epidemiologists and anthropologists co-developed culturally appropriate interventions to prevent person-to-person transmission of the Nipah virus in villages in Bangladesh. Practical, simple, and culturally appropriate messages were developed, including strong messages on (1) washing hands at key times, such as before eating, after feeding a patient, and after cleaning patient saliva, vomit, urine, phlegm, or feces; (2) keeping caregivers' and patients' food in separate bowls, not sharing leftovers; and (3) sleeping in separate beds, sleeping in head-to-foot position to avoid contamination, or sleeping on the floor. Pictorial cards were developed for caregivers taking care of adult and child patients. Responses to the messaging were assessed; communities emphasized the importance of clearly explaining the benefits of these measures, including social approbation (clean people praised by other caregivers), economic benefits (averting the costs of illness affecting the entire family), and health (benefits to both caregiver and patient).

Outcome: This research was helpful in designing public health intervention for communities where close contact with the sick is the norm (Islam et al. 2013) (◘ Fig. 2).

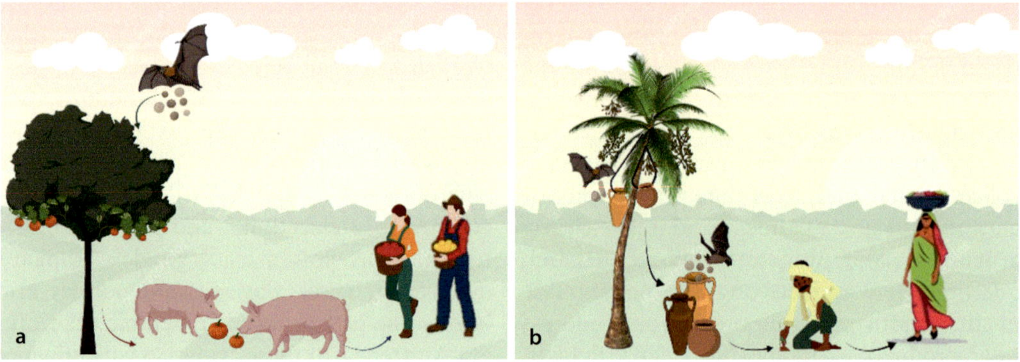

◘ **Fig. 2** Public material explaining transmission of Nipah virus in Malaysia and Bangladesh. **a** Shows the mode of transmission in Malaysia; bats roosting in fruit trees contaminate fruits, which are in turn are consumed by pigs, then pig to human transmission occurs. **b** Shows mode of transmission in Bangladesh, during the winter months, the season of harvesting date palm sap. The fruit bats contaminate the date palm sap stream and sap collection containers with saliva or urine. Consumption of contaminated raw date palm sap leads to human infection. (Hassan et al. 2022)

Case Study 2

Social Science Research to Inform Risk Communication during the Zika Virus Epidemic in Brazil, 2016

Operational challenge: The Zika virus epidemic erupted in 2015 with Brazil at its epicenter. To effect a fast response, most institutions generated, packaged, and disseminated recycled risk communications from past dengue campaigns, since both diseases are primarily spread via *Aedes aegypti* mosquito. This resulted in one-sided health communications targeting women and ignoring the underlying sociocultural and behavioral determinants limiting the feasibility of Zika virus prevention.

Research: A team of public health practitioners, anthropologists, and clinicians in Fortaleza, Brazil, used a rapid anthropological assessment (RAA) to explore how the prevention recommendations resonated with the target population. The RAA included (1) free-listing questions, where respondents provide as many answers as they can think of; (2) ranking prevention methods; (3) scenario discussions; (4) conversations with community members; (5) in-depth, semi-structured interviews with women of reproductive age; and (6) community observations. Findings were aimed at improving risk communications.

Outcome: This study provided insights into why disease prevention seemed ineffective during the outbreak. It highlighted how the repurposed dengue messaging fed complacency, as the information did not give Zika-specific instructions for prevention. The priority population did not believe the recommendations were realistic, as the messaging did not consider wealth disparities, sociocultural barriers, environmental issues, or interpersonal factors impeding the prevention of mosquito bites, pregnancy, or sexual transmission of the disease. Recommendations were then revised to create actionable, tailored, issue-specific messaging to best support disease prevention during the Zika outbreak (Stolow et al. 2020) (◘ Fig. 3).

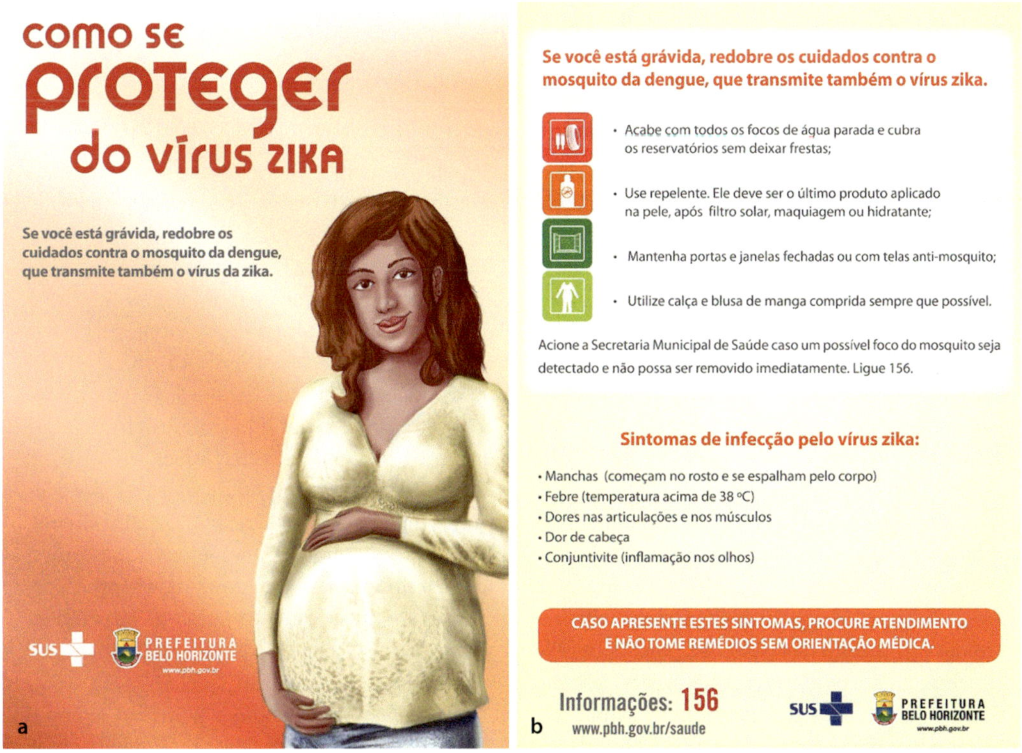

◘ **Fig. 3** A Brazilian Zika prevention brochure. As noted by Coutinho et al. (2021), there was much Zika prevention messaging but the burden of action was on women rather than advocating a community-wide response

Case Study 3

Social Science Research to Understand the Effects of a Financial Incentive to Increase Reporting of Ebola Cases, Liberia 2014

Operational challenge: During the Ebola epidemic in Liberia the World Bank planned to introduce incentivized contact tracing by suggesting that for each suspect case reported to officials, US$5 would be paid. It was assumed that such payment would increase the reporting of Ebola cases.

Research: A team of two epidemiologists and one anthropologist were asked to assess whether local communities would accept an incentivized contact tracing scheme. This information was needed rapidly to inform further emergency response interventions. It was decided that a rapid qualitative assessment with focus-group discussions would be the best and most feasible methodology and give communities the opportunity to openly air their opinion. Contact tracers, community leaders, women, and youth were invited to participate.

Outcome: The planned scheme was rejected by the study participants; they argued that it would create social disruptions in families and communities in already stretched social relations. Moreover, the study leads were able to provide operational ideas from the community on how the outbreak could be curbed. The investigation also demonstrates how interdisciplinary rapid qualitative assessments which strive to engage communities can prevent missteps in emergency response (Kutalek et al. 2015).

Case Study 4

Social Science Research to Inform Guidelines for Infection Prevention in a Home Where a Person with Confirmed COVID-19 Is Living

Operational challenge: During the COVID-19 pandemic, households were important sites for transmission of severe acute respiratory syndrome coronavirus 2 (SARS-CoV-2). Preventive measures were recommended. However, these measures focused on biomedical aspects of infection prevention and control and did not account for the lived experience of household members, including, for example, the very human desire to express care for loved ones when they were unwell.

Research: An observational mixed-methods study was conducted. Households with a person with confirmed SARS-CoV-2 infection were recruited via drive-through testing sites of municipal health services, healthcare worker screening, hospital emergency visits, primary care physicians, or preoperative screening. The research team recorded household characteristics, including those of all individual household members. In a subset of households, one adult household member was interviewed. The findings highlighted that all households reported implementing some preventive measures; however, the use of face masks was least frequently reported. Importantly, respondents reported that they adapted measures based on pragmatic constraints, perceived severity of illness of the index patient, and the extent to which they were willing to limit social interaction. Respondents did not believe in the effectiveness of wearing face masks within the house due to influences from media, impracticality, and stigma. Interviewees reported that quarantine had a high emotional burden and wanted more information about the exact duration of quarantine, their own COVID-19 status, symptoms, and when to seek medical help.

Outcome: These findings informed national and regional guidelines related to prevention of SARS-CoV-2 transmission in the home (Verberk et al. 2021).

Case Study 5

Social Science Research to Integrate Healthcare Worker Perceptions and Practice into Improved Infection Prevention and Control Strategies for Ebola Virus Disease (EVD)

Operational challenge: During the 13th (October–December 2021) EVD outbreak in the Democratic Republic of the Congo (DRC), the first confirmed cases in children under 5 years were nosocomial infections at healthcare facilities. Although infection prevention and control (IPC) scorecards were being used to evaluate risks, understanding of specific practices and risks of infection among children was limited (a phenomenon which had also been identified and analyzed during the 10th EVD outbreak [August 2018 to June 2020]).

Research: The Integrated Analytics Cell (CAI) conducted healthcare worker surveys based on tools developed during the 10th and 11th (June–November 2020) EVD outbreaks, including targeted questions to understand how healthcare workers perceived their roles in infection prevention and control and their understanding and ability to identify risks specific to small children in healthcare facilities (UNICEF 2022).

Outcome: Survey results highlighted that the problems were not simple lack of knowledge about transmission. They arose from real and perceived shortfalls in capacity to identify risks and take measures needed to stop infection. For example, healthcare workers were aware of the need to disinfect beds, but the types of mattresses available in the facilities made disinfection impossible. The surveys also found limited awareness that non-sterilization, or use of the same bed by multiple children and their family members, can be a source of nosocomial infection. Healthcare workers were more likely to see their role as raising alerts, rather than in disinfection, decontamination, and sterilization to stop infection. The results were immediately translated into targeted training on sterilization and decontamination, as well as increased distribution of protected mattresses and training materials developed to help minimize child-to-child nosocomial infection risks (Mossoko and Kombe 2022).

2 Who Conducts Social Science Research in a Public Health Emergency Response?

Social scientists bring conceptual frameworks, methodological skill, and rigor to field research. However, evidence related to social dynamics of disease transmission prevention and control is often developed by responders from many disciplines, including clinicians, epidemiologists, and community health workers. In an emergency, research is also performed by multi-disciplinary teams, local government authorities, and frontline response workers. Rapid training for research teams and pre-developed resources, including protocols and research tools that are pragmatic, easily understood, and adaptable to local contexts and particular outbreak patterns (e.g., modes of pathogen transmission), can advance integration of social science research into public health emergency response (WHO 2021). Further, post-epidemic structures to promote and sustain local and national social practitioners are essential foundations for in-country capacity for future responses.

3 Rapid Research for Emergency Response

A shared challenge for all research conducted in an emergency is producing evidence quickly enough to be useful for response efforts during the acute phase of the crisis (Gobat et al. 2019). Research approaches that require long lead times to develop protocols, collect and analyze data, and share results through reports or peer-reviewed publication often cannot provide such urgently needed evidence in time. Over the past decades, many rapid research methodologies and practical recommendations for emergency research have been developed (► Chap. 31) (Nuffield Council on Bioethics 2020; Sigfrid et al. 2020; WHO 2022b). During the COVID-19 pandemic, further innovations accelerated and diversified data collection, analysis, and reporting.

This section sets out some practical considerations for rapid social science research in an emergency response. It is an introduction to readers who may be new either to rapid methods or to social science research methods more broadly.

3.1 A Starting Point: Clarify Research Questions and How Findings Will Be Used

For research to inform acute phases of the emergency, there should be a clear "line of sight" as to how evidence will be used and by whom. Research questions should be grounded in the realities of those involved, for example, policy makers, practitioners, or clinicians working in the response. The outcome of research should have clear benefit to these stakeholders, to patients, and/or to others in affected communities. One way to think about this is to consider the different pillars of response and their functions and the ways in which evidence can be used by people working in these pillars. For example, those working to improve infection prevention and control would see value in understanding social and behavioral drivers of nosocomial infection. Those working in public health response would value understanding barriers and enablers for improved contact tracing. Ideally, questions should be formulated, prioritized, and adjusted to circumstances and cultural norms in collaborations with end users and decision makers to ensure results will be applied. Purely theoretical questions and those driven by academic self-interest are unlikely to produce useful short-term results and are, therefore, ethically dubious when resources are scarce.

There are some broad common areas of questioning that surface repeatedly at the start of new disease outbreaks. These include, among others:

- How do affected communities understand the outbreak? How do they perceive their risk of becoming infected? How does their perception of risk influence the choices they make in preventing infection and transmission?
- What social practices or behaviors might be driving, preventing, or mitigating disease transmission?
- How is the outbreak affecting people's lives in aspects like access to services, socio-economic status, health, gender-based violence, etc.?
- How, when, and where do people seek care and treatment when unwell? What stands in the way of people seeking or accessing care when unwell?
- How, when, and where do people seek access to essential health services, such as those for sexual and reproductive health, maternal and child health, or non-communicable diseases?
- How do inequalities, inequities, governance, and power structures influence the behavior of affected populations? How can understanding these dynamics drive inclusive, equitable response policies and practices? (Carter et al. 2020)

At the start of the COVID-19 pandemic, for the first time in a global health crisis, world leading experts rapidly convened to forge consensus on priority evidence gaps to inform response (WHO 2020a). The COVID-19 Research Roadmap included three urgent priority areas for evidence from social and behavioral sciences to inform the acute phase of the pandemic:

1. Evidence to drive feasible, relevant, and acceptable policies that enable uptake of, and adherence to public health and social measures[1] (PHSM) for COVID-19 prevention and control
2. Evidence to drive patient-centered care in clinical and community settings and protect health workers
3. Evidence to promote risk communication that is informed by science and able to reach intended audiences, and that counters misinformation and disinformation

1 PHSM include personal protective measures (e.g., physical distancing, avoiding crowded settings, hand hygiene, respiratory etiquette, mask-wearing); environmental measures (e.g., cleaning, disinfection, ventilation); surveillance and response measures (e.g., testing, genetic sequencing, contact tracing, isolation, and quarantine); physical distancing measures (e.g., regulating the number and flow of people attending gatherings, maintaining distance in public or workplaces, domestic movement restrictions); and international travel-related measures.

Further, this research agenda highlighted biomedical and social vulnerability and the differential impacts of the pandemic on vulnerable groups. The research agenda was revisited and adjusted throughout the pandemic. However, these broad priorities remained relevant throughout the pandemic, and indicate key areas where social science research can contribute to effective response in new health emergencies.

New questions will arise during every outbreak in response to unforeseen events and knowledge gaps. For example, in 2015 during the Ebola epidemic in Liberia, anthropologists conducted a rapid assessment of community-based Ebola response efforts and documented factors that delayed care-seeking for EVD (Allen and Lacson 2015). Systematically collected feedback from communities can help responders understand community needs, shape and adapt response approaches, and identify next steps for research (Baggio et al. 2019). Researchers should also consider work others are doing, coordinate with them, minimize duplication, and share data and research outputs for mutual benefit. These steps will pay dividends in research outcomes: questions relevant to affected communities and responders are more likely to bring positive changes and have salience and value to these stakeholders and the communities themselves.

Case Study 6

Social Sciences Analytics Cell (CASS) and the Integrated Analytics Cell (CAI)

The Cellule d'Analyse en Science Sociale (CASS) was established during the Ebola outbreak in eastern DRC in 2018–2020. This research unit was embedded in the national response structure and focused on supporting response teams with evidence and analytics to inform decision-making. A multi-disciplinary team drew from social epidemiology, epidemiology, anthropology, social science, and health demography in their work. In March 2019 the Ministry of Health (MoH) Ebola Response Coordination Unit signed off on terms of reference for CASS to operate as a support unit alongside the MoH Epidemiological Cell.

CASS was staffed by six international, four national, and 18 local researchers. It also included team members from WHO, Médecins Sans Frontières, and the U.S. Centers for Disease Control and Prevention (CDC). Under MoH, CASS included and coordinated with university and non-governmental organization (NGO) partners and researchers. All data were made freely available online as agreed with the MoH.

CASS identified operational research priorities in the following four ways.

1. Regular analysis of key health behavior indicators, which can identify potential risks and improve understanding of the epidemiological situation. For example, analysis of the perceptions and practices of health workers has provided insights into nosocomial infections (▶ Case Study 5) and identified correlations between higher rates of nosocomial infection and high-risk perceptions and behaviors.
2. Epidemiological data, such as changes in community death rates, changes in health seeking behaviors, etc. Social science research questions were then developed to help explain the epidemiological situation and adapt response interventions.
3. Response interventions: before or after specific response interventions and changes in interventions, CASS conducted analyses to understand the impact and perceptions of the intervention or change.
4. On request from response pillars and their programmatic data managers: to support any pillar to better understand the barriers to and enablers for response interventions, or to better explain data related to their program (e.g., healthcare worker behavior and nosocomial infection; barriers to willingness to participate in safe and dignified burials).

Individual CASS studies had single page terms of reference (ToR) documents that had been approved by the MoH response coordination unit, usually within 24–48 h. The ToRs set out study objectives, methodology, and how anticipated results would inform the response. ToRs were prepared and where the study was conducted and were reviewed with relevant stakeholders before the study began. For example, a rapid study looking at questions on perceptions and trust in EVD treatment centers would be first shared with the teams running the centers. Such stakeholder consultation facilitated response pillar and coordination ownership of results and better use of evidence. All studies were conducted within 3 days to 3 weeks, depending on the question(s) and method(s) applied (Carter et al. 2021).

Following the 10th EVD outbreak, the CASS and Epidemiological Cell integrated approach was modeled (Carter et al. 2021) and, together with key partners and the MoH in the DRC, the CASS was converted into the Integrated Analytics Cell (CAI). This approach brought together social sciences, program data (including surveillance and epidemiological data), and health information systems data, as well as socio-economic, environmental, and other data sources to systematically support outbreak and public health emergencies (including, to date, COVID-19, EVD, measles, malnutrition, plague, and cholera).

3.2 Have a Toolbox of Rapid Research Methods

Research methods define the tools, techniques, and approaches to answer a well-articulated research question. Qualitative and quantitative methods differ in the questions they address, the way they collect data, and the form of the data collected, as well as in the data analysis tools they use (Mack et al. 2015). Social science research lends itself particularly well to qualitative research, producing rich, detailed insights into the values, beliefs, and behaviors of individuals, families, communities, and populations. Quantitative and mixed methods are equally useful and widely used. Meaningful research often requires ample preparation and time for implementation, analysis, and dissemination, but rapid methodologies for urgent research have been developed. These methods are neither a short cut to results that would be obtained through longer-term methods nor an excuse for lower-quality research. Rather, rapid methods provide tools adapted for diverse situations to provide credible and trustworthy data for decision-making in an emergency.

Qualitative methods include participant observation, informant interviews, focus group discussions, participatory approaches, rapid assessments, and focused ethnographic work. New methods and tools, such as photo narratives and peer interviews, may also be of value. Knowledge, attitude, and behavior surveys are the most common quantitative methods used in social science research. These kinds of surveys, conducted over time, provide insight into self-reported understanding, beliefs, risk perceptions, behaviors, and norms related to a wide range of preventative behaviors and how these change over time (Collis et al. 2022; Betsch et al. 2020). Mixed methods research takes advantage of the complementarity of differing methodologies, recognizing that some questions cannot be answered with qualitative or quantitative methods alone (Shorten and Smith 2017).

While interdisciplinary teams will be familiar with quantitative data, they may be less accustomed to using qualitative data. Criticisms of qualitative data include that the numbers of respondents are usually smaller than for large quantitative approaches, that the data captured are "anecdotal," or that the data are not representative. These criticisms often reflect a misunderstanding of the nature and potential utility of qualitative data. Qualitative research does not ask for numbers (how many, how often, how many in box A and how many in box B) but asks how and why questions to provide rich, in-depth understanding of certain phenomena (Moser and

Korstjens 2017). Observations of trends and the outcomes of quantitative methods, including, for example, health services utilization data, household surveys, and surveillance data can inform key questions best addressed using qualitative methods. Conversely, observations arising in qualitative data, including interviews and focus group discussions, may give rise to questions that are best addressed using quantitative methods. A defining feature of social science research is the attention paid to social dimensions of disease transmission prevention and control, rather than the biological transmission of pathogens.

3.3 Planning and Conducting Field Work

It is good practice to document research plans in advance, ideally as a research protocol setting out each step of the research. Protocols, even when they are not obligatory as they are in clinical research, improve quality, credibility, and transparency and can be helpful to other research groups trying to replicate a study during current or future outbreaks. Stand-alone research projects usually have a detailed protocol, which requires local ethics review board approval and sometimes other reviews and approvals before research can begin. Research rapidly conceived and conducted as part of the response should ideally also document a project plan, although these are often brief. For example, ▶ Case Study 5 notes the single-page ToRs reviewed for each study.

Data collection must follow the context and realities of the emergency and the response. Principles of good participatory practice provide guidance for involving affected communities in research (▶ Chap. 18). This involves engaging and obtaining feedback from key stakeholder groups to ensure the research is designed in a way that is culturally acceptable in the context in which it will be conducted. Some practical suggestions include understanding the best places, times, and methods of communications for recruiting research participants; offering proportionate reimbursement (e.g., for travel or to compensate for any loss of earnings); coordinating data collection with other response partners; and adjusting research tools to be flexible and mindful of participant burden. Local partners are practically indispensable for this kind of community engagement and sensitivity to cultural norms.

4 Making an Impact

Rapid operational research is designed to address key operational challenges or emerging issues. When planning research, it is important to think about who needs to know the results and how the results can be both useful to and useable by decision-makers. Knowing how to convey research findings to different audiences is an essential research skill that is often neglected in the formal training of research scientists but is essential if the research is to be useful to adjust and align response actions (▶ In Practice 32.1). This requires researchers to understand the structure of the response, including the roles of national, local, and community governance, the WHO Incident Management System, NGOs, partner governments, and other response participants. Essential communication must be tailored to key decision makers, and national or local officials, civilian or military, will require different kinds of presentations than those running clinical research programs or emergency health response. All these stakeholders may need to be involved to interpret findings and co-develop recommendations or follow-up actions. It is unethical to withhold findings that could shape a more community-appropriate or humane response.

Publishing the results of social science emergency research—after sharing with response partners and other stakeholders—is important both for knowledge generation and for disseminating methodological and operational lessons learned. There has been justified criticism of some researchers from high-income countries who "parachute" in to affected regions and then publish their research in an international journal without involving or acknowledging in-country collaborators (Lancet Glob Health Int Advisory Board 2018). As in other disciplines, there should be an agreed publication policy and clear, fair criteria for authorship from the start.

5 Reflexivity: Being Aware of the Lens Through Which You Conceive and Conduct Research

Reflexivity is a core concept in some social science disciplines (Hopf et al. 2001). Briefly stated, reflexivity is the concept that who the researcher is and how the researcher interacts with research participants plays a role in how research findings are constructed. This means that social scientists often consider their findings in relation to themselves as researchers and as human beings with their own social context, one that can be very different from that of the research participants. Therefore, researchers consider how their background, culture, religion, moral convictions, and assumptions influence what they see and how they interpret it. This analysis requires self-awareness, unpacking unconscious bias, and acknowledging and challenging preconceptions and stereotypes about countries and communities. It also means recognizing one's own limits, cultivating curiosity about what lies beyond those limits, humility about one's own perspective, and listening to understand, not to confirm pre-existing ideas.

Reflexivity enhances credibility of research by acknowledging the potential for personal bias. When reporting the outcomes of qualitative studies, it is good practice to include information about the researchers and their relationship with research participants (Tong et al. 2007) and to consider the impact of these factors on the research. Ways to moderate potential cross-cultural bias include:

- Ensuring that all analyzed data are presented back to local research teams for feedback and consensus
- Coding data in teams and reviewing codes and coded data with local researchers
- Triangulating data with other studies and with community feedback
- Ensuring diversity in the composition of research teams
- Presenting research findings to other members of response teams, such as government workers, surveillance teams, or infection prevention and control teams

6 Ethics of Social Science Public Health Emergency Research

Researchers in all fields have a responsibility to ensure that their practice upholds accepted ethical principles (▶ Chaps. 4 and 33, In Practice 33.2 and 33.3). As with other research disciplines working with human subjects, ethical principles are foundational in the design and conduct of social science research. Guidelines for ethical practice have been promulgated by WHO (2016b), Médecins Sans Frontières (Schopper et al. 2015) and the Council for International Organizations of Medical Sciences (CIOMS 2016). Seeking formal ethical clearance at (emergency) review boards provides some assurance for researchers and their participants that research plans meet ethical standards, but researchers remain responsible for ensuring their research is planned and implemented ethically. This includes ensuring that

- Research questions have value for the response and affected communities
- Research participants are fully informed before deciding to participate in research
- Consent is obtained at all necessary levels
- The privacy of participants is respected
- All data collected are analyzed
- The outcome of research is effectively communicated to inform response decision-making

Some practical social science considerations of ethical research conduct during a public health emergency response follow.

6.1 Community Entry

Communities or individuals in the midst of a disease outbreak may be vulnerable on many levels— physically, mentally, emotionally, and economically (Zafar et al. 2016; IASC Reference Group on Mental Health and Psychosocial Support in Emergency Settings 2015; WHO 2016a). Gaining their trust may be difficult but remains imperative (▶ Chaps. 18 and 30) (Stellmach et al. 2018). Especially in emergencies, interviewers must consider possible harm to human subjects. For example, it may be wise to avoid large focus group discussions that could lead to disease transmission, potential intracommunity violence, or community disapproval. Researchers should proactively seek locally relevant information regarding referral response procedures if they witness or suspect coercion or abuse. They should also be ready to signpost local services or NGOs if participants ask for support. Psychosocial and protection teams trained all researchers working in CASS, for example, on referral mechanisms and pathways for managing serious incidents. Researchers should also look beyond local experts and gatekeepers in communities to engage with marginalized groups where appropriate. However, in an emergency response, where rapid assessment is a necessity, community access and trust among marginalized groups is often challenging.

6.2 Informed Consent

From the perspective of social sciences, adaptations to consent processes that account for contextual realities are both appropriate and desirable. For example, while in Western medical practice the ethical principle of individual autonomy is considered of primary importance, in other contexts the individual may take second place to the family or community. This does *not* mean that individual informed consent need not be obtained, but that consent is understood as a broader construct that includes social partners, such as family or community (Appiah 2020).

One practical example that demonstrates how informed consent processes can be adapted to include both individual and community consent is as follows: In clinical research projects on malaria in Mali, novel approaches for obtaining informed consent were developed by getting the permission of both the community and the individual families taking part in the research. Challenges with documenting consent arose, since written documents could prevent illiterate people from taking part. In this project, many participants were opposed to signing a document because they believed that their word should be sufficient. The study lead emphasized "how different the informed consent process needs to be in different places in the world" (Doumbo 2005). These clinical studies were not conducted in emergencies, but they offer an insight into how the consent processes can be adapted.

The following examples relate to appropriateness of spoken rather than written consent. In Bangladesh, particularly in very poor areas and urban informal settlements, many potential research participants are illiterate and may be afraid to sign documentation, fearing that they are signing away rights (i.e., land, home, access to services). To record consent, the researcher signs and notes a verbal consent, which is documented for the record. Voice recording was considered by research teams; however, feedback from local communities was that this was also not acceptable, particularly if they are sharing views about the health service, weak governance, or violations of rights. Following the liberation of Mosul from the Islamic State in Iraq and Syria in 2017, household surveys were conducted to understand community reconstruction and reconciliation needs. However, any documentation of participation in the study was not trusted, many reporting that providing a name felt like a death sentence (Lafta et al. 2018). Taking notes and filling in forms or recording, especially when not in the local language, can be confusing and may seem to conflict with assurances of confidentiality, as some may wonder why something confidential is being documented and for whom. This latter example illustrates how researchers working in complex humanitarian crises must be prepared to work without paper and pens and, rather, listen and document notes following discussions.

6.3 Incentives and Reimbursement

Especially in resource-poor settings, study participants appreciate incentives and reimbursements. However, overly generous payments can become undue inducements to participate in research (Bentley and Thacker 2004), thus increasing inequity, or at least the perception of inequity, in the research process. This can also create conflict within communities when some people are selected and receive gifts, money, and incentives in kind (Rashid 2007). It is important "to add value to the lives of the people" who participate in research, "recognizing them as subjects in the process and not simply as sources of data" (Pittaway et al. 2010). At the same time, researchers must be sensitive to the local, social, and moral worlds participants inhabit. Just as the boundary between reasonable and excessive compensation is uncertain, so is that between researcher and community, insider versus outsider, academic versus applied research, professional versus personal. One must take care to understand one's own position in any interaction (Dilger et al. 2015).

The critical question of the unpaid burden on study participants also arises. Researchers often request that participants be available during the researcher's time availability, which are working hours for many participants. In low and middle-income countries (LMICs), many people work in informal settings and earn nothing if they miss working hours, so study participation may mean loss of income for people whose economic status is already marginal. The CASS/CAI researchers in the DRC would meet women where they were, at 6:00 AM before church, or after church at water collection points. Focus groups could thus be organized easily among women without interfering with their daily activities. Other options that CASS/CAI researchers used were to bring food and/or provide support with meal preparation to free time for women to participate in interviews of focus groups. The best approaches (time, location, method) for data collection should be identified together with local research teams and remain flexible based on the community group or individuals.

6.4 Ethical Review Boards and Processes

Much rapid social science research has been conducted during health emergencies without prior approval from ethical review boards (► Chap. 33). While procedures vary across time and place, some types of rapid research conducted as a part of response may be viewed as exempt from the formal processes expected of more academic health-related research. Despite possible reservations about this pragmatic approach, it is important to be critically reflective about the messy realities in which one conducts research. Ethical review board processes do not always take into account the "larger moral and human dimensions of the political and economic structures" in which people live (Bourgois 1990). Researchers need to be flexible and responsive and tolerate different approaches to practice. In the field, issues can arise unexpectedly; for example, a violent encounter may be sparked by certain questions, or the sudden eviction of an informal settlement. Research training needs to emphasize the role of researchers in such circumstances, including their own actions, power, and position (Rashid 2007). It is not the narrow definitions of ethical protocols, which may not speak to the complexity of the crisis, that are foundational, but the wisdom and judgment to keep the ethical principles to the forefront. Local ownership of the research is crucial to practical ethics: protocols written for high-income countries may fit poorly with the community where research is being conducted; written informed consent may be inappropriate, for example, if one is investigating sexual abuse and violence in a patriarchal society or a conflict-ridden place. It should be noted here that clinical research to assess medical interventions, with its inherent uncertainties and potential risks to bodily integrity, always requires rigorous ethical review, as specified in generally accepted guidelines like Good Clinical Practice and the Declaration of Helsinki (ICH 2016; WMA 2013).

7 Getting the Best Results from Social Science Research in the Field

7.1 Choose the Right Social Science and the Right Social Scientist

Social science is an exceptionally wide field encompassing multiple professions, but one dividing line, often within separate disciplines and even within individual scientists' careers, is theoretical vs applied. While theoretical social scientists primarily try to *understand and explain* social processes, applied social scientists use concepts, theories, and practical experience to resolve problems in the real world or to critically reflect on and adapt the application of social science.

Social science expertise may be central both to an infectious disease emergency response considered generally and to the research element of the response, especially when the social realities and cultural meanings of health, disease, birth, life, and death need to be understood. When seeking a social scientist for a response team, finding the *right* one is important. This will generally be someone working in applied social science who

- Has worked with and understands the professional language of interdisciplinary teams that include epidemiologists and infectious disease experts
- Has performed research in a similar response
- Knows how to act in a health emergency
- Is familiar with rapid research methods
- Can think flexibly and adapt research methods without sacrificing rigor
- Knows how to work with other disciplines to communicate outside their own field and to the public
- Has experience of the affected geographic region and is sensitive to local cultures, contexts, and the heterogeneity of communities

Social scientists with a background in outbreak or public health response programs may be more easily placed to support response teams turning evidence into action. In the case of CASS/CAI, all researchers hired are expected to have had some emergency response experience, to "speak" the language of programs, and to propose actions based on evidence produced.

Social scientists trained in different disciplines bring different perspectives and have different skill sets. To identify the best fit for a research team, it is important to consider the information needs of the response. For example, ethnographers and anthropologists contributed to the surveillance team investigation during the 2021 EVD outbreak in Guinea. They were able to map family trees to better understand transmission chains. Expertise in epidemiology and health communication may be needed when investigating a population's knowledge of disease transmission in order to develop communication strategies. Researchers with experience in large scale surveys and using corresponding software (SPSS[2] or equivalents) may be well suited to analyze data of this kind.

7.2 Understanding Social Science Data and Approaches: Strengths and Limits

How and why questions are usually complex. It may be challenging for social scientists to articulate this complexity in emergencies when time is a rare resource. They may face difficulties being heard when meetings need to be short, and all response pillars must present their data, which in most cases is quantitative. More than their colleagues, social scientists must be able to articulate

2 A widely used software program for statistical analysis in the social sciences.

their contributions clearly, without using social science jargon, and reduce complexity without being simplistic. A social scientist with a 5-min slot at the end of a coordination meeting may feel disadvantaged vis-à-vis colleagues presenting surveillance, epidemiological, statistical, or biomedical data. Strong narratives usually resonate with an audience, because they provide real stories and experience from the field and lived experience, adding a more nuanced perspective than that conveyed by numbers. When and where possible, it is very useful to coach and work with researchers in response coordination roles to help them better understand how social science data contributes to decision-making. CASS started this process during the 10th DRC EVD outbreak in 2018 with the MoH; 3 years later, the MoH absorbed the CASS into their CAI. In the four subsequent EVD outbreaks, integrated social sciences data has not only been included but has been requested and expected to guide response strategy.

Leaders and managers of response teams need to understand what social science researchers can bring to the table, support their activities, and give them a voice in the team and time to present their findings. Make time and space for critical perspectives and for discussion of innovative methodology. Anthropologists involved in the 2014–2016 West Africa Ebola epidemic took on vital roles in adapting essential public health interventions to local cultural norms even while facing questions about their legitimacy vis-à-vis communities, other responders who viewed themselves as "firefighters," and even colleagues in academia. While these anthropologists were able to conduct their research and draw on anthropological knowledge to inform the response, questions were also raised about the legitimacy of such roles (Lees et al. 2020).

Case Study 7

Voice from the Field: Ask the Right Questions, Collect the Right Data to Guide Response

Operational challenge: A key goal of an EVD response is to encourage those experiencing symptoms to seek care as early as possible, in part to stem further transmission in the community. During the first 6 months of the 10th EVD outbreak in the DRC, delays in treatment seeking (time between symptom onset and seeking care at a facility where an EVD alert could be raised) were 5–7 days or more, thereby increasing the risk that even if EVD was detected and patients received care, their chances of recovery would fall even as they (potentially) spread the disease. Preliminary community surveys sought to find out if community members could list three EVD symptoms, which over 90% of respondents were able to do. The survey also included the question, "If you believe you had Ebola, would you seek care?" Over 80% of respondents said they would. This discrepancy between data captured in community surveys and clinical data from EVD patients related to care seeking was difficult to interpret. Those leading the response were confused and accused communities of being resistant to seeking care. They also criticized the quality of the survey data, hypothesizing that respondents said they would seek care because of their perception that this was the "right" or socially desirable answer, rather than reporting their own inclinations.
Research: CASS worked with clinical teams to develop better surveys by looking at health behavior and specific knowledge required to improve the chances that infected people would seek health care. These surveys asked communities which symptoms would induce them to seek care and after how many days. They also asked respondents to list all the EVD symptoms they knew about. The results were compared with biomedical data provided by clinical teams on the most commonly presented EVD symptoms among patients.

Outcome: Survey results highlighted that the most common symptoms (e.g., body aches and pains, low fever) were not known to be EVD symptoms and, therefore, did not result in healthcare seeking. Rather, the EVD symptoms (bleeding, vomiting, and high fever) presented on posters around the communities were cited as reasons for seeking treatment. Following these studies, all communication materials were adapted to better present the more common, less severe EVD symptoms and to encourage people to get early treatment. Continued analysis of delays to treatment seeking eventually saw the delays drop from 5–7 to 2–3 days (CASS 2019, 2020; Groupe de Recherche Sciences Sociales (GRSS), 2019–2020, unpublished).

7.3 Employ the Right Social Scientists in Time

In all health emergencies, human behavior is crucial for the success or failure of a response. It is important to assess how behavior is driven by cultural, social, economic, and structural circumstances, and to look at how and why the background and circumstances lead to observed behaviors. This assessment must take place *with* the affected communities, in the form of community participation or community engagement (Bedson and Abramowitz 2018; WHO 2017; Burtscher 2013). For global medical research, "researchers need to develop an understanding of the unique ways in which different cultural groups make decisions" (Doumbo 2005). As with many other aspects of response, preparedness pays off, and it is useful to employ social scientists *before* problems arise, i.e., before community "resistance" (Cohn and Kutalek 2016; Anoko 2014; Fairhead 2016) or vaccine hesitancy or refusal derail response plans (Sobo 2015). Usually there are several factors involved and a social logic that influences community response to external support, researchers, and interventions. All too often pervasive mistrust and suspicion about the motives and actions of perceived authority figures play a central role, by no means in developing countries alone, but in high-income setting as well (Nguyen 2019; Viswanath et al. 2021). Trust, rapport, and engaging communities in these discussions early helps researchers get their research questions right. Social scientists can draw from the lessons of previous outbreaks and provide useful material for a variety of research contexts, especially when they co-design their research with implementers, fieldworkers, and communities (Islam et al. 2013). Social scientists are critical to successful research in health emergencies because they have valuable perspectives to share and important data to contribute (Giles-Vernick et al. 2019).

8 Conclusions

Just as clinical research was not fully accepted as a core part of the response to public health emergencies until fairly recently, the vital role of social science research has not always been understood and accepted (Lees et al. 2020). Emergency research response is conducted in a human context, among people whose understanding and reactions may be quite different from those of the medical scientists planning and implementing a research program. Aside from being transparent, ethical, and methodologically rigorous, research, and especially public communications about research, must be in a form that is acceptable to the community where it takes place. The urgency of bringing evidence and analytics to inform response operations means that social science research, like public health and clinical research, should also be rapidly conducted.

As the emerging field of social science emergency response research develops, what methodological rigor in rapid research response means in practice is becoming clearer. Research questions must follow a clear logic to align with the goals of accountable and community-based outbreak response, as well as the cultural context in which they are asked. Questions should address what responders need to know to deliver a community-centered and effective response, rather than what would be interesting to know from an academic research perspective. Research design, delivery, and dissemination should be less top-down in approach and include co-development with multiple stakeholders, including local and operational partners. Collaboration with the community is not only a practical necessity during an emergency response but an increasingly recognized ethical imperative (► Chap. 18). Research methods can and should adapt to the local contexts where emergencies occur, but methodological transparency and rigor are still essential to credibility, particularly when research results will inform high-level strategic decision-making. Finally, while we have focused on social science research in this chapter, it is important to note that not everything can be solved with research. Being aware of the limits of social science is as important as championing its contributions.

Discussion Questions

1. Human needs and realities are often highly dynamic and localized: what worked last year may not be successful now, and what is effective in one community will not necessarily work in the next one down the road. Provide some examples of how evidence from social science can help tackle operational challenges and inform emergency responses.
2. Who is responsible for ensuring that social science research informs a public health emergency response?
3. Although new questions will arise in response to emerging events and knowledge gaps, what are some common, practical questions social science researchers might ask at the start of an infectious disease outbreak? What tools can researchers use to rapidly answer some of these questions?
4. Explain the concept of reflexivity and how understanding the concept can enhance credibility.
5. Applied social scientists use concepts, theories, and practical experience to resolve real world problems, such as understanding the social realities and cultural meanings of health and disease during an infectious disease emergency. Discuss the background and expertise needed for a social scientist to become a valuable member of a response team.
6. A social scientist's assessment of how human behavior is driven by cultural, social, economic, and structural circumstances may be crucial to the success of an emergency response. Discuss what such assessments can contribute and some of the limits of social science input.

References

Afifi RA, Novak N, Gilbert PA, Pauly B, Abdulrahim S, Rashid SF, Ortega F, Ferrand RA. 'Most at risk' for COVID19? The imperative to expand the definition from biological to social factors for equity. Prev Med. 2020;139:106229.

Albrecht D. Vaccination, politics and COVID-19 impacts. BMC Public Health. 2022;22:96.

Allen D, Lacson R. Understanding why Ebola deaths occur at home in urban Montserrado County, Liberia. U.S. CDC, Liberia MOH; 2015.

Andreas M, Iannizzi C, Bohndorf E, Monsef I, Piechotta V, Meerpohl JJ, Skoetz N. Interventions to increase COVID-19 vaccine uptake: a scoping review. Cochrane Database Syst Rev. 2022;8:Cd015270.

Anoko JN. Communication with rebellious communities during an outbreak of Ebola virus disease in Guinea: an anthropological approach. Atlanta: Ebola Response Anthropology Platform; 2014.

Appiah R. Community-based participatory research in rural African contexts: Ethico-cultural considerations and lessons from Ghana. Public Health Rev. 2020;41:27.

Atkinson P, Gobat N, Lant S, Mableson H, Pilbeam C, Solomon T, Tonkin-Crine S, Sheard S. Understanding the policy dynamics of COVID-19 in the UK: early findings from interviews with policy makers and health care professionals. Soc Sci Med. 2020;266:113423.

Baggio O, Camara CA, Prue C. Bringing community perspectives to decision-making in the Ebola response in the Democratic Republic of Congo. Humanit Exchange. Humanitarian Practice Network; 2019.

Bavel JJ, Van KB, Boggio PS, Capraro V, Cichocka A, Cikara M, Crockett MJ, Crum AJ, Douglas KM, Druckman JN, Drury J, Dube O, Ellemers N, Finkel EJ, Fowler JH, Gelfand M, Shihui Han S, Haslam A, Jetten J, Kitayama S, Mobbs D, Napper LE, Packer DJ, Pennycook G, Peters E, Petty RE, Rand DG, Reicher SD, Schnall S, Shariff A, Skitka LJ, Smith SS, Sunstein CR, Tabri N, Tucker JA, van der Linden S, van Lange P, Weeden KA, Wohl MJA, Zaki J, Zion SR, Willer R. Using social and behavioural science to support COVID-19 pandemic response. Nat Hum Behav. 2020;4:460–71.

Bedford J, Farrar J, Ihekweazu C, Kang G, Koopmans M, Nkengasong J. A new twenty-first century science for effective epidemic response. Nature. 2019;575:130–6.

Bedson J, Abramowitz S. Minimum quality standards for community engagement (draft). New York: UNICEF; 2018.

Bedson J, Skrip LA, Pedi D, Abramowitz S, Carter S, Jalloh MF, Funk S, Gobat N, Giles-Vernick T, Chowell G, de Almeida JR, Elessawi R, Scarpino SV, Hammond RA, Briand S, Epstein JM, Hébert-Dufresne L, Althouse BM. A review and agenda for integrated disease models including social and behavioural factors. Nat Hum Behav. 2021;5:834–46.

Bentley JP, Thacker PG. The influence of risk and monetary payment on the research participation decision making process. J Med Ethics. 2004;30:293–8.

Betsch C, Wieler LH, Habersaat K. Monitoring behavioural insights related to COVID-19. Lancet. 2020;395:P1255–6.

Bourgois P. Confronting anthropological ethics: ethnographic lessons from Central America. J Peace Res. 1990;27:43–54.

Burtscher D. Involving communities: guidance document for approaching and cooperating with communitites. Médecins Sans Frontières; 2013.

Carter SE, Gobat N, Zambruni JP, Bedford J, van Kleef E, Jombart T, Mossoko M, Nkakirande DB, Colorado CN, Ahuka-Mundeke S. What questions we should be asking about COVID-19 in humanitarian settings: perspectives from the social sciences analysis cell in The Democratic Republic of the Congo. BMJ Glob Health. 2020;5:e003607.

Carter SE, Ahuka-Mundeke S, Pfaffmann Zambruni J, Navarro Colorado C, van Kleef E, Lissouba P, Meakin S, le Polain de Waroux O, Jombart T, Mossoko M, Nkakirande DB, Esmail M, Earle-Richardson G, Degail MA, Umutoni C, Anoko JN, Gobat N. How to improve outbreak response: a case study of integrated outbreak analytics from Ebola in eastern Democratic Republic of the Congo. BMJ Glob Health. 2021;6:e006736.

CASS. Briefing notes CASS 2019. Cellule D'analyse en Sciences Sociales (Cass); 2019.

CASS. Breifing notes 2020. Cellule D'analyse en Sciences Sociales (Cass); 2020.

Chan EY, Yang NG, Kim JH, Newnham EA, Huang Z, Hung H, Dubois C, Hung KKC, Wong ELY, Wong SYS. Informal home care providers: the forgotten health-care workers during the COVID-19 pandemic. Lancet. 2020;395:1957–9.

CIOMS. International ethical guidelines for health-related research involving humans. Geneva: Council for International Organisations of Medical Sciences; 2016.

Cohn S, Kutalek R. Historical parallels, Ebola virus disease and cholera: understanding community distrust and social violence with epidemics, PLOS Curr Outbreaks. 2016:1.

Collis A, Garimella K, Alex Moehring M, Rahimian A, Stella Babalola N, Gobat DS, Stolow J, Aral S, Eckles D. Global survey on COVID-19 beliefs, behaviours and norms. Nat Hum Behav. 2022;6:1310–917.

Coutinho RZ, Montalvo AV, Weitzman A, Marteleto LJ. Zika virus public health crisis and the perpetuation of gender inequality in Brazil. Reprod Health. 2021;18:40.

Dilger H, Huschke S, Mattes D. Ethics, epistemology, and engagement: encountering values in medical anthropology. Med Anthropol. 2015;34:1–10.

Doumbo OK. It takes a village: medical research and ethics in Mali. Science. 2005;307:679–81.

Fairhead J. Understanding social resistance to the Ebola response in the Forest region of the Republic of Guinea: an anthropological perspective. ASR. 2016;59:7–31.

Farmer P. Social inequalities and emerging infectious diseases. Emerg Infect Dis. 1996;2:259–69.

Giles-Vernick T, Kutalek R, Napier D, Kaawa-Mafigiri D, Dückers M, Paget J, Ahmed SM, Cheah PY, Desclaux A, De Vries D, Hardon A, MacGregor H, Pell C, Rashid SF, Rodyna R, Schultsz C, Sow K, Wilkinson A. A new social sciences network for infectious threats. Lancet Infect Dis. 2019;19:461–3.

Gobat NH, Amuasi J, Yazdanpanah Y, Sigfrid L, Davies H, Byrne J-P, Carson G, Butler C, Nichol A, Goossens H. Advancing preparedness for clnical research during infectious disease epidemics. Eur Respir J Open. 2019;5:00227-2018.

Gostin LO, Mundaca-Shah CC, Kelley PW. Neglected dimensions of global security: the global health risk framework commission. JAMA. 2016;315:1451–2.

Hassan D, Ravindran R, Hossain A. Nipah virus mystery: insights into transmission and mechanism of disease progression. J Pure Appl Microbiol. 2022;16:26–34.

Hopf T, Kratochwil FV, Lebow RN. Reflexivity: method and evidence. In: Smelser NJ, Baltes PB, editors. International encyclopedia of the social & behavioral sciences. Elsevier (Pergamon); 2001. p. 82–7.

Hrynick TA, Ripoll Lorenzo S, Carter SE. COVID-19 response: mitigating negative impacts on other areas of health. BMJ Glob Health. 2021;6:e004110.

IASC Reference Group on Mental Health and Psychosocial Support in Emergency Settings. Mental health and psychosocial support in ebola virus disease outbreaks: a guide for public health programme planners. Geneva: Inter-Agency Standing Committee (IASC) Reference Group on Mental Health and Psychosocial Support in Emergency Settings; 2015.

ICH. Good clinical practice: ICH harmonised guideline. Integrated addendum to ICH E6(R1): guideline for good clinical practice ICH E6(R2) ICH consensus guideline. Geneva: International Council for Harmonisation of Technical Requirements for Pharmaceuticals for Human Use (ICH); 2016.

Islam MS, Luby SP, Gurley S. Developing culturally appropriate interventions to prevent person to person transmission of Nipah virus in Bangladesh: cultural epidemiology in action. In: Banwell C,

Ulijaszek S, Dixon J, editors. When culture impacts health. Academic Press: London; 2013.
Kutalek R, Wang S, Fallah M, Wesseh CS, Gilbert J. Ebola interventions: listen to communities. Lancet Glob Health. 2015;3:e131.
Lafta R, Cetorelli V, Burnham G. Living in Mosul during the time of ISIS and the military liberation: results from a 40-cluster household survey. Confl Heal. 2018;12:31.
Lancet Glob Health Int Advisory Board. Closing the door on parachutes and parasites. Lancet Glob Health. 2018;6:e593.
Lees S, Palmer J, Procureur F, Blanchet K. Contested legitimacy for anthropologists involved in medical humanitarian action: experiences from the 2014-2016 West Africa Ebola epidemic. Anthropol Med. 2020;27:125–43.
Lindahl JF, Grace D. The consequences of human actions on risks for infectious diseases: a review. Infect Ecol Epidemiol. 2015;5:30048.
Mack N, Woodsong C, MacQueen KM, Guest G, Namey E. Qualitative research methods: a data collector's field guide. Research Triangle Park, NC: Family Health International; 2015.
Martindale AM, Pilbeam C, Mableson H, Tonkin-Crine S, Atkinson P, Borek A, Lant S, Gobat N, Solomon T, Sheard S. Perspectives on COVID-19 testing policies and practices: a qualitative study with scientific advisors and NHS health care workers in England. BMC Public Health. 2021;21:1216.
Mello MM, Opel DJ, Benjamin RM, Callaghan T, DiResta R, Elharake JA, Flowers LC, Galvani AP, Salmon DA, Schwartz JL, Brewer NT, Buttenheim AM, Carpiano RM, Clinton C, Hotez PJ, Lakshmanan R, Maldonado YA, Omer SB, Sharfstein JM, Caplan A. Effectiveness of vaccination mandates in improving uptake of COVID-19 vaccines in the USA. Lancet. 2022;400:535–8.
Moser A, Korstjens I. Series: practical guidance to qualitative research. Part 1: introduction. Eur J Gen Pract. 2017;23:271–3.
Mossoko M, Kombe J. Use of healthcare worker (HCW) surveys in recent Ebola outbreaks in The Democratic Republic of the Congo (DRC). Integrated outbreak analytics field exchange GOARN. 2022.
Nguyen V-K. An epidemic of suspicion—Ebola and violence in the DRC. N Engl J Med. 2019;380:1298.
Norton A, Bucher A, Antonio E, Advani N, Grund H, Mburu S. Living mapping review for COVID-19 funded research projects. Ukcdrorguk. 2021.
Nuffield Council on Bioethics. Research in global health emergencies: ethical issues. Oxford, UK: Nuffield Council on Bioethics; 2020.
Pittaway E, Bartolomei L, Hugman R. 'Stop stealing our stories': the ethics of research with vulnerable groups. J Hum Rights Pract. 2010;2:229–51.
Rashid SF. Accessing married adolescent women: the realities of ethnographic research in an urban slums environment in Dhaka, Bangladesh. Field Methods. 2007;19:369–83.
Rashid SF, Aktar B, Farnaz N, Theobald S, Ali S, Alam W, Ozano K. Fault-lines in the public health approach to Covid-19: recognizing inequities and ground realities of poor residents lives in the slums of Dhaka City, Bangladesh. Social Sciences and Humanities Open; 2020.
Ryan RE, Parkhill A, Schonfeld L, Walsh L, Lowe D, Merner B, Nelson N, Hill SJ. What are relevant, feasible and effective approaches to promote acceptance, uptake and adherence to physical distancing measures for COVID-19 prevention and control? In health evidence network (HEN) synthesis report 72. Copenhagen. 2021.
Saker L, Lee K, Cannito B, Gilmore A, Campbell-Lendrum D. Globilisation and infectious disease: a review of the linkages. In: Special programme for research and training in tropical diseases (TDR). Geneva: UNICEF/UNDP/World Bank/WHO; 2004.
Schopper D, Dawson A, Upshur R, Ahmad A, Jesani A, Ravinetto R, Segelid MJ, Sheel S, Singh J. Innovations in research ethics governance in humanitarian settings. BMC Med Ethics. 2015;16:10.
Seale H, Dyer CEF, Abdi I, Rahman KM, Sun Y, Qureshi MO, Dowell-Day A, Sward J, Saiful Islam M. Improving the impact of non-pharmaceutical interventions during COVID-19: examining the factors that influence engagement and the impact on individuals. BMC Infect Dis. 2020;20:607.
Shorten A, Smith J. Mixed methods research: expanding the evidence base. Evid Based Nurs. 2017;20:74–5.
Sigfrid L, Maskell K, Bannister PG, Ismail SA, Collinson S, Regmi S, Blackmore C, Harriss E, Longuere KS, Gobat N, Horby P, Clarke M, Carson G. Addressing challenges for clinical research responses to emerging epidemics and pandemics: a scoping review. BMC Med. 2020;18:190.
Sobo EJ. Social cultivation of vaccine refusal and delay among Waldorf (Steiner) school parents. Med Anthropol Q. 2015;29:381–99.
Stellmach D, Beshar I, Bedford J, du Cros P, Stringer B. Anthropology in public health emergencies: what is anthropology good for? BMJ Glob Health. 2018;3:e000534.
Stolow J, Kendall C, Pinheiro FML, da Rocha Feitosa MC, de Almeida Furtado KA, Martins AF, dos Santos MPA, Ellery AEL, Dias L, de Holanda Barreto IC, Moses L, Castro A, Dunn C, Kerr L. Women's perceptions of Zika virus prevention recommendations in Fortaleza, Brazil. JPHP. 2020;1:288–314.
Tong A, Sainsbury P, Craig J. Consolidated criteria for reporting qualitative research (COREQ): a 32-item checklist for interviews and focus groups. Int J Qual Health C. 2007;19:349–57.
UNICEF. Integrated Analytics Cell (CAI): the integration and use of multidisciplinary and integrated analysis to better understand and respond to epidemics. UNICEF; 2022. https://www.unicef.org/

drcongo/en/integrated-analytics-cell. Accessed 5 Oct 2022.
van der Westhuizen H-M, Kotze K, Tonkin-Crine S, Gobat N, Greenhalgh T. Face coverings for covid-19: from medical intervention to social practice. BMJ. 2020;370:m3021.
Verberk JDM, Anthierens SA, Tonkin-Crine S, Goossens H, Kinsman J, de Hoog MLA, Bielicki JA, Bruijning-Verhagen PCJL, Gobat NH. Experiences and needs of persons living with a household member infected with SARS-CoV-2: a mixed method study. PLoS One. 2021;16:e0249391.
Vickery J, Atkinson P, Lin L, Rubin O, Upshur R, Yeoh E-K, Boyer C, Errett NA. Challenges to evidence-informed decision-making in the context of pandemics: qualitative study of COVID-19 policy advisor perspectives. BMJ Glob Health. 2022;7:e008268.
Viswanath K, Bekalu M, Dhawan D, Pinnamaneni R, Lang J, McLoud R. Individual and social determinants of COVID-19 vaccine uptake. BMC Public Health. 2021;21:818.
Voo TC, Reis AA, Thomé B, Ho CW, Tam CC, Kelly-Cirino C, Emanuel E, Beca JP, Littler K, Smith MJ, Parker M, Kass N, Gobat N, Lei R, Upshur R, Hurst S, Munsaka S. Immunity certification for COVID-19: ethical considerations. Bull World Health Organ. 2021;99:155–61.
Wanat M, Hoste M, Gobat N, Anastasaki M, Böhmer F, Chlabicz S, Colliers A, Farrell K, Karkana MN, Kinsman J, Lionis C, Marcinowicz L, Reinhardt K, Skoglund I, Sundvall PD, Vellinga A, Verheij TJ, Goossens H, Butler CC, van der Velden A, Anthierens S, Tonkin-Crine S. Transformation of primary care during the COVID-19 pandemic: experiences of healthcare professionals in eight European countries. Br J Gen Pract. 2021;71:e634–e42.
WHO. Clinical care for survivors of Ebola virus disease: interim guidance. Geneva: World Health Organization; 2016a.
WHO. Guidance for managing ethical issues in infectious disease outbreaks. Geneva: World Health Organization; 2016b.
WHO. Community engagement framework for quality, people-centred and resilient health services. Geneva: WHO; 2017.
WHO. A coordinated global research roadmap. 2020a.
WHO. A coordinated global research roadmap: 2019 novel coronavirus. Geneva: World Health Organization; 2020b.
WHO. Perceptions of Health workers regarding health facility IPC for COVID-19: a research template. 2021.
WHO. COVID-19 research and innovation: powering the world's pandemic response—now and in the future. 2022a.
WHO. Strengthening pandemic preparedness planning for respiratory pathogens. Geneva: World Health Organization; 2022b.
WHO. Strengthening the global architecture for health emergency preparedness, response and resilience. WHO; 2022c.
WMA. World medical association declaration of Helsinki: ethical principles for medical research involving human subjects (2013). JAMA. 2013;310:2191–4.
Zafar A, Talati C, Graham E. 2014–2015 West Africa Ebola crisis: impact update. Washington, DC: World Bank; 2016.

Governance, Institutions, and Partnerships

Nicole Lurie

Oveview of Book Section VI: Global governance is a puzzlement in a political world based on nation-states. In a few areas, say posts and telecommunications, there are effective, binding global standards. Infectious diseases are an inherently global issue, but truly global infectious disease response remains elusive.

Nicole Lurie and Gerald T. Keusch (► Chap. 27) propose a possible framework for improving global health emergency response, especially to ensure that research to develop, assess, produce, and distribute medical countermeasures can begin expeditiously, accompanied by outreach to public audiences to convey understanding and minimize suspicion and misinformation. Building better research capacity to detect and respond to novel pathogens, along with support for more consistent resources, coordination, and governance should become an ongoing project for nation-states and the global community in interpandemic periods.

Muhammad Ali Pate and Sulzhan Bali (► Chap. 28) examine how International Financial Institutions support preparedness through initiatives by the World Bank and others to provide financing and incentives to strengthen disease response systems and bolster core capacity, benefiting both national health systems and clinical research capacity. Amanda Rojek and Gail Carson (► Chap. 29) articulate the benefits of global collaborative organizations for research response to public health emergencies, discuss stumbling blocks that limit collaboration, and propose measures to better prepare and implement international collaboration in future outbreaks.

Yazdan Yazdanpanah et al. (► Chap. 30) draw lessons about health research partnerships from their crisis experience, including the importance of common goals, mutually respectful relationships, and combining complementary strengths into strong, functional whole. Rebecca F. Grais and Emmanuel Baron (► In Focus 30.1) note the research efforts of medical humanitarian NGOs like Médecins Sans Frontières (MSF), and how they contribute to medical research by integrating research into their patient-centered response to infectious disease emergencies. Finally, Chuen-Yen Lau et al. (► In Practice 30.2) describe the contributions a long-running research partnership between the Indonesia Ministry of Health and the U.S. National Institute of Allergy and Infectious Diseases has made to Indonesian and U.S. readiness to respond to novel diseases.

Contents

27 A Global Framework for Research Preparedness and Response

Nicole Lurie and Gerald T. Keusch

Contents

Learning Track Note: This chapter appears in Learning Tracks: Global Health; Global Health Law; Health Policy, Multilateral Cooperation, International Governance

E. S. Higgs and R. A. Sorenson (eds.), *Principles and Practice of Emergency Research Response*,
https://doi.org/10.1007/978-3-031-48408-7_40

Learning Objectives

This chapter should enable readers to understand and discuss:

- Primary elements of the global research and development ecosystem for response to infectious disease.
- Opportunities to counter EID emergencies that have been missed because of weaknesses in response capabilities.
- How global infectious disease response could be made more equitable, given that
  - Sovereignty resides in nation-states which tend to put their own citizens first.
  - The wealthiest states generally have the greatest capacity to respond to infectious disease emergencies.
  - It is far harder to mobilize resources for preparedness than for response.

1 Introduction

Over the last two decades a series of infectious disease public health emergencies has impelled scientists and governments around the world to study new pathogens and their clinical presentation, identify treatment alternatives, and develop approaches to their prevention or control—and to do so with the urgency befitting a crisis with many lives at stake. At the beginning of the twenty-first century research was not viewed as an essential element of infectious disease response. As a result, the inclusion of research as an integral component of response to public health emergencies has lagged far behind global recognition of the threat of newly identified infectious diseases. The advent of severe acute respiratory syndrome (SARS) in 2002 was a call to action for strengthening global surveillance and early warning systems, but the felt urgency for research on medical countermeasures (MCMs) rapidly waned when public health measures stopped the outbreak before new therapies or vaccines could be developed and tested (Brim and Wenham 2019). When the H1N1 influenza pandemic began in 2009 (▶ Chap. 30), improved global surveillance systems allowed it to be detected relatively quickly. Seasonal influenza vaccines were rapidly adapted to include the new pandemic strain, although emergency vaccine deployment was too late to blunt the peak of the pandemic's trajectory (Fineberg 2014).

There have been many missed opportunities in the past for research response to address other aspects of disease control (e.g., effectiveness of school closures or use of masks) and improved diagnosis and treatment (e.g., unrecognized superinfection with Methicillin-resistant *Staphylococcus aureus*, a major cause of death in children) (Long et al. 2010). The slow global production and inequitable distribution of H1N1 influenza vaccines around the world and the limited willingness by developed nations to make some of their supply quickly available to other countries, whether through the World Health Organization (WHO) or bilateral arrangements, limited the overall impact these vaccines could have produced. The disparity was amplified by both legal liability issues and vaccine hesitancy, which was more pronounced in historically underserved populations. This contributed to global as well as domestic inequalities in H1N1 influenza vaccine uptake (Mesch and Schwirian 2015), problems that reappeared during the coronavirus disease 2019 (COVID-19) pandemic as stumbling blocks for effective vaccine distribution (Halabi et al. 2020).

The 2014–2016 Ebola outbreak in West Africa (▶ Chap. 30) brought with it a new series of challenges and missed opportunities to improve the research response (Rojek and Horby 2017). As the disease spiraled out of control, scientists struggled to develop new types of rapid diagnostic tests for use in austere environments, and to design and test novel therapeutics, repurposed older drugs, and vaccines. A slow start, disagreements on study designs, a dearth of clinical research-ready sites, and the limited power of clinical trials to document efficacy as Ebola case numbers began to wane all led to a slow start for research during that outbreak. Inadequate preparedness, financing, and governance for conducting research in an emergency were related to the low priority global health and emergency response communities assigned to clinical research. This can be clearly seen in the exclusion of research from initiatives to improve global health security and infectious disease response, such as the Global Health Security Agenda, which held its first ministerial meeting in 2014 as the Ebola outbreak was becoming the center of worldwide attention.

There was considerable skepticism at that time that clinical research could produce results in a fast-moving epidemic and controversy over conducting randomly controlled trials when patient mortality was near 50%. There was also resistance in the humanitarian response community to adding research to the extraordinary burden of patient care in full personal protective gear in the tropics, or even allowing others to get in the way of patient care to do their research (Adebamowo et al. 2014; Levine 2016). A report from the U.S. National Academies of Science, Engineering, and Medicine (NASEM 2017) made a series of important recommendations aimed at preventing similar research response problems from occurring again. These were reinforced by reports from multiple other groups around the world with recommendations addressing preparedness, governance, and financing to control outbreaks of emerging infectious diseases. Unfortunately, many of these recommendations still had not been adequately implemented when the COVID-19 pandemic began, 5 years after the Ebola outbreak was over.

As depicted in Fig. 1, the global research and development (R&D) ecosystem, with its multiple actors interacting in a constantly changing environment, was continuously evolving during the decade before the COVID-19 pandemic emerged (Lurie et al. 2021). In 2010, the pharmaceutical industry was seeking new models of partnership to accelerate translation of scientific discoveries into treatments that would benefit populations and create markets. By 2020, a rich network of collaborations between traditional competitors in private-sector companies, governments, and academia had emerged to help expedite the development and delivery of new products, with much of the initial effort focused on chronic disease and on cancer.

The Ebola outbreak of 2014–2016 in West Africa was a major impetus for change in the approach towards research in the midst of an

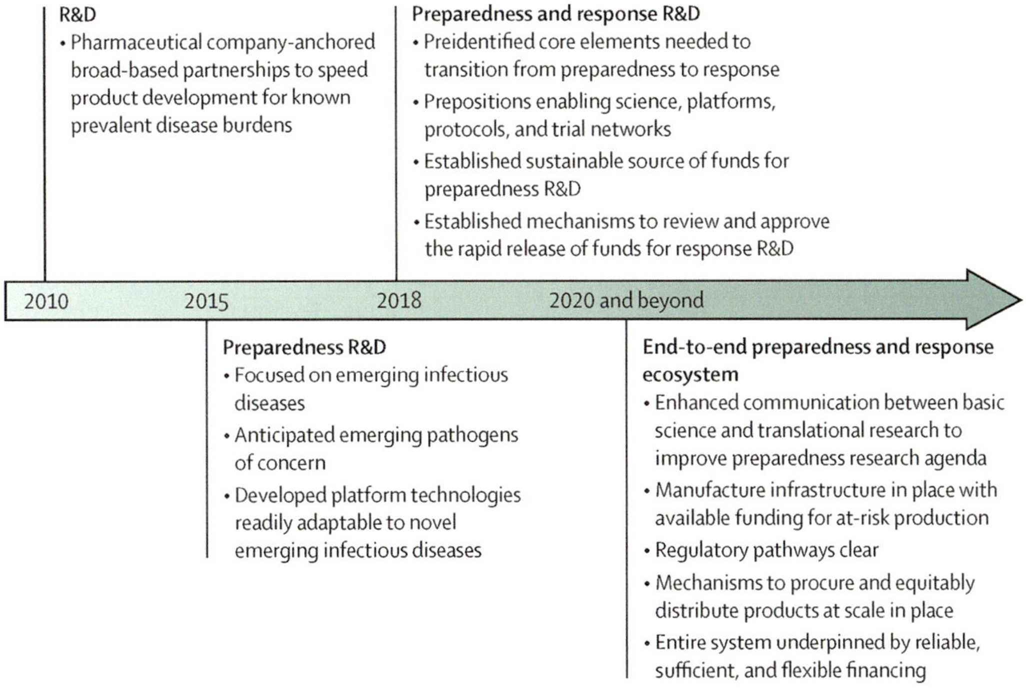

Fig. 1 Elements of the biomedical R&D ecosystem (Lurie et al. 2021)

EID emergency. When it began there were two Ebola vaccine candidates available to move quickly into clinical trials (Kennedy et al. 2017). Both vaccine candidates began trials in Liberia in early 2015, supported by the U.S. National Institute of Allergy and Infectious Diseases (NIAID) in partnership with the Liberian Ministry of Health, but transmission of the Ebola virus was already dropping below the numbers needed to gather interpretable data for Phase III results because basic public health measures to prevent exposure had been put into place. A further trial, using a ring strategy akin to that used in smallpox eradication, was undertaken in Guinea (Henao-Restrepo et al. 2017). Lessons learned during the West Africa trials were then applied during the substantial Ebola outbreak in the Democratic Republic of the Congo in 2018–2020, allowing rapid initiation of vaccine delivery together with a system for data collection, which further demonstrated the vaccine's efficacy and provided additional evidence of its safety, consistent with the suggestive findings previously obtained in West Africa. This new work facilitated ultimate licensure of one of the vaccines 18 years after development started and 5 years after the outbreak in which clinical trials began (Wolf et al. 2021). This success reinforces the notion that the first step to promote improvements in the global pandemic preparedness and response system is to both learn from the past and apply those lessons to the future.

2 Learning from Experience: Adaptations and Creativity in Global Research Response to Epidemics

Vowing that the world should learn from prior shortcomings, and in collaboration with multiple experts around the globe, in 2016 the WHO created its R&D Blueprint to reorganize how it would prepare and respond to pandemic threats (WHO 2016). It was envisioned as a global coordination mechanism that would "reduce the time between the declaration of a public health emergency of international concern and the availability of effective tests, vaccines, and medicines that can be used to save lives and avert crisis," both by improving preparedness for such events and improving global coordination of emergency research response (WHO 2016). As the WHO argued in its prospectus for the R&D Blueprint, "the Ebola epidemic has demonstrated that it is possible to accelerate R&D during emergencies and that it is feasible to safely and effectively implement research interventions in affected countries. It also highlighted the imperative to advance R&D preparedness and effective collaboration frameworks ahead of any new epidemic" (WHO 2016). The R&D Blueprint also aimed to increase support and capacity for necessary research, including clinical research capacity and clinical trials of new MCMs. This provided motivation for global partners to consider research capacity as part of their development efforts and pandemic preparedness planning, and to push the development, testing, and ultimate availability of these products to move more rapidly through the R&D process. Innovative ideas included the identification of priority pathogens for countermeasure development efforts—and flexible platform strategies adaptable to whatever pathogen was subsequently involved in an outbreak of concern—that could be developed during an interepidemic period, and crafting approaches to coordinate multiple aspects of clinical research before and in the course of an outbreak. One result of energized new thinking was the establishment of the Coalition for Epidemic Preparedness Innovations (CEPI) in 2017, with the mission of facilitating development of vaccines for potentially epidemic pathogens (Ingstad Sandberg et al. 2020).

The COVID-19 pandemic has led to increasing interest in creating a new global health security or pandemic preparedness convention or equivalent binding instrument, together with governance reforms that would make global action, including research, more responsive and effective (Gostin et al. 2021). Based on the limited success of the only recent stand-alone treaty related to health, the Framework Convention on Tobacco Control, which went into effect in 2005, not only will this require a major effort to enact, but its effectiveness cannot be assured without the full support and compliance of all states that have joined with the spirit as well as the letter of the document.

With regard to effective research response, it should be axiomatic that research cannot proceed without trained researchers (▶ Chap. 42), prepared clinical research networks (▶ Chap. 31), well-equipped laboratory (▶ Chap. 9) and clinical research facilities (▶ Chap. 40), information technology expertise and equipment (▶ Chap. 34), and a competent administrative system (▶ Chap. 32) to support the research enterprise across all of its necessary domains: from scientific and ethical review of proposals (▶ Chap. 5), data management capacities (▶ Chap. 35), training of researchers and staff, experience in compliance with international standards in the conduct of clinical research, expertise in pharmacovigilance (▶ Chap. 36), appropriate oversight of biosafety and biosecurity (▶ Chap. 41), and strong linkages to the health and public health needs of the country (▶ Chap. 18).

In the face of numerous, unfulfilled recommendations concerning how the world should improve its ability to address future outbreaks, WHO and the World Bank created an independent Global Preparedness Monitoring Board (GPMB) to monitor and advocate for their implementation. In its first annual report in September 2019, the GPMB noted that many recommendations following the 2009 H1N1 influenza and 2014 Ebola pandemics had been "poorly implemented, or not implemented at all, and serious gaps persist … [and] for too long, we have allowed a cycle of panic and neglect when it comes to pandemics: we ramp up efforts when there is a serious threat, then quickly forget about them when the threat subsides. It is well past time to act" (GPMB 2019). The need to improve the R&D ecosystem for pandemics was a major theme of the report, but the most specific proposal was for "donors, countries and multilateral institutions to develop a multiyear plan and approach for strengthening R&D research capacity, in advance of and during an epidemic" by September 2020.

One year later, nine months into the COVID-19 pandemic, GPMB observed in its second annual report that "while progress on the coordination of R&D has been made during the pandemic, this progress is fragile" (GPMB 2020). Operating within a political context for global action as GPMB does, the second report called on "Researchers, research institutions, research funders, the private sector, governments, the World Health Organization and international organizations [to] improve coordination and support for research and development in health emergencies and establish a sustainable mechanism to ensure rapid development, early availability, effective and equitable access to novel vaccines, therapeutics, diagnostics and non-pharmaceutical interventions for health emergencies, including capacity for testing, scaled manufacturing and distribution." This was an important call to action, which in context challenges the research community itself to identify the continuing gaps in the research response ecosystem and propose milestones for the conduct of R&D, and on governments and international organizations to establish a suitable enabling mechanism alongside the leadership of the health and public health systems, both nationally and internationally. Like many components of the R&D ecosystem for potential pandemic diseases, particularly those for which there are few or no safe, effective, and approved countermeasures, bold action is essential to catalyze progress on development, production, distribution, access, affordability, and delivery of countermeasures to people everywhere.

Fortunately, there has been improvement in at least some aspects of the global R&D architecture. For example, when a large Lassa fever virus outbreak erupted in 2018 in Nigeria, WHO and the government of Nigeria co-convened a group to identify research priorities for managing it. The outbreak was controlled before it spread widely, but new observational research improved understanding of the epidemiology of Lassa fever virus as a disease primarily transmitted by rodents, with relevance to future control of the disease (Siddle et al. 2018). There were failures as well; for example, ribavirin, an expensive antiviral of questionable efficacy in the treatment of Lassa fever, was administered to the vast majority of patients, wherever available, without any rigorous studies having been done to assess its effectiveness because there was no pre-agreed methodology for such studies. In part this was because of widespread resistance to conducting a placebo-controlled trial during an emergency, even though many global actors had reached a broad ethical consensus that such trials are in fact essential at the time of the West Africa Ebola outbreak (London et al. 2018; Salam et al. 2021). CEPI had already begun to support the development of a Lassa vaccine, but there were no candidate products sufficiently advanced for trials during this outbreak. Nonetheless, the outbreak and attention to a research agenda facilitated the identification of a set of research activities needed to support the ultimate development of countermeasures (Hatchett and Lurie 2019).

Another post-Ebola innovation was the launch of the WHO Health Emergencies Program, incorporating research as an essential component of its command structure (Council on Foreign Relations 2020; Independent Panel for Pandemic Preparedness and Response 2021). The new leadership and structure to address health emergencies contributed significantly to the improved performance of WHO during the COVID-19 pandemic, although opportunities for continued improvement abound (Boyd and Wilson 2021; Kuznetsova 2020). It is worth noting that infectious disease emergencies are not the only crises for which research responses are required; environmental, climate, chemical, and nuclear emergencies also stand to benefit from improvements in research preparedness and response, global engagement, adequate resources, and informed leadership.

The conceptual shift to a preparedness R&D ecosystem in the decade preceding COVID-19 has already paid off in important ways. Development of the messenger RNA (mRNA) vaccine platform, in part through research on the two novel coronavirus outbreaks preceding the severe acute respiratory syndrome coronavirus 2 (SARS-CoV-2)—SARS-CoV-1 and Middle East respiratory syndrome coronavirus (MERS-CoV)—and critical science preparedness activities led to an understanding of how to stabilize the prefusion form of the spike protein and a prototype mRNA coronavirus vaccine potentially adaptable to any future emerging pandemic coronavirus (Corbett et al. 2020). This is among the innovations that enabled the rapid development of safe and effective SARS-CoV-2 vaccines. Similarly, other groups took up adaptation of both new and traditional technologies to "the new pathogen on the block" (Ura et al. 2021). In short, prior insights and technology combined with the quick initiation of targeted preclinical research rapidly led directly to clinical trials and ultimately to regulatory approval (▶ Chap. 6) via Emergency Use Authorizations of two mRNA vaccines in Europe and the United States and a viral vectored vaccine in Europe, less than a year after the outbreak was recognized. Further authorizations and in some cases full licensure of these and other vaccines have followed, as clinical trials have generated sufficient information for regulatory action.

On the other hand, the inability to produce COVID vaccines and other useful products at sufficient scale and the lack of commitment and financial resources to buy and distribute them everywhere needed, both efficiently and equitably, perpetuated profound global inequalities. The need for an end-to-end, truly global R&D preparedness and response ecosystem for emerging pandemic infectious diseases, with their attendant social, economic, and political consequences, has been recognized (Lurie et al. 2021). The issue remains, as always, how to translate lessons learned into enduring solutions.

In truth, by the time the COVID-19 pandemic took the world by storm in the early months of 2020, many of the key scientific elements required for an end-to-end approach to R&D were known (Higgs et al. 2017). Newer and more agile research coordination and support mechanisms were nominally in place, at least in the infectious disease arena. WHO and a coalition of national health research funding agencies around the world comprising the Global Research Collaboration For

Infectious Disease Preparedness (GLOPID-R) convened a research agenda setting meeting six weeks after COVID-19 was recognized, defined key research requirements for the pandemic, and called on scientists around the world to join what has become an unprecedented example of scientific discovery and collaboration. Many of the gaps in the end-to-end R&D ecosystem that have slowed or inhibited progress relate to a lack of clarity on roles and responsibilities for development of countermeasures and the inability to pre-position and rapidly fund researchers with the capability to conduct critical elements of the research response. Often the paucity of research resources in lower-income countries has left gaps in our understanding as well.

A 2020 report for the GPMB on the R&D preparedness ecosystem clearly identified the concern that "research" has often been conceived too narrowly, and that a comprehensive system is critically needed, beginning with MCM discovery and ending with the delivery of the right countermeasures to the right people at the right time, equitably, and in relation to global public health impact rather than economic and/or political power (Keusch and Lurie 2020). The ecosystem gaps have led to a haphazardly coordinated pandemic research response, one that was underfunded in all but the wealthiest and most capable countries, which then prioritized the protection of their own populations, further exacerbating global inequality. Inadequate or inefficiently available financing, even when there was a will to act, has meant that organizations in many affected countries have had to divert precious time and energy from research response as such to a constant scramble for funds and vaccine doses, leaving poorer nations at the end of the line when it comes to providing input into developing life-saving measures and to much-delayed access to successful MCMs. Ongoing gaps in global research coordination and the lack of a pre-established system of governance, particularly with regard to clinical research coordination and design, have wasted research resources and delayed the generation of evidence about what actually works and in what settings or contexts.

On top of the barriers to research on MCMs, an inadequate understanding of human behavior in a prolonged pandemic, including how people get and use information, how they calculate risk and assess benefits, and how these factors figure into issues such as skepticism about both public health and MCMs including vaccines, have meant that products that are developed are not optimally used to save lives and diminish morbidity and long-term consequences of the disease. In many countries a wide-ranging distrust of government and authority underlies poor public response (COVID-19 National Preparedness Collaborators 2022).

There are certainly triumphs that should be acknowledged, applauded, and amplified, such as the rapid sharing and curation of gene sequences by GISAID, the development and deployment—albeit inequitably—of vaccines in less than a year, some pre-positioned clinical research networks adaptable to a variety of clinical research needs, and the use of adaptive trial designs to identify effective therapeutics more rapidly. In the COVID-19 pandemic even the much-maligned regulatory agencies around the world have recognized the need to move more rapidly, resist political interference, and make evidence-based decisions to authorize the use of these new products outside of research studies when circumstances warrant, even when the evidence is not strong enough to permit full licensure.

3 Key Elements of Research Response Needed for the Future

At the same time the health and humanitarian response needs to be rolled out, a critical, early activity during any crisis is to define and execute a research agenda (NASEM 2017). In a prolonged emergency, research priorities will evolve over time and therefore should be regularly revisited, with the full understanding that time remains of the essence. A research agenda does not need to be developed de novo with each event; it can evolve from a pre-scripted checklist or agenda of critical activities and prepositioned capabilities necessary to execute these activities. It is critical that such a checklist be flexible and adaptable to the situation and affected region, and that capabilities to execute anticipated activities are prepositioned in each region, particularly to ensure that the result is co-developed with local and regional scientists and leadership and not just international experts and the current global R&D and manufacturing sectors.

From an infectious disease perspective, a checklist can start with key elements enabling a public health and biomedical science response needed for an MCM-oriented research response, one which addresses the set of issues and needs generated before and during the first year of the COVID-19 pandemic. Responsibility for executing these research activities was poorly defined at the outset of the pandemic. However, during the COVID response CEPI envisioned and implemented a global laboratory network capable of running standardized assays to assess immune responses to vaccines (and future pathogens) and to develop and conduct testing in animal models (CEPI 2020). Maintaining (and expanding) such networks as core, prepositioned global capabilities for the future would make sense and be invaluable. This needs to include assignment of responsibilities and availability of funding even before there are emergency situations. Maintaining expertise, continuity of funding, and enhancement of infrastructure is a requirement to avoid catastrophic events like COVID-19, because research systems cannot immediately function if they are not already in place when they are needed. Two chronically underdeveloped areas of research readiness are the organization, approval and execution of clinical trials, and the study of human behavior relevant to emergency outbreak situations including the perception of and response to risk.

The recently expressed global ambition to develop vaccines available for use within 100 days of a recognized need (CEPI 2022; Pandemic Preparedness Partnership 2021; Saville et al. 2022), in part through developing prototype vaccines in each potentially high-consequence viral family, will require an additional set of elements for research response, based in structural biology, immunology, and manufacturing innovations to advance technology and platforms before knowing the specifics to which they will be adapted. These should be defined and developed as soon as possible to be ready when needed.

3.1 Clinical Trials

It is increasingly possible to accelerate development of multiple classes of therapeutics, as well as vaccines, with the advances in structural biology, development of bioactive chemical and small molecule libraries, rapid throughput screening of compounds, methods for producing monoclonal antibodies, and the development of new in vitro and in vivo animal models representative of human disease pathogenesis for emerging infectious agents. However, the speed of translation to actual human use depends on their rapid, parallel clinical evaluation. Fortunately, there has been progress applicable to potentially pandemic emerging infectious diseases. Adaptive trial designs, in which "accumulating evidence is used to modify the trial's course in accordance with preset rules" (Pallmann et al. 2018), can allow the early termination of trials or arms of trials because sufficient data are available to conclude there is either no effect or the intervention is in fact effective. While most clinical trials conducted during the COVID-19 pandemic, especially in the early months, were either underpowered or too poorly designed to draw conclusions, several adaptive trials, notably the Randomised Evaluation of COVID-19 Therapy (RECOVERY) trial in the UK and the later WHO-sponsored global SOLIDARITY trial, both of which tested multiple products simultaneously, were quickly able to identify products that worked, e.g., dexamethasone, and those that did not, e.g., hydroxychloroquine. The former exemplifies the benefits of an available UK government-funded network, which linked academic centers with a healthcare system and patient base (the National Health Service) under a partnership with the

National Institute for Health Research (RECOVERY Trial 2022) (▶ In Practice 14.1). The UK Clinical Research Network had been established in 2008, and while it was originally envisioned as a mechanism to address common, chronic health problems, it was a well-functioning, pre-positioned platform for clinical research (workforce, clinical care, laboratory, coordinated information systems) when COVID-19 emerged and able to rapidly pivot to the new urgent problem.

Going forward, functioning clinical trial networks will be needed in multiple areas of the world, within a global "network of networks" that agrees to a set of clinical trial design principles and pre-established interim or prototype protocols. These sites must be ready to not only conduct trials but contribute to integrating research into the roll-out of interventions and public health measures in a crisis. One example of such a trial network was REMAP-CAP, a global network studying community acquired pneumonia that had a pre-defined emergency response arm (Goossens et al. 2021). To be viable, such networks will need ongoing funding and involvement in trials during interpandemic periods to maintain skills and systems. It is hard to envision such a global network without support from those nations with abundant and available resources, in full collaboration with nations where outbreaks are most likely to begin. There will be additional challenges to address before these networks can serve as clinical trial first responders to test innovations in clinical care as well as assess investigational products in clinical trials. Foremost among them will be a rapid system of Research Ethics Committee/Institutional Review Board (REC/IRB) approval and country regulatory authorization for the conduct of trials by local, regional, and international partners. The move to a single IRB for multi-center trials in the United States may be a promising model to explore for multi-country research networks (Gordon et al. 2017). An independent, expert global coordination or governance system will also need to be established so that products that are most promising or fit for purpose can be prioritized, and others are unable to "hijack" clinical trial resources through political or financial influence. The provision of core financing for such networks to do other valuable work when they are not needed for emergency response (to stay "warm") in exchange for their agreement to participate in the global system of cooperation and equitable access is one possible mechanism to underwrite the enterprise. Realizing such a vision will take an enormous amount of work but is a worthy and frankly essential goal to pursue; respected expert leadership will matter.

A global clinical research infrastructure will be needed for clinical care, therapeutics, and vaccines. For example, during COVID-19, each vaccine developer executed its own clinical trial design using its own networks, although NIAID insisted on some common designs and endpoints for the trials it funded. Because each vaccine was tested against its own placebo control group, the number of trial participants receiving placebo was large, and it was impossible to directly compare one vaccine to another.

4 Understanding Human Behavior

Every public health emergency touches people in many communities, and multiple forces shape their understanding of the crisis and how to protect themselves. Prior experience, future expectations, and the trust placed by communities in leadership are all pertinent, whether political, scientific, or healthcare and public health leaders. While misinformation and anti-vaccine propaganda go back to at least the mid-nineteenth century (Larson 2020), the propagation of misinformation and its deleterious effect on crisis management and public health response has reached new heights. Large minorities of the population in many countries fell prey to false narratives about etiology and epidemiology of disease, medical countermeasures, and the intentions of public health, medical, and scientific practitioners. Such narratives have been aided and abetted by nations, social media, misinformation provided by friends, family, or celebrities from one or another sector of society, and wide dissemination of messages without reliable screening or fact-checking (Briand et al. 2021).

It is critically important to have a better understanding of human behavior in the face of a crisis, in particular the way people assess and respond to risks, and how such understanding can be applied to help mitigate potentially counterproductive effects. As we have seen in both the Ebola epidemic and COVID-19 pandemic, the need for behavioral science research to inform many aspects of the end-to-end response and the deployment and acceptance of lifesaving countermeasures is, like the need for research response during an outbreak, more evident now than it has ever been. Most countries do not have a surge workforce of anthropologists, sociologists, or behavioral scientists, or even a sizeable enough contingent of practicing social scientists to operate under the levels of stress and uncertainty routine in an emergency. This suggests a clear need to determine how to provide the "just in time" training of a workforce to interview community members, take the pulse of a community's understanding and attitudes, and provide reliable sources of information for locally or nationally known leaders the community will trust. The usual approach in low- and middle-income countries has been to "parachute" in anthropologists or other social scientists and public health personnel from developed countries, who may or may not know the languages, cultural heritage, educational level, and morés of a society, and whose style of engagement is different and palpably foreign. There is no strong global effort to plan and facilitate such an effort as far as the authors are aware. However, it is worth noting that many non-governmental and humanitarian organizations have in-country staff who have at least some familiarity with the local culture and different groups within populations who could potentially be mobilized for these efforts; countries have robust networks of community health workers who could be similarly engaged. As with clinical, laboratory, epidemiology, and specimen collection resources, planning for and ideally pre-positioning individuals and systems for such an effort will undoubtedly be a key ingredient of research responses in the future. Planning and resources that are ideally linked to community needs in the interepidemic period are, as ever, essential precursors if the need is to be addressed in real time and from the beginning of an outbreak.

5 Developing a Health Research System to Support Evidence-Based National Health Priorities

There are many challenges for nations deciding to build a health research infrastructure able to support initiatives to improve the health of the population. Beyond the obvious, that individuals' health and quality of life are inextricably intertwined, multiple analyses over the past three decades have documented that a healthier population is critical for economic stability and growth in both the short and the long term (Bloom and Canning 2008). COVID-19 has brought this message home and has helped nudge the health development paradigm away from a top-down approach, investing in infrastructure to increase the wealth of a nation and provide a trickle-down health benefit when all citizens can afford better health care, toward a bottom-up approach whereby investments to improve the health of the poor yield substantial dividends all the way up the economic ladder as worker productivity increases. In this strictly economic assessment, the role of health research is central to provide information on the most impactful investments government and societal leaders can opt for. Information derived from many types of research, from basic epidemiology to MCM validation to better understanding of how social determinants affect a nation's health, must be translated into health policies and public investments across the whole of society, leading to downstream impacts on individual and societal wealth.

The first step in this paradigm, building a research system in all countries capable of providing relevant and reliable information to inform and improve decision-making, has been highlighted as essential for well over three decades, beginning with the seminal 1990 Evans Commission report (Commission on Health Research for Development 1990). Two fundamental requirements for creating an essential national health research (ENHR) system emerge from such reports: researchers and the necessary research infrastructure to sustain the research agenda, ranging from laboratory and clinical capabilities to policy questions, and good linkages to a network of worldwide peers. Every country needs an ENHR program, albeit at varying levels of sophistication. Previous expert groups have recommended that countries target 2% of their gross national product as the minimum investment needed to develop their science and technology capabilities, with at least 5–10% of that allocated specifically to health research. Such investments can be financed through the World Bank or other mechanisms; as noted in a recent World Bank report, the Bank itself should help lay out the investment case for countries to commit such funds (International Vaccines Task Force 2018).

To achieve the ENHR goal, researchers need to be educated and trained across a broad spectrum of disciplines. Some of these educational inputs must be provided at the national level, supplemented as appropriate through advanced training in other countries which have the necessary institutions and are willing to support education and training for foreign students and more advanced trainees. But to attract those receiving education and training abroad back to their home country requires an infrastructure that permits these individuals to use acquired research strengths to a sufficient degree to warrant their decision to return home. Many, especially the most able and creative, will have the opportunity to remain where they have been learning their profession, often in a developed country with much higher income levels (Dohlman et al. 2019; Kasprowicz et al. 2020).

Infrastructure needs vary from simple but comprehensive and accurate systems to generate health, disease, and demographic data necessary to identify priority health concerns to highly technical, instrumentation-dependent molecular biology and genetics research, or higher order information technology and computing capabilities to collect and analyze big data sets of population-level information. Regardless, the ENHR concept includes establishing a minimum research base to understand prevalent health problems, prioritizing limited resources to maximize impact, and promoting self-sufficiency and efficiency in health strategies (Evans 1990; Weisz and Tousignant 2019). At a minimum, the research base must include the ability to evaluate whatever crises the country is faced with, so that appropriate decisions on how to address them can be taken at the country level—though in the case of a novel pathogen, as we have seen, answers may not be immediately forthcoming, even with a large proportion of the world's research resources going to the problem. The required research base does not mean that every country must be involved in the pre-clinical R&D for MCMs. It does, however, extend to the need to ensure that whatever countermeasures are employed are fit for purpose, and that their impact on the crisis can be evaluated in real time.

6 Financing an End-to-End Research Response

Policymakers have begun to consider sustainable financing mechanisms (▶ Chap. 28) to strengthen preparedness for emerging infectious disease outbreaks, including R&D preparedness, with much of it focusing on the interpandemic period (Pandemic Preparedness Partnership 2021). This will require both planning and resources to pre-position research groups and their capabilities, whether they are using advanced genomics to better define epidemiology, resources for collecting human specimens, development and testing of novel diagnostics, vaccine platforms to jump start vaccine development against novel pathogens, or building clinical trial networks and manufacturing capacity that can pivot to urgently needed products when a crisis threatens. As plans for funding mechanisms evolve, however, they must recognize the critical necessity of end-to-end, or "lab to jab" capabilities of an R&D preparedness and response ecosystem.

There is increasing recognition that population needs go beyond developing countermeasures, readiness to test them wherever they will be deployed, manufacturing the products at scale, and ensuring delivery and deployment to those in need. For example, such efforts cannot efficiently proceed without pre-existing agreements on who accepts the financial and liability risks, and who has responsibility to manufacture, procure, and equitably distribute and deliver MCMs. If the goal expounded in 2021 to develop and distribute vaccines within 100 days of identifying a need is to be achieved (Saville et al. 2022), manufacturing at risk, that is without scientific or financial guarantees of success, would need to start within 30–45 days into a pandemic to impact its trajectory early in its course. Without major reforms and flexible, realistic financial commitments, it is unlikely that national and global financing institutions could move quickly enough to support the ability to manufacture, procure, and deploy needed vaccines. Moreover, countries will still need to execute their part of the end-to-end response and ensure these countermeasures, whether diagnostics, therapeutics, or vaccines, reach the intended recipients. Operational and behavioral science research will be badly needed at every step in this process. It seems doubtful that low- and many middle-income countries will be able to finance these activities on their own, so they will require at least some level of external financial support.

Following the West Africa Ebola outbreak, the World Bank created a Pandemic Emergency Financing Facility to help the least resourced countries. However, it was not much utilized, either before or during the COVID-19 pandemic, and closed down in April 2021; its mechanism proved to be too cumbersome and slow to be practical (Brim and Wenham 2019; Saville et al. 2022; World Bank 2021). Regardless of the mechanism ultimately identified, it must be able to support operational and behavioral research for pandemic control, support end-to-end countermeasure development and deployment, provide immediate access to funds, be able to make investments upfront and at financial risk, and be governed by a politically independent body of experts, including economists and bankers, with significant senior science, health, and public health expertise. These individuals should also be committed to the challenges full time, authorized to make decisions rapidly and be prepared to act on them without delay; this must be considered a serious and deep commitment. It should be evident that financing must be closely tied to governance of the research response because activities approved and financed early are likely to get done and have the greatest chance to succeed, as well as blazing the trail for later continuing research.

7 Creating a Research Response and End-to-End Needs

There is a cliché that says what gets measured gets done, meaning measuring key factors provides the information needed to focus on achieving the goal (Henderson 2016). Operationalizing a research response not only means outlining critical steps, responsibilities, and performance indicators, but also developing sufficient accountability to ensure milestones are met. That, in turn, requires measuring performance. COVID-19 has proven once again that the R&D response to a pandemic is neither simple nor monolithic. There are many interrelated and interdependent parts that are executed by various distinct actors, sometimes in sequence and sometimes at the same time. To keep this functioning optimally needs a system for oversight, flexible tools to promote action, and operational expertise on the part of its managers. A future research response will need to delineate the critical roles and responsibilities as early in the process as possible, and preferably pre-event, identify milestones for each component and actor, and monitor and report regularly on progress or the lack of it. Then it becomes possible to focus on the problems, identify gaps, eliminate barriers, and ensure what is working continues to do so. While no such system currently exists, the global architecture in place suggests that the existing Global Preparedness Monitoring Board could be reformed in its next iteration to take on such an effort. Doing so would, of course, need the backing of the sponsors, authority, and access to resources, both expert personnel and finances.

8 Governance

The lack of an existing governance system for end-to-end R&D processes during the COVID-19 pandemic led the major global organizations to create the Access to Covid Tools Accelerator, or ACT-A (WHO 2021). These public and private sector organizations came together to first discuss and share plans on diagnostics, therapeutics, and vaccines, as well as an integrated effort to strengthen health systems. Neither ACT-A nor COVAX, the WHO-established vaccines pillar to promote vaccine R&D, procurement, allocation, and deployment of at least emergency authorized products, are established legal entities. Over time, the coordination system has evolved as the needs of the pandemic have shifted further downstream to delivery and use of products, but research needs continue. Indeed, the entire continuum of R&D requirements and what coordination will look like as immediate response shifts to preparation for a new pandemic or a recrudescence of COVID-19 remain uncertain.

Conceptually, the effort has many attributes of a strong governance system, with participation from key actors and a commitment to problem solving. However, as Moon et al. (2015) have pointed out, a future governance system must have a clear system for decision-making, transparency about how decisions are reached, and mutual understanding among the various parties about definitions and boundaries for their roles and responsibilities.

9 The Way Forward for Global Governance of R&D Preparedness and Response

There is considerable evidence that a global framework for R&D must take an end-to-end approach, with research elements needed at every point along the continuum from basic science to administration of safe, effective products to people. It is also clear that different abilities, actors, and actions are needed at different points in the process. But key roles and responsibilities have to be defined across the entire ecosystem, so that no essential elements of preparedness and response are neglected. The economic concept of comparative advantage is a useful metaphor here, but the world must not depend on uncoordinated nation-states or other actors to meet all requirements. All the elements needed for research response must be coordinated, strengthened, globalized, and prepositioned to the extent possible. In addition, capacities must be in active use in inter-crisis periods, with core business functions and sustainable, equitable financing, supported by a strong system of governance and accountability. One cannot simply build a clinical research site or a vaccine plant and put it in storage till the next crisis. While the ideal structure has yet to be envisioned or financed, a set of normative principles with regard to R&D ecosystem governance emerges from the recent COVID-19 pandemic experience:

1. The R&D ecosystem, or its conceptualization, must expand to cover the entire "lab to jab" spectrum and include R&D as well as product manufacturing, procurement, and access. Indeed, research is critical to achieving faster manufacturing and making current capacities fit for purpose to better achieve access goals (e.g., vaccine thermostability).
2. As an axiom of governance, in a potential crisis when the consequences of the emergency are still unclear there must be a strong commitment to at-risk investment of necessary resources for a full-scale, immediate response. The response must include development and manufacture of potential countermeasures before it is certain they will work, with rapid de-escalation of effort as the situation warrants.
3. The R&D ecosystem must involve countries at all levels of income and development. Many aspects of this system can be strengthened in interpandemic periods, and core capabilities can be prepositioned

regionally. However interpandemic R&D is financed, it must pursue this goal. Emergency response R&D cannot proceed unless and until all the essential elements for scientifically and ethically sound implementation are available.
4. Access to the products derived from the R&D system must be equitable in terms of both scope and timing. Major research funders and international financing instruments can incorporate commitments to product access into both intellectual property rights (IPR) arrangements and funding agreements to ensure products also become available to low and middle-income countries as they are produced during a health emergency. A system for financing the R&D system must cover both the interpandemic period as well as provide rapid (close to day 0) emergency financing in a global crisis.
5. Development and manufacturing of the products derived from the R&D system should be geographically distributed, both to provide equity of opportunity as well as to protect as much of the world as possible from export controls and nationalism. No small group of countries should be expected to manufacture products for the entire world. By the same token, when supply is scarce, it is essential to allow companies other than intellectual property rights holders to manufacture patented products in an emergency. While difficult, it is essential to make authorized MCMs widely available in an emergency.
6. A global process to bring together and enhance coordination among the diverse actors involved in pandemic preparedness and response is essential. For example, high-level decision-making could be guided by a board, chaired by a senior, experienced, neutral individual (or co-chairs), and include representatives of the key organizations involved across the spectrum from global product R&D to product use, ensuring appropriate representation from all sectors and regions. Critical response steps will require many decisions from managers in particular organizations across different sectors. For example, an emergency use authorization for a vaccine or therapy will trigger guidance to medical providers and the public, higher-volume production, distribution to health facilities, arrangements for delivery to end-users, Phase IV observations of product safety and effectiveness, etc. High-level decisions will need to be coordinated with those making the operational calls on these and many other response actions.

Previous crises have been met with recurrent cycles of panic and neglect. It is both possible and essential to improve the R&D preparedness and response ecosystem to meet future challenges. It is high time to do the hard work to make these rational changes happen and actually function as intended if we are to avoid another COVID-19 tragedy *when we could have taken steps to prevent or sharply mitigate the impact.*

? Discussion Questions

1. What are the primary elements of the global R&D ecosystem for response to infectious disease? What is the origin of this ecosystem, in general terms?
2. Name a few opportunities that have been missed because of weaknesses in response capabilities.
3. How can global infectious disease response be made more equitable, considering that
   (a) The nation-state is the primary locus of sovereignty, and nation-states tend to put their own citizens first.
   (b) The wealthiest states tend to have the most capacity to respond to infectious disease.
   (c) It is far harder to mobilize resources for preparedness than for response.

References

Adebamowo C, Bah-Sow O, Binka F, Bruzzone R, Caplan A, Delfraissy J-F, et al. Randomised controlled trials for Ebola: practical and ethical issues. Lancet. 2014;384(9952):1423–4. https://doi.org/10.1016/S0140-6736(14)61734-7.

Bloom DE, Canning D. Population health and economic growth. Washington, DC: Commission on Growth and Development; 2008. Report No.: Working Paper No. 24.

Boyd M, Wilson N. Failures with COVID-19 at the international level must not be repeated in an era facing global catastrophic biological risks. Aust N Z J Public Health. 2021;45(2):184. https://doi.org/10.1111/1753-6405.13082.

Briand SC, Cinelli M, Nguyen T, Lewis R, Prybylski D, Valensise CM, et al. Infodemics: a new challenge for public health. Cell. 2021;184(25):6010–4. https://doi.org/10.1016/j.cell.2021.10.031.

Brim B, Wenham C. Pandemic emergency financing facility: struggling to deliver on its innovative promise. BMJ. 2019;367:l5719. https://doi.org/10.1136/bmj.l5719.

CEPI. CEPI creates new collaborative taskforce to assess impact of emerging viral strains on effectiveness of COVID-19 vaccines. Oslo: Coalition for Epidemic Preparedness Innovations; 2020. https://cepi.net/news_cepi/cepi-creates-new-collaborative-taskforce-to-assess-impact-of-emerging-viral-strains-on-effectiveness-of-covid-19-vaccines/. Accessed 15 Apr 2022.

CEPI. A world in which epidemics and pandemics are no longer a threat to humanity. Oslo: Coalition for Epidemic Preparedness Innovations; 2022. https://cepi.net/about/whyweexist/. Accessed 14 Nov 2022.

Commission on Health Research for Development. Health research: essential link to equity in development. New York: Commission on Health Research for Development; 1990.

Corbett KS, Edwards DK, Leist SR, Abiona OM, Boyoglu-Barnum S, Gillespie RA, et al. SARS-CoV-2 mRNA vaccine design enabled by prototype pathogen preparedness. Nature. 2020;586(7830):567–71. https://doi.org/10.1038/s41586-020-2622-0.

Council on Foreign Relations. Improving pandemic preparedness: lessons from COVID-19. New York: Council on Foreign Relations; 2020.

COVID-19 National Preparedness Collaborators. Pandemic preparedness and COVID-19: an exploratory analysis of infection and fatality rates, and contextual factors associated with preparedness in 177 countries, from Jan 1, 2020, to Sept 30, 2021. Lancet. 2022;399:1489. https://doi.org/10.1016/s0140-6736(22)00172-6.

Dohlman L, DiMeglio M, Hajj J, Laudanski K. Global brain drain: how can the Maslow theory of motivation improve our understanding of physician migration? Int J Environ Res Public Health. 2019;16(7) https://doi.org/10.3390/ijerph16071182.

Evans JR. Essential national health research. A key to equity in development. N Engl J Med. 1990;323(13):913–5. https://doi.org/10.1056/nejm199009273231311.

Fineberg HV. Pandemic preparedness and response—lessons from the H1N1 influenza of 2009. N Engl J Med. 2014;370(14):1335–42. https://doi.org/10.1056/NEJMra1208802.

Goossens H, Derde L, Horby P, Bonten M. The European clinical research response to optimise treatment of patients with COVID-19: lessons learned, future perspective, and recommendations. Lancet Infect Dis. 2021;22:e153. https://doi.org/10.1016/s1473-3099(21)00705-2.

Gordon VM, Culp MA, Wolinetz CD. Final NIH policy on the use of a single institutional review board for multisite research. Clin Transl Sci. 2017;10(3):130–2. https://doi.org/10.1111/cts.12447.

Gostin LO, Halabi SF, Klock KA. An international agreement on pandemic prevention and preparedness. JAMA. 2021;326(13):1257–8. https://doi.org/10.1001/jama.2021.16104.

GPMB. A world at risk: annual report on global preparedness for health emergencies. Geneva: Global Preparedness Monitoring Board, World Health Organization; 2019.

GPMB. A world in disorder 2020. Global preparedness monitoring board annual report 2020. Geneva: Global Preparedness Monitoring Board; 2020.

Halabi S, Heinrich A, Omer SB. No-fault compensation for vaccine injury—the other side of equitable access to COVID-19 vaccines. N Engl J Med. 2020;383(23):e125. https://doi.org/10.1056/NEJMp2030600.

Hatchett R, Lurie N. Outbreak response as an essential component of vaccine development. Lancet Infect Dis. 2019;19(11):e399–403. https://doi.org/10.1016/s1473-3099(19)30305-6.

Henao-Restrepo AM, Camacho A, Longini IM, Watson CH, Edmunds WJ, Egger M, et al. Efficacy and effectiveness of an rVSV-vectored vaccine in preventing Ebola virus disease: final results from the Guinea ring vaccination, open-label, cluster-randomised trial (Ebola Ca Suffit!). Lancet. 2017;389(10068):505–18. https://doi.org/10.1016/S0140-6736(16)32621-6.

Henderson R. What gets measured gets done. Or does it? Forbes; 2016.

Higgs ES, Dubey SA, Coller BAG, Simon JK, Bollinger L, Sorenson RA, et al. Accelerating vaccine development during the 2013-2016 West African Ebola virus disease outbreak. Curr Top Microbiol Immunol. 2017;411:229–61. https://doi.org/10.1007/82_2017_53.

Independent Panel for Pandemic Preparedness & Response. Building on the past: background paper 1. Geneva: Independent Panel for Pandemic Preparedness & Response; 2021.

Ingstad Sandberg K, Andresen S, Gopinathan U, Hustad Hembre BS. The formation of the Coalition for Epidemic Preparedness Innovations (CEPI): an empirical study. Wellcome Open Res. 2020;5 https://doi.org/10.12688/wellcomeopenres.16284.1.

International Vaccines Task Force. Money and microbes: strengthening clinical research capacity to prevent epidemics. Washington, DC: World Bank; 2018.

Kasprowicz VO, Chopera D, Waddilove KD, Brockman MA, Gilmour J, Hunter E, et al. African-led health research and capacity building—is it working? BMC Public Health. 2020;20(1):1104. https://doi.org/10.1186/s12889-020-08875-3.

Kennedy SB, Bolay F, Kieh M, Grandits G, Badio M, Ballou R, et al. Phase 2 placebo-controlled trial of two vaccines to prevent Ebola in Liberia. N Engl J Med. 2017;377(15):1438–47. https://doi.org/10.1056/NEJMoa1614067.

Keusch GT, Lurie N. The R&D preparedness ecosystem: preparedness for health emergencies: report to the Global Preparedness Monitoring Board. Geneva: Global Preparedness Monitoring Board; 2020.

Kuznetsova L. COVID-19: the world community expects the World Health Organization to play a stronger leadership and coordination role in pandemics control. Front Public Health. 2020;8:470. https://doi.org/10.3389/fpubh.2020.00470.

Larson HJ. Stuck: how vaccine rumors start—and why they don't go away. New York: Oxford University Press; 2020.

Levine AC. Academics are from Mars, humanitarians are from Venus: Finding common ground to improve research during humanitarian emergencies. Clin Trials (London, England). 2016;13(1):79–82. https://doi.org/10.1177/1740774515617935.

London AJ, Omotade OO, Mello MM, Keusch GT. Ethics of randomized trials in a public health emergency. PLoS Negl Trop Dis. 2018;12(5):e0006313. https://doi.org/10.1371/journal.pntd.0006313.

Long CB, Madan RP, Herold BC. Diagnosis and management of community-associated MRSA infections in children. Expert Rev Anti-Infect Ther. 2010;8(2):183–95. https://doi.org/10.1586/eri.09.127.

Lurie N, Keusch GT, Dzau VJ. Urgent lessons from COVID 19: why the world needs a standing, coordinated system and sustainable financing for global research and development. Lancet. 2021;397(10280):1229–36. https://doi.org/10.1016/S0140-6736(21)00503-1.

Mesch GS, Schwirian KP. Social and political determinants of vaccine hesitancy: lessons learned from the H1N1 pandemic of 2009-2010. Am J Infect Control. 2015;43(11):1161–5. https://doi.org/10.1016/j.ajic.2015.06.031.

Moon S, Sridhar D, Pate MA, Jha AK, Clinton C, Delaunay S, et al. Will Ebola change the game? Ten essential reforms before the next pandemic. The report of the Harvard-LSHTM Independent Panel on the Global Response to Ebola. Lancet. 2015;386(10009):2204–21.

NASEM. Integrating clinical research into epidemic response: the Ebola experience. Washington, DC: The National Academies Press, National Academies of Sciences Engineering and Medicine Publications; 2017.

Pallmann P, Bedding AW, Choodari-Oskooei B, Dimairo M, Flight L, Hampson LV, et al. Adaptive designs in clinical trials: why use them, and how to run and report them. BMC Med. 2018;16(1):29. https://doi.org/10.1186/s12916-018-1017-7.

Pandemic Preparedness Partnership. 100 days mission to respond to future pandemic threats: reducing the impact of future pandemics by making diagnostics, therapeutics and vaccines available within 100 days: a report to the G7. London: G7 United Kingdom 2021; 2021.

RECOVERY Trial. University of Oxford, Oxford. 2022. https://www.recoverytrial.net/. Accessed 15 Apr 2022.

Rojek AM, Horby PW. Offering patients more: how the West Africa Ebola outbreak can shape innovation in therapeutic research for emerging and epidemic infections. Philos Trans R Soc Lond B Biol Sci. 2017;372(1721) https://doi.org/10.1098/rstb.2016.0294.

Salam AP, Cheng V, Edwards T, Olliaro P, Sterne J, Horby P. Time to reconsider the role of ribavirin in Lassa fever. PLoS Negl Trop Dis. 2021;15(7):e0009522. https://doi.org/10.1371/journal.pntd.0009522.

Saville M, Cramer JP, Downham M, Hacker A, Lurie N, Van der Veken L, et al. Delivering pandemic vaccines in 100 days—what will it take? N Engl J Med. 2022;387:e3. https://doi.org/10.1056/NEJMp2202669.

Siddle KJ, Eromon P, Barnes KG, Mehta S, Oguzie JU, Odia I, et al. Genomic analysis of Lassa virus during an increase in cases in Nigeria in 2018. N Engl J Med. 2018;379(18):1745–53. https://doi.org/10.1056/NEJMoa1804498.

Ura T, Yamashita A, Mizuki N, Okuda K, Shimada M. New vaccine production platforms used in developing SARS-CoV-2 vaccine candidates. Vaccine. 2021;39(2):197–201. https://doi.org/10.1016/j.vaccine.2020.11.054.

Weisz G, Tousignant N. International health research and the emergence of global health in the late twentieth century. Bull Hist Med. 2019;93(3):365–400. https://doi.org/10.1353/bhm.2019.0049.

WHO. An R&D blueprint for action to prevent epidemics: plan of action 2016. Geneva: World Health Organization; 2016.

WHO. ACT now, ACT together: 2020–2021 impact report. Geneva: World Health Organization. Accelerator AtC-TA; 2021.

Wolf J, Jannat R, Dubey S, Troth S, Onorato MT, Coller B-A, et al. Development of pandemic vaccines: ERVEBO case study. Vaccines (Basel). 2021;9(3):190. https://doi.org/10.3390/vaccines9030190.

World Bank. Pandemic emergency financing facility. Washington, DC: World Bank; 2021. https://www.worldbank.org/en/topic/pandemics/brief/pandemic-emergency-financing-facility. Accessed 9 Feb 2022.

28 Financing Emergency Research Response During Infectious Disease Outbreaks: Lessons from the World Bank and Other International Financial Institutions

Muhammad Ali Pate and Sulzhan Bali

Contents

Learning Track Note: This chapter appears in Learning Tracks: Global Health; Health Policy, Multilateral Cooperation, International Governance

E. S. Higgs and R. A. Sorenson (eds.), *Principles and Practice of Emergency Research Response*,
https://doi.org/10.1007/978-3-031-48408-7_41

Learning Objectives

This chapter will help readers understand and describe:

- The role of international financial institutions (IFIs) in financing preparedness and response for emerging infectious diseases
- How IFIs can support emergency response research
- How IFI initiatives complement other global efforts to strengthen disease surveillance and response systems
- How IFIs effectively contribute to partnerships
- How IFIs have used development lending to bolster core capacity of health systems and clinical research
- Constraints faced by IFIs in financing clinical research
- Examples of lessons learned in recent pandemics
- The potential for IFIs to further improve investment in emergency research preparedness and response

1 Introduction: International Financial Institution Investments in Health Security

International financial institutions (IFIs) began to play an increasingly crucial role in health security financing after the 2014–2016 West Africa Ebola virus disease (EVD) epidemic. Since then, diverse actors in the global health field, including large foundations, regional players, and IFIs have increasingly assumed major roles in global health, health security, and integrating research into emergency response.

Box 1: What Are International Financial Institutions?

IFIs are financial institutions, established or chartered by more than one country, which provide financial support for development projects via grants and loans. The owners (shareholders) of IFIs are typically governments of sovereign countries, but also include other multilateral institutions and international organizations. Each IFI has its own independent legal and operational status (Bhargava 2006). IFIs include the International Monetary Fund (IMF) and the five multilateral development banks: the World Bank Group (WBG), the African Development Bank (AfDB), the Asian Development Bank (ADB), the Inter-American Development Bank (IDB), and the European Bank for Reconstruction and Development (EBRD) (Bhargava 2006). IFIs have broad country membership, including both borrowing and lending countries. While IMF and WBG are global institutions and are considered specialized but independent agencies in the United Nations (UN) system, the other four focus on a single world region and are often called regional development banks.

Other publicly owned international banks also provide lending for development; these are often clustered together as multilateral financial institutions rather than IFIs, as they usually have narrower membership structures and/or focus on specific sectors or activities (Bhargava 2006). A few global public-private international partnership organizations, such as the Global Fund to Fight AIDS, Tuberculosis and Malaria (Global Fund), also serve as international financing organizations by mobilizing, managing, and disbursing financing, albeit with a narrower focus on ending the epidemics of HIV/AIDS, tuberculosis, and malaria to attain the corresponding Sustainable Development Goals (SDGs) for health (Bartsch 2007). While this chapter primarily focuses on IFIs, it also highlights the role of these global financing partnerships, such as the Global Fund and Gavi, the Vaccine Alliance, in strengthening emergency response research for infectious diseases.

During and after the West Africa EVD outbreak, several commissions and task forces offered recommendations on how the global community could better prepare for crises. They included investing more in preparedness, leveraging new funding mechanisms for emergency response, such as an insurance model, and establishing a global research and development (R&D) facility to develop drugs for outbreaks (Gostin et al. 2016; GPMB 2019; Moon et al. 2015). In response, the international development community took several steps to strengthen the capacity to prevent, detect, and respond to outbreaks (GPMB 2019). They included establishing the World Health Emergencies (WHE) Programme and Contingency Fund for Emergencies (CFE) at the World Health Organization (WHO), the African Union's Africa Centres for Disease Control and Prevention (Africa CDC), the African Risk Capacity (ARC) Group, and the Coalition for Epidemic Preparedness Initiatives (CEPI). These changes include initiatives by the World Bank Group and other IFIs to strengthen both preparedness and response aspects of health security (African Risk Capacity (ARC) Group 2022; CEPI 2020; Nkengasong et al. 2017; WHO 2017).

2 International Financial Institution Initiatives to Strengthen Emergency Response: Leveraging Insurance, Contingency Financing, and Institutional Changes

IFIs were heavily engaged in financing the emergency response to the EVD outbreak. For example, AfDB was among the first to support EVD-affected countries, with a grant of US$3 million in April 2014 and overall financing of US$223 million. During the epidemic, IFIs distributed over US$1 billion to affected countries for outbreak response (Office of the UN Special Envoy on Ebola 2016). The WBG provided US$518 million for immediate response and US$650 million in International Development Association (IDA) grants and loans (Reynolds 2015; World Bank 2019c). However, delays in detection of Ebola cases, resource mobilization, and financing hindered a swift and effective response.

Since then, there has been notable progress in creating new financing mechanisms, approaches, and funding commitments for response. These include the World Bank's expansion of the eligibility criteria for its Crisis Response Window (CRW) and adoption and adaptation of the Contingent Emergency Response Component (CERC) and the Catastrophic Demand Drawdown Option (Cat-DDO), which permits access to funds within WBG-financed projects and budget support during crises, respectively.[1] Further, in 2016 the World Bank launched its Pandemic Emergency Financing Facility (PEF), in consultation with WHO and other partners, to rapidly finance surge response (World Bank 2019c). When the coronavirus disease 2019 (COVID-19) pandemic struck, several IFIs responded early and vigorously to support Ministries of Health (MoHs).

On March 17, 2020, the World Bank approved the COVID-19 Fast-Track Facility to help countries prevent, detect, and respond to the rapid viral spread of severe acute respiratory coronavirus-2 (SARS-CoV-2). On April 2, 2020, the World Bank approved the global COVID-19 Strategic Preparedness and Response Program, using the multi-programmatic approach (MPA) to provide up to US$6 billion for response from its International Bank for Reconstruction and Development (IBRD) and IDA funds to focus on the COVID-19 health response. Up to US$4.4 billion of these funds have been committed across all seven World Bank regions. In October 2020, additional financing of US$12 billion was approved for COVID-19 vaccine

1 CERC enabled WBG to release US$2.5 million during the 2018 Nigerian Lassa epidemic within 9 days and US$40 million to Yemen twice for cholera response. Similarly, activation of CERC in the Health System Strengthening for Better Maternal and Child Health Results Project resulted in release of US$80 million twice to DRC to respond to its tenth EVD outbreak. Similarly, in 2020 Romania became the first country to request Cat-DDO activation to ensure readiness to respond to the 2019-nCoV (interim name for COVID-19) epidemic.

acquisition and deployment. As of January 17, 2022, the Bank had approved 83 operations totaling US$7.6 billion to support vaccine procurement and rollout in 69 countries.

Similarly, other IFIs provided crucial support for country response. For example, AfDB created a US$10.2 billion Crisis Response Facility (CRF) to provide a flexible range of support to African countries to help manage pandemic impacts (African Development Bank 2021). A US$3 billion "Fight COVID-19" social bond was successfully marketed to make resources available immediately. The Islamic Development Bank (IsDB) also approved five health-sector projects with an overall allocation of US$172.3 million in Benin, Chad, Côte d'Ivoire, Guinea, and Pakistan to help mitigate COVID-19. The Bank also contributed US$72.5 million toward the International Vaccine Access Center (IVAC) Covid-19 Vaccine Support for Pakistan (Islamic Development Bank 2021). In 2021, ADB committed US$4.9 billion through rapid-disbursing operations, including policy-based lending (US$4.6 billion) and the COVID-19 Pandemic Response Option (US$250 million), to help countries fight COVID-19 (ADB 2021). To address gaps in continuity of essential health services and enhance resilience to future pandemics, ADB provided US$1.3 billion for programs and projects supporting COVID-19 response in education, public health, and social protection (ADB 2021).

IFI financing during recent health emergencies, including COVID-19, has focused on curbing the impact of health crises while also leveraging response efforts and strengthening pandemic preparedness. Given the speed with which countries needed to mount a response and the long-standing fragility of many health systems, the focus was on supporting countries in delivering COVID-19 interventions.

3 Mobilizing International Financial Institution Investment to Bolster Preparedness

In 2016, the World Bank, in partnership with the Wellcome Trust, launched the International Working Group (IWG) for Financing Preparedness to recommend innovative measures for development partners and governments to finance preparedness (WBG 2017). To monitor the state of global preparedness, WHO and the World Bank also launched the Global Preparedness Monitoring Board (GPMB) in 2018 (GPMB 2021) (◘ Fig. 1).

IFIs are increasingly contributing to country preparedness. For example, World Bank-funded emergency response projects have often embedded health-system strengthening and preparedness activities together. Between 2020 and 2022, the World Bank committed more than US$15 billion in the health sector towards the Strategic Preparedness and Response Program (SPRP) using the multi-programmatic approach (MPA). Many of these COVID-19 health response operations also include a focus on longer-term prevention and preparedness (World Bank 2023). Even prior the COVID-19 pandemic, the World Bank committed an average of US$133 million per year to strengthen preparedness in the period from FY2015 to FY2019. During the COVID-19 pandemic (FY2020 to FY2022), the World Bank's financing for preparedness increased more than six-fold, reaching US$882.2 million per fiscal year on average—representing an increase in commitment to support preparedness. Through their core funding mechanisms, IFIs have become the largest source of external financing for pandemic prevention, preparedness, and response (PPPR). For example, in Ghana, the US$35 million World Bank operation includes support for strengthening national laboratories to provide real-time disease surveillance and outbreak reporting systems.

Furthermore, multi-donor trust fund (MDTF) programs, such as the World Bank's Health Emergency Preparedness and Response (HEPR) Umbrella Program, can serve as critical tools in the arsenal of IFIs for promoting PPR. The World Bank launched HEPR in 2021 to provide financing and technical assistance for pandemic preparedness in low-income countries with weak health emergency preparedness and response capabilities, including countries that are unable to access regular World Bank financing because they

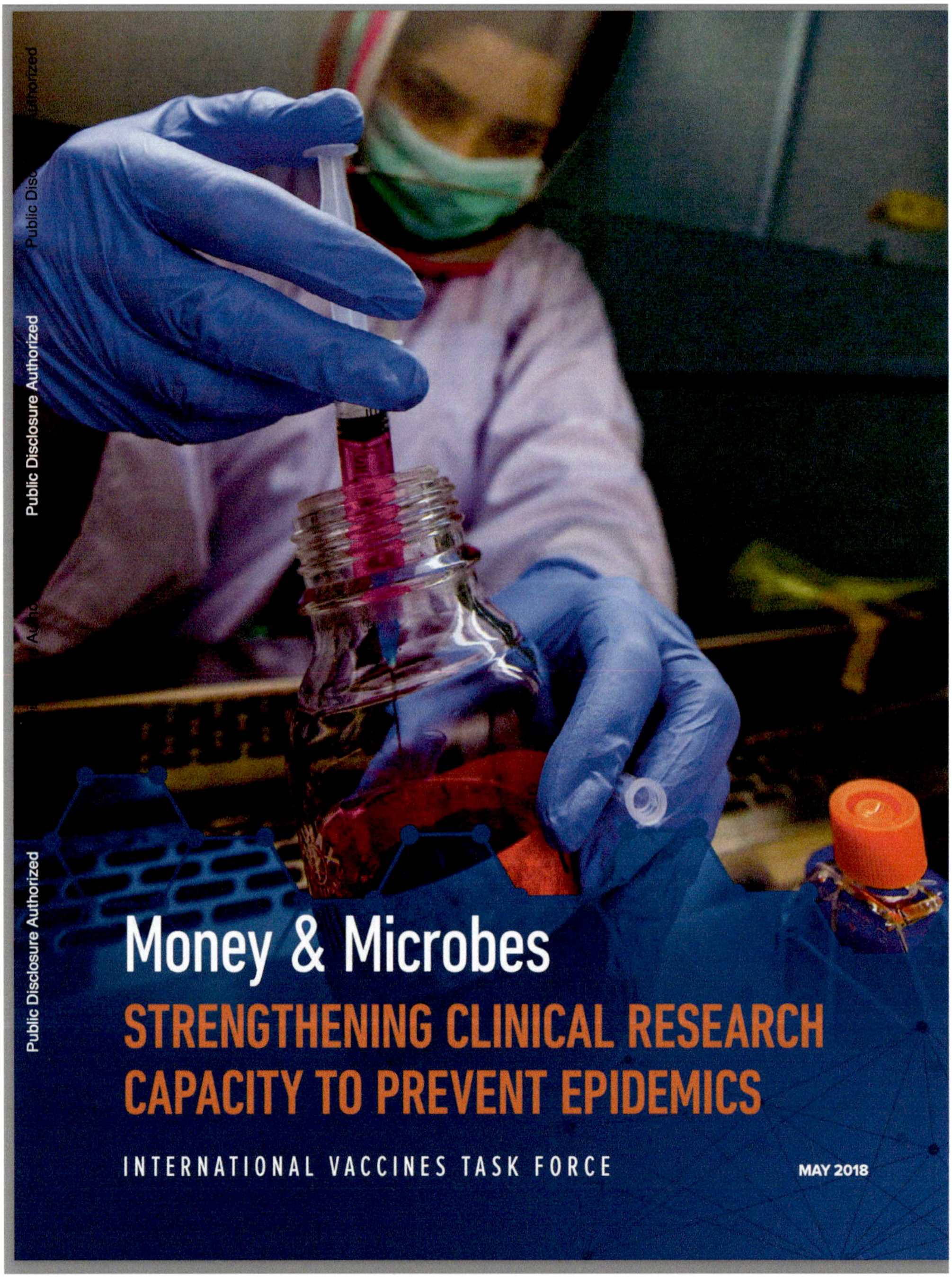

Fig. 1 The Money & Microbes report, supported and published by the World Bank, was an important step in recognition of the need for financing research as an integral element of infectious disease response. (International Vaccines Task Force 2018)

are in arrears with their payments to the IDA (World Bank 2021).

IFIs have also supported regional investments in preparedness, such as the East Africa Public Health Laboratory Network, the Southern Africa Tuberculosis Health Systems project, the Regional Disease Surveillance Systems Enhancement (REDISSE) Program,

Africa CDC, and ADB's Greater Mekong Sub-region Health Security project and Pacific Regional Systems Strengthening project.

3.1 Emergency Research for Emerging or Re-emerging Infectious Diseases (EIDs) Limited by Weak Country Research Capacity

Research is a crucial building block for emergency response. It spans epidemiological, virological, and disease course research on pathogens and the diseases they cause to development and assessment of medical countermeasures (MCMs). It includes fundamental research for development of diagnostics, vaccines, and therapeutics, and applied research, such as emergency response implementation research, evaluations, and social research. These research domains are critical to understanding and stopping epidemics (Hall et al. 2019).

The 2014–2016 Ebola epidemic in West Africa underscored the urgent need to strengthen the mobilization of rapid, robust research during epidemics and the importance of access to effective therapeutics, vaccines, and personal protective equipment (PPE) (NASEM 2017). Ebola had not been identified in West Africa previously, and reliable systems for sharing epidemiological, genomic, and clinical data were absent. Multiple analyses of the Ebola response highlighted the need to develop a framework of norms and rules for conducting research during epidemics, ensure equitable benefit, and develop a global R&D financing facility for drugs, diagnostics, and PPE.

Since then, some strengthening of epidemic response research has occurred. These include WHO's R&D Blueprint, a global strategy that includes 10 prioritized EIDs, a roadmap of action, and a structure for coordinating research during emergencies. The R&D Blueprint was instrumental in supporting the deployment of rVSV-ZEBOV vaccine for Ebola, prioritization of R&D activities for Zika virus vector control interventions, and the use of GeneXpert to augment diagnostic capacity during the ninth and tenth EVD epidemics in the Democratic Republic of the Congo (DRC) (WHO 2019).

Another major milestone has been the launch of the Coalition for Epidemic Preparedness Innovations (CEPI)—a partnership of bilateral donors, philanthropy, civil organizations, and IFIs such as the World Bank—to stimulate, finance, and coordinate vaccine development against prioritized diseases with epidemic potential (▶ Chap. 13). CEPI was launched in January 2017, with US$500 million initial funding from the Bill and Melinda Gates Foundation, Wellcome Trust, Norway, Japan, and Germany (Hatchett and Lurie 2019; Leigh et al. 2018). CEPI raised US$800 million to invest in vaccine candidates for diseases like Lassa fever, Middle East respiratory syndrome (MERS), Nipah, chikungunya, and Rift valley fever.

Other R&D initiatives include the Global Research Collaboration for Infectious Diseases Research (GloPID-R), European and Developing Countries Clinical Trial Partnership (EDCTP), U.S. Biomedical Advanced Research and Development Authority (BARDA), U.S. National Institutes of Health (NIH) R&D investments, and several new networks for research collaboration (e.g., the Joint West Africa Research Group and the African Coalition for Epidemic Research, Response, and Training). Recently, the Global Virome Project was established to find and sequence viruses circulating in wildlife that could spill over to humans.

COVID-19 further underscores the importance of R&D and innovation as key enablers of response not only to the COVID-19 pandemic as such, but also to its health, economic, and social disruptions. Research has progressed during the pandemic at an unprecedented speed and scale, and gains in understanding the virus and developing and assessing countermeasures have been impressive. When the SARS-CoV-2 virus was identified in early 2020, researchers shared its entire genetic sequence online within 42 days. Rapid research and dissemination of results were vital to vaccine development. Research on related coronaviruses and mRNA vaccine platforms underway long before COVID-19 appeared was instrumental in speeding up trials and developing timely interventions (Bloom et al. 2021).

Vaccine development often takes many years, but during COVID-19 there were nearly 100 vaccines in development and eight in clinical trials within 6 months, with the first emergency use authorizations coming from the U.S. Food and Drug Administration (FDA) and the European Medicines Agency (EMA) in December 2020. In the first weeks of the outbreak, WHO activated the R&D Blueprint and established the Solidarity international clinical trials aimed at rapidly assessing the relative effectiveness of COVID-19 treatments (WHO 2022b, c). As the need for strengthened international coordination of the COVID-19 R&D effort became evident, major global health organizations—WHO; CEPI; the Foundation for Innovative New Diagnostics, a global alliance for diagnostics; Gavi, the Vaccine Alliance; the Global Fund; Unitaid; the Wellcome Trust; and the World Bank—established the Access to COVID-19 Tools Accelerator (ACT-A) with additional support from governments, manufacturers, and other funders (WHO 2022a).

Despite such efforts to improve coordination of R&D during the pandemic, progress has still been ad hoc at best. GPMB reports in 2020 and 2021 have called on countries to invest in R&D, enable data sharing (especially genome sequences), and create an "end-to-end mechanism for research, development, and equitable access to common goods" (GPMB 2021). The momentum created by the pandemic is an opportunity to establish effective and sustainable mechanisms to support the R&D necessary to confront health emergencies.

3.2 The Market Is Failing to Support R&D for Emerging or Re-emerging Infectious Diseases

Without the prospect of profit, it is difficult to find private-sector partners to fund the research, including clinical trials, required for licensing vaccines, therapeutics, and diagnostics (VTDs) to fight epidemics (Leigh et al. 2018). Despite a large potential market, there is a market failure for pharmaceutical investment in innovation for EID VTD: the development process is risky; lengthy (typically up to 10 years); and costly (on the order of US$1 billion or more until licensure, with the success rate of interventions that enter trials historically less than 12% (NASEM 2017). Given profit maximization driving the private sector, investments in R&D tend to go to diseases with a high potential return on investment—often those prevalent in high-income countries (HICs), especially chronic diseases for which patients need to take medications over the long term.

This suggests that market mechanisms do not generate sufficient incentives for companies to invest in drug discovery or development for EIDs or diseases prevalent in low- and middle-income countries (LMICs). Despite the high social impact, vaccines and point-of-care diagnostics are also less profitable than drugs and laboratory assays, resulting in lower incentive to invest in R&D to prevent EIDs. As a result, few companies invest in emergency response research, particularly for VTD (Perkins et al. 2017). Reliable incentives are lacking for mechanisms that incentivize international collaboration to develop VTD outside of emergencies.

3.3 Rationale for Public Investment in Emergency Response Research

Given the high social impact, research on EIDs (including the development of VTD and research on delivery and acceptance of countermeasures) is considered a global public good (GPG). As a general rule, public goods are considered to be non-rival (one person's consumption of the good does not diminish another person's access to it) and non-excludable (a person must not be denied access to that good). While the knowledge generated by medical research could be considered a GPG, even access to that knowledge comes with a price and a delay (e.g., payment to a journal for access to an article that has taken time to write and review). GPGs are items available to all (air and water), abstractions like knowledge or human rights, or services like national defense or (in many developed countries) health care (Reiss 2021).

In this context, actions aimed at improving health, including (1) knowledge generation, (2) fostering global health leadership and stewardship, and (3) activities controlling negative and regional externalities, such as pandemic preparedness, can be viewed as global public goods (McDade et al. 2019). While the rationale for public investment in emergency response research is strong, the results of that research, for example in the form of VTD, are often distributed based on ability to pay and thus not non-excludable and are in limited supply and thus not non-rivalrous (Lie and Miller 2020).

Gaps in health research capacity, VTD production, and distribution networks impact not only the availability of VTD to lower income countries, but they directly affect decision-making and may undermine public trust, both of which are integral to an effective emergency response. A lack of information and evidence during a health shock can generate misinformation, as with the promotion of hydroxychloroquine, an anti-malarial drug, for COVID-19 treatment without sound clinical evidence—the drug turned out be non-beneficial for COVID-19 and appeared to be associated with heart arrhythmias (Infante et al. 2021). Evidence-based decision-making is critical to public trust and hinges on well-designed research during emergencies, including biomedical and epidemiological research, data modeling, R&D, and clinical trials. In the aftermath of recent epidemics, including Ebola outbreaks in West Africa, DRC, and Uganda, Zika largely in South America, and of course during the COVID-19 pandemic, investment in emergency response research as a GPG has been recognized as essential to attain SDGs and health security (Lurie et al. 2021).

3.4 Research During Emergencies Requires Prior Investment in Research Systems

In addition to insufficiently focusing on R&D, several LMICs have weak research and regulatory systems. An analysis of global health security capacity in all countries found that 76% have limited capacity to test and approve new medical countermeasures (MCMs), and 50% and 80% have low capacity to acquire MCMs and to dispense MCMs during emergencies, respectively (GHS Index 2021).

Striking gaps in R&D investments and capacities persist between HICs and LMICS, which are more vulnerable to the threat of epidemics in part because of weaker health systems. Lack of adequate research infrastructure and equipment, coupled with limited research capacity, results in a significant research disparity. For example, less than 0.5% of global publications in health research comes from Africa. Analysis by WHO reveals that the number of research grants for health research in the United States in 2016 was 53,114, with only 450 and 122 for Africa and Southeast Asia, respectively (Ralaidovy et al. 2020).

Research is essential not only for developing VTD but also for understanding their effects, both desired and undesired, in diverse populations. In addition to fundamental research—required for pathogen detection, identification, and development of diagnostics, therapeutics, and vaccines—there is also a need to strengthen applied research capabilities. This includes implementation research, evaluation methods, and social research during emergencies to understand attitudes, barriers, and enablers for interventions. Research for understanding population differences and disparities in access to and demand for vaccines proved critical in the response to COVID-19. Research during COVID-19 also highlighted the issue of mistrust in governments and pharmaceutical companies, hindering the uptake of vaccines and leading to defiance of physical distancing guidelines and masking mandates. Research on new SARS-CoV-2 strains via genome sequencing also informed decisions on MCM composition and administration, on physical distancing, travel guidelines, and isolation periods for patients and community.

3.5 International Financial Institutions and Research Financing

While IFIs are among the largest multilateral funders of global health and GPGs (Sridhar et al. 2017), they were not established with research financing as a primary goal and have not been much involved in financing research until recently. Direct investments by IFIs are subject to demand generation by countries and regions, requiring high-level political commitment by the ministry of finance (MoF) and often the head of government. Strong advocacy has often been needed to ensure research investments are high on their agenda. Further, given the risks of MCM development, investing in research can have reputational risks for both governments and IFIs, which often raise funds on capital markets through issuance of bonds and from member states. Additionally, governance of research directly supported by IFIs (there are often no ethical review boards set up for IFIs) can be challenging as the IFIs would have to rely on national institutions.

While IFIs typically are not set up to directly fund R&D for EIDs, they still have a strong comparative advantage and role in supporting emergency response research (McDade et al. 2019). First, IFIs such as the World Bank are well placed to deliver on GPGs (Sridhar et al. 2017). With their strong convening power, IFIs can steer global and regional agendas by bringing donors together for consensus-building, harmonization of priorities, and resource mobilization. This includes regional data sharing, harmonization of regulatory processes, and investments in centers of excellence for cutting edge research.

Second, the comparative advantage of IFIs includes knowledge sharing and technical assistance for policy advice. For example, the World Bank in its role as a "knowledge bank" can strengthen knowledge generation and exchange to support emergency response research.

Third, IFIs have longstanding relationships with MoFs and other ministries, such as agriculture and education, which can strengthen cross-sectoral advocacy and collaboration for investments in emergency response research. IFIs can further make an investment case for preparedness for emergency response research.

Fourth, global public-private financing partnerships, such as the Global Fund and Gavi, and to some extent IFIs, can shape markets to incentivize research on MCMs for EIDs through advanced market commitments (AMC). For example, Gavi provided US$5 million to develop Ebola vaccines. During COVID-19, IFIs helped LMICs finance and distribute vaccines. The World Bank partnered with COVAX, the vaccine distribution arm of WHO's COVID-19 response, and the African Union (through the Africa Vaccine Acquisition Task Team) to help countries purchase and deploy vaccines, thus helping shape the market for COVID-19 vaccines.

Fifth, IFIs have a strong comparative advantage in fund management, including trust funds, for major global private-public partnerships that invest in emergency response research. For example, the World Bank serves as the trustee for CEPI.

Finally, IFIs support emergency response research through their routine approach to lending for projects that strengthen research systems and policy lending that provides budgetary support to countries contingent on policy reforms. Transport and electricity are as necessary to clinical research efforts as experimental medicinal products (▶ Chap. 39).

Consequentially, although IFIs are not structured to finance research, there are innovative examples wherein IFIs financing can be leveraged to strengthen research capacity by integrating investments in research capabilities and research systems in projects. For example, for the COVID-19 multiprogrammatic approach (MPA), the template used by projects included components for monitoring and evaluation as well as learning agendas to support research on forecasting, social behaviors including compliance with and impact of social distancing measures under different contexts, etc. Furthermore, research requires not just direct research financing but also capabilities such as sequencing capacity, trained molecular biologists and scientists, quality laboratories, training in clinical trials and evaluations, strong public health institutions, knowledge exchange, regional hubs—all requiring long-term country investments that IFIs can support. The following section highlights some innovative examples wherein IFIs can be leveraged to promote investments in research capacity especially for health emergencies.

3.6 How International Financial Institutions Can Support Emergency Response Research: Examples from the World Bank

IFIs partner with major institutions to manage funds and can bring donors together to support R&D. As partners, IFIs can strengthen financial management, coordination, resource mobilization, and financing of emergency response research through multi-donor trust funds (MDTFs) and small trust funds, which provide targeted funding for World Bank (or other agency) implementation and supervision, and Financial Intermediary Fund (FIF) partnerships, which provide large-scale funding under independent governance (World Bank 2019a).

3.6.1 Convening Global Partnerships During Emergencies

IFIs, in their role as convenors, can advocate for investments in GPGs. For example, the World Bank co-convened the Access to COVID-19 Tools Accelerator (ACT-A)'s Health System Connector (HSC) as a time-limited global collaboration to accelerate the development, production, and equitable access to COVID-19 tests, treatments, and vaccines to expedite the end of the acute phase of the pandemic. ACT-A brought together diverse stakeholders, including multilateral institutions and IFIs, academic researchers, and the private sector to speed development and delivery of COVID-19 interventions.

3.6.2 Leveraging Trust Funds for R&D

IFIs can leverage trust funds to support research. For example, the International AIDS Vaccine Initiative (IAVI) was among the first product development partnerships for R&D. IAVI aimed to accelerate R&D for HIV vaccines while supporting affordability and access to data, and the World Bank supported IAVI in developing its investment case. The partnership with the World Bank enabled IAVI to facilitate a conference on R&D for global health research,[2] where participants shared lessons on vaccine development and galvanized efforts to mobilize private-sector financing for vaccine development for high-priority, epidemic-prone diseases (World Bank 2019b). Japanese government funding, coupled with management of internal and external expectations, helped minimize reputational risk: it had to be clear to stakeholders that supporting basic science research might or might not result in a viable vaccine, but would still yield significant knowledge.

IAVI provides a successful model of how IFI partnership and co-financing can help leverage small trust funds by reducing transactional costs for supervision, knowledge sharing, and financial management. This model can be replicated to improve cost effectiveness of other official development assistance (ODA) through small or multi-donor trust funds for emergency response research with reduced transactional costs.

It is important to recognize that successful development of COVID-19 vaccines in record time was largely possible because of decades of HIV research, vaccine development and clinical research capacity building. Investment in HIV research also informed strategies on how to reach the most impacted communities, with the most widely used guidance for community engagement, Good Participatory Practice, growing out of HIV/AIDS research (UNAIDS and AVAC 2007; UNAIDS and WHO 2021).

2 IAVI organized a forum called "*Strategic Investment in Global Health Vaccine R&D: Strengthening collaboration among global health initiatives and harnessing private sector engagement*," with CEPI and the Global Health Innovative Technology (GHIT) Fund at the Universal Health Coverage (UHC) Forum in 2017. The meeting was co-hosted by the Japanese Government, the World Bank, WHO, and UNICEF to launch a process for further international collaboration and coordination.

3.6.3 Multi-Donor Trust Funds Strengthening Research Systems

Multi-donor trust funds (MDTF) focused on pandemic preparedness and response (PPR) can also strengthen research systems. For example, the Health Emergency Preparedness and Response (HEPR) Multi-Donor Fund, supported by Japan, Australia, and Germany, brings together different sectors to support preparedness activities in the health sector (e.g., expanding surveillance efforts, training health and laboratory staff, developing contingency plans, and strengthening laboratory networks) and preparedness support activities in other sectors (World Bank 2022a). HEPR has strengthened research systems in several countries and regions, including Africa. For example, it is advancing Africa's genomics surveillance network, coordinated by Africa CDC, through grant support for the Centre for Epidemic Response and Innovation in South Africa and the African Centre of Excellence for Genomics of Infectious Disease (ACEGID) (World Bank 2022a). In Zimbabwe and São Tomé and Príncipe, the HEPR Umbrella Program is supporting training of laboratory technicians, availability of climate-friendly cold chain equipment, and installation and maintenance of solar systems in health facilities—all activities that also support a broader research system (World Bank 2022a).

3.7 Leveraging Routine Lending to Accelerate Research

IFIs can use routine development assistance lending to build core country capacities for prevention, detection, and response as well as research on outbreaks. Mobilizing rapid, robust research during outbreaks depends on investments during non-crisis periods. However, there continue to be major gaps even in funding core capacities required of all countries under the International Health Regulations (2005), which are less demanding than research capacity requirements (WHO 2016). IFIs can also use development lending to accelerate innovation of infectious disease VTD when countries prioritize commitment to research.

3.7.1 Financing Research on Emerging or Re-emerging Infectious Diseases by Strengthening Public Health

The following six major capacity challenges hindered research during the West Africa EVD epidemic

1. Lack of clinical experience with Ebola
2. Poor surveillance and laboratory capacity
3. Deficiency of crucial health system infrastructure and health care workers
4. Small pool of clinical research experts and very limited prior experience in the conduct of clinical research
5. Ethics review boards lacking the resources, experience, and information management systems needed to evaluate an unprecedented number of clinical research proposals
6. Lack of experience and expertise on complex legal and bureaucratic steps in clinical trial conduct, e.g., contract negotiations (NASEM 2017)

Multiple studies have emphasized the importance of knowledge sharing, specimen transport, infrastructure (e.g., cold chain), a functional health care system, and a qualified health and epidemiology workforce as cornerstones for accelerating response research and clinical trials (Hatchett and Lurie 2019; NASEM 2019). For example, the Sierra Leone Trial to Introduce a Vaccine against Ebola (STRIVE) faced grave challenges, including a lack of −80 °C freezers, cold chain, basic equipment (e.g., centrifuges), Good Clinical Practice (GCP) training, and laboratories in smaller towns (Widdowson et al. 2016). A lack of laboratory infrastructure also undermined initial clinical trials in Liberia by fueling mistrust when investigational Ebola virus vaccines had to be stored in the U.S. Embassy in Monrovia due to lack of cold storage capacity elsewhere (NASEM 2017). Strengthening research capacity for epidemic threats cuts across many aspects of preparedness and requires a legal framework, strong country and regional systems for scientific, ethical, and regulatory review, good laboratories, human resources, and equipment.

The development of sustainable disease surveillance and response capacities during inter-epidemic periods is essential for countries to conduct foundational research and prepare for future threats. IFIs can provide financing to build core capacity for health-system research, including surveillance, diagnostic capacity, rehabilitation of facilities, laboratory equipment for clinical and epidemiological research, and research supplies. The World Bank finances multiple regional and country projects to

- Strengthen regional and country assets and infrastructure by improving surveillance systems, laboratory networks, and regional biobanks.
- Strengthen regional and national institutions for project management and public-health research.
- Improve capacity building through interdisciplinary training opportunities, such as field epidemiology training programs (FETP).
- Foster knowledge sharing between countries.

World Bank lending projects that have strengthened key elements of emergency response research include:

3.7.2 The East Africa Public Health Laboratory Network

The East Africa Public Health Laboratory Network shows how an IFI-funded project on laboratory strengthening for tuberculosis can support overall research systems strengthening and anti-microbial resistance (AMR) surveillance. Launched in 2010, the US$129 million project established a network of efficient, high-quality, accessible public-health laboratories in Burundi, Kenya, Rwanda, Tanzania, and Uganda (World Bank 2017). The project has helped 32 laboratories become centers of excellence and increased access to laboratories for poor and vulnerable populations. The project strengthened diagnostic and surveillance capacity, laboratory worker training, and operational research. These included multi-country research on patterns of drug resistance to newly prescribed antibiotics, renovation and construction of laboratories, roll-out of molecular technology for multi-drug resistant tuberculosis (MDR-TB), financing to support certification of the Uganda National TB Reference Lab as a WHO supranational reference lab, training over 10,000 health personnel, strengthening cross-border disease surveillance, and emergency response gap analysis, which enabled swift response to Marburg and EVD outbreaks.

3.7.3 The Southern Africa Tuberculosis Health Systems Support Project

The Southern Africa Tuberculosis Health Systems Support (SATBHSS) project was conceptualized as a disease-specific project[3] to address tuberculosis (TB), including antimicrobial resistant or multi-drug resistant TB [AMR or MDR-TB]), as well as TB/HIV coinfection, in Southern Africa. SATBHSS also supports investments in health systems, strengthening disease surveillance, response to infectious disease outbreaks in cross-border areas, and occupational health interventions in the mining and labor sectors. MDR-TB is one of the world's biggest AMR challenges, and the project systematically supports coordinated regional investment to control MDR-TB. The project also supports pilot programs for health care worker screening and strengthening laboratories. SATBHSS has also coordinated simulations for EVD preparedness and response, which helped contain a 2018 cholera outbreak in six Southern Africa Development Community countries. The project has supported key innovations in TB care and control and proven to be a valuable resource for countries in responding to public health threats (Fig. 2).

3 The development objectives of SATBHSS are to (a) improve coverage and quality of TB control and occupational lung disease services in targeted geographic areas of participating countries and (b) strengthen regional capacity to manage the burden of TB and occupational diseases. The project is active in Lesotho, Malawi, Mozambique, and Zambia with the East, Central, and Southern Africa Health Community and the New Partnership for Africa's Development as its regional implementation partners.

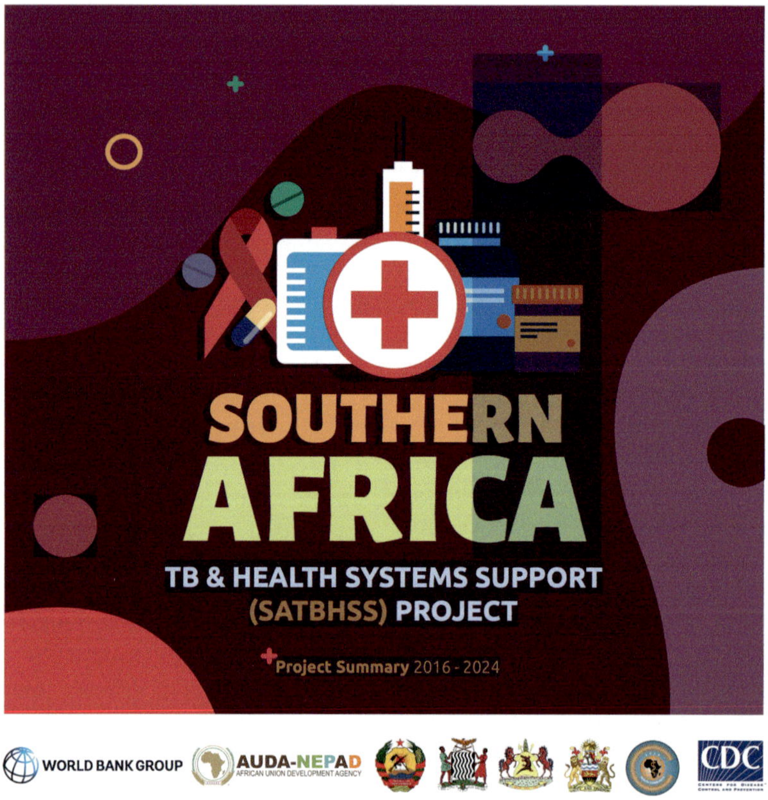

Fig. 2 Southern Africa TB and Health Systems Support Project summary. (SATBHSS Project Brochure 2021)

3.7.4 The Regional Disease Surveillance Systems Enhancement Program

The Regional Disease Surveillance Systems Enhancement (REDISSE) program is a series of projects established after the 2014–2016 West Africa Ebola outbreak to address systemic weaknesses in national and regional capacity for disease surveillance and response. Developed jointly by the Health, Nutrition, and Population and Agriculture Global Practices of the World Bank, REDISSE is a flagship regional One Health program focusing on the human-animal-environment interface where many novel diseases arise (▶ Chap. 10). REDISSE supports 16 countries in West Africa, the West African Health Organization (WAHO), and the Economic Community of Central African States, and has helped establish regional and multisectoral partnerships to

1. Promote collaboration.
2. Reduce the economic burden caused by epidemics.
3. Extend efficiency gains through resource sharing.
4. Bolster health security as a global public good.
5. Address common research needs.
6. Improve rapid response.

3.7.5 The Africa CDC Project

The Africa CDC project strengthened the all-Africa CDC and public-health assets in Ethiopia and Zambia. The project supports transnational surveillance networks, emergency-response mechanisms, training for laboratory workers and field epidemiologists, equipment maintenance, and other health functions to manage epidemic risks across the continent, including sentinel and reference laboratories in Ethiopia and Zambia which can be utilized regionally. Reference laboratories, including bio-safety level (BSL) 2+ laboratories, are crucial for emergency research on pathogens that pose risks to laboratory personnel and surrounding communities. In many countries, lack of adequate BSL-2 and BSL-3 laboratories limits research on such pathogens, or samples may be handled with limited biosecurity measures, posing a risk to workers and communities. Establishment of regional facilities will facilitate research, buttress biosafety, and speed detection of outbreaks. Support of institutions such as Africa CDC can facilitate IFI financing for development of broad capacities and policies for research, such as continent-wide material transfer agreements (MTAs) for expedited sample identification and sequencing, development of research priorities, etc.

3.8 Financing Academic Capacity Building for Research

Lack of research capacity, including high-quality laboratories, is among the most critical challenges to emergency response research. Investments by IFIs in programs such as REDISSE are strengthening regional knowledge exchange and capacity building and enhancing country capacity to conduct health research. Among the needs is training in budget management, grant acquisition, and procurement to make capacity sustainable. Sustainable research capacity also requires strong scientific talent, high-quality universities, and career paths for researchers. Despite being hotspots for emerging epidemics, Southeast Asia and Africa have proportionately very low levels of health research. For example, Africa represents 15% of the global population and 25% of global disease burden but only 2% of global research output and 0.1% of patents (Lan et al. 2014; Schemm 2013; Simpkin et al. 2019). As highlighted by severe acute respiratory syndrome coronavirus (SARS-CoV), Ebola virus, and SARS-CoV-2, strengthening international collaboration between universities can facilitate the development of diagnostics and MCMs during epidemics.[4] Private-sector collaboration with universities also increases the propensity of firms to introduce new products (Marotta et al. 2007).

IFIs have been able to provide development financing for strengthening academic research, research partnerships, and innovation. The African Higher Education Centers of Excellence (ACE) Program provides financing to strengthen the quality of post-graduate education and build collaborative research capacity across Africa (ACE 2022). Under ACE, IFIs have encouraged regional specialization, so participating universities can deliver better specialized training and research support. Subject areas have been selected through a competitive process in key priority disciplines, including health.[5] These centers address development challenges in infectious disease management, public health, and drug development by providing postgraduate training and research experience in molecular biology, analytical epidemiology, traditional medicine, and pharma-biotechnology. They also provide a regional platform for innovative drug development, including exploring the use of traditional medicine, and support equitable access to medications and diagnostics in the region. Since 2014, ACE Health Centers have been leaders in applied research, with the Africa Center for Infectious Genomics and Diseases (ACEGID) playing a central role in the 2014 Ebola response by leading the diagnostics and testing of the first Ebola sample collected in Lagos, Nigeria, and more recently the first genomic sequencing of SARS-CoV-2 in Africa.

4 For example, the early publication of the SARS-CoV-2 genome sequence by China and the immediate and continued agreement by major journals to publish related papers with open access have facilitated development of COVID-19 public health measures, therapeutics, vaccines, and diagnostics.

5 In West Africa, successful Health ACEs include the West Africa Center for Biology of Infectious Diseases at the University of Ghana and the Africa Center for Genomics of Infectious Diseases (ACEGID) at Redeemer's University in Nigeria. In East and Southern Africa, health ACEs are in Ethiopia, Malawi, Tanzania, Uganda, and Zambia.

The ACE project has led to international accreditation of several health-related programs, increased enrollment in health postgraduate programs across Africa, and several memoranda of understanding (MoUs) on research and training collaborations between ACE centers and other regional and international universities and research institutions.

Box 2: Examples of How the World Bank's Investment in Africa Higher Education Centers of Excellence (ACE) Is Strengthening Emergency Response Research

The ACE Center for Genomics of Infectious Diseases in Nigeria (ACEGID), supported through the ACE Program, played a key role in Nigeria during the 2014–16 Ebola outbreak in West Africa, testing the first Ebola patient identified there within 6 h of receiving the blood sample. This proved to be critical for the successful containment of Ebola in the country. The Center also played a crucial role in the investigation of a yellow fever outbreak in the Edo State of Nigeria. The blood samples of patients received at the Irrua Teaching Hospital were sent to the ACEGID laboratory at Redeemer's University because of the Center's track record in rare and dangerous pathogen diagnosis. Using a novel metagenomic sequencing technology that was developed at ACEGID, the pathogen was swiftly identified as a yellow fever virus strain different from all other known yellow fever strains in Nigeria for the last 96 years (Ajogbasile et al. 2020). Twenty-nine of 50 samples were confirmed positive for yellow fever virus by reverse transcriptase-quantitative polymerase chain reaction, 14 of which resulted in genome assembly. The results were swiftly communicated to the Nigeria Centre for Disease Control and Prevention and enabled a quick response and mass vaccination in Edo State that contained the outbreak. ACEGID also sequenced the first African SARS-CoV-2 genome from the first known Nigerian COVID-19 case.

3.9 Lending for Innovation, and R&D for Public Health

IFIs support emergency response research by leveraging development financing for co-financing innovative R&D for MCMs in LMICs. The pharmaceutical sector is critical in R&D for EIDs. However, market failures and the long-standing disconnect between R&D investments and needs in LMICs result in limited research on public-health priorities for LMICs, particularly on neglected tropical diseases and emerging infectious diseases, though there have been several recent partnerships established to remedy the situation (Chatelain and Ioset 2011; Ioset and Chang 2011; Sunyoto 2020). A mix of regulatory and financial barriers to commercialization, lack of capacity for product design and clinical trials, weak intellectual property rights, lack of basic infrastructure, and a shortage of experienced researchers disincentivize private-sector investment in R&D in LMICs. Despite growing capacity for Phase III clinical trials, the production and manufacturing phase of the value chain also remains weak (Simpkin et al. 2019). These inequalities are reflected in the mismatch of R&D outputs with needs. For example, between 1975 and 1999, just over 1% of the 1393 new chemical entities marketed by the pharmaceutical industry were for use in tropical diseases and TB, despite these diseases accounting for 12% of the global disease burden (Torreele et al. 2004; Trouiller et al. 2002). Incentivizing investment in R&D through collaborative financing mechanisms is crucial to stimulate research capacity and future research output in LMICs.

An example is the World Bank's Innovate in India for Inclusiveness project, a US$250 million project established in 2017 and co-financed by the World Bank and government of India (World Bank 2022b). The project helped unlock India's potential for R&D by facilitating innovation in biopharmaceutical products and medical devices to address India's public-health priorities. India has displayed immense growth and capacity for manufacturing generic drugs and vaccines, but research on diseases that largely affect people with lower incomes remains limited. Innovate in India for Inclusiveness was established to promote innovative, early development of biopharmaceuticals and medical devices to address India's public health priorities according to disease burden rather than commercialization potential. The project targets critical gaps in infrastructure, human capital and skills, and technology transfer with the goal of strengthening the pilot-to-market innovation ecosystem. Grant funding is provided to support centers of excellence for validation, early-stage bio-manufacturing, clinical development, training, and technology transfer. Grantees are selected from among top institutions in both the public and private sectors, those that already have a successful track record in the biotechnology space but may lack specific capabilities to enable faster, lower-cost validation through preclinical and clinical development and early-stage manufacturing. It provides grant funding to consortia of private, public, and academic institutions to accelerate development of low-cost vaccines, biopharmaceuticals, diagnostics and medical devices targeted to public health priorities in India (World Bank 2018).

By extending financing to consortia, the project seeks to foster a more collaborative R&D environment and link micro, small, and medium enterprises with larger companies. By engaging vaccine development ethicists from its early stages, the project has minimized reputational risks associated with clinical trial failures. Further, a partnership with NIH has facilitated capacity building for clinical trials and a collaborative environment for R&D investment in India. Two COVID-19 vaccines supported by the project during Phase I/II clinical trials received emergency authorization in 2021 (World Bank 2022b). The project has surpassed its goal of creating a more robust pipeline for affordable products and spurred greater public-private collaboration for research, and is also supporting development of vaccines for other diseases including influenza, dengue, chikungunya, and cholera (Swarup et al. 2019).

3.10 The World Bank's Comparative Advantage in Financial Management

IFIs often partner with other parts of the international community to support large initiatives that are not sufficiently supported by existing funds or mechanisms. Apart from MDTF or single-donor trust funds, IFIs can use their financial and administrative management advantage with financial intermediary funds (FIFs). These are independently governed financial partnership platforms that fund projects implemented by multiple entities, such as other multilateral banks or UN agencies. In FIFs, the World Bank acts as a limited trustee, providing well-established financial, investment management, and accounting platforms, along with specialized legal and treasury services (WBG 2019). In some instances, the Bank also acts as the secretariat or serves as an implementing entity for FIF. While their governance structures vary, all FIFs have external governing bodies responsible for funding decisions. FIFs can incorporate innovative financing and governance arrangements and flexible designs, allowing funds to come through multiple channels and from the private sector, bilateral donors, and foundations (WBG 2014).

Examples of such partnerships include the Onchocerciasis Control Program, which was the first FIF-type partnership, the Global Fund to Fight AIDS, Tuberculosis, and Malaria, CEPI, and PEF. At the end of the financial year 2018 (FY18), there were 27 FIF-type partnerships in operation with cumulative funding of US$97.4 billion. These FIF partnerships transferred US$6.7 billion for development projects in FY2018 (WBG 2019).

FIFs particularly add value when a global call for collective action for GPGs requires long-term, large-scale funding, closely coordinated decision-making, and joint implementation across several multilateral organizations. FIF partnerships allow the World Bank to use its advantage in financial services, including receiving, holding, and investing funds; transferring funds as directed by the FIF governing body; and providing treasury management. Beyond its trustee role, the World Bank can provide secretariat services, donate to a FIF, provide advisory support, or serve as an implementing entity for FIF funds. Engagement of the World Bank in such partnerships raises their profile, ensures due diligence, and increases trust by donors, which helps mobilize resources. Partnership with the World Bank also reduces transactional costs for holding, investing, and disbursing funds.

As a partner, the World Bank has leveraged several of the following FIF-type partnerships (◘ Table 1) that have facilitated research or shaped markets to advance research.

3.10.1 Coalition for Epidemic Preparedness Innovations (CEPI)

The World Bank helped launch CEPI and facilitate resource mobilization for vaccine development to combat emerging infectious disease, including identified pathogens with pandemic potential and the unknown pathogen X—of which the first turned out to be SARS-CoV-2. The Bank also serves as a trustee for CEPI. CEPI's goal is to move new vaccines through late pre-clinical studies to proof of concept and safety in humans before epidemics happen or very rapidly after they are identified. Its current aspiration is to develop and assess vaccines for initial use within 100 days after a new pathogen is sequenced (Pandemic Preparedness Partnership 2021).

CEPI also supports vaccine platforms that can be readily adapted and deployed against known and unknown pathogens. As a trustee, the World Bank manages contributions, investments, cash transfers, accounting, and financial reporting. When CEPI was in its start-up phase, partnership with the World Bank facilitated swift resource mobilization, so that CEPI had already raised US$800 million of its US$1 billion target before COVID-19 struck, enabling it to invest in vaccine candidates for Lassa fever, MERS, Nipah, and more recently chikungunya, Rift Valley fever, and COVID-19.

3.10.2 Gavi, the Vaccine Alliance

The World Bank's partnership in FIFs for the International Finance Facility for Immunization (IFFIm) and Advance Market Commitments (AMC) enabled the establishment of Gavi as the largest contributor to childhood immunization in lower-income countries, and now as an important actor in emergency response. IFFIm, the frontloading mechanism that supports Gavi, has received over US$6.3 billion in pledges from nine donors over a period of 23 years. These commitments were used to issue vaccine bonds in capital markets, which helped raise US$4.5 billion from investors to provide Gavi with greater flexibility beyond donor funding. The AMC partnership helps accelerate the global rollout of vaccines against pneumococcal diseases, a leading cause of child mortality in 60 of the poorest countries. AMC financial commitments provide vaccine manufacturers with incentives to invest in vaccine research and expand manufacturing capacity for affordable vaccines. Donors commit funds to guarantee a low price for vaccines to qualifying countries. The World Bank assumed financial risk for AMC and reputational risk for both AMC and IFFIm.

Gavi has played a key role in advancing emergency response research though its efforts in market shaping, surge response, and implementation research (Gavi 2019; Malhame et al. 2019). For example, Gavi supports diagnostic development for yellow fever through provision of market pull incentives for test kits and maintains diagnostics stockpiles for yellow fever, meningitis, and cholera (Johnson 2018; Zerhouni 2019). In 2016, with a global shortage of yellow fever vaccine, Gavi and WHO pioneered fractional dosing of yellow fever vaccine.[6] Further, Gavi provided US$5 million in AMC to the private sector for the development of the first licensed Ebola vaccine (rVSV-ZEBOV), which was used during the 2018–2020 Ebola epidemic in DRC (Oroxom and Glassman 2019; Schnabel and Glassman 2019). Gavi also supports malaria

6 Research showed that one-fifth of standard doses still provided protection from yellow fever for at least 12 months (► Case Study 25.1).

Table 1 Examples of Financial Intermediary Fund-type partnerships. In the latter half of 2022, the World Bank launched the Financial Intermediary Fund for Pandemic Prevention, Preparedness, and Response to improve preparedness and response for future pandemics (WBG 2022) (authors)

FIF	Type of FIF-funded program	The Bank's role(s) in the governing body	The Bank's role(s) in FIF-funded partnership programs			Number of implementing entities/donors	
			Trustee	Implementing entity	Secretariat services	Implementing entities	Donors
Advance Market Commitment	Supports the Gavi Alliance	Member of AMC Stakeholders Committee	Yes (Financial manager)	–	–	–	6
Coalition for Epidemic Preparedness Innovations	Global Partnership	Observer (Dfi) as Trustee	Yes	–	–	1	5
Global Fund to Fight AIDS, Tuberculosis, and Malaria	Global Partnership	Nonvoting member of the Board and its committees (Dfi) as trustee	Yes	–	–	–	63
International Finance Facility for Immunization	Global Financing Mechanism/UK Charity	Observer (Dfi)	Yes (Treasury manager)	–	–	–	9
Pandemic Emergency Financing Facility	Global Partnership	Co-chair (HNP) and Observer as Trustee (Dfi)	Yes	Yes	Yes	3	4

vaccine development and implementation research on MCM delivery.

3.10.3 The Global Fund to Fight AIDS, Tuberculosis, and Malaria

The Global Fund to Fight AIDS, Tuberculosis, and Malaria is an innovative financing partnership among governments, the private sector, civil society, and communities that provides funding for programs to prevent and treat people with HIV/AIDS, tuberculosis, and malaria. The Global Fund is funded by 55 donor countries, the Bill & Melinda Gates Foundation, European Commission, UN Foundation, WHO, and the private sector. The World Bank serves as its trustee and is a non-voting ex-officio member of its Board. The Global Fund raises and invests nearly US$4 billion annually in its 3-year replenishment cycles to support its programs, including emergency response research, by providing catalytic investments for facilitating market entry of new MCMs through a revolving fund that makes advanced commitments to manufacturers to reduce market entry risk (Global Fund 2019).

Box 3: Financial Intermediary Funds for Pandemic Prevention, Preparedness, and Response: The Pandemic Fund (Fig. 3)

With broad support from the G20 and beyond, on June 30, 2022, the World Bank's Board of Directors approved the proposal to establish the Pandemic Fund—a Financial Intermediary Fund (FIF) for pandemic prevention, preparedness, and response (PPPR). FIFs are an important tool in the development finance toolbox, offering customized financing platforms for multi-stakeholder partnerships. The new FIF for PPPR will provide a dedicated stream of additional, long-term financing to strengthen critical PPPR capabilities in low- and middle-income countries through investments and technical support at the national, regional, and global levels.

Fig. 3 Pandemic Fund logo. (Courtesy World Bank)

Pandemic Fund's investments in PPPR, including to address gaps in surveillance, laboratory capacity, risk communication, zoonotic disease, risk management and more, will help avert the much larger costs that the world would incur in a future pandemic. These investments at regional and country-level will also strengthen the research system through investments in laboratory systems, knowledge sharing, workforce capacity, information sharing, and public health assets sharing.

4 Lessons Learned

4.1 Develop Emergency Research Capacity in Synergy with Capacity for Ongoing Health Research

Building research capacity is an essential component of preparedness. Clinical research (particularly during epidemics) requires strong laboratory infrastructure and systems, human resources, information technology, project and financial management, bio-banking, and ethical review board and regulatory capacity (Gostin et al. 2016; Moon et al. 2015; World Bank 2018). To maximize the impact of emergency research, International Health Regulations (IHR)-required capacities must be strengthened in LMICs, which are often most vulnerable to epidemics. Unfortunately, many LMICs lack adequately trained workforces, laboratory facilities and research infrastructure, and regulatory and ethical review capacities. Strong laboratory systems assist in detection and contribute to critical research, and investments in human resources (including field epidemiology training) support local capacity building for epidemiological research (Beyeler et al. 2019; Carpenter and Bhadelia 2019). Limited access to public health infrastructure and facilities, such as laboratories, research institutions, and advanced training, poses a critical challenge to emergency research and requires upfront investments. By investing in core IHR capacities and disease surveillance and detection systems during non-crisis periods, IFIs can strengthen surge capacity for emergency research response. IFI investments in laboratories and human resources can be optimized for research by integrating applied and clinical research training with field epidemiology training, by conducting clinical research on locally endemic diseases when there is not an outbreak emergency, and by bringing laboratories into the research endeavor. A service model with the private sector can also be explored where laboratories have partnership with the pharmaceutical sector for conducting clinical trials.

4.2 Promote Research Collaboration Among Countries and Stakeholders

Lack of coordination and formal governance, absence of priority setting, insufficient information sharing, and transparency issues are major challenges that can hinder resource mobilization and implementation of emergency response research (Beyeler et al. 2019). Despite new initiatives, resources for research remain fragmented, and there is information asymmetry and insufficient transparency on sources of funding and results of clinical trials, which can lead to duplication of efforts. In such scenarios, the World Bank (or other IFIs) are strategically well placed to bring together countries, regional partners, and developmental partners and use its consensus-building processes and coordination and advocacy functions to enable prioritization and resource mobilization for research. IFIs also typically have fewer challenges working regionally than bilateral players and demonstrate greater legitimacy to ensure trust for resource mobilization.

4.3 Countries Can Leverage International Financial Institution Financing for Research by Ensuring Demand for Investment in Research Is Voiced at the Highest Levels of Government

Policy commitments to preparedness, including research, facilitate emergency response and require advocacy and macroeconomic justifications at the highest levels. Through regular efforts to make the investment case with country leadership, it is possible to ensure research financing is prioritized in the national agenda and subsequently in IFI financed projects. The World Bank's internal processes of Country Policy Institutional Assessment, Systematic Country Diagnosis, and Country Partnership Framework can also be used to encourage such investments. Mainstreaming the importance of research, innovation, and PPR into these country-specific processes can help make research funding a greater priority and generate demand for research investment to unlock financing for research. In addition to IFI investment projects, countries can also request financing from the Pandemic Fund to strengthen investments in surveillance, laboratory systems, human resources—all of which strengthen research systems as well.

4.4 Provide Incentives for Investing in Preparedness and Regional Collaboration

The World Bank's Regional Program for the International Development Association (IDA) provides regional funds along with country

IDA allocations for projects that meet regional criteria.[7] Incentives to countries for using IFI financing or domestic financing for regional approaches to health security and research, such as via matching funds or schemes like the Regional Program for IDA, can facilitate establishment of regional assets and promote cross-border collaboration essential to EID research in emergencies. Further, regional partnerships and programs can enable efficiency gains in research through sharing assets.

4.5 Include Research-Related Indicators in Monitoring and Evaluation

Tracking progress in R&D at a global systems level and project level can guide efforts to strengthen emergency response research. The Global Preparedness Monitoring Board (GPMB), established jointly by the World Bank and WHO, regularly monitors system-wide progress on research and development for EIDs, thereby ensuring accountability. Including research-specific indicators in development projects that report detailed results more systematically helps to ensure research needs are prioritized in preparedness projects. Without such research-linked indicators, investments in research capacity are not likely to meet emergency needs.

4.6 Share Information and Investment Plans Between Epidemics

Preparedness for emergencies can become more robust with planning; pre-approved clinical trial designs; prepositioned MTAs, ethical review protocols and procedures; and regional platforms for vaccine research (Gobat et al. 2019; Gostin et al. 2016). An example is the regional Partnership for Research on Ebola Vaccines in Liberia (PREVAIL), which was set up for ZMapp and vaccine trials during the West Africa Ebola epidemic and enabled swift trials (Kennedy et al. 2016). Similarly, swiftly sharing information stimulates collaboration and implementation of emergency response research, as was seen during the COVID-19 outbreak, where sharing of the genomic sequence and open-access publication of research findings were instrumental in the development of diagnostic tests, vaccines, and therapeutics.

4.7 Develop Additional Incentives to Encourage Investment in R&D

Accelerating development of MCMs, especially in LMICs, requires technical and financial support to successfully navigate the development process and clinical trials. Engagement with the pharmaceutical industry and institutions such as U.S. National Institutes of Health (NIH) can improve sustainability of initiatives and provide technical support needed to stimulate R&D for MCMs.

IFIs can help mobilize investments in clinical research by incorporating components and indicators for research into development assistance lending operations and health security investments. Research-sensitive investments in preparedness that both bolster research systems and regional research networking (including in countries experiencing fragility, conflict, and violence) and favor regional and country-level investments in clinical research for MCMs can stimulate emergency response research. Greater investments in regional institutions, such as West African Health Organization (WAHO) and Africa CDC, would build the capacity of the research institutions to be competitive for research financing.

The IAVI project provides a successful model in which IFI partnership and co-financing can help leverage small trust funds by reducing transactional costs for supervision, knowledge sharing, and financial

7 Including (a) participation of three or more countries and institutions, (b) clear evidence of country and regional ownership, (c) regional benefits through generation of positive externalities and mitigation of negative externalities beyond countries, and (d) provision of a platform for policy harmonization.

management. This model can be replicated to enable utilization of other Official Development Assistance (ODA) through small trust funds or MDTF for emergency response research with reduced transactional costs. The World Bank's HEPR Program and the new FIF for PPR can also be leveraged to strengthen research systems and provide catalytic investments for generating demand for greater investment in research. A trust fund can facilitate consultations and country mechanisms to strengthen prioritization and resource alignment for research, provide technical assistance to invest in research for PPR, and subsidize country investments in research through concessional financing and buy-downs.

World Bank innovative financing mechanisms and FIFs (including CEPI) can be used to stimulate R&D, enable tech transfer, and build capacity. These FIFs can be leveraged to finance clinical trials and scale up MCM production during emergencies (Yamey et al. 2020). Use of FIFs to finance R&D would mitigate fragmentation of resources and improve reaction time, reduce transaction costs, and speed resource mobilization for research during emergencies.

? Discussion Questions

1. Discuss the IFI role in financing preparedness and response for EIDs and how IFIs can more effectively contribute.
2. IFIs are not traditionally purpose-built to finance research but have a strong comparative advantage in strengthening systems and coordinating research. Provide examples from the World Bank of how IFIs can support emergency response research.
3. The development of sustainable disease surveillance and response capacities during inter-epidemic periods is essential for countries to conduct ongoing research and prepare for future threats. How do IFI initiatives complement other global efforts to strengthen disease surveillance and response systems?
4. IFIs often partner with other organizations to respond to pressing needs that are not sufficiently addressed by existing funds or mechanisms. What are IFIs especially good at contributing to such partnerships or consortia?
5. How have IFIs used development lending to bolster core capacity at the intersection of health systems and clinical research? How does this contribute to research during emergencies?
6. What are some constraints faced by IFIs in financing clinical research?
7. Briefly list and discuss some lessons we have learned in recent outbreaks and pandemics. In light of this experience, what opportunities can you identify for IFIs to improve their investments in emergency research preparedness and response?

References

ACE. The ACE impact project. Accra-North: Association of African Universities; 2022. https://ace.aau.org/#:~:text=The%20Africa%20Higher%20Education%20Centers,%2C%20Agriculture%2C%20applied%20Social%20Science%20%2F. Accessed 22 Nov 2022.

ADB. Annual report 2021: toward a green and inclusive recovery. Manila: Asian Development Bank; 2021. Report No.: ISBN: 978-92-9269-422-7 (print); 978-92-9269-423-4 (electronic); 978-92-9269-424-1 (ebook).

African Development Bank. Evaluation of the Bank Group's support to RMCs in the face of COVID-19. 2021.

African Risk Capacity (ARC) Group. African Risk Capacity (ARC) Group. Johannesburg: African Risk Capacity (ARC) Group; 2022. https://www.arc.int/. Accessed 17 Nov 2022.

Ajogbasile FV, Oguzie JU, Oluniyi PE, Eromon PE, Uwanibe JN, Mehta SB, et al. Real-time metagenomic analysis of undiagnosed fever cases unveils a yellow fever outbreak in Edo state, Nigeria. Sci Rep. 2020;10(1):1–6. https://doi.org/10.1038/s41598-020-59880-w.

Bartsch S. The global fund to fight AIDS, tuberculosis and malaria. Global health governance and the fight against HIV/AIDS. Springer; 2007. p. 146–71.

Beyeler N, Fewer S, Yotebieng M, Yamey G. Improving resource mobilisation for global health R&D: a role for coordination platforms? BMJ Glob Health. 2019;4(1):e001209.

Bhargava VK. The role of the international financial institutions in addressing global issues. Global issues for global citizens: an introduction to key development challenges. Washington, DC: World Bank; 2006.

Bloom DE, Cadarette D, Ferranna M, Hyer RN, Tortorice DL. How new models of vaccine development for COVID-19 have helped address an epic public health crisis. Health Aff (Millwood). 2021;40(3):410–8. https://doi.org/10.1377/hlthaff.2020.02012.

Carpenter S, Bhadelia N. Maximum containment infectious disease laboratories as an integral part of emergency preparedness and emergency response. In: Singh SK, Kuhn J, editors. Defense against biological attacks. 1st ed. New York: Springer; 2019. p. 125–44.

CEPI. CEPI creates new collaborative taskforce to assess impact of emerging viral strains on effectiveness of COVID-19 vaccines. Oslo: Coalition for Epidemic Preparedness Innovations; 2020. https://cepi.net/news_cepi/cepi-creates-new-collaborative-taskforce-to-assess-impact-of-emerging-viral-strains-on-effectiveness-of-covid-19-vaccines/. Accessed 15 Apr 2022.

Chatelain E, Ioset JR. Drug discovery and development for neglected diseases: the DNDi model. Drug Des Devel Ther. 2011;5:175–81. https://doi.org/10.2147/dddt.S16381.

Gavi. Market shaping goal. 2019. https://www.gavi.org/our-alliance/strategy/phase-4-2016-2020/market-shaping-goal. Accessed 19 Feb 2020.

GHS Index. 2021 Global health security index. Washington, DC: Nuclear Threat Initiative; 2021. https://www.ghsindex.org/. Accessed 19 Nov 2022.

Global Fund. Market shaping strategy. 2019. https://www.theglobalfund.org/media/5798/core_market-shaping_strategy_en.pdf?u=637166000390000000. Accessed 4 Aug 2024.

Gobat N, Amuasi J, Yazdanpanah Y, Sigfid L, Davies H, Byrne J-P, et al. Advancing preparedness for clinical research during infectious disease epidemics. ERJ Open Res. 2019;5:00227-2018.

Gostin LO, Mundaca-Shah CC, Kelley PW. Neglected dimensions of global security: the global health risk framework commission. JAMA. 2016;315(14):1451–2.

GPMB. A world at risk: annual report on global preparedness for health emergencies. Geneva: Global Preparedness Monitoring Board, World Health Organization; 2019.

GPMB. From worlds apart to a world prepared: Global Preparedness Monitoring Board report 2021. Geneva: World Health Organization, GPM Board; 2021.

Hall W, Jamieson A, Wardle G. Advancing epidemics R&D to keep up with a changing world: progress, challenges, and opportunities. London: Wellcome Trust; 2019.

Hatchett R, Lurie N. Outbreak response as an essential component of vaccine development. Lancet Infect Dis. 2019;19(11):e399–403. https://doi.org/10.1016/s1473-3099(19)30305-6.

Infante M, Ricordi C, Alejandro R, Caprio M, Fabbri A. Hydroxychloroquine in the COVID-19 pandemic era: in pursuit of a rational use for prophylaxis of SARS-CoV-2 infection. Expert Rev Anti Infect Ther. 2021;19(1):5–16.

International Vaccines Task Force. Money and microbes: strengthening clinical research capacity to prevent epidemics. Washington, DC: World Bank; 2018.

Ioset J-R, Chang S. Drugs for neglected diseases initiative model of drug development for neglected diseases: current status and future challenges. Future Med Chem. 2011;3(11):1361–71. https://doi.org/10.4155/fmc.11.102.

Islamic Development Bank. Development effectiveness report. 2021.

Johnson H. GAVI support for yellow fever diagnostic capacity. Geneva: Gavi, the Vaccine Alliance; 2018.

Kennedy SB, Neaton JD, Lane HC, Kieh MWS, Massaquoi MBF, Touchette NA, et al. Implementation of an Ebola virus disease vaccine clinical trial during the Ebola epidemic in Liberia: design, procedures, and challenges. Clin Trials (London, England). 2016;13(1):49–56. https://doi.org/10.1177/1740774515621037.

Lan G, Blom A, Kamalski J, Lau G, Baas J, Adil M. A decade of development in sub-Saharan African science, technology, engineering and mathematics research. Elsevier, World Bank; 2014.

Leigh J, Moon S, Garcia E, Fitzgerald G. Is global capacity to manage outbreaks improving? The Graduate Institute of International and Development Studies, Global …; 2018.

Lie RK, Miller FG. Allocating a COVID-19 vaccine: balancing national and international responsibilities. Milbank Q. 2020;99:450. https://doi.org/10.1111/1468-0009.12494.

Lurie N, Keusch GT, Dzau VJ. Urgent lessons from COVID 19: why the world needs a standing, coordinated system and sustainable financing for global research and development. Lancet. 2021;397(10280):1229–36. https://doi.org/10.1016/S0140-6736(21)00503-1.

Malhame M, Baker E, Gandhi G, Jones A, Kalpaxis P, Iqbal R, et al. Shaping markets to benefit global health—a 15-year history and lessons learned from the pentavalent vaccine market. Vaccine X. 2019;2:100033.

Marotta D, Mark M, Blom A, Thorn K. Human capital and university-industry linkages' role in fostering firm innovation: an empirical study of Chile and Colombia. Washington, DC: World Bank, Latin American and the Caribbean Region HDSU; 2007. Report No.: 1813-9450, Contract No.: 4443.

McDade KK, Kraus J, Petitjean H, Schrade C, Fewer S, Beyeler N, et al. Aligning multilateral support for global public goods for health under the Global Action Plan. Durham, NC: Center for Policy Impact in Global Health; 2019.

Moon S, Sridhar D, Pate MA, Jha AK, Clinton C, Delaunay S, et al. Will Ebola change the game? Ten essential reforms before the next pandemic. The report of the Harvard-LSHTM Independent Panel on the Global Response to Ebola. Lancet. 2015;386(10009):2204–21.

NASEM. Integrating clinical research into epidemic response: the Ebola experience. Washington, DC: National Academies of Sciences Engineering and Medicine Publications, The National Academies Press; 2017.

NASEM. Exploring lessons learned from a century of outbreaks: readiness for 2030: proceedings of a workshop. Washington, DC: National Academies of Sciences Engineering and Medicine Publications, The National Academies Press; 2019.

Nkengasong JN, Maiyegun O, Moeti M. Establishing the Africa Centres for Disease Control and Prevention: responding to Africa's health threats. Lancet Glob Health. 2017;5(3):e246–7. https://doi.org/10.1016/s2214-109x(17)30025-6.

Office of the UN Special Envoy on Ebola. Resources for results V. 2016 (1 Sep 2014–31 Oct 2015).

Oroxom R, Glassman A. Vaccine introduction and coverage in Gavi-supported countries 2015–2018: implications for Gavi 5.0. 2019.

Pandemic Preparedness Partnership. 100 days mission to respond to future pandemic threats: reducing the impact of future pandemics by making diagnostics, therapeutics and vaccines available within 100 days: a report to the G7. London: G7 United Kingdom 2021; 2021.

Perkins MD, Dye C, Balasegaram M, Bréchot C, Mombouli J-V, Røttingen J-A, et al. Diagnostic preparedness for infectious disease outbreaks. Lancet. 2017;390(10108):2211–4.

Ralaidovy AH, Adam T, Boucher P. Resource allocation for biomedical research: analysis of investments by major funders. Health Res Policy Syst. 2020;18(1):20. https://doi.org/10.1186/s12961-020-0532-0.

Reiss J. Public goods. In: Zalta EN, editor. Stanford encyclopedia of philosophy. Stanford, CA: Metaphysics Research Lab, Stanford University; 2021.

Reynolds CA. World Bank Group's support to the Ebola virus response effort. BMJ. 2015;350:h1283.

SATBHSS Project Brochure. African Union Development Agency, Johannesburg. 2021.

Schemm Y. Africa doubles research output, moves toward knowledge-based economy-what factors are driving the increase in scientific research being conducted by African scientists. Res Trends. 2013;35:1–4.

Schnabel L, Glassman A. Gavi from the country perspective: assessing key challenges to effective partnership. Center for Global Development; 2019.

Simpkin V, Namubiru-Mwaura E, Clarke L, Mossialos E. Investing in health R&D: where we are, what limits us, and how to make progress in Africa. BMJ Glob Health. 2019;4(2):e001047. https://doi.org/10.1136/bmjgh-2018-001047.

Sridhar D, Winters J, Strong E. World Bank's financing, priorities, and lending structures for global health. BMJ. 2017;358:j3339.

Sunyoto T. Partnerships for better neglected disease drug discovery and development: how have we fared? Expert Opin Drug Discov. 2020;15(5):531–7. https://doi.org/10.1080/17460441.2020.1736550.

Swarup R, Sharma A, Logani JM. Building a robust ecosystem for vaccine research in India. Int J Infect Dis. 2019;84:S7–9.

Torreele E, Usdin M, Chirac P. A needs-based pharmaceutical R&D agenda for neglected diseases. Geneva: World Health Organization; 2004.

Trouiller P, Olliaro P, Torreele E, Orbinski J, Laing R, Ford N. Drug development for neglected diseases: a deficient market and a public-health policy failure. Lancet. 2002;359(9324):2188–94. https://doi.org/10.1016/S0140-6736(02)09096-7.

UNAIDS, AVAC. Good participatory practice: guidelines for biomedical HIV prevention trials. Geneva: Joint United Nations Programme on HIV/AIDS (UNAIDS); 2007.

UNAIDS, WHO. Ethical considerations in biomedical HIV prevention trials: UNAIDS/WHO guidance document. Geneva: Joint United Nations Programme on HIV/AIDS (UNAIDS); 2021. p. 70.

WBG. Financial intermediary funds in the World Bank Group. In: Finance WBGD, editor. World Bank Group; 2014.

WBG. From panic and neglect to investing in health security: financing pandemic preparedness at a national level. Washington, DC: World Bank. Preparedness IfF; 2017.

WBG. Financial intermediary funds: a unique instrument in the aid architecture. Trust fund reform brief. World Bank Group; 2019.

WBG. Pandemic Fund. Washington, DC: World Bank Group; 2022. https://www.worldbank.org/en/programs/financial-intermediary-fund-for-pandemic-prevention-preparedness-and-response-ppr-fif. Accessed 22 Nov 2022.

WHO. International Health Regulations (2005). 3rd ed. Geneva: World Health Organzation; 2016.

WHO. A strategic framework for emergency preparedness. Geneva: World Health Organization; 2017.

WHO. WHO's work in emergencies: prepare, prevent, detect and respond: annual report 2018. World Health Organization; 2019.

WHO. The Access to COVID-19 Tools (ACT) accelerator. Geneva: World Health Organization; 2022a. https://www.who.int/initiatives/act-accelerator. Accessed 19 Nov 2022.

WHO. WHO COVID-19 solidarity therapeutics trial. Geneva: World Health Organization; 2022b. https://www.who.int/emergencies/diseases/novel-coronavirus-2019/global-research-on-novel-coronavirus-2019-ncov/solidarity-clinical-trial-for-covid-19-treatments. Accessed 7 Sep 2022.

WHO. WHO COVID-19 solidarity trial vaccines. Geneva: World Health Organization; 2022c. https://

www.who.int/emergencies/diseases/novel-coronavirus-2019/global-research-on-novel-coronavirus-2019-ncov/solidarity-trial-of-covid-19-vaccines. Accessed 7 Sep 2022.

Widdowson MA, Schrag SJ, Carter RJ, Carr W, Legardy-Williams J, Gibson L, et al. Implementing an Ebola vaccine study—Sierra Leone. MMWR Suppl. 2016;65(3):98–106. https://doi.org/10.15585/mmwr.su6503a14.

World Bank. Drug-resistant infections: a threat to our economic future. World Bank Group; 2017.

World Bank. Money and microbes: strengthening clinical research capacity to prevent epidemics. Washington, DC: World Bank Group; 2018.

World Bank. FIF framework update. Washington, DC: World Bank; 2019a.

World Bank. Implementation completion and results report on a small grant in the amount of usd 3,593,757 to the International AIDS Vaccine Initiative for support to research and development at the International AIDS Vaccine Initiative. Washington, DC: Health NPGP; 2019b. Report No.: <TF0A4434>, Contract No.: ICR00004605.

World Bank. Pandemic emergency financing facility. Washington, DC: World Bank; 2019c. https://www.worldbank.org/en/topic/pandemics/brief/pandemic-emergency-financing-facility. Accessed 15 Jan 2020.

World Bank. Health emergency preparedness and response (HEPR) umbrella program. 2021.

World Bank. Annual report 2021—health emergency preparedness and response umbrella program. 2022a.

World Bank. Innovate in India for inclusiveness. Washington, DC: World Bank; 2022b. https://projects.worldbank.org/en/projects-operations/project-detail/P156241. Accessed 22 Nov 2022.

World Bank. Preventing, preparing for, and responding to disease outbreaks and pandemics—future directions for the World Bank Group. Washington, DC: World Bank; 2023.

Yamey G, Schaferhoff M, Pate M, Chawla M, Ranson K, Zhao F, et al. Funding the development and manufacturing of COVID-19 vaccines. Brookings Institution; 2020.

Zerhouni E. GAVI, the Vaccine Alliance. Cell. 2019;179(1):13–7.

29 International Collaboration to Advance Research Preparedness and Response

Amanda Rojek and Gail Carson

Contents

Learning Track Note: This chapter appears in Learning Tracks: Global Health; Health Policy, Multilateral Cooperation, International Governance; Preparedness
Case studies: Kenneth Ballie, Lennie Derde, Alice Norton and Lina Moses

E. S. Higgs and R. A. Sorenson (eds.), *Principles and Practice of Emergency Research Response*,
https://doi.org/10.1007/978-3-031-48408-7_42

Principiis obsta; sero medicina paratur cum mala per longas convaluere moras.
Stop it at the start; it is late to prepare medicine when disease has grown strong by long delay.
—Ovid, "Remedia Amoris," ll. 91–92

Learning Objectives

This chapter should enable readers to understand and discuss:

- The value of international collaborations in research responses to public health outbreaks.
- Barriers to optimal collaboration and mechanisms to overcome them, based on lessons from COVID-19 and earlier pandemics.
- Factors that limit international and intersectoral collaboration.
- Risks associated with inadequate infrastructure for response to health emergencies.
- Conclusions of a systemic review of clinical research efforts during the 2009 H1N1 influenza pandemic.
- Some design features of the International Severe Acute Respiratory and Emerging Infection Consortium (ISARIC) Clinical Characterization Protocol (CPP).
- Examples of adaptive clinical trial platforms.

1 Introduction

Outbreak responses are interdisciplinary by nature; therefore, preparedness for a research response must be interdisciplinary and multisectoral. Since our continued global vulnerability to infectious diseases is clear, collaborations to coordinate solutions across traditional geographical and specialty boundaries are critical. Preparedness and response, too, must be approached not as separate domains but as a spectrum of required activities, evolving as we develop new tools, countermeasures, and methodologies. At the heart of our efforts are the affected communities, especially those deemed vulnerable or hard to reach.

At their best, such international collaborations can provide rapid and robust answers to key scientific questions because they:

- Use the breadth of experience and expertise of the collaborators, including practitioners who are the first to treat patients afflicted with a new or re-emerging infection and those who have global expertise in a pathogen family or in clinical trial design or conduct. Diverse investigators working together are not only more likely to devise an effective approach to problems; they also help ensure that study data and samples meet shared aims and standards of different disciplines without duplication.
- Harness larger populations for research recruitment and adapt to shifts in disease epidemiology during enrollment periods (e.g., international spread of cases or changing viral phenotype). Furthermore, the faster study recruitment requirements can be met, the faster a vaccine, therapy, or diagnostic device (VTD) in development can be adopted if found safe and effective—or abandoned for the next most promising option if not.
- Prevent unnecessary duplication. Better collaboration and coordination in a future outbreak could prevent some of the mishaps of the early COVID-19 pandemic, such as the uncoordinated proliferation of trials, many of them either poorly designed or without enough research participants to reach statistically valid conclusions (Bugin and Woodcock 2021), leading to subsequent use of therapies like hydroxychloroquine and ivermectin, which better-designed trials found not to be efficacious (Lee et al. 2021; Naggie et al. 2022).
- Produce inclusive evidence that represents all populations, especially vulnerable populations and those often overlooked in data collection.

2 The Reality of Insufficient International Collaboration

2.1 Uncoordinated, Inequitable Use of Resources

During the COVID-19 pandemic, the initial level of international collaboration was less than ideal, with unwise and uncoordinated use of research resources characterizing much of the early research response. Over time, the initiative of several leading global health agencies brought better planning and coordination to bear on the developing COVID-19 research agenda. These included the World Health Organization (WHO); Gavi, the Vaccine Alliance; and the Coalition for Epidemic Preparedness Innovations (CEPI), all of which cosponsored the Access to COVID-19 Tools Accelerator (ACT-A) and COVID-19 Vaccines Global Access (COVAX). WHO convened COVID-19 research agenda meetings, the first of them in collaboration with the Global Research Collaboration for Infectious Disease Preparedness and Response (GloPID R) (WHO 2020). WHO also led several clinical research studies under the name Solidarity, bringing together numerous sites from all over the world under one protocol (WHO 2022a, b).

There is no single answer to the question of what limits international collaboration. At a study level, investigators—particularly those from resource-poor settings or new to outbreak research—may in some instances not be linked into or even aware of international consortia or coordination and standardization mechanisms, such as those available through WHO. Unfortunately, traditional academic paradigms for recognizing contributions to scientific articles can motivate investigators or institutions to limit collaboration and the number of listed authors to improve their academic standing. Even large consortia may have jurisdictional limitations. Funders, for example, may limit their remit to a particular geographical area; incompatible regulatory requirements for trials or for drug or vaccine licensing between regions may also limit collaboration. Underlying inequity between rich and poor, both within and among nations, manifested itself in various ways from the start of the COVID-19 pandemic. While it can be argued that national governments' first obligation is to their citizens, some higher-income countries acted to secure *excess* COVID-19 vaccine supplies through market power and export controls to an extent dubbed vaccine nationalism (Bollyky and Brown 2020; Emanuel et al. 2020; Lie and Miller 2020).

2.2 Political Tensions and Lack of Trust

Moreover, political tensions between countries and lack of trust between countries and multi-lateral institutions can also limit collaboration, particularly for drug and vaccine pre-clinical and clinical research and subsequent equitable access to VTD. The global scientific enterprise should be able to rise above parochialism to benefit the global health ecosystem comprehensively. Some of the WHO and 2022 World Bank–proposed frameworks may facilitate a lift for science and specifically address the spectrum of preparedness into an early response.

2.3 Lack of Standardized Case Report Forms for Disease Characterization and Identification of Prognostic Indicators in Observational Research

The risks of a fractured research infrastructure and delayed research implementation are clear. With respect to observational data, the 2014–2016 Ebola virus disease (EVD) epidemic in West Africa demonstrates the benefits of standardized and harmonized case report forms and the harmful clinical implications of their absence. During this outbreak, WHO used standardized case reporting forms for listing symptoms at presentation, which helped improve historical descriptions of the Ebola virus disease phenotype (e.g., correcting overemphasis on hemorrhagic manifestations and rash). They have also been instrumental in recalibrating incubation periods, serial intervals, and case fatality rate (Agua-Agum et al. 2015). However, these forms were almost exclusively used for admission and outcome, not to follow the progression of symptoms or development of complications; that is, they had an epidemiological rather than clinical focus. A systematic review and meta-analysis of *clinical* data from that outbreak revealed a striking duplication of effort and lack of harmonization. Over 80% (28/34) of articles reviewed reported duplicate or overlapping data, something acknowledged in only one of the publications. Individual patient data was rarely available (two articles), and pooling of data was impossible due to heterogeneity in categorization of data. For example, age ranges were defined differently across all but two articles; among 15 peer-reviewed manuscripts that reported viral load, 10 different categorization systems were used (Rojek et al. 2019). The consequences include a lack of clarity about important clinical indices, such as predictors of mortality. ◘ Figure 1 shows

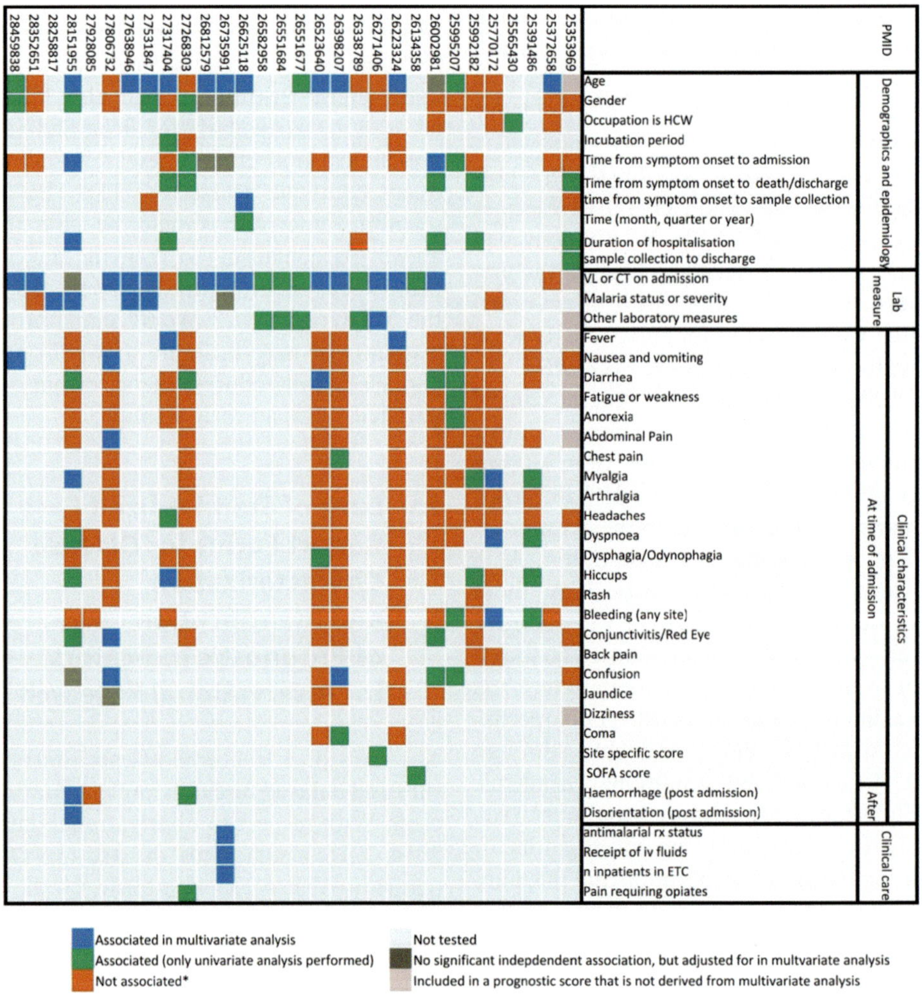

◘ **Fig. 1** Reported predictors of mortality for patients with laboratory confirmed Ebola virus disease (EVD). Asterisk indicates if an association on univariate analysis is not supported by multivariate analysis. *VL* viral load, *Ct* cycle threshold, *Rx* treatment (Rojek et al. 2019)

the diversity of reporting methods for predictors of mortality in patients with EVD from the West Africa outbreak.

2.4 Fractured Response to the 2009 H1N1 Influenza Pandemic

With respect to clinical trials, the 2009 H1N1 influenza pandemic illustrates the risks of a fractured response. During this pandemic, various treatments, including neuraminidase inhibitors (e.g., oseltamivir), were widely used to treat patients. However, a systematic review of clinical research outputs (Fig. 2) strikingly found that despite the large number of patients treated, fewer than 600 hospitalized patients were enrolled in clinical trials that published their results; none of the results were available before the public health emergency ended over a year later (Rojek et al. 2020). All the studies were insufficiently sized and had inadequate power for assessing antiviral efficacy. Consequently, considerable controversy remains regarding the efficacy of these drugs, with implications not only for clinical practice but also for decisions about stockpiling potential pandemic influenza treatments. Notably, most of the few patients enrolled in these clinical trials were also enrolled in already established seasonal influenza or severe acute respiratory infection studies, a model which has been built upon significantly in the following years.

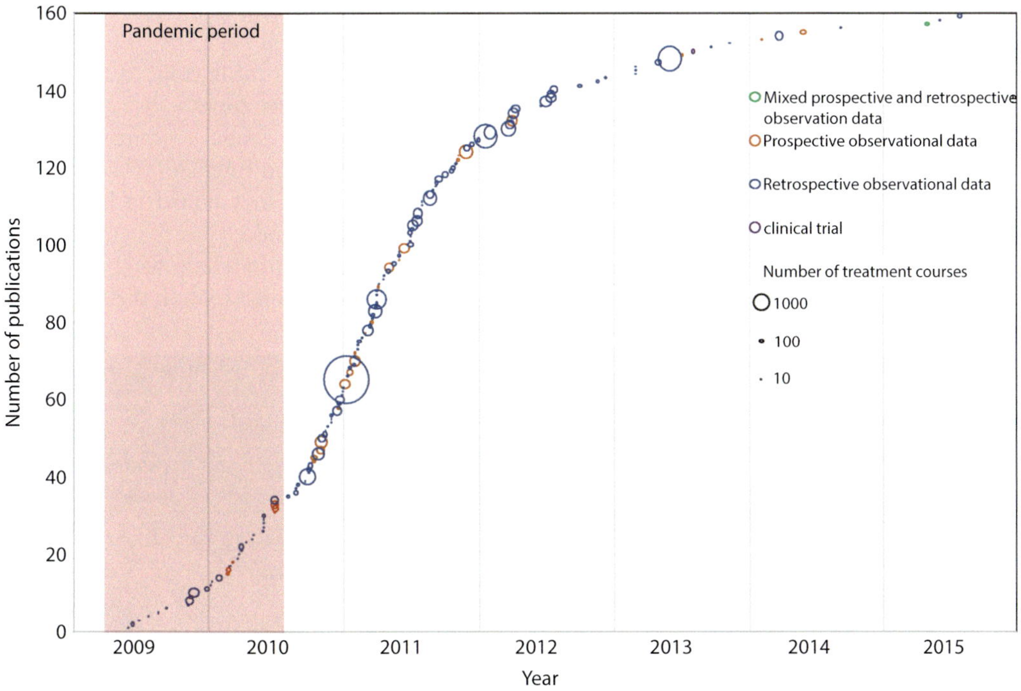

Fig. 2 Findings from a systematic review of clinical studies describing treatment of H1N1 pandemic influenza. Studies are shown according to type of study and number of treatment courses described. The pandemic period ranges from April 1, 2009, to the end of the PHEIC on August 10, 2009. Previously published (Rojek et al. 2020). (CC 4.0 Open)

3 Improved Clinical Research Through International Collaboration

There has been substantive progress in international collaboration since the 2009 H1N1 influenza pandemic. In the rest of this chapter, we examine several examples (case studies) of impactful clinical research during the COVID-19 pandemic and draw conclusions highlighting how international collaboration to improve preparedness is a key driver for an improved clinical research response.

3.1 "Sleeping" Protocol Model

During the WHO clinical management research prioritization meeting for COVID-19 held in January 2020, the priority was identified as harmonized clinical characterizations research (ISARIC 2020b). The International Severe Acute Respiratory and Emerging Infection Consortium (ISARIC) case-reporting forms are an example of success in this space. ISARIC was born in 2011 in the aftermath of the inadequate clinical research response to the 2009 H1N1 influenza pandemic. The ISARIC model uses a "sleeping" protocol model (whereby the protocol is approved but awaits disease outbreak patients to be "woken up"). The first ISARIC pre-approved observational study protocol is the ISARIC-WHO Clinical Characterization Protocol (CCP) (ISARIC 2020a). The CCP has been implemented in response to various emerging pathogen threats since 2012. It was adapted for COVID-19 and launched via the ISARIC Web site on January 24, 2020 (Fig. 3).

The following design features of the ISARIC CCP encourage international collaboration and offer benefits and advantages.

- Use of a modular protocol adaptable to available resources.
- Recognizing and citing all data-contributing sites as manuscript contributors.
- Mandate for all analyses using international data to be led by or to include one or more investigators from low- or middle-income countries.
- Frequent collaborator calls to accommodate multiple time zones.
- Preparation of some resources in languages other than English.
- A scientific advisory board to help define the research agenda.
- A data-sharing model allowing contributing sites to continue to own their data.

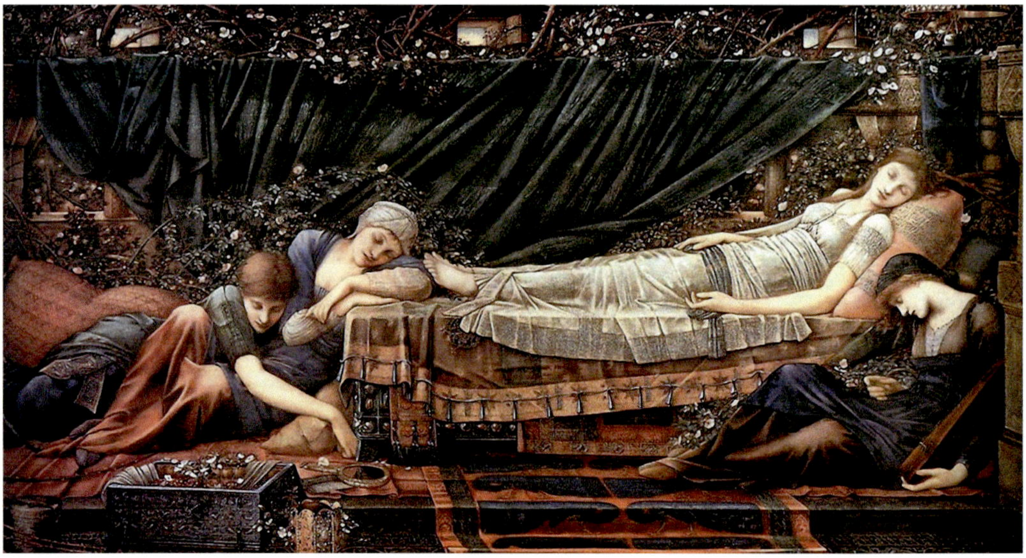

Fig. 3 Unlike fairy-tale princesses, sleeping protocols are not meant to slumber for a century. (Edward Burne-Jones, ca. 1890)

- Annual collaborator meetings during interpandemic periods to share research and build collaboration and interpersonal connections.
- Opportunities for academic exchange.
- Focus on core research activities and outbreak research response.
- Strong, enduring links with WHO and national public health institutions.

The UK branch, known as ISARIC4C (Comprehensive Clinical Characterization Collaboration), has undertaken the COVID-19 research efforts described in ▶ Case Study 1, illustrating how research preparedness embedded within a health system—the UK National Health Service (NHS) and the National Institute for Health Research (NIHR)—responded effectively (ISARIC 2020a).

Case Study 1

Initial COVID-19 Observational Research in the UK

In 2012, after years of international and cross-specialty consensus-building, a single, standardized generic research protocol was created for clinical characterization of any emerging infection (Dunning et al. 2014). These tools were released under an open-source license so anyone may download and use, adapt, or distribute them.

The original reports on COVID-19 clinical findings utilized these harmonized data collection tools (Huang et al. 2020; Yang et al. 2020). We established the CCP as a "sleeping protocol" across the majority of hospitals in the UK in 2012, obtaining approval from both the institutional review board (IRB), aka research ethics committee (REC), and hospital management. The protocol was activated in February 2020 under the banner of the ISARIC4C COVID-19 Clinical Information Network, in time to recruit the first cases of COVID-19 in the UK (Docherty et al. 2020).

This rapid activation enabled the ISARIC4C study to obtain critical samples to facilitate vaccine development, define international standards for serology assays, and record initial observations on disease course and patient response to symptomatic treatment. By establishing data collection across much of the NHS, with contemporaneous data analytics at the UK Outbreak Data Analysis Platform, the ISARIC4C study enabled outbreak monitoring in UK hospitals and identification of disease key clinical features, prognostic markers, transmission in hospitals, and host genetics underlying susceptibility. By November 2021, the ISARIC4C study had obtained structured data on 253,181 cases and published over 40 peer-reviewed papers.

The primary reason for the study's success was not only the preparation but the active maintenance of the study during the interpandemic period through periodic trial activations of the protocol for other infectious diseases, enabling the team to identify technical and logistical challenges and overcome them. Some of the activations were planned, e.g., to capture severe acute respiratory infection (SARI) data; others were in response to diseases that met the eligibility criteria, e.g., Middle East respiratory syndrome (MERS) and mpox. The coordination and motivation of the UK National Health Service (NHS) to assist with research was a critical factor. The success of the study required a great deal of human labor to manually transcribe clinical details into case report forms. The investigators sincerely hope that before the next major pandemic a technological solution can automate this process.

Kenneth Baillie

3.2 Adaptive Platform Clinical Trials

Adaptive platform clinical trials have been used for some time in oncology. For outbreaks, this trial design has the advantages of adaptability to emerging evidence on potential therapies and parallel enrollment, which meets urgent recruitment needs during sometimes brief outbreak periods. An example of years of international collaboration involving data experts, statisticians, and critical care doctors focused on delivering for a pandemic is the Randomized Embedded Multifactorial Adaptive Platform Trial for Community-Acquired Pneumonia (REMAP-CAP).

Case Study 2

REMAP-CAP

REMAP-CAP (▶ Chap. 15) was set up with seed funding from the European Union Platform for European Preparedness Against [Re-] emerging Epidemics Consortium and had been enrolling patients using a novel type of randomized controlled trial (RCT) since soon after it began in 2014 (Angus et al. 2020). It was specifically designed to pivot during a pandemic and investigate a novel or re-emerging causative pathogen, making any necessary adaptations to the trial design. REMAP-CAP focused on international collaboration early on and was already active in 13 countries by January 2020 when the severe acute respiratory syndrome coronavirus 2 (SARS-CoV-2) emerged.

Before the COVID-19 pandemic, REMAP-CAP studied both new treatments and the comparative effectiveness of existing treatments for community-acquired pneumonia (CAP). The underlying idea was to have a RCT running in "peacetime" and adapt it to the specific research needs of a future pandemic. To this end, an adaptive platform trial (APT) design was used as conventional RCT designs lack flexibility. The platform aspect of APT design means that under a single master protocol, multiple interventions can be investigated in parallel, rather than in series, improving efficiency and reducing costs. The adaptive design features allow quick learning, dropping ineffective interventions as soon as they reach a prespecified futility threshold and immediately adding interventions that reach prespecified thresholds for superiority to the standard of care. Novel interventions or groups of interventions ("domains") can be added. Another adaptive feature that can be incorporated is updating the weights of randomization frequencies so that more patients are randomized to interventions that show evidence of greater promise, known as "response adaptive randomization." The trial uses a Bayesian statistical framework to support the design (▶ Chaps. 22 and 23).

By early 2020, REMAP-CAP was active across 52 sites in Europe (including the UK), Australia, New Zealand, and Canada and was recruiting into four different domains (empiric antibiotics, macrolides, influenza antivirals, and corticosteroids) investigating CAP treatments. About 450 patients had been enrolled globally. The study adapted, as planned, for the COVID-19 pandemic. The first COVID-19 patient was included on March 9, 2020, 2 days before WHO declared the outbreak a pandemic.

By December 2021, REMAP-CAP has investigated a total of 50 current or completed interventions in 330 sites across the globe. In addition to the pre-pandemic regions, recruitment is ongoing in the United States, Japan, Colombia, India, Nepal, and Pakistan. Over 9000 patients have been randomized. The trial has contributed significantly to the treatment of hospitalized patients with COVID-19 as several platform conclusions were reached.

Lennie Derde

4 Preparedness for Global Research Response

Although at the time of writing the world remains in the pandemic response phase, the threat of other epidemics never goes away, and the frequency of novel and re-emerging pathogens in humans is increasing (Morens and Fauci 2020). Research readiness and preparedness must continue for diseases other than COVID-19. Nevertheless, some questions arise. Is it sufficient to prepare by implementing a sleeping protocol, or is ongoing integration of the research into healthcare more effective? The success of RECOVERY in the UK is witness to a pre-existing system with research integrated in the NHS and NIHR (Agua-Agum et al. 2015) at no cost to the UK public.

4.1 Coordination of Research Funding

Research does not happen without funding (► Chap. 28 and In Focus 32.2). Here too, uncoordinated funding or funding by well-meaning organizations without the expertise to ensure good trial design can result in duplicative or wasteful resource use. The Global Research Collaboration for Infectious Disease Preparedness (GloPID-R) is a consortium of funders of research from all over the world. ► Case Study 3 provides an example of their work during the pandemic. The COVID-19 Project Tracker jointly developed by the UK Collaborative on Development Research (UKCDR) and GloPID-R shows how a tool can help with research funding coordination, which may in turn lead to research collaboration (GLOPID-R 2022).

Case Study 3

Organizing Funders to Avoid Duplication of Effort

Research funders recognize the need to coordinate research funding to prevent duplicative research and improve the positive impact of their investments. Such coordination should not be limited to the COVID-19 pandemic but should occur during future infectious disease epidemics and pandemics as well as in other continuing medical research. UKCDR and GloPID-R established the COVID-19 Project Tracker early in the pandemic to improve the visibility of research funding and its alignment with research priorities identified through the joint WHO and GloPID-R Research Forum and the resulting roadmap (WHO 2020). The tracker collates projects relating to COVID-19 from funders around the world and codes these based on the WHO COVID-19 Roadmap. Launched in April 2020, the COVID-19 Research Tracker is an online database that has grown to contain data on over 14,000 COVID-19 research projects, representing more than $5.5 billion in funding from over 200 organizations worldwide. By providing an overview of research projects mapped against the priorities identified in the COVID-19 Roadmap, the tracker aims to help funders and researchers collaborate in the interest of a more effective and coherent global research response. ◘ Figure 4 suggests measures to better prepare for the next outbreak with pandemic potential.

A comprehensive, cross-cutting analysis of the COVID-19 Research Project tracker data was established in the form of a living mapping review published on the Wellcome Open Research platform to improve data use (Bucher et al. 2023). The tracker has been viewed over 35,000 times and has informed funding decisions across the globe. "R&D Preparedness Ecosystem" (Keusch and Lurie 2020) cited the COVID-19 Project Tracker as instrumental "to insure maximum scientific output results,"

Enhancing international collaborations, clinical trials recruitment, study design, and advocacy
Mechanisms to engage, support, and benefit from international collaborations: ➢ Agreed data ownership rules. ➢ Agreed authorship rules. ➢ Plan for proportionate representation in management structure.
Preparatory mechanisms to maximize recruitment during an outbreak: ➢ Pre-approvals for likely bottlenecks (protocol finalization, contractual agreements, ethics approvals). ➢ Consider opportunities for data collection activities between epidemics to test system in an epidemic focused project. Alternatively, build on pandemic modules to primarily non-epidemic studies to ensure 'match readiness' when an outbreak occurs. ➢ Specifically fund ongoing administrative (project and financial management of grants) and data support.
Study design that is resilient to a multi-country outbreak: ➢ Consider tiered data-collection and sampling requirements to account for differences in resources between sites and countries or provide scope to add additional modules for sites with advanced capabilities in a specific area (such as viral culture). ➢ Simplify studies to key outcomes to prevent additional regulatory hurdles in different jurisdictions.
Advocacy work: ➢ Encourage regulators to streamline, simplify, and harmonize multi-country approvals. ➢ Advocate for efficient systems that minimize data collection requirements of healthcare workers. ➢ Support institutions with lower resource levels to develop expertise & infrastructure capacity (e.g., laboratory). ➢ Integration of research into health systems.

Fig. 4 Preparedness measures for researchers to consider. (Authors)

while "COVID-19 Research and Innovation Achievements" noted its usefulness for "reaching global funding decisions" (WHO 2021). With some funders now taking a longer-term view, we are collaborating with the Canadian Institutes of Health Research to map the COVID-19 Project Tracker to the UN Research Roadmap for the COVID-19 recovery research priorities and to support the coordination of the research response to that framework (UN 2020). The tracker data is also being used to further learn from the COVID-19 global funding response and improve global research policies and processes for future epidemics and pandemics.

Alice Norton

4.2 Interdisciplinary Collaboration

Community engagement, partnership building, political support, coordination, and preparedness for primary care research studies, follow-up studies, and trial recruitment are critical to research success and will be covered in another chapter of this volume (▶ Chap. 18). Another form of outreach that is sometimes neglected is inter-disciplinary collaboration, a primary goal of the Global Outbreak Alert and Response Network (GOARN).

Case Study 4

GOARN Operational Research

GOARN is a network of over 270 institutions and agencies dedicated to infectious disease outbreak response. For over 20 years, GOARN has leveraged the skills and resources of the network to provide technical and operational support for health emergencies all over the globe. Recent health emergencies, including the COVID-19 pandemic and the 2014–2016 Ebola epidemic in West Africa, have shown us that systematic studies embedded in response are not only feasible but an essential component of effective, evidence-based response (NASEM 2017). This experience has also shown us that during health emergencies, research studies that are not embedded with local partners (researchers and responders) can undermine local health research systems and lead to mistrust in research practices in local communities (Heymann et al. 2016). Recognizing the important role that research can play in improving outbreak response and the vulnerabilities in ensuring equitable and collaborative research during crises, GOARN has expanded its mission in 2017 to include operational research. The goal of GOARN Research is to leverage our multidisciplinary and multisectoral global network to support local and contextualized research to enable the best evidence-based practices in health emergency response. At the heart of this approach is enabling frontline responders and local communities experiencing the epidemic to generate and address their own evolving research priorities.

While research to develop MCMs (vaccines, therapeutics, and diagnostics) is important to combat epidemics, GOARN Research focuses on how these MCMs and other non-pharmaceutical interventions are best implemented in outbreak response using approaches from operational research and implementation science. GOARN Research activities support:

- Mobilization of researchers to conduct operational research support during health emergencies.
- Utilization evidence from research findings to improve operationalized and implementable action.
- Identification of evidence gaps in response activities and country- and region-level research prioritization.
- Advocacy for operational research and implementation science with policy makers and funding agencies.

With its diverse partner institutions—public health agencies, large international humanitarian organizations, and local academic partners—GOARN is uniquely positioned to work with frontline responders and communities to identify research needs, link with GOARN members to support locally partnered research, and operationalize the link between research findings and feasible, effective action. This requires GOARN Research to support mechanisms to identify operational research questions at local, country, region, and global levels. It also requires a system to identify existing and current research capacities across GOARN and match research expertise with local researchers and responders to quickly roll out research that can have a timely impact on improving preparedness, mitigating morbidity and mortality, curbing disease transmission, and ending outbreaks (hopefully before they become epidemics and pandemics). This collaborative system must meet many requirements, including equitable research partnerships, ethical review, data sharing, dissemination of findings and publications, and operationalization of research findings to improve response. GOARN Research aims to elevate community- and country-led research that will rapidly and responsively transform operations. Such research may not make novel discoveries captured in the highest impact journals, but it can identify pragmatic, innovative, and adaptive improvements that can shift the tide of an epidemic.

Lina Moses

5 Conclusion

One key lesson from the COVID-19 pandemic is that implementing harmonized research is easier than establishing isolated independent studies (ISARIC 2020b)—at least once the necessary preparedness steps have been taken. Furthermore, funding and support must be directed in a strategic manner to properly support the research that has the best chance of finding definitive solutions to pressing clinical and public health questions. ◘ Figure 4 proposes some measures researchers can undertake to better prepare to facilitate international collaboration in future outbreaks.

Discussion Questions

1. At their best, how do international collaborations improve the timeliness and reliability of research response in order to answer key scientific questions, whether or not there is an infectious disease emergency? Discuss some of the factors that limit international and intersectoral collaboration.
2. Discuss some risks associated with lack of research infrastructure for response to health emergencies, as in the 2014–2016 Ebola virus disease epidemic in West Africa.
3. The research efforts during the 2009 H1N1 influenza pandemic did not generally implement well-designed and sufficiently powered clinical trials. Why not? What did a systematic review of clinical research outputs for this pandemic reveal?
4. List some of the design features of the ISARIC CCP, which encourages international collaboration. Provide and discuss an example of (a) an adaptive platform for clinical trials or (b) research funders organizing to avoid duplication of efforts during a pandemic research response.

References

Agua-Agum J, Ariyarajah A, Aylward B, Blake IM, Brennan R, Cori A, et al. West African Ebola epidemic after one year—slowing but not yet under control. N Engl J Med. 2015;372(6):584–7. https://doi.org/10.1056/NEJMc1414992.

Angus DC, Berry S, Lewis RJ, Al-Beidh F, Arabi Y, Bentum-Puijk WV, et al. The REMAP-CAP (Randomized Embedded Multifactorial Adaptive Platform for Community-acquired Pneumonia) study. Rationale and design. Ann Am Thorac Soc. 2020;17(7):879–91. https://doi.org/10.1513/AnnalsATS.202003-192SD.

Bollyky TJ, Brown CP. The tragedy of vaccine nationalism: only cooperation can end the pandemic. Foreign Affairs. Sep/Oct 2020.

Bucher A, Antonio E, Grund H, Jabin N, Jones C, Kifle M, et al. A living mapping review for COVID-19 funded research projects: two year update. Wellcome Open Res. 2023;5:209. https://doi.org/10.12688/wellcomeopenres.16259.9.

Bugin K, Woodcock J. Trends in COVID-19 therapeutic clinical trials. Nat Rev Drug Discov. 2021; https://doi.org/10.1038/d41573-021-00037-3.

Docherty AB, Harrison EM, Green CA, Hardwick HE, Pius R, Norman L, et al. Features of 20,133 UK patients in hospital with covid-19 using the ISARIC WHO Clinical Characterisation Protocol: prospective observational cohort study. BMJ. 2020;369:m1985. https://doi.org/10.1136/bmj.m1985.

Dunning JW, Merson L, Rohde GGU, Gao Z, Semple MG, Tran D, et al. Open source clinical science for emerging infections. Lancet Infect Dis. 2014;14(1):8–9. https://doi.org/10.1016/s1473-3099(13)70327-x.

Emanuel EJ, Persad G, Kern A, Buchanan A, Fabre C, Halliday D, et al. An ethical framework for global vaccine allocation. Science. 2020; https://doi.org/10.1126/science.abe2803.

GLOPID-R. COVID-19 research project tracker. Oxford: International Severe Acute Respiratory and Emerging Infection Consortium; 2022. https://www.glopid-r.org/articles-newsletter/covid-19-research-project-tracker/. Accessed 8 Sep 2022.

Heymann DL, Liu J, Lillywhite L. Partnerships, not parachutists, for Zika research. N Engl J Med. 2016;374(16):1504–5. https://doi.org/10.1056/NEJMp1602278.

Huang C, Wang Y, Li X, Ren L, Zhao J, Hu Y, et al. Clinical features of patients infected with 2019 novel coronavirus in Wuhan, China. Lancet. 2020; https://doi.org/10.1016/S0140-6736(20)30183-5.

ISARIC. Clinical Characterisation Protocol (CCP). International Severe Acute Respiratory and Emerging Infection Consortium (ISARIC), Oxford. 2020a. https://isaric.org/research/covid-19-clinical-research-resources/clinical-characterisation-protocol-ccp/#:~:text=The%20Clinical%20Characterisation%20Protocol%20(CCP,in%20a%20globally%2Dharmonised%20manner. Accessed 8 Sep 2022.

ISARIC. Global outbreak research: harmony not hegemony. Lancet Infect Dis. 2020b;20(7):770–2. https://doi.org/10.1016/s1473-3099(20)30440-0.

Keusch GT, Lurie N. The R&D preparedness ecosystem: preparedness for health emergencies: report to the Global Preparedness Monitoring Board. Geneva: Global Preparedness Monitoring Board; 2020.
Lee Z, Rayner CR, Forrest JI, Nachega JB, Senchaudhuri E, Mills EJ. The rise and fall of hydroxychloroquine for the treatment and prevention of COVID-19. Am J Trop Med Hyg. 2021;104(1):35–8. https://doi.org/10.4269/ajtmh.20-1320.
Lie RK, Miller FG. Allocating a COVID-19 vaccine: balancing national and international responsibilities. Milbank Q. 2020; https://doi.org/10.1111/1468-0009.12494.
Morens DM, Fauci AS. Emerging pandemic diseases: how we got to COVID-19. Cell. 2020;182(5):1077–92. https://doi.org/10.1016/j.cell.2020.08.021.
Naggie S, Boulware DR, Lindsell CJ, Stewart TG, Gentile N, Collins S, et al. Effect of ivermectin vs placebo on time to sustained recovery in outpatients with mild to moderate COVID-19: a randomized clinical trial. JAMA. 2022;328(16):1595–603. https://doi.org/10.1001/jama.2022.18590.
NASEM. Integrating clinical research into epidemic response: the Ebola experience. Washington, DC: The National Academies Press; 2017.
Rojek AM, Salam A, Ragotte RJ, Liddiard E, Elhussain A, Carlqvist A, et al. A systematic review and meta-analysis of patient data from the West Africa (2013–16) Ebola virus disease epidemic. Clin Microbiol Infect. 2019;25(11):1307–14. https://doi.org/10.1016/j.cmi.2019.06.032.
Rojek AM, Martin GE, Horby PW. Compassionate drug (mis)use during pandemics: lessons for COVID-19 from 2009. BMC Med. 2020;18(1):265. https://doi.org/10.1186/s12916-020-01732-5.
UN. UN research roadmap for the COVID-19 recovery: leveraging the power of science for a more equitable, resilient and sustainable future. New York: United Nations. COVID-19 UCRt; 2020.
WHO. A coordinated global research roadmap: 2019 novel coronavirus. Geneva: World Health Organization; 2020.
WHO. COVID-19 research and innovation achievements. Geneva: World Health Organization; 2021.
WHO. WHO COVID-19 solidarity therapeutics trial. Geneva: World Health Organization; 2022a. https://www.who.int/emergencies/diseases/novel-coronavirus-2019/global-research-on-novel-coronavirus-2019-ncov/solidarity-clinical-trial-for-covid-19-treatments. Accessed 7 Sep 2022.
WHO. WHO COVID-19 solidarity trial vaccines. Geneva: World Health Organization; 2022b. https://www.who.int/emergencies/diseases/novel-coronavirus-2019/global-research-on-novel-coronavirus-2019-ncov/solidarity-trial-of-covid-19-vaccines. Accessed 7 Sep 2022.
Yang X, Yu Y, Xu J, Shu H, Xia J, Liu H, et al. Clinical course and outcomes of critically ill patients with SARS-CoV-2 pneumonia in Wuhan, China: a single-centered, retrospective, observational study. Lancet Respir Med. 2020;8(5):475–81. https://doi.org/10.1016/s2213-2600(20)30079-5.

30 Organizational Partnerships for Preparedness and Response to Emerging and Re-emerging Infectious Diseases

Yazdan Yazdanpanah, Claire Madelaine, Nicolas Pulik, and Yves Souteyrand

Contents

Learning Track Note: This chapter appears in Learning Tracks: Global Health; Clinical Research; Preparedness; Health Policy, Multilateral Cooperation, International Governance

E. S. Higgs and R. A. Sorenson (eds.), *Principles and Practice of Emergency Research Response*,
https://doi.org/10.1007/978-3-031-48408-7_43

Learning Objectives

This chapter will help readers understand and describe:

- How partnerships including multi-national and inter-disciplinary stakeholders should be configured to address emerging infectious diseases emergencies
- Successful partnership principles and recommendations for future research partnerships
- The roles of stakeholders in developing and conducting research in response to emerging infectious disease outbreaks
- The main points of the Council on Health Research for Development (COHRED) (2000) guidelines to promote fairness in research collaboration and partnership
- Issues that have hindered past partnerships and areas for improvement
- Integration and implementation successes and failures in the COVID-19 pandemic
- Recommendations drawn by the authors from previous crises
- Principles of efficient, equitable research partnerships

1 Introduction

Emerging and re-emerging infectious diseases (EIDs) can be defined as "infections that have newly appeared in a population or have existed but are rapidly increasing in incidence or geographic range" (Morse 1995). EIDs can be classified as newly emerging, re-emerging/resurging, or deliberately introduced (Morens et al. 2004).

Despite continual, impressive progress in the development of new vaccines, diagnostics, and therapeutics, emerging infectious diseases remain a major health threat to human populations. The global response to these diseases has in recent decades been reactionary rather than precautionary, in part because they have not been seen as major threats in high- and middle-income countries. But even before the coronavirus disease 2019 (COVID-19) crisis, the past decade had seen an increasing number of outbreaks:

- Middle East respiratory syndrome coronavirus (MERS-CoV) was identified in the Arabian Peninsula in 2012 and continues to be detected.
- Chikungunya, formerly an Old-World disease, appeared in the Caribbean and South America in 2013 and now appears to be established in the Americas.
- Ebola virus disease had not been detected in West Africa until the 2014–2016 epidemic there.
- Zika virus seems to have spread relatively slowly from Africa to East Asia, island hopped across the Pacific, and caused an epidemic in South America from 2015 to 2016.

Despite the clear warning provided by these recent events, the severe acute respiratory syndrome coronavirus 2 (SARS-CoV 2) demonstrated that no country was prepared to face such a pandemic, despite assessments that showed high adherence to the International Health Regulations (2005) and other preparedness measures to respond effectively to infectious disease threats (Haider et al. 2020). Further investments and coordination are clearly needed to enable a robust public health response and accelerated research into a pathogen of concern. Research covering a broad range is needed, including detection, mathematical modeling, disease diagnosis and characterization, and transmission. Preparations for coordinated, rigorous clinical research are also essential, especially since technical advances now allow for accelerated production of medical countermeasure (MCM) candidates. Behavioral and social sciences provide guidance for implementing research and interventions. However, limited skills, expertise, and finance can inhibit lower-resource countries from carrying out such necessary research. Broader societal and cultural factors need to be carefully addressed to ensure international partnership based on confidence, fairness, and mutual benefit.

2 Partnership in Research

Public health crises demand partnerships on multiple dimensions:

- Interdisciplinary, multi-sectoral
- Entire government (within governments)

- Multi stakeholder
  - Non-governmental organizations
  - Academia
  - Healthcare professionals
  - Community health and humanitarian workers
  - People in the community—the response backbone and the source of research participants
  - International organizations (World Health Organization [WHO] and others)
  - Private sector including pharmaceutical companies

Partnership in health can be defined as a collaborative relationship between two or more parties for the common goal of improving the health of populations based on mutually agreed roles and principles, while sharing risks as well as benefits. Partnerships can range from legally incorporated entities with specific governance arrangements to simpler collaborations with varied stakeholders, using diverse terms such as "partnership," "alliance," "network," "coalitions," "consortium," "program," or "collaboration."

Partnerships for global health and global health research have become an important mechanism for health development for the past several decades, with increasing joint initiatives that involve stakeholders from different sectors, including governments, academia, industry, and civil society organizations (Kickbusch and Quick 1998; Larkan et al. 2016). This has resulted in the production of new, vital health data and scientific advancement, yet the progress of global health research activity has been insufficient. The reasons for this are complex and multifaceted – as noted by Ward et al. (2018), "this is not so much a limitation in the science (although this remains a factor in respect of some diseases) but also an outcome of social and structural inequality."

In general, global health research has demonstrated that partnership approaches, with some exceptions, have done little to combat, and may even have perpetuated, longstanding issues, such as: Global North-South dependency, the legacy of colonialism, distorted health research priorities, weak and unprepared healthcare systems, underutilized local professionals and knowledge, unfair distribution of risks and benefits, and insufficient access to life-saving interventions for the populations most in need (Franzen et al. 2017; Petryna 2007). The increasing prevalence of EIDs has highlighted the need to bring new and differently arrayed forces together to fight outbreaks, contribute to research, and play new roles in meeting specific pandemic related challenges.

2.1 Key Partnership Actors

Key players for developing and conducting research in EID outbreaks include the affected or potentially affected communities, national authorities and health systems, research organizations, academic centers, non-governmental organizations (NGOs), pharmaceutical companies, international funders, and WHO.

First, conducting research during an outbreak requires acceptance from the community from which research participants will come (▶ Chap. 18). As has been evident during many outbreaks and pandemics, national governments and international agencies addressing health security threats sometimes struggle to understand popular reactions to infectious disease emergence and outbreaks, complicating their efforts to control deadly diseases. A necessary though not sufficient measure to minimize popular delusions is to make affected population groups partners in research, creating communications interchange between community and biomedical perspectives. Developing and implementing effective models for engaging communities and integrating the social sciences into preparedness and response strategies for infectious disease threats must become a priority element in research programs (Giles-Vernick et al. 2019).

Research carried out in the field during outbreaks needs implementation partners, especially when the field is lacking the needed physical and human infrastructure. Some of this infrastructure can be provided by emergency front-line health care organizations providing care, often NGOs like Médecins Sans Frontières, International Medical Corps, or the Alliance for International Medical Action. Effective responses to EID outbreaks should focus first on a robust public health response provided by these front-line health care workers, including isolation of suspected cases, contact tracing, implementation of preventive measures such as vaccination if available, and safe care for infected individuals. Local health systems and healthcare providers are thus important partners. To accomplish research goals, such as candidate medical countermeasure (MCM) evaluation, it is important to involve these actors in research. Their role can strongly depend on in-country capacity for research with respect to existing infrastructure and human resources, experience, and expertise. It is therefore essential, and even an ethical obligation, to identify and train local investigators, improve existing physical and trial infrastructure, and collaborate on needed research. Unused assets atrophy, so ongoing collaborative work and ultimately funding for fully independent research is essential to long-term sustainability (▶ Chap. 14) (Yozwiak et al. 2016).

It is also essential to include local regulatory and ethics agencies. Conducting research, especially clinical trials involving humans, requires evaluating plausible benefits and risks of research and resulting MCMs for trial participants and their communities. Ethical approval of trials and licensure or emergency approval of MCMs is the prerogative of each sovereign country and its institutions. Local regulatory and ethical committee reinforcement thus needs to be part of capacity building plans. The objective of capacity building is to "develop individuals, organizations and societies (individually and collectively) to perform functions, effectively, efficiently, and in a sustainable manner" (UNDP 1998), "to leave tangible benefits and not just creat[e] a dependency on external resources" (Lau et al. 2014). Fulfilling capacity building objectives in a partnership is key and ensures that local health research is increasingly able to respond to local health needs and assure the safety and health of local and global populations (Ward et al. 2017; Yozwiak et al. 2016).

When outbreaks overwhelm the capacities of local health systems or develop into complex emergencies, as has been the case in many countries challenged by the COVID-19 epidemic, international humanitarian organizations often play a crucial role in providing care. They are well positioned to help implement research programs, given their interactions with patients and the community. It is important to improve understanding of the place of research in infectious disease response, as well as research expertise within these organizations, to facilitate the conduct of clinical research. Relationships between humanitarian organizations and research institutions have occasionally been difficult in the past, mainly because of differing perspectives (Caplan et al. 2015; WHO 2014a). In the long term, strengthening the research capacities of humanitarian organizations should also underpin cooperation outside of times of crisis and make for more productive North-South research collaborations (▶ Chaps. 18 and 29).

National research institutions are of course essential partners for research conducted during an epidemic. They bring unique local expertise and ensure the scientific quality of the studies, although conducting research alongside response to an outbreak is quite different from the usual conduct of research. Because there are frequently important constraints on conducting research in countries and regions where an outbreak occurs, international research institutions' involvement, and international collaborative research partnerships are important to bridge health research gaps. These partnerships are essential to provide funding and expertise but are even more important for building capacities (Petryna 2007).

Government organizations are essential in research partnerships, as national governments, in particular ministries of health, bear first responsibility for responding to epidemics and protecting the health of the population. They are consequently a major stakeholder for leading discussions and implementation of preparedness and response, including research. Due to the potential global spread of EIDs, and especially when authorities face conflicts, political instability, or lack of preparedness, appropriate multisectoral partnerships should be developed.

Private sector companies, although they do not always have market incentives to proactively develop lifesaving products for EID, can form partnerships during an outbreak to share risks and benefits in order to bring vaccines, therapeutics, or diagnostic tests into the field for clinical trials, not to mention their primary role in manufacturing validated MCMs. Companies must be included in collaborative preparedness, including plans for research and development directions (R&D roadmaps) and product profiles of vaccines, medicines, and diagnostics for pathogens families with pandemic potential. This involvement will help guide research and quality, safety, and efficacy parameters in line with good manufacturing practices (Bok et al. 2021).

Funders are also necessary partners in global EID research (▶ Chap. 28). They can facilitate a rapid, coordinated approach to funding research on pathogens or pathogen families with pandemic potential (Matthiessen et al. 2016). They can also contribute to a capacity building agenda for preparedness and response to a public health emergency.

WHO is the lynchpin of international response to outbreaks of emerging infectious diseases. It is the international body responsible for coordinating health aspects of outbreak response, including coordination of research. "To fulfil its mandate, WHO has a core responsibility in the area of research and coordination of research. WHO will use its convening capacity to fulfil this responsibility. Although WHO is not a funding agency nor in general a major implementer of research activities, it has a global mandate to set evidence-based priorities and standards for research, ensuring that all voices are heard and avoiding conflicts of interests" (Kieny et al. 2016). WHO is the global coordinating center for preparedness and for responding to epidemics. After its widely criticized response to the 2014–2016 West Africa Ebola epidemic, WHO undertook an overhaul of its emergency preparedness and response functions. Most relevant for research is the Research & Development Blueprint, a global strategy and preparedness plan to improve preparedness and rapid activation of research and development of countermeasures during public health emergencies (WHO 2020a).

2.2 Principles for Successful Research Partnerships

Partnerships are critical to effectively implement programs and improve health. They are essential to raise visibility of an unmet need, support coordination, provide financial support to countries, and provide common platforms for working together. One of the greatest strengths of partnerships is their ability to combine the complementary strengths of different stakeholders to achieve common objectives. However, development research often has a problem with how tasks and rewards are allocated:

> The predominant model tends to be one in which data collection happens in the global south—often by local enumerators—with researchers in the global north conducting all the analysis and delivering the final, fully-baked report. While this type of research model can produce useful insights, it may get limited uptake if it fails to respond to local needs or isn't developed from a partnership based in mutual trust (Rose and Estes 2021).

The criteria for a successful partnership in research and the principles that should govern its development and implementation have been under discussion by academics, research organizations, and WHO for decades. Most past analyses have not considered the specific context of research implemented in crisis environments, but their analytical framework is relevant for these contexts. Just as the COVID-19 pandemic took hold, the Nuffield Council on Bioethics (2020) published a book-length synthesis of the ethics of research in an emergency, while WHO has also provided updated guideline documents for research during emergencies (WHO 2016a, 2020c, d, e).

John et al. (2016) conducted a survey of research partners from Uganda, Kenya, and the United States who had extensive global health research experience about what they considered the top three factors that strengthened or impeded successful international research collaborations. All interviewed research partners came from academic or research institutions and had more than 10 years of global health research experience. Although the questions were open-ended, responses were highly consistent. Four key factors for successful partnerships were identified: (1) mutual respect and benefit, (2) trust, (3) good communication, and (4) clear partner roles and expectations.

The myriad disciplines, perspectives, contexts, and practical applications or experiences of partners involved in international global health research present challenges to building successful partnerships. However, some core concepts must be considered. To identify these concepts, Larkan et al. (2016) built an evidence-based framework using an inductive exploratory research process. A total of 17 partners were involved in this research, of which nine were Southern and eight Northern-based partners. These partners came from research institutions, civil society organizations, private companies, and networks. Seven core concepts emerged that are consistent with the findings of John and collaborators: focus, values, equity, benefit, communication, leadership, and resolution. Larkan et al. (2016) suggest, "while objectives are important, they are not in and of themselves sufficient to ensure focus. Common goals and minimum common programs among partners were identified as essential attributes," adding that values refer "to understanding the organizational culture of each partner and the underlying societal norms within which each partner operates." Trust was identified as a prerequisite to successful partnership. Equity was a core concept and in particular mutual respect and openness to learning from each other. Moreover, respondents agreed on the importance of research programs providing benefits to communities and/or partner organizations beyond the immediate partnership. Skill generation and capacity building are particularly important indicators of project success.

In their paper "International Collaborative Research Partnerships: Blending Science with Management and Diplomacy," Lau et al. (2014) note that "the assumption that people choose to conduct research to investigate interesting questions or improve community health is common, but may be incorrect. Partners may perceive training needs, revenue, or infrastructure establishment as the primary goal." Having a transparent, open, honest, and unambiguous communication strategy is crucial for research partnerships to succeed. Finally, resolution and leadership were found to be core concepts.

In further exploration of the kind of leadership needed for successful partnerships, Lau et al. (2014) emphasize that delegation of roles and responsibilities, shared management and accountability, and balance and diplomacy are essential; leadership development and careful planning should be given high priority. Governance plans, memoranda of understanding (MoU), or principles of partnership documents are extremely helpful in defining the parameters of the collaboration and establishing realistic expectations for both parties. An MoU, Lau et al. find, "forces a project to set mutual goals with measurable success outcomes so that tasks can be defined to enable projects to attain desired operational results." It is also important to agree on strategies that will minimize conflicts or challenges that may arise over the course of the partnership.

The Research Fairness Initiative, an initiative by the Council on Health Research for Development (COHRED) is aimed at improving fairness, efficiency, and impact of research collaboration globally. COHRED (2000) published a reporting guide to promote and measure fairness in research collaboration and partnership. The report identifies three domains to investigate when developing collaborative research, each including five topics and related indicators to monitor. The three domains are the following:

1. *Fairness of opportunity* "aims to improve the participation of all concerned at relevant stages of research development, often

well before research even begins." It includes relevance to communities in which research is done, early engagement of partners, and the need to make contributions of partners explicit.
2. *Fair process* "aims to improve fairness in how research is conducted and research partnerships and programs are implemented," including fair local hiring, training and sourcing, respect of local ethics review system, and data ownership.
3. *Fair sharing of benefits, costs, and outcomes*, includes research system capacities, technology transfer, and environmental, social, and cultural impacts.

3 Selected Recent Major EIDs: Lessons Learned

Before the 2014–2016 West Africa Ebola epidemic, research conducted during EID outbreaks was limited. An early effort occurred in 2002–2003, during the severe acute respiratory syndrome (SARS) outbreak, a life-threatening disease for which no treatments were available. The scientific community could not launch a multi-sectoral, interdisciplinary coordinated research effort. Nucleic acid sequencing abilities were relatively primitive compared to now (the first draft of the human genome having been completed in 2000 at a cost about 6 orders of magnitude greater than it is currently). Nevertheless, the scientific community reacted quickly to identify and characterize the novel virus, with a genetic sequence completed about 6 months after the first cases, and a candidate vaccine was ready to begin animal trials by a year after the outbreak began (Finlay et al. 2004).

WHO convened international response consultations, and scientists from Canada, China, and the United States were especially active in launching research programs. ◘ Figure 1 shows some of the achievements of this effort in the relatively brief period before SARS was contained through public health and infection control methods. The research response to SARS was a dress rehearsal for a play that fortunately closed early but provided essential experience for the actors and stage crew. It also started continued research on the zoonotic potential of coronaviruses (Song et al. 2019).

Therapeutics trials posed considerably greater difficulties. Stockman et al. (2006) note the inability to implement properly designed trials, the heterogeneity in treatment regimens used, and the non-standardized collection of clinical information, which were major obstacles to evaluating potential treatments and to clearly interpreting collected data.

The emergence and global spread of 2009 A(H1N1) influenza prompted the largest pandemic response ever mounted at that time (▸ Chap. 29). Many aspects of this response were positive. However, Abelin et al. (2011) identified several areas where improvements would facilitate an expedited response:

- Technical enhancements
- Enhancing decision-making processes
- Pre-establishing supply agreements
- Streamlining regulatory processes
- Regional collaboration
- Overcoming communications challenges

Other matters related to vaccine development, evaluation, supply, and coverage were also of concern. The 2009 H1N1 influenza pandemic provided opportunities for international research cooperation that were not seized upon. Although Europe-wide effectiveness studies were conducted, they were not combined in a centralized, coordinated manner with European efficacy and safety studies. The pandemic also illustrated the need to reinforce regional virus epidemiology capabilities including biosurveillance, particularly in less developed countries and regions. The initial stages of H1N1 inactivated vaccine virus development and production scale-up proved highly challenging (Robertson et al. 2011). This highlighted the need for close collaboration between academic, government, and industry researchers, along with WHO network colleagues and decision makers to determine vaccine standardization. During both the SARS and H1N1 epidemics, obstacles to research response included delays in

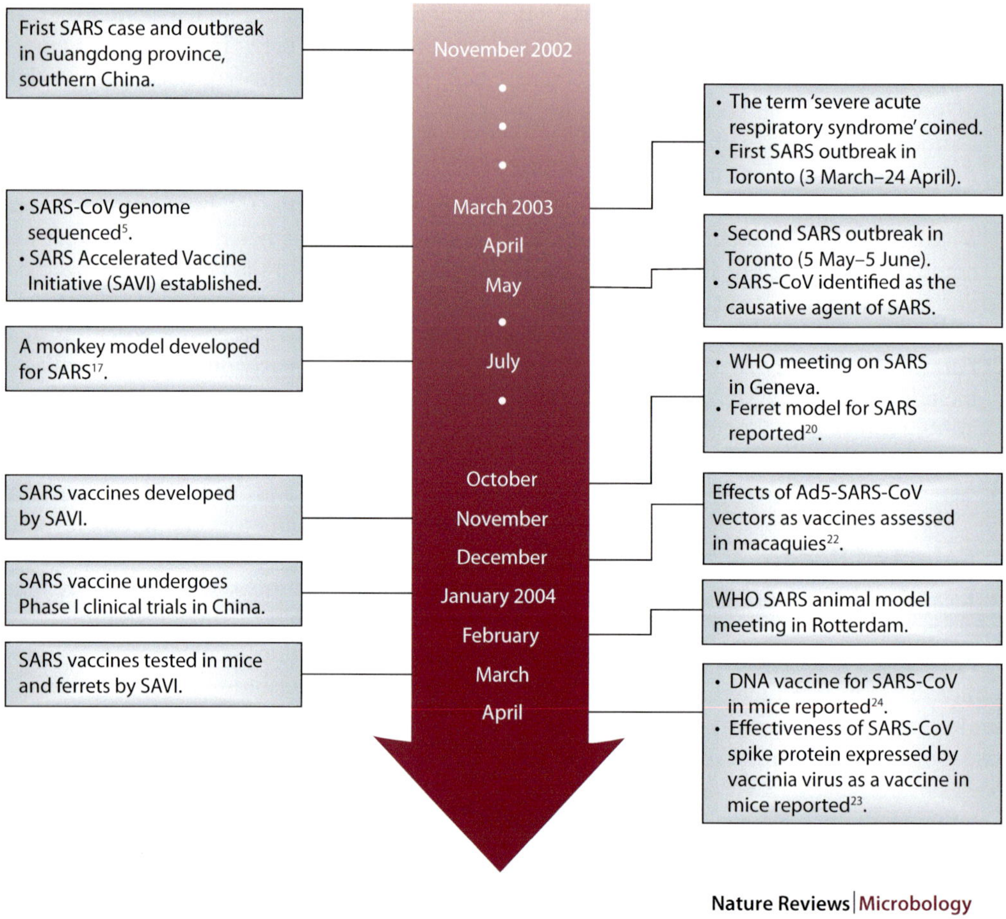

Fig. 1 Achievements of research response to the 2002–2003 SARS pandemic through early 2004. (Finlay et al. 2004)

political commitment, funding, and mobilization of researchers; insufficient coordination among stakeholders, both nationally and internationally; and administrative, regulatory, and ethical impediments.

3.1 The West Africa Ebola Outbreak (2014–2016)

The 2014–2016 West Africa Ebola outbreak marked a turning point in the global preparedness and response to epidemics (▶ Chap. 17). It was different from all previous Ebola outbreaks, moving fast, crossing borders, affecting large numbers of people, and killing many. Its unprecedented scale triggered a multifaceted response, including money from foreign governments for building care facilities (Ebola Treatment Units [ETUs]), expanding laboratory capacity for diagnosis, and mobilizing foreign volunteers, from health care workers to public health outbreak control experts, to help with patient care and stop the epidemic. The role of NGOs was particularly important in response to this epidemic. Alongside the humanitarian emergency, a scientific emergency appeared, which was characterized by awareness of the urgent need for experimental treatments and vaccines. The magnitude and duration of the outbreak seemed to allow research teams, for the first time, to plan clinical research protocols for evaluating the efficacy of experimental vaccines and treatments. The outbreak prompted the initiation and implementation of comprehensive research programs, including clinical trials conducted during the epidemic. These met with varying degrees of success, but demonstrated the ability of researchers, regulators, scientific and ethics review boards, governments and health authorities, sponsors, NGOs, and communities to work together.

The index Ebola case in West Africa was retrospectively identified as a child in the remote Guinean village of Meliandou, Guéckédou Prefecture who became ill in December 2013. Only after August 8, 2014, when WHO declared the Ebola outbreak a public health emergency of international concern (PHEIC) (WHO 2014b), did the international community recognize the critical importance of engaging in a global public health response that included research. Several meetings were organized to discuss the use of potential Ebola therapeutics and vaccines, which were in various stages of development, and consider the related scientific, ethical, and regulatory issues of conducting clinical trials. In the following months, the different stakeholders started working together and building partnerships to launch the first therapeutic and vaccine trials. Through their logistical support, humanitarian organizations and NGOs not usually involved in research contributed greatly to the implementation of clinical trials. Trial teams benefited from ETUs and their infrastructure already established and run by international NGOs, and from existing relationships between organizations, local officials, and community members (Levine 2016) (▶ In Practice 40.1). Partnerships also benefited from existing relationships between scientists and research institutions and authorities of affected countries.

In 2014, the WHO convened meetings to coordinate the planning of clinical trials for candidate Ebola vaccines. Under pressure from the outbreak, protocol development timelines and scientific and ethics approvals were compressed. To address requests from clinical trial investigators in Africa, Phase I studies were conducted in high-income countries before vaccine trials (Phase II and III) were launched in Africa by February 2015. Several international collaborative partnerships were built to launch the vaccine trials during the epidemic, including (1) the Ebola Ça Suffit Ring Vaccination Trial, a collaboration between the government of Guinea, WHO, Médecins Sans Frontières (MSF), and the Norwegian Institute of Public Health launched in Guinea in April 2015 (Henao-Restrepo et al. 2017); and (2) the Partnership for Research on Ebola Vaccines in Liberia (PREVAIL), part of an agreement between the Liberian and U.S. governments for a long-term collaborative partnership in clinical research between the two countries; its first trial, PREVAIL I, started in Liberia in February 2015 (Kennedy et al. 2017, 2016).

During the Ebola outbreak in West Africa, real, effective partnerships were built. Governments and foundations mobilized funds, companies brought therapeutic and vaccine candidates into the field, and collaborations among WHO, research institutions, national health authorities, NGOs, and civil society enabled advances through accelerated clinical trials. In addition, research launched was multisectoral, multidisciplinary, and multi-partner and covered diagnosis and pathogen characterization, clinical research for evaluating potential countermeasures, and social science. However, despite successes and generation of new Ebola information, the overall scientific harvest of the trials has been described as "thin" (Cohen and Enserink 2015). As Kennedy et al. (2017) note, "Finally, we could not establish whether either vaccine was effective in preventing EVD [Ebola virus disease] since the number of cases of EVD declined drastically in Liberia owing to a concerted public health effort that succeeded in ending the outbreak in Liberia before the PREVAIL I trial could be expanded to its phase 3 component." This applied to a greater or lesser degree to several clinical trials implemented during the outbreak.

Several elements contributed to this outcome, including the shortcomings of the surveillance systems, inadequate involvement of funders and researchers before WHO declared the PHEIC, and the delay in declaring the PHEIC that prompted the global response. In addition, the disparate goals and missions of international partners created a conflict between the perspectives of medical science and humanitarian medicine. At first, stakeholders debated the ethics of conducting randomly controlled clinical trials during a public health emergency with high mortality. Some stakeholders responding to the massive humanitarian crisis claimed that experimental drugs should be given to as many patients as possible, while others argued for an ethical obligation to conduct formal clinical trials during an epidemic to quickly and efficiently identify beneficial MCMs. Disputes arose about randomized trials versus nonrandomized alternative designs, the use of a standard-of-care control arm, and the fair distribution of limited products (Adebamowo et al. 2014; Cox et al. 2014; Lanini et al. 2015). Although the debate among health-care workers and researchers was considered fruitful, leading to the adaptation of clinical research methods (Dunning et al. 2016), too much time was spent debating trial design, rather than quickly implementing trials and investigating the safety and efficacy of MCMs in time to fight the epidemic.

Community acceptance of research programs also proved to be challenging. Clinical trials require volunteer participants, but a good relationship between researcher and participant, which depends on mutual trust, was difficult to achieve in West Africa where a context of fear and mistrust of outsiders, along with a lack of knowledge about clinical research, may be aggravated by limited understanding among international researchers of local culture and social traditions (▶ Chap. 18).

Experiences gained from clinical trials and research projects conducted as part of the Ebola outbreak response clearly demonstrated some of the difficulties of designing successful clinical trials and coordinating among all stakeholders to reach consensus on implementation. To mitigate these issues, some stakeholders argued that WHO should have played a stronger role coordinating the multitude of disparate efforts. However, the overwhelming problem was lack of preparedness (Cohen and Enserink 2015).

3.2 The Zika Outbreak (2015–2016)

On February 1, 2016, WHO declared its fourth PHEIC in response to clusters of microcephaly and Guillain-Barré syndrome in the Americas, which were suspected to be associated with the ongoing 2015–2016 Zika virus epidemic (WHO 2016c). Many lessons learned from the response to the West Africa Ebola outbreak helped in the response to the Zika virus outbreak (▶ Chap. 21). Importantly, general agreement emerged on the need for international collaboration on regulatory issues, research, and data sharing (Haug et al. 2016). During the epidemic's first stages, the scientific community expended titanic efforts to rapidly understand Zika virus biology and pathology, improve diagnostic methodologies, and develop specific therapeutic and prophylactic alternatives (Martin-Acebes and Saiz 2019). Important collaborative work has been achieved, thanks to the rapid involvement of donors and the opening of calls for proposals, which allowed the creation of international partnerships. These partnerships include three multinational and multi-disciplinary research consortia funded by the European Union (EU): ZikAlliance, ZikaPlan, and ZikAction (TGHN 2022).

As during the West Africa Ebola epidemic, delays in developing practical diagnostic tests for the right population at the right time were a costly barrier to disease control and prevention during the Zika epidemic (Peeling et al. 2019). To mitigate these issues, meetings were organized to define research priorities and determine if products could be tested in clinical trials. In general, though, the Zika epidemic highlighted continued lack of preparedness and of available agents for efficacy testing.

3.3 Recent Democratic Republic of the Congo (DRC) Ebola Outbreaks

When an Ebola outbreak began in the Equateur province of the DRC in May 2018,

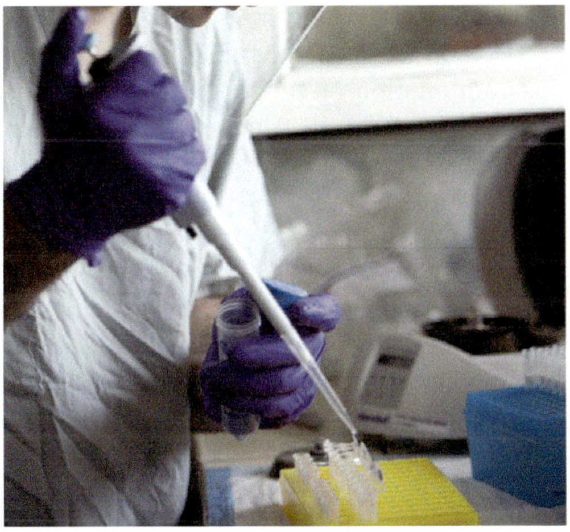

■ **Fig. 2** Testing samples for Ebola in the DRC. (Courtesy of WHO)

collaborative efforts to implement research started immediately (▶ In Practice 16.1). These efforts capitalized on the experience and results obtained from clinical trials launched during previous Ebola outbreaks. The response of humanitarian and scientific actors to containing the virus relied on results of the Ebola Ça Suffit and other trials in West Africa and included ring vaccination with the rVSV-ZEBOV vaccine. In addition, they rapidly administered multiple novel therapies under a WHO framework for Monitored emergency use of unregistered and investigational interventions (MEURI) (WHO 2016b, 2018). These two actions were possible thanks to preparedness, prior knowledge of vaccines and treatments, and availability of protocols that were ready to use or adapt. Once again, as in West Africa, a rapid decline in Ebola cases prevented researchers from drawing statistically sound conclusions about the efficacy of therapeutic products through randomized controlled trials (■ Fig. 2).

When another Ebola outbreak started in the DRC in August 2018, in the northeastern province of North Kivu, ring vaccination under MEURI was initiated within only 7 days after the declaration of the outbreak. The ability to mount such a rapid response underlines how crucial the involvement of all stakeholders, including national health authorities, is from the outset of discussions, including national health authorities. Clear, strong leadership focused on scientifically sound objectives—but including stakeholders at all levels—is essential to success. The northeastern DRC Ebola response exemplifies the need for strong organizational partnerships from the earliest stages of planning (Mulangu et al. 2019). Organizational strength was especially needed because the northeastern DRC response took place in a region not only vulnerable to Ebola virus disease but beset by ongoing violent conflict, food insecurity, and lack of functional health infrastructure—little infrastructure of any kind, in fact, including electrical power, paved roads, and clean water. The response has also highlighted the necessity of broad-based organizational partnerships to implement research programs and access vulnerable populations, even when scientists are facing violence (Maxmen 2019).

3.4 The COVID-19 Pandemic: What Lessons Can Be Drawn?

The COVID-19 pandemic has underlined the fundamental roles of partnerships and coordination in global health. Continents, regions, and countries have undertaken different measures, and their populations have responded with varying degrees of acceptance as they have faced the recurring waves of SARS-CoV-2 variants. Organizational partnerships have determined the success or failure of mitigating the spread of the epidemic and limiting its impact on populations. While the pandemic has shown that previous lessons regarding preparedness and response had not been fully integrated and implemented, some successes must be highlighted (▶ Chap. 31).

For instance, research mobilization on COVID-19 has been unprecedented. On January 30, 2020, following the recommendations of the Emergency Committee, the WHO Director-General declared that the new Coronavirus outbreak, first identified in China, constituted a PHEIC. Two weeks after the declaration, WHO and the Global Research Collaboration for Infectious Disease Preparedness and Response (GloPID-R), an international network of funders to facilitate coordination and information sharing, jointly organized a COVID-19 Global Forum on research and innovation. This forum aimed at "assessing the current level of knowledge about the new virus, agreeing on critical research questions that need to be answered urgently, and finding ways to work together to accelerate and fund priority research to curtail this outbreak and prepare for those in the future" (WHO 2020b). As the conclusions of the forum were published in March 2020, the WHO R&D Blueprint began facilitating a coordinated response to COVID-19 to "accelerate diagnostics, vaccines and therapeutics for this novel coronavirus" (WHO 2020f). GloPID-R, in partnership with the United Kingdom (UK) Collaborative on Development Research (UKCDR), has developed a database connected to the WHO R&D Blueprint, which compiles member research projects in relation to COVID-19 (Norton et al. 2021). The database maps research areas to projects and available funding to guide international research (UKCDR and GloPID-R 2022). The database also classifies projects by countries, showing a continuing clear imbalance towards funding and research in high-income countries.

As of August 2022, the WHO database on scientific publications includes more than 667,000 publications on COVID-19 collected since the beginning of the epidemic (WHO 2022c), reflecting scientific collaboration that has been one of the bright spots of the global pandemic response. Without basic research and established networks of trust, we would not have been able to understand and react to this crisis as rapidly as we did. Examples of this effective scientific collaboration, and the underlying challenges, illustrate both progress and shortcomings in global research capacity.

The devastating impact of the SARS-CoV-2 outbreak rapidly highlighted the urgent need for effective therapies to control the spread of the disease and alleviate life-threatening symptoms and disorders. Although many drugs have in vitro activity against various coronaviruses, no reliable clinical evidence at the beginning of the outbreak supported the efficacy and safety of any drug against coronaviruses in humans, including SARS-CoV-2. Thus, the rapid and simultaneous combination of supportive care and randomized controlled trials (RCT's) quickly emerged as the only way to find effective and safe treatments for COVID-19 and improve patient management. WHO recommended that researchers around the world systematically evaluate experimental therapeutics in RCT's and generate data from large trials to provide strong evidence of drug safety and effectiveness. Conversely, WHO and others also noted the unreliability of small and poorly designed trials that appeared to find benefit in, for example, hydroxychloroquine, early in the pandemic (Bugin and Woodcock 2021; Cochrane Collaborative 2020).

Clinical trials initially focused on drug repurposing strategies that offered an attractive, immediate, and realistic approach to tackle the growing pandemic. Large collaborative studies have been rapidly set up, showing unprecedented ability to bring together different national and international actors, and overcome obstacles that can delay the start of clinical trials. As early as March 2020, WHO and its partners launched the SOLIDARITY trial. WHO provided a master protocol and simplified procedures to enable hospitals from many countries to participate. Between March 2020 and January 2021, 14,304 potentially eligible patients were recruited from 454 hospitals in 35 countries in all 6 WHO regions. The study subsequently demonstrated little or no effect of tested therapeutics on hospitalized COVID-19 patients (WHO Solidarity Trial Consortium 2021, 2022). Other adaptive platform trials were rapidly organized as well, as shown in ◘ Table 1.

Through their navigation of regulatory, legal, and financial obstacles that could have significantly slowed down the conduct of clinical trials (Diallo et al. 2022), these large trials and trial consortia can be considered examples of partnership successes on national and international levels. However, better preparedness and stronger coordination could have minimized the many small, disparate studies worldwide that evaluated identical therapeutic candidates, assessed drugs without in vitro or in vivo data, and frequently had method-

Table 1 Selected collaborative trials of therapeutics for COVID-19 and its consequences (authors)

Name	Start (end)	Location	Sponsors	Participants	Investigating	Reference
RECOVERY	March 2020	UK, later international	UK National Institutes of Health Research, UK National Health Service	Patients hospitalized with COVID-19	COVID-19 therapeutics	Horby (2024)
REMAP-CAP (Randomized, Embedded, Multifactorial Adaptive Platform Trial for Community-Acquired Pneumonia)	April 2016 (COVID-19 as of February 2020)	13 countries	University Medical Center Utrecht	Intensive care unit patients with pneumonia (COVID-19)	Therapeutics	Angus et al. (2020)
DisCoVeRy	March 2020	Europe	INSERM	Hospitalized patients with COVID-19 in need of oxygen therapy	Therapeutics	Ader (2020)
ANTICOV	September 2020	13 African countries + Brazil	Drugs for Neglected Diseases initiative	Patients with mild to moderate COVID-19 symptoms	Therapeutics	ANTICOV (2022)
ACTIV (Accelerating COVID-19 Therapeutic Interventions and Vaccines)	April 2020	United States	National Institutes of Health, pharmaceutical industry	COVID-19 patients, people at high risk from COVID-19	Therapeutics, vaccines	Wholley (2024)
SOLIDARITY	March 2020	Global	WHO	Various	Therapeutics, vaccines	WHO (2022d)

ological weaknesses (i.e., statistically underpowered or yielding inappropriate/inconclusive outcomes) (Bugin and Woodcock 2021; Cochrane Collaborative 2020).

Vaccine R&D has been dynamic and productive. Safe and effective COVID-19 vaccines, especially effective against severe forms of the disease, have been developed in record time. Vaccine trials, based on various technological platforms, were initiated in the first quarter of 2020, and vaccination deployment in populations started in December 2020. As of August 2022, 11 vaccines were registered on the WHO Emergency Use List, 170 vaccines were in clinical development and 198 vaccines in pre-clinical development (WHO 2022b). These emergency approvals were made possible by a combination of different factors, including the enormous resources devoted to the COVID-19 pandemic, cooperation between a wide range of public and private stakeholders, previous research on coronavirus vaccines and on vaccine platforms, and other innovations in technology and R&D (Bloom et al. 2021). Funds allocated for vaccine development, trials, and manufacturing have been exceptionally high.

First, the U.S. government committed up to 13 billion USD for vaccine developers, including 2.5 billion to support vaccine development efforts, in addition to purchase agreements. The EU, UK, and others similarly committed to fund R&D and accelerate vaccine availability. Second, the intense cooperation between governments, public research institutions, and private industry has been critical for achieving rapid vaccine development. Enlisting the cooperation of private industry to help meet the key economic challenges of investing in the development of a vaccine was crucial, because in the absence of government intervention the private sector is not generally predisposed to fully absorb the risk of investing in vaccines. Third, innovation in vaccine R&D relied on emerging technologies and well-designed clinical vaccine trials. Vaccines registered in the WHO Emergency Use Listing Procedure (EUL) used several different technological platforms. Some relied on well-established approaches (e.g., inactivated whole-virus and protein-based vaccines), while others relied on new vaccine technologies (e.g., messenger RNA [mRNA] vaccines) approved for the first time as vaccine for humans. Therefore, the process of vaccine trials implementation has been dramatically accelerated. The need to speed up the development and delivery of a vaccine has introduced new approaches with many phases executed in parallel rather than sequentially. Developers have combined clinical trial phases, started subsequent clinical phases before confirming the success of previous trials, or conducted parallel clinical trials.

However, the distribution of vaccines at the global level was very unequitable. By May 2022, around 11.7 billion doses of COVID-19 vaccines had been administered worldwide, with 59.5% of the population fully vaccinated against COVID-19 (Our World in Data 2022). In subsequent months, more than 75% of people living in high income countries were fully vaccinated, but this rate was about 17% on the African continent and only 12.5% among low-income countries (Ritchie et al. 2022, ◘ Fig. 3).

The COVID-19 Vaccines Global Access (COVAX) Facility was created by WHO; Gavi, the Vaccine Alliance; and the Coalition for Epidemic Preparedness Innovations (CEPI) to reduce inequality in access to vaccine by maximizing the chances of people, wherever they live, of getting quick, fair, and safe access to COVID-19 vaccinations. CEPI leads the R&D component of COVAX and has identified a portfolio of suitable vaccine candidates. COVAX works with manufacturers to secure investment and incentives to expand production capacity for vaccines "at risk" before they receive regulatory authorization, thus ensuring that mass dose production can begin immediately after or even before vaccine authorization. The COVAX objective for 2021 was to provide 1.4 billion doses of free vaccines to eligible low-income and lower-middle income countries, enough to fully vaccinate 20% of their populations. However, by January 2022, these countries received only 1 billion doses through COVAX, far fewer than the planned objective (WHO 2022a). By November 2022 COVAX had shipped 1.83 billion doses, and along with the commercial availability of lower-price COVID-19 vac-

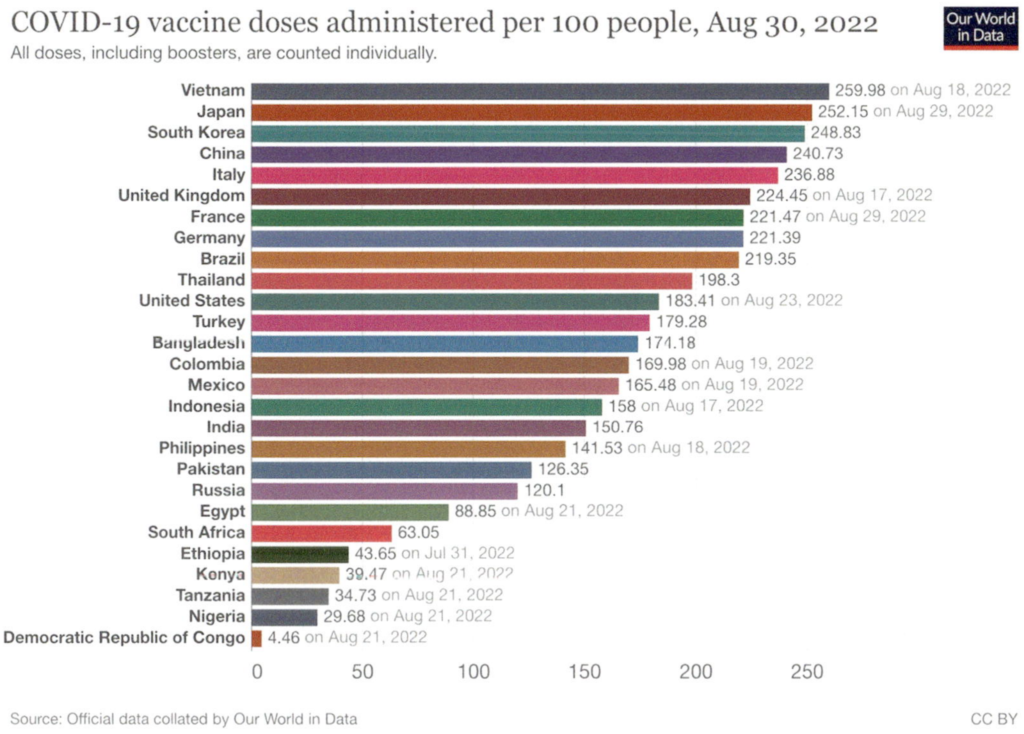

Fig. 3 Coronavirus vaccine doses administered in the world's 30 largest countries. (Our World in Data 2022; CC BY 4.40, downloaded 31 Aug 2022)

cines, that enabled people in most countries who wanted vaccination to obtain them, except in very remote areas.

The shortfalls have had several causes, such as lack of resources, the export ban from producer countries, including India, due to domestic outbreaks, and, above all, vaccine nationalism and related bilateral deals at higher prices between high income countries and manufacturers to ensure preferential access (Bollyky and Brown 2020; Lie and Miller 2020). To mitigate such a breach in global solidarity and a fundamentally unbalanced global context of vaccine production, various initiatives have been undertaken to ensure the convergence between production and populations in need. For instance, the African Union and Africa Centres for Disease Control and Prevention (Africa CDC) have launched the Partnerships for African Vaccine Manufacturing (2022) framework for action, with the ambitious goal of having not the current 1% but rather 60% of all vaccines needed in Africa produced on the continent.

Furthermore, a recent WHO initiative aims to respond to the vaccine production challenge by supporting technology transfer, human resources capacity building, and technological skill strengthening in low and middle resources countries. In April 2021, WHO launched a global call for Expression of Interest (EOI) to establish mRNA vaccine technology transfer hubs that can scale up production and access to COVID vaccines (WHO 2021). Following this call, the establishment of the first hub was announced in South Africa, relying on a partnership involving WHO and the COVAX partners, Africa CDC, and a network of universities and private companies. In total, 15 countries in Africa, Asia and Latin America will be recipients of mRNA technology from the WHO mRNA technology transfer hub (WHO 2022e). Other initiatives are underway to strengthen capacities to manufacture vaccines in African countries, including Senegal and Rwanda. In Senegal, CEPI and the Institut Pasteur de Dakar (IPD) have signed a memo-

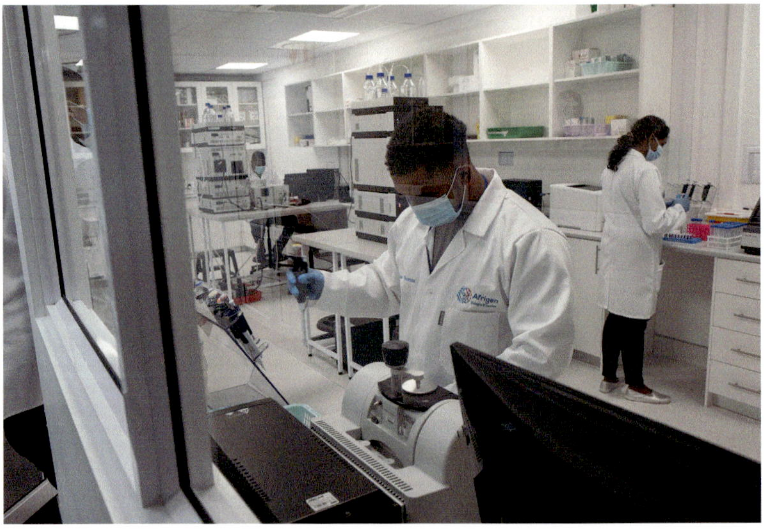

Fig. 4 Lab technicians work in laboratories in Afrigen, a company in Cape Town that has been selected as the WHO Vaccine Hub, in South Africa, on 11 February 2022. (Courtesy WHO; Photo by Rodger Bosch for MPP/WHO mRNA hub)

randum of understanding (MoU) to formalize the partnership between the two organizations to advance the MADIBA project, a regional manufacturing hub for COVID-19 and other vaccines (CEPI 2022) (Fig. 4).

Although the partnership between public and private sectors has been a catalyst for rapid discovery, development, and dissemination of vaccines, this partnership has been unbalanced in favor of the private sector, with a lack of transparency regarding pricing and the terms of bilateral contracts at a time of urgent global need. Furthermore, the issue of intellectual property and patent rights continues to obstruct vaccine production in LMICs and the movement toward making vaccines a global public good (Lancet COVID-19 Commission 2021).

In the area of genomic surveillance, technological advances allowing sequencing in real time have had a tremendous positive impact on public health and the pandemic response. Indeed, prompt sharing of genome sequences has enabled rapid identification of the novel pathogen SARS-CoV-2 and the development of diagnostic tests and vaccines. Simultaneously, large-scale genome sequencing has allowed monitoring of virus evolution and identification of viral transmission chains. Widespread distribution of sequencing capacities and genomic surveillance systems is thus essential to state-of-the-art global biosurveillance.

In addition to existing or newly created national genomic surveillance networks, international initiatives have been launched. For example, the open-access platform GISAID, created as the Global Initiative on Sharing Avian Influenza Data in 2006 to facilitate data sharing on influenza viruses, has now been used to share SARS-CoV-2 sequences. As early as January 10, 2020, the first whole-genome sequences of SARS-CoV-2 were made available on GISAID, facilitating global responses to the pandemic including rapid creation of mRNA vaccine candidates. GISAID has maintained the world's largest repository of SARS-CoV-2 sequences. By November 2022, the GISAID database contained 13.7 million SARs-CoV-2 sequences (GISAID 2022). However, the preponderance of sequences is coming from a few developed countries, while the proportion coming from low- and middle-income countries (LMICs) is low. International initiatives are working to increase sequencing capacities in LMICs (Helmy et al. 2016).

In 2019, the Africa CDC, in collaboration with more than 20 international and national organizations, launched the Institute of Pathogen Genomics to provide rapid and timely response to infectious disease threats in Africa (Africa CDC 2022). Eighteen countries on the continent are providing support for SARS-CoV-2 sequencing, with an increasing

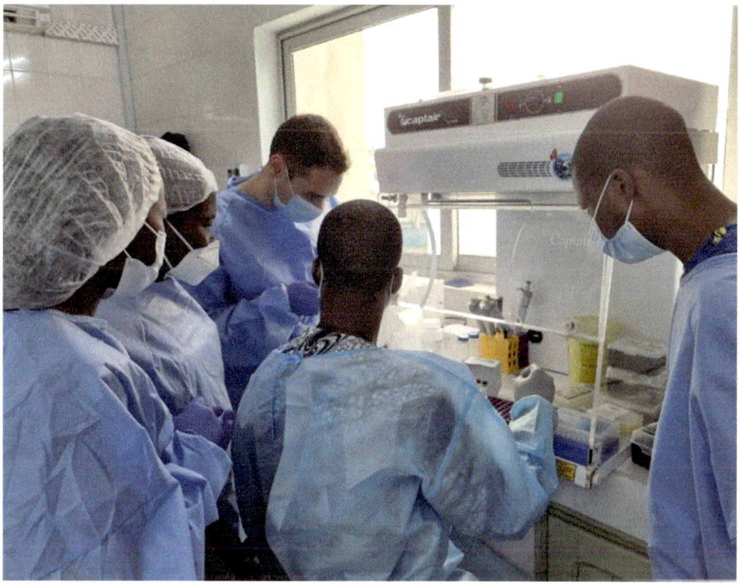

Fig. 5 Training laboratory staff in West Africa on detecting mutations in SARS-CoV-2 virus. (AFROSCREEN 2023)

number of laboratories being leveraged for this activity and accounting for more than 115,000 identified SARS-CoV-2 sequences by August 2022.

Another initiative in the field of genomic surveillance is AFROSCREEN, a multi-institutional sequencing capacity building project in Africa financed by the French Agency for Development (AFD) and coordinated by ANRS Maladies Infectieuses Emergentes (Emerging Infectious Diseases) (AFROSCREEN 2023). AFROSCREEN has been designed in conjunction with the national authorities of each country to meet urgent surveillance needs for emergent SARS-CoV-2 variants. It aims to reinforce each country's genomic surveillance system and facilitate development of such systems where they do not yet exist. AFROSCREEN demonstrates a commitment to inter-institutional and international collaborations to tackle major research and public health challenges. This project is implemented by a consortium comprising three French research institutes (ANRS MIE, Institut Pasteur and the Research Institute for Sustainable Development (IRD) and their partner laboratory networks in 13 sub-Saharan African countries, with Africa CDC, the West African Health Organization (WAHO), and WHO as formal partners (Fig. 5).

4 Conclusion and Recommendations

In conclusion, the COVID-19 pandemic saw the emergence of new and effective forms of research partnerships among various stakeholders and in multiple research disciplines. Cooperative research efforts sometimes encountered forms of biomedical nationalism, a barrier that hindered efforts undertaken to ensure global coordination and partnerships. Furthermore, community involvement seemed limited to COVID-19 research partnerships when compared to efforts for other diseases (e.g., Ebola and HIV/AIDS).

Critically, research partnerships are efficient, performant, and enduring only if they involve all relevant partners: affected communities, national health and governmental authorities, health professionals, research organizations, academic centers, NGOs, pharmaceutical companies, international funders, and WHO. Finally, as highlighted by the COVID-19 pandemic, efficient research partnerships must abide by key principles, such as mutual respect and benefit, fair process, clear roles and expectations, trust, and good communication.

Going forward, the following recommendations, drawn from knowledge gained from previous crises and principles of efficient research partnerships, need to be implemented. First, preparedness must be improved through partnerships during inter-epidemic phases to coordinate international efforts in R&D for infectious disease pathogens, including priority pathogens, a One Health approach to prevent emerging infectious disease occurrence, therapeutic and vaccine identification, pre-clinical studies, Phase I and Phase II trials, and generic clinical trial design templates. Second, to improve the response during epidemic phases, rapid financing must be made available through funding partnerships and efficient coordination of organizations and stakeholders. Research programs need to ensure that vaccines and therapeutic products are prioritized, suitable trial designs are developed and selected, and trials are monitored and evaluated. Third, research needs to be embedded into reinforced national health systems, with clear leadership and division of labor. Research capacities must be strengthened and made sustainable. In this context, human resources and infrastructure, including those needed for clinical trials, should be a priority for all partners. Furthermore, surveillance, data management, and regulatory systems must be strengthened, and ethical considerations, including the need for greatly improved risk communication, must be highlighted. Fourth, it is essential to develop human resources and workforce capacities, including fellowships and training programs. This is a condition for being able to quickly activate research networks during times of crisis, keeping outbreaks from becoming large-scale epidemics, and enabling work on long-term preparedness during inter-epidemic phases. Fifth, international partners should support an interdisciplinary, multisectoral approach that integrates epidemiological, diagnostic, clinical, and socio-behavioral research into the outbreak response. Innovative partnerships between scientists and policy and programs decision-makers can translate science into policy and programmatic decisions.

Discussion Questions

1. What makes for an effective partnership in health emergencies?
2. How can health partnerships do more to address longstanding inequality and inequity?
3. Major stakeholders for the conduct of research response in health emergencies include affected communities, national authorities and health systems, research organizations, academic centers, NGOs, pharmaceutical companies, international funders, and WHO. Choose two of these key players and discuss their roles.
4. COHRED (2000) published guidelines to promote and measure fairness in research collaboration and partnership. What three domains does COHRED consider essential to consider in the development of collaborative research?
5. The emergence and global spread of 2009 A(H1N1) influenza prompted the largest pandemic response ever mounted at that time. What areas for improvement were identified in retrospect?
6. Looking back on the COVID-19 response, what are some integration and implementation successes derived from applying previous lessons? What about less successful initiatives and unanticipated problems?
7. Are your country and the global infectious disease response system currently taking the steps needed to coordinate research response to the next pandemic?
8. Discuss the recommendations made by the authors. Do you have additional recommendations?

References

Abelin A, Colegate T, Gardner S, Hehme N, Palache A. Lessons from pandemic influenza A(H1N1): the research-based vaccine industry's perspective. Vaccine. 2011;29(6):1135–8. https://doi.org/10.1016/j.vaccine.2010.11.042.

Adebamowo C, Bah-Sow O, Binka F, Bruzzone R, Caplan A, Delfraissy J-F, et al. Randomised controlled trials for Ebola: practical and ethical issues. Lancet. 2014;384(9952):1423–4. https://doi.org/10.1016/S0140-6736(14)61734-7.

Ader F. Protocol for the DisCoVeRy trial: multicentre, adaptive, randomised trial of the safety and efficacy of treatments for COVID-19 in hospitalised adults. BMJ Open. 2020;10(9):e041437. https://doi.org/10.1136/bmjopen-2020-041437.

Africa CDC. Institute of Pathogen Genomics (IPG). Addis Ababa: Africa CDC; 2022. https://africacdc.org/institutes/ipg/#:~:text=Africa%20PGI%20is%20an%20initiative,genomics%20and%20bioinformatics%20across%20Africa. Accessed 26 Aug 2022.

AFROSCREEN. Sequencing capacity-building in Africa. Paris: ANRS Maladies infectieuses émergentes; 2023. https://www.afroscreen.org/en/. Accessed 4 Aug 2023.

Angus DC, Berry S, Lewis RJ, Al-Beidh F, Arabi Y, van Bentum-Puijk W, et al. The REMAP-CAP (Randomized Embedded Multifactorial Adaptive Platform for Community-Acquired Pneumonia) study. Rationale and design. Ann Am Thorac Soc. 2020;17(7):879–91. https://doi.org/10.1513/AnnalsATS.202003-192SD.

ANTICOV. Platform trial to find early treatment options for COVID-19 in low-resource settings. Geneva: Drugs for Neglected Diseases initiative (DNDi); 2022. Accessed 25 Aug 2022.

Bloom DE, Cadarette D, Ferranna M, Hyer RN, Tortorice DL. How new models of vaccine development for COVID-19 have helped address an epic public health crisis. Health Aff (Millwood). 2021;40(3):410–8. https://doi.org/10.1377/hlthaff.2020.02012.

Bok K, Sitar S, Graham BS, Mascola JR. Accelerated COVID-19 vaccine development: milestones, lessons, and prospects. Immunity. 2021;54(8):1636–51. https://doi.org/10.1016/j.immuni.2021.07.017.

Bollyky TJ, Brown CP. The tragedy of vaccine nationalism: only cooperation can end the pandemic. Foreign Affairs, Sep/Oct 2020.

Bugin K, Woodcock J. Trends in COVID-19 therapeutic clinical trials. Nat Rev Drug Discov. 2021;20:254. https://doi.org/10.1038/d41573-021-00037-3.

Caplan AL, Plunkett C, Levin B. Selecting the right tool for the job. Am J Bioeth. 2015;15(4):4–10. https://doi.org/10.1080/15265161.2015.1010993.

CEPI. CEPI and Institut Pasteur de Dakar partner to advance COVID-19 vaccine manufacturing in Africa. CEPI; 2022.

Cochrane Collaborative. Targeted update: safety and efficacy of hydroxychloroquine or chloroquine for treatment of COVID-19. London: World Health Organizaton R&D Blueprint Cochrane Collaborative; 2020.

Cohen J, Enserink M. As Ebola epidemic draws to a close, a thin scientific harvest. Science. 2015;351(6268):12–3. https://doi.org/10.1126/science.351.6268.12.

COHRED. Priority setting for health research: lessons from developing countries. The Working Group on Priority Setting. Health Policy Plan. 2000;15(2):130–6. https://doi.org/10.1093/heapol/15.2.130.

Cox E, Borio L, Temple R. Evaluating Ebola therapies—the case for RCTs. N Engl J Med. 2014;371(25):2350–1. https://doi.org/10.1056/nejmp1414145.

Diallo A, Trøseid M, Simensen VC, Boston A, Demotes J, Olsen IC, et al. Accelerating clinical trial implementation in the context of the COVID-19 pandemic: challenges, lessons learned and recommendations from DisCoVeRy and the EU-SolidAct EU response group. Clin Microbiol Infect. 2022;28(1):1–5. https://doi.org/10.1016/j.cmi.2021.10.011.

Dunning J, Longuet C, Salam A. Ebola research: an encounter between science and humanitarian action. Alternatives Humanitaires—Humanitarian Alternatives; 2016.

Finlay BB, See RH, Brunham RC. Rapid response research to emerging infectious diseases: lessons from SARS. Nat Rev Microbiol. 2004;2(7):602–7. https://doi.org/10.1038/nrmicro930.

Franzen SR, Chandler C, Lang T. Health research capacity development in low and middle income countries: reality or rhetoric? A systematic meta-narrative review of the qualitative literature. BMJ Open. 2017;7(1):e012332. https://doi.org/10.1136/bmjopen-2016-012332.

Giles-Vernick T, Kutalek R, Napier D, Kaawa-Mafigiri D, Dückers M, Paget J, et al. A new social sciences network for infectious threats. Lancet Infect Dis. 2019;19(5):461–3. https://doi.org/10.1016/S1473-3099(19)30159-8.

GISAID. GISAID Freunde von GISAID e.V., Munich. 2022. Accessed 22 Aug 2022.

Haider N, Yavlinsky A, Chang Y-M, Hasan MN, Benfield C, Osman AY, et al. The Global Health Security index and Joint External Evaluation score for health preparedness are not correlated with countries' COVID-19 detection response time and mortality outcome. Epidemiol Infect. 2020;148:e210. https://doi.org/10.1017/S0950268820002046.

Haug CJ, Kieny MP, Murgue B. The Zika challenge. N Engl J Med. 2016;374(19):1801–3. https://doi.org/10.1056/nejmp1603734.

Helmy M, Awad M, Mosa KA. Limited resources of genome sequencing in developing countries: challenges and solutions. Appl Transl Genom. 2016;9:15–9. https://doi.org/10.1016/j.atg.2016.03.003.

Henao-Restrepo AM, Camacho A, Longini IM, Watson CH, Edmunds WJ, Egger M, et al. Efficacy and effectiveness of an rVSV-vectored vaccine in preventing Ebola virus disease: final results from the Guinea ring vaccination, open-label, cluster-

randomised trial (Ebola Ca Suffit!). Lancet. 2017;389(10068):505–18. https://doi.org/10.1016/S0140-6736(16)32621-6.
Horby P. In practice: the RECOVERY trial. 2024.
John CC, Ayodo G, Musoke P. Successful global health research partnerships: what makes them work? Am J Trop Med Hyg. 2016;94(1):5–7. https://doi.org/10.4269/ajtmh.15-0611.
Kennedy SB, Neaton JD, Lane HC, Kieh MWS, Massaquoi MBF, Touchette NA, et al. Implementation of an Ebola virus disease vaccine clinical trial during the Ebola epidemic in Liberia: design, procedures, and challenges. Clin Trials (London, England). 2016;13(1):49–56. https://doi.org/10.1177/1740774515621037.
Kennedy SB, Bolay F, Kieh M, Grandits G, Badio M, Ballou R, et al. Phase 2 placebo-controlled trial of two vaccines to prevent Ebola in Liberia. N Engl J Med. 2017;377(15):1438–47. https://doi.org/10.1056/NEJMoa1614067.
Kickbusch I, Quick J. Partnerships for health in the 21st century. World Health Stat Q. 1998;51(1):68–74.
Kieny MP, Rottingen J-A, Farrar J. The need for global R&D coordination for infectious diseases with epidemic potential. Lancet. 2016;388(10043):460–1. https://doi.org/10.1016/s0140-6736(16)31152-7.
Lancet COVID-19 Commission. Global diplomacy and ooperation in pandemic times: lessons and recommendations from COVID-19. 2021.
Lanini S, Zumla A, Ioannidis JPA, Caro AD, Krishna S, Gostin L, et al. Are adaptive randomised trials or non-randomised studies the best way to address the Ebola outbreak in West Africa? Lancet Infect Dis. 2015;15(6):738–45. https://doi.org/10.1016/s1473-3099(15)70106-4.
Larkan F, Uduma O, Lawal SA, van Bavel B. Developing a framework for successful research partnerships in global health. Global Health. 2016;12(1):17. https://doi.org/10.1186/s12992-016-0152-1.
Lau CY, Wang C, Orsega S, Tramont EC, Koita O, Polis MA, et al. International collaborative research partnerships: blending science with management and diplomacy. J AIDS Clin Res. 2014;5(12) https://doi.org/10.4172/2155-6113.1000385.
Levine AC. Academics are from Mars, humanitarians are from Venus: Finding common ground to improve research during humanitarian emergencies. Clin Trials (London, England). 2016;13(1):79–82. https://doi.org/10.1177/1740774515617935.
Lie RK, Miller FG. Allocating a COVID-19 vaccine: balancing national and international responsibilities. Milbank Q. 2020;99:450. https://doi.org/10.1111/1468-0009.12494.
Martin-Acebes MA, Saiz JC. The scientific response to Zika virus. J Clin Med. 2019;8(3) https://doi.org/10.3390/jcm8030369.
Matthiessen L, Colli W, Delfraissy J-F, Hwang E-S, Mphahlele J, Ouellette M. Coordinating funding in public health emergencies. Lancet. 2016;387(10034):2197–8. https://doi.org/10.1016/s0140-6736(16)30604-3.
Maxmen A. Science under fire: Ebola researchers fight to test drugs and vaccines in a war zone. Nature. 2019;572(7767):16–7. https://doi.org/10.1038/d41586-019-02258-4.
Morens DM, Folkers GK, Fauci AS. The challenge of emerging and re-emerging infectious diseases. Nature. 2004;430(6996):242–9. https://doi.org/10.1038/nature02759.
Morse SS. Factors in the emergence of infectious diseases. Emerg Infect Dis. 1995;1(1):7–15. https://doi.org/10.3201/eid0101.950102.
Mulangu S, Dodd LE, Davey RT Jr, Tshiani Mbaya O, Proschan M, Mukadi D, et al. A randomized, controlled trial of Ebola virus disease therapeutics. N Engl J Med. 2019;381(24):2293–303. https://doi.org/10.1056/NEJMoa1910993.
Norton A, Bucher A, Antonio E, Advani N, Grund H, Mburu S, et al. A living mapping review for COVID-19 funded research projects: three-month update. Wellcome Open Res. 2021;5:209. https://doi.org/10.12688/wellcomeopenres.16259.2.
Nuffield Council on Bioethics. Research in global health emergencies: ethical issues. Oxford: Nuffield Council on Bioethics; 2020.
Our World in Data. Coronavirus (COVID-19) vaccinations. Oxford: Our World in Data; 2022. https://ourworldindata.org/covid-vaccinations. Accessed 20 May 2022.
Partnerships for African Vaccine Manufacturing. Partnerships for African vaccine manufacturing (PAVM): framework for action. Addis Ababa: Partnerships for African Vaccine Manufacturing; 2022.
Peeling RW, Murtagh M, Olliaro PL. Epidemic preparedness: why is there a need to accelerate the development of diagnostics? Lancet Infect Dis. 2019;19(5):e172–e8. https://doi.org/10.1016/s1473-3099(18)30594-2.
Petryna A. Clinical trials offshored: on private sector science and public health. BioSocieties. 2007;2(1):21–40. https://doi.org/10.1017/s1745855207005030.
Ritchie H, Mathieu E, Rodés-Guirao L, Appel C, Giattino C, Ortiz-Ospina E, et al. Coronavirus pandemic (COVID-19). Oxford: Our World in Data; 2022. https://ourworldindata.org/coronavirus. Accessed 26 Aug 2022.
Robertson JS, Nicolson C, Harvey R, Johnson R, Major D, Guilfoyle K, et al. The development of vaccine viruses against pandemic A(H1N1) influenza. Vaccine. 2011;29(9):1836–43. https://doi.org/10.1016/j.vaccine.2010.12.044.
Rose S, Estes J. Creating effective research-policy partnerships for COVID response and beyond. Center for Global Development talks. Washington, DC: Center for Global Development; 2021.
Song Z, Xu Y, Bao L, Zhang L, Yu P, Qu Y, et al. From SARS to MERS, thrusting coronaviruses into the

spotlight. Viruses. 2019;11(1) https://doi.org/10.3390/v11010059.

Stockman LJ, Bellamy R, Garner P. SARS: systematic review of treatment effects. PLoS Med. 2006;3(9):e343. https://doi.org/10.1371/journal.pmed.0030343.

TGHN. Zika consortia. The Global Health Network; 2022. https://zikainfection.tghn.org/zika-consortia/. Accessed 25 Aug 2022.

UKCDR, GloPID-R. COVID-19 research project tracker. London: UK Collaborative on Development Research; 2022. https://www.ukcdr.org.uk/covid-circle/covid-19-research-project-tracker/. Accessed 25 Aug 2022.

UNDP. Capacity assessment and development in systems and strategic management context. New York: UN Development Programme. Management Development and Governance Division BfDP; 1998. Report No.: Technical Advisory Paper No. 3, Contract No.: Technical Advisory Paper No. 3.

Ward CL, Shaw D, Anane-Sarpong E, Sankoh O, Tanner M, Elger B. The ethics of health care delivery in a pediatric malaria vaccine trial: the perspectives of stakeholders from Ghana and Tanzania. J Empir Res Hum Res Ethics. 2017;13(1):26–41. https://doi.org/10.1177/1556264617742236.

Ward CL, Shaw D, Sprumont D, Sankoh O, Tanner M, Elger B. Good collaborative practice: reforming capacity building governance of international health research partnerships. Global Health. 2018;14(1):1. https://doi.org/10.1186/s12992-017-0319-4.

WHO. Ethical issues related to study design for trials on therapeutics for Ebola virus disease: WHO Ethics Working Group meeting 20–21 October, summary of discussion. Geneva: World Health Organization; 2014a. Contract No.: WHO/HIS/KER/GHE/14.2.

WHO. Statement on the 1st meeting of the IHR Emergency Committee on the 2014 Ebola outbreak in West Africa. Geneva: World Health Organization; 2014b.

WHO. Good participatory practice guidelines for trials of emerging (and re-emerging) pathogens that are likely to cause severe outbreaks in the near future and for which few or no medical countermeasures exist (GPP-EP). Geneva: World Health Organization; 2016a. p. 53.

WHO. Guidance for managing ethical issues in infectious disease outbreaks. Geneva: World Health Organization; 2016b.

WHO. WHO statement on the first meeting of the International Health Regulations (2005) (IHR 2005) Emergency Committee on Zika virus and observed increase in neurological disorders and neonatal malformations. Geneva: World Health Organization; 2016c.

WHO. Consultation on monitored emergency use of unregistered and investigational interventions (MEURI) for Ebola virus disease (EVD). Geneva: World Health Organization; 2018. Contract No.: 25 Aug.

WHO. About the R&D blueprint. Geneva: World Health Organization; 2020a. https://www.who.int/blueprint/about/en/. Accessed 19 Aug 2022.

WHO. A coordinated global research roadmap: 2019 novel coronavirus. Geneva: World Health Organization; 2020b.

WHO. Ethical standards for research during public health emergencies: distilling existing guidance to support COVID-19 R&D. Geneva: World Health Organization. COVID-19 WWGoE; 2020c. Contract No.: WHO reference number: WHO/RFH/20.1.

WHO. Guidance for research ethics committees for rapid review of research during public health emergencies. Geneva: World Health Organization; 2020d.

WHO. Prioritizing diseases for research and development in emergency contexts. Geneva: World Health Organization; 2020e. https://www.who.int/activities/prioritizing-diseases-for-research-and-development-in-emergency-contexts. Accessed 9 Dec 2020.

WHO. R&D blueprint and COVID-19. Geneva: World Health Organization; 2020f. https://www.who.int/teams/blueprint/covid-19. Accessed 30 Aug 2022.

WHO. Call for expression of interest to: contribute to the establishment of a COVID-19 mRNA vaccine technology transfer hub. 2021.

WHO. COVAX calls for urgent action to close vaccine equity gap. Geneva: World Health Organization; 2022a.

WHO. COVID-19 vaccine tracker and landscape. Geneva: World Health Organization; 2022b. https://www.who.int/publications/m/item/draft-landscape-of-covid-19-candidate-vaccines. Accessed 25 Aug 2022.

WHO. COVID-19: global literature on coronavirus disease. Geneva: World Health Organization; 2022c. https://search.bvsalud.org/global-literature-on-novel-coronavirus-2019-ncov/. Accessed 25 Aug 2022.

WHO. Global research on coronavirus disease (COVID-19). Geneva: World Health Organization; 2022d. https://www.who.int/emergencies/diseases/novel-coronavirus-2019/global-research-on-novel-coronavirus-2019-ncov. Accessed 26 Aug 2022.

WHO. The mRNA vaccine technology transfer hub. Geneva: World Health Organization; 2022e. https://www.who.int/initiatives/the-mrna-vaccine-technology-transfer-hub#:~:text=The%20mRNA%20vaccine%20technology%20transfer%20hub&text=Announced%20on%2021%20June%202021,the%20mRNA%20vaccine%20technology%20hub. Accessed 13 Dec 2022.

WHO Solidarity Trial Consortium. Repurposed antiviral drugs for Covid-19—interim WHO Solidarity trial results. N Engl J Med. 2021;384(6):497–511. https://doi.org/10.1056/NEJMoa2023184.

WHO Solidarity Trial Consortium. Remdesivir and three other drugs for hospitalised patients with COVID-19: final results of the WHO Solidarity ran-

domised trial and updated meta-analyses. Lancet. 2022;399(10339):1941–53. https://doi.org/10.1016/S0140-6736(22)00519-0.
Wholley D. ACTIV: a U.S. public-private partnership responds to COVID-19. 2024.
Yozwiak NL, Happi CT, Grant DS, Schieffelin JS, Garry RF, Sabeti PC, et al. Roots, not parachutes: research collaborations combat outbreaks. Cell. 2016;166(1):5–8. https://doi.org/10.1016/j.cell.2016.06.029.

30.1 In Focus: Research and Medical Humanitarian NGOs

Rebecca F. Grais and Emmanuel Baron

Contents

Learning Track Note: This chapter appears in Learning Tracks: Global Health; Health Policy, Multilateral Cooperation, International Governance; Preparedness

E. S. Higgs and R. A. Sorenson (eds.), *Principles and Practice of Emergency Research Response*,
https://doi.org/10.1007/978-3-031-48408-7_44

Learning Objectives

This chapter will help readers understand and describe:

- How an infectious diseases emergency should be defined.
- The fundamentals of the Epicentre model and how it compares to academic, private sector, and government models.
- Some assumptions people make about what medical issues matter.

1 Why Epicentre?

Medical humanitarian non-governmental organizations (NGOs), among which Médecins Sans Frontières (MSF) is perhaps the best known, aim primarily to provide medical care to populations affected by conflict or disaster or for whom access to care is absent or limited. MSF often operates in emergency and disaster situations and has developed medical, logistics, and financial systems to respond quickly and effectively, meaning that MSF is among the first organizations to provide a medical response. Along with care provision, advocacy for patients and populations is a core component of MSF's mission. It has become increasingly accepted that clinical research is an integral part of emergency response to any pathogen for which there are inadequate medical countermeasures (MCMs) (London 2018; CIOMS 2016). Balancing the immediate provision of vital medical care with the need to contribute to research for the development of effective therapies and vaccines is not a simple task, either ethically or logistically. What, for example, is the ethical responsibility of medical humanitarian responders to contribute to research on MCMs that may only be useful in future outbreaks? How can MSF and other first-response organizations most effectively achieve what appear to be the separate and possibly incompatible goals of ending an outbreak and developing countermeasures that may not be ready for use until after the outbreak has ended? We do not have ready answers to all these questions, and indeed many will have to be answered case by case, based on our experience, the pathogen, the population affected, the resources available, and many other aspects of each event (◘ Fig. 1).

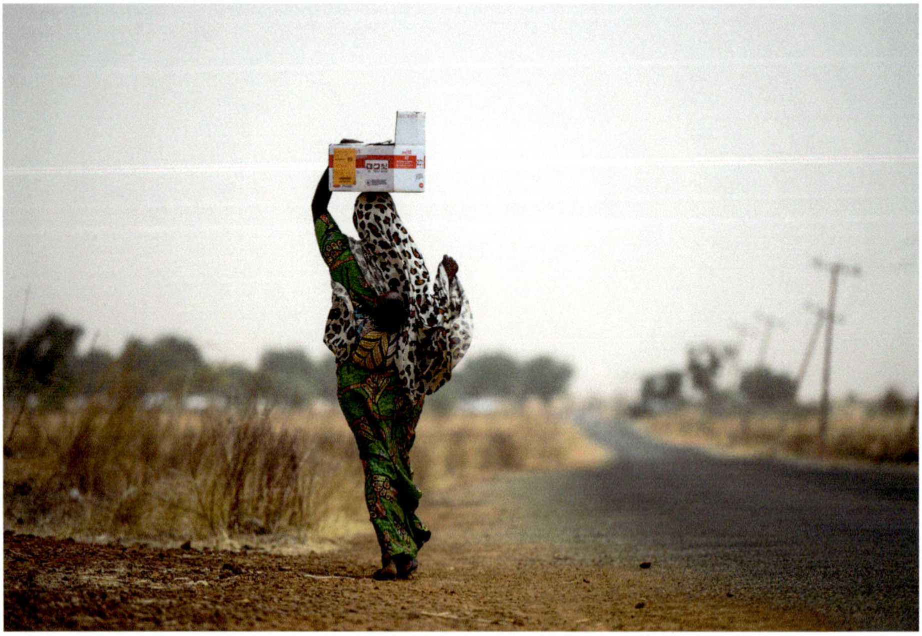

◘ **Fig. 1** A woman with her malnourished child, near Sokoto, Nigeria, enrolled in a trial comparing different treatment distribution strategies. (Photo: Taylor Glenn)

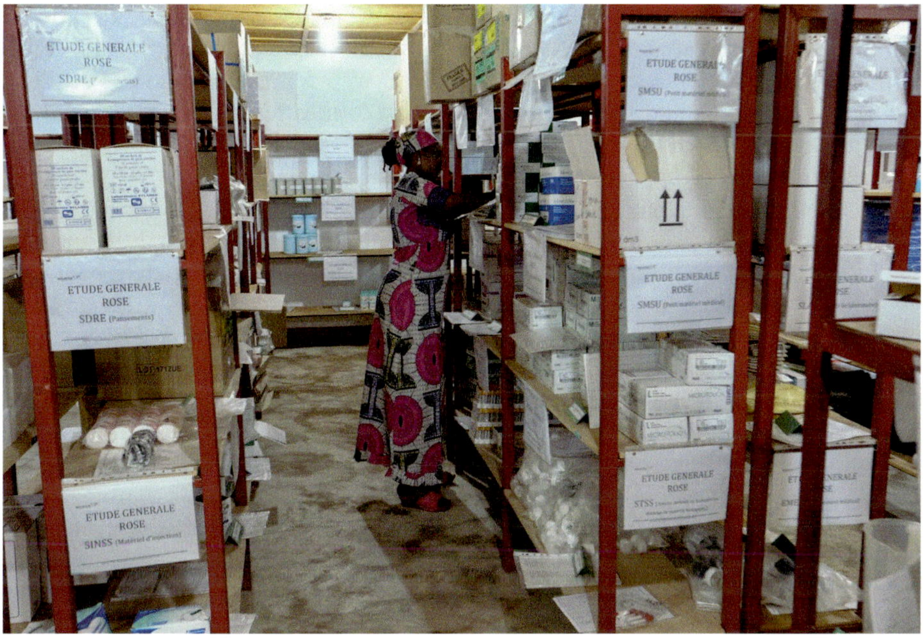

Fig. 2 Epicentre pharmacist supporting a clinical trial on a heat-stable rotavirus vaccine in Maradi, Niger. (Photo: Eric Bouvet)

Health research, whether basic, translational, clinical, field, operational, or applied, has not been a primary function of humanitarian NGOs. In the case of MSF, for example, with its primary focus on care provision, our satellite (spinoff) organization known as Epicentre, adhering to the same core principles as MSF but with a focus on research, was created in 1986. Epicentre was the first group of its kind, established within MSF, but with a distinct governance structure to preserve the distinction between care provision and research. Although there has been renewed Western scientific and media attention and interest in conducting emergency epidemic research, Epicentre and many other actors in low-income countries have implemented research for many decades, if not more. Here, we describe Epicentre as an alternative model to the academic, private business, and governmental approach to medical research in emergencies (Fig. 2).

2 What Is an Emergency?

Emergency response research during an outbreak can have different meanings to different actors (▶ Chap. 16). Depending on their background, culture, education, responsibilities, and interests, actors may have differing medical, epidemiological, social, and political perspectives, with varying degrees of appreciation for a larger picture. Today, there are over 70 million forcibly displaced persons and about 1 billion people living in about 40 different fragile states—many of them living in a permanent state of vulnerability (UNHCR 2020; World Bank 2020). Billions more live in a greater or lesser degree of poverty. Social vulnerability generally means vulnerability to disease as well, setting the stage for outbreaks and other infectious disease events that may receive little international or even national attention, with several important implications (WHO 2021) (▶ Chaps. 5 and 16). Four different meanings of "emergency" have implications for inclusion of research response.

First, emergencies are perceived as exceptional, unexpected events that serve as a trigger for international mobilization, but how emergencies are defined and declared varies greatly. In a country like Niger, where rigorous research has been successfully conducted for many years, there has been little international interest in outbreaks of meningitis, cholera, measles, or Rift Valley fever. Though the population considers some of these events emergencies and research is conducted to find new solutions to medical problems, results are rarely applied to emergencies in other locations. This is a failure in generalizing research results when they do not catch the attention of high-income countries.

Second, until recently, pivotal phase II or III trials of a novel vaccine, drug, or diagnostic test during an emergency have been relatively rare and even more so among vulnerable populations. The design and implementation of trials during an epidemic may be more complex as well as more urgent than comparable trials in high-income countries (► Chap. 22 and In Focus 22.1). For example, while exclusion of participants suffering from malnutrition may be routine, malnutrition is prevalent in many contexts where disease outbreaks occur, and understanding the effects of investigational products in malnourished patients may be essential for future use. Other criteria, such as access to high-quality care, may not be applicable, especially if an already poorly resourced health system is under stress. Much of the research done in outbreaks in the past has been for the purpose of evaluating an alternative care delivery strategy or therapeutic regimen, rather than for the purpose of generating evidence to inform licensure of a novel medical countermeasure.

Third, research in emergencies is often aimed at a new or reemerging threat where there is a lack of existing medical countermeasures. The emergency-focused approach often overshadows well-known, high-burden diseases such as cholera or measles, both of which can lead to large-scale epidemics, as recently seen in the Democratic Republic of the Congo (DRC) and Yemen. In 2019, international media coverage of the DRC Ebola outbreak far exceeded that of the concurrent measles epidemic there, even as deaths attributable to measles far exceeded the number of cases of Ebola (Ducomble and Gignoux 2020). The emergence of drug-resistant tuberculosis and delays in polio eradication have likewise received relatively little media coverage. Infectious diseases that could directly threaten high-income countries, or which may be potential weapons of bioterrorism, arouse greater interest in wealthy countries (Hoffman and Silverberg 2018).

Fourth, working through governmental channels has some limitations. Decisions to allocate resources to an outbreak response can be conditioned on geographical, historical, or geopolitical considerations. The responses to outbreaks of Ebola in West and Central Africa, for example, have in large part followed historical and linguistic ties. Funding by rich countries, when needed for a robust outbreak response in low-income countries, is often contingent on high-level political will. And while governments can provide unparalleled resources if the will is there, they can also be perceived as supporting unstable or illegitimate governments, whatever their intentions. Medical response workers during recent Ebola outbreaks in the DRC, for example, came under attack from local people who perceived them as part of a distrusted authority structure (Kraemer et al. 2020; Dyer 2019).

3 A Different Model for Research in Health Emergencies

Epicentre was created in 1986 by MSF to support epidemiology and research within the daily medical care programs of MSF. Epicentre's structural and organizational model ensures a constant, direct connection between MSF clinicians and research teams, whose engagement in public health events ensures that research is not ad hoc but a matter of course.

For practitioners, this provides a direct channel to describe their difficulties and translate them into research questions. This can lead, for example, to evaluation of different means to treat and follow up HIV-infected patients in high-incidence rural areas, the best ways to use imprecise diagnostic tests to diagnose tuberculosis, and measures to improve oral vaccine performance in infants in sub-Saharan Africa. Moreover, practitioners in situations where access to information and the time to absorb it are limited can turn to Epicentre personnel to keep up to date on recent scientific advances, thus improving care through the application of new knowledge.

Epicentre provides a research model different from an academic or governmental model. At its creation, MSF made a strategic choice to ensure core funding for Epicentre via its own fundraising. This means that from project inception to dissemination of results and translation of results into access, Epicentre focuses more on the research question and less on the career and publication requirements of academia or the budget cycle and political constraints that may come with government funding. Epicentre may also be able to provide longer-term opportunities for research staff from low-resource countries, who may otherwise have no access to dependable academic or governmental institutions to pursue a career in research. Today, the financial commitment from MSF remains, but Epicentre also receives additional research-specific funds for specific studies, professional development, and laboratory infrastructure to keep pace with evolving research methods (◘ Fig. 3).

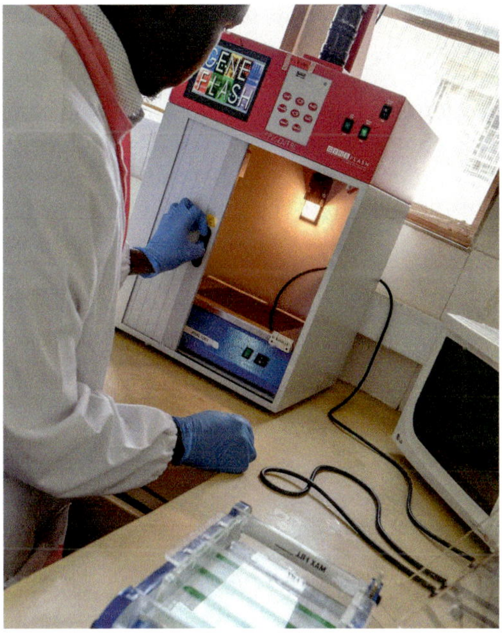

◘ **Fig. 3** Laboratory staff performing PCR for anti-malarial resistance in a drug efficacy trial in Mbarara, Uganda. (Photo: Eric Bouvet)

There have been times when humanitarian medical responders have seen the arrival of researchers planning a clinical trial as detrimental to their goal of saving as many lives as possible (Dunning et al. 2016). Others have questioned the ethics of placebo-controlled trials during a high-mortality outbreak (Adebamowo et al. 2014). But the justification for urgent research, including clinical trials, during high-mortality emergencies in low-income countries is exemplified by the licensure of vaccines and therapies for Ebola following clinical trials in West Africa and then the DRC (FDA 2019, 2020), to say nothing of the rapid development of vaccines during the coronavirus disease 2019 (COVID-19) pandemic. Measures to improve readiness for such research in the event of an epidemic or pandemic have become a standard feature of preparedness planning (Gobat et al. 2019) (▶ Chap. 26). Epicentre, as a long-standing epidemiology and research body with a deep understanding of emergency infectious disease response, is well placed to facilitate potentially useful research in an emergency.

Moreover, the development and widespread availability of new medical tools can too often rely heavily on business interests rather than on population needs. Since Epicentre remains largely independent from influential donors, it can provide a platform to advocate for research needs that lack a market incentive. Partnerships and contributions to multicenter trials add expertise and opportunities to expand the portfolio as well.

The Epicentre model also has its limitations. Research scientists may find this approach unfamiliar. Epicentre is not quite a Western organization or a low-income country NGO. Compensation is deliberately low by Western standards, and all staff members, irrespective of their origins, travel and work routinely in insecure settings, which provide unique opportunities but also come with inherent risk. Epicentre challenges the conventional model of research institutions in rich countries providing funding and oversight to implementing partners in poor ones. This may be an oversimplification, especially since research partnerships of all kinds have been changing in recent years, but it provides an idea as to how Epicentre sees its role.

4 Some Lessons Learned

First, security and economic threats at a global scale, or the perception thereof, must not remain the sole drivers of international mobilization for research in emergencies. With ad hoc mobilization and intermittent assistance, the needs of populations and the need to develop medical countermeasures for diseases of epidemic potential often remain unanswered. Medical NGOs provide critical support in many situations, and MSF had the foresight to ensure that research could be integrated into this support. Second, including local actors in the response to epidemics as equals has not always been a priority, but it is now generally accepted that community involvement in framing research is neither optional nor a mere formality (▶ Chap. 18). Practical difficulties, like English-language dominance and working habits based on Anglo-Saxon culture, can stand in the way. Even aside from language barriers, this can lead to de facto exclusion or junior status for some partners, due to their lack of experience of international cooperation. Without full partnership, however, both the benefits and the beneficiaries of research may be limited, and an extra effort to include partners who lack experience is essential (▶ Chap. 30).

Third, research needs, study design, and implementation can vary depending upon epidemiological, social, economic, and political contexts, among other factors. The future seems especially difficult to predict at this historical moment, and diverse experiences in emergency response research create a broader set of options that can be applied in uncharted terrain. Existing guidelines for good practices are useful in familiar situations, and increasing recognition of the importance of coping with emergencies has sparked several efforts to produce corresponding guidance (CIOMS 2021; IASC 2019; Nuffield Council on Bioethics 2020; WHO 2020a, b). Nevertheless, adapting to changing realities and new methods requires a more substantial set of skills. While many of them are described in this volume, with an effort to elucidate both principles and practice, making good decisions in complex situations with a high degree of uncertainty is a skill that requires experience, education, and training. It is a problem without any simple solutions, like those we face repeatedly in every emergency research response.

? Discussion Questions

1. Who and what do you think determines which research questions are addressed?
2. What is different about the Epicentre model, compared to an academic, private sector, or governmental model?
3. How do you think an emergency should be defined?
4. What assumptions are made about what medical problems matter?

References

Adebamowo C, Bah-Sow O, Binka F, Bruzzone R, Caplan A, Delfraissy J-F, et al. Randomised controlled trials for Ebola: practical and ethical issues. Lancet. 2014;384(9952):1423–4. https://doi.org/10.1016/S0140-6736(14)61734-7.

CIOMS. International ethical guidelines for health-related research involving humans. Geneva: Council for International Organisations of Medical Sciences; 2016.

CIOMS. Clinical research in resource-limited settings. A consensus by a CIOMS Working Group. Geneva: Council for International Organizations of Medical Sciences (CIOMS); 2021.

Ducomble T, Gignoux E. Learning from a massive epidemic: measles in DRC. Lancet Infectious Diseases. 2020;20(5):542.

Dunning J, Longuet C, Salam A. Ebola research: an encounter between science and humanitarian action. Alternatives Humanitaires—Humanitarian Alternatives; 2016.

Dyer O. MSF suspends Congo Ebola effort after deadly clinic attacks. BMJ. 2019;364:l1010. https://doi.org/10.1136/bmj.l1010.

FDA. First FDA-approved vaccine for the prevention of Ebola virus disease, marking a critical milestone in public health preparedness and response. Washington, DC: U.S. Food and Drug Administration; 2019.

FDA. FDA approves treatment for Ebola virus. Washington, DC: U.S. Food and Drug Administration; 2020.

Gobat N, Amuasi J, Yazdanpanah Y, Sigfrid L, Davies H, Byrne J-P, et al. Advancing preparedness for clinical research during infectious disease epidemics. Eur Respir J Open. 2019:5. https://doi.org/10.1183/23120541.00227-2018.

Hoffman SJ, Silverberg SL. Delays in global disease outbreak responses: lessons from H1N1, Ebola, and Zika. Am J Public Health. 2018;108(3):329–33. https://doi.org/10.2105/ajph.2017.304245.

IASC. Humanitarian system-wide scale-up activation protocol for the control of infectious disease events. Geneva: Inter-Agency Standing Committee; 2019.

Kraemer MUG, Pigott DM, Hill SC, Vanderslott S, Reiner RC Jr, Stasse S, et al. Dynamics of conflict during the Ebola outbreak in the Democratic Republic of the Congo 2018–2019. BMC Med. 2020;18(1):113. https://doi.org/10.1186/s12916-020-01574-1.

London AJ. Social value, clinical equipoise, and research in a public health emergency. Bioethics. 2018;33(3):326–34. https://doi.org/10.1111/bioe.12467.

Nuffield Council on Bioethics. Research in global health emergencies: ethical issues. Oxford: Nuffield Council on Bioethics; 2020.

UNHCR. Figures at a glance. Geneva: UNHCR, The UN Refugee Agency; 2020. https://www.unhcr.org/en-us/figures-at-a-glance.html. Accessed 1 Mar 2020.

WHO. Ethical standards for research during public health emergencies: distilling existing guidance to support COVID-19 R&D. Geneva: World Health Organization. COVID-19 WWGoE; 2020a. Contract No.: WHO reference number: WHO/RFH/20.1.

WHO. Good Participatory Practice for COVID-19 clinical trials—a toolbox. Geneva: World Health Organization; 2020b.

WHO. Social determinants of health. In: Health topics. 2021. https://www.who.int/health-topics/social-determinants-of-health#tab=tab_1. Accessed 18 Jul 2021.

World Bank. Classification of fragile and conflict-affected situations. Washington, DC: World Bank Group; 2020. Accessed 1 Mar 2020.

30.2 In Practice: Building and Maintaining Preparedness for a Rapid Research Response in Indonesia

Chuen-Yen Lau, Louis Grue, Aaron Neal, and Muhammad Karyana

Contents

Learning Track Note: This chapter appears in Learning Tracks: Global Health; Health Policy, Multilateral Cooperation, International Governance

E. S. Higgs and R. A. Sorenson (eds.), *Principles and Practice of Emergency Research Response*,
https://doi.org/10.1007/978-3-031-48408-7_45

Learning Objectives

This chapter will help readers understand and describe:

- The value of standing research partnerships, drawing on the example of INA-RESPOND activities during the COVID-19 pandemic
- How research partnerships such as INA-RESPOND are established and maintained
- Essential elements for sustainable international research networks

1 Introduction

Establishing research capacity in sentinel areas where zoonotic diseases are most likely to jump to humans is crucial for the early detection of emerging pathogens and public health emergency preparedness (▶ Chaps. 8 and 10) (Salyer et al. 2017). Improving research capacity strengthens health systems and ensures that in-country partnerships and institutions are already in place to build upon when an emerging infectious disease requires an urgent research response. When trained research staff and functioning laboratories are supporting established research sites, researchers can write study protocols more quickly, adapt them to specific conditions with their local partners, and implement them through tested infrastructure. Such capacity building cannot be performed once and then left dormant. Ongoing research, focused on pathogens of local and international public health priority, is needed for personnel to remain trained and for infrastructure to remain ready (◘ Fig. 1).

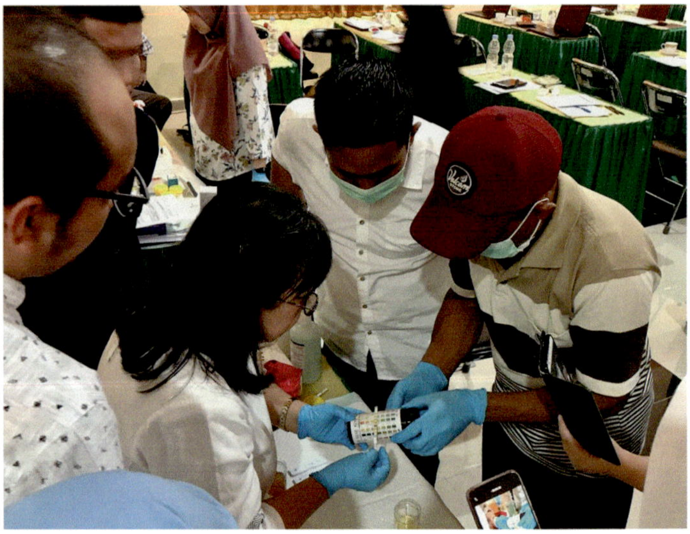

◘ **Fig. 1** INA-RESPOND laboratory staff demonstrating dipstick urinalysis during a clinical study training session in Central Sulawesi, Indonesia. (Photo: Aaron Neal)

2 The Indonesia Research Partnership on Infectious Diseases

Through the Indonesia Research Partnership on Infectious Diseases (INA-RESPOND), U.S. and Indonesian governments collaboratively conduct scientific studies and maintain a nationwide clinical research network in readiness. The partnership is a joint venture of the Indonesia Ministry of Health (MOH) and the National Institute of Allergy and Infectious Diseases (NIAID) of the U.S. National Institutes of Health (NIH). Following a long history of scientific cooperation between Indonesia and the United States, INA-RESPOND was formally established in 2010 through the signing of a bilateral Agreement on Scientific Cooperation and an official visit to the NIH campus in Bethesda, Maryland, by the Minister of Health of Indonesia (INA-RESPOND 2022). Today, INA-RESPOND conducts observational and interventional clinical research consistent with MOH priorities, laying the groundwork for evidence-based public health policy decisions and building sustainable research capacity in Indonesia. Network staff publish and present findings that ultimately affect treatment, diagnosis guidelines, and health policy for Indonesia. One example includes an INA-RESPOND study on patients hospitalized with an acute febrile illness of unknown origin, which found an unexpected burden of undiagnosed rickettsiosis and led the MOH to issue a policy brief to increase awareness and promote approaches that would improve diagnosis and reduce misdiagnosis during hospitalization, since rickettsiosis had often been misdiagnosed. The study also produced (◘ Fig. 2) several peer-reviewed papers (Lokida et al. 2020).

INA-RESPOND works under the governance of a central steering committee comprising representatives from Indonesian and U.S. governments, network hospitals, and other stakeholders. All activities across the network of 20 sites are coordinated centrally by a secretariat located at the MOH in Jakarta. The secretariat has developed and houses expertise in research site development and management, monitoring, protocol development and implementation, financial oversight, regulatory support, agreements and contracts, data management, data analysis, and dissemination of results. Network staff coordinate closely with the MOH, NIAID, the academic and hospital sites that compose the network, and RSU Kabupaten Tangerang, a district hospital west of Jakarta that houses the INA-RESPOND central reference laboratory. These bodies support ongoing research that maintains network capacity between outbreaks, provides ongoing staff training and opportunities for potential partners, and develops and tests laboratory capacity so that detection, diagnosis, and emergency response capacity continually improve. Unlike the individual grant- or project-centered model of research collaboration typically seen in the academic research community, INA-RESPOND is sustained at a fundamental level by its government partners. This means that when a particular project ends, the partnership persists and moves on to the next research area of interest as it remains ready to respond to an outbreak or epidemic.

With over 10 years of capacity building and clinical research experience, INA-RESPOND was well prepared to serve as a critical element of the Indonesian MOH's national COVID-19 response when the virus was first detected in the country on March 2, 2020. Prior to the first identified case, INA-RESPOND reference laboratory staff were able to secure scarce, experimental diagnostic reagents through the Network's partnership with NIAID. This allowed the lab to immediately begin testing suspected cases and serve as the central testing authority for Banten province and its population of approximately 13.16 million. As COVID-19 spread, the MOH relied on INA-RESPOND to assess policies on serological diagnostic tests, validate neutralizing antibody assays, and coordinate international research study activities, including for the WHO Solidarity Trial in Indonesia. At the same time, INA-RESPOND worked with existing partners at NIAID and the International Network for Strategic Initiatives in Global HIV Trials (INSIGHT) to implement multi-site COVID-19 observa-

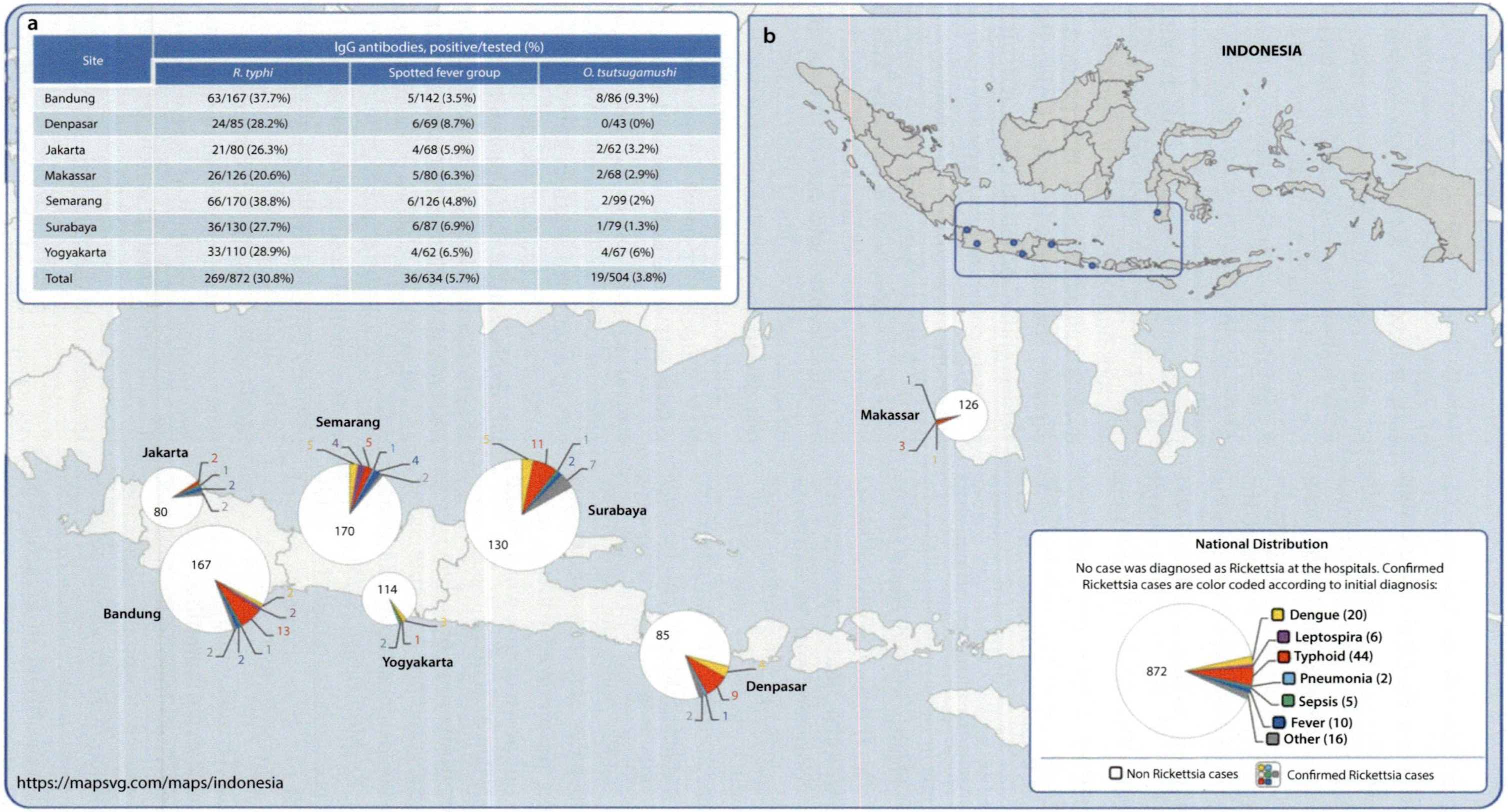

Site	IgG antibodies, positive/tested (%)		
	R. typhi	Spotted fever group	*O. tsutsugamushi*
Bandung	63/167 (37.7%)	5/142 (3.5%)	8/86 (9.3%)
Denpasar	24/85 (28.2%)	6/69 (8.7%)	0/43 (0%)
Jakarta	21/80 (26.3%)	4/68 (5.9%)	2/62 (3.2%)
Makassar	26/126 (20.6%)	5/80 (6.3%)	2/68 (2.9%)
Semarang	66/170 (38.8%)	6/126 (4.8%)	2/99 (2%)
Surabaya	36/130 (27.7%)	6/87 (6.9%)	1/79 (1.3%)
Yogyakarta	33/110 (28.9%)	4/62 (6.5%)	4/67 (6%)
Total	269/872 (30.8%)	36/634 (5.7%)	19/504 (3.8%)

Fig. 2 Map and figures from Lokida et al. (2020) showing misdiagnosed cases of rickettsiosis at eight tertiary hospitals in Indonesia and distribution. **a** Prevalence of IgG antibodies to *R. typhi*, spotted fever group, and *O. tsutsugamushi* (positive IgG/subject tested). **b** Geographical distribution of acute rickettsia cases in AFIRE study. (Mapfree source MapSVG)

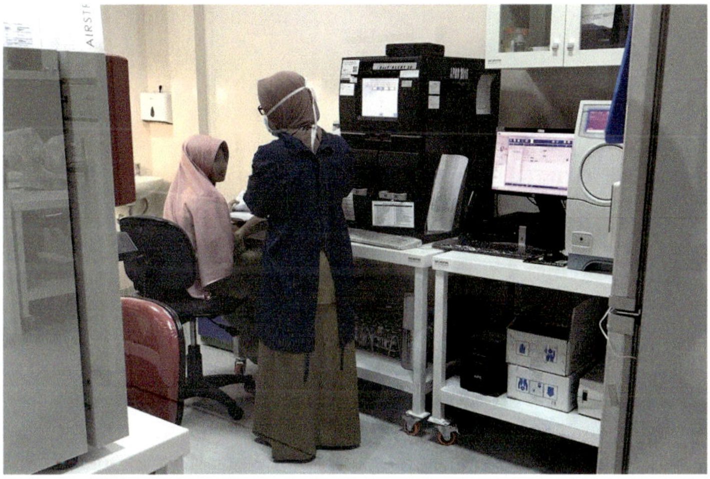

Fig. 3 Laboratory capacity built at RSU Kabupaten Tangerang through the INA-RESPOND partnership. (Photo: Chuen-Yen Lau)

tional and interventional studies, including a double-blind randomized controlled trial of hyperimmune intravenous immunoglobulin in patients hospitalized with COVID-19 (INA-RESPOND 2022). In every case, the ability of INA-RESPOND to substantially enhance Indonesia's response to COVID-19 was the direct product of long-term, sustained research capacity building (Fig. 3).

3 Essential Elements for a Stable International Research Network

Our experience in Indonesia highlights several essential elements for a stable international research network. A formal agreement between sponsoring governments imparts authority and credibility, as well as ensuring that officials responsible for funding decisions, necessary permits, and authorizations will be engaged. This was essential in the rapid response to COVID-19, where import permits, regulatory permits, and formal review processes were expedited. Involving high-level stakeholders also permits direct and sanctioned access to the most relevant institutions for conducting research. Clinical trials targeting specific populations, directed specimen collection efforts from at-risk communities, or surveillance activities focused on specific disease areas require access to hospitals, clinics, and field sites that may be otherwise inaccessible to non-government entities, like foreign academic researchers. A relationship at the government-to-government level supports clear communication channels between institutional leaders in both nations, allowing research results, experiences, and scientific or clinical guidance to be disseminated rapidly to public health decision-makers. In any arrangement, both partner countries must benefit: the host country gains the benefit of improved infrastructure for research, clinical care, and health policy guidance, while the external partner benefits from refined prevention strategies to keep an epidemic from spreading globally or at least mitigating the impact if it does spread. Bilateral investment gives both sides a sense of ownership.

Strong relationships built on trust, transparency, and honest give-and-take compromises make it easier to manage challenges or conflicts, such as cultural differences, funding shortfalls, political changes, or an emergency response to a new outbreak. A history of NIAID and Indonesian MOH personnel working side by side builds collaboration and relationships to support a coordinated emergency research response in case of need, facilitating development of medical countermeasures like vaccines and therapeutics for the partners and ultimately the world. This could not be more apparent during the COVID-19 pandemic, where the years of relationship and trust building that had gone into INA-RESPOND were able to sustain the partnership during times of significant uncertainty, immense pressure, and long-distance engagement.

Should an emerging infection be detected, INA-RESPOND would collect clinical information and analyze related specimens through an active general infectious disease research protocol. Protocols and sub-studies to examine specific aspects of the outbreak could be rapidly developed and initiated, as was the case with COVID-19. INA-RESPOND's already active general surveillance protocol ORCHID, which was designed to be both comprehensive and flexible, was immediately repurposed to target suspected COVID-19 cases. Ongoing studies on febrile illnesses, tuberculosis, HIV, parasitic diseases, and pediatric pneumonia ensure that the necessary personnel, infrastructure, and relationships are functioning. In the course of a research response, partners would start with their existing roles in the network and tailor their work to the disease at hand. Ongoing partnerships can help prevent impeded responses due to differences between nation states over intellectual property rights or data ownership. Pathogens are unaffected by borders, but responses can be hindered by legal and political obstacles to sharing samples and data.

4 Conclusion

We expect INA-RESPOND to continue over the long term and expand by bringing in additional partners. The network has already undertaken collaborations with the Kirby Institute at the University of New South Wales on options for treatment of HIV. This growth, while directly beneficial for future HIV care in Indonesia, has helped move the network from hypothesis-generating observational studies to interventional studies in a natural, mentored way. The results from this study will provide data on the efficacy of antiretroviral drugs not yet licensed in Indonesia, potentially leading to licensure and improved access to lifesaving medications. During the COVID-19 pandemic, the existing capacity of the INA-RESPOND reference laboratory attracted interest from external groups, including scientists at Columbia University interested in collaborating on pathogen sequencing. Though the short-term focus of the collaboration is on immediate capacity building and identifying SARS-CoV-2 variants in Indonesia, the long-term vision is to include Indonesia in a global network of research sites focused on pathogen surveillance by sequencing.

Advanced development and maintenance of a research network, coupled with continuous enhancement of its research capacity, is a strategic approach to epidemic preparedness and response. It averts much of the chaos and wasted resources that come with trying to mount a rapid research response from nothing during an epidemic. Indonesia, with both middle-income and less developed areas, and INA-RESPOND can serve as a model for creating research capacity in more challenging environments (Karyana et al. 2021).

Discussion Questions

1. Discuss the advantages of pre-existing research partnerships.
2. How are research partnerships established and maintained?

References

INA-RESPOND. INA-RESPOND network's website. Jakarta: INA-RESPOND; 2022. https://ina--respond.net/. Accessed 14 Nov 2022.

Karyana M, Kosasih H, Neal AT, Lau CY. Maintaining international research collaborations in the setting of a pandemic: approach in Indonesia. J Glob Health. 2021;11:03087. https://doi.org/10.7189/jogh.11.03087.

Lokida D, Hadi U, Lau C-Y, Kosasih H, Liang CJ, Rusli M, et al. Underdiagnoses of Rickettsia in patients hospitalized with acute fever in Indonesia: observational study results. BMC Infect Dis. 2020;20(1):364. https://doi.org/10.1186/s12879-020-05057-9.

Salyer S, Silver R, Simone K, Behravesh CB. Prioritizing zoonoses for global health capacity building—themes from one health zoonotic disease workshops in 7 countries, 2014–2016. Emerg Infect Dis J. 2017;23(13):S55. https://doi.org/10.3201/eid2313.170418.

Research Operations

Laura A. McNay

Parts I–VI of this volume provide broad perspectives on the principles and practice of emergency research response. Part VII puts us on the ground, as it were, from the perspective of those facilitating and conducting emergency clinical research operations, both in the United States during the COVID-19 pandemic and in West and Central Africa during Ebola emergencies. Most of Part VII describes how research teams met the requirements for a scientifically and ethically sound clinical research program in low resource and sometimes insecure settings, describing some of the obstacles they had to overcome and providing future response teams with a sense of how the elements of high-quality clinical research can be brought together relatively quickly even when almost none are there to begin with.

Gregg Larson and coauthors (► Chap. 31) recount some of the obstacles they encountered during the urgent research response to the COVID-19 pandemic in the United States and advise on future preparedness measures. Larson and Laura McNay (► Chap. 32) bring their professional experience to bear on launching clinical research operations where there is little research capacity and meager healthcare infrastructure, setting the stage for the rest of Part VII. Larson (► In Focus 32.2) also provides a primer on insurance and liability, lack of which can delay or prevent essential research. Jerome Pierson begins ► Chap. 33 with the requirements for ethical review where existing research ethics committees may have limited capacity. Fatorma Bolay (► In Practice 33.1) narrates the strengthening of Liberian ethical review capacity during the Ebola emergency there. Susan Vogel and Pierson (► In Practice 33.2) explain how independent monitoring was ensured during the West Africa Ebola response. Barbara Sina and John Tierney (► In Practice 33.3) revisit capacity building, this time specifically for research ethics review.

Mike Galcik and David Parrish (► Chap. 34) delineate the essential information and communication technology requirements for a research response, along with workarounds when infrastructure leaves something to be desired. Laurie K. Doepel and Hassan Kiawu (► Case Study 32.1) discuss another aspect of communications and interactions with the press and broadcast media. Data management (► Chap. 35) is sometimes neglected but indispensable part of clinical research, as Harry van Loen and colleagues explain. Pharmacovigilance (► Chap. 36)—monitoring for unexpected or untoward adverse effects of an investigational medicine—ensures one of the two basic assessment goals of clinical research and safety; Marc Teitelbaum et al. explain the concept and provide recommendations for successfully managing pharmacovigilance in emergencies.

Logistical support for clinical research sites (► Chap. 37) can be problematic in countries with relatively few transport options, especially when some of them may be suspended during an infectious disease emergency. Beth Baseler et al. summarize the needs, including strong partnerships; export–import, transportation, supply, and equipment management; waste management; and in-country logistics staff. Introducing chapters with a more specific focus, Matt Kirchoff (► Chap. 38) describes what the pharmacy operation of a clinical research program needs and how to get one set up when supplies and equipment may have to come from another continent. Dan Littlefield (► Chap. 39) elucidates the cold chain required to get pharmaceuticals, especially investigational new drugs, from a producer to a remote clinical research site, and explains the electrical supply obstacles at some sites and how to address them.

Olivier Tshiani Mbaya et al. (► Chap. 40) describe site selection criteria, provide checklists for site activation, and lay out criteria to ensure that trial protocols can be implemented. Essential for both site selection and ongoing operations is a security assessment and appropriate security management, as explained by Billy Sivahera and colleagues (► Chap. 41). Finally, Beth Baseler et al. (► Chap. 42) provide an adaptable framework based on team communications, collaboration, partnership, and mutual respect for identifying, hiring, and training staff. The reader should complete this section with an even greater sense of the complexity of a clinical trial, especially when we consider many things taken for granted in developed countries, like clean water and power, fast internet, and an array of existing clinical trials sites and other medical infrastructure.

Contents

31 Operational Recommendations for Streamlining Emergency Research Responses to Pandemics

Gregg Larson, Rachel Harrigan, and Laura A. McNay

Contents

Learning Track Note: This chapter appears in Learning Tracks: Emergency Research Response, Research Operations; Health Policy, Multilateral Cooperation, International Governance

E. S. Higgs and R. A. Sorenson (eds.), *Principles and Practice of Emergency Research Response*, https://doi.org/10.1007/978-3-031-48408-7_46

Learning Objectives

This chapter will help readers understand and describe:

- Why a national or global research agenda is needed for optimal operational planning for clinical research in response to an infectious disease emergency.
- Operational disciplines essential for supporting clinical trials during an emergency research response.
- Factors facilitating the rapid design and implementation of the Randomised Evaluation of COVID-19 Therapy Trial (RECOVERY).
- Based on implementation and conduct of the ACTIV-3 research program, measures that can:
  - Accelerate the start of a research study
  - Expedite prudent clinical site selection and activation
  - Streamline compliance with regulatory requirements
  - Clarify and expedite essential agreements and documents
  - Simplify agreement on adequate research liability coverage
  - Establish beneficial pharmaceutical collaboration

1 Background

Experience with both the Ebola and coronavirus disease 2019 (COVID-19) responses recounted here may help researchers anticipate, avoid, and overcome barriers to research mobilization in future outbreaks. Operations in the research response to the Ebola outbreaks of 2014–2016 in West Africa and 2018–2020 in the Democratic Republic of the Congo (DRC) foreshadowed operations in the COVID-19 research response. The experience gained during the Ebola outbreaks in West Africa and the DRC was informative, and research conducted then helped win broad acceptance of clinical research as an integral part of emergency response to an infectious disease outbreak (NASEM 2017). The hope that safe and effective vaccines, therapeutics, and diagnostics (VTDs) could be developed in time for distribution during an emergency was realized during the COVID-19 pandemic. At the same time, implementing a vastly larger research response in high-income countries meant overcoming other obstacles associated with coordination of multiple countries and governments, clinical trial networks, and industry partners.

The massive resources directed to accelerated COVID-19 emergency response research in 2020 focused on the safety and efficacy of numerous VTDs. The effort was successful, yielding essential data for their authorization, approval, or a finding of little or no benefit. While it ultimately reduced pandemic morbidity and mortality, limited planning for accelerated research on such a scale hindered a rapid, coherent response. Moreover, COVID-19 adaptive platform trial designs added complexity not found in traditional Phase III clinical trials that compare a single intervention with a control arm. The response research demonstrated the need to prepare for VTD development, clinical assessment, and implementation while the world is not facing a pandemic emergency and to respond coherently from the moment a novel, re-emerging, or significant new variant of a pathogen with pandemic potential is identified. In a world where novel infectious disease outbreaks appear to be increasing, thanks in part to climate change and human encroachment on wildlife habitat, planning for a rapid research response must be an integral part of global health security preparedness (Bedford et al. 2019; Carter et al. 2021; Finlay et al. 2004; Goossens et al. 2022; Hashem et al. 2020; Lurie et al. 2013; NASEM 2017; Olliaro and Torreele 2022; Sigfrid et al. 2020).

Operational challenges and recommendations for future emergency research response are illustrated with examples from the Randomised Evaluation of COVID-19 Therapy (RECOVERY) study in the UK (▶ In Focus 14.1 and 15.1), the U.S.-based Accelerating COVID-19 Therapeutic Interventions and Vaccines (ACTIV) public-private partnership (Goossens et al. 2022; LaVange et al. 2021) (▶ Chap. 15), and the Strategies and Treatment for Regulatory and Viral Emergencies (STRIVE) protocol proposal developed by the International Network for Strategic Initiatives in Global HIV Trials (INSIGHT) for the ACTIV partnership (STRIVE 2023).

2 Key Operational Considerations

2.1 Planning During an Emergency

Despite early steps during the severe acute respiratory syndrome coronavirus (SARS-CoV, retronym SARS-CoV-1) outbreak in 2003–2004 and progress during the 2009 H1N1 influenza pandemic, clinical trials during the Ebola virus disease outbreaks from 2014 to 2020, and more than two decades of stepped-up efforts to prepare for a pandemic, the world was not ready for COVID-19. Recognition among scientists and health agencies that future pandemics were likely did not lead to effective preparedness planning for clinical research that could be implemented concurrently with development of clinical trial protocols or adaptation of advance protocols (Abelin et al. 2011; Angus et al. 2020; Hatchett et al. 2007; Madhav et al. 2017; Marston et al. 2017; Rojek and Horby 2016; WBG 2017).

During an emergency research response, rapid generation of a coordinated, rigorous national or global research agenda is needed as soon as possible to inform clinical trial designs and guide operational planning. The clinical research operational response needs to proceed in parallel with agenda and protocol development and should commence *as soon as a protocol concept is identified.* Delaying essential operational decisions because a protocol is not finalized sets the stage for a multitude of woes. The many factors involved in implementing a protocol require that planning and implementation go hand in hand. The typical, sequential cadence of clinical trial implementation, absent an emergency, is not sufficient. A quick start will mean more trial modifications as plans and protocols change, but this is an emergency cost that must be borne. In addition, prospective consideration of scientific and operational requirements will inform decisions about what is essential versus what can be elided during an emergency. Substantive ethical and scientific standards, however, must never be loosened or compromised (▶ Chap. 4) (◘ Fig. 1).

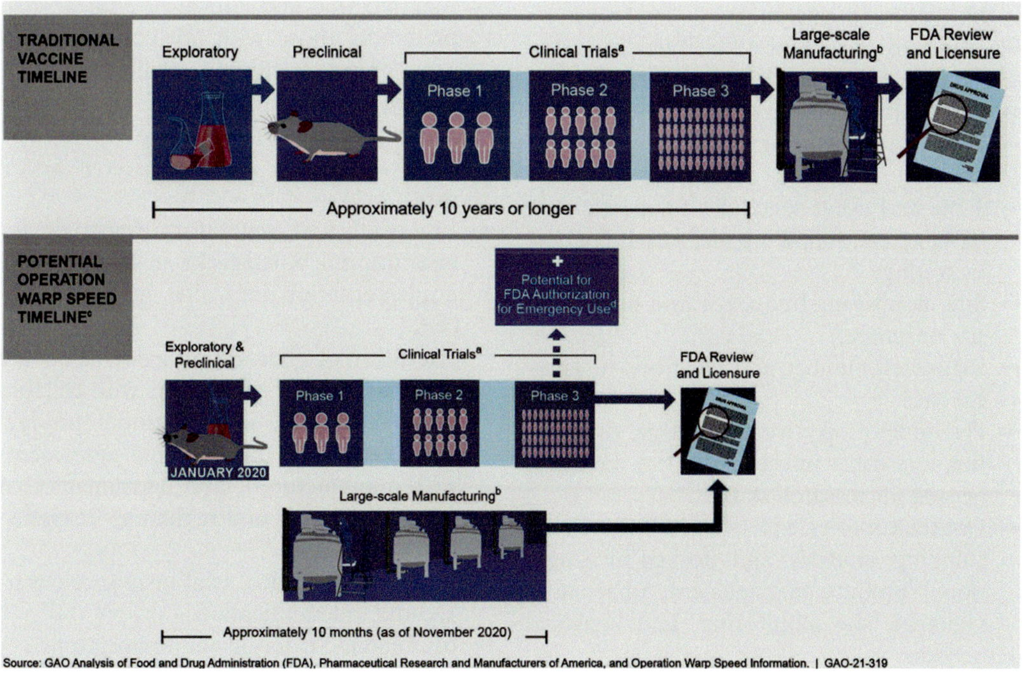

◘ **Fig. 1** Timeline of accelerated research response in Operation Warp Speed. (GAO 21-319, USG public domain)

2.2 Parallel Scientific and Operational Actions

Many activities must be conducted simultaneously to support the development and implementation of an emergency research program. The need for single, multiple, or platform trial design protocols will broadly determine the complexity of the research structure. Once protocol concepts receive approval, scientific and operational teams should begin to concurrently develop the actual protocol. Presumably, these teams will already have been assembled from the statistical, data management, and operations centers assigned responsibility for the emergency research response. Operations personnel should participate in scientific discussions to ensure that science and operational planning are synchronized as much as possible, and both should benefit from an understanding of each other's expectations and needs. The ground covered during these scientific discussions will be both broad and shifting as the protocol concept advances to a fully developed protocol. A list of likely scientific topics, while hardly exhaustive, follows. Operational aspects of many of these topics are also described in greater detail in this section of this book.

- Standard of care for all trial participants
- Investigational medicinal product(s)
- Trial participant recruitment targets
- Participant inclusion and exclusion criteria
- Time and event schedules for participant baseline and follow-up visits and diagnostic testing
- Site monitoring frequency and mode (on-site or remote)
- Estimated number and locations of clinical sites
- Personnel protective equipment, diagnostics, and other infection control measures needed for research staff
- Contractor roles, e.g., laboratory specimen shipping, analysis, and storage investigational product management, pharmacovigilance, site monitoring, and logistical services
- Clinical site pharmacy requirements and supply needs
- Data collection methodology (hard copy or electronic), management, reporting, and security needs
- Data and safety monitoring board (DSMB) organizational plans and review schedules
- Safety monitoring and reporting requirements
- Access to investigational product data
- Human subject protections and participant consent language that addresses unspecified future uses of research samples
- Access to trial data and publication of study results

As it gains an understanding of the scientific team's expectations and needs, the operations team can concurrently proceed to develop plans for:

- Contractual support as needed, e.g., from contract research organizations (CROs)
- Vendors able to supply goods and services, including both global CROs and more limited, specialty services (e.g., outpatient phlebotomy, contract nurses, etc.)
- Funding, including sources and distribution of funds to clinical sites
- Identification and launch of clinical sites, preferably those with adequate facilities, experienced staff, and ability to enroll research participants
- Adequate support staffing of teams and sites, with quick augmentation if necessary
- Financial and regulatory remedies for institutional bottlenecks in the protocol implementation and site initiation process
- Execution of clinical trial agreements and material transfer agreements with collaborating countries, investigational product agreements and data sharing agreements with manufacturers, and agreements that transfer sponsor and regulatory responsibilities
- Purchase of clinical trial insurance coverage and indemnification
- Internal and external communications
- Overall project management, communication, and Web site development

Well-synchronized planning should enable the operational team to create a dynamic checklist of implementation items by each operational discipline as the protocol evolves. The team should prospectively define paths for decision-making and quickly identify and elevate issues that require higher-level resolution (e.g., study objectives for achieving product registration or emergency use authorization or the potential that multiple studies could compete for participants).

3 The RECOVERY Trial

The following key elements facilitated the remarkably rapid design and initiation of the RECOVERY study in the UK, with an emphasis on trial simplicity (Flanagan 2020; Kupferschmidt 2020; RECOVERY Trial 2022). The first participant was enrolled 9 days after the full protocol was written and 2 days after it was approved. The first 1000 participants were enrolled in 16 days (Goossens et al. 2022) (► In Practice 14.1 and 15.1). Noteworthy features of the trial included the following:

- A short, 20-page protocol with an adaptive design and a very limited number of primary endpoints.
- Accelerated (9 days) ethical and regulatory approval.
- All documents freely available online, including the protocol, approvals, prior meeting slides and minutes, and training materials.
- A five-page consent form and one-page case report form completed at bedside by clinicians.
- Accelerated data collection and processing through the UK National Health Service (NHS) Digi Trials.
- Fast publication of adaptive, platform trial results as trial arms were stopped for efficacy, safety, or futility and new arms started (RECOVERY Collaborative Group 2020, 2021).
- Simplified credential verification requirements for investigators—any qualified staff member could act as a principal investigator (PI), waiving the need for the PI to provide a curriculum vitae and a good clinical practice (GCP) certificate (while no GCP training was required, all staff completed study background training).
- Any doctor with a prescribing license (General Medical Council credentials) could prescribe.
- Simplification of site identification, with any hospital caring for eligible patients considered suitable to take part in the trial.
- Outreach to all doctors by UK Chief Medical Officers to strongly encourage participation in COVID-19 trials.
- A facile consent process with PIs authorized to determine that staff members (e.g., medical students) had the necessary experience and training to obtain informed consent.
- A single, non-negotiable, non-commercial site contract, with site email confirmation sufficient to proceed.

The RECOVERY study team expedited protocol development by using existing protocols developed for Middle East respiratory syndrome (MERS) research. Besides the efficiencies of the centralized and standardized NHS structure, the team capitalized on routine NHS data collection, with key events such as death and intensive care unit admission extracted directly from existing data streams.

4 The ACTIV-3 Trials

4.1 Background on the National Institutes of Health (NIH) Clinical Research Infrastructure

The COVID-19 emergency made it imperative for multiple NIH institutes and centers (ICs) and their extramural clinical trial networks to overcome barriers that hindered collaboration. While there are common U.S. government and NIH policies that apply to all, the 27 ICs have considerable autonomy to develop additional guidelines and policies that meet their specific research needs. Even within a single institute, such as the National Institute

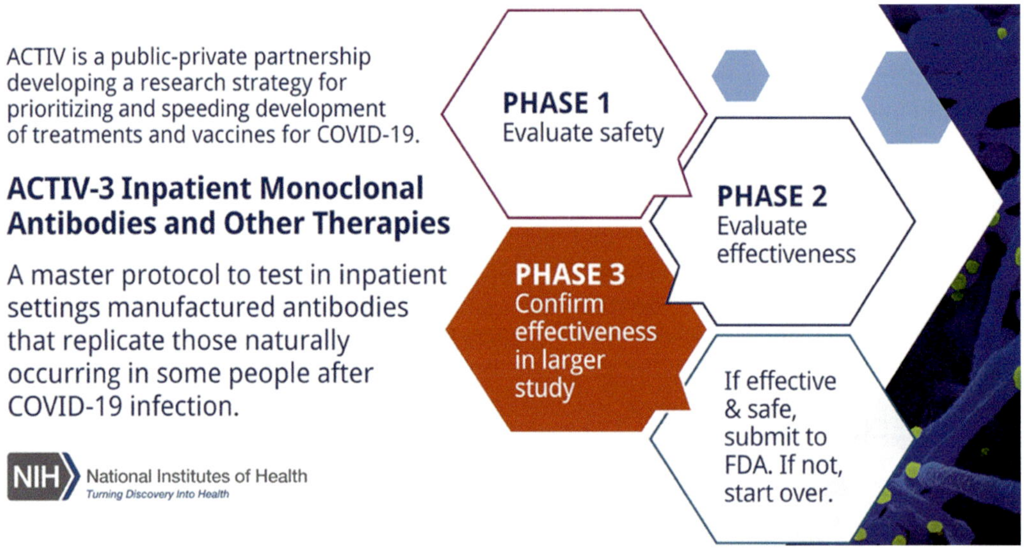

Fig. 2 Summary of ACTIV-3 trial of inpatient monoclonal antibodies and other therapies. (NIH, USG public domain)

of Allergy and Infectious Diseases (NIAID), several divisions conduct extramural research, each with slightly different internal procedures and contract support mechanisms.

This diversity of approach works well absent an overriding emergency. When multiple NIH networks sought to collaborate and implement the ACTIV clinical research portfolio, however, integration was challenging. The ACTIV portfolio consisted of six platform clinical trials that targeted distinct, sometimes overlapping patient populations with different treatments. Some sites hosted multiple trials, occasionally with conflicting recruitment priorities (NIH 2021a) (▶ Chap. 15).

By harnessing NIH clinical trial networks addressing human immunodeficiency virus (HIV), heart and lung research, and more, ACTIV tapped experienced clinical trialists familiar with government and regulatory requirements in the USA and internationally. Their networks of existing clinical research sites were supplemented by community hospitals and clinics, scientific input from industry and the NIH, and support from non-profits. This approach enabled ACTIV to enroll the trial populations needed to answer important research questions and assess therapeutic interventions at different points in disease progression. Despite these advantages, the NIH community had to overcome numerous administrative, contracting, and bureaucratic obstacles that hindered rapid implementation.

4.2 ACTIV-3

The lessons learned from the ACTIV research program are still a work in progress, subject to future analysis in government reports and academic papers. Even without polished conclusions, a microcosm of experience can be related on the implementation and conduct of ACTIV-3 (NIH 2021b). ACTIV-3 was a collaboration of two NIH institutes[1] and five clinical trial networks.[2] The ACTIV-3 master protocol, TICO (Therapeutics for Inpatients with COVID-19), was an in-patient, adaptive platform trial that assessed six investigational products for safety and efficacy (Fig. 2). It

1 National Heart, Lung, and Blood Institute (NHLBI) and National Institute of Allergy and Infectious Diseases (NIAID).

2 International Institute for Strategic Initiatives in Global HIV Trials (INSIGHT), Cardiothoracic Surgical Trials Network (CTSN), Prevention and Early Treatment of Acute Lung Injury (PETAL), the U.S. Department of Veterans Affairs (VA), and the NIAID Division of Clinical Research (DCR).

opened in August 2020 and enrolled 2753 participants at 115 clinical research sites affiliated with collaborating networks spanning five continents. Although TICO enrollment closed in April 2022, other ACTIV-3 research followed:

- ACTIV-3b Therapeutics for Severely Ill Inpatients with COVID-19 (TESICO), a study evaluating the safety and efficacy of investigational agents aimed at improving the outcomes of participants with COVID-19-related acute respiratory failure (NIH 2021c). This study closed in November 2022.
- Vaccination for Recovered Inpatients with COVID-19 (VATICO), a sub-study of recovered TICO participants who had received certain investigational agents or placebo in TICO. They were offered open-label Moderna and Pfizer vaccinations and followed for 48 weeks to determine durability of response (NIH 2021d). This study closed in December 2022.

4.3 Surmounting Obstacles in ACTIV-3

The following sections focus on recommendations to accelerate emergency research response in several specific areas. Past infectious disease research conducted by NIH in West Africa during Ebola outbreaks, as well as COVID-19 research during the pandemic, have informed these recommendations. While diseases, incidence, interventions, and environments differed, many similar organizational, financial, bureaucratic, and regulatory barriers hindered the emergency research response. The documentation of such barriers in reports and articles is extensive and includes recommendations to avert repetition, but practical solutions still seem to demand reinvention in successive outbreaks.

Improved preparedness and response after COVID-19 needs to build on continued COVID-19 research, as well as the effort to develop candidate VTDs for other virus families known to infect humans (Cassetti et al. 2022). "Warm-base" functioning clinical trial networks responsive to U.S. government and coordinated research agendas are essential to a rapid research response distinguished by speed, flexibility, quality, and efficiency. In October of 2022, NIH asked the INSIGHT research network to develop a master protocol for prospective respiratory and viral trials in hospitalized participants. The resulting Strategies and Treatment for Respiratory and Viral Emergencies (STRIVE) protocol is a collaborative effort with other U.S. and international trial networks and the NIH (NIH 2022). In addition to the rapid implementation benefits of this approach, STRIVE also promises more demographic diversity, with reliance on a suite of international coordinating centers able to build infrastructure when and where it might be needed.

4.3.1 Accelerated Research Start-Up

A variety of steps can be taken to speed up preparations for clinical trial research during a public health emergency. There are two basic, easily understood approaches for doing so:

1. During an emergency, requirements for response research and funding get top priority with the entities responsible for them.
2. Steps normally conducted sequentially are conducted in parallel (e.g., scientific and ethical reviews are pursued simultaneously), while operational arrangements proceed apace without waiting for final protocol approval.

One principle, however, must be paramount when departures from standard research practice are undertaken. There can be no compromise of scientific or ethical principles that would jeopardize participant safety or reliable study results (▶ Chap. 3). Recommendations:

- Collaborations of multiple research networks, countries, and sites should quickly establish a high-level combined working group with funder, sponsor, regulator, researcher, national, and international representatives to overcome legal and regulatory hurdles and institutional barriers.

- Early agreement on a research concept that can serve as the basis for accelerated development of a final protocol is essential. This requires scientific and operational leadership committed to an accelerated development schedule commensurate with the emergency and availability of resources. An uncomplicated, effective trial design, and trial mechanics sufficient to answer the basic research question should be employed.
- A well-designed protocol, with broad participant eligibility criteria, is a necessary condition for short case report forms and other streamlined data collection instruments. Research documents that can be quickly prepared and are limited in number will simplify clinical staff training and expedite regulatory review.
- Harmonization of safety reporting, standard of care, diagnostic testing, specimen collection, and site registration requirements (e.g., GCP and GPP training, informed consent requirements, etc.), generally under International Conference on Harmonisation of Technical Requirements for Pharmaceuticals for Human Use (ICH) guidelines, should bring common standards to the collaborating clinical trial networks.
- Multiple ethics committee reviews could delay trials and need to be expedited or consolidated, preferably as a preparedness step rather than during an emergency response.
- Centralized leadership, statistical and data management, operations, pharmaceutical distribution, and a specimen repository are interdependent. To the extent possible, their co-location under unified management can enhance communication, streamline progress, and reduce institutional barriers.
- An independent data and safety monitoring board should be immediately established to regularly review research results.
- Construction of a research website also should begin immediately. It will be modified over time to foster communications, disseminate documents and vital information, and track research progress.

4.3.2 Prudent Clinical Site Selection

Pandemic emergency clinical trials will require multiple clinical sites to recruit and follow enough participants for statistically robust results. Geographic diversity will help ensure that trial results are broadly generalizable and applicable to populations that differ by gender, income, race, ethnicity, or other characteristics. Clinical site recruitment effectiveness will depend on multiple variables, such as research experience, relations with the surrounding communities, location relative to disease incidence, essential research capabilities (e.g., pharmacy, laboratory, imaging, specialized treatment resources), institutional and national government support, transportation infrastructure, and alliances with established research networks (▶ Chap. 40). Recommendations include the following:

- A directory of experienced clinical trial networks should be established and maintained. Infectious disease networks that bring multiple countries and sites to a research endeavor are particularly valuable for coordination of research programs and expedited implementation. Other experienced research networks, not focused on infectious diseases, also can significantly contribute if they are able to quickly repurpose and adapt to work on pandemic trials. In addition to publicly funded networks, the directory should include pharmaceutical industry networks engaged in VTD development and production research.
- Because research sites cannot be mothballed and easily brought back to life, network clinical sites should be engaged in ongoing, high-quality research during interpandemic periods. Ideally such research will either contribute to pandemic preparedness or develop VTD for diseases of concern at the research locations. As a preparedness measure, public funding for clinical trial networks and ongoing trials should be conditioned on a written understanding that clinical sites will transition from interpandemic research to emergency research as specified in the funding documents.

- While it was necessary to bring in new sites during the COVID-19 pandemic (McNay et al. 2021), those with a solid track record in clinical trials and participant recruitment should be favored over those with eagerness and enthusiasm, but little experience. When time is limited, sites lacking research history are difficult to integrate into an urgent, complex research program.
- Assess prospective site recruitment potential. The likelihood of emerging infectious disease outbreaks in particular places should be considered when selecting and funding clinical research sites (▶ Chap. 10). With a new outbreak, the current and potential geographic incidence of the disease under study is a primary concern. An expanding outbreak will affect trial implementation, including the need for additional sites, locations, and participant recruitment. An outbreak could also wane faster than expected, whether on its own or due to a successful public health or clinical research response (Kennedy et al. 2016).
- Recognize that existing networks, clinical sites, and investigators may have preferred methodologies and differing approaches to clinical trials. There is little room, however, for substantial deviation from standards (e.g., ICH Good Clinical Practice) that are recognized by stringent regulatory authorities. Research that does not meet those standards will not produce results acceptable to regulators for VTD authorization or approval.
- Ensure that the proposed research is fully supported by institutional and site investigators and will not be adversely affected by conflicting priorities or ongoing research that recruits from similar populations.
- Potential networks, sites, and partner institutions should understand and concur with proposed financial arrangements. Compensation usually covers a mix of fixed costs (e.g., start-up investigator compensation, other staffing, pharmacy, and monitoring expenses) and variable costs, based on projected study enrollment and actual documentation of participant care. Reasonable compensation should be set by trial leadership at the outset of site recruitment. Despite differences in institutional settings and locations, reimbursement should be standardized to avoid time-consuming negotiations, dissatisfaction over unequal funding, and lack of transparency.
- Give preference to sites that will rely on central research ethics committees or institutional review boards (RECs or IRBs), rather than requiring separate reviews.
- Build a logistics checklist and give preference to sites able to implement the research with the least assistance. Prospective clinical sites must demonstrate that they have the necessary technical and logistical resources to conduct the trial, collect data, and enter data into a central database. Required resources may include administrative, laboratory, and imaging support, a functional pharmacy, communication and data collection capacity, specialized medical treatment, language services, security, and sufficient, functional space for staff and participants.
- Give preference to sites that have comprehensive, flexible capabilities that can be swiftly reallocated and sites that can access additional staff, expertise, and resources when necessary for the research effort.
- Within each country, leadership should be centralized at a single institution with a responsible lead investigator. Competing national leadership centers will complicate and delay trial implementation.

4.3.3 Timely Clinical Site Activation

Before a clinical site can be activated to recruit, enroll, and follow trial participants, many tasks must be undertaken by the trial operations center (▶ Chap. 32), the institution hosting the site, and the site itself. The primary task will be establishment of formal financial relationships between institutions hosting eligible clinical sites, or their affiliated networks, and the research operations center. Logistical requirements should have largely been satisfied during site selection, although there may be some consequential financial matters related to logistics that must be addressed at this stage. Other regulatory and pharmaceutical requirements must also be satisfied after site selection, but before activation; they are addressed separately in the sections that follow.

Contracts must be negotiated that define financial compensation for the research conducted in accordance with statements of work. Presumably, the clinical research sites would have already concurred with the compensation policies during site selection. Under such contracts, funding and work requirements normally go through various intermediate levels of administration and coordination. For example, an international site in the INSIGHT network might receive funding from the research operations center that passes through a regional coordinating center and/or a country coordinating center. Other networks may have unique hierarchical structures that must be reflected in their layered contracts, while stand-alone, non-network sites may have direct, single-institution contractual relationships with the research operations center. Recommendations include the following:

- Begin development of standardized operations center contracts that reflect the fixed and variable compensation amounts established for all sites participating in the research.
- Provide some upfront funding to sites for costs related to international and national regulatory compliance and other preparatory needs before they commence research.
- Operations centers should have broad implementation authority (likely from the national government) that obviates the need for multiple approvals from lower-level authorities. Examples might include authority to hire personnel, import needed equipment and pharmaceuticals, set up communications networks, etc.
- Establish a special funding mechanism to address unanticipated or unavoidable resource shortcomings that could delay site activation (e.g., site renovations, power and water supply, vehicle procurement, etc.).
- Develop incentives for sites that exceed expectations for rapid enrollment of eligible research participants, data quality, and timely submission of specimens and reports.
- Contracts and compensation should come with funding assurances that cover the entire research period foreseen, minimizing the need for extensions, amendments, further negotiations, or institutional hesitancy to continue research work.

4.3.4 Streamlined Regulatory Compliance

The RECOVERY trial demonstrated how quickly trial design and implementation can occur in an emergency, particularly within the structure of a single, unified healthcare system serving the participating sites, under a single regulator, all with a common language (► In Practice 14.1 and 15.1). Global and, in many cases, national pandemic preparedness requires establishing broad regulatory harmonization across multiple jurisdictions. The most widely accepted standards for harmonization are those promulgated by ICH. For more than 30 years, the ICH has worked together with the world's regulatory authorities to develop detailed guidelines for clinical trial design and implementation (ICH 2023). The U.S. Food and Drug Administration (FDA), the European Medicines Agency (EMA), and other regulatory authorities incorporate ICH guidance documents into their national regulatory systems. ICH guidelines are well positioned to serve as the basis for clinical research network standards. Recommendations include the following:

- Consider modification of FDA forms for international research, so that a single template is used as the basis to collect essential information required by the FDA and other regulators and then modified as necessary for specific trial needs. Basing the forms on ICH guidelines, for example, could streamline paperwork.
- Simplify site registration. Review checklists for successful site registration, and remove any tasks that are not necessary to maintain participant safety and trial integrity.

- Eliminate requirements for advance submission of the following documents, with the understanding that documentation will still be eventually required and verified:
  - Signed and dated curriculum vitae (CV) and medical license for PI and sub-investigators and signed and dated CV for Pharmacist of Record (ICH Good Clinical Practice (GCP) also requires that these documents be on-file at the clinical site).
  - Documentation of human subjects protection and GCP initial training and refresher dates, the timing of which can vary by institution and location.
  - Documentation of clinical research site training dates on protocol.
  - For pharmaceutical interventions, pharmacy training documentation before shipment of investigational new drugs.
  - For pharmaceutical interventions, financial conflict-of-interest forms signed by investigators.
- According to the U.S. Common Rule for human subject protections (OHRP 2021), a single REC/IRB ethical review, rather than separate reviews by all involved institutions, is now required for U.S. sites participating in multi-site research funded by the U.S. government. Implementation of single REC review should preclude any duplication of local review, and institutions should cede privacy and ethics review to the single REC. Unfortunately, the single REC rule has not been easy to implement (Serdoz et al. 2022). International clinical research partnerships are still likely to require ethical review by at least one REC/IRB in each participating country, but it is important to keep additional reviews to a minimum. Also:
  - Reject efforts by local review boards to impose informed consent alterations.
  - Reject efforts by local institution human subject protection offices to impose nonessential conditions or ancillary reviews for data/specimen access or for other research activities.
- Following receipt of investigator reports, the statistical and data management center will send their analysis to regulatory agencies. Safety data collection should emphasize key clinical events that matter. Non-essential data collection should be minimized (▶ Chap. 36).
- Assess whether the impact of confidentiality and data-privacy regulation (e.g., the Health Insurance Portability and Accountability Act [HIPAA] in the United States or General Data Protection Regulation [GDPR] in the European Union) could delay site registration and seek remedies.
- Prepare for remote monitoring, with restricted access to sites where security and transport are problematic or where bureaucratic and complicated site authorizations are needed for each on-site visit.

4.3.5 Prompt Negotiation of Essential Research Agreements and Documents

Before research can begin, formal written agreements may need to be negotiated between collaborating research partners. The inclusion of functioning clinical trial networks in pandemic preparedness should limit the need for negotiations during an infectious disease emergency. In the United States, for example, delegation of authorities held by a federal government agency may be pursued when U.S. government-funded research is implemented by a non-governmental clinical trial network. Such agreements can be difficult to reach on the fly. Research partners may seek agreed terms for the transfer, custody, and use of biological specimens collected during the research—a complex and unsettled area of international law. Recommendations include the following:

- Insofar as possible, partners should negotiate high-level agreements to define roles and responsibilities for research on which they may collaborate in advance of any emergency.

  - ICH GCP allows a sponsor to "transfer any or all of the sponsor's trial-related duties and functions to a [contract research organization] CRO" (ICH 2016), although the ultimate responsibility for meeting standards remains with the sponsor. Regulatory authorities that follow ICH guidelines, like FDA and EMA, require assurances that the research is performed in accordance with controlling study documents, GCP, applicable regulatory and monitoring requirements, investigational new drug (IND) management requirements, and safety directives.
  - ICH also authorizes CROs to transfer selected responsibilities to other partners. A delegation of sponsor responsibilities (DSR) provided by NIH authorizes designated parties to act on behalf of a research sponsor, liaise with international health authorities, and assume international regulatory responsibilities related to research.
- Research sponsors and networks should prepare model agreements, reviewed and approved by legal representatives, for domestic and international coordinating centers and sites. Accepted model agreements will be extremely important to collect documentation and promote timely implementation of the emergency response research, but it should be noted that this is easier said than done.
  - Clinical Trial Applications (CTAs) must be submitted to national regulatory agencies. Support by international coordinating centers should be enlisted to collect national CTAs from their respective collaborating countries.
  - Material Transfer Agreements (MTAs) address the ownership, transfer, use, longer-term custody, related research publication, commercial use, and disposition of biological material (e.g., pathogen samples, blood components, other bodily fluids, and swabs) collected by a clinical site. The parties to the MTAs may be research operations centers, other collaborating network coordinating centers, country-based international organizations that manage one or more clinical sites, or stand-alone site institutions.

4.3.6 Liability Coverage

Collaborating countries and institutions will demand that liability coverage be provided for clinical sites and participants (▶ In Focus 32.2). This is particularly important for research conducted during a pandemic when the risk associated with possible injuries or deaths of staff or participants is magnified by scientific uncertainties (e.g., disease transmissibility, tentative and limited morbidity and mortality data, new and untested interventions, etc.) and public fear. Liability coverage is an early operational requirement, and securing coverage from insurers can be complicated by uncertainty about risks, trial sponsors' inability or reluctance to assume financial responsibility, a limited number of insurance underwriters, and differing assurances sought by various stakeholders. Recommendations include the following:

- Make early and fundamental risk management determinations.
  - What level and scale of risk can be anticipated in connection with the research?
  - Is there an international source for emergency response liability coverage (e.g., the World Bank Pandemic Emergency Fund)?
  - If not, is the trial sponsor financially able and willing to offer liability coverage?
  - If not the trial sponsor, can risk management be transferred to other responsible parties (e.g., a government agency, educational institution, or insurance company)?
  - Will liability coverage with clinical trial insurance be sufficient, or will indemnification also be sought, e.g., by one party agreeing to cover the losses of third parties?
- If one of the collaborating parties (e.g., the sponsor or funder) provides liability coverage, determine whether the risk management framework is sufficient or seek supplemental coverage on the commercial market.

- If the existing, internal risk management framework is sufficient, initiate negotiations and prepare documents needed to provide assurances of coverage to collaborating governments/institutions and their clinical sites.
- Risk underwriters in the commercial market will require detailed descriptions of the research. The underwriters will then provide country-specific insurance certificates, usually in the country language, describing the scope and period of coverage, and will invoice the trial's sponsor or operations center.

4.3.7 Collaboration with the Pharmaceutical Industry

Research with a pharmaceutical intervention—an investigational new drug or candidate vaccine—usually requires the cooperation of a private sector producer; early agreement on the scientific, operational, and regulatory structure of the research; access to proprietary and confidential IND documents; details on product labeling, supply, shipping, and post-trial disposition; clinical site pharmaceutical management; and publication of research results. The parties must recognize that interests and expectations will differ and should seek early resolution of as many potential issues as possible. Recommendations include the following:

- Establish a high-level public-private partnership or working group with scientific, operational, and regulatory representatives that can agree on key logistical steps and are committed to quickly clear unexpected obstacles (▶ Chap. 15). As a condition for collaboration, the working group should obtain industry assurances that proprietary and confidential documents will be provided as needed for investigational products.
- Establish a drug logistics subgroup for each investigational product, and identify therapeutics and supplies needed to achieve the specified standard of care. Note that the standard of care could change during the trial, especially with a novel pathogen. The subgroup should complete the following tasks:
  - Map out the production and supply chain to determine how the investigational product and other supplies will be shipped to research sites.
  - Develop critical timelines based on projected clinical trial initiation, production capacity, participant recruitment, and product shelf life to maintain uninterrupted research supplies.
  - Monitor establishment of procedures for labeling, supply, shipping to receiving depots, and release by specified persons ("qualified persons" in the European Union).
- Negotiate and implement clinical trial agreements between the research sponsor and manufacturer, recognizing that the sponsor and principal investigator have primary authority over the conduct of the trial and resulting publications.
- Develop plans for distribution, review, and publication of trial results.
- If necessary, engage a pharmaceutical CRO with receiving depots, quality control, and management capabilities for the labeling, storage, and distribution of the investigative product and other needed therapeutics and related supplies to clinical sites.
- Identify and compile a master file with all essential regulatory documents (e.g., investigational medical product dossiers, investigational brochures, etc.) that will be supplied by the manufacturer and accessible to collaborators and regulators.
- Ensure standardized investigational product and standard of care labeling that meets research and regulatory needs across all countries participating in the research.

4.3.8 High-Level Contract Management Flexibility

The funders and sponsors of emergency response research will most likely depend on prime contractors to assist them with operations support (▶ Chap. 29). These contractors can provide many different services, including management and oversight of research network and institutional subcontractors, subcontracting to specialized CROs, logistics support, and funding of exceptional or unexpected needs. Because contractor selection and negotiations can contribute to delays, prime contractors need the flexibility to modify customary procedures for an emergency. This flexibility needs to extend to subcontractors responsible for the conduct of the research and their coordinating centers and sites, as provided for under ICH guidelines (ICH 2016). Recommendations include the following:

- Research funds must be available early so subcontractors can initiate trial operation activities.
- Subcontracting institutions tasked with early work will want assurances that compensation will cover costs incurred, especially if work proceeds while execution of contracts is pending. The parties should be prepared with "authorizations to proceed" or simplified letter contracts with budget limits. These instruments would be replaced following execution of more traditional contracts.
- Prime contractors should seek early operational approvals from funders that balance urgency with reduced, but still transparent, oversight. Early oversight should not burden subcontractors with non-essential reporting when they need to focus on building operational capabilities. The following measures will lessen the probability of adverse outcomes for prime contractors with this approach:
  - Known entities already under contract, or with a history of satisfactory performance, should be preferred.
  - Pre-qualification of prospective contractors will cut vetting time. Broad statements of terms and conditions should be sought with indefinite delivery/indefinite quantity contracts or similar mechanisms.
  - Rigorous evaluation of contractor proposals can then focus on budgets and technical proposals rather than contractor qualifications for the work.
  - Work timelines should provide for retrospective reporting and documentation when time allows.
- Prime contractors must ensure that their subcontractors have funds in time to meet their obligations.
- Emergency response research will generally be affected by location and rate of disease incidence and available scientific information. Simplified subcontracts, broad statements of work, and flexible delegation of responsibilities are advisable.
- Novel diseases and interventions can pose surprising and costly difficulties. Contingency funding could cover unforeseen expenses, but may not be authorized. If so, alternate funding mechanisms should be identified as soon as difficulties are encountered.
- Consider adaption of existing contract mechanisms before introducing new ones.
- Prime contractors should prioritize emergency response research funding and logistical support over their other obligations.

5 Conclusion

Clinical research operational challenges and solutions during the COVID-19 pandemic and Ebola outbreaks of 2014–2016 in West Africa and 2018–2020 in the DRC provided experience in emergency research operations to hundreds of research staff, including the authors, and were a proving ground for rapid integration and implementation of emergency clinical research for infectious disease outbreaks (NASEM 2017). Adapting solutions that have worked in past emergencies and conducting scientific research and operational support activities in parallel rather than in sequence are the best-known ways to accelerate assessment of VTDs and mitigation of pandemic morbidity and mortality. A swift, coherent, and flexible research response to future public health emergencies must build on the lessons of accelerated research programs already implemented: accelerated start-up, prudent clinical site selection, timely clinical site activation, streamlined regulatory compliance, prompt execution of fundamental agreements, adequate research liability coverage, collaboration with pharmaceutical manufacturers, and flexible contract management. It is especially important to build in early flexibility within network payment systems to ensure that a safety net can accommodate unforeseen expenditures. Continued work on pandemic preparedness can help reduce the burden of urgent tasks, but flexibility, experience, and creative thinking will be critical to responding to the next outbreak with pandemic potential. The STRIVE trial is a good example of scientific action that promotes pandemic preparation by building and sustaining a research framework based on the recent past but poised to function now and in the future.

Discussion Questions

1. Why is a national or global research agenda needed? When does operational planning for emergency response research need to begin? How can operational planning proceed in parallel with protocol development?
2. List and discuss some of the disciplines essential for emergency clinical research.
3. What are some of the key elements that facilitated the rapid design and initiation of the RECOVERY study?
4. How can the lessons learned from the ACTIV-3 research program facilitate a swift, flexible research response?
   (a) Speed and brevity are goals that many trials seek but few realize. Discuss some recommendations that can accelerate research start-up and implementation.
   (b) Clinical research may entail the participation of many clinical sites. Discuss some recommendations for prudent site selection.
   (c) What tasks must be undertaken before a clinical site can be activated to recruit, enroll, and follow trial participants.
   (d) How can regulatory compliance for international emergency research be streamlined?
   (e) What can be done to accelerate negotiations between collaborating research partners?
   (f) What can be done to ensure functional clinical research collaboration with industry?

References

Abelin A, Colegate T, Gardner S, Hehme N, Palache A. Lessons from pandemic influenza A (H1N1): the research-based vaccine industry's perspective. Vaccine. 2011;29(6):1135–8. https://doi.org/10.1016/j.vaccine.2010.11.042.

Angus DC, Berry S, Lewis RJ, Al-Beidh F, Arabi Y, van Bentum-Puijk W, et al. The REMAP-CAP (Randomized Embedded Multifactorial Adaptive Platform for Community-Acquired Pneumonia) study. Rationale and design. Ann Am Thorac Soc. 2020;17(7):879–91. https://doi.org/10.1513/AnnalsATS.202003-192SD.

Bedford J, Farrar J, Ihekweazu C, Kang G, Koopmans M, Nkengasong J. A new twenty-first century science for effective epidemic response. Nature. 2019;575(7781):130–6. https://doi.org/10.1038/s41586-019-1717-y.

Carter SE, Ahuka-Mundeke S, Pfaffmann Zambruni J, Navarro Colorado C, van Kleef E, Lissouba P, et al. How to improve outbreak response: a case study of integrated outbreak analytics from Ebola in Eastern Democratic Republic of the Congo. BMJ Glob Health. 2021;6(8) https://doi.org/10.1136/bmjgh-2021-006736.

Cassetti MC, Pierson TC, Patterson LJ, Bok K, DeRocco AJ, Deschamps AM, et al. Prototype pathogen approach for vaccine and monoclonal antibody development: a critical component of the NIAID plan for pandemic preparedness. J Infect Dis. 2022;227:1433. https://doi.org/10.1093/infdis/jiac296.

Finlay BB, See RH, Brunham RC. Rapid response research to emerging infectious diseases: lessons from SARS. Nat Rev Microbiol. 2004;2(7):602–7. https://doi.org/10.1038/nrmicro930.

Flanagan BM. Quality by design in the RECOVERY trial (randomized evaluation of COVID-19 therapy). Clin Res. 2020;34(10):9–17.

Goossens H, Derde L, Horby P, Bonten M. The European clinical research response to optimise treatment of patients with COVID-19: lessons learned, future perspective, and recommendations. Lancet Infect Dis. 2022;22(5):e153–e158. https://doi.org/10.1016/s1473-3099(21)00705-2.

Hashem H, Abufaraj M, Tbakhi A, Sultan I. Obstacles and considerations related to clinical trial research during the COVID-19 pandemic. Front Med (Lausanne). 2020;7:598038. https://doi.org/10.3389/fmed.2020.598038.

Hatchett RJ, Mecher CE, Lipsitch M. Public health interventions and epidemic intensity during the 1918 influenza pandemic. Proc Natl Acad Sci USA. 2007;104(18):7582–7. https://doi.org/10.1073/pnas.0610941104.

ICH. Good clinical practice: ICH harmonised guideline. Integrated addendum to ICH E6(R1): guideline for good clinical practice ICH E6(R2) ICH consensus guideline. Geneva: International Council for Harmonisation of Technical Requirements for Pharmaceuticals for Human Use (ICH); 2016.

ICH. Mission: harmonisation for better health. Geneva: International Council for Harmonisation of Technical Requirements for Pharmaceuticals for Human Use; 2023. https://www.ich.org/page/mission. Accessed 20 Jul 2023.

Kennedy SB, Neaton JD, Lane HC, Kieh MWS, Massaquoi MBF, Touchette NA, et al. Implementation of an Ebola virus disease vaccine clinical trial during the Ebola epidemic in Liberia: design, procedures, and challenges. Clin Trials (London, England). 2016;13(1):49–56. https://doi.org/10.1177/1740774515621037.

Kupferschmidt K. One U.K. trial is transforming COVID-19 treatment. Why haven't others delivered more results? Science. 2020; https://doi.org/10.1126/science.abd6417.

LaVange L, Adam SJ, Currier JS, Higgs ES, Reineck LA, Hughes EA, et al. Accelerating COVID-19 therapeutic interventions and vaccines (ACTIV): designing master protocols for evaluation of candidate COVID-19 therapeutics. Ann Intern Med. 2021;174:1293. https://doi.org/10.7326/m21-1269.

Lurie N, Manolio T, Patterson AP, Collins F, Frieden T. Research as a part of public health emergency response. N Engl J Med. 2013;368(13):1251–5. https://doi.org/10.1056/nejmsb1209510.

Madhav N, Oppenheim B, Gallivan M, Mulembakani P, Rubin E, Wolfe N. Pandemics: risks, impacts, and mitigation. In: Jamison DT, Gelband H, Horton S, Jha P, Laxminarayan R, Mock CN, et al., editors. Disease control priorities: improving health and reducing poverty. Washington, DC: The International Bank for Reconstruction and Development/The World Bank; 2017.

Marston HD, Paules CI, Fauci AS. The critical role of biomedical research in pandemic preparedness. JAMA. 2017;318(18):1757–8. https://doi.org/10.1001/jama.2017.15033.

McNay LA, Arnoczy G, Martell M, Mock P, Wright ME, Simpson S, et al. Community-based hospitals: new partners for government-sponsored clinical research during public health emergencies. Vaccine. 2021;39(42):6183–5. https://doi.org/10.1016/j.vaccine.2021.09.008.

NASEM. Integrating clinical research into epidemic response: the Ebola experience. Washington, DC: National Academies of Sciences Engineering and Medicine Publications, The National Academies Press; 2017.

NIH. Accelerating COVID-19 therapeutic interventions and vaccines (ACTIV). 2021a. https://www.nih.gov/research-training/medical-research-initiatives/activ. Accessed 20 Feb 2023.

NIH. ACTIV-3: therapeutics for inpatients with COVID-19 (TICO). Bethesda, MD: National Institutes of Health; 2021b. https://clinicaltrials.gov/ct2/show/NCT04501978. Accessed 20 Feb 2023.

NIH. ACTIV-3b: therapeutics for severely ill inpatients with COVID-19 (TESICO). Bethesda, MD: National Institutes of Health; 2021c. https://clinicaltrials.gov/ct2/show/NCT04843761. Accessed 20 Feb 2023.

NIH. Vaccination for recovered inpatients with COVID-19 (VATICO). Bethesda, MD: National Institutes of Health; 2021d. https://clinicaltrials.gov/ct2/show/NCT04969250. Accessed 20 Feb 2023.

NIH. Strategies and treatments for respiratory infections and viral emergencies (STRIVE). Bethesda, MD: National Institutes of Health; 2022. https://clinicaltrials.gov/ct2/show/NCT04969250. Accessed 20 Feb 2023.

OHRP. Revised common rule educational materials. Rockville, MD: Office for Human Research Protections; 2021. https://www.hhs.gov/ohrp/education-and-outreach/revised-common-rule/index.html. Accessed 28 Feb 2023.

Olliaro P, Torreele E. Global challenges in preparedness and response to epidemic infectious diseases. Mol Ther. 2022;30(5):1801–9. https://doi.org/10.1016/j.ymthe.2022.02.022.

RECOVERY Collaborative Group. Dexamethasone in hospitalized patients with Covid-19. N Engl J Med. 2020;384(8):693–704. https://doi.org/10.1056/NEJMoa2021436.

RECOVERY Collaborative Group. Tocilizumab in patients admitted to hospital with COVID-19 (RECOVERY): a randomised, controlled, open-label, platform trial. Lancet. 2021;397(10285):1637–45. https://doi.org/10.1016/s0140-6736(21)00676-0.

RECOVERY Trial. UK Research and Innovation. 2022. https://www.ukri.org/news-and-events/tackling-the-impact-of-covid-19/vaccines-and-treatments/recovery-trial-identifies-covid-19-treatments/. Accessed 20 Feb 2023.

Rojek AM, Horby PW. Modernising epidemic science: enabling patient-centred research during epidemics. BMC Med. 2016;14(1):212. https://doi.org/10.1186/s12916-016-0760-x.

Serdoz ES, Edwards T, Pulley J, Beadles J, Ozier J, Harris P, et al. The IRB Reliance Exchange (IREx): a national web-based platform for operationalizing single IRB review. J Clin Transl Sci. 2022;6(1):e39. https://doi.org/10.1017/cts.2022.376.

Sigfrid L, Maskell K, Bannister PG, Ismail SA, Collinson S, Regmi S, et al. Addressing challenges for clinical research responses to emerging epidemics and pandemics: a scoping review. BMC Med. 2020;18(1):190. https://doi.org/10.1186/s12916-020-01624-8.

STRIVE. Strategies and Treatments for Respiratory Infections and Viral Emergencies (STRIVE). Bethesda, MD: National Institutes of Health; 2023. https://www.clinicaltrials.gov/study/NCT05822583?term=STRIVE%20&cond=respiratory&page=1&rank=1. Accessed 4 Aug 2023.

WBG. From panic and neglect to investing in health security: financing pandemic preparedness at a national level. Washington, DC: World Bank; 2017. Preparedness IfF, Dec 2017.

32 Launching a Clinical Research Operation

Gregg Larson and Laura A. McNay

Contents

Learning Track Note: This chapter appears in Learning Tracks: Clinical Research; Global Health Law; Preparedness; Research Ethics; Emergency Research Response, Research Operations

E. S. Higgs and R. A. Sorenson (eds.), *Principles and Practice of Emergency Research Response*,
https://doi.org/10.1007/978-3-031-48408-7_47

Learning Objectives

This chapter will help readers understand and describe:

- Requirements for launching an international clinical research program in an impoverished region of a developing country
- Major obstacles that may arise in an emergency research response
- The response of high-income countries to the COVID-19 pandemic and lessons that could be drawn from it
- If a person who is impoverished and has no other access to adequate medical treatment can give true informed consent to participate in a research study

1 Introduction

In recent years, it has become increasingly clear that an infectious disease outbreak can require emergency research on an expedited basis. Since the outbreak of Ebola in West Africa and the identification of the severe acute respiratory syndrome coronavirus 2 (SARS-CoV-2), debate on this point has shifted from whether it should be done to how it can be done. The next infectious disease outbreak with pandemic potential is just as likely to occur in a resource-poor area with very little medical research capacity as in a country with more technical capacity (Allen et al. 2017). It will occur in a world of vastly increased connectivity over the last few decades (Morand and Walther 2020). Prudence thus requires that the world be prepared to rapidly implement an emergency research response at the site of the outbreak. As long as the outbreak remains geographically limited, many studies can only be done in this limited area: this includes natural history studies of modes of transmission, the course of the disease, development of diagnostics, and clinical trials of medical interventions focused on prevention (e.g., vaccines or pre-exposure/post-exposure prophylaxis) or treatment (e.g., drugs, devices, or therapies) (NIH 2017).

This and the following chapters lay out what is needed to conduct such research, based largely on the concrete experience of the authors in implementing needed research during the Ebola outbreaks in West Africa (2014–2016) and in the Democratic Republic of the Congo (DRC) (2018–2020). Under the then-prevailing circumstances, logistical, pharmacy, laboratory, data management, communications, regulatory, and healthcare operations infrastructure had to be strengthened or built from the ground up. In describing what must be done in such an emergency to implement scientifically sound, ethical research in a challenging environment, this material will also suggest what infrastructure, institutional, and human resource preparations ought to be made in advance to facilitate the next emergency response. These lessons may be especially pertinent now, as the COVID-19 pandemic has repeatedly underscored our institutional and societal difficulties in dealing with a new pathogen that repeatedly evolves significant variants, an experience demonstrating that nations thought to be best prepared for Pathogen X were not necessarily so. For example, most of the early research studies in the United States and Western Europe were not well designed to produce interpretable, regulatory level results, and they contributed to public confusion about some hypothetical therapies for COVID-19 (hydroxychloroquine and ivermectin) that have continued to interfere with sound response measures (Bugin and Woodcock 2021).

2 Launching a Clinical Research Operation

Launching a research operation to support a clinical trial in the midst of an infectious disease emergency is a daunting task. Although we know that disease outbreaks and epidemics will occur, the time, place, and pathogen are virtually never foreseen. The emergency might be a sudden outbreak of a previously unknown pathogen, a new variant of a known one, or an uncontrolled outbreak of a familiar disease. Its etiology may not be understood, and early assessments of its geographic incidence, rate of progression, transmissibility, and morbidity and mortality may be unreliable (Cori et al. 2017). The duration of the emergency may be unpredictable, the setting unfamiliar, and knowledge of local medical capacity scanty while the research team needs results as soon as possible. Use of an investigational product that has been little tested in humans will require careful safety monitoring in an environment that can hinder efficient data collection (NASEM 2017).

Inadequate research and health system capacity where the outbreak occurs may limit the scope, speed, and effectiveness of response. Because infectious disease incidence is higher where poverty and illiteracy are prevalent, the research may have to be conducted in a resource-poor environment, requiring more investment than it would in developed-country settings. Countries with meager healthcare infrastructure often lack dependable communications, electrical power, clean water, and transportation. Biosurveillance, regulatory and ethical oversight, and research capacity are often weak and political and societal stability questionable (Global Preparedness Monitoring Board 2019). There are likely to be few medical personnel with research experience. Populations in such settings may resist both nonpharmaceutical and medical response, including research, while popular reliance on traditional medicine may further complicate matters. Past or active armed conflict; ineffective governance; tribal, ethnic, sectarian, or caste divisions; or displaced populations can present formidable logistical and security challenges for both response and research staff and study participants.

An emergency research design implemented in a resource-poor setting either will be shaped by the challenges described above or will need to shape the research environment and provide what is necessary to implement the study (Medical Research Council 2006). Usually, there is an interplay between these alternatives. A research program may need to renovate space, import equipment, bring in expatriate staff, and otherwise fill gaps in infrastructure and capacity, as detailed in this section of *Principles and Practice of Emergency Research Response*. Some consideration can be given beforehand to the possibility that innovative trial designs, such as adaptive randomized trials, may reduce trial duration and be more productive and cost-effective. They also might lead to greater community acceptance by including a potentially beneficial agent in every arm of the trial, thereby overcoming resistance to the use of a placebo in research on a disease with high mortality, such as Ebola (Cooper et al. 2015; Kazanjian 2020; Thorlund et al. 2018).

Even though each new outbreak is unexpected and has its own unique characteristics, past experience must inform preparedness and our capacity to effectively implement research (Lurie et al. 2013). This chapter addresses how to launch research during an infectious disease emergency, with the understanding that the diseases, settings, and research objectives will neither repeat themselves nor be static. Our framework applies broadly to most emergency scenarios, including the most challenging—resource-poor settings with minimal infrastructure and ongoing civil or military strife. We also assume very limited advance planning suited to the particular outbreak; broad community mistrust of health officials, central government, and unfamiliar organizations; and limited access to or trust in modern medicine. We try to follow the Global Preparedness Monitoring Board (2019) recommendation that countries, donors, and multilateral institutions "must be prepared for the worst." If the setting is less challenging, the precautions, actions, and checklist included here should still help responders account for the many operational elements required for a robust research program based on the proposed research questions, setting, and evolving outbreak.

3 Frameworks and Partners

At the outset, a proposed emergency research agenda must consider what international, regional, national, and local frameworks are relevant to the proposal, and whether support structures, including everything from space and supplies for research sites to an in-country research ethics committee (REC) and research consortium, might have to be established or strengthened (▶ Chap. 27). Organizations, collaborators, and allies that can move the proposed research forward will need to be identified and enlisted, both internationally and locally (▶ Chap. 18).

3.1 International

Consideration of international resources should address the following:

- What are the key organizations responsible for emergency response and who are the key individuals within them (NASEM 2017)?
- Are international organizations already present and functioning in the local setting?
- Is response research part of their mandate, or is their titular role peacekeeping, humanitarian response, or development?
- Has the World Health Organization (WHO) declared a public health emergency of international concern (PHEIC)?
- Are other multinational organizations involved (e.g., the United Nations [UN], international financial institutions, United Nations Children's Fund [UNICEF], or regional organizations like the Economic Community of West African States or the Association of Southeast Asian Nations)?
- Will they support a research program?
- Does the research sponsor have a voice at WHO and other relevant bodies, directly or indirectly, and leverage that can influence implementation of the research?

Making sense of the international context requires understanding existing relationships between the research sponsors and WHO, as well as treaties and agreements relevant to the proposed research (Kaiser Family Foundation 2019). It is also important to recognize bilateral, regional, and institutional relationships. Are there historic ties (e.g., France and Guinea, the United Kingdom and Sierra Leone, the United States and Liberia) or institutional links (e.g., among the National Institutes of Health [NIH], the UK Medical Research Council [MRC], the French National Institute of Health and Medical Research, or the Wellcome Trust) that should be considered? Developed-country embassies may provide particularly useful information on the host country's government agencies and individual contacts and may assist with negotiation of needed agreements. They may also be able to provide logistical assistance. If the research sponsor is a government agency, other agencies may provide support. In the case of a U.S.-led response, these would often include the U.S. Centers for Disease Control and Prevention (CDC) and the U.S. Agency for International Development (USAID) and possibly the Defense Department (Margesson 2015). Research sponsored by other governments could also be supported by their government agencies (▶ Chap. 29).

3.2 National

We live in a world where national sovereignty prevails. A constructive relationship with the national government(s) where the research is proposed is a necessary and immediate priority. This should start with a high-level understanding. For example, an invitation from the Liberian Minister of Health to the U.S. Secretary of Health and Human Services initiated the U.S.-supported Ebola research in Liberia (Lane et al. 2016). An advance team would then arrive; it should be able to knowledgeably negotiate basic issues, commit funding and expertise on behalf of the research sponsor, and lay the groundwork for research. Early talks must identify key agencies and decision-makers in the host government and assess their reception of the proposed research. This could include public health, healthcare, medical education, ethical and regulatory, and public safety and national security agencies. An understanding of the government's policy making, relevant decisions, and implementation effectiveness is essential (▶ Chaps. 30 and 33) (◘ Fig. 1).

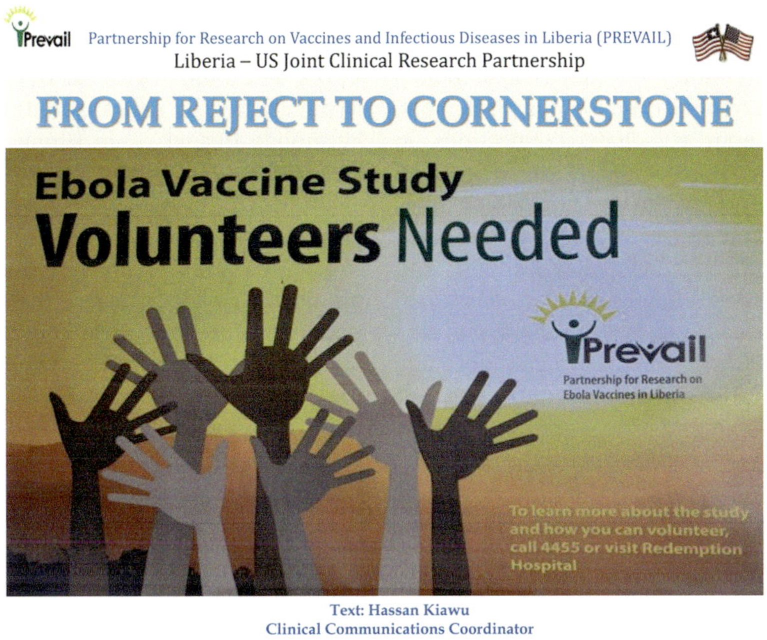

Fig. 1 PREVAIL presentation with poster seeking to recruit clinical study volunteers. (Courtesy U.S.-Liberia PREVAIL partnership)

In some cases, national governments may not be able to impose rule of law or enforce public health decisions. This was true to an extent in Liberia during the 2014–2016 West Africa Ebola outbreak and indeed in the United States during the COVID-19 pandemic. Blair et al. (2017) found that a high level of mistrust toward government correlated with lower compliance with disease-control measures; moreover, those who experienced hardship during the epidemic were less likely to trust the government. A national lack of response, or a heavy-handed one (e.g., curfews, quarantines, martial law), may alienate the affected population and create resistance to public health measures that can only be overcome with intense community engagement efforts (Calain and Poncin 2015; Chandler et al. 2015). Whatever the de facto strength of the national government, no response or research is likely to be carried out without its agreement, although Ooms and Hammonds (2014) point out some rare potential exceptions.

Assuming national government support for the research program, many questions arise:

- What memorandums of understanding or other written agreements are needed to define commitments, responsibilities, and joint undertakings? Who will negotiate and draft such documents?
- Does the national legislature need to take actions to provide a legal or regulatory framework or budgetary support for the proposed research?
- Does the national government need to strengthen its regulatory and ethical review capacity?
- How can state and non-state organizations, such as ministries with health-related portfolios, laboratories, pharmaceutical suppliers, hospitals, universities, and other health care institutions, be integrated into the research?

3.3 Higher Education

Universities, especially medical schools, can be valuable allies, particularly if they have research programs; they may also host a research ethics committee (REC) (▶ Chap. 33

and In Practice 33.1). They should be able to provide background on the overall disease burden in the country and may be able to help with clinical monitoring. Senior professors, many of whom will have connections in national government and with their local community or ethnic group, can lend credibility and help quell suspicions about the source of the epidemic, the emergency response, and research interventions. Medical students can fill staffing needs, and both students and faculty may seek research employment, especially if their institutions are closed during an epidemic (Carter et al. 2018). Moreover, collaboration helps build research capacity at partner institutions, improving future preparedness and creating openings for future collaboration (Sands et al. 2016). The relationship between the NIH, the government of Liberia, and the University of Liberia developed during the Ebola epidemic continues to benefit all parties and has sparked research beyond the initial vaccine trial.

3.4 Local Institutions

An immediate necessity for research planning is to assess potential research sites; these may be existing medical facilities, emergency treatment centers established by medical nongovernmental organizations (NGOs), or sites that must be adapted or rebuilt. Local government officials should be brought into the conversation early to build support for the research. Local leaders who are not part of formal government, including traditional and religious leaders, teachers, respected artists, performers, craftworkers, etc., can be very helpful in the conduct of research, as can local press. Leaders trusted by the community can lend credibility to messages that counter rumors and unfounded fears about the outbreak, response, and research—rumors that may have been spread by the press, social media, traditional healers, or parties involved in a conflict (Ives 2016; Spinney 2019). Trusted leaders and community members can also help craft and distribute tailored messages. In the case of Liberia, these included "print and electronic media through press releases, talk shows, and radio jingles," as well as "dialogue, written materials, songs, and dramas enacted by mobile theater … in simple English and local vernacular" (Doe-Anderson et al. 2016).

Violence rooted in hostility toward national and local government and the presence of paramilitary and criminal groups in the northeast DRC, where the August 2018 Ebola outbreak arose, was a concern throughout the 2018–2020 DRC Ebola response. Violence interrupted an Ebola therapeutics trial and hindered response efforts following health worker injuries and killings in targeted attacks on treatment centers (Ilunga Kalenga et al. 2019; Mulangu et al. 2019). Such violence often reflects deep-seated alienation on the part of vulnerable and often victimized populations (Nguyen 2019; Stearns 2012). While careful outreach may help secure safety for medical personnel, patients, and research participants, underlying problems cannot be resolved by a medical response or research program.

3.5 NGOs

International medical NGOs are indispensable for emerging and re-emerging infectious disease (EID) response and important partners in research. NGOs are likely to be treating patients and promoting transmission control measures before researchers can start trials. Their facilities are potential research sites. NGOs involved in emergency response have sometimes been leery of clinical research on unproven medical countermeasures (MCMs), which they may see as a coldly scientific and even commercial enterprise incompatible with their humanitarian mission. Randomly controlled trials (RCTs), some have suggested, unethically deny lifesaving medical interventions to patients in a placebo control arm (Adebamowo et al. 2014; Delisle et al. 2005; Levine 2016). After the successes of response research in the West Africa and DRC Ebola outbreaks, there was a growing willingness on the part of NGOs to cooperate with research teams (▶ In Practice 17.1 and In Focus 30.1). In any case, NGOs should be fully informed of research activities relevant to their response efforts.

Local NGOs, if they exist, can be particularly valuable because of their knowledge of the setting, language, culture, and infrastructure. In addition, they may operate clinics, hospitals, or laboratories that could host research, assist with recruitment of research participants and staff, provide logistical support, or help with other tasks where local knowledge is needed.

3.6 Contractors

International or in-country contractors with research management, logistics, security, construction, staffing, or emergency response expertise can often act more quickly than governments to hire experienced personnel and get them into the field. Still, contract negotiation during the Ebola epidemic in West Africa seriously delayed the beginning of some trials (Lang 2015). Contractors already supporting clinical research, if available, bring the additional advantages of experience, access to materiel, and often a flexible hiring mechanism. To the extent qualified local contractors are available, they will come with better knowledge of the immediate environment and very likely lower costs, as well as the potential for building local support by providing employment.

Contractors played an important role during the West Africa Ebola epidemic and the more recent outbreaks in the DRC. NIH contractors based primarily in the United States brought needed logistical, communications, laboratory, and transportation skills and did not require lengthy procurement processes because their contracts were already in place. In-country contractors were especially helpful for construction; hiring, training, and management of local staff; and social mobilization and communication.

3.7 Pharmaceutical, Device, or Diagnostic Companies

While clinical trial protocols will define scientific questions, methodology, and procedures, pharmaceutical, device, or diagnostic companies also play an essential role in many studies. Medical interventions will usually require purchased or donated products and related scientific data and documentation, from the firms that develop, manufacture, and distribute them. In addition to agreements on product supplies, clear communications with points of contact at the company and any relevant subunits or contractors become especially vital in an emergency response. On-site pharmacies are needed to receive, prepare, and distribute products and supplies (▶ Chap. 38).

From an operational standpoint, the following questions will need to be answered regarding the companies and products:

- Are the products investigational or licensed? How will this impact the research timeline?
- Will the products be donated or purchased? If the products are purchased, are financial resources sufficient?
- Are there sufficient inventories, or are supplies dependent on manufacturing schedules or otherwise limited?
- Who is responsible for delivery of the products to research sites? Is a cold chain required?
- Do the products entail other supply needs (e.g., freezers, temperature monitors, biosafety cabinets, etc.)?
- Is clinical trial insurance or indemnification necessary to protect pharmaceutical companies, research collaborators and staff, and research participants (▶ In Focus 32.2).

4 Organizational Requirements

The research team must accomplish four interdependent tasks to establish a support structure. The team must execute necessary agreements and develop three basic management tools: an organization chart, timeline, and budget. The process will vary with the circumstances and should not be expected to end before the research project itself—all these elements can change as the work progresses, activities scale up, and unanticipated difficulties are resolved.

4.1 Formalize Needed Agreements

Negotiated agreements, even interim or tentative ones, are essential for avoiding misunderstandings, shaping viable partnerships, and providing clarity about fundamental organizational and research issues. High-level bilateral and multilateral agreements between international entities and national governments establish basic understandings about the roles of the parties. These may cover, among other topics, financing; waiver of import and customs duties; logistics; data access; specimen collection, control, and destruction; research participant insurance or indemnification; ethics and regulatory oversight; the extended future of the research endeavor; provision of post-research vaccines, therapeutics, or other research products to affected research participants and communities; and authorization for foreign personnel to care for research participants. A good example is the scientific and technological cooperation agreement on the response to Ebola between the United States and Liberia signed in Monrovia on November 19, 2014. Lower-level agreements or memorandums of understanding between national and local bodies and organizations conducting the research can further delineate commitments (Cutts et al. 2006).

4.2 Create an Organization Chart

An organization chart is an essential document for sorting out and mapping relationships among individuals and sub-units of the research program. An administrative hierarchy identifies the key individuals leading the research and their roles (▶ Chap. 42). Ideally, there will be explicit pairings of national and international partners to strengthen collaboration, foster communications, and build local research capacity. Formally acknowledged parity between partners should boost team building and lessen potential tensions over external vs. local control (Cutts et al. 2006). The organization chart will clarify expected interactions between distant and local partners and, in part, determine communications needs. It will need to be updated to ensure that research organizational or personnel changes are reflected over the duration of the project. The chart and sub-charts are also planning documents for both hiring and day-to-day staffing schedules (◘ Fig. 2).

4.3 Develop a Research Timeline

A critical path timeline depends on the course of the outbreak, study design, and the expertise of the investigators (Kumar and Chakraborty 2016; NASEM 2017). It should be broken down by milestones, tasks, and subtasks, showing the parties responsible for them (i.e., a Gantt Chart), and should highlight interdependencies between tasks. Timeline milestones should serve as interim research goals. Like the organization chart, the timeline is a key document for research planning and implementation; it should be revisited frequently and revised as circumstances warrant.

4.4 Prepare a Budget

With an organization chart and timeline in place, preparing a line-item budget becomes feasible. The sequence of these tasks is iterative, in that a budget needs both direction from the top and reporting from the field to be a workable financial instrument. Financial contributors need to be consulted, especially if multiple funding sources have differing goals, obligations, and constraints. There are tools available to assist with building a budget (Global Health Network 2022; Nevens et al. 2019).

A key step in the budget process is preparation of participant enrollment projections

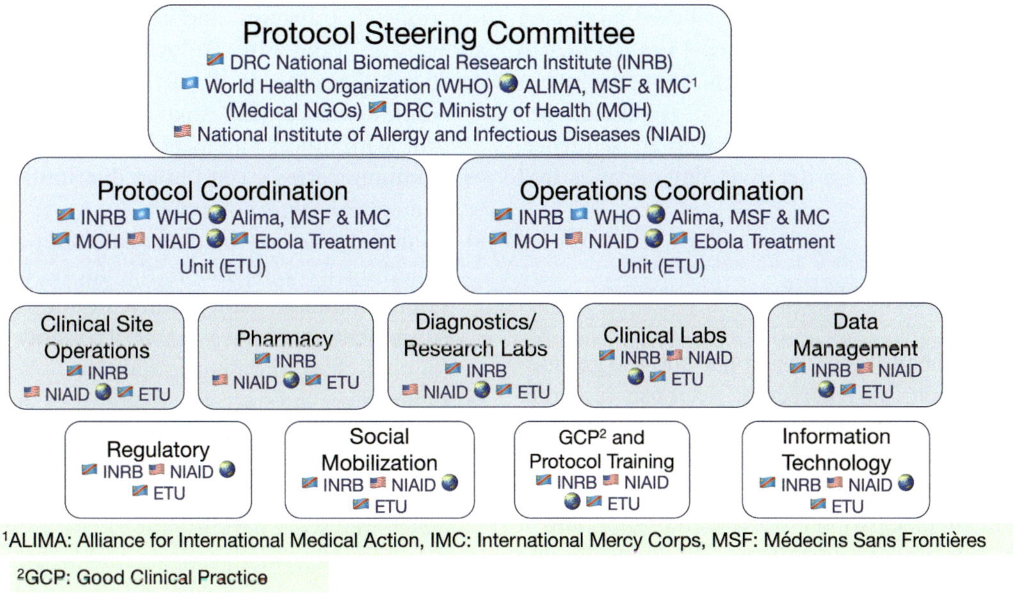

Fig. 2 In this organization chart, positions are shared between the DRC and NIAID, with representatives of other institutions included as appropriate. Institutions shown are likely to represented by different individuals in the various management groups. This is a sample draft chart by the authors modified for this chapter to illustrate the principle and does not necessarily reflect the actual organizational structure of the study. (Authors)

and visit schedules that can be meshed with per-visit compensation, yielding estimated cash requirements over time that can be integrated into the budget (Larson et al. 2017). Compensation for research participants can be a significant research cost. Other major line items include research staff lodging, per diem, and transportation needs; local hiring and payroll; equipment and supply purchases; shipping; leasing, renovating, or constructing facilities; local contracting; insurance; and communications. Funding must be nimble, and budget adaptations will be necessary as research scope and implementation evolve, the number of participants and research support staff varies, and key activities progress.

Ancillary documents for internal management of funds are also needed. They include a chart of accounts; procedures for local bidding and procurement; designation of individuals responsible for oversight, authorizations, and disbursements; and documentation requirements.

Finally, international and local banking arrangements must be set up. A local bank should be selected to process international and local money transfers, manage staff payroll, and ensure security when cash for participant compensation is disbursed. While electronic transfer of funds to participants is frequently proposed, it is not always feasible where participants are unfamiliar with such transfers (Carter et al. 2018).

5 Establish a Research Operations Center

A research operations center is an essential component. It may be limited to hosting administrative staff with management and communication responsibilities, or it may also include pharmaceutical and laboratory functions, data management, logistics, and participant clinical care. Its size, composition, and function depend on the scope of the research, the location of collaborators and potential research participants, the setting and infrastructure, financial resources and budget, etc. There is little discussion in the scientific literature of such operations centers for emergency response research, very likely due to their relative novelty. What follows is based largely on the authors' experience during the 2014–2016 Ebola outbreak in Liberia. Establishing a research operations center can be divided into three major steps, undertaken in sequence, although with an iterative dimension as well (► Chap. 40).

5.1 Assess Needs

Once the protocol design has laid the groundwork for the emergency response research, necessary agreements have been formulated, an organizational structure and timeline built, and a budget prepared, the crucial elements are in place to set up research sites and a research operations center. While ideally one would have full detail on the research requirements beforehand, operations center planning must begin as soon as possible during an emergency, requiring flexibility and a facility or facilities that can accommodate growth. More than any other single source of information, the research protocol will provide the planning team with the information it needs to prepare a detailed listing of the essential physical components needed for the research. These can include facilities for pharmacy functions, biosafety equipment, laboratory analysis, specimen collection and storage, data management, supply storage, triage space, robing and disrobing space for personal protective equipment, identification badging, secure disbursement for participant compensation, and participant recruitment and care facilities for baseline and follow-up visits. These components may all be in a centralized location, in dispersed locations, or in more remote locations (data management could be outside the country altogether).

5.2 Determine Functions and Synergies

Research needs and information about resources available in various locations will inform space and facilities requirements and decisions to concentrate or disperse functions. Efficiency may favor centralization of some functions if transport and communications allow. The range of co-located functions could include some, or all, of the following:

- Administrative and financial coordination, with offices and meeting space
- Communications, cell phone distribution, and conferencing equipment
- Pharmacy, device, or diagnostic support, including freezers and refrigerators, biosafety cabinets, temperature monitoring equipment, barcode readers, and storage for cold-chain shipping containers
- Laboratory support for diagnostics and clinical care, specimen collection, temperature-controlled specimen storage, barcode readers, portable equipment, lab tables, and workstations
- Supply receipt, management, and distribution, with adequate space and shelving for handling and storing a wide variety of research supplies and materials, power transformers, and generators
- Local or international procurement and distribution logistics
- Transportation, including drivers, vehicles, and fuel storage
- Data management coordination with provision for servers, barcode readers, tablets, laptops, printers, scanners, and paper forms
- Records repository for electronic or paper files
- Clinical site staff offices, informed consent rooms, and instruction space
- Security infrastructure, including guard force training and equipment, master keys and combinations, safes and vaults, locks, and secure rooms for participant compensation
- Identification badging equipment for staff and participants
- Triage and infection control capabilities, and participant care space

5.3 Choose a Location

When there has been sufficient determination of operations center functions, site assessments to choose its location can begin in earnest. Some information may be readily accessible at the outset to rapidly winnow alternatives, but other data, such as spatial patterns of disease prevalence and progress on social mobilization, may not yet be available. Consultation with research partners and other knowledgeable individuals on potential sites, followed by in-person visits, should consider the following questions:

- Are there existing facilities that can be quickly renovated or repurposed?
- Do the timeline and budget allow for the design and construction of new or substantially renovated facilities?
- Can synergies with other collaborators be realized at prospective sites?
- Are there political considerations that enhance or disqualify certain sites?
- Are there security considerations that enhance or disqualify certain sites?
- Will operations center functions be co-located with participant/clinical activities?
- Must the site be near air, water, or land transport?
- Must the site location be central to research facilities and clinical sites or close to collaborator facilities?
- Should the site accommodate fuel storage for generators or vehicles?
- Will spatial epidemiology, population mobility, and access to research participants influence the location?
- To what extent can staff be hired from the surrounding community?
- Is there a reliable clean water supply?
- Is the power supply sufficient and reliable, or will generators be needed?
- Is the communications infrastructure sufficient and reliable?

6 Implementation Checklist

It may be that clinical research "is now widely accepted as an essential element of the response to epidemics and preparedness" (Hall et al. 2019) and "research has to be embedded in the immediate response to an outbreak and not come as an afterthought" (Kelland 2015). That does not mean that obstacles have been swept away. The checklist below assumes that a great many difficulties will need to be overcome. It follows the same general order as the chapter text. Because each research endeavor will be unique, the checklist may or may not include the items required in particular cases, but it can be adapted to the user's needs.

Checklist

	NA	Pending	Done
3. Identify Potential Partners			
Assess Roles of International Organizations	☐	☐	☐
Assess Foreign Government Relationships	☐	☐	☐
Identify Diplomatic Assets	☐	☐	☐
Assess Roles of National Government and Agencies	☐	☐	☐
Assess Roles of Higher Education Institutions	☐	☐	☐
Assess Roles of Local Government and Organizations	☐	☐	☐
Establish Communication with Parties in Conflict Zones	☐	☐	☐
Assess Roles of International NGOs	☐	☐	☐
Assess Roles of National or Local NGOs	☐	☐	☐
Identify Potential International Contractors	☐	☐	☐

	NA	Pending	Done
Identify Potential Local Contractors	☐	☐	☐
Determine Pharma, Device, or Diagnostic Company Roles	☐	☐	☐
4. Organizational Structure			
4.1. Agreements			
High-Level			
Border Controls	☐	☐	☐
Security Clearances	☐	☐	☐
Financial Assistance	☐	☐	☐
Import, Customs, and Tax Waivers	☐	☐	☐
Data Access	☐	☐	☐
Specimen Collection, Custody, and Transfer	☐	☐	☐
Research Participant Insurance/Indemnification	☐	☐	☐
Medical Care and Evacuation of Research Personnel	☐	☐	☐
Conflict Resolution	☐	☐	☐
Ethics/Regulatory Oversight	☐	☐	☐
Post Emergency Research	☐	☐	☐
Post Emergency Vaccines, Therapeutics, Devices, Diagnostics	☐	☐	☐
Lower-Level			
Local Governments	☐	☐	☐
Local Contractors	☐	☐	☐
Tribal, Sectarian, Ethnic, and Community Entities	☐	☐	☐
4.2. Organization Chart			
Determine Overall Governance of Research	☐	☐	☐
Build Administrative/Research Relationships	☐	☐	☐
Identify Relevant External/Internal Parties	☐	☐	☐
Identify and Pair Key External/Internal Individuals	☐	☐	☐
Integrate Working Groups	☐	☐	☐
4.3. Develop a Research Timeline			
Define Major Tasks/Milestones	☐	☐	☐
Define Critical Path/Dependencies	☐	☐	☐
Assign Responsible Parties	☐	☐	☐
Integrate Important Time/Schedule Considerations	☐	☐	☐
Create Timeline	☐	☐	☐
4.4. Prepare a Budget			
Prepare Line-Item Budget	☐	☐	☐
Integrate Funding Sources and Timing	☐	☐	☐

	NA	Pending	Done
Develop Participant Enrollment and Visit Projections	☐	☐	☐
Determine Participant Compensation	☐	☐	☐
Develop Ancillary Budget Documents	☐	☐	☐
Complete Banking Arrangements	☐	☐	☐
5. Establish a Research Operations Center			
5.1. Assess Needs			
Establish Multi-Disciplinary Team	☐	☐	☐
Review Research Protocol/Design Requirements	☐	☐	☐
Identify Essential Research Components	☐	☐	☐
5.2. Determine Functions and Synergies			
Administrative Coordination	☐	☐	☐
Financial Coordination	☐	☐	☐
Communications	☐	☐	☐
Pharmacy, Device, or Diagnostic Support	☐	☐	☐
Laboratory Support	☐	☐	☐
Supply Receipt and Management	☐	☐	☐
Procurement	☐	☐	☐
Distribution Logistics	☐	☐	☐
Transportation Support	☐	☐	☐
Data Management	☐	☐	☐
Records Repository	☐	☐	☐
Clinical Space Needs	☐	☐	☐
Identification Badging	☐	☐	☐
Security	☐	☐	☐
Clinical Triage	☐	☐	☐
Participant Care	☐	☐	☐
5.3. Choose a Location			
Space Needs Have Been Determined	☐	☐	☐
New or Substantially Renovated Facility	☐	☐	☐
Existing As-Is Facility, Minimal Alteration	☐	☐	☐
Possible Siting Synergies with Collaborators Identified	☐	☐	☐
Political Considerations Identified	☐	☐	☐
Security Considerations Identified	☐	☐	☐
Colocation of Operations and Clinical Care Functions	☐	☐	☐
Proximity to Air, Water, or Land Transport Infrastructure	☐	☐	☐
Centrality to Other Research and Medical Facility Locations	☐	☐	☐

	NA	Pending	Done
Fuel Supply and Storage	☐	☐	☐
Spatial Epidemiology/Access to Research Participants	☐	☐	☐
Fulfillment of Staffing Needs	☐	☐	☐
Review Social Mobilization Activity	☐	☐	☐
Access to Water Supply Infrastructure	☐	☐	☐
Access to Power Supply Infrastructure	☐	☐	☐
Access to Communications Infrastructure	☐	☐	☐

? Discussion Questions

1. Would you be interested in joining an international research and emergency treatment program in an impoverished region of a developing country? Why? Why not?
2. What do you think is the most difficult part of setting up such an operation in the middle of an infectious disease outbreak?
3. How well do you think the rich nations of the world handled the breakout and spread of COVID-19? What did we learn from it?
4. Can you get true informed consent from a person who may be illiterate, impoverished, and uninformed about present-day medicine?

References

Adebamowo C, Bah-Sow O, Binka F, Bruzzone R, Caplan A, Delfraissy J-F, et al. Randomised controlled trials for Ebola: practical and ethical issues. Lancet. 2014;384(9952):1423–4. https://doi.org/10.1016/S0140-6736(14)61734-7.

Allen T, Murray KA, Zambrana-Torrelio C, Morse SS, Rondinini C, Di Marco M, et al. Global hotspots and correlates of emerging zoonotic diseases. Nat Commun. 2017;8(1):1124. https://doi.org/10.1038/s41467-017-00923-8.

Blair RA, Morse BS, Tsai LL. Public health and public trust: survey evidence from the Ebola virus disease epidemic in Liberia. Soc Sci Med. 2017;172:89–97. https://doi.org/10.1016/j.socscimed.2016.11.016.

Bugin K, Woodcock J. Trends in COVID-19 therapeutic clinical trials. Nat Rev Drug Discov. 2021;20:254. https://doi.org/10.1038/d41573-021-00037-3.

Calain P, Poncin M. Reaching out to Ebola victims: coercion, persuasion or an appeal for self-sacrifice? Soc Sci Med. 2015;147:126–33. https://doi.org/10.1016/j.socscimed.2015.10.063.

Carter RJ, Idriss A, Widdowson M-A, Samai M, Schrag SJ, Legardy-Williams JK, et al. Implementing a multisite clinical trial in the midst of an Ebola outbreak: lessons learned from the Sierra Leone trial to introduce a vaccine against Ebola. J Infect Dis. 2018;217(Suppl_1):S16–23. https://doi.org/10.1093/infdis/jix657.

Chandler C, Fairhead J, Kelly A, Leach M, Martineau F, Mokuwa E, et al. Ebola: limitations of correcting misinformation. Lancet. 2015;385(9975):1275–7. https://doi.org/10.1016/S0140-6736(14)62382-5.

Cooper BS, Boni MF, Pan-ngum W, Day NP, Horby PW, Olliaro P, et al. Evaluating clinical trial designs for investigational treatments of Ebola virus disease. PLoS Med. 2015;12(4):e1001815. https://doi.org/10.1371/journal.pmed.1001815.

Cori A, Donnelly CA, Dorigatti I, Ferguson NM, Fraser C, Garske T, et al. Key data for outbreak evaluation: building on the Ebola experience. Philos Trans R Soc Lond B Biol Sci. 2017;372(1721) https://doi.org/10.1098/rstb.2016.0371.

Cutts FT, Enwere G, Zaman SMA, Yallop FG. Operational challenges in large clinical trials: examples and lessons learned from the Gambia pneumococcal vaccine trial. PLoS Clin Trials. 2006;1(3):e16. https://doi.org/10.1371/journal.pctr.0010016.

Delisle H, Roberts JH, Munro M, Jones L, Gyorkos TW. The role of NGOs in global health research for development. Health Res Policy Syst. 2005;3(1):3. https://doi.org/10.1186/1478-4505-3-3.

Doe-Anderson J, Baseler B, Driscoll P, Johnson M, Lysander J, McNay L, et al. Beating the odds: successful establishment of a phase II/III clinical research trial in resource-poor Liberia during the largest-ever Ebola outbreak. Contemp Clin Trials Commun. 2016;4:68–73. https://doi.org/10.1016/j.conctc.2016.06.008.

Global Health Network. Downloadable templates and tools for clinical research. Oxford: Global Health Training Centre; 2022. https://globalhealthtrials.tghn.org/articles/downloadable-templates-and-tools-clinical-research/. Accessed 26 Jan 2022.

Global Preparedness Monitoring Board. A world at risk: annual report on global preparedness for health emergencies. Geneva: Global Preparedness Monitoring Board; 2019.

Hall W, Jamieson A, Wardle G. Advancing epidemics R&D to keep up with a changing world: progress, challenges, and opportunities. London: Wellcome Trust; 2019.

Ilunga Kalenga O, Moeti M, Sparrow A, Nguyen V-K, Lucey D, Ghebreyesus TA. The ongoing Ebola epidemic in the Democratic Republic of Congo, 2018–2019. N Engl J Med. 2019;381(4):373–83. https://doi.org/10.1056/nejmsr1904253.

Ives M. When epidemics go viral. Atlantica. 18 Oct 2016.

Kaiser Family Foundation. The US government engagement in global heath: a primer. San Francisco: The Henry J. Kaiser Family Foundation; 2019. Contract No.: #8508-05.

Kazanjian P. Polio, AIDS, and Ebola: a recurrent ethical dilemma. Clin Infect Dis. 2020;70(2):334–7. https://doi.org/10.1093/cid/ciz662.

Kelland K. MERS, Ebola, bird flu: science's big missed opportunities. 2015.

Kumar A, Chakraborty BS. Application of critical path analysis in clinical trials. J Adv Pharm Technol Res. 2016;7(1):17–21. https://doi.org/10.4103/2231-4040.173263.

Lane HC, Marston HD, Fauci AS. Conducting clinical trials in outbreak settings: points to consider. Clin Trials (London, England). 2016;13(1):92–5. https://doi.org/10.1177/1740774515618198.

Lang T. Ebola: embed research in outbreak response. Nature. 2015;524(7563):29–31. https://doi.org/10.1038/524029a.

Larson GS, Baseler BR, Hoover ML, Pierson JF, Tegli JK, Johnson MP, et al. Conventional wisdom versus actual outcomes: challenges in the conduct of an Ebola vaccine trial in Liberia during the international public health emergency. Am J Trop Med Hyg. 2017;97(1):10–5. https://doi.org/10.4269/ajtmh.16-1015.

Levine AC. Academics are from Mars, humanitarians are from Venus: finding common ground to improve research during humanitarian emergencies. Clin Trials (London, England). 2016;13(1):79–82. https://doi.org/10.1177/1740774515617935.

Lurie N, Manolio T, Patterson AP, Collins F, Frieden T. Research as a part of public health emergency response. N Engl J Med. 2013;368(13):1251–5. https://doi.org/10.1056/nejmsb1209510.

Margesson R. International crises and disasters: U.S. humanitarian assistance response mechanisms. Washington, DC: Congressional Research Service; 2015. Contract No.: RL33769.

Medical Research Council. Developing and evaluating complex interventions. Swindon, Wilts: Medical Research Council; 2006.

Morand S, Walther BA. The accelerated infectious disease risk in the anthropocene: more outbreaks and wider global spread. BioRxiv. 2020; https://doi.org/10.1101/2020.04.20.049866.

Mulangu S, Dodd LE, Davey RT Jr, Tshiani Mbaya O, Proschan M, Mukadi D, et al. A randomized, controlled trial of Ebola virus disease therapeutics. N Engl J Med. 2019;381(24):2293–303. https://doi.org/10.1056/NEJMoa1910993.

NASEM. Integrating clinical research into epidemic response: the Ebola experience. Washington, DC: National Academies of Sciences Engineering and Medicine Publications, The National Academies Press; 2017.

Nevens H, Harrison J, Vrijens F, Verleye L, Stocquart N, Marynen E, et al. Budgeting of non-commercial clinical trials: development of a budget tool by a public funding agency. Trials. 2019;20(1):714. https://doi.org/10.1186/s13063-019-3900-8.

Nguyen V-K. An epidemic of suspicion—Ebola and violence in the DRC. N Engl J Med. 2019;380:1298. https://doi.org/10.1056/NEJMp1902682.

NIH. NIH clinical trials and you. Washington, DC: US National Institutes of Health; 2017. https://www.nih.gov/health-information/nih-clinical-research-trials-you/basics. Accessed 14 Feb 2020.

Ooms G, Hammonds R. Global constitutionalism, responsibility to protect, and extra-territorial obligations to realize the right to health-time to overcome the double standard (once again). Int J Equity Health. 2014;13:68. https://doi.org/10.1186/s12939-014-0068-4.

Sands P, Mundaca-Shah C, Dzau VJ. The neglected dimension of global security—a framework for countering infectious-disease crises. N Engl J Med. 2016;374(13):1281–7. https://doi.org/10.1056/nejmsr1600236.

Spinney L. Fighting Ebola is hard. In Congo, fake news makes it harder. Science. 2019; https://doi.org/10.1126/science.aaw6657.

Stearns J. North Kivu: the background to conflict in North Kivu province of eastern Congo. Usalama Project. London: Rift Valley Institute; 2012.

Thorlund K, Haggstrom J, Park JJ, Mills EJ. Key design considerations for adaptive clinical trials: a primer for clinicians. BMJ. 2018;360:k698. https://doi.org/10.1136/bmj.k698.

32.1 Case Study: Clinical Research Communications during an Outbreak: Media Outreach Supporting Liberia–U.S. Research Partnership

Hassan Kiawu and Laurie K. Doepel

Contents

Learning Track Note: This chapter appears in Learning Tracks: Emergency research response, research operations; Public health and epidemiology

E. S. Higgs and R. A. Sorenson (eds.), *Principles and Practice of Emergency Research Response*,
https://doi.org/10.1007/978-3-031-48408-7_48

1 Introduction

In October 2014, during the Ebola outbreak in West Africa that had spread to Liberia earlier that year, the Minister of Health and Social Welfare (MoH) of the government of Liberia, Walter T. Gwenigale, wrote to the U.S. Department of Health and Human Services (HHS) Secretary, Sylvia M. Burwell, proposing the establishment of a clinical research partnership to meet the urgent need to assess candidate medical countermeasures (MCMs) for their safety and efficacy against Ebola virus disease (EVD) (Kennedy et al. 2016; Prevail II Writing Group 2016). As described elsewhere in this volume, a bilateral agreement was signed soon after to establish the Partnership for Research on Ebola Virus in Liberia (PREVAIL). This agreement reflected the mutual commitment of the two countries to cooperation and shared responsibility. Overall responsibility rested with the Liberian MoH and the U.S. Ambassador to Liberia. Since its inception, the ongoing clinical research program, primarily funded by the U.S. National Institutes of Health (NIH), has been led by Liberian and U.S. scientists and clinicians (Massaquoi et al. 2016).

2 The Communications Pillar in PREVAIL's Social Mobilization and Communications Working Group

An initial organizational structure for PREVAIL was established that included a Social Mobilization and Communications (SMC) working group. The initial SMC team comprised four pillars:

- Advocacy
- Community engagement
- Communications
- Monitoring and evaluation

This case study briefly describes key considerations in the organization and functions of the PREVAIL SMC Communications Pillar during the first Ebola clinical trials conducted by PREVAIL.

2.1 Optimizing Media Messages

The success of PREVAIL in Liberia, a low-resource country with little clinical research experience before 2014, depended on a robust program of social mobilization, communications, and community engagement (SMC). SMC is broadly equivalent to good participatory practice (GPP), the term more often used outside Africa. Under either name, the purpose is to promote public understanding of clinical research, build trust in research program objectives, facilitate enrollment in clinical trials, and meet the ethical requirement that research participants be treated as partners in rather than subjects of research. The Communications Pillar was responsible for several unique and critical functions integral to the SMC team. These functions included

1. Conveying information about PREVAIL to the Liberian public through local and international media outlets
2. Ensuring that information disseminated to and through the media was accurate and appropriate for intended audiences
3. Promptly correcting misinformation and disinformation about PREVAIL and its research reported in the media or otherwise circulating publicly in Liberia or internationally
4. Highlighting significant progress achieved in PREVAIL clinical trials for local and global audiences
5. Assisting the SMC team, in collaboration with MoH health promotions team, to develop messages and materials regarding Ebola for pre-testing and subsequent dissemination to the public

The Communications Pillar was headed by co-leads from Liberia and from the United States and included up to four other members. Because the Liberian co-lead had been a reporter for the BBC during the country's civil war and subsequently had worked as a communications professional with a Liberia-based corporation, he already had extensive knowledge and contacts with the media in Liberia. This proved to be particularly valuable. Building trusted relationships with reporters and other news and information sources is critical for communication professionals involved in the research response during a public health emergency and proved especially valuable early on in correcting erroneous information about PREVAIL as reported by the media.

Although the Liberian co-lead had been educated in communications and worked as a journalist, he had no experience in science communications. The U.S. co-lead had complementary skills to her co-lead's in-country expertise: graduate-level training in science communications and a 30-year career writing for laypersons about biomedical research, primarily supported by the National Institute of Allergy and Infectious Diseases (NIAID) at NIH. In the early 2000s, she also had contributed communications expertise to a bilateral HIV clinical research project, Phidisa, between NIH and the South African military (Motumi et al. 2007).

While NIAID had been tapped by HHS to partner with Liberia in PREVAIL, another component of HHS, the Centers for Disease Control and Prevention (CDC), was preparing to launch a clinical trial of an experimental Ebola vaccine in neighboring Sierra Leone. To help harmonize communications about these two efforts, HHS public affairs staff initiated regular teleconferences with the research project communications teams from NIH and CDC to build cross-agency awareness and collaboration on best practices and lessons learned as the trials got underway.

Once the clinical infrastructure for PREVAIL had been built and staffed, the first urgent objective was to launch a randomized, placebo-controlled clinical trial of two experimental Ebola vaccines in Liberia to test their safety and efficacy. The first clinical trial, PREVAIL 1, was launched on February 2, 2015, shortly after the Liberian communications co-lead had been hired. PREVAIL did not have video or camera equipment at that time, but we requested and gratefully received support from U.S. Embassy public affairs staff, who took video and photographs of the initial trial launch and helped us disseminate the press release the PREVAIL team had prepared to describe it.

NIAID's communications office in Bethesda, Maryland, issued a complementary press release at the same time to its U.S. and international media contacts in coordination with the U.S. and Liberian co-leads for PREVAIL communications. The draft NIAID press release was initially vetted through the PREVAIL leadership and NIH and HHS experts. The main differences between the two releases were that the PREVAIL release was intended primarily for Liberian and African audiences. It featured Liberian scientists from PREVAIL and in-country spokespersons, such as the Liberia Minister of Health. The NIAID release included quotes from Liberian scientists and from Anthony Fauci, the NIAID Director, who became a primary U.S. government spokesperson on the Ebola pandemic (Fig. 1).

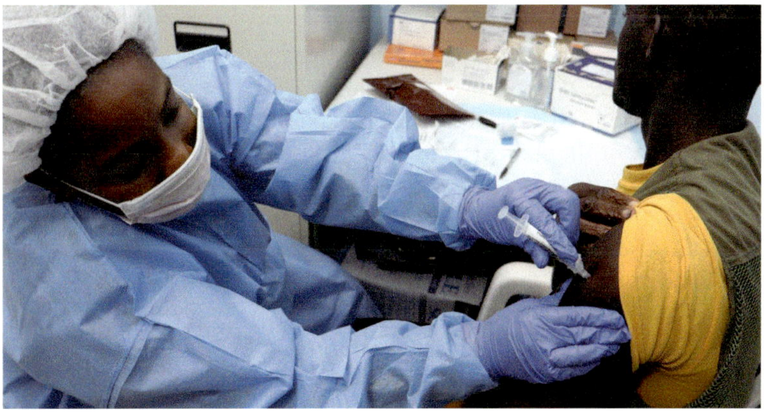

Fig. 1 A participant in the PREVAIL vaccine trial receiving an injection. (Credit: NIAID)

3 Key Considerations for the PREVAIL Communications Pillar

3.1 Establishing Relationships with Partner Organizations

The PREVAIL communications co-leads quickly built relationships with communications liaisons for key partner organizations, such as the U.S. Embassy, the Liberia MoH, other organizations managing the emergency response to the outbreak, and with reporters and news organizations. The U.S. Embassy was especially helpful in reviewing and helping to disseminate PREVAIL news releases. The Liberia MoH also reviewed PREVAIL news releases, and it was critical to coordinate with them the timing for launching certain studies or components of the studies so as not to jeopardize other ongoing or planned public health initiatives in Liberia, such as a measles immunization campaign. The Liberian communications co-lead's relationships with reporters were a key factor in correcting a serious error in the initial reporting about PREVAIL 1 that mischaracterized study participants' modest reimbursement for inconvenience and travel as unethical inducement.

3.2 Developing Standard Operating Procedures (SOPs) for Communications

We developed SOP checklists for communications activities and followed them to uphold the integrity of the clinical trials; to make processes as smooth as possible during the emergency response; and to involve all persons needed for review or oversight of a particular activity. Examples of SOPs developed by the PREVAIL Communications Pillar include

- Coordinate international media inquiries between the Liberia and U.S. communications co-leads to determine the best spokespersons.
- Develop and review PREVAIL news releases.
- Arrange for Liberia Ministry of Information, Culture, and Tourism (MICAT) press conferences.
- Obtain informed consent for patient interviews or filming requested by news media representatives. Note: The original informed consent form signed by the patient, their PREVAIL physician, and the media representative is filed in the patient's medical record, and the communications liaison was present during such interviews.
- Review, approve, and coordinate responses to requests by the media or others to tour PREVAIL facilities. Note: Media was always accompanied by the communications liaison when touring PREVAIL facilities to make sure no patient identifiers or off-limit areas or people are included in the filming.

3.3 Media Training Sessions

- *For in-country journalists*: Most Liberian journalists had no experience reporting on science, much less clinical research specifically. So early on, it was critical to hold media training sessions to familiarize reporters with PREVAIL, its overall mission, and its clinical research objectives. These sessions also offered an opportunity to describe how clinical research is conducted and how clinical trial results are evaluated. It also enabled us to introduce and familiarize reporters with the scientists leading PREVAIL. In these sessions, the communications liaisons and PREVAIL researchers explained the science in language understandable to non-scientist members of the public. Recurrent sessions were held before the introduction of each new clinical trial to give reporters a better understanding of what the trial was about before they reported on it.
- *For PREVAIL spokespersons*: Media training sessions were also used to allow Liberian scientists who would be spokespersons to practice describing the research and its

importance using language the public could understand. We anticipated difficult questions they might be asked and practiced with them how best to respond. The Liberian co-lead also provided additional coaching for spokespersons on how to address the media.

3.4 Arranging Media Interviews and Press Conferences

- The Liberia communications co-lead arranged for in-country press conferences conducted through the Ministry for Information, Culture, and Tourism. In consultation with the identified PREVAIL spokesperson(s), the communications staff prepared opening statements and talking points for the PREVAIL spokespersons and used these opportunities to disseminate PREVAIL news releases. Radio interviews were also arranged with PREVAIL scientists because in Liberia radio is the medium through which most people get their news.
- Because of scarce and unreliable Internet connectivity in Liberia at the time and the work and cost of creating a social media presence, a social media platform for PREVAIL was not initiated during the Ebola outbreak. PREVAIL has subsequently transitioned out of an emergency mode to a sustainable clinical research organization whose social media presence is being implemented.

3.5 Communications Principles for Spokespersons

- *Transparency*: Share what PREVAIL is doing and what has been learned in a timely manner.
- *Honesty*: Always be honest. Admit when you do not know something and always speak the truth, even if that might be uncomfortable or inconvenient.
- *Clarity*: Use clear, simple descriptions anyone can understand. Use language appropriate to Liberian culture. Communicate for understanding, and avoid using medical, technical, or public health jargon. Focus on what you say, what the public needs to understand about what PREVAIL is doing, and why it matters.

4 Conclusion

As indicated by the Liberia experience, high-quality, rigorous clinical research can be effectively implemented during outbreaks in countries with limited resources and minimal clinical research experience. However, the process must occur within the framework of a collaborative research partnership (such as PREVAIL), which employs robust and honest communication and social mobilization skills that strengthen ethical and regulatory systems, harness cultural competencies, and support the development of enhanced clinical research infrastructure and capacity.

Discussion Questions

1. List four pillars of PREVAIL's Social Mobilization and Communications (SMC) Working Group.
2. List and discuss the Communications Pillar's several unique and critical functions integral to the SMC team.
3. Key considerations for the PREVAIL Communications Pillar were (1) establishing relationships with key partner organizations, (2) developing SOPs and SOP checklists, (3) holding recurrent media training sessions, (4) arranging media interviews and press conferences, and (5) emphasizing key communication principles with spokespersons. Discuss how these considerations help to effectively implement rigorous clinical research during outbreaks in countries with limited resources and minimal clinical research experience, such as Liberia.

References

Kennedy SB, Neaton JD, Lane HC, Kieh MWS, Massaquoi MBF, Touchette NA, et al. Implementation of an Ebola virus disease vaccine clinical trial during the Ebola epidemic in Liberia: design, procedures, and challenges. Clin Trials (London, England). 2016;13(1):49–56. https://doi.org/10.1177/1740774515621037.

Massaquoi MBF, Kennedy SB, Tegli JK, Bolay FK, Kateh FN. Fostering collaboration on post-Ebola clinical research in Liberia. Lancet Glob Health. 2016;4(4):e239. https://doi.org/10.1016/S2214-109X(15)00323-X.

Motumi N, Emery S, Lane HC. Project Phidisa: development of clinical research capacity within the South African National Defence Force. Curr Opin HIV AIDS. 2007;2(1):69–76. https://doi.org/10.1097/COH.0b013e328011e9c0.

Prevail II Writing Group. A randomized, controlled trial of ZMapp for Ebola virus infection. N Engl J Med. 2016;375(15):1448–56. https://doi.org/10.1056/NEJMoa1604330.

32.2 In Focus: Clinical Trial Insurance and Indemnification

Gregg Larson

Contents

Learning Track Note: This chapter appears in Learning Tracks: Global Health Law; Emergency Research Response, Research Operations

E. S. Higgs and R. A. Sorenson (eds.), *Principles and Practice of Emergency Research Response*,
https://doi.org/10.1007/978-3-031-48408-7_49

Learning Objectives

This chapter will help readers understand and describe:

- The meaning of "insurance" and "indemnification" as applied to risk management during an emergency response
- How emergency response circumstances affect cost–risk analysis and allocation
- Why the commercial insurance market finds it difficult to estimate the risk associated with experimental interventions
- Alternative risk management strategies from the 2014–2016 Ebola epidemic in West Africa
- What assurances of healthcare or evacuation may be necessary to ensure recruitment of medical and research personnel during health emergencies

1 Background

When planning or conducting clinical research in an emergency response setting, there will be concerns about the allocation of costs from possible injuries or deaths that might be associated with the research. Administration of investigative vaccines, pharmaceuticals, or treatments poses potential risks to health, while history, inaccurate press coverage, or unsubstantiated rumors may engender perceived risk (Halabi et al. 2020; Halabi and Monahan 2015).

It is important to preface any discussion of risk management by defining two key terms that are often confused, insurance and indemnification. Both are forms of protection against financial loss due to a perceived risk, and both seek to compensate a verified affected party or restore it to its financial status prior to an occurrence that triggers a claim or liability (Gassner 2020; Halabi and Monahan 2015).

- **Insurance** will transfer risk from one party to another in exchange for an advance financial payment (the insurance premium), which may be paid by those at risk or by another party on their behalf. The insured party is protected from financial loss in accordance with the terms specified in the insurance policy.
- **Indemnification** allocates risk, usually between contracting parties, by altering the legal rights and obligations of the parties, with one party accepting all, or more, of the risk of loss than it would otherwise bear, on behalf of the other party.

2 Risk Management Alternatives and Allocation

There is a variety of alternatives for risk management in clinical trials. The level of risk, the scale of the emergency, applicable government laws and regulatory requirements, the amount of funding needed, the financial resources of sponsors and research partners, adherence to Good Clinical Practice and Good Participatory Practice (ICH 2016; WHO 2016, 2020) (▶ Chaps. 6 and 18), and ethical considerations can all influence the choice of a risk management alternative (▶ Chap. 5).

Participants in clinical trials customarily receive assurances of cost-free, standard-of-care treatment[1] for a research-related injury due to the intervention or to ancillary trial activities (e.g., blood tests, or an injury from a fall at the research site) (Steinbrook 2006). This commitment is usually set forth in the protocol and in the informed consent document reviewed with, and given to, trial participants. Trial sponsors (e.g., a pharmaceutical manufacturer, an educational institution, or a government agency) can either directly absorb these costs or, if they are unable or unwilling to do so, may transfer the financial risk. If sponsors choose to transfer the risk, they or another party can purchase clinical trial insurance in the commercial insurance market, or the sponsors can seek a party that will con-

1 There is of course a great deal of debate about what the standard of care is in various circumstances: is it the best care available in developed countries, the best care normally available locally, or the best care that can be provided locally given limitations in infrastructure, facilities, and personnel available (Lie et al. 2004; Schuklenk 2004)?

tractually agree to indemnification of the sponsor's risk. Advance determination of where treatment of research-related injuries will occur and arrangements to provide for reimbursement of treatment costs and compensation (if specified) will generally be needed for an insurance policy.

Emergency response circumstances can affect risk allocation choices. The commercial insurance market may find it difficult to estimate the risk associated with an intervention, and truncated safety testing may render sponsors or manufacturers more reluctant to accept responsibility for possible injuries (The Economist 2014), and local procedures for adjudicating claims may be unacceptable to sponsors or insurers. In such instances, government may step in to cover treatment or insurance costs or offer indemnification contracts to sponsors, especially if the manufacturer requires such coverage before providing the investigational product. Costs could be borne directly by a government, or possibly by a dedicated funding source established with either budgetary allocations or capital from other sources (Henry et al. 2015). The U.S. government has had a long-standing mechanism for indemnification of claims brought in U.S. courts against vaccine manufacturers: the Public Readiness and Emergency Preparedness Act (PREP) (HHS/ASPR 2019). The U.S. Secretary of Health and Human Services authorized Ebola vaccine coverage under PREP in 2014 and did the same for COVID-19 vaccines in 2020 (Halabi and Monahan 2015). However, governments where emergency response research is likely, often in developing countries, may offer little or no protection for manufacturers, especially when the interventions are not licensed and government indemnification could unduly burden countries that lack financial resources (Ebola Vaccine Team B 2017).

Beyond treatment, compensation is seldom offered for injuries or deaths attributable to a clinical trial, especially after it has concluded (Steinbrook 2006). Such compensation could be demanded by national governments, by nongovernmental organizations (NGOs), or by local healthcare advocacy groups. Again, there are a variety of ways to address this risk (e.g., commercial insurance, indemnification contracts, or self-insurance funds), although all involve expenses that can be substantial. Establishing a compensation mechanism can also entail complex negotiations and processes for determinations of fault, attribution to a clinical trial intervention, cost of coverage, the period of coverage, levels of compensation, and dispute resolution.

3 Examples of Risk Management Alternatives

Some considerations with regard to these various risk management alternatives are illustrated in the following examples. The examples relate to both commercial insurance and self-funding of injury and death claims.

During the 2014–2015 Ebola epidemic in West Africa, research sponsors and the Sierra Leone government explored purchase of commercial insurance coverage for vaccine trial injury or death compensation. While the provision of insurance was expected to allay participant fears about the study, it also sparked "worried conversations about the likelihood that if the trial provided insurance it meant the trialists expected people to die in the process" (Enria et al. 2016).

The Liberian government wanted assurances of compensation for injury or death claims attributable to Partnership for Research on Ebola Vaccines in Liberia (PREVAIL) I vaccine trial participation and ancillary activities. Initial contacts with commercial insurance companies indicated that coverage would be expensive. A 2015 quote for PREVAIL I from the ACE Illinois Union Insurance Company estimated the annual cost at a minimum of US$65,000–$100,000, plus about $14.16 per participant over the first 1000 enrolled, depending on the amount of coverage and deductibles. Despite the cost, commercial insurance was attractive because it was competitive, was based on a large risk pool, and could be activated more quickly. Purchase of commercial liability insurance, however, was rejected because Liberian representatives lacked faith in the coverage and commitments offered by the international carriers (Larson et al. 2017).

Instead, Liberian representatives proposed a broad-scope, self-insurance fund based in Liberia. The fund would be capitalized by the U.S. government and pharmaceutical firms and would be managed by Liberia's National Social Security and Welfare Corporation, the government entity responsible for the administration of the country's social security system.

Both Liberia and the U.S. National Institutes of Health (NIH) engaged in lengthy negotiations to resolve differences regarding the source and amount of fund capitalization, the appropriate entity to adjudicate claims, third-party dispute arbitration, and another fundamental issue—the scope of coverage. The NIH supported coverage for study-related injuries but was unwilling to agree to Liberian requests for treatment and compensation for unrelated diseases that were diagnosed in research participants. Discussions continued as the PREVAIL study opened in late February 2015, but differences over the source and amount of capitalization, claims adjudication, dispute arbitration, and scope of coverage proved insurmountable. Initial PREVAIL I follow-up concluded in May 2016 without agreement but also without any subsequent trial claims of injury or death (Larson et al. 2017).

Early in the West African Ebola epidemic, the World Bank and some governments discussed emergency indemnification, but made no progress in developing an overall structure for clinical trials. Anticipating similar demands for liability compensation in future disease outbreaks, the World Bank launched a Pandemic Emergency Financing Facility (PEF) in 2017 to finance insurance funds and provide for more equitable risk-sharing (Ebola Vaccine Team B 2017; Gostin and Friedman 2015; World Bank 2019). PEF did not attract enthusiastic support from potential funders (Brim and Wenham 2019). However, the fund was activated three times between 2018 and 2019 for the ninth and tenth Ebola outbreaks in the Democratic Republic of the Congo at the request of its government, in the amount of US$61.4 million. In 2020, the PEF was again activated and allocated $195.84 million to 64 of the world's poorest countries for COVID-19. In these instances, the funds were intended for surge response in emergency outbreaks and did not provide for research liability financing (World Bank 2019).

4 Insurance for Medical and Research Personnel

Other insurance issues in emergency response research include in-country medical care and medical evacuation insurance for local and international medical and research personnel. Coverage may be based on an individual's personal health insurance, but policy language may limit the coverage, or insurers may add specific disease exclusions to new or renewal policies (Cohn et al. 2014). Ultimately, responsibility for gaps in medical care or evacuation insurance will likely rest with governments, NGOs, or institutions employing the research personnel that respond to the health emergency. Otherwise, it may be more difficult to recruit or reposition personnel for research settings absent such assurances of care or evacuation.

5 Conclusions

While we have sketched out some options and potential solutions above, much work remains to ensure adequate insurance and indemnity coverage for clinical research during an emergency in developing countries.

Discussion Questions

1. Define "insurance" and "indemnification" in the context of risk management during an emergency response.
2. Discuss how emergency response circumstances can affect choices of cost risk allocation.
3. What happens if the commercial insurance market finds it difficult to estimate the risk associated with an intervention?
4. Discuss the examples of alternative risk management strategies from the 2014–2015 Ebola epidemic in West Africa.

5. What assurances of care or evacuation may be necessary to ensure optimal recruitment and temporary re-assignment of medical and research personnel during health emergencies? Who can, or should, provide such assurances?

References

Brim B, Wenham C. Pandemic emergency financing facility: struggling to deliver on its innovative promise. BMJ 2019;367:l5719. https://doi.org/10.1136/bmj.l5719.

Cohn C, Naidu R, Das A. As virus spreads, insurers exclude Ebola from new policies. Reuters Business. 2014. https://www.reuters.com/article/idUSL3N0SG69X/. Accessed 24 July 2024.

Ebola Vaccine Team B. Completing the development of Ebola vaccines. Report. Minneapolis: University of Minnesota; 2017.

Enria L, Lees S, Smout E, Mooney T, Tengbeh A, Leigh B, et al. Power, fairness and trust: understanding and engaging with vaccine trial participants and communities in the setting up the EBOVAC-Salone vaccine trial in Sierra Leone. BMC Public Health. 2016;16(1):1140. https://doi.org/10.1186/s12889-016-3799-x.

Gassner S. Indemnities vs. insurances: do you understand the difference? Grosvenor Performance Group; 2020. https://www.grosvenor.com.au/resources/indemnities-versus-insurances-do-you-understand-the-difference/. Accessed 27 Jan 2020.

Gostin L, Friedman E. A retrospective and prospective analysis of the West African Ebola virus disease epidemic: robust national health systems at the foundation and an empowered WHO at the apex. Lancet. 2015;385(9980):1902–9. https://doi.org/10.1016/S0140-6736(15)60644-4.

Halabi S, Monahan J. Sharing the burden of Ebola vaccine related adverse events. Tulane J Int Comp Law. 2015;24:131.

Halabi S, Heinrich A, Omer SB. No-fault compensation for vaccine injury—the other side of equitable access to Covid-19 vaccines. N Engl J Med. 2020;383(23):e125. https://doi.org/10.1056/NEJMp2030600.

Henry L, Larkin M, Pike E. Just compensation: a no-fault proposal for research-related injuries. J Law Biosci. 2015;2(3):645–68. https://doi.org/10.1093/jlb/lsv034.

HHS/ASPR. PREP (Public readiness and emergency preparedness act). Washington, DC: Office of the Assistant Secretary for Preparedness and Response, US Department of Health and Human Services; 2019. https://www.phe.gov/Preparedness/legal/prepact/Pages/default.aspx. Accessed 25 Jan 2020.

ICH. Good clinical practice: ICH harmonised guideline. Integrated addendum to ICH E6(R1): guideline for good clinical practice ICH E6(R2) ICH consensus guideline. Geneva: International Council for Harmonisation of Technical Requirements for Pharmaceuticals for Human Use (ICH); 2016.

Larson GS, Baseler BR, Hoover ML, Pierson JF, Tegli JK, Johnson MP, et al. Conventional wisdom versus actual outcomes: challenges in the conduct of an Ebola vaccine trial in Liberia during the international public health emergency. Am J Trop Med Hyg. 2017;97(1):10–5. https://doi.org/10.4269/ajtmh.16-1015.

Lie RK, Emanuel E, Grady C, Wendler D. The standard of care debate: the Declaration of Helsinki versus the international consensus opinion. J Med Ethics. 2004;30(2):190–3. https://doi.org/10.1136/jme.2003.006031.

Schuklenk U. The standard of care debate: against the myth of an "international consensus opinion". J Med Ethics. 2004;30(2):194–7. https://doi.org/10.1136/jme.2003.006981.

Steinbrook R. Compensation for injured research subjects. N Engl J Med. 2006;354(18):1871–3. https://doi.org/10.1056/NEJMp068080.

The Economist Business. Giving it a shot. 2014. https://www.economist.com/business/2014/10/30/giving-it-a-shot. Accessed 25 January 2020.

WHO. Good participatory practice guidelines for trials of emerging (and re-emerging) pathogens that are likely to cause severe outbreaks in the near future and for which few or no medical countermeasures exist (GPP-EP). Geneva: World Health Organization; 2016. p. 53.

WHO. Good Participatory Practice for COVID-19 clinical trials—a toolbox. Geneva: World Health Organization; 2020.

World Bank. Pandemic emergency financing facility. Washington, DC: World Bank; 2019. https://www.worldbank.org/en/topic/pandemics/brief/pandemic-emergency-financing-facility. Accessed 15 Jan 2020.

33 Ethical Review of Clinical Research During an Emergency Response

Jerome F. Pierson

Contents

Learning Track Note: This chapter appears in Learning Tracks: Clinical Research; Research Ethics; Emergency Research Response, Research Operations

E. S. Higgs and R. A. Sorenson (eds.), *Principles and Practice of Emergency Research Response*,
https://doi.org/10.1007/978-3-031-48408-7_50

Learning Objectives

This chapter will help readers understand and describe:

- Core elements of ethical research during a pandemic response
- Ethical and scientific review requirements to ensure that risks to research participants are appropriately accounted for and minimized
- Primary responsibilities of research ethics committees and scientific and safety reviewers
- Organizations most likely to have the capacity to support and implement effective research response, including needed reviews, during disease outbreaks
- WHO MEURI process that provides guidance for the use of investigational products outside research and potential disadvantages of using investigational products this way
- Vulnerable populations whose special requirements researchers must consider when planning research

1 Introduction

This chapter focuses on the ethical review of clinical research implemented as part of an emergency response carried out in partnership between two countries. However, much of the material below could also apply to other partnerships. ▶ In Practice 4.2 discusses ethical review for the massive, worldwide research effort to understand and counter severe acute respiratory syndrome coronavirus 2 (SARS-CoV-2). As a matter of context, emergency research oversight requires a concerted effort by all partners involved to ensure that the entire process is well documented, well understood, and transparent. Oversight needs to be thorough, but that does not have to mean formal and bureaucratic. Lane et al. (2016) provide a roadmap for investigators and planners in an emergency research response that describes key considerations, including ethical ones, for planning and oversight in the emergency response setting.

Following the principles discussed in Lane et al. (2016) and in ▶ Chap. 4 in this volume, the design and implementation of the research should include the following:

1. The design of any research is done in partnership with officials, scientists, and physicians, including clinical investigators, as well as representatives of affected communities from the country or countries where the research program will be conducted. An assessment of existing research infrastructure in the host country is also essential for research planning, which may require ethical review training and capacity building.
2. All research designs undergo rigorous, independent scientific review to ensure their validity, including the plausibility of benefits from candidate vaccines, therapies, or other interventions.
3. Initial and continuing ethical review is conducted by Research Ethics committees (REC),[1] both in the host country and by the sponsoring institution(s), to ensure that the research protocol meets global ethical standards, takes local context into account appropriately, and complies with laws and regulations governing research in the country where research will occur and those of the sponsoring organization(s). The REC will also take into account one or more of the broadly accepted international guideline documents, like *Guidance for Managing Ethical Issues in Infectious Disease Outbreaks*; *International Ethical Guidelines for Health-Related Research Involving Humans*; and *Good Participatory Practice: Guidelines for Biomedical HIV Prevention Trials* (▶ Chaps. 4 and 5)

1 Research ethics committee (REC) is the preferred term in this book because it is more descriptive than the usual term used in the United States, institutional review board (IRB), as well as more familiar globally. Other frequently used terms in English include medical research ethics committee (MREC), research ethics board (REB), and human research ethics committee (HREC).

(CIOMS 2016; UNAIDS and AVAC 2011; WHO 2016, 2019).
4. When the study involves randomization to a masked intervention, whether a placebo or alternate medical countermeasure, initial and periodic review is undertaken by an independent Data and Safety Monitoring Board (▶ Chap. 23), with representation from the population affected by the outbreak, to ensure the safety of research participants and proper consideration and integration of host-country perspectives.
5. Research planners must commit to making the data supporting reported results broadly available as soon as practically possible.
6. From the outset, planners need to keep in mind other bodies that need to be involved in a review of the research (e.g., is a radiation safety committee or an institutional biosafety committee review needed).
7. The research must be scientifically and ethically acceptable to regulatory authorities who will ultimately be responsible for approval or licensing of interventions found to be safe and efficacious (▶ Chap. 6).

2 Scientific Review

While this chapter deals primarily with ethical review, independent assessment of the scientific basis for the research is no less essential. Indeed, research must be scientifically sound to be ethical in an emergency, for it would otherwise be diverting scarce resources to no useful purpose, as well as subjecting participants to risk without the likelihood of findings regulators will be able to use. So fundamental is this requirement that the first sentence of the first guideline in the widely respected (CIOMS 2016) guidelines is "the ethical justification for undertaking health-related research involving humans is its scientific and social value."

While the requirement for scientific review is not necessarily codified to the extent that REC requirements are, the REC depends on a formally constituted scientific review committee or another scientific peer review to assess the scientific rationale and design of the research. Scientific review is normally undertaken by a properly qualified committee of peers in the scientific discipline of the study, which evaluates the available pre-clinical and clinical data to ensure that risks to research participants are appropriately accounted for and minimized. The scientific review must include host-country representation to ensure that the planned research benefits the impacted community. Like RECs, scientific review bodies periodically reconvene to evaluate related literature and interim study results that may bear upon the relevance or safety of the study. This is an ongoing process to consider and recommend changes to the study if indicated by the findings or to recommend discontinuation in some circumstances.

Depending on the scope of an infectious disease outbreak, dialogue on study design may involve discussions at the level of the World Health Organization (WHO) and with other sponsoring governments or organizations. For example, in 2018, under the aegis of their Research and Development Blueprint, WHO convened an ad hoc expert consultation on clinical trials for Ebola therapeutics. Experts in trial design and infectious diseases from around the globe, including experts from the Democratic Republic of the Congo (DRC), where the country's most serious Ebola outbreak to date had begun in August 2018, discussed the merits of a proposed randomized controlled trial of Ebola therapeutic candidates (Mulangu et al. 2019; WHO 2018a). The transparency of this process generated confidence in the proposed research, both in the region affected by the outbreak and in the research community planning the implementation of the study.

3 Research Ethics Committee Review

The regulatory requirements for REC review are well codified in U.S. and other regulatory frameworks (Council of the European Union and European Parliament 2006; FDA 2023; HHS 2023; WHO 2020). The challenging part of the REC review process, especially in multinational research with more than one sponsoring organization, is determining precisely what REC reviews are required. Ethical review in accordance with the laws and regulations of the country or countries where the research will take place is indispensable. In the case of EID outbreak research, that often means places where the health systems, very likely under-resourced in any case, are stressed well beyond capacity. In addition, many institutions require that the RECs overseeing their research review the research if their staff or faculty are actively engaged in any given research project, at the very least for the portion of the research in which their researchers are participating. If, for example, a clinical research study is funded or linked to funding with U.S. federal funds, then U.S. requirements apply—that is, review by an appropriately constituted REC in the United States with authority to oversee the research in the setting where it takes place. In the case of research sponsored in whole or part by a U.S. institution that uses federal funding, the REC must be registered with the HHS Office for Human Research Protections and approved for a Federal-Wide Assurance for the partner research institution (HHS 2023).

Thus, multiple RECs may need to approve the research. Multiple reviews and revisions may strengthen the scientific and ethical rigor of the research program and the safety of participants but obviously have the potential to generate confusion and delay. Aside from multiple committees that must meet their deadlines, they could make incompatible stipulations that require further time and effort to resolve. Research teams must be aware of the various national and institutional requirements—another reason for the necessity of collaboration with in-country investigators. Online tools such as the NIH ClinRegs Web site (NIAID 2023) and the European Clinical Research Information Network (2023) are platforms used to access, analyze, and compare requirements in selected countries. Further work to extend the coverage of such platforms is one of many seldom-mentioned actions needed to improve global preparedness for emergency research response (NASEM 2017).

In addition to planning for multiple REC reviews, it is important to consider the potential pool of research participants. Research that may involve potentially vulnerable populations such as children, pregnant women, or prisoners has special requirements that investigators must consider in planning their research. The CIOMS (2016) guidelines, to take one example, include a chapter on research involving vulnerable people, which is introduced by a strong normative statement: "When vulnerable individuals and groups are considered for recruitment in research, researchers and research ethics committees must ensure that specific protections are in place to safeguard the rights and welfare of these individuals."

While an emergency response to an outbreak is a less-than-optimal time to embark on REC capacity building, it is surely a test of the adequacy and adaptability of existing ethical review capacity in the country of the outbreak and the ability of its medical system to rise to the challenge. The lessons of the emergency experience should become the basis for sustainable, long-term planning to build medical ethics expertise and corresponding institutional structures (► In Practice 33.3).

Longer-term capacity building aside, a REC in the country where emergency research will be conducted may need more immediate guidance on critical ethical considerations for the research. One approach used in the response to the 2014–2016 West Africa Ebola outbreak was the provision of meeting minutes from the National Institute of Allergy and Infectious Diseases (NIAID) IRB to the newly established Liberian National Research Ethics Board (► In Practice 33.1). The minutes documented the controverted issues considered by the NIAID IRB and in effect provided the Liberian REC with a shortcut through the discussion of the more general ethical issues, allowing them to proceed more quickly to consideration of the local context when evaluating the risks and benefits of the proposed research.

4 Regulatory Mechanisms for Investigation of Unlicensed Medical Interventions

While ► Chap. 6 focuses on regulatory factors for the conduct of research on investigational medical countermeasures (MCMs) in an outbreak setting, the policy guidance of research funders must also be considered. For example, while research on investigational products conducted outside the United States is not typically subject to the requirements of the U.S. Food and Drug Administration (FDA), it has been common practice at NIAID to conduct research with an FDA Investigational New Drug (IND) approval when applicable. As such, planners need to provide sufficient time in the planning horizon for review by the applicable regulatory bodies. Timelines for reviews such as this, both in the United States and internationally, typically span months versus weeks.

Regarding the policy position of NIAID and international research with investigational drugs, an understanding of the organizational link between NIAID and FDA provides a window into the potential synergy from their common U.S. Department of Health and Human Services (HHS) lineage. As related organizations, they have the common goal of advancing overall U.S. response to disease outbreaks and work collaboratively on U.S. government inter-agency teams, discussing the merits of various products and the associated study designs. Moreover, FDA works with multinational pharmaceutical partners and countries where outbreaks occur to ensure that all parties are informed about and support any necessary FDA assistance to the nascent regulatory bodies reviewing dossiers associated with investigational drug and vaccine studies. (The role of stringent regulatory authorities in capacity building is described in greater detail in ► Chap. 6.)

Similar procedural requirements will apply when WHO or other developed-country sponsors are supporting or overseeing the research. WHO has a procedure called Emergency Use Listing (EUL), which covers investigational use of new products (WHO 2019) and is primarily intended for use in Public Health Emergencies of International Concern (PHEIC). Another WHO process that may need to be considered in the research context is called Monitored Emergency Use of Unregistered and Investigational Interventions (MEURI), which provides guidance for use of investigational products outside research—when, for example, there is impetus to use unlicensed products during a high-mortality outbreak like Ebola (WHO 2018b).

5 Institutional Biosafety Committees

For research involving recombinant or synthetic nucleic acid molecules, consideration of an institutional biosafety committee (IBC) is also required, according to NIH guidelines (NIH 2019). This requirement is substantially more challenging for outbreak countries to comply with but it was effectively satisfied during the 2014–2016 West African Ebola outbreak. As the concepts associated with convening an IBC are not universally understood and rarely practiced in resource-limited settings, uncommon solutions were sought to comply with the requirement. The executive secretary of the NIH Intramural IBC invited representatives from West Africa to take part in a conference call meeting with the IBC. The combined group was chartered as a new entity responsible for the protection of the research participants, study team, and local community from any potentially adverse consequences of the spread of replicating portions of one of the vaccines used in the first Partnership for Research on Ebola Vaccines in Liberia (PREVAIL) study (Kennedy et al. 2017). The collective discussion provided all parties with a better understanding of the challenges associated with the conduct of the trial in that setting and resulted in a better appreciation of the relative risks associated with the vaccine in the environment where the study took place. While the role of the IBC is tied directly to funding from the NIH in the United States, those funded by other sources should consult directly with respective funders about any such requirements.

6 Conclusion

Navigating the labyrinth of reviews required to initiate clinical research can seem an overwhelming task. Establishing a pathway for a clinical research study during an epidemic is even more daunting. However, embarking on that path with realistic expectations and a sound project management approach can reduce frustrations and delays and ensure that all reviews achieve their overall regulatory purpose of protecting research participants. As noted, the review process may seem overly bureaucratic at times. In emergency response, a degree of creative adaptability may be essential, but such creativity must be applied to satisfy essential ethical requirements, not to skirt them. However fraught the circumstances, researchers should never lose sight of their goal: ethically and scientifically sound research that leads to better medical care for people suffering from disease.

? Discussion Questions

1. Why do clinical trials need to be reviewed for compliance with ethical and scientific standards?
2. What platforms are available for accessing, analyzing, and comparing national and institutional regulatory requirements in selected countries?
3. What might make a social group or population especially vulnerable, so that researchers need to consider their special circumstances in research planning and review?
4. What organizations have roles in supporting and implementing research response to disease outbreaks?
5. What is the WHO process that provides guidance for use of investigational products outside research? What are the potential disadvantages of using experimental products outside a research setting?

References

CIOMS. International ethical guidelines for health-related research involving humans. Geneva: Council for International Organisations of Medical Sciences; 2016.

Council of the European Union, European Parliament. Decision No. 1982/2006/EC of the European Parliament and of the Council of 18 December 2006 concerning the seventh framework programme of the European Community for research, technological development and demonstration activities (2007–2013). Luxembourg: The Publications Office of the European Union; 2006.

European Clinical Research Information Network. European Clinical Research Information Network. 2023. http://campus.ecrin.org. Accessed 27 Jan 2023.

FDA. Institutional review boards (IRBs) and protection of human subjects in clinical trials. Silver Spring, MD: U.S. Food and Drug Administration; 2023. https://www.fda.gov/about-fda/center-drug-evaluation-and-research-cder/institutional-review-boards-irbs-and-protection-human-subjects-clinical-trials. Accessed 27 Jan 2023.

HHS. Office for Human Research Protections. Washington, DC: U.S. Department of Health and Human Services; 2023. https://www.hhs.gov/ohrp/. Accessed 27 Jan 2023.

Kennedy SB, Bolay F, Kieh M, Grandits G, Badio M, Ballou R, et al. Phase 2 placebo-controlled trial of two vaccines to prevent Ebola in Liberia. N Engl J Med. 2017;377(15):1438–47. https://doi.org/10.1056/NEJMoa1614067.

Lane HC, Marston HD, Fauci AS. Conducting clinical trials in outbreak settings: points to consider. Clin Trials (London, England). 2016;13(1):92–5. https://doi.org/10.1177/1740774515618198.

Mulangu S, Dodd LE, Davey RT Jr, Tshiani Mbaya O, Proschan M, Mukadi D, et al. A randomized, controlled trial of Ebola virus disease therapeutics. N Engl J Med. 2019;381(24):2293–303. https://doi.org/10.1056/NEJMoa1910993.

NASEM. Integrating clinical research into epidemic response: the Ebola experience. Washington, DC: National Academies of Sciences Engineering and Medicine Publications, The National Academies Press; 2017.

NIAID. ClinRegs: aggregating clinical research regulations from around the globe. 2023. https://clinregs.niaid.nih.gov/. Accessed 27 Jan 2023.

NIH. NIH guidelines for research involving recombinant or synthetic nucleic acid molecules. Washington, DC: U.S. National Institutes of Health, Office of Science Policy; 2019.

UNAIDS, AVAC. Good participatory practice: guidelines for biomedical HIV prevention trials. Geneva: UNAIDS (Joint United Nations Programme on HIV/AIDS); 2011.

WHO. Guidance for managing ethical issues in infectious disease outbreaks. Geneva: World Health Organization; 2016.
WHO. WHO R&D Blueprint: ad-hoc expert consultation on clinical trials for Ebola therapeutics: deliberations on design options for randomized controlled clinical trials to assess the safety and efficacy of investigational therapeutics for the treatment of patients with Ebola virus disease. Geneva: World Health Organization; 2018a.
WHO. WHO supports Ebola vaccination of high risk populations in the Democratic Republic of the Congo. 2018b. https://www.who.int/news/item/21-05-2018-who-supports-ebola-vaccination-of-high-risk-populations-in-the-democratic-republic-of-the-congo.
WHO. Yellow fever. Geneva: World Health Organization; 2019. https://www.who.int/news-room/fact-sheets/detail/yellow-fever. Accessed 23 Jan 2020.
WHO. Ethics review committee: review process. Geneva: World Health Organization; 2020. https://www.who.int/ethics/review-committee/review_process/en/. Accessed 20 Jan 2020.

33.1 In Practice: Ethical Review During Emergencies: The Liberian Experience

Fatorma Bolay and Robert A. Sorenson

Contents

Learning Track Note: This chapter appears in Learning Tracks: Research Ethics; Emergency Research Response, Research Operations

E. S. Higgs and R. A. Sorenson (eds.), *Principles and Practice of Emergency Research Response*,
https://doi.org/10.1007/978-3-031-48408-7_51

Fatorma Bolay was Director of the Liberia Institute for Biomedical Research when he passed away in March 2021. He reviewed a near-final version of this text before his death, but some subsequent changes have been made by the editors.

Learning Objectives

This chapter will help readers understand and describe:

- Ethical review guidelines and implementation challenges during EID emergencies, especially in low-resource countries experiencing social disruption.
- How the agencies responsible quickly built ethical review capacity in Liberia during the West Africa 2014–2016 Ebola epidemic and what training was required.
- Factors that facilitated an agile response by the National Research Ethics Board of Liberia to the re-emergence of the Ebola virus in 2015.

1 Emergency Ethics Review

Ethical review for clinical research, always a careful exercise in balancing inviolable human subject protections with potential risks of novel medical interventions, faces heightened challenges in an infectious disease emergency like the 2014–2016 Ebola outbreak in West Africa (▶ Chap. 5). Strong pressures to mitigate morbidity and mortality and stop disease transmission combine with resource shortages and disorganization common to emergencies to present an ethics review board with tough choices that need quick decisions. The task is even more difficult when a country like Liberia—with little research capacity and institutions still recovering from a long civil war—is suddenly faced with an epidemic that threatens its social fabric (NASEM 2017). Even during the 2003 outbreak of SARS in Toronto, clinical researchers noted that slow approvals from research ethics boards had resulted in "delays and missed opportunities" (Muller et al. 2004).

2 Ethical Review Capacity in Liberia Before the 2014–2016 Ebola Outbreak

After 14 years of civil war in Liberia, the Liberia Institute for Biomedical Research (LIBR) reestablished its Institutional Review Board (IRB, equivalent to REC or Research ethics committee) to support health research in 2007. While the LIBR IRB was rebuilding its capabilities with partners dedicated to improving research and ethical review capacity in Africa,[1] it had only undertaken two protocol reviews of research proposals before the Ebola outbreak struck in 2014. Since Liberia had no official national ethical review body, continual requests soon followed for the LIBR IRB to conduct ethical reviews of research proposals that would not otherwise have involved LIBR. In response, the Liberian Ministry of Health and Social Welfare (MOH) recognized the LIBR IRB as the official IRB for the MOH, with a name change to the National Health Science and Research Ethics Committee (NHSRC). At that time there was another nascent ethical review board known as UL PIRE, a collaborative agreement between the University of Liberia and the Atlantic Center for Research & Evaluation (PIRE) based in the United States (UL-PIRE 2012).

3 Ethical Review During the EVD Outbreak

On March 30, 2014, the first two Ebola virus disease (EVD) cases were confirmed in Liberia, and on April 7 the first EVD case was confirmed in the capital, Monrovia; many additional cases soon followed (WHO 2015). During the EVD outbreak, the NHSRC was

1 Partners included the Pan African Bioethics Initiative (PABIN), Strategic Initiative for Developing Capacity in Ethical Review (SIDCER), and Mapping African Research Ethics Review Capacity (MARC).

reconstituted and directed to conduct Ebola-related ethical reviews. Board members included epidemiologists, clinicians, sociologists, anthropologists, public health experts, religious and local community elders, and other subject matter experts as the need arose. Many of the members, although experts in their own fields, had little or no experience with ethical review of research proposals.

In order to legitimize the newly reconstituted NHSRC, which became the National Research Ethics Board (NREB) in December 2014, the Ministry of Health issued official appointment letters to the members pending national legislation. NREB members immediately began to undertake training, supported by NIH and WHO, on principles of research ethics in complex emergencies, concentrating on expedited protocol review, amending protocols, protocol resubmission, protocol continuation, etc. Thanks to the training and institution-building supported by NIH and WHO, Liberia quickly built capacity to carry out ethical reviews during the Ebola outbreak.

4 Ebola Outbreak Response

In collaboration with the World Health Organization, UNICEF, and the U.S. Centers for Disease Control and Prevention (CDC), the Liberia MOH first initiated response measures that included public health interventions, sanitary protections, contact tracing, and isolation to hinder the spread of infection. In August 2014, the MOH requested research cooperation from the U.S. Department of Health and Human Services, resulting in a collaboration between the Liberian MOH and the U.S. National Institute of Allergy and Infectious Diseases (NIAID). The first clinical trial of this partnership to undergo ethical review by the reconstituted NREB was the PREVAIL-1 vaccine study, a phase 2 randomized clinical trial testing two vaccines (rVSV-ZEBOV and ChAd3-EBO-Z) against a placebo in a total of 1500 participants (Kennedy et al. 2017) (▶ Chap. 17).

5 November 2015 Cluster Study

After Liberia was first declared Ebola-free in May 2015, the virus resurfaced in June and November 2015. In the November case, a 15-year-old boy and two additional family members were diagnosed with Ebola (WHO 2016). Based on interim results from cluster trials (also known as ring trials) in Guinea (Henao-Restrepo et al. 2015), a modified protocol for a single-arm cluster vaccination trial using the rVSV-ZEBOV vaccine came to the NREB with a request for approval within 2 days, given the urgency of ensuring that the re-emergence of the Ebola virus remain limited (Bolay et al. 2019; Henao-Restrepo et al. 2017). The NREB demonstrated how it had evolved into a functional, effective body by ensuring compliance with ethical principles under the deadline. This made it possible for the amended study to begin vaccinating contacts just 4 days after the new protocol was received. While the virus reappeared once more in Liberia, in March–April 2016, the NREB approval speeded the cluster vaccination response and Liberia's subsequent Ebola-free status. The governance of ethical practices at the National Research Ethics Board of Liberia (NREB) continues to evolve as the types of review and structures for monitoring research ethics in Liberia have evolved in parallel with the types and quantity of research conducted over the last several years.

In the post-Ebola period, the NREB made significant strides in the protection of human subjects in research and the review of rigorous clinical trials, ensuring the safety of research participants in line with best practices for upholding ethical norms. The NREB has also continued with human resource development at the national and international levels; over the last 5 years, NREB members have benefited from both local and international training in research ethics, bioethics, and research conducted in emergency settings. Nevertheless, capacity strengthening must continue, as well as work on clear definition of objectives and functions, particularly in the context of post-Ebola changes in the Liberian health sector.

Discussion Questions

1. How do ethical review guidelines apply, and how is their implementation more complex, during emergency response research in low-income countries experiencing social unrest?
2. Many National Research Ethics Board (NREB) members during the Liberia Ebola epidemic of 2014 were experts in their own fields but had little experience with ethical review of research proposals. What agencies and what training helped build ethical review capacity during the Ebola outbreak?
3. Liberia was first declared Ebola-free in May 2015, but the virus resurfaced later in the same year. To limit the re-emergence of the Ebola virus, NREB approved a modified protocol for a single-arm cluster vaccination trial using the rVSV-ZEBOV within 2 days. What factors were crucial to this agile response?

References

Bolay FK, Grandits G, Lane HC, Kennedy SB, Johnson MP, Fallah MP, et al. PREVAIL I Cluster Vaccination Study with rVSVΔG-ZEBOV-GP as part of a public health response in Liberia. J Infect Dis. 2019;219(10):1634–41. https://doi.org/10.1093/infdis/jiy698.

Henao-Restrepo AM, Longini IM, Egger M, Dean NE, Edmunds WJ, Camacho A, et al. Efficacy and effectiveness of an rVSV-vectored vaccine expressing Ebola surface glycoprotein: interim results from the Guinea ring vaccination cluster-randomised trial. Lancet. 2015;386(9996):857–66. https://doi.org/10.1016/s0140-6736(15)61117-5.

Henao-Restrepo AM, Camacho A, Longini IM, Watson CH, Edmunds WJ, Egger M, et al. Efficacy and effectiveness of an rVSV-vectored vaccine in preventing Ebola virus disease: final results from the Guinea ring vaccination, open-label, cluster-randomised trial (Ebola Ca Suffit!). Lancet. 2017;389(10068):505–18. https://doi.org/10.1016/S0140-6736(16)32621-6.

Kennedy SB, Bolay F, Kieh M, Grandits G, Badio M, Ballou R, et al. Phase 2 placebo-controlled trial of two vaccines to prevent Ebola in Liberia. N Engl J Med. 2017;377(15):1438–47. https://doi.org/10.1056/NEJMoa1614067.

Muller MP, McGeer A, Straus SE, Hawryluck L, Gold WL. Clinical trials and novel pathogens: lessons learned from SARS. Emerg Infect Dis. 2004;10(3):389–94. https://doi.org/10.3201/eid1003.030702.

NASEM. Integrating clinical research into epidemic response: the Ebola experience. Washington, DC: National Academies of Sciences Engineering and Medicine Publications, The National Academies Press; 2017.

UL-PIRE. UL-PIRE Africa, Africa center, a prevention research center. Monrovia: UL-PIRE; 2012. https://www.ul-pireafrica.org/. Accessed 16 Dec 2020.

WHO. One year into the Ebola epidemic: a deadly, tenacious and unforgiving virus. Geneva: World Health Organization; 2015.

WHO. Ebola situation report, March 30, 2016. Geneva: World Health Organization; 2016.

33.2 In Practice: Independent Monitoring of Emergency Response Clinical Trials

Susan Vogel and Jerome F. Pierson

Contents

Learning Track Note: This chapter appears in Learning Tracks: Research Ethics; Emergency Research Response, Research Operations

E. S. Higgs and R. A. Sorenson (eds.), *Principles and Practice of Emergency Research Response*,
https://doi.org/10.1007/978-3-031-48408-7_52

Learning Objectives

This chapter will help readers understand and describe:

- The reason for independent monitoring and the clinical trial elements included.
- When and how the independent monitoring team should identify risks to the trial process and data integrity.
- Considerations for site assessment.
- Resources required for a clinical research program to monitor a study.
- Essential elements of adverse and unexpected events as they are reported.

1 The Need for Monitoring

Regardless of where a study is conducted and under what conditions (e.g., limited resources, security threats, poor transport, spotty communications), independent monitoring is essential to help ensure participants' rights, safety, and welfare. Data integrity and compliance with the protocol approved for the clinical trial by the research ethics committee (REC) and trial sponsors must be monitored from beginning to end. Moreover, regulatory bodies, such as the U.S. Food and Drug Administration (FDA) and European Medicines Agency (EMA), mandate that clinical research with investigational products be conducted in accordance with the good clinical practice (GCP) guidelines of the International Council for Harmonisation of Technical Requirements for Pharmaceuticals for Human Use (ICH GCP) (2016). If a risky environment or inaccessibility means on-site monitoring is not operationally feasible, sponsors need to creatively identify approaches to independent monitoring. Sponsors of research on investigational medicinal products need to identify the critical processes and data required for verification of efficacy as well as the risks of the products, both at the overall program level and the individual research site. The independent monitors need to be an integral part of the research planning process in order to devise a feasible and effective mechanism for verifying key information, and yet they need to be independent enough that they are not unduly influenced by trial managers—independent enough to be the bearers of bad news if that turns out to be necessary.

2 Identifying Risks

During an emergency response, the opportune time for the monitoring team to identify foreseeable risks to the trial process and data integrity is during the initial protocol planning process and site readiness assessments. The site assessment needs to consider all applicable regulatory and protocol requirements. The assessment report then details how implementing tasks will be performed and with what staffing profile at that particular site. These assessments should be done by responsible research team members at the site who have seen and walked through the location, talked to existing staff if it is a medical facility, ascertained transportation links, etc. An on-the-spot assessment offers the best opportunity to strategize how to manage staff, equipment, research participants, clinical samples, and data. However, if the security risk is such that supervisory monitors cannot visit the study site, the team will have to rely on staff at the site to complete a monitoring assessment with immediate follow-up, either by teleconference or at a central location in a safer region of the country where all parties can discuss the assessment.

3 Resource Needs

Of course, the success of a trial relies on more than a well-constructed protocol. As discussed elsewhere in this volume (► Chap. 32), the site needs to have the wherewithal to manage the study, including necessary structures to see participants, provide medical care if they are inpatients, and house a pharmacy, laboratory, and data management area. The functional areas will require corresponding equipment as well as Internet, running water, and reliable electricity, either through the grid or from generators. In some cases, staff housing could also be required.

Site planning needs to begin while the protocol is still in development, since the limitations of a study site can impact the development of the protocol and affect how source documentation and case reports are formatted and recorded. Communication and transportation shortfalls and the constraints on study staff, who may need to work in an isolation unit and heavy personal protective equipment to prevent transmission of the disease under investigation, are among the factors that can require adaptations in reporting processes (► Chap. 35).

4 Regulatory Requirements

Understanding all the applicable layers of regulatory review is also indispensable. The study cannot begin until all RECs and scientific reviewers have agreed on the same version of the protocol. This can be challenging if there are simultaneous submissions of the protocol to several RECs and they respond with differing stipulations. Understanding the critical pathway for the various required approvals is essential in an urgent research response. The research team will need to pursue scientific and REC reviews, regulatory approvals, logistics requirements, etc. on parallel paths rather than sequentially as might be done in "peacetime" research.

A related need, vital to the monitoring function, is understanding exactly what all the regulatory and oversight bodies require for reporting adverse and unexpected events and deviations once the study is underway (► Chap. 6). For timely reporting, it is essential to know:

- What kind of events must be reported
- When to report—at regular intervals or immediately after certain events
- To which organization
- Through what channel
- In what format

5 Qualifications and Training

Before the study begins, it is also important to ensure that on-site investigators are qualified as required by ICH GCP and other applicable regulatory and oversight bodies. For example, the four-arm PALM Ebola Therapeutics randomized controlled trial (RCT) took place in the North Kivu Province of the Democratic Republic of the Congo (DRC), an area with multiple security threats that included direct, violent attacks on Ebola treatment units (ETU) (Nguyen 2019). The Congolese study team there worked with international nongovernmental organization (NGO) partners who were providing care in Ebola treatment units to enroll participants and conduct the RCT (► In Practice 17.1) (Aruna et al. 2019; Mulangu et al. 2019). To help mitigate the risk of frequently moving staff on the dangerous road system, training was carried out to the extent possible before the study began, with follow-up as needed throughout study implementation. This included study protocol and protocol implementation training, ICH GCP, and focused group training in pharmacy, laboratory, and other specialized competencies. Independent monitors ensured staff were trained and appropriately delegated responsibilities before beginning any study-related activities. Regular, transparent communication with the study team was fundamental to ensuring new staff were properly trained and assigned to the right tasks.

Independent monitoring lends itself to continuous quality improvement efforts by all involved in the research response. This becomes evident as the response progresses and new challenges unfold. Flexibility and openness to a documented and well-communicated continuous quality improvement effort are essential. On the other hand, an expectation of perfection that may inform a workable strategy in a developed country could be unrealistic and potentially disastrous in an emergency that requires improvisation and adaptability.

Training site personnel is a critical element for positive outcomes of independent monitoring. Research partnerships are expected to include an element of capacity building where applicable, which means that training and development of personnel on independent monitoring and evaluation need to be included in the overall capacity building plan.

Discussion Questions

1. What is the purpose of independent monitoring? What are the factors that must be overseen through the clinical trial?
2. During an emergency response, when should the monitoring team identify risks to the trial process and data integrity? What must the site assessment consider, and how can supervisory monitors obtain this information if they cannot visit the site due to security risks?
3. What resources does a clinical research program need to monitor a study?
4. What are the essential elements for reporting adverse and unexpected events?

References

Aruna A, Mbala P, Minikulu L, Mukadi D, Bulemfu D, Edidi F, et al. Ebola virus disease outbreak—Democratic Republic of the Congo, August 2018-November 2019. MMWR Morb Mortal Wkly Rep. 2019;68(50):1162–5. https://doi.org/10.15585/mmwr.mm6850a3.

ICH. Good clinical practice: ICH harmonised guideline. Integrated addendum to ICH E6(R1): guideline for good clinical practice ICH E6(R2) ICH consensus guideline. Geneva: International Council for Harmonisation of Technical Requirements for Pharmaceuticals for Human Use (ICH); 2016.

Mulangu S, Dodd LE, Davey RT Jr, Tshiani Mbaya O, Proschan M, Mukadi D, et al. A randomized, controlled trial of Ebola virus disease therapeutics. N Engl J Med. 2019;381(24):2293–303. https://doi.org/10.1056/NEJMoa1910993.

Nguyen V-K. An epidemic of suspicion—Ebola and violence in the DRC. N Engl J Med. 2019; https://doi.org/10.1056/NEJMp1902682.

33.3 In Practice: Capacity Building for Research Ethics Review in Low- and Middle-Income Countries

Barbara Sina and John Tierney

Contents

Learning Track Note: This chapter appears in Learning Tracks: Global Health; Research Ethics; Social Science Response Research; Emergency Research Response, Research Operations

E. S. Higgs and R. A. Sorenson (eds.), *Principles and Practice of Emergency Research Response*, https://doi.org/10.1007/978-3-031-48408-7_53

Learning Objectives

This chapter will help readers understand and describe:

- Essential partnership elements that enable a research program to urgently conduct sound ethical review of clinical research proposals
- The place of review mechanisms in forming an international emergency research response partnership
- Measures that can be taken to build sustainable research ethics review capacity over the longer term
- Some conclusions the global bioethics community has made in light of the COVID-19 pandemic. How these lessons might help strengthen the research review infrastructure of low- and middle-income countries

1 Introduction

International research ethics guidelines, national legislation in most countries, and the policies of most research funders require that all research with human participants undergo ethical review by a research ethics committee (REC)[1] with jurisdiction over the location of a proposed research study. Since World War II, globalization of biomedical research has gone hand in hand with development of international and national guideline documents, for example, the Declaration of Helsinki in 1964 and the International Ethical Guidelines for Health-Related Research Involving Humans in 1982 (CIOMS 2016; Grady 2019; WMA 1964). However, relatively little global health research funding and resources have supported development of research ethics review system capacities in low- and middle-income countries (LMICs). A dearth of well-qualified ethics committee members, staff, and administrative support is common even at national research institutions and regulatory authorities in LMICs (Saxena et al. 2019). International research funders have begun to offer more support for research ethics capacity needs in LMICs over the last two decades (Mokgatla et al. 2018), but recent global infectious disease outbreaks have exposed shortcomings in even well-functioning ethical review systems in developed countries when they must meet the demands of outbreak research (Faust et al. 2021). Countries with less robust ethics review systems and limited current support, less pertinent expertise, and lower administrative capabilities have been even more affected (Marzouk et al. 2021).

Any emergency outbreak that the World Health Organization declares a Public Health Emergency of International Concern (PHEIC) is likely to generate multiple research proposals, resulting in a surge of applications for ethical review under enormous time pressure (Meyer et al. 2021). Among the multiple protocols submitted, there may well be duplicative studies from research groups with little relevant field experience acting with little coordination with other researchers. Initial proposals may lack critical details due to the many uncertainties of an emerging pathogen or a pathogen emerging in a new environment. Quality of study design may be uneven. Knowledge about disease transmission, safety procedures, and standards of patient care is likely to change over time during the outbreak. Depending on local circumstances, ethics reviewers may need to increase scrutiny of participant vulnerability, potential stigma, and other psychosocial impacts of proposed research. Reviewers could also face increased tension over the ethics of using placebos in randomly controlled trials (RCTs) during high-mortality outbreaks, alternative research designs, inclusion of children and pregnant women, and whether risk-benefit analysis has been properly conducted (Macklin 2021).

On a practical level, the review committee members with the greatest expertise will likely be juggling many additional professional and personal obligations. Ethical review processes may lack needed flexibilities, authority, staff-

1 Research ethics committee (REC) is the preferred term in this book because it is more descriptive than the usual term used in the United States, institutional review board (IRB), as well as more familiar globally. Other frequently used terms in English include medical research ethics committee (MREC), research ethics board (REB), and human research ethics committee (HREC).

ing, electronic applications, tracking, and communication systems. Information resources for committee members, researchers, and other stakeholders may be inadequate. A number of these issues may be exacerbated by mandated isolation measures and closures at universities, research institutions, and government agencies, not to mention society at large (Hashem et al. 2020).

An essential element of genuine partnership with the country, health system, and communities hosting the research program is immediate capacity building to ensure reasonably adequate review of response research proposals by affected stakeholders. Looking beyond the crisis, research partners must make every effort to continue sustainable strengthening of local resources and institutions, so they can continue oversight of ongoing research, review new research proposals, and be better prepared for the next outbreak or other public health emergency (▸ Chaps. 4 and 5). To that end, this chapter will concentrate on three areas:

1. Evaluation of existing research ethics review capacity
2. Partnering and exchange to immediately address gaps and needs
3. Developing future research infrastructure and capacity

2 Evaluation of Existing Research Ethics Review Capacity

One of the first tasks for a research team setting up an emergency research response partnership is to determine what national laws, guidelines, and procedures govern the conduct and oversight of research. For example, shortly before the 2014–2016 Ebola outbreak in West Africa, both the Liberia Medicines and Health Products Regulatory Authority (2014) and the Pharmacy Board of Sierra Leone (2019) had established or updated national guidelines for the conduct of clinical trials. Documents such as these provide a starting point for determining what steps needed to be undertaken to initiate a clinical trial, including an early understanding of what REC reviews and other regulatory steps are required (▸ Chap. 26).

Several efforts have been made to collate and analyze detailed information about LMIC REC capacity and make this information available to the scientific community. For example, the MARC (Mapping African Research Ethics Review and Medicines Regulatory Capacity) initiative collected data about available REC infrastructure, protocol submission methods, review procedures, and membership and administrative staff including bioethics training backgrounds. This initiative recently expanded to include the PAHO (Pan-American Health Organization) region and covers over a thousand RECS (see Health Research Web below). Analysis of MARC data on African REC member training by Mokgatla et al. (2018) found evidence of strengthened ethical review across the continent: 49% of RECs had members who had completed short courses in research ethics, 28% of RECS included members with related degrees, and only 11% did not have any members with relevant bioethics training.

Box 1

Information on international research regulations, ethics review systems, and accreditation in many countries may be found through Web sites and publications cited here:

The *U.S. Office on Human Research Protection International Program* maintains several relevant resources for finding relevant information:

- The International Compilation of Human Research Standards lists over 1000 laws, regulations, and guidelines on human subjects protections in 133 countries and from many international organizations (OHRP 2020).
- A searchable database lists institutions that have qualified for a Federal-wide assurance

(FWA) that the institution is in compliance with U.S. Protection of Human Subjects regulations (OHRP 2021). An FWA is required for U.S. federally funded research wherever it takes place.

The *Health Research Web*, maintained by the Council on Health Research for Development, includes country information about governance, policies, research ethics review, medicines regulation, etc. (Health Research Web 2021).

There is a WHO list of National Research Ethics Committees (WHO 2015).

The Association for the Accreditation of Human Research Protection Programs, Inc. (AAHRPP) lists accredited organizations, accreditation standards, and resources (AAHRPP 2023).

The Forum for Ethical Review Committees in the Asia and Western Pacific region recognizes RECs in compliance with WHO Operational Guidelines for Ethics Committees Reviewing Biomedical Research (SIDCER-FERRCAP Foundation 2022).

The multinational Caribbean Public Health Agency hosts both a Caribbean Network of Research Ethics Committees and a Network of Caribbean Regulatory Systems, which work together to improve ethical and regulatory review in the region (CARPHA 2023).

The FDA International Office works in partnership with foreign governments, regulatory coalitions, development organizations, and academic institutions on regulatory systems strengthening (FDA 2023).

FDA also makes medical countermeasure (MCM) cooperative agreements to assist the regulatory agencies of other countries when they are faced with an emerging infectious disease outbreak (FDA 2019). During the 2014–2016 West Africa Ebola outbreak, for example, the FDA developed and implemented confidentiality agreements with their regulatory counterparts in each of the countries most affected by the outbreak (FDA 2020). This allowed the FDA to share non-public information about the investigational MCMs with the local authorities, facilitating their review and providing experience that should enhance their ability to evaluate studies of other products used in clinical trials in the future.

The European Medicines Agency (EMA) implements bilateral interactions with non-EU regulators (EMA 2023).

The International Coalition of Medicines Regulatory Authorities has published a "Framework for the Involvement of Health Regulatory Authorities in the Management of Global Health Crises" (ICMRA 2019).

The Pan-American Health Organization has a List and System for Evaluation of the National Regulatory Authorities for Medicines (PAHO 2018).

In an emergency, some countries may waive some of the requirements set forth in their regulations or guidance to expedite a rapid research response. Nevertheless, it must be clear that only procedural steps can be elided; substantive ethical review still needs to meet institutional, national, and international standards. Even if one reached the conclusion that ethical review could be weakened, as a practical matter, authorities including the U.S. Food and Drug Administration, European Medicines Agency, and WHO will not accept research results for the purpose of pre-certification, emergency authorization, or licensing unless they are satisfied that the research demonstrably satisfies ethical requirements (EMA 2021; FDA 2021; WHO 2020a). For many years, and especially since the clinical trials carried out during the 2014–2016 Ebola outbreak in West Africa, reflection on ethical issues and ethical review practice for research conducted during emergencies have served as foundations for specific ethical guidance issued for health emergencies, including COVID-19 research (Nuffield Council on Bioethics 2020; Saxena et al. 2019; WHO 2020b, c, d, e). Some LMICs also issued their own emergency research ethics regulations, guidance, or action plans for the COVID-19 epidemic (Mathur 2020; Reyes 2020; Tibenderana et al. 2021; Zhang et al. 2020).

3 Partnership, Information, and Action

Ethics review during a pandemic must navigate between the Scylla of compromising essential standards and the Charybdis of delay. As is likely with any novel pathogen, initial uncertainties about transmission and disease course with SARS-CoV-2 complicated ethical and scientific review, as did the haste with which countries mobilized resources to mount a research response. Changing conclusions about SARS-CoV-2 transmission made it difficult to know how best to protect research participants, medical workers, and community members, even as evolving public health messaging engendered mistrust among many populations. Dramatic differences in mortality rates between socially secure and disadvantaged populations made it clear that health equity needed to be a priority in research as in healthcare. A multitude of early trials that were not well designed to produce robust results sharpened the question of how to ensure trials were scientifically as well as ethically sound; the related issues of whether to publish flawed results and how quickly are still difficult to answer (Dean et al. 2020; Lumeng et al. 2020).

The questions above applied everywhere COVID-19 research was done, though the bulk of emergency research was done in developed countries with strong biomedical research capacity and with the repurposing of a great proportion of biomedical research capacity from other questions to COVID-19. In LMICs, researchers and research organizations can seek to build capacity to meet the extraordinary demands and limitations imposed by the current epidemic and future outbreaks and to ensure excellence in ethics review through:

1. Commitment to partnership and coordination (▶ Chap. 30)
2. Ensuring access to expert consultation and focused training
3. Urgent improvements in information and communications technology (▶ Chap. 34)

3.1 Partnership and Coordination

It is widely accepted that true collaborative partnership between researchers and sponsors in developed countries and researchers, policy makers, and communities in developing countries helps make research ethical; in fact, Emanuel et al. (2004) make it the first principle in their influential article, "What Makes Research in Developing Countries Ethical?" Intensive collaboration and coordination among all researchers, regulatory agencies, and health institutions involved in any response initiative are critical to effective epidemic response. Partnerships with LMIC ethical review committees must both support independent decision-making as required by country sovereignty and institutional autonomy and meet the urgent need to validate countermeasures against the outbreak by beginning research as soon as possible (▶ Chap. 30).

Mentorship and advisory consultations are one relatively expeditious approach to fill any gaps in REC member expertise. For example:

- A REC more experienced with reviewing clinical research in an emergency could provide advice and training on how to modify standard operating procedures (SOPs) to decrease the length of time for reviews.
- An experienced REC could recommend electronic application and protocol submission systems and videoconferencing platforms for virtual review meetings appropriate for LMIC Internet capacity and provide training in their use.

- Expert independent consultants could be provided to advise on alternative trial designs, statistical calculations for sample size, biosafety precautions, informed consent, and other research requirements.

Collaborations between ethics committees reviewing the same protocol—often one at the sponsoring organization and another at the research location—to help streamline the approval process could be arranged. For example, sharing the minutes of deliberations to better understand the most salient risk/benefit considerations and assess their applicability in the local context could be useful. If technology, regulations, and timing allow, it may be possible for RECs to conduct a simultaneous joint review so that the perspectives of both bodies are mutually understood, potentially allowing for more timely feedback to the research team. Ravinetto et al. (2011) suggest that dual ethical review by two RECs serves a useful purpose by ensuring thorough review in light of "universal" standards and "a better informed and comprehensive assessment of both the clinical sites and the sponsoring organization" by a "culturally close ethics committee" (◘ Fig. 1).

An enormous contribution to the ethical conduct of research during an epidemic is early coordination and agreement for collaboration among researchers working at the same site(s). It is common practice in epidemics to isolate infected individuals in one or a small number of treatment units, which then become the site(s) for enrolling participants for many research studies (Marzouk et al. 2021). Without clear coordination among research groups, RECs must consider how to handle duplicative studies, the risks of the same patient being involved in more than one study, different definitions of severity of disease and standard of care, and additional pressures on already stressed healthcare and clinical laboratory staff in the treatment unit. Research ethics committees may be forced to recommend prioritization among multiple, competing research protocols. Yeoh and Shah (2021) describe the trade-offs and prioritization of COVID-19 studies based on clinical urgency among the following types of studies: (1) studies that aim to have an immediate impact

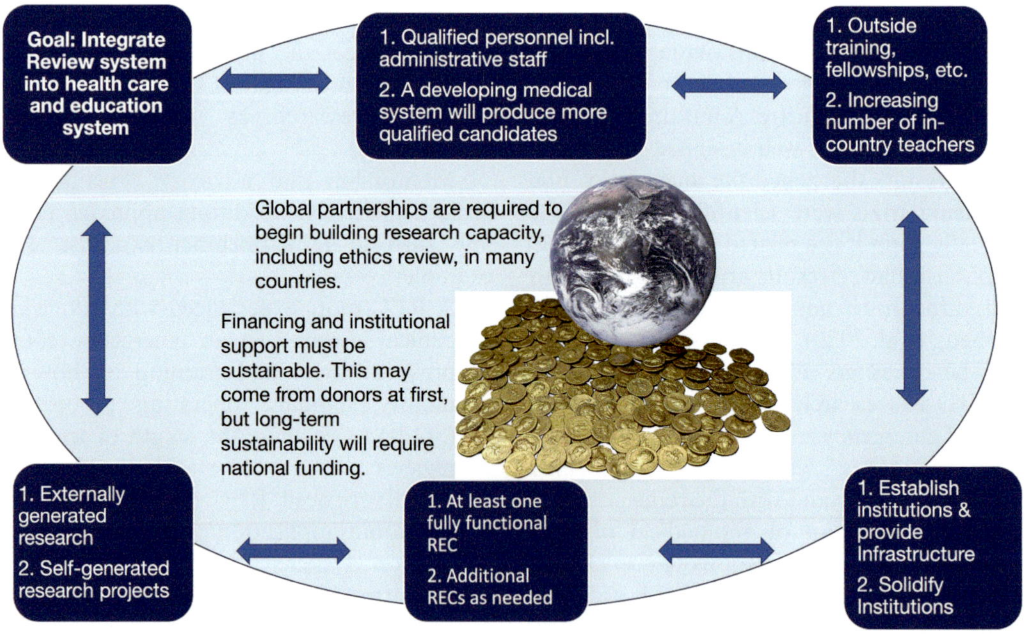

◘ **Fig. 1** Some of the iterative requirements for building research ethics review capacity. Initial steps designated 1, further steps 2. (Photo credits: 1. NASA and 2. Tiia Monto)

on containing the spread of the epidemic or optimizing treatments for those affected; (2) studies with mid- to long-term goals during the epidemic, such as research and development, as well as providing equitable access to diagnostics, therapeutics, and vaccines; and (3) continuation and codification of other ongoing research on life threatening or highly stigmatized conditions. Collaborative agreements between research groups can be used to set common criteria for compassionate use of experimental treatments and set up effective remote processes for consent, patient monitoring, data collection, and clinical management. These agreements can also harmonize how research findings will be conveyed to participants and to all stakeholders involved in the epidemic response.

3.2 Access to Ethics Expertise and Focused Training

While similar ethical issues arise in each new epidemic, specific ethical issues and research policies also evolve as medical science and standards of care progress and as the unique elements of each epidemic unfold. Researchers and ethics review committees can now call on ethics experts from many countries for consultation and epidemic-focused ethics training, as well as up-to-date information resources. Epidemic Ethics, for example, is a global community of bioethicists (led by the World Health Organization and supported by the Fogarty International Center, Global Forum on Bioethics in Research, Global Health Network, Global Network of WHO Collaborating Centers, and Wellcome Trust) building on pre-existing expertise and resources to provide real-time, trusted, contextual support to communities, policy makers, researchers, and responders in relation to the ethical issues arising out of global health emergencies, with a current focus on the COVID-19 pandemic (Epidemic Ethics 2023). Their Web site includes a resource page with a continuously updated worldwide compilation of guidance and policies, training courses and tools, ethics journal publications, etc. The Web site also maintains a registrar for bioethicists from all countries, an ethics advisory platform for consultation, and blog discussions on emerging ethical issues and recordings of their virtual seminar series. Other university-based and independent bioethics centers maintain Web sites with international epidemic ethics resources and access to international bioethics experts (Berman Institute of Bioethics 2023; Center for Bioethics and Health Law 2023; Hastings Center 2021; Nuffield Council on Bioethics 2021; Pandemic Ethics Resources 2021).

Research review committees also need continuously updated information feedback on research, clinical, and public health aspects of the epidemic disease, including safety considerations, new clinical risk findings, disease-related stigma, psychosocial support mechanisms, health facility staffing and admissions status, etc., to make well-informed decisions on research protocols, to monitor implementation, and to approve modifications as the situation unfolds. While a number of these issues may be considered in the scientific review of protocols, few models for how to effectively include ethics review committees in epidemic professional information flow have emerged. Streamlining ethical review through a concentration of member effort and expertise may mean that REC members are already receiving professional updates through other channels. This approach has sometimes been strengthened by forming subcommittees of the most expert members of an REC or creation of a specific REC composed of expert representatives from all RECs of multiple research sites in a country to review epidemic research protocols. To cope with rapidly changing understanding of the pathogen, disease course, and public health characteristics of an epidemic, ethics committees should follow emerging guidance and research results and monitor studies they have approved as research proceeds (▶ In Practice 4.2).

3.3 Strengthening Electronic Systems and Communication Infrastructure

Research ethics committees may lack sufficient institutional and technical support for interactive Web sites, electronic application and research protocol tracking, and secure virtual conferencing that would increase the efficiency of their processes (▶ Chap. 34). In LMICs, research ethics committees may lack paid staff, a dedicated securable facility, computers, and dependable access to the Internet. These needs will likely be amplified during epidemic lockdowns, further constraining attempts to streamline and adapt review processes. While international research grant funding often cannot directly support these needs, indirect costs paid through grants to institutions are meant to support related infrastructure, such as that needed for ethical review committees. Researchers should note whether a country's regulations require RECs to meet in person with a large quorum, use paper copies with official signatures, or limit consultation with outside experts, researchers, etc. This is the sort of requirement that may need to be reviewed for modification or waivers during an emergency.

4 Developing Future Research Review Infrastructure and Capacity: Ethics Preparedness

Among many reflections on the Ebola virus outbreak in West Africa, ethics preparedness was identified as foundational to timely and effective research response (Bioethics Commission 2015). Research ethics committees are thought to play an essential role in building trust and protecting societal values in epidemic research (Mathur 2020). In 2018, WHO convened an international workshop that identified areas where enhanced practices and procedures for ethical preparedness could facilitate rapid, sound ethical review. Needed steps include preparation of ethics committee SOPs for emergency response review; procedures for communication with oversight and public health authorities; pre-reviewed, pre-approved template or example protocols and consent forms; mechanisms for multi-country or regional emergency ethical consultation to support rapid review; requirements for benefits; and data and sample sharing plans (Saxena et al. 2019). Having such preparations in place would enhance the capacity of LMICs to mobilize more quickly and coordinate more effectively in the event of a future outbreak, regardless of the specific disease (Bain et al. 2018; Silaigwana and Wassenaar 2015). For example, in the aftermath of research conducted during the Ebola virus outbreak, Liberia hosted conferences on bioethics in 2017 and 2018 that resulted in organizational changes and revised guidelines for medical research that proved useful during the COVID-19 pandemic (National Research Ethics Board of Liberia 2019).

Developing infrastructure and clinical research capacity, including capacity for ethical and regulatory review, requires a substantial investment of time and capital, especially human capital, based on thoughtful consideration of the short- and long-term needs of the particular research environment. In addition to the physical infrastructure and logistical support needs described above, the human resource capacity of the research ethics system should be a long-term commitment of an LMIC and its development partners as an integral part of building research capacity. Unfortunately, as the World Bank-supported International Vaccines Task Force (2018) report concludes, "Committing domestic resources for epidemic preparedness, and the clinical research needed to support it, can be a huge challenge for resource-constrained economies that struggle to meet more proximate and immediate demands." Some international research funders have recognized the specific needs for developing research ethics systems and provide support for bioethics education, ethics review capacity, and research on high-priority ethical issues in LMICs (EDCTP 2021; Fogarty International Center 2021; Wellcome Trust 2021). It is not enough, however, to provide training and capacity development without institutional support for ethicists and their activities. They must have long-term positions, salaries, office space, and all essential attributes of a valued entity in research and regulatory institutions if research capacity in LMICs, including ethical review, is to be viable over the longer term and available for emergency response (Potter and Brough 2004). Based on their analysis of African REC information, Mokgatla et al. (2018) reported that 91% had access to computers, 84% had dedicated office space, 81% had telephones, 78% had Internet access, 59% had a photocopier, and a quarter of all RECs had access to all these critical tools. Also reflecting growing institutional support, 59% reported an organizational budget for running the REC although most did not yet remunerate their members. In the end, it is hard to build sustainable research ethics review capacity without building the other elements of a functional medical research ecosystem and ultimately a fully functional health and healthcare system.

Discussion Questions

1. What are some essential elements of genuine partnership with the country, health system, and communities hosting an emergency research program?
2. In the emergency context, how does one ensure adequate review of response research proposals by all affected stakeholders? Note three actions that allow researchers and research organizations to build research ethics review capacity.
3. What are some options for strengthening electronic systems, clinical research capacity, and communication infrastructure of low- and middle-income countries?

References

AAHRPP. Association for the Accreditation of Human Research Protection Programs. Washington, DC: Association for the Accreditation of Human Research Protection Programs; 2023. https://www.aahrpp.org. Accessed 22 Mar 2023.

Bain LE, Ngwain CG, Nwobegahay J, Sumboh JG, Nditanchou R, Awah PK. Research Ethics Committees (RECs) and epidemic response in low and middle income countries. Pan Afr Med J. 2018;31:209. https://doi.org/10.11604/pamj.2018.31.209.17076.

Berman Institute of Bioethics. Johns Hopkins University, Baltimore. 2023. https://bioethics.jhu.edu/. Accessed 22 Mar 2023.

Bioethics Commission. Ethics and Ebola: public health planning and response. Washington, DC: Presidential Commission for the Study of Bioethical Issues; 2015.

CARPHA. Caribbean Public Health Agency. Port of Spain, TT: Caribbean Public Health Agency; 2023. https://www.carpha.org. Accessed 22 Mar 2023.

Center for Bioethics and Health Law. University of Pittsburgh, Pittsburgh. 2023. http://bioethics.pitt.edu/. Accessed 22 Mar 2023.

CIOMS. International ethical guidelines for health-related research involving humans. Geneva: Council for International Organisations of Medical Sciences; 2016.

Dean NE, Gsell P-S, Brookmeyer R, Crawford FW, Donnelly CA, Ellenberg SS, et al. Creating a framework for conducting randomized clinical trials during disease outbreaks. N Engl J Med. 2020;382(14):1366–9. https://doi.org/10.1056/NEJMsb1905390.

EDCTP. Funding clinical research for medical tools to detect, treat and prevent poverty-related infectious diseases in sub-Saharan Africa. The Hague: European and Developing Countries Clinical Trials Partnership; 2021. https://www.edctp.org/. Accessed 19 Dec 2021.

EMA. Good clinical practice. Amsterdam: European Medicines Agency; 2021. https://www.ema.europa.eu/en/human-regulatory/research-development/compliance/good-clinical-practice. Accessed 27 May 2021.

EMA. Partners and networks: bilateral interactions with non-EU regulators. Amsterdam: European Medicines Agency; 2023. https://www.ema.europa.eu/en/partners-networks/international-activities/bilateral-interactions-non-eu-regulators. Accessed 22 Mar 2023.

Emanuel EJ, Wendler D, Grady C. What makes clinical research in developing countries ethical? The benchmarks of ethical research. J Infect Dis. 2004;189:930–7.

Epidemic Ethics. 2023. https://epidemicethics.tghn.org. Accessed 22 Mar 2023.

Faust A, Sierawska A, Krüger K, Wisgalla A, Hasford J, Strech D. Challenges and proposed solutions in making clinical research on COVID-19 ethical: a status quo analysis across German research ethics committees. BMC Med Ethics. 2021;22(1):96. https://doi.org/10.1186/s12910-021-00666-8.

FDA. MCM-related cooperative arrangements. Washington, DC: U.S. Food and Drug

Administration; 2019. https://www.fda.gov/emergency-preparedness-and-response/mcm-legal-regulatory-and-policy-framework/mcm-related-cooperative-arrangements. Accessed 23 Feb 2020.

FDA. MCM-related cooperative arrangements. Washington, DC: U.S. Food and Drug Administration; 2020. https://www.fda.gov/emergency-preparedness-and-response/mcm-legal-regulatory-and-policy-framework/mcm-related-cooperative-arrangements. Accessed 2 Dec 2020.

FDA. Clinical trials and human subject protection. Washington, DC: Food and Drug Administration; 2021. https://www.fda.gov/science-research/science-and-research-special-topics/clinical-trials-and-human-subject-protection. Accessed 27 May 2021.

FDA. Partnerships and collaboration. Silver Spring, MD: U.S. Food and Drug Administration; 2023. https://www.fda.gov/international-programs/partnerships-and-collaboration. Accessed 22 Mar 2023.

Fogarty International Center. International bioethics training. Bethesda, MD: National Institutes of Health; 2021. https://www.fic.nih.gov/Programs/Pages/bioethics.aspx. Accessed 17 Dec 2021.

Grady C. Bioethics in the oversight of clinical research: institutional review boards and data and safety monitoring boards. Kennedy Inst Ethics J. 2019;29(1):33–49. https://doi.org/10.1353/ken.2019.0009.

Hashem H, Abufaraj M, Tbakhi A, Sultan I. Obstacles and considerations related to clinical trial research during the COVID-19 pandemic. Front Med (Lausanne). 2020;7:598038. https://doi.org/10.3389/fmed.2020.598038.

Hastings Center. The Hastings Center, Garrison, NY. 2021. https://www.thehastingscenter.org/. Accessed 17 Dec 2021.

Health Research Web. Council on Health Research for Development (COHRED). 2021. https://healthresearchweb.org/en/home. Accessed 21 Nov 2021.

ICMRA. Framework for the involvement of health regulatory authorities in the management of global health crises. London: International Coalition of Medicines Regulatory Authorities; 2019.

International Vaccines Task Force. Money and microbes: strengthening clinical research capacity to prevent epidemics. Washington, DC: World Bank; 2018.

Liberia Medicines and Health Products Regulatory Authority. In: (LMHRA) LMaHPRA, editor. Guideline for application to conduct of clinical trials in Liberia. Monrovia: Liberia Medicines and Health Products Regulatory Authority (LMHRA); 2014. p. 60.

Lumeng JC, Chavous TM, Lok AS, Sen S, Wigginton NS, Cunningham RM. Opinion: a risk-benefit framework for human research during the COVID-19 pandemic. Proc Natl Acad Sci USA. 2020;117(45):27749–53. https://doi.org/10.1073/pnas.2020507117.

Macklin R. Double standards redux. Indian J Med Ethics. 2021;VI(2):1–7. https://doi.org/10.20529/ijme.2021.021.

Marzouk D, Sharawy I, Nakhla I, El Hodhod M, Gadallah H, El-Shalakany A, et al. Challenges during review of COVID-19 research proposals: experience of Faculty of Medicine, Ain Shams University Research Ethics Committee, Egypt. Front Med (Lausanne). 2021;8:715796. https://doi.org/10.3389/fmed.2021.715796.

Mathur R. Ethics preparedness for infectious disease outbreaks research in India: a case for novel coronavirus disease 2019. Indian J Med Res. 2020;151(2 & 3):124–31. https://doi.org/10.4103/ijmr.IJMR_463_20.

Meyer MN, Gelinas L, Bierer BE, Hull SC, Joffe S, Magnus D, et al. An ethics framework for consolidating and prioritizing COVID-19 clinical trials. Clin Trials (London, England). 2021:1740774520988669. https://doi.org/10.1177/1740774520988669.

Mokgatla B, IJsselmuiden C, Wassenaar D, Kasule M. Mapping research ethics committees in Africa: evidence of the growth of ethics review of health research in Africa. Dev World Bioeth. 2018;18(4):341–8. https://doi.org/10.1111/dewb.12146.

National Research Ethics Board of Liberia. Operational guidelines (amended version 2019). Monrovia: National Research Ethics Board of Liberia (NREB); 2019. p. 24.

Nuffield Council on Bioethics. Research in global health emergencies: ethical issues. Oxford: Nuffield Council on Bioethics; 2020.

Nuffield Council on Bioethics. Nuffield Council on Bioethics, London. 2021. https://www.nuffieldbioethics.org/. Accessed 17 Dec 2021.

OHRP. International compilation of human research standards. Washington, DC: Office of Human Research Protection, U.S. Department of Health and Human Services; 2020.

OHRP. Database for registered IORGs & IRBs, approved FWAs, and documents received in last 60 days. Silver Spring, MD: U.S. Food and Drug Administration; 2021. https://ohrp.cit.nih.gov/search/docsearch.aspx. Accessed 21 Nov 2021.

PAHO. System for evaluation of the national regulatory authorities for medicines. Washington, DC: Pan-American Health Organization; 2018. https://www3.paho.org/hq/index.php?option=com_content&view=article&id=1615:2009-sistema-evaluacion-autoridades-reguladoras-nacionales-medicamentos&Itemid=0&lang=en#gsc.tab=0. Accessed 22 Mar 2023.

Pandemic Ethics Resources. University of Miami, Miami. 2021. https://bioethics.miami.edu/education/public-health-ethics/pandemic-resources/index.html. Accessed 17 Dec 2021.

Pharmacy Board of Sierra Leone. In: Pharmacy Board of Sierra Leone, editor. Guidelines for application and authorisation of clinical trials of medicines,

vaccines, medical devices and food supplements. Freetown, SL: Pharmacy Board of Sierra Leone; 2019. p. 43.
Potter C, Brough R. Systemic capacity building: a hierarchy of needs. Health Policy Plan. 2004;19(5):336–45. https://doi.org/10.1093/heapol/czh038.
Ravinetto R, Buve A, Halidou T, Lutumba P, Taliduna A, Juffrie M, D'Alessandro U, Boelaert M. Double ethical Review of North-South collaborative clinical research: hidden paternalism or real partnership? Tropical Medicine and International Health. 2011;16(4):527–30. https://doi.org/10.111/j.1365-3156.2011.02732.x.
Reyes M. Research in the time of COVID-19: challenges of research ethics committees. J ASEAN Fed Endocr Soc. 2020;35(1):29–32. https://doi.org/10.15605/jafes.035.01.07.
Saxena A, Horby P, Amuasi J, Aagaard N, Kohler J, Gooshki ES, et al. Ethics preparedness: facilitating ethics review during outbreaks—recommendations from an expert panel. BMC Med Ethics. 2019;20(1):29. https://doi.org/10.1186/s12910-019-0366-x.
SIDCER-FERRCAP Foundation. Strategic Initiative for Developing Capacity in Ethical Review (SIDCER)-Forum for Ethical Review Committees in the Asian and Western Pacific Region (FERCAP) Foundation. Bangkok: Strategic Initiative for Developing Capacity in Ethical Review (SIDCER)-Forum for Ethical Review Committees in the Asian and Western Pacific Region (FERCAP) Foundation; 2022. https://www.sidcer-fercap.org/pages/research.html. Accessed 22 Mar 2023.
Silaigwana B, Wassenaar D. Biomedical Research Ethics Committees in sub-Saharan Africa: a collective review of their structure, functioning, and outcomes. J Empir Res Hum Res Ethics. 2015;10(2):169–84. https://doi.org/10.1177/1556264615575511.
Tibenderana J, Hamade P, Marasciulo M, Nakwagala F, Magumba G, Nuwa A, et al. Challenges and strategies for conducting clinical research during the COVID-19 pandemic: experiences from resource limited settings. Eur J Clin Med. 2021;2(1):1–6. https://doi.org/10.24018/clinicmed.2021.2.1.9.
Wellcome Trust. Research development awards in humanities, social science and bioethics. London: Wellcome Trust; 2021. https://wellcome.org/grant-funding/schemes/research-development-awards-humanities-social-science-and-bioethics. Accessed 27 Aug 2022.
WHO. List of national ethics committees. Geneva: World Health Organization; 2015.
WHO. Emergency use listing procedure. Geneva: World Health Organization; 2020a.
WHO. Ethical standards for research during public health emergencies: distilling existing guidance to support COVID-19 R&D. Geneva: World Health Organization. COVID-19 WWGoE; 2020b. https://apps.who.int/iris/handle/10665/331507. Contract No.: WHO reference number: WHO/RFH/20.1.
WHO. Good Participatory Practice for COVID-19 clinical trials—a toolbox. Geneva: World Health Organization; 2020c.
WHO. Guidance for research ethics committees for rapid review of research during public health emergencies. Geneva: World Health Organization; 2020d.
WHO. Integrating ethics in infectious disease outbreaks. Geneva: World Health Organization; 2020e. https://extranet.who.int/ethics/home. Accessed 6 Oct 2020.
WMA. Declaration of Helsinki: recommendations guiding doctors in clinical research. Helsinki: World Medical Association; 1964.
Yeoh KW, Shah K. Research ethics during a pandemic (COVID-19). Int Health. 2021;13(4):374–5. https://doi.org/10.1093/inthealth/ihaa054.
Zhang H, Shao F, Gu J, Li L, Wang Y. Ethics committee reviews of applications for research studies at 1 hospital in China during the 2019 novel coronavirus epidemic. JAMA. 2020;323(18):1844–6. https://doi.org/10.1001/jama.2020.4362.

34 Information and Communications Technology to Support Research in Low-Resource Settings

Mike Galcik and David Parrish

Contents

Learning Track Note: This chapter appears in Learning Tracks: Emergency Research Response, Research Operations

E. S. Higgs and R. A. Sorenson (eds.), *Principles and Practice of Emergency Research Response*,
https://doi.org/10.1007/978-3-031-48408-7_54

Learning Objectives

This chapter will help readers understand and describe:

- In what circumstances can "traditional" information and communications technology be superseded by more cost-effective and sustainable options?
- Factors to consider when replacing one communications platform with another
- How ICT can help effectively utilize the diverse skills of the entire research team
- Five key response stages involved in applying ICT in emergency research response
- Aspects of ICT that most require coordination with the local and site teams

1 Overview

1.1 Communications Styles and Tools

Information and communications technology (ICT) networks are, or at least should be, tightly coupled with how collaborations are organized and managed. Patterns of contact among team members define the communications network supporting the needed flow of information and decision-making processes. Communication networks can be characterized based on these patterns into general categories that will facilitate the selection and implementation of ICT tools (◘ Fig. 1). These tools can range widely, from email for document sharing to the implementation of project-based web sites and collaboration portals. As the roles and structure of the response evolve, it is important to continually reassess the information and communication pathways; some redundancy is a good thing as a backstop, but unplanned changes can also result in the coexistence of multiple patterns of communication and consequent confusion and missed messages.

The deployment of ICT tools as part of the overall research support effort requires, in addition to understanding the necessary patterns of team communication, establishing technical capacity and training for competencies, especially in areas of the world that may not have them available locally. Additionally, ICT strategies, methods, and implementation need to correspond with the drivers, goals,

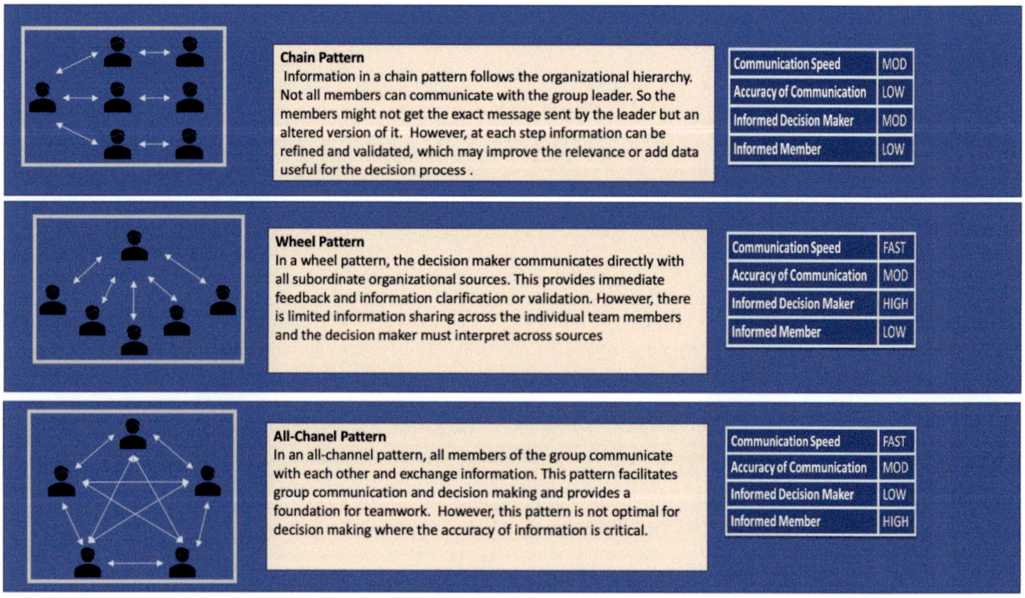

◘ **Fig. 1** Understanding patterns of communication is foundational to setting up the right kind of ICT network. (Authors)

and constraints in play at each stage of the response lifecycle. Responsibilities of the ICT team at the successive stages of response are categorized below. These response stages are used throughout the chapter and include.

1. *Initiation.* Collect and organize key measures and indicators to support the planning and decision-making process for the site selection and corresponding deployment of ICT resources.
2. *Planning.* Determine operational partners, draft and finalize partnership agreements. Quantify and provide preliminary data on resource needs. Establish strategy for coordination and execution of ICT to support outbreak response.
3. *Implementation.* Leverage resources and integrate both operational and organizational assistance from external partners into the outbreak area. As in emergencies in general, efficiency and cost may have to be sacrificed for expedience and reliability. Once research capabilities are established, many of the choices for deployment and support should be reevaluated.
4. *Monitoring and control.* Following the establishment of ICT and information technology (IT) staff, re-evaluate decisions and structures to support long-term capabilities and governance. As research organization management becomes fully operational and ICT working groups establish oversight, shift ICT efforts to transferring skills and technical capacity to the local team, building on its skills and resources while enhancing internal controls. As part of the refactoring, emphasize automation and cost containment to support the research, including potential future research, in the local environment. Local capacity building may also comprise local supply chains, technological support teams, long-term maintenance and support for infrastructure, communications, equipment, and other systems and equipment. Explore cooperative arrangements with other outbreak responders to encourage local capacity development. If establishing a local research capability is not a priority or not possible, monitoring and control can remain centralized with the response organization and provided remotely.
5. *Closing.* Transfer resources and operational control to the local ICT team or partner research organization network. Although exceptions may arise, most research studies will have a significant operational transition from an immediate response to establishing local research capabilities and ultimately transfer of programs to local partners.

1.2 Establishing Emergency Capabilities

Even when the goal is to help establish independent, sustainable research capacity in the area of the outbreak, low-resource areas will seldom have the initial technical capability or infrastructure to support a research response. From a pandemic preparedness perspective, this is another reason for development partners in general to support communications and technological capacity building in underserved areas (Wilson and Jumbert 2018). Given limited infrastructure, larger, better established and better resourced external partners will implement the early stages of a research response, relying on their own technical infrastructure and capabilities. The goal of establishing local research capacity may limit the tools and platform to be established to those sustainable in the local environment with local resources and ultimately may require some refactoring once the initial response stabilizes.

The sections below take a pragmatic approach in describing setup, execution, and continued support for the ICT capabilities. Pragmatism and flexibility are watchwords in any emergency response and, all the more so, in areas with limited infrastructure and other resources.

The fundamental role of ICT in infectious disease research response can be seen clearly in the coronavirus disease 2019 (COVID-19) pandemic. The next time a pathogen with pandemic potential emerges in a less-developed country, as is likely (Morens and

Fauci 2020), there will be little or no debate about the need for an immediate research response, and the ICT team will need to mobilize early. The team setting up the means of communications and collaboration across the research response requires a breadth of skills and resources, and especially so when capacities in the area of the outbreak are lacking. The team must be ready to plan, develop, and deploy core networking, data center, and clinical management systems and potentially cope with transport delays, uncertain electrical power, physical and cyber-security threats, lack of local skilled personnel, and corruption. Keeping in mind the phases of the response and the ultimate transition to the host organization, we will describe five key aspects of this effort.

1. Establish an ICT framework and define policies and practices.
2. Create a physical technical infrastructure.
3. Select and procure the equipment to access infrastructure.
4. Provide access and interoperability with communication tools and platforms for the entire research team and for external communications.
5. Establish local systems to support information collection, processing, and storage.

These elements must work together symbiotically, meaning that system components in one area will be required to advance capabilities in another. This in turn requires that key managers of the ICT ecosystem have oversight and the skills to identify, deploy, configure, and stabilize the needed systems. As such, a shared vision and set of objectives for the depth and breadth of ICT implementation requires not only monitoring the status of each component but continued assessment and mitigation of the following assumptions, constraints, and risks.

- Assumptions
  - Critical infrastructure components either exist in the operational area, or there is funding to develop, procure, and deploy them.
  - Key stakeholders, partners, and collaborators have been identified and are authorized to provide funding and support for initiatives.
  - All local, domestic, and international laws governing export and import control have been considered or are on track for completion; arrangements have been made for compliance or waivers (▶ Chaps. 32 and 37).
- Constraints
  - Limited local resources, including critical infrastructure, equipment, and personnel
  - Supply chain and logistical limitations, including
    - (Possible) transport service cuts due to the outbreak
    - Import/export and customs regulations and procedures
    - Transporting goods and materials to remote locations
    - In a global pandemic, shortages of key goods and reduced transport options
  - Change in scope or funding of project
  - Discontinuity of personnel or loss of critical knowledge experts
- Risks
  - Background risks
    - Operation within a country classified as a high-security risk to personnel, information systems, or both
    - Export/import control and regulatory risks, such as those related to foreign vendor agreements
    - Lack of skilled or properly qualified IT personnel
  - Security incidents
    - Cyber-security intrusion resulting in system or data compromise or loss
    - Catastrophic equipment failure
    - Loss of funding for Internet service provider or electricity costs
    - Loss of critical physical infrastructure, such as electricity and Internet connectivity
    - Theft, loss, or damage of equipment, systems, or platforms

2 Technology Assessment, Procurement, and Operations

2.1 Technology Requirements Assessment

Defining an operational strategy and technical landscape as early as possible will allow for the selection of the appropriate tools, equipment, and IT resources (▶ Chap. 35). When possible, templates and standard operating procedures (SOPs) should be predefined as part of research response planning and capacity building in low-income countries. This will facilitate rapid, organized information collection, analysis, and dissemination, both for disease surveillance and to support planning and decision-making. We are likely to see considerable impetus to improve biosurveillance and research capacity around the world once the COVID-19 pandemic is under better control; taking clinical research ICT needs into account during such capacity building efforts will contribute to a sustainable research enterprise in countries and a better global response to future infectious disease outbreaks. The initial technology assessment is the cornerstone for strategic planning, and a sound assessment of ICT requirements will support local adaptations and reduce costs later when it is operationally feasible and appropriate.

2.2 Technology Assessment Outline

The technology assessment process should be guided by data collection forms, based on prepared templates, that focus on key areas outlined below.

- For area of operations (AO), evaluate
  - Operational environment, including
    - Language requirements
    - Security posture
    - Transport options
  - Existing technical infrastructure
  - Electrical power availability and stability
  - Area telecommunications company (phone services and Internet)
  - Technology companies available in AO
  - Technology staff skills in AO
  - Assess area equipment availability and quality standards
- Partners and collaborators
  - Determine the roles of partners and collaborators
  - Identify and establish communication systems interfaces
- For site selection, determine
  - Number of sites
  - Location of sites (domestic, international, cyberspace)
  - Technical infrastructure at sites
  - Technical expertise at sites
  - Electrical power availability and stability at sites
  - Security at sites
  - Facilities at sites
  - Equipment at sites
  - Local Internet/mobile telephony providers at sites
- Supply chain
  - International technology constraints
  - Identify technology vendors in AO
  - Shipping and import requirements applicable to the AO
  - Evaluate local supply chain and how to obtain equipment
- Telecommunications
  - Identify locality capabilities for telecommunications backbones (landlines, cellular, satellite, cable, fiber optics)
  - Identify key contacts and project collaborators
  - Evaluate roaming agreements and cost implications for initial travelers
  - Evaluate teleconferencing and videoconferencing capabilities at sites

The data captured in the assessment (◘ Fig. 2) will provide the basis for actions and decisions on how to deploy ICT to support the research response and the phased implementation of technology and technical resources in the five core areas. The output of these decisions or actions provides the basis to support the initial conduct of the study. As additional information becomes available and the study progresses, operational plans will change accordingly.

INITIAL INFORMATION TECHNOLOGY SITE ASSESSMENT REPORT

SITE VISIT DATE	
ASSESSOR	
LOCATION	

I FACILITY TOUR / PHYSICAL INSPECTION			
A. Describe physical location			
B. Does the site currently have internet connectivity?	YES ☐	NO ☐	N/A ☐
C. Describe internet connection			
D. Describe the internet connection options			
Recommendations and Additional Comments:			

II DATA INFRASTRUCTURE			
A. Does the site have an existing data center or similar dedicated IT room?	YES ☐	NO ☐	N/A ☐
B. Fire protection systems present?	YES ☐	NO ☐	N/A ☐
C. Type of fire protection system?			
D. Separate temperature and humidity controls?	YES ☐	NO ☐	N/A ☐
E. Redundant network backbones?	YES ☐	NO ☐	N/A ☐
F. Describe data center			
G. Data Management Room Dimensions			
Recommendations and Additional Comments:			

Fig. 2 Sample page from technology needs assessment. (Authors/USG public domain)

3 ICT Operational Framework

The ICT team will define how to manage the policies, practices, and resources needed to provide communications solutions in the environment of each research project, based on the changing objectives outlined above. Practical implementation will initially be driven by the lead partner organization, with the goal of making the local research organization an equal partner as expeditiously as possible and transferring leadership and operational control over time. In this process, many of the policies, practical constraints, and modes of operation established at the outset will carry over through the transition. The early stage of the response will be driven by the urgent need to begin the research; therefore, efficiency, cost-effectiveness, and process automation will not be the top priorities. Over time, and with increasing operational proficiency, ICT team operations and deployment of ICT equipment and networks will become better suited to the research organization as it evolves to support the outbreak response. Ultimately, operational control may shift from the study team to an ICT working group under the purview of a steering committee and supported by local vendors and technologists. The response (◘ Fig. 3) will occur in phases that can be summarized along with the key actions the ICT team must undertake.

1. *Initiation.* Collect and evaluate key scoping data on the extent and complexity of the ICT operational framework for the planned response. While research project management specifies its data and communications needs, the ICT team will define technical requirements and implement installation and support structures for communications within and outside the study team. Scoping data will include detailed information on the area where studies will be conducted and capabilities at each particular site, most critically the availability and stability of Internet and telecoms access and electricity. The ICT capacity of locally based partners is also a vital term of the equation.
2. *Planning.* Based on this information, the ICT team will establish regular dialogue and information exchange among part-

IT Framework				
Initiation	**Planning**	**Implementation**	**Monitoring and Control**	**Closing**
• Identify key areas needed (equipment /communication/infrastructure/systems.) **• Identify partners and collaborators.** **• Conduct site visits.** **• Determine availability of critical components in locality.** **• Identify internet service providers.** **• Evaluate systems and applications available and/or needed.** **• Evaluate operational environments and language needs.**	• Evaluate acquisition options (build/buy /lease/partner). • Establish and review service level agreements. • Identify critical positions and personnel. • Define project scopes. • Evaluate clinical processes and determine where suitable ICT solutions can be leveraged to enhance activities. • Establish communication mechanisms to facilitate informed decisions. •Assess supply chain limitations.	• Manage and provide guidance to local teams. • Establish regular meetings. • Respond to ad hoc inquiries for information sharing and collaboration.	• Develop regular maintenance and support windows. • Interface with local support teams. • Respond to outages, system changes, equipment failures, and new technology requests. • Share information and exchange knowledge on ongoing basis. •Address supply chain challenges.	• Determine strategy for hand-off to partners. • Develop methodologies for transfer of knowledge, equipment, and licenses.
Tools:	IT site assessment template			

◘ **Fig. 3** Actions for creation of an ICT operation capable of reacting to and maturing along with evolving response needs. (Authors) ners, collaborators, and stakeholders; it will review project plans, establish deadlines, and identify resource needs. The ICT team will most likely be staffed by and will draw policies and practices from the more experienced partner organization. Through the course of study implementation, operations will be adapted and augmented to support the concrete needs of the outbreak response in the local environment. The output of the planning stage should provide a general inventory of scope and tasks, which ICT staff will manage and coordinate.

3. *Implementation.* With initial plans based on the technical assessment, operational activities by the ICT staff will at first be more reactive than strategic—recall the military adage that no plan survives contact with the enemy. As unforeseen problems and emergencies are overcome, and the team establishes the ICT systems and personnel needed to support a functional organization, a more prospective, stable, and strategic approach can be nurtured, along with the formal organizational documentation describing it.
4. *Monitoring and control.* Once the operational framework, the functional organization, and the organogram are in synch, a stable ICT presence capable of supporting the communications and information needs of the clinical study should require fewer resources, even though ad hoc solutions and single-issue decisions may continue to be needed. With ongoing experience, the team should develop standard operating procedures to make such decisions routine.
5. *Closing.* Transition of ICT operations to the local research partner organization will require another round of meetings with partners, customers, and stakeholders to determine a suitable mechanism for hand-off of ICT hardware, software, systems, and infrastructure. The build-up of a local ICT working group as part of the host research organization—which then serves as an ICT counterpart for the transition process—is essential for identifying linkages among action items to ensure funding, seamless transition, and avoiding any hard cutoffs. The teams will then work out and implement migration plans for licensing account management, knowledge transfer, etc.

4 Equipment Selection and Procurement

Based on the project scope, including the number of sites, staffing numbers, laboratories, and clinical equipment requiring computer interfaces, the team will need to procure computers (laptops, desktops, tablets), mobile devices (phones, tablets, hot spots), printers, ID card printers, storage devices (USB flash drives, external hard drives, network attached storage), cameras, bar code readers, communications infrastructure (routers, switches, access points, network cabling), temperature monitoring devices, uninterruptible power supply (UPS) devices, voltage regulators (power adapters), and projectors (◘ Fig. 4). Although the ICT team will likely not be responsible for procuring them, generators and fuel may well be necessary to power systems, at least as a backup (▶ Chap. 9). Information requirements and data linkages to other research elements are also important, including integration of clinical, laboratory, and pharmaceutical equipment, processes, and personnel (▶ Chap. 35).

1. *Initiation.* The technology assessment and scope will be a preliminary determination of the quantity and specifications of equipment required, based on end users identified in the clinical protocol and support documents. This leads into a structured process for procurement, transport, accountability, and configuration. The availability of clean power, local support, and access to a local supply chain for pur-

	CONFIGURATION CHECKLIST
☐	Install operating system
☐	Install antivirus software and verify auto-update setting enabled
☐	Install productivity software
☐	Install web browser(s)
☐	Perform operating system and application updates
☐	Set device name conforming to naming convention
☐	Enable encryption of hard drive(s)
☐	Create local account(s), as appropriate
☐	Create domain account(s), as appropriate
☐	Configure user specific settings, as appropriate

Fig. 4 Selection and maintenance actions to support ICT response needs. (Authors)

chase and distribution must also be detailed to support the planning process.

2. *Planning.* Leverage or establish a suitable supply chain (possibly already in place in association with the partnering organization) to ensure timely delivery of items needed to start the study. An approval and procurement methodology based on the study protocol should be established. Local procurement is advantageous if (a) standardization of equipment is possible and (b) information security configuration and safeguards can be put into place in accordance with industry standards. International procurement is likely to increase lead time considerably.
3. *Implementation.* Manage configuration and installation of equipment, including electronic naming and labeling of equipment for identification on networks, where applicable. Prepare and use a standard configuration checklist (Fig. 5) to ensure appropriate configuration of devices. Ensure property accountability asset tags are applied and coordinate shipment, delivery, and deployment with local ICT or operations staff.
4. *Monitoring and control.* Establish a communication channel for user technical support and incident management, including escalation abilities. Establish periodic audits of equipment to ensure proper property accountability. Monitor equipment lifecycle dates, develop support budgets, and facilitate lifecycle replacement.
5. *Closing.* Determine the time remaining in the lifecycle of the equipment and evaluate whether it can be repurposed. Determine whether to return to lead organization, transfer to partners, donate, or dispose of. Ensure any data storage devices are appropriately sanitized before transfer. In conjunction with property and operations management staff, facilitate all final property assignment records.

5 Flexible Communications

The primary objective of ICT is to facilitate communication among the team, with partners, and with the outside world (Fig. 6). Access to and maintenance of communications platforms are essential in providing this capability (▶ Chap. 32.1). Many commercial solutions for communication and collaboration may require bandwidth and platform stability unattainable in remote or underserved regions. While solutions like satellite-based communications or premium cellular access are available for a price, costs may limit the level of service that can be provided. However, as infrastructure develops—something that

Equipment				
Initiation	**Planning**	**Implementation**	**Monitoring and Control**	**Closing**
• Identify needs (laptops, desktops, phones, tablets, printers, mobile hotspots, UPS devices, projectors, etc.). • Identify custodians of record. • Develop independent acquisition mechanism or integrate into supply chain. • Identify local IT support team and distribution system. • Assess environmental and operational considerations (power, ruggedized models). • Determine time constraints to prevent manufacturer supply delays.	• Develop requestor and approval matrix to ensure consistency and that appropriate equipment is procured. • Evaluate local supply chain and efficiencies of obtaining locally vs shipping. • Prevent bottlenecks by providing ability to track status and disposition of orders. • Standardize platforms. • Ensure remote support session capabilities. • Consider export control restrictions.	• Coordinate deployment with shipments. • Establish small supply of loaners, with applicable loaner SOP. • Confirm compliance with appropriate information security standards (encryption/antivirus/ etc.). • Determine whether to configure equipment at point of origin or locally. •Ensure sufficient site security for equipment.	• Tier 1 basic technical support provided locally, Tier 2 intermediate, and Tier 3 advanced technical support via remote support sessions. • Manage software patches and antivirus updates. • Effect warranty repairs. Monitor and resupply consumables (toner/ID cards). • For long-term studies, account for lifecycle replacement of equipment.	• Abandon or transfer equipment in place or return. • Document sanitization of hard drives.
Tools:	Deployment and configuration guides; equipment estimates; property management tracking			

Fig. 5 Standard configuration checklist. (Authors)

can happen rapidly in a major international response—continual reassessment may allow for additional options and major improvements in existing ones like cellular service. A rundown on the pluses and minuses of many equipment and configuration options is available in the UNICEF Emergency telecommunications handbook (2017).

1. *Initiation.* Determine the availability of platforms for communication, including land-based phone lines, cellular service, fiber optic, or cable service providers for voice-over-Internet-protocol (VOIP) offerings. Satellite telephony is available virtually everywhere, but while not nearly as costly as it once was, is not a practical solution for voluminous data transfer. Evaluate web and videoconferencing solutions available at sites and assess interoperability with clinical sites and research partner platforms. Consider cost impact for phone, texting, and data plans, especially for international projects. Identify all partners and partner locations.
2. *Planning.* Meet with project stakeholders to define deliverables and determine budget. Contact communication service providers to determine offerings. Develop a statement or scope of work and solicit requests for proposals. Assemble project team to review proposals, including Service Level Agreements (SLAs), which define the level of service a customer expects from a supplier, specify how the service is monitored, and set any remedies or penalties for non-fulfillment. Provide recommendations to the project management team for approval.
3. *Implementation.* Facilitate application (app) configuration and installation on mobile devices. Evaluate roaming rates and agreements with local providers and provide local phones and usage guidance to traveling team members. Coordinate provisioning of roaming plans with service providers to control communications costs during travel. Train local IT staff on setup and support of web- and videoconferencing platforms.
4. *Monitoring and control.* Monitor account usage and add/remove accounts as needed. Mobile apps change frequently, so consider new variations as they are released (e.g., Skype was originally used in early rapid response, followed by Vonage, and then WhatsApp to reduce costs and improve performance). Tomorrow's best option may be different, and network

Communications				
Initiation	**Planning**	**Implementation**	**Monitoring and Control**	**Closing**
• Identify local capabilities for telecommunications backbone (landlines, cellular, satellite, cable, fiber optics). Identify key contacts. • Evaluate roaming agreements and cost implications for initial travelers. • Evaluate tele- and videoconferencing capabilities, including room design.	• Establish service agreements with service providers. • Ensure SLAs are agreed and in effect. • Develop guidance documents and instructions on alternate communication methods. • Consider costs of roaming compared to local carriers. • Establish group email and phone lists. • Unify email platform for external traffic.	• Install common apps on mobile devices and provide guidance on use. • Deploy video-conference units and integrate with meeting platforms. • Procure domain names. • Establish phone access arrangements for visiting personnel.	• Review contracts periodically to manage costs and ensure best service. • Account management, including creation and deletion of user accounts.	• Terminate or transfer agreements. • Return, transfer, or dispose of equipment.
Tools:	Traveler mobile communication guidance docs; online coverage maps and costing calculators			

Fig. 6 Actions to establish tools and strategies for communications for the research organization. (Authors)

effects are important (i.e., which platform is predominant in the area of operations). Evaluate Internet service providers (ISPs) and wireless carrier costs against SLA performance and potential competitors. Request reductions or change providers when appropriate.

5. *Closing.* Determine equipment status and deposition in consultation with local partners and collaborators. Coordinate termination or transfer of licenses, agreements, accounts, and domain names. Ensure study-related materials contained within any hosting platform are properly accounted for, transferred, or sanitized.

6 Infrastructure

Infrastructure at a country level, among the research partners, and at each site is a critical functional element, based on which ICT and information systems must be planned and implemented (Fig. 7). Aspects of infrastructure include the presence and reliability of electrical power (▶ Chaps. 32, 37, and 39), prevailing telecommunications, fiber and other networks, and commercial service availability for communication and infrastructure support. Networking and communication infrastructure are essential to study implementation, and both simplicity and redundancy are of value. Manual curation and a very high support-to-end-user ratio should be planned for and expected, especially at the outset.

1. *Initiation.* Based on the technical assessment and site surveys, establish the technical infrastructure needs for the project data center, local area networking, and ICT facility needs. Evaluate technologies in place and determine whether partner relationships can be leveraged to supplement existing commercially available infrastructure or if new infrastructure is needed.
2. *Planning.* Design the physical and/or logical layout of the site and project networks. Review existing data centers (generally at partner site or cloud-based) to ensure appropriate physical, environmental, and logical safeguards are in place. Provide recommendations and direction for sensitive data leaving country of origin (▶ Chap. 7) and security practices (▶ Chap. 41). Identify vendors and providers of Internet bandwidth (which can often be a rate-limiting factor) and the best

Infrastructure				
Initiation	**Planning**	**Implementation**	**Monitoring and Control**	**Closing**
• Identify core technologies available (fiber, IEEE 802.11 LAN protocols, cable, copper, dish). **• Identify partners and collaborators.** **• Request site drawings and building layouts.** **• Conduct site survey.**	• Design site network topology. • Ensure appropriate level of fault tolerances. • Add redundancies (cabling, power). Develop disaster recovery plan. • Ensure suitable spare (backup) equipment is available. • Determine proper correlation of cost for reducing outage risk with impact of outage.	• Coordinate with local installation teams. • Evaluate business requirements and develop management policies to ensure appropriate use.	• Establish remote and local monitoring. • Refine policies to optimize performance. • Ensure immediate response to cybersecurity or inappropriate use incidents.	• Terminate or transfer agreements and cloud licensing. • Determine transfer or disposition of equipment.
Tools:	Network topology maps; cloud-based controllers			

Fig. 7 Actions to establish core technical infrastructure. (Authors)

feasible networking and telecommunications capacity to sites and study team activities.

3. *Implementation.* Provide direction and oversight of final construction stages, including power connections and cabling if applicable. Install and configure equipment together with local staff to ensure adherence to quality standards. Perform verification and acceptance testing of equipment. Identify a site liaison for operations input into network traffic-shaping policies and data segregation. Utilize local ICT or operations staff to convey local Wi-Fi connection information.
4. *Monitoring and control.* Train local ICT staff on remote monitoring of network infrastructure, including incident alerts and remediation. Ensure critical components remain secured, with access limited to authorized personnel (using a combination of physical locks and logical logins, as required). Consider offsite storage and chain of custody of physical keys to prevent unauthorized access.
5. *Closing.* Evaluate equipment and determine disposition. Coordinate the termination or transfer of licenses, agreements, and accounts. Ensure study-related materials contained within any hosting platform are properly accounted for, transferred, or sanitized. Facilitate the transfer of physical keys and account credentials, where appropriate.

7 Information Systems

Information systems vary from paper files to a single, stand-alone computer with software applications to networks with multiple software applications, databases, and supporting hardware platforms. During early response phases (Fig. 8), consider the longer-term implications of utilizing off-the-shelf, conventional temporary products, such as spreadsheets, to perform functions that will ultimately be better fulfilled by a database. Consider and evaluate pathways to bridge or pull data into a more robust, permanent solution. Discuss with the study team and investigators what languages might need to be included in the study protocol and other documents for use by partner organizations and locally hired study staff (▶ Chap. 42). Evaluate any potential interfaces or data interchanges that might be needed for core clinical data management or supporting systems.

1. *Initiation.* Identify critical stakeholders and conduct needs analysis. Determine functional requirements and cross walk against existing systems used by the part-

Information Systems				
Initiation	**Planning**	**Implementation**	**Monitoring and Control**	**Closing**
• Assemble stakeholder team. **• Identify needs, current capabilities, and partner/collaborator systems.** **• Plan for, inter alia, inventory management, participant scheduling, biometric identification, social media, websites, storage, and backups.** **• Evaluate infrastructure and determine if locally or remote hosting is more appropriate.**	• Develop user and system requirements. • Consider configurable commercial software vs custom built. • Evaluate costs, including licensing and hosting. • Develop training materials and user guides. • Conduct system walkthroughs and pilot exercises prior to going live.	• Phase rollouts and interface with teams to ensure suitable integration into process flows. • Designate tech leads/power users. • Ensure communication channels are in place for planned outages or upgrades.	• Ensure local and remote technical support available 24/7, with escalation as needed. • Respond promptly to system service or change requests.	• Transfer ownership or dispose. • Data migration to stakeholders.
Tools:	IT Governance templates (business needs, project process agreement, change management log, communication matrix, risk management log, security approach, requirements definition, contingency plan, design, interface control, test plans)			

Fig. 8 Actions to select and deploy information systems. (Authors)

ner organization. Develop conceptual and preliminary design models. Consider the process and workflows and incorporate into the model.

2. *Planning.* Review concepts and business cases provided by stakeholders. Evaluate the availability of solutions that can meet needs, be quickly deployable, and be optimally usable by study staff. Consider open-source solutions and short and longer-term implications of creating custom applications compared with a configurable, commercially available product. Hardware platforms used in support of systems in rural or remote locations should be durable and able to function for extended periods with unreliable power supplies.
3. *Implementation.* Coordinate testing and trial runs with stakeholders. Evaluate application use cases in development environments during acceptance testing. Identify required changes and categorize into a prioritization matrix for immediate or phased implementation, depending on importance. Finalize training and guidance materials and provide in different formats for various learner styles (written, visual, kinesthetic). Establish procedures for providing help desk inquiries and support.
4. *Monitoring and control.* Establish a communication channel for user technical support and incident management, including escalation ability on a tiered service model ranging from basic help to advanced, expert-level support, with the latter provided by research program headquarters or more likely an overseas location—another reason for strong communications. When installing new software releases, functions, and system changes, the project ICT team must communicate changes to all key stakeholders and conduct iterative training and review to ensure users accept and can use the new functionality, and that it operates as expected.
5. *Closing.* Coordinate the termination or transfer of licenses, agreements, and accounts. Ensure study-related materials contained within any hosting platform are properly accounted for, transferred, or sanitized, as appropriate. Develop and review data migration pathways.

8 Conclusion

Meeting the technology and communication needs of a clinical research project from conception to closing is challenging even when infrastructure and supply systems are well developed and functioning as needed. In an emergency infectious disease response, urgency, the unpredictability of a new pathogen or an uncoordinated research response can lead to errors, some avoidable and others less so. We have seen many such missteps in the COVID-19 research response, some of them with enduring consequences, like the promotion of hydroxychloroquine or ivermectin as medical countermeasures for severe acute respiratory syndrome coronavirus 2 (SARS-CoV-2) infection and COVID-19 disease.

Add the constraints of operating in a low-resource environment, as with the emergence of Ebola in West Africa in 2014 and the eastern Democratic Republic of the Congo in 2018, and the task requires even greater dedication, experience, and flexibility. The basic takeaway from the experiences described above is to start simple, with the most essential requirements, and build out as technology, technical staff, and infrastructure allow. The challenges of establishing a coherent, cohesive approach to a robust network for communications, data-storage and analysis, and program management depend to a great extent on how and when they can be introduced, to say nothing of scientific and technological progress, including, for example, gene-sequencing methods. The approaches described above are meant as general guidelines which will require tailoring for each EID response, as well as continuing technological development. One hopes we will be better prepared for the next emerging infectious disease outbreak than we have been in the recent past.

? Discussion Questions

1. Describe a scenario in which initial ICT tool(s) could be substituted by those that might be more cost-effective and/or sustainable in the local environment.
2. Describe the ways to effectively utilize the available skillsets of the entire research program team to meet project goals.
3. Of the five key response stages (initiation, planning, implementation, monitoring and control, and closing) discussed throughout the chapter, which one requires the most coordination with the local team? Why?
4. Provide an example of a situation in which the original communication platform was replaced by another. What factors should be considered before making such a change?

References

Morens DM, Fauci AS. Emerging pandemic diseases: how we got to COVID-19. Cell. 2020;182(5):1077–92. https://doi.org/10.1016/j.cell.2020.08.021.

UNICEF. Emergency telecommunications handbook. New York: UNICEF, Division IaCT; 2017. https://www.scribd.com/document/444100858/Emergency-Telecommunications-Handbook-pdf. Accessed 3 Aug 2024.

Wilson C, Jumbert MG. The new informatics of pandemic response: humanitarian technology, efficiency, and the subtle retreat of national agency. J Int Humanit Action. 2018;2018, 3(1) https://doi.org/10.1186/s41018-018-0036-5.

35 Data Management in Emergency Response Research

Harry van Loen, Moses Badio, and Yven Van Herrewege

Contents

Learning Track Note: This chapter appears in Learning Tracks: Biostatistics; Clinical Research; Emergency Research Response, Research Operations

E. S. Higgs and R. A. Sorenson (eds.), *Principles and Practice of Emergency Research Response*,
https://doi.org/10.1007/978-3-031-48408-7_55

Learning Objectives

This chapter will help readers understand and describe:

- Understand the essential role of proper data management in ensuring the validity and quality of clinical research and its impact on analysis, results, reporting, and study conclusions.
- Learn key concepts and central elements of sound data management to be employed during emergency clinical research.
- Describe the following:
  - Data management and the role of a data management plan in a clinical research study
  - The roles and responsibilities of dedicated data managers
  - The advantages and disadvantages of electronic data capture
  - The principles of ALCOA+
  - Access to clinical trial data
  - Regulations and guidelines for the Ebola-TX study
  - Specific data challenges in EID outbreaks
  - Experience-based guidelines for good project management practices
  - Factors preventing rapid, open dissemination of research data
  - The meaning and importance of data lock
  - Methods of clinical trial data dissemination and the benefits of data sharing
  - Obstacles to efficient data archiving and retrieval
  - Measures that contribute to greater data reliability

1 Introduction

Proper data management in emergency clinical research is essential for ensuring the validity and quality of research. It is a key aspect of good clinical practice (GCP) guidelines (ICH 2016; WHO 2005). Adherence to these guidelines is mandated by ethics review committees and international regulatory authorities. Requirements include planning and use of validated data management tools and processes to ensure research data is collected according to standardized, verifiable procedures and based on reliable, accurate data resources which will allow analysis, reporting, and dissemination of study results of the highest quality (Manghani 2011). Note that while the following discussion focuses on clinical research, as the most data-intensive research requiring the most statistical analysis, the principles and practical requirements apply to other types of emergency research as well.

Data management is not merely the development of a study database for the collection of "data," defined as quantitative or qualitative variables, signs, and observations collected from various sources. Instead, it should be seen as a process stretching from the preparation and initiation of a project or study, over the conduct of the study, through to the analysis and reporting of study results and sharing the underlying data. Several essential concepts in data management related to data quality and data integrity deserve to be looked at carefully, including necessary precautions to protect the rights, privacy, and safety of often vulnerable research participants and communities—especially so when considering research in emergency settings and vulnerable populations (▶ Chap. 5).

Treating data management as a fundamental part of emergency clinical research helps ensure sufficient resources can be allocated not only to ensure adherence to GCP guidelines, governmental regulations, and data management standards but also to support timely reporting of high-quality research results, the main objective of any research project. Unfortunately, data management is often sorely neglected, poorly supported, and suboptimally conducted (Haug et al. 2011; Pandav et al. 2002). Especially in noncommercial, academic programs with limited funding and human resource capacity, data management requirements are not self-fulfilling. Moreover, conducting research (including state of the art clinical trials) in emergency and/or resource-poor settings can pose additional, serious challenges: scant financial and human resources and technical obstacles such as poor Internet connectivity, electrical power outages and voltage fluctuations, limited information technology (IT) infrastructure, etc. may hinder operations. In these circumstances, as exemplified by the Ebola virus outbreak in West Africa in 2014–2016 and the 2018–2020 Ebola outbreak in the Democratic Republic of Congo (DRC), data management must adapt to specific, unique circumstances in which regulatory requirements need to be balanced against real-life feasibility in emergency settings (Hossmann et al. 2019; Mulangu et al. 2019).

In these settings, a rather pragmatic approach should be considered. No one-size-fits-all recommendations can be given for (1) the setup and organization of the data management team; (2) the preparation and execution of a data management plan; (3) specific data management requirements tailored to research, technical, and user needs; or (4) the selection and implementation of data capture tools. All of these topics are discussed below. A generic outline of data capture and data review processes during the conduct of such research is also presented. Finally, we briefly discuss database lock and data extraction as a preparatory step for data archiving and data sharing. In general, this chapter aims to introduce key concepts in good data management practices, using examples from emergency research studies, rather than attempting to provide an exhaustive technical overview. Although as authors we regularly refer to our specific experience with Ebola clinical trials, the principles described in this chapter can be applied to any clinical or other type of emergency research.

2 Roles and Responsibilities in Data Management

Over the past three decades, clinical research and in particular clinical data management (CDM) have become an established discipline with specific roles and responsibilities for individuals and groups working with data, as illustrated in Fig. 1 (Krishnankutty et al. 2012; Lu and Su 2010; Prokscha 2012). However, academic, noncommercial clinical research programs, especially in infectious disease emergency response research, often lack the resources to hire one or more dedicated

Role	Responsibilities	Reports to
Data Entry Clerk	• Enters study data into an electronic Case Report Form (eCRF) (the study database)	• Principal Investigator or Data Manager
Data Reviewer/Quality Control Officer	• Reviews data quality • Queries sites on data inconsistencies	• Data Manager
Data Manager	• Ensures overall CDM of the study/project (data integrity, quality, confidentiality, security) • Designs Data Management Plan and other relevant CDM documentation and tools • Represents CDM at project team meetings • Supervises the other CDM team members	• Principal Investigator • Project/Study coordinator
Database Administrator	• Designs and develops the study database and eCRF • Maintains authorized access and security to the database and eCRF	• Principal Investigator (sometimes) • IT manager
Programmer	• Programs and tests the edit checks on the study database or eCRF	• Principal Investigator (sometimes) • IT manager
Medical Coder	• Standardizes the study medical terms (e.g., adverse events, concomitant medications)	• Principal Investigator or Data Manager

Fig. 1 A non-exhaustive overview of roles and responsibilities in data management. (Authors)

professionals responsible for data management. As such, it is crucial to outline to all study members their specific roles and responsibilities in data management. Note that these roles and responsibilities may differ depending on the study and the data management team involved.

Collaborating in a multinational or multisite study poses additional challenges and requires a clear differentiation of activities conducted at a coordinating center versus those at the local sites. It is good study practice to assign a dedicated data manager for the study and, if possible, to identify a supervising, central data manager at the coordinating center and one or more site data managers at each clinical site. In addition, data entry clerk(s) and data reviewer(s) as well as a medical coder should be identified as part of the site team and central team, respectively. Assuring data management is performed by qualified and well-trained staff is equally important.

Figure 2 shows the data management setup and the assigned data management roles for the Ebola-TX study "Emergency Evaluation of Convalescent Plasma for Ebola Virus Disease (EVD) in Guinea" (van Griensven et al. 2016; van Griensven and Haba 2019). An Ebola treatment center (ETC) located in Conakry, Guinea, acted as a site where EVD patients were recruited. A site data manager, supervising a site team of two data entry clerks, handled the daily capture and management of clinical and lab data. Daily communication was set up between the site data manager and the central data manager at the coordinating Institute of Tropical Medicine in Antwerp, Belgium (ITM). An information technology (IT) manager sent by ITM to the site supported both data managers in implementing the electronic data capture system in the challenging circumstances of the 2014–2016 West Africa Ebola emergency.

Furthermore, the central data manager oversaw CDM for the study as a whole, represented CDM at regular trial management meetings where all essential study stakeholders were represented, and supervised the activities of the two data reviewers/quality control officers. The central data manager also functioned as a first-line IT helpdesk (e.g., assigning passwords to users), while collaboration with the IT department ensured further support for more complex IT issues. Moreover, the central data manager collaborated, especially on data quality, with ITM's quality assurance manager, monitor, and statistician (Fig. 2).

In recent years, new roles in data management have been introduced. Figure 3 illustrates some of these newer roles with their specific responsibilities, highlighting the flexibility required of a data management team to adapt to changes in data management processes.

As highlighted above, data management in (clinical) research clearly requires specific

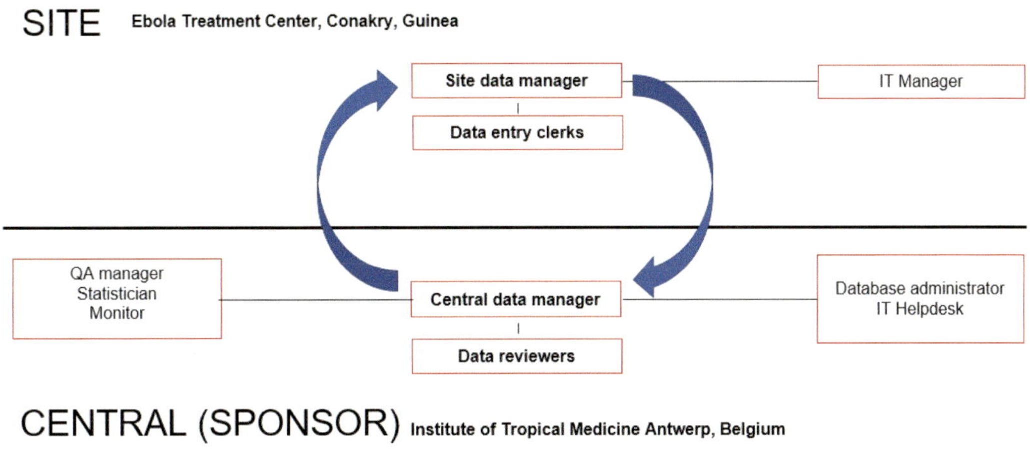

Fig. 2 Data management setup and data management roles during the Ebola-TX study. (Authors)

Fig. 3 Additional roles in (clinical) data management. (Authors)

Role	Responsibilities
Data Custodian	• Ensures consistent data storage, processing, and transmission. • Ensures database security. • Duties overlap with database administrator (Fig. 1).
Data Steward	• Ensures quality of data and metadata. • Duties overlap with data manager (Fig. 1). • Focus on data sharing in academic environments.
Data Scientist	• Provides specialized knowledge and analysis of data. • Recommends solutions that meet business needs. • Duties overlap with study statistician.
Data Protection Officer	• Ensures compliance with data protection standards, e.g., GDPR (EU General Data Protection Regulation).

expertise, based on education and on-the-job training. In this regard, it is important to ensure sustainable capacity-building mechanisms in order to maintain this expertise and keep it up to date (Chap. 8).

3 Data Management Plan

The importance of a data management plan (DMP) to support research has attracted considerable interest from research stakeholders in recent years, as exemplified by a 2018 editorial in *Nature* highlighting the DMP as a prerequisite for good data management (Anon 2018). Funders such as Horizon 2020, the European Commission's 2014–2020 research funding mechanism, require a DMP outlining how project data will be managed and shared (EC 2020). Similarly, both UK research funders and the U.S. National Science Foundation stipulate when projects must have a DMP (Digital Curation Centre 2021; NSF 2018). Digital tools that provide a generic DMP template users may modify as desired are also now available, with DMPonline and DMPTool as the best known (DMPonline 2021; DMPTool 2021; Jones et al. 2020; Sallans and Donnelly 2012).

Although much of this interest seems recent, Smale et al. (2020) note that published evidence of data management plans in research goes back to 1966. Since then, DMPs have been around with various names, contents, shapes, and foci. We define a DMP as a formal document to plan pre-study, study, and post-study data practices and processes. We distinguish the following DMP purposes:

- Documenting essential preparations for and processes of data handling
- Ensuring traceability from data collection to analysis, reporting, and sharing
- Assuring compliance with sponsor and regulatory requirements for data management
- Providing guidance to all study stakeholders involved in data management
- Organizing timelines, roles, and responsibilities for data management and related study tasks

In addition, we propose an outline of a DMP as shown in Table 1.

In emergency clinical research, a DMP has clear added value in improving the quality of the study and the results generated. For the Ebola-TX study, planning and preparation eventually succeeded with a timely database lock. This was due to successful communications between the study partners, in particular the coordinating ITM center in Antwerp and the ETC in Conakry where the study was conducted, and to prompt responses to resolve various bottlenecks. Challenges included the data collection form design, which had to be adapted several times before and during the study. These adaptations had to be documented to ensure a validated system. Another challenge was setting up a local area network to support data capture and transfer between the high-risk red zone where patients infected with EVD were treated and stringent infection prevention was needed and the low-risk green zone where personal protective equipment was not required for healthcare workers. Rapid deployment of an experienced ITM IT man-

Table 1 Contents of a data management plan (authors)

DMP component	Clarification/description
Introduction	• Reference to study protocol/project identification • Document title • Name of author(s) and date
Documentation of approval	• Names, signatures, and date of approval by stakeholders
Version history	• A DMP should be considered as a living document • Section keeping track and control of the various DMP versions
Table of contents	• List of all sections by page number
Definitions and acronyms	• Glossary of words, definitions, and abbreviations
Pre-study (study setup)	
General DMP information	• Aim and purpose of the DMP
Study protocol summary	• Brief summary of the study. This should include dataflows and/or workflows
Communication	• Clear procedures on communication and on the contacts or focal points for data management (DM)
Documentation	• Procedures and requirements for DM documentation
Pre-study project management	
Roles/responsibilities	• List of personnel, roles, responsibilities, study access rights, training, and other qualifications
Timelines	• List of essential DM milestones and deliverables
Risk management.	• Identification of processes or data critical to ensure reliable results and protection of human participants
Regulatory and funder requirements and standards	• Compliance with ethical procedures and regulations covering safety and privacy of human participants and data safety, security, and confidentiality. Compliance with discipline-specific standards
Data types and sources	• Description of types of data, formats, volume, origin, and location. Should be documented in data dictionaries, annotated data collection forms, and data flows
Data collection form design	• Design of collection forms with strict adherence to the study protocol and good design practices • Specification of paper or electronic data capture tools or both • Programming edit checks and branching logic on electronic data capture tools
System design	• Defining software and hardware (server, internet, devices) • Keeping track of software and system versions in use; update/upgrade policy • Compliance with regulatory requirements on data integrity and confidentiality
System validation	• Documentation that both software and hardware are fit for purpose of data collection and management • Ensuring that changes in systems are implemented in a controlled manner (change control)
System security	• Administrative, technical, and physical safeguards in place

(continued)

Table 1 (continued)

DMP component	Clarification/description
Backup and recovery	• Implementation of regular backups of servers, devices, and databases • Plan for recovery in case of disaster or data loss
Training	• Documented evidence of training on DM (what, who, when, and by whom)
During the study	
Data capture	• Compliance with data collection and entry guidelines
Data review	• Verifying the accuracy, consistency, and completeness of data and compliance with study protocol • Manual checking • Automatic checking, by programmed edit checks • Discrepancy handling and resolution of queries
Data tracking	• Keeping timely track of study data, source, and status
Data coding	• Ensuring reference to coding conventions, by using the WHO Drug Dictionary (for standardizing medicines) and MedDRA, the ICH Medical Dictionary for Regulatory Activities (for standardizing medical events)
Data storage	• Specification of paper retention, electronic data and files storage, or both • Policy on storage at coordinating center versus local study sites
Data transfer	• Transfer of data between stakeholders of a study • Transfers during and after study • Ensuring security measures
IT support	• Assigning role of IT helpdesk • Providing IT maintenance and problem-solving
Post-study	
Database lock	• Ensuring data security and integrity following data capture and review • Following a checklist and organizing a final data quality control before approval for database lock • Specify circumstances for unlocking a locked database (approved reasons only) • Removal of access rights from users to the database or system as their roles end
Data management report	• Final updated DMP • Describe quality issues • List all deviations from the DMP
Archiving	• Long-term storage to ensure security and confidentiality of the data, to allow comprehensive reconstruction of the completed work, and to fulfill regulatory requirements
Data sharing	• Promoting secondary research and reuse of study data • Meeting regulatory, funder, or publisher requirements • Sharing data as openly as possible, as closed as necessary (removing personally identifiable data) • Implementing a data-sharing governance mechanism for personal data, sensitive data, and medical data

ager was critical to timely resolution of data collection and transfer issues as they arose at the study site. Also, having an experienced and motivated investigator as a site data manager was of incalculable value for the successful implementation of study and DM processes.

Emergency response research is urgent by definition, and the time required to prepare well-designed data collection and entry documents is a potential bottleneck. It is a clear advantage to use generic, readily available templates for DMPs. Such generic templates, for example, those provided by the African Coalition for Epidemic Research, Response and Training (ALERRT), could be part of a library of study documentation templates, combining sections likely to be needed in any study with sections to be adapted to specific studies (ALERRT 2024). Making DMPs machine-actionable or automatically generated and shared insofar as practical is another way to reduce administrative burden (Miksa et al. 2019).

► Sections 4–7 of this chapter will discuss some essential DMP topics in more detail.

4 Data Management Requirements

Emergency response research for infectious disease outbreaks should be viewed as a heterogeneous research area or cluster of various disciplines rather than as one well-defined type of expertise or research. It involves stakeholders with different backgrounds, active in different research fields, and working with a variety of discipline-specific tools, systems, regulations, standards, and guidelines. As such, the challenges for DM and IT are diverse. Owada et al. (2016) describe procedures for epidemiological data management during an Ebola outbreak in Sierra Leone, with a focus on data collection and data handling, mentioning several problems related to DM organization, including lack of supervision and inadequate training of DM staff.

Note that strictly regulated clinical trials require specific tools such as an electronic audit trail for tracking changes in the database, as well as restricted access to the database. As a result, software tools or IT systems for use in one type of study (e.g., epidemiological studies or basic research studies) are often inappropriate for use in clinical trials without technical modifications. Another concern in an emergency, especially one occurring in a low-resource environment, is that time constraints could prevent adequate validation of the IT system and might compromise regulatory standards and quality (Hossmann et al. 2019). In this section, we will consider key requirements for DM related to the type of research conducted and the requirements from a regulatory, technical, and project management point of view.

4.1 Types of Research

Different types of research usually have different requirements, which also holds true for DM. The EVD outbreak in West Africa during 2014–2016 was a good indicator of the diversity of emergency research. Several systematic reviews reported a variety of emergency response research at the cellular or genetic level, patient level, and population level (Abramowitz et al. 2018; Cori et al. 2017; Holmes et al. 2016; Lee et al. 2019). The coronavirus disease 2019 (COVID-19) pandemic has of course prompted a deluge of diverse research programs (Anon 2021).

DM of an observational study versus DM of a clinical trial differs in several respects. For example, clinical research on a new drug needs to comply with stringent regulations, while non-interventional studies are less strictly regulated (including observational studies but also social science and anthropological studies). Some principles of DM are (or should be) common for all types of research, such as the need for data integrity, data quality, and ensuring data security. Other DM norms can be quite different, such as how crucial data are collected, data-handling tools and processes, and the qualifications required of data personnel. Understanding the type of research being performed is a first step to organize DM and then to define the requirements from ethical, regulatory, technical, and project management viewpoints.

For this chapter, and in keeping with the thematic focus of the book, we mostly refer here to good practices, guidelines, and regulations for preparing, conducting, and reporting a clinical trial. As noted, these are in some cases more stringent than would be required in case of nonclinical (non-interventional) research, but even the latter could benefit from adhering to the same principles or at least referring to them and thinking through why they may not be required.

4.2 Regulatory Requirements

All clinical research, including emergency response research on infectious diseases, must be carried out in compliance with international and local regulations (▶ Chap. 6)*, guidelines, standards, and funder requirements concerning DM.* Rather than trying to detail all national regulatory and other requirements, which depend on the type of research and where it is conducted, we refer to European Union (EU) and U.S. regulatory requirements on the main aspects of DM. As a concrete example, we refer to the Ebola-TX study, an emergency clinical trial sponsored by the Institute of Tropical Medicine Antwerp (Belgium), with EVD patients recruited from February 2015 to July 2015 in an Ebola treatment center managed by Médecins Sans Frontières (MSF) in Conakry, Guinea (van Griensven and Haba 2019). For the Ebola-TX study alone, the following regulations, guidelines, standards, and funder requirements were applicable to DM:

1. **EU Directive 2001/20/EC on clinical trials**. The Ebola-TX study adhered to this directive by ensuring that the trial subject data, information, and documents were properly generated, recorded, and reported (EC 2021b).[1]
2. **EU Directive 95/46/EC** refers to the rights of the subject to physical and mental integrity, to privacy, and to the protection of the subject data (EU 1995).[2] Ebola-TX measures to ensure security and confidentiality include controlled access to study computers, sponsor servers, study binders, offices, and server locations. Private information of trial participants must be handled confidentially, with personal identifying information omitted from electronic case report forms (eCRFs), other paper and electronic files, and publications. Ebola-TX trial data were properly anonymized before data sharing.
3. **U.S. Food and Drug Administration (FDA) 21 Code of Federal Regulations (CFR) part 11** defines the criteria under which electronic records and electronic signatures are considered trustworthy, reliable, and equivalent to paper records (FDA 2018). The Ebola-TX study used MACRO, a specific CDM system to comply with these criteria.
4. **The European Medicines Agency (EMA) incorporates Guidelines on Good Manufacturing Practice (GMP; see next paragraph)-Annex 11**, with specific requirements on the use of computerized systems. Ebola-TX ensured that its computer software, as well as the eCRFs used for data collection and management, were validated for their intended use, conforming to an established validation protocol and procedure (EC 2011).
5. **The International Council for Harmonisation of Technical Requirements for Pharmaceuticals for Human Use (ICH)** promulgates guidance for many aspects of clinical trials and pharmaceutical production. Many of these, e.g., GMP, are incorporated by stringent regulatory authorities like FDA and EMA into their own guidance. This also includes **good clinical practice (GCP)**, a foundational international guideline for designing, conducting, recording, and reporting clinical trials. GCP is designed to be used in conjunction with about 60 separate, detailed ICH

1 EU Regulation No. 536/2014 on clinical trials officially superseded EU Directive 2001/20/EC on January 31, 2022. There will be a 3-year transition period to full implementation and phaseout of the older procedures.

2 EU Directive 95/46/EC was replaced in 2018 by the EU General Data Protection Regulation.

guideline documents for many aspects of clinical trials. As above, these guidelines govern the conduct of clinical research in the EU, the United States, and many other countries (ICH 2022). Ebola-TX assigned a unique identification code to each participant, documented validation of the electronic data processing system, maintained standard operating procedures (SOPs) and data entry guidelines, provided an electronic audit trail and data traceability by maintaining an updated list of system users, as well as maintained adequate backup of the study data (ICH 2016).

6. **The Clinical Data Interchange Standards Consortium (CDISC)** publishes standards, such as CDASH (Clinical Data Acquisition Standards Harmonization), SDTM (Study Data Tabulation Model), and Operational Data Model-XML, to enhance the clinical trials process on data collection, data tabulation, and data transfer, respectively (CDISC 2021). Ebola-TX examined the feasibility of adhering to these standards, which are primarily used by the pharma industry for regulatory submission in the United States. Despite the time constraints and lack of previous experience with CDISC, Ebola-TX implemented CDASH for its CRFs and thereby facilitated future data sharing.
7. **Medical Dictionary for Regulatory Activities (MedDRA)**. The Ebola-TX study standardized its reporting of adverse events in accordance with this widely used international reference (MedDRA 2021).
8. **Funder requirements**. The EU, in particular its Horizon 2020 Research and Innovation Programme (EC 2021a), was the main funder for the Ebola-TX study. Since 2016, they have required adherence to the FAIR data principles for scientific DM to improve findability, accessibility, interoperability, and reuse of research data and metadata (Wilkinson et al. 2016). Since 2016, these requirements have been taken into consideration when providing Ebola-TX data for secondary research.

4.3 Technical and User Requirements

Appropriate tools and systems should be chosen for collecting, managing, and handling research data during and after a study. Acquiring and configuring the IT infrastructure to support research in resource-limited settings is often challenging, especially where Internet connectivity is lacking or unreliable, mains electric power supply is intermittent or of poor quality, computer use is uncommon, and skilled local IT support personnel are scarce. The COVID-19 pandemic has triggered a call for further global data standardization and harmonization (Ros et al. 2020) and better planning and preparation in health informatics (Basit et al. 2021).

Over the years, there has been a gradual shift from paper to electronic systems for data collection, both in industry and academic settings (Tufts University and Veeva Systems 2017; Wilcox et al. 2012). Compared to traditional pen and paper data collection, electronic data capture has improved quality and reduced time and cost (Fleishmann et al. 2017; Le Jeannic et al. 2014; Walther et al. 2011). Replacing paper data collection with electronic data capture can also be achieved in resource-poor settings (Seebregts et al. 2009; Thriemer et al. 2012; Zeleke et al. 2019). However, no single information and communications technology (ICT) solution seems to fit every setting. The architecture of a system for health data capture in a remote area depends on integrating its three main components: networks, data capture devices, and data capture applications (Ashar et al. 2010). The choice of ICT solution will depend on user requirements, available infrastructure in the location of the study, and procurement of necessary hardware (► Chap. 34).

There has also been a rapid evolution from static computers to mobile alternatives, such as personal digital assistants (already obsolete), laptops, cell phones, smartphones, and tablets. Users may find a tablet more convenient than a laptop or choose a rugged device to withstand severe field conditions, rather than an office-use version. Additional devices like mobile printers, scanners, barcode readers, portable medical diagnostics, smart watches, and biometric trackers have made their appearance as ICT solutions in health research settings. Application software has evolved in tandem with hardware components. There is growing interest in so-called apps, software applications designed to run on mobile devices to support healthcare and emergency response research. Ensuring reliable electrical power to support these ICT solutions becomes more essential than ever (▶ Chap. 37). ICT technologies also help enable electronic medical records (Clifford et al. 2008; Shaffer et al. 2019), disease surveillance and response systems (Groseclose and Buckeridge 2017; Hussain-Alkhateeb et al. 2018; Randrianasolo et al. 2010), and the use of mobile data capture tools and software applications (Brinkel et al. 2014; de Visser et al. 2015; eHealth Africa 2021; El-Khatib et al. 2018; Karimuribo et al. 2017; Ming et al. 2019; Mohanty et al. 2019).

Aside from commercial clinical data management systems (MACRO, Castor, Medidata Rave, Inform, etc.) which require payment by the user, other options are available for academic institutions, including no-cost licenses for nonprofit users and open-source software. These include the free software REDCap and OpenClinica (until recently open-source), both with a particular use in clinical research (Fegan and Lang 2008; Harris et al. 2009, 2019; Omollo et al. 2014; Tom-Aba et al. 2015; Voysey et al. 2021). Open Data Kit, another open-source software program, is often used for surveillance studies and epidemiological research (Fornace et al. 2018; Maduka et al. 2017; Wamwenje et al. 2019).

The 2014–2016 EVD outbreak in West Africa produced many lessons learned for DM and the use of ICT. A remarkable improvement was recorded in the reporting of daily follow-up of contacts of EVD patients, using technology based on Open Data Kit (Tom-Aba et al. 2015). In addition, the use of smartphones or tablets for recording patient information in an ETC was shown to be more efficient and safer than paper-based methods (MSF 2016). Electronic data capture also has less potential for delays or errors than paper forms, which require subsequent manual reentry for digitization (Cori et al. 2017).

Aside from the shift from paper to electronic data collection, data quality challenges have been addressed by hiring information management officers and by using some of the many tools, platforms, and systems available for data collection, sharing, and mapping. In a report for the U.S. Agency for International Development, Fast and Waugaman (2016) discuss proliferation of platforms and tools, among them the following:

- EpiInfo Viral Hemorrhagic Fever Module
- Open Data Kit
- KoboToolboxVozanoo
- OpenMRS
- OpenHie
- District Health Information Software 2
- Magpi
- Sense FOLLOW-up/ID
- Tableau
- iForm
- Go.Data (WHO)

There are many papers describing tools available in this fast-moving field, and there will no doubt be continued development in this area as the COVID-19 response shifts out of high gear and into sustained research for preparedness and response. Both medical care and clinical research see a growing interest in health informatics and/or digital health, with technologies as diverse as the forecasting of outbreaks, use of big data, biometrics, wearables, the Internet of things, and artificial intelligence (George et al. 2019; Manteghinejad and Javanmard 2021; Tilahun et al. 2021; Woo 2019).

In addition, it should be noted that the platforms and tools very useful for one study could be inapplicable to another (see ▶ Sect. 4.1). For example, while a classical retrospective research study might use spreadsheets such as Excel or epidemiological software such as EpiData or EpiInfo, these tools are not suitable (and should be avoided) for collecting data in prospective clinical studies, for which specific clinical data management systems are more suitable. Such systems are designed to comply with the regulatory requirements discussed above, such as GCP (see ▶ Sect. 4.2). Moreover, these systems will have varying technical specifications for operating systems, networks, hardware, and compatibility with other devices and applications and will need to be chosen in consultation with ICT personnel (Kuchinke et al. 2010).

There are specific data challenges and requirements in infectious disease research, as seen in both recent large Ebola outbreaks and the COVID-19 response. For example, collection and transfer of patient data from high-risk "red zone" areas where potentially infectious patients are isolated to the low-risk "green zone" are likely to be safer using electronic transfer rather than moving paper or hardware from one to the other. Initial methods for data transfer in ETCs in West Africa imposed compromises on the quality, quantity, and confidentiality of patient data (Oza et al. 2017). Difficult working conditions, challenges in efficiently documenting patient history and progress, lack of harmonization in data collection between ETCs, and unreliable Internet connectivity at ETCs have been mentioned as key bottlenecks potentially interfering with study conduct (Jobanputra et al. 2016). These challenges may be even more acute for emergency clinical trials where the following considerations for the technical setup of the CDM system apply:

- Paper and electronic tools are potentially "dirty" (contaminated with an infectious pathogen) and must not be routinely transferred from the high-risk zone to the low-risk zone.
- Personal protective equipment (PPE) used by the staff involved in patient care and research, such as heavy-duty gloves, may pose a challenge to collecting or entering data.
- Time constraints. The time medical staff can spend in the high-risk zone of the treatment center may be strictly limited by the heat stress of working in PPE in a tropical environment. As time is prioritized for giving care to patients and for obligatory procedures such as donning and doffing PPE and cleaning specific equipment, time left over for research is restricted, though recent innovations have eased that constraint (▶ In Practice 40.1).
- Disinfectants used for regularly cleaning patient rooms, surfaces, and equipment may have a corrosive effect on data collection and management devices and hardware.

The Ebola-TX study sought to overcome such challenges even while collecting source data on paper case report forms (CRFs). Although heavy-duty hand gloves had to be worn by the medical staff, it was still feasible to make photographs of each CRF page with a smartphone in the high-risk zone. Agreements were made with the site on using ethanol instead of chlorine for disinfecting smartphones. Data were then transferred via a local area network to a "data center" (a laptop functioning as a server) in the low-risk zone. Each page was then printed out and entered on a study laptop loaded with electronic CRFs, using the GCP-compliant CDM software MACRO. MACRO was used offline to overcome possible Internet connectivity issues and then regularly synchronized with the central server at ITM, the study sponsor (◻ Fig. 4). This approach differed from other studies where the transfer of source data from red to green zone was performed by other means such as "shouting over the fence," by using walkie talkies, or by showing the paper at the "fence," as in ◻ Fig. 5.

4.4 Project Management Requirements

Research projects have several components, from describing the research question or hypothesis through analyzing the study data to the publication of the findings. Practicalities, such as a timely study start, consequent follow-up, and coming to conclusions, can be challenging, especially in low-resource settings. Proper research management includes assigning appropriate human, financial, and technical resources, adherence to strict and sometimes short timelines (especially in emergency research), and ensuring quality throughout the study. Success depends on how well the project is planned, organized, implemented, and managed, and

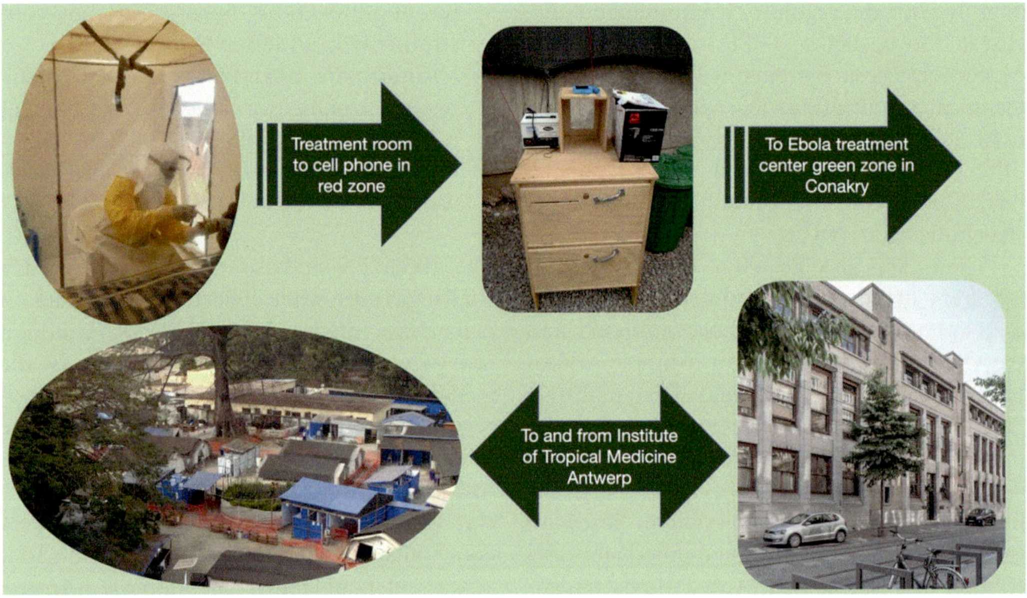

Fig. 4 Some of the data locations important in the Ebola-TX study: the first photo shows medical care and research performed in the high-risk, red zone; the second is a small cabinet in the red zone jury-rigged with a smartphone (blue) on top to precisely frame a full A4 size paper case report form; the third is the Ebola Treatment Center in Conakry and the fourth is the Institute of Tropical Medicine in Antwerp, between which Ebola-TX study data had to flow efficiently and reliably. (Photos: ITM Antwerp)

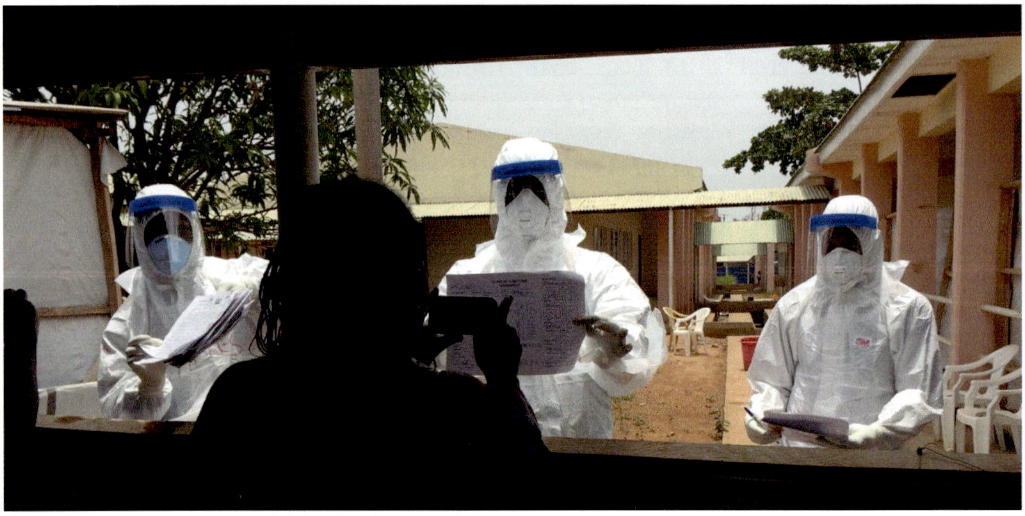

Fig. 5 Another way of transferring case information from the red zone. (Photo: Jerry Pierson)

DM in particular is an essential element of successful research that can benefit from better management (Parvathaneni et al. 2018).

Inadequate understanding of DM and the processes required often leads to underestimating the workload. Whereas data capture might be an obvious process, data validation and the often labor-intensive and time-consuming process of querying to ensure the data are clean and reliable are frequently overlooked. Quite often study databases are not ready to be released at study start; this can

Fig. 6 Basic phases of data management during a clinical study. (Authors)

1. Project initiation (pre-study phase)
• Assign (a) study data manager(s) and other DM roles (see also Section 2).
• Implement a DM Plan (DMP) & relevant DM standard operating procedures (SOPs) (see also Section 3).
• Use tools such as a Gantt chart or process and data flow charts to visualize research projects rapidly with deliverables, milestones, and processes.
• Set FPFV (First patient first visit), LPLV (Last patient last visit), and database lock as essential points of reference in time.
• Implement risk assessment.
• Ensure appropriate communication. o Appointing focal point(s) for DM (at sponsor and at site[s]). o Schedule regular study meetings. o Include a data manager at study meetings. • Utilize meeting minutes template to document decisions.
• Employ a TMF template (Trial Master File = organization of study paper documentation & electronic files, at a central level and at sites).
• Prepare a DM Contact Log with name, function/role, email, phone number.
2. Project execution (study phase)
• Assure compliance with the DMP and all relevant study phase DM SOPs.
• Adhere to timelines on FPFV, LPLV, Database Lock.
• Communicate the project/study progress at the regular study meetings.
• Document any relevant changes in DM on the study/project in meeting minutes or in an updated DMP.
3. Project closure (post-study phase)
• Ensure compliance with the DMP and all relevant post-study phase DM SOPs.
• Prepare a data management report: this document will list the information from the DMP, with deviations and possible additional information.
• Report the deviations which have an impact on the analysis to the relevant study stakeholders (investigator, statistician).

lead to downstream delay and a postponed database lock (Tufts University and Veeva Systems 2017). Sometimes databases or systems have not been tested or validated on their functionality before data capture begins or may not have been tested at all.

In academic clinical research, especially in low-resource settings, one person may wear many hats and be responsible for diverse activities and deliverables, such as designing the case report form and other documentation, database design and programming, testing, training, data cleaning, medical coding, organizing an IT helpdesk, archiving, and data sharing. Moreover, that person may even be involved in several simultaneous studies. However, little seems to have been published on the project management of clinical research or of academic research in general. The authors, therefore, provide the following guidelines (Fig. 6) for good project management practices based on their own experience.

5 Selection and Implementation of Data Capture Tools

The choice of the method for data capture, including collection tools, is based on several factors, as described in ► Sect. 4. The examples below are typical for clinical trials, and there may be other approaches with other kinds of research, but selecting a robust data capture system and tools is critical to the successful implementation of high-quality research. In resource-limited settings, this decision includes but is not limited to available resources (e.g., Internet, equipment, and related supplies), skilled personnel, and the conditions in which the research is being conducted, which may include the widespread danger of infection, poor infrastructure, and security concerns.

Fig. 7 Advantages and disadvantages of paper data collection (Authors)

Nº	Advantages of a paper-based system	Disadvantages of a paper-based system
1.	Suitable for resource-limited settings where technology is not widely assessable	Time-consuming in organizing, depending on the scale of the research
2.	Easily understandable, with limited training needs.	High level of effort, time, and labor required to correct errors in data collection
3.	The lack of technical glitches associated with electronic data capture	Record/questionnaire retention

Fig. 8 Advantages and disadvantages of EDC. (Authors)

Nº	Advantages of an electronic data capture (EDC) system	Disadvantages of anEDC system
1.	Database is readily available for cleaning or analysis, depending on how rigorously the system has been set up.	Logistical and infrastructural requirements: reliable electric power, internet connectivity, device security, and suitable locations for device storage should be considered. However, many devices run on battery power, and EDC systems can support offline data collection at remote places without internet connectivity for later synchronization.
2.	Questionnaires can be quickly modified based on experience during implementation.	More training may be required, especially in resource-limited settings.
3.	Quick data entry process with fewer errors after entry (enhanced by real-time edit checks).	

5.1 Paper-Based Data Capture

A paper-based data capture system is the traditional method for collecting research data in resource-limited settings. Collecting data on paper forms and transferring them to a location where the data will be entered in the study database minimize the need for ICT systems at some study sites. In a paper-based study, questionnaires are designed, printed, and organized in binders assigned to each study participant. The binder will include all the forms to be completed by study staff or participants. Figure 7 lists some of the advantages and disadvantages of paper-based data collection and transfer.

5.2 Electronic Data Capture

An electronic data capture (EDC) system is a computerized system for the collection of clinical research data using electronic questionnaires or electronic case report forms (eCRFs). With EDC systems, study staff primarily enter data directly into a database via computer, mobile phone, or tablet. An EDC provides immediate organization and retrieval of electronic data for each study participant (Fig. 8).

5.3 Selection of Data Capture System and Software

The selection of a system and software to capture and manage data depends on several factors. An important criterion is that the system meets all regulatory requirements as indicated in ▶ Sect. 4.2 and 4.3. During a health emergency, the quick deployment of a robust data management system for research is pivotal for understanding the epidemic, let alone a pandemic, and developing countermeasures. Selection of user-friendly software or a system that is known to local end users or easily learned helps increase efficiency and improves data quality. Where there are existing research institutes or programs pivoting their work to meet the health emergency, harmonization with existing DM systems can help keep disruptions to a minimum. In August 2020, during the COVID-19 outbreak in Liberia, the Partnership for Research on Ebola Vaccines in Liberia (PREVAIL) (a clinical research partnership established by the United States and Liberian governments) rapidly rolled out a COVID-19 observational study at the country's biggest treatment center. Although initially the idea was to set up an EDC system, data capture was initiated on paper, followed by data entry in REDCap. The decision to use paper forms was reached because it was difficult to use electronic devices while wearing PPE in an infectious environment. Paper CRFs were completed and photographed in the high-risk zone and then electronically transmitted to a secured computer in the low-risk zone for quality control and data entry. REDCap software was chosen because many of the research staff were already familiar with the system (NIH 2021).

5.4 Study Settings and Available Resources

As outlined in previous sections (▶ Sects. 4.3 and 5.3) and other chapters, the study settings and available technologies are critical factors for the selection of a DM system and software (▶ Chaps. 34, 37, and 40). In resource-limited settings, human resource capacity is vital for effectively implementing a robust DM system. Implementing a DM system is not limited to DM or IT-related staff. It incorporates a wide range of clinical and nonclinical staff, many of them involved in the collection and review of data. There are specific roles and responsibilities of members of the DM as well as the clinical and nonclinical study teams. In compliance with GCP, the entire research team should be trained to use the data collection tools (paper based or eCRF) to ensure compliance with the GCP standard. The training of clinical staff is mainly focused on CRF completion and queries management, while DM staff receive similar training in addition to learning the functionality of the DM system (▶ Chap. 42).

5.5 Development of Standard Operating Procedures (SOPs)

As required by GCP guidelines, an electronic DM system should have clear and succinct SOPs covering system setup, installation, use, and troubleshooting. These SOPs are used as training manuals, user guidelines, and reference tools as the system is implemented. Some of the most common SOPs for use of these systems are shown in ◘ Fig. 9.

5.6 System Validation: Testing Software, Data Collection Tools, and Systems

For GCP-compliant studies using electronic DM systems, the sponsor should ensure and document that systems conform to the sponsor's established requirements for completeness, accuracy, reliability, and consistent intended performance. This includes the following:

1. Validating the software and system (e.g., REDCap installation and operational functioning online at server and at mobile device)

◘ **Fig. 9** SOPs for data collection. (Authors)

№	Name of SOP	Scope of SOP
1.	CRF completion	Instructions on how to complete the CRF (paper or electronic)
2.	Quality control	Instructions on how to review CRFs after completion, perform quality control and assurance, ensure data completeness and validity, etc.
3.	Resolving queries	Instructions on how to handle queries generated during or after data entry
4.	Data entry and validation	Instructions on how to electronically capture and validate data

2. Validating study electronic questionnaires or eCRFs (operational functioning of a study-specific database design, its edit checks and skip logic)

Both (1) and (2) should be in place and verified before data capture starts.

3. Validating upgrades of software, changes to the system, updates of the eCRF/database design during the study
4. Documentation including validation plan, user requirements specifications, installation qualification, operational qualification, and validation reports

If at all possible given time pressures, simulated or pilot studies to test paper or electronic questionnaires before the research study begins are invaluable for ensuring that a DM system is properly structured and robust. Whether or not such a "shakedown cruise" is possible, all study instruments must be finalized and the database put into production mode for the actual study, whereupon only actual study data can be entered.

A trial run can

- Identify errors on the questionnaires or CRFs including skip logic and instructions for completion.
- Ensure that the study database is functional and robust and that its edit checks and logic are properly programmed.
- Test the data transmission procedure, Internet connectivity, and strength where applicable.
- Provide hands-on staff training on the system.

6 Data Capture and Data Review

6.1 Data Flow

A well-defined DM system has a clear flow of information from data capture to analysis. Research studies are designed with specific data flow depending on the environment, study design, and the type of data collection system. Active data tracking is essential for an up-to-date overview of the accumulating data.

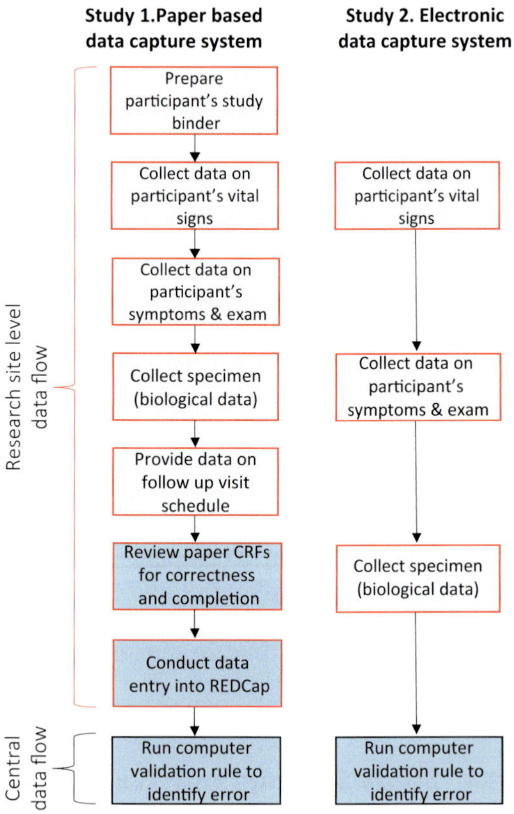

Fig. 10 Data flow process for a paper-based and an electronic data capture system, as used in a study conducted in Liberia. (Authors)

The data flow of a paper-based system will vary from that of an EDC system because the needs and requirements for each system differ. CRF tracking—the identification of missing or blank paper pages—before sending data from the site to the location where data entry is done is an important aspect of ensuring efficient data flow. Figure 10 illustrates data flow in paper-based and electronic data capture processes for studies conducted in Liberia. Study 1 is a natural history study of Ebola survivors conducted from 2015 to 2021, while Study 2 is a malaria incidence study (Duffy 2022; PREVAIL III Study Group 2019). During Study 1, the participants' binders were prepared with blank CRFs that were completed at each of the stations before the review phase began. At the end of data collection during each participant visit, the folder was sent for data review/quality control before the participant left the site. At the end of the review, applicable corrections were made and the folder was sent for data entry. At the end of each day at the central office, an automated program checked the data for accuracy, consistency, completeness, and logic violation. Inconsistencies identified were sent back to the site as queries. This cycle was repeated throughout the implementation of the study. The data flow in Study 2 indicates how EDC and transfer can simplify the steps required.

6.2 Data Capture

6.2.1 Paper-Based Data Capture

In a paper-based system, physical forms are completed, reviewed, and validated before they are sent for data entry. This means checking for and resolving missing data, sections, or pages; missing signatures if applicable; and inaccurate and inconsistent data. In Study 1, a REDCap database was set up at the research site to manage the data. Two data clerks each independently entered the same paper CRF into the REDCap database. One of the two data clerks then reviewed the data for consistency between the entries. If there was any inconsistency, the paper form was reexamined, and the appropriate correction was made in the database. This kind of double data entry is often mentioned as the gold standard for processing paper-based data collection systems in a clinical research setting. This improves data accuracy and reduces the need for unnecessary data cleaning post entry.

6.2.2 Electronic Data Capture

As described in ► Sect. 5.2, direct entry into an EDC system is normally more efficient than first recording data on paper and then reentering them into a digital system. Some EDC systems can be used with mobile devices like phones and tablets and be configured for offline data collection when connections are down, with synchronization once the connections are restored.

EDC systems also allow for "edit checks," which auto-review data for validity and tell the user to recheck the entry by showing a message such as "Value is out of range. Please examine." The system thus facilitates rapid resolution of accuracy issues. Other useful programming includes branching or skip logic (e.g., when gender/sex is entered as male, references applicable only to females will be skipped or inactivated automatically). By such means, the system helps ensure that single data entry supports robust, high-quality data (◘ Fig. 11). In addition, these systems use status icons to indicate the quality and progress of data capture and to show when data is almost ready or final for analysis. This gives an EDC system a further advantage over a paper-based system by obviating much of the post-entry effort and time required with a paper-based system.

6.3 Data Review, Quality Assurance, and Quality Control

Data review, data validation, data cleaning, and quality control are terms used interchangeably to describe the processes needed to assure valid or clean data. The ultimate assurance for data validation and data integrity is to adhere to the ALCOA+ principles (Bargaje 2011), ensuring that data are

- Attributable
- Legible
- Contemporaneous
- Original
- Accurate

Plus

- Complete
- Consistent
- Enduring
- Available

Actions to achieve ALCOA+ principles include the edit checks designed to identify inaccurate or invalid data using ranges, but also computer functions to pick out duplicate data, incomplete or inconsistent data, and protocol violations. In addition to programmed automatic review, manual review of data may be considered. Where resources permit, specific staff members, such as data mon-

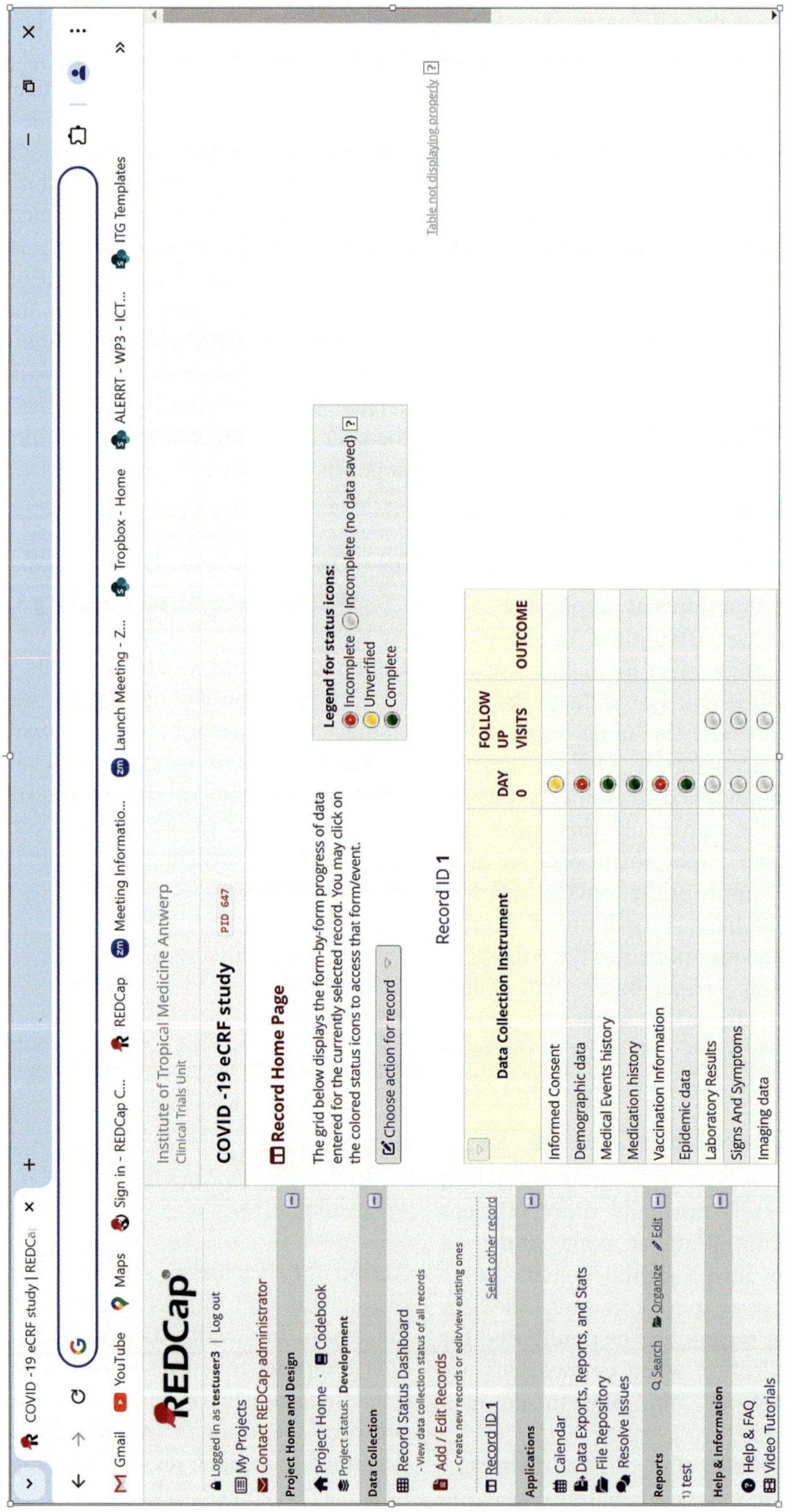

Fig. 11 Screenshot from REDCap showing progress of data entry for study participant 1, indicated by colored status icons. (Courtesy REDCap)

itors, local data managers, quality control officers at the clinical sites, and central data managers and statisticians at a central location may all validate data. Quality control should occur throughout a study. As shown in ◻ Fig. 10, data review and quality control occur at each stage of the data flow. At the end of data collection and before the participant leaves the site, detailed quality control is performed. This process provides a comprehensive look at all the data collected for that study visit and allows for initial corrections, while the participant is still at the site for verification.

6.4 Database Queries: Generation and Resolution

Generation of queries and ensuring corresponding database updates are important tasks of data review/quality control. Electronic DM systems include validation rules that specify normal ranges for numerical variables, logic checks between variables to evaluate data consistency and missing data, and similar cross-checking. Automatic queries are enhanced by indicators within the system (e.g., REDCap's red status icons indicating incomplete data on a data capture form). A central DM team implements this process in close collaboration with the study staff doing data collection and entry. Depending on the software and DM system, additional "manual" queries may be sent to the clinical team by the staff members checking the data (◻ Fig. 12).

Paper-based systems require that queries written on paper data clarification forms be sent to the clinical teams and returned with an answer or clarification. With a paper-based system, tracking, overview, and overall organization of these queries and paper forms are very labor-intensive.

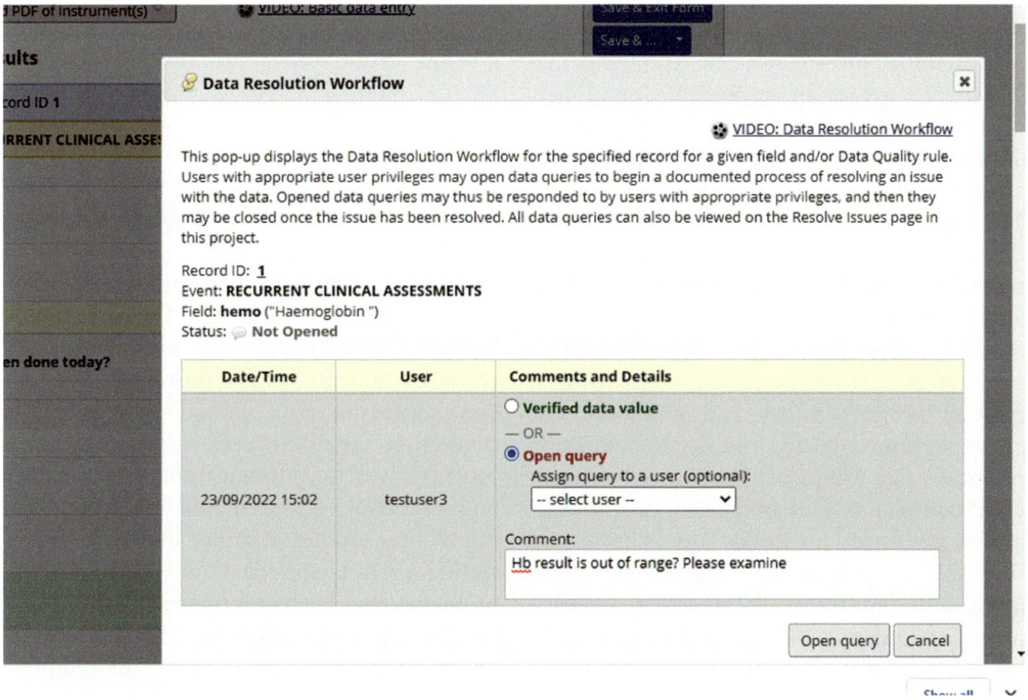

◻ **Fig. 12** Tools for checking data entries are integrated into some electronic clinical data management systems, e.g., REDCap. The pop-up window presents the query "Hb result is out of range? Please examine" and allows assignment to a staff member who will examine the value given, respond, and correct if applicable. (Courtesy REDCap; Harris et al. 2009, 2019)

7 Database Lock

The goal of any clinical research study is the timely reporting and analysis of all data collected throughout the study. Before data analysis can start, the database is expected to be complete, clean, accurate, and consistent, with all queries resolved and final quality control performed. Subsequently, the database is locked, either at predefined time points during the study (intermediate lock) and/or at the study end (final lock), to prevent unauthorized or unintentional changes to the data as statistical analysis takes place. Database lock should be carefully planned and described in the study protocol and DM plan and finally agreed upon at a dedicated database lock meeting, during which the integration of data from various types, sources, and locations should be considered.

Several stakeholders are involved in database lock, as part of either the sponsor team or the clinical site team. After all data entry by the data entry clerks, and after final quality checks by the data reviewers, the data manager, the study statistician, and either the coordinating investigator or the principal investigator are jointly responsible for approving the database lock. Following approval, the data can be locked in the EDC software, and all edit rights to the database will be removed. The formal locking of the database and the date on which the edit access rights were removed should be documented in a database lock approval form.

Due to limited resources, including technical and regulatory expertise, many clinical research projects in low- and middle-income countries have collected and stored data using programs like Microsoft Excel or other non-GCP-compliant software that does not meet global standards for good DM. The use of such software makes database lock harder to implement, and the availability of free access tools for DM (e.g., REDCap) should make use of noncompliant software unnecessary.

Interim database locks and subsequent interim analyses allow for early decisions on the need to adapt or halt the study for reasons of clear efficacy, futility, or unacceptable side effects. This aspect can be of special importance in emergency research, where timely decisions to proceed with one or more specific, potentially lifesaving interventions over other, less beneficial interventions can save lives even during the study. For example, the interim data analysis of a randomized controlled trial of EVD therapeutics conducted in the Democratic Republic of Congo indicated superiority of two out of four treatments evaluated, upon which it was decided to limit further treatment of new study participants to these two most promising therapies for the remainder of the trial (Mulangu et al. 2019).

Following database lock, all study data are secured on the server of either the study sponsor or the host institution, ready for extraction for statistical analysis. Even in emergency research settings, the electronic study database can often be stored on a centralized, secured server in preparation for analysis as planned in the statistical analysis plan. In the DRC EVD trial reported by Mulangu et al. (2019), study data were collected on bar-coded paper case report forms at the bedside, scanned and digitally sorted into electronic patient folders at the ETC, and subsequently entered into a web-based REDCap database by trial staff at a remote data coordinating center.

8 Data Archiving and Data Sharing

Once study data have been analyzed and all outcomes described in the study protocol have been reported, the data set and all essential study documents (study protocol, informed consent forms, etc.) should be retained in binders or folders in safe, appropriate long-term facilities for future use and in accordance with regulatory requirements. When considering clinical studies, whether in an emergency setting or not, specific guidelines related to archiving have been described as part of ICH-GCP E6 (R2), which states, "The sponsor and investigator/institution should maintain a record of the location(s) of their respective essential documents including source documents. The storage system used during the trial and for archiving (irrespective of the type of media used) should provide for document identification, version history, search, and retrieval" (ICH 2016). EMA guidelines on the content, management, and archiving of the clinical trial master file are similar (EMA 2018). An appropriate storage area should be available to maintain the documents, so they remain complete and legible throughout the trial and the required retention period and can be made available to the competent authorities. The storage facilities should be of an appropriate size and secured throughout the entire archiving period, which can be more than 30 years (EMA 2018). Access to archived data should be restricted either by user access levels to the archive area of a server and/or by access controls to the storage location where the records are retained.

Research data can be archived locally, at institutional or university level, but online data repositories also offer solutions, some of them cost-free, if the needed capacity is not available within the research framework. Examples of such repositories are listed in ◘ Fig. 13.

Sharing the results of clinical research and the underlying data contributes to the advance of scientific knowledge, including novel research designs and the testing of new hypotheses (Rani and Buckley 2012). The focus on data sharing gained momentum when Wilkinson et al. (2016) published the FAIR data principles to improve the *findability*, *accessibility*, *interoperability*, and *reuse* of research data. Other authors propose that effective data sharing can be promoted by more clearly crediting the researchers who generated the original data (Pierce et al. 2019). GloPID-R (2018), a network of research funders, elaborated principles for data sharing in public health emergencies. ALERRT and the Pan-African Network For Rapid Research, Response, Relief and Preparedness for Infectious Disease Epidemics (PANDORA) research networks, both funded by the European and Developing Countries Clinical Trials Partnership (EDCTP), have developed a set of data-sharing principles (ALERRT and PANDORA 2019).

These principles may be of special interest in low-resource settings because they promote equity and fairness toward researchers and communities which provide the data, particularly those in developing countries. For research programs responding to public health emergencies, some funders require that data be shared within 30 days after it has been generated, entailing a well-organized database lock, within a few days after the last patient data is gathered (EDCTP 2018).

Rapidly and openly sharing research data in public health emergencies helps maximize the utility of clinical studies and minimize duplication of effort—both matters of key importance for a timely, effective emergency research response (Bugin and Woodcock 2021; Chretien et al. 2016; Hanahoe et al. 2021; Langat et al. 2011; Yozwiak et al. 2015). Lessons learned from past outbreaks, in particular the West Africa EVD emergency, provide insight for better tackling the numerous

◘ **Fig. 13** Selected data repositories/databases. (Authors)

Name	Data Type	Provider	URL
Zenodo	General research data	EU	https://zenodo.org/
Data Archiving and Networked Services	General research data	Netherlands	https://dans.knaw.nl/en/
Infectious Diseases Data Observatory	Clinical and observational study data	Independent coalition based in UK	https://www.iddo.org/
UK data archive	Social science data	UK	https://ukdataservice.ac.uk/
NIAID Clinical Trials Data	Human genomic and clinical data	USA	https://www.niaid.nih.gov/research/accessing-clinical-data

challenges to optimal data sharing (Georgetown University Medical Center 2018; Pisani et al. 2018). Overcoming some of the barriers requires the promotion of a data-sharing culture, encouraging collaboration across research disciplines and communities, developing data-sharing platforms, promoting data standardization, and refining public health and decision-making infrastructure. The COVID-19 pandemic has drawn further attention to the need for rapid data sharing during an infectious disease emergency, in part because of scientific and technological advances that have made it possible to develop medical countermeasures faster than ever before (Cosgriff et al. 2020; Moorthy et al. 2020; Van Noorden 2021).

In 1997, a collaboration of scientific bodies concluded that "The value of data lies in their use. Full and open access to scientific data should be adopted as the international norm for the exchange of scientific data derived from publicly-funded research" (National Research Council 1997). This is nowadays also reflected in the guidelines of the International Committee of Medical Journal Editors (ICMJE), which rightly promotes the ethical obligation to responsibly share data generated by interventional clinical trials, in part because trial participants have put themselves at risk, and for the benefit of patients, investigators, sponsors, and society (ICMJE 2021; Taichman et al. 2016).

The benefits of data sharing are multiple, but data sharing is only possible when the data is well-managed and systematically archived. However, many databases, especially those of studies conducted in an emergency setting, are not well archived, and access for secondary use is limited, thereby reducing the return on (often public) research investment. Various obstacles can block efficient data archiving and retrieval:

- Unclear organizational responsibility
- Inadequate infrastructure
- Limited staff with appropriate DM and analysis skills
- Limited data review and cleaning
- Researchers' reluctance to share "their" data
- No formal database identified
- Lack of institutional data archiving and data-sharing policies

For relevant discussions and further insight into several aspects related to data sharing, see ► Chap. 7 in this book.

Discussion Questions

1. What is data management?
2. Why does a clinical research study need a data management plan (DMP)?
3. It is crucial to outline to all members of the study team their specific roles and responsibilities in data management. List and discuss roles and responsibilities of dedicated professionals in data management.
4. What are the advantages and disadvantages of electronic data capture versus collecting data on paper forms?
5. A useful set of principles for data validation and data integrity is called ALCOA+. What does ALCOA stand for, and what does the + mean? Are there additional principles you think should be added?
6. Who should have access to clinical trial data and when?
7. Discuss some regulations, guidelines, standards, and funder requirements that were applicable for the Ebola-TX study.
8. Discuss some specific data challenges and requirements in infectious disease research, as seen in both recent large Ebola outbreaks and the COVID-19 response.
9. Describe some empirical guidelines for good project management.
10. What are some of the factors preventing rapid, open dissemination of research data?
11. Briefly discuss the importance and process of data lock.
12. Many databases, especially those of studies conducted in an emergency set-

ting, are not well archived, and access for secondary use is limited, thereby reducing the return on research investment. Discuss various obstacles that can block efficient data archiving and retrieval.

References

Abramowitz SA, Hipgrave DB, Witchard A, Heymann DL. Lessons from the West Africa Ebola epidemic: a systematic review of epidemiological and social and behavioral science research priorities. J Infect Dis. 2018;218(11):1730–8. https://doi.org/10.1093/infdis/jiy387.

ALERRT, PANDORA. ALERRT and PANDORA data sharing principles. ALERRT and PANDORA; 2019.

ALERRT. Outbreak Research Data Management: The Global Health Network; 2024 [Available from: https://alerrt.tghn.org/elearning/doi-26/; https://doi.org/10.48060/tghn.26.

Anon. Everyone needs a data-management plan. Nature. 2018;555(7696):286. https://doi.org/10.1038/d41586-018-03065-z.

Anon. COVID research: a year of scientific milestones. Nature. 2021; https://doi.org/10.1038/d41586-020-00502-w.

Ashar R, Lewis S, Blazes DL, Chretien JP. Applying information and communications technologies to collect health data from remote settings: a systematic assessment of current technologies. J Biomed Inform. 2010;43(2):332–41. https://doi.org/10.1016/j.jbi.2009.11.009.

Bargaje C. Good documentation practice in clinical research. Perspect Clin Res. 2011;2(2):59–63. https://doi.org/10.4103/2229-3485.80368.

Basit MA, Lehmann CU, Medford RJ. Managing pandemics with health informatics: successes and challenges. Yearb Med Inform. 2021;30(1):17–25. https://doi.org/10.1055/s-0041-1726478.

Brinkel J, Krämer A, Krumkamp R, May J, Fobil J. Mobile phone-based mHealth approaches for public health surveillance in sub-Saharan Africa: a systematic review. Int J Environ Res Public Health. 2014;11(11):11559–82. https://doi.org/10.3390/ijerph111111559.

Bugin K, Woodcock J. Trends in COVID-19 therapeutic clinical trials. Nat Rev Drug Discov. 2021;20:254. https://doi.org/10.1038/d41573-021-00037-3.

CDISC. CDISC standards in the clinical research process. Austin, TX: Clinical Data Interchange Standards Consortium; 2021.

Chretien J-P, Rivers CM, Johansson MA. Make data sharing routine to prepare for public health emergencies. PLoS Med. 2016;13(8):e1002109. https://doi.org/10.1371/journal.pmed.1002109.

Clifford GD, Blaya JA, Hall-Clifford R, Fraser HS. Medical information systems: a foundation for healthcare technologies in developing countries. Biomed Eng Online. 2008;7:18. https://doi.org/10.1186/1475-925x-7-18.

Cori A, Donnelly CA, Dorigatti I, Ferguson NM, Fraser C, Garske T, et al. Key data for outbreak evaluation: building on the Ebola experience. Philos Trans R Soc Lond B Biol Sci. 2017;372(1721) https://doi.org/10.1098/rstb.2016.0371.

Cosgriff CV, Ebner DK, Celi LA. Data sharing in the era of COVID-19. Lancet Digit Health. 2020;2(5):e224. https://doi.org/10.1016/s2589-7500(20)30082-0.

de Visser EJ, Freedy E, Payne JJ, Freedy A. AREA: a Mobile application for rapid epidemiology assessment. Proc Eng. 2015;107:357–65. https://doi.org/10.1016/j.proeng.2015.06.092.

Digital Curation Centre. Funders' data policies. Edinburgh: Digital Curation Centre; 2021. https://www.dcc.ac.uk/guidance/policy/funders-data-policies. Accessed 20 Dec 2021.

DMPonline. Plan to make data work for you: data management plans that meet institutional funder requirements. Edinburgh: Digital Curation Centre; 2021. https://dmponline.dcc.ac.uk/. Accessed 20 Dec 2021.

DMPTool. Welcome to the DMPTool: create data management plans that meet institutional and funder requirements. Oakland, CA: University of California Curation Center (UC3); 2021. https://dmptool.org/. Accessed 20 Dec 2021.

Duffy PE. Plasmodium and other parasites in pregnant women and children around Margibi and Montserrado Counties, Liberia. Bethesda, MD: National Library of Medicine; 2022. https://clinicaltrials.gov/ct2/show/NCT03719599. Accessed 10 Jan 2022.

EC. Good manufacturing practice: medicinal products for human and veterinary use: annex 11: computerised systems, SANCO/C8/AM/sl/ares(2010)1064599. 2011.

EC. Data management—H2020 online manual. In: Funding and tenders portal. Brussels: European Union; 2020. https://ec.europa.eu/research/participants/docs/h2020-funding-guide/cross-cutting-issues/open-access-data-management/data-management_en.htm. Accessed 28 Mar 2022.

EC. Horizon 2020. Brussels: European Commission; 2021a. https://ec.europa.eu/programmes/horizon2020/en. Accessed 20 Dec 2021.

EC. Medicinal products: EudraLex—volume 10—clinical trials guidelines. Brussels: European Commission; 2021b. https://ec.europa.eu/health/documents/eudralex/vol-10_en. Accessed 20 Dec 2021.

EDCTP. EDCTP2 policy on clinical trials registration, publication and data sharing. 2018.

eHealth Africa. eHealth Africa, Kano, NG. 2021. https://www.ehealthafrica.org/. Accessed 29 Dec 2021.

El-Khatib Z, Shah M, Zallappa SN, Nabeth P, Guerra J, Manengu CT, et al. SMS-based smartphone application for disease surveillance has doubled completeness and timeliness in a limited-resource setting—evaluation of a 15-week pilot program in Central African Republic (CAR). Confl Heal. 2018;12:42. https://doi.org/10.1186/s13031-018-0177-6.

EMA. Guideline on the content, management and archiving of the clinical trial master file (paper and/or electronic). 2018.

EU. Directive 95/46/EC of the European Parliament and of the Council of 24 October 1995 on the protection of individuals with regard to the processing of personal data and on the free movement of such data. Off J Law. 1995;281:31.

Fast L, Waugaman A. Fighting Ebola with information: learning from data and information flows in the West Africa Ebola response. Washington, DC: USAID; 2016.

FDA. Part 11, electronic records; electronic signatures—scope and application. Silver Spring, MD: U.S. Food and Drug Administration; 2018.

Fegan GW, Lang TA. Could an open-source clinical trial data-management system be what we have all been looking for? PLoS Med. 2008;5(3):e6. https://doi.org/10.1371/journal.pmed.0050006.

Fleishmann R, Decker AM, Kraft A, Mai K, Schmidt S. Mobile electronic versus paper case report forms in clinical trials: a randomized controlled trial. BMC Med Res Methodol. 2017;17:153. https://doi.org/10.1186/s12874-017-0429-y.

Fornace KM, Surendra H, Abidin TR, Reyes R, Macalinao MLM, Stresman G, et al. Use of mobile technology-based participatory mapping approaches to geolocate health facility attendees for disease surveillance in low resource settings. Int J Health Geogr. 2018;17(1):21. https://doi.org/10.1186/s12942-018-0141-0.

George DB, Taylor W, Shaman J, Rivers C, Paul B, O'Toole T, et al. Technology to advance infectious disease forecasting for outbreak management. Nat Commun. 2019;10(1):3932. https://doi.org/10.1038/s41467-019-11901-7.

Georgetown University Medical Center. Data sharing during the West Africa Ebola public health emergency. Washington, DC: Georgetown University Medical Center, Security CfGHSa; 2018.

GloPID-R. Principles of data sharing in public health emergencies. Global Research Collaboration for Infectious Disease Preparedness; 2018.

Groseclose SL, Buckeridge DL. Public health surveillance systems: recent advances in their use and evaluation. Annu Rev Public Health. 2017;38:57–79. https://doi.org/10.1146/annurev-publhealth-031816-044348.

Hanahoe H, Austin CC, Shanahan H. Sharing COVID data? Check these recommendations and guidelines. Nature. 2021;592(7855):507. https://doi.org/10.1038/d41586-021-01028-5.

Harris PA, Taylor R, Thielke R, Payne J, Gonzalez N, Conde JG. Research electronic data capture (REDCap)—a metadata-driven methodology and workflow process for providing translational research informatics support. J Biomed Inform. 2009;42(2):377–81. https://doi.org/10.1016/j.jbi.2008.08.010.

Harris PA, Taylor R, Minor BL, Elliott V, Fernandez M, O'Neal L, et al. The REDCap consortium: building an international community of software platform partners. J Biomed Inform. 2019;95:103208. https://doi.org/10.1016/j.jbi.2019.103208.

Haug A, Zachariassen F, Liempd DV. The costs of poor data quality. J Ind Eng Manag. 2011;4(2):26. https://doi.org/10.3926/jiem.v4n2.p168-193.

Holmes EC, Dudas G, Rambaut A, Andersen KG. The evolution of Ebola virus: insights from the 2013-2016 epidemic. Nature. 2016;538(7624):193–200. https://doi.org/10.1038/nature19790.

Hossmann S, Haynes AG, Spoerri A, Diatta ID, Aboubacar B, Egger M, et al. Data management of clinical trials during an outbreak of Ebola virus disease. Vaccine. 2019;37(48):7183–9. https://doi.org/10.1016/j.vaccine.2017.09.094.

Hussain-Alkhateeb L, Kroeger A, Olliaro P, Rocklöv J, Sewe MO, Tejeda G, et al. Early warning and response system (EWARS) for dengue outbreaks: recent advancements towards widespread applications in critical settings. PLoS One. 2018;13(5):e0196811. https://doi.org/10.1371/journal.pone.0196811.

ICH. Good clinical practice: ICH harmonised guideline. Integrated addendum to ICH E6(R1): guideline for good clinical practice ICH E6(R2) ICH consensus guideline. Geneva: International Council for Harmonisation of Technical Requirements for Pharmaceuticals for Human Use (ICH); 2016.

ICH. Quality guidelines. Geneva: International Council for Harmonisation; 2022. https://www.ich.org/page/quality-guidelines. Accessed 22 Feb 2022.

ICMJE. Clinical trials. 2021. http://www.icmje.org/recommendations/browse/publishing-and-editorial-issues/clinical-trial-registration.html. Accessed 31 Dec 2021.

Jobanputra K, Greig J, Shankar G, Perakslis E, Kremer R, Achar J, et al. Electronic medical records in humanitarian emergencies—the development of an Ebola clinical information and patient management system. F1000Res. 2016;5:1477. https://doi.org/10.12688/f1000research.8287.3.

Jones S, Pergl R, Hooft R, Miksa T, Samors R, Ungvari J, et al. Data management planning: how requirements and solutions are beginning to converge. Data Intell. 2020;2(1–2):208–19. https://doi.org/10.1162/dint_a_00043.

Karimuribo ED, Mutagahywa E, Sindato C, Mboera L, Mwabukusi M, Kariuki Njenga M, et al. A smartphone app (AfyaData) for innovative one health disease surveillance from community to national levels in Africa: intervention in disease surveillance. JMIR Public Health Surveill. 2017;3(4):e94. https://doi.org/10.2196/publichealth.7373.

Krishnankutty B, Bellary S, Kumar NB, Moodahadu LS. Data management in clinical research: an overview. Indian J Pharmacol. 2012;44(2):168–72. https://doi.org/10.4103/0253-7613.93842.

Kuchinke W, Ohmann C, Yang Q, Salas N, Lauritsen J, Gueyffier F, et al. Heterogeneity prevails: the state of clinical trial data management in Europe—results of a survey of ECRIN centres. Trials. 2010;11:79. https://doi.org/10.1186/1745-6215-11-79.

Langat P, Pisartchik D, Silva D, Bernard C, Olsen K, Smith M, et al. Is there a duty to share? Ethics of sharing research data in the context of public health emergencies. Public Health Ethics. 2011;4(1):4–11. https://doi.org/10.1093/phe/phr005.

Le Jeannic A, Quelen C, Alberti C, Durand-Zaleski I. Comparison of two data collection processes in clinical studies: electronic and paper case report forms. BMC Med Res Methodol. 2014;14:7. https://doi.org/10.1186/1471-2288-14-7.

Lee JS, Adhikari NKJ, Kwon HY, Teo K, Siemieniuk R, Lamontagne F, et al. Anti-Ebola therapy for patients with Ebola virus disease: a systematic review. BMC Infect Dis. 2019;19(1):376. https://doi.org/10.1186/s12879-019-3980-9.

Lu Z, Su J. Clinical data management: current status, challenges, and future directions from industry perspectives. Open Access J Clin Trials. 2010;2:93–105. https://doi.org/10.2147/OAJCT.S8172.

Maduka O, Akpan G, Maleghemi S. Using Android and Open Data Kit Technology in data management for research in resource-limited settings in the Niger Delta Region of Nigeria: cross-sectional household survey. JMIR Mhealth Uhealth. 2017;5(11):e171. https://doi.org/10.2196/mhealth.7827.

Manghani K. Quality assurance: importance of systems and standard operating procedures. Perspect Clin Res. 2011;2(1):34–7. https://doi.org/10.4103/2229-3485.76288.

Manteghinejad A, Javanmard SH. Challenges and opportunities of digital health in a post-COVID19 world. J Res Med Sci. 2021;26:11. https://doi.org/10.4103/jrms.JRMS_1255_20.

MedDRA. MedDRA: medical dictionary for regulatory activities. Geneva: International Council for Harmonisation of Technical Requirements for Pharmaceuticals for Human Use; 2021. https://www.meddra.org/. Accessed 20 Dec 2021.

Miksa T, Simms S, Mietchen D, Jones S. Ten principles for machine-actionable data management plans. PLoS Comput Biol. 2019;15(3):e1006750. https://doi.org/10.1371/journal.pcbi.1006750.

Ming D, Rawson T, Sangkaew S, Rodriguez-Manzano J, Georgiou P, Holmes A. Connectivity of rapid-testing diagnostics and surveillance of infectious diseases. Bull World Health Organ. 2019;97(3):242–4. https://doi.org/10.2471/blt.18.219691.

Mohanty B, Chughtai A, Rabhi F. Use of mobile apps for epidemic surveillance and response—availability and gaps. 2019.

Moorthy V, Henao Restrepo AM, Preziosi MP, Swaminathan S. Data sharing for novel coronavirus (COVID-19). Bull World Health Organ. 2020;98(3):150. https://doi.org/10.2471/blt.20.251561.

MSF. MSF-supported research on Ebola. Brussels: Médecins Sans Frontières; 2016.

Mulangu S, Dodd LE, Davey RT Jr, Tshiani Mbaya O, Proschan M, Mukadi D, et al. A randomized, controlled trial of Ebola virus disease therapeutics. N Engl J Med. 2019;381(24):2293–303. https://doi.org/10.1056/NEJMoa1910993.

National Research Council. Bits of power: issues in global access to scientific data. Washington, DC: National Academies Press; 1997.

NIH. Ebola virus disease survivors: clinical and immunologic follow-up. Bethesda, MD: National Institutes of Health, National Library of Medicine; 2021. https://clinicaltrials.gov/ct2/show/NCT02431923. Accessed 29 Dec 2021.

NSF. Data management plans guidance for principal investigators. Alexandria, VA: National Science Foundation; 2018.

Omollo R, Ochieng M, Mutinda B, Omollo T, Owiti R, Okeyo S, et al. Innovative approaches to clinical data management in resource limited settings using open-source technologies. PLoS Negl Trop Dis. 2014;8(9):e3134. https://doi.org/10.1371/journal.pntd.0003134.

Owada K, Eckmanns T, Kamara KB, Olu OO. Epidemiological data management during an outbreak of Ebola virus disease: key issues and observations from Sierra Leone. Front Public Health. 2016;4:163. https://doi.org/10.3389/fpubh.2016.00163.

Oza S, Jazayeri D, Teich JM, Ball E, Nankubuge PA, Rwebembera J, et al. Development and deployment of the OpenMRS-Ebola electronic health record system for an Ebola treatment center in Sierra Leone. J Med Internet Res. 2017;19(8):e294. https://doi.org/10.2196/jmir.7881.

Pandav R, Mehta A, Belle SH, Martin DE, Chandra V, Dodge HH, et al. Data management and quality assurance for an international project: the Indo-US Cross-National Dementia Epidemiology Study. Int J Geriatr Psychiatry. 2002;17(6):510–8. https://doi.org/10.1002/gps.650.

Parvathaneni M, Pattarkine M, Chappidi DY. Implementation of project management in clinical research. Inventi Rapid Clin Res. 2018;2018(1):1.

Pierce HH, Dev A, Statham E, Bierer BE. Credit data generators for data reuse. Nature. 2019;570(7759):30–2. https://doi.org/10.1038/d41586-019-01715-4.

Pisani E, Ghataure A, Merson L. Data sharing in public health emergencies: a study of current policies, practices and infrastructure supporting the sharing of data to prevent and respond to epidemic and pandemic threats. London: Wellcome Trust; 2018.

PREVAIL III Study Group. A longitudinal study of Ebola sequelae in Liberia. N Engl J Med. 2019;380(10):924–34. https://doi.org/10.1056/NEJMoa1805435.

Prokscha S. Practical guide to clinical data management. 3rd ed. Boca Raton, FL: CRC Press; 2012.

Randrianasolo L, Raoelina Y, Ratsitorahina M, Ravolomanana L, Andriamandimby S, Heraud JM, et al. Sentinel surveillance system for early outbreak detection in Madagascar. BMC Public Health. 2010;10:31. https://doi.org/10.1186/1471-2458-10-31.

Rani M, Buckley BS. Systematic archiving and access to health research data: rationale, current status and way forward. Bull World Health Organ. 2012;90(12):932–9. https://doi.org/10.2471/blt.12.105908.

Ros F, Kush R, Friedman C, Gil Zorzo E, Rivero Corte P, Rubin JC, et al. Addressing the Covid-19 pandemic and future public health challenges through global collaboration and a data-driven systems approach. Learn Health Syst. 2020;5(1):e10253. https://doi.org/10.1002/lrh2.10253.

Sallans A, Donnelly M. DMP online and DMPTool: different strategies towards a shared goal. Int J Digit Curation. 2012;7(2):123–9. https://doi.org/10.2218/ijdc.v7i2.235.

Seebregts CJ, Zwarenstein M, Mathews C, Fairall L, Flisher AJ, Seebregts C, et al. Handheld computers for survey and trial data collection in resource-poor settings: development and evaluation of PDACT, a Palm Pilot interviewing system. Int J Med Inform. 2009;78(11):721–31. https://doi.org/10.1016/j.ijmedinf.2008.10.006.

Shaffer JG, Schieffelin JS, Gbakie M, Alhasan F, Roberts NB, Goba A, et al. A medical records and data capture and management system for Lassa fever in Sierra Leone: approach, implementation, and challenges. PLoS One. 2019;14(3):e0214284. https://doi.org/10.1371/journal.pone.0214284.

Smale NA, Barr D, Magatova E, Denyer G, Unsworth K. A review of the history, advocacy and efficacy of data management plans. Int J Digit Curation. 2020;15(1) https://doi.org/10.2218/ijdc.v15i1.525.

Taichman DB, Backus J, Baethge C, Bauchner H, de Leeuw PW, Drazen JM, et al. Sharing clinical trial data: a proposal from the International Committee of Medical Journal Editors. Lancet. 2016;387(10016):e9–e11. https://doi.org/10.1016/s0140-6736(15)01279-9.

Thriemer K, Ley B, Ame SM, Puri MK, Hashim R, Chang NY, et al. Replacing paper data collection forms with electronic data entry in the field: findings from a study of community-acquired bloodstream infections in Pemba, Zanzibar. BMC Res Notes. 2012;5:113. https://doi.org/10.1186/1756-0500-5-113.

Tilahun B, Gashu KD, Mekonnen ZA, Endehabtu BF, Angaw DA. Mapping the role of digital health technologies in prevention and control of COVID-19 pandemic: review of the literature. Yearb Med Inform. 2021;30(1):26–37. https://doi.org/10.1055/s-0041-1726505.

Tom-Aba D, Olaleye A, Olayinka AT, Nguku P, Waziri N, Adewuyi P, et al. Innovative technological approach to Ebola virus disease outbreak response in Nigeria using the open data kit and form hub technology. PLoS One. 2015;10(6):e0131000. https://doi.org/10.1371/journal.pone.0131000.

Tufts University, Veeva Systems. Tufts-Veeva 2017 eClinical landscape study. Boston: Tufts University, Tufts Center for the Study of Drug Development; 2017.

van Griensven J, Haba N. Emergency evaluation of convalescent plasma for Ebola viral disease (EVD) in Guinea (Ebola-Tx). Bethesda, MD: National Librarry of Medicine; 2019. https://clinicaltrials.gov/ct2/show/NCT02342171. Accessed 20 Dec 2021.

van Griensven J, Edwards T, de Lamballerie X, Semple MG, Gallian P, Baize S, et al. Evaluation of convalescent plasma for Ebola virus disease in Guinea. N Engl J Med. 2016;374(1):33–42. https://doi.org/10.1056/NEJMoa1511812.

Van Noorden R. Scientists call for fully open sharing of coronavirus genome data. Nature. 2021;590(7845):195–6. https://doi.org/10.1038/d41586-021-00305-7.

Voysey M, Clemens SAC, Madhi SA, Weckx LY, Folegatti PM, Aley PK, et al. Safety and efficacy of the ChAdOx1 nCoV-19 vaccine (AZD1222) against SARS-CoV-2: an interim analysis of four randomised controlled trials in Brazil, South Africa, and the UK. Lancet. 2021;397:99. https://doi.org/10.1016/S0140-6736(20)32661-1.

Walther B, Hossin S, Townend J, Abernethy N, Parker D, Jeffries D. Comparison of electronic data capture (EDC) with the standard data capture method for clinical trial data. PLoS One. 2011;6(9):e25348. https://doi.org/10.1371/journal.pone.0025348.

Wamwenje SAO, Wangwe II, Masila N, Mirieri CK, Wambua L, Kulohoma BW. Community-led data collection using Open Data Kit for surveillance of animal African trypanosomiasis in Shimba hills, Kenya. BMC Res Notes. 2019;12(1):151. https://doi.org/10.1186/s13104-019-4198-z.

WHO. Handbook for good clinical research practice (GCP): guidance for implementation. Geneva: World Health Organization; 2005.

Wilcox AB, Gallagher KD, Boden-Albala B, Bakken SR. Research data collection methods: from paper to tablet computers. Med Care. 2012;50(Suppl):S68–73. https://doi.org/10.1097/MLR.0b013e318259c1e7.

Wilkinson MD, Dumontier M, Aalbersberg IJ, Appleton G, Axton M, Baak A, et al. The FAIR guiding principles for scientific data management and stewardship. Sci Data. 2016;3(1):160018. https://doi.org/10.1038/sdata.2016.18.

Woo M. Trial by artificial intelligence. Nature. 2019;573:S100.

Yozwiak NL, Schaffner SF, Sabeti PC. Data sharing: make outbreak research open access. Nature. 2015;518(7540):477–9. https://doi.org/10.1038/518477a.

Zeleke AA, Worku AG, Demissie A, Otto-Sobotka F, Wilken M, Lipprandt M, et al. Evaluation of electronic and paper-pen data capturing tools for data quality in a public health survey in a health and demographic surveillance site, Ethiopia: randomized controlled crossover health care information technology evaluation. JMIR Mhealth Uhealth. 2019;7(2):e10995. https://doi.org/10.2196/10995.

36 Safety and Pharmacovigilance in Emergency Research Response

Marc Teitelbaum, Negin Atri, and Kelly Cahill

Contents

Learning Track Note: This chapter appears in Learning Tracks: Clinical Research; Emergency Research Response, Research Operations

E. S. Higgs and R. A. Sorenson (eds.), *Principles and Practice of Emergency Research Response*,
https://doi.org/10.1007/978-3-031-48408-7_56

Learning Objectives

This chapter will help readers understand and describe:

- What pharmacovigilance (PV) is, key goals of a PV program, and some PV methods
- How safety assurances in the development of medical countermeasures (MCMs) overlap to create intentional redundancy
- Pharmacovigilance (PV) roles that must be incorporated into a protocol's safety section
- How emergency response research protocols differ from typical protocols
- Factors to consider when developing PV standard operating procedures in areas where healthcare system capacity is overwhelmed during an outbreak
- Meeting the training needs of overworked research and clinical care staff with widely varying degrees of experience
- Safety data collection during a high-risk public health emergency and some factors that may hinder data collection during outbreaks
- Recommendations for collaboration, adaptability, and adherence to principles to ensure that PV can be successfully managed in emergencies

1 Introduction

In early 2020, the world became aware of an still-unnamed virus that would soon change people's daily lives. As the coronavirus disease 2019 (COVID-19) pandemic has come to have more dramatic effects on our social lives and livelihoods than any infectious disease event in a century, the public at large has learned many previously unfamiliar terms:

- Diagnostics and testing
- Isolation
- Airborne transmission
- Ventilators
- Personal protective equipment
- Hospital capacity
- Front-line workers
- Therapeutics

Although pharmacovigilance (PV) is still not a broadly understood term, much of its terminology now is, thanks to the COVID-19 pandemic:

- Vaccine safety
- Adverse events reporting system
- Adverse events and reactions
- Serious adverse events
- Adverse events of special interest
- Mortality risk
- Monitoring
- Statistical significance
- Placebo arm
- Clinical trial
- Regulatory review and approval
- Emergency use authorization
- Off-label use

Terms that those working in pharmacovigilance (PV) use every day have been heard on the nightly news, particularly during the worst of the pandemic, yet pharmacovigilance as a subject and those who practice it remain largely unfamiliar to the average person. As the world desperately sought a "magic bullet" for treatment, hoped for an effective vaccine, and argued over herd immunity, one question kept rising to the top of conversation, from blogs to scientific and lay press articles, to the highest podiums of power, "Is it safe?" In that one question, we have the beginnings of a definition of pharmacovigilance, both in normal times and in the response to a pandemic, where preventives and therapeutics are pushed forward with special urgency. At best, some will prove highly efficacious and safe when administered to large populations. At worst the harm done will exceed any benefit—not only physical harm, but damage to the trust of millions of people in scientific research, the regulatory process, and the pharmaceutical industry. Many research products will likely fall into some middle ground, where the critical ratio of harm or risk vs. efficacy or benefit will be indeterminate, subject to argument, or require restrictive usage rules. We have seen and, as of this writing, continue to see this range of outcomes during the COVID-19 pandemic.

One of the many characteristics that differentiates safety and pharmacovigilance practice in a pandemic setting from routine practice is urgency, public attention, and above all scale. In response to outbreaks and

Age group	Females			Males		
	TTS cases	Doses admin	Reporting rate† (per million)	TTS cases	Doses admin	Reporting rate† (per million)
18-29 yrs old	5	1,089,649	4.59	3	1,565,212	1.92
30-39 yrs old	11	1,037,386	10.60	3	1,443,900	2.08
40-49 yrs old	10	1,108,495	9.02	6	1,392,990	4.30
50-64 yrs old	9	2,002,984	4.49	5	2,338,263	2.14
65+ yrs old	2	1,096,923	1.82	0	1,004,285	0

Fig. 1 Reported rates of thrombosis with thrombocytopenia syndrome (TTS) with Janssen (Johnson & Johnson) COVID-19 vaccine when 14.1 million doses had been administered. The overall reporting rate was 3.83 cases per million Janssen COVID-19 vaccine doses. However, the reporting rates for females were much higher than males, particularly for females 30–49 years of age. (See 2021; USG public domain)

pandemics of emerging and re-emerging infectious diseases, while standards remain broadly the same, pressure, publicity, pace, and scope intensify with the number of people affected. When it comes to diseases and conditions that are not spreading rapidly, novel medical countermeasures (MCMs) are assessed under relatively low pressure, with all due caution and limited publicity, exposing only the number of individuals necessary to power statistically sound studies. Without careful management, this may translate to an increase in actual harm or misperceptions about the safety of a new vaccine or therapeutic. For example, if a drug has an intrinsic flaw that will cause a serious adverse event (SAE) in 1 person out of 1000 exposed to it, a normally paced development program may identify and perhaps successfully mitigate the danger posed by that flaw after only one or two SAEs. In a pandemic setting, if pressure to introduce the drug leads to rapid distribution and widespread use, exposure of many thousands simultaneously could lead to scores of the 1:1000 SAEs. Even though the event rate is the same, the pressures, public attention, and stakes in a pandemic response could make the SAE into a headline story, which might easily overshadow impressive efficacy data on the agent. Figure 1 shows an SAE with an occurrence rate far below 1:1000, which nevertheless received wide coverage and led to the suspension of the use or rollout of the Janssen vaccine for a time in several countries around the world (BBC News 2021).

The relevant question in drug development safety and PV (Fig. 2) in any setting, and particularly in a pandemic, is not simply, "Is the drug safe?" but "Are the anticipated risks acceptable when balanced against the harm of the disease and the efficacy of the drug in mitigating that harm?" If the harm of the pandemic disease itself decreases along the two primary axes of frequency and severity (i.e., infections are less common and symptoms less severe), the acceptability of any toxicity due to a proposed therapeutic agent also decreases. One would not use a drug, no matter how effective it might be, that was very likely to cause a serious adverse event (SAE) to counter a pandemic of a relatively mild and self-limited upper respiratory infection. Conversely, drugs with significant toxicity may reasonably be deployed if they can stem an outbreak of a highly fatal disease with no good alternative treatment.

It is those in the field of pharmacovigilance who will ascertain the numerator (risk) for the most essential equation (risk/benefit) governing effective response to emerging diseases. Viewed through the lens of the COVID-19 pandemic, the pharmacovigilance teams at pharmaceutical companies, government research institutes, teaching hospitals, health ministries, and elsewhere have been charged with ensuring the complete collection and analysis of every negative or untoward event associated with medical countermeasures, in both research and authorized emergency use. Their work produces actionable

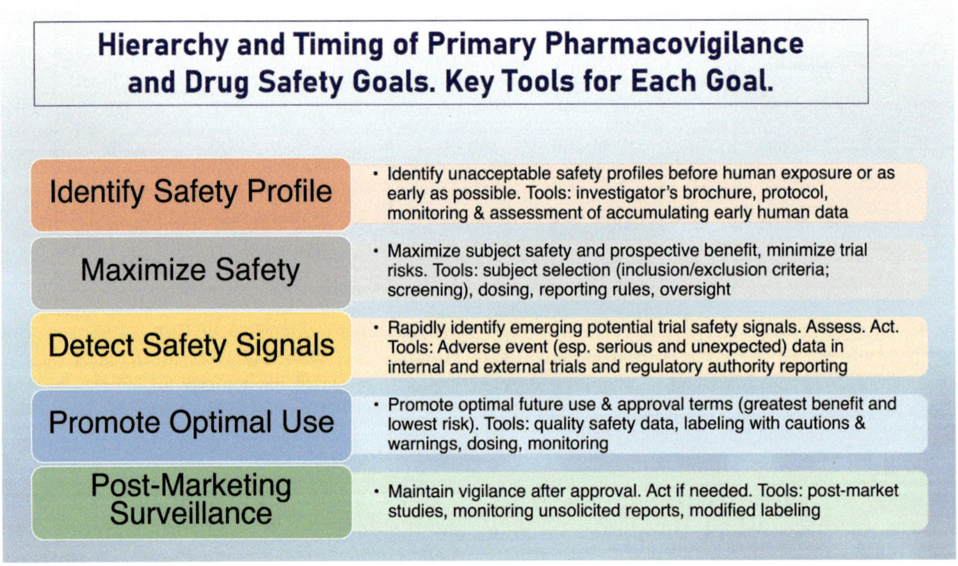

Fig. 2 The key goals of pharmacovigilance and some of the tools for achieving them. (Authors)

information for oversight bodies, reviewers, regulators, and decision-makers. It has permitted the development and deployment of therapeutics and especially vaccines with unprecedented speed and remarkable effectiveness.

All safety data—whether gathered from human or animal models, cell cultures, assays, or biochips—make up the global safety and pharmacovigilance building block of pandemic response. The nature and probability of the events that these data reflect inform human clinical trial design, monitoring plans, stopping rules for trials, and ultimately end use. It will be the pharmacovigilance practitioners, in close cooperation with clinical study teams, who will monitor safety as candidate prevention or treatment measures move from bench to bedside and into broader populations, focused on the question, "Is it safe?"

2 What Is Pharmacovigilance?

2.1 Definitions and Goals

WHO (2004) defines pharmacovigilance as "the science and activities relating to the detection, assessment, understanding and prevention of adverse events (AE) or any other possible drug-related problems." There are four classical minimum elements to a pharmacovigilance report:

1. An identifiable adverse event (AE)
2. An identifiable patient
3. An identifiable reporter
4. An identifiable drug[1]

In routine practice, patients who are affected by an AE, their guardian, or their medical care provider report the AE to the healthcare system and the pharmacovigilance system. In clinical studies, investigators compile data on all adverse events in research participants.

The regulations and the practice of pharmacovigilance vary significantly from one drug category to another, a difference most pronounced in the way safety is assessed for vaccines compared to therapeutics (Cobert et al. 2019; Waller and Harrison-Woolrych 2017). The Global Health Training Centre (2021) has a freely accessible course, "Introduction to Collecting and Reporting

1 In this chapter, we will use the term drug to refer to a range of pharmaceutical products, including vaccines, therapeutics, and other interventions intended to prevent, treat, or resolve disease.

Adverse Events," which reviews the fundamentals of the subject.

The two sides to the drug evaluation coin, efficacy and safety, are abundantly clear in the U.S. Food and Drug Administration's (FDA) criterion for drug approval: "the drug is determined to provide benefits that outweigh its known and potential risks for the intended population" (FDA 2022). This risk/benefit ratio may play out on many levels. In human subjects research, the projected risk/benefit ratio, the risks to individual research participants, and minimization of anticipated risks through good study design are the criteria for regulatory approval of a clinical trial. In practice, even approved drugs, available on the market for a given purpose or purposes, must be assessed for individual patients and populations. Will the magnitude and likelihood of benefit to people prove to be worth the anticipated risks?

Note that the benefit—the denominator of this equation—can never be zero, at least not to society or some population at risk of a disease. The direct benefit may be zero to healthy individuals undergoing initial human testing of the intervention, but there must be a prospect of benefit to others. Otherwise, as in a mathematical equation, the risks would become metaphorically infinite, even if they were relatively rare and trivial. If aspirin did not ease aches and pains, there would be no reason to take it, even if it were nearly benign—the smallest safety issue would be unacceptable if there were no known benefit.

Pharmacovigilance is necessary because even though a clinical trial is predicated on the hypothesis that the intervention being tested will provide benefits that outweigh the risks, that hypothesis may turn out to be wrong. It may not even be shown to be wrong until the drug gets past the approval stage. There are many well-known cases of drugs receiving regulatory approval and then causing serious harm: perhaps most notoriously thalidomide in the late 1950s and early 1960s. That case, where a drug was found to cause terrible fetal harm that clearly outweighed any benefit in pregnant women, led to major improvements in regulation and pharmacovigilance (Fornasier et al. 2018). Still, even in the twenty-first century, the balance between adverse events and benefits may not be fully assessed until well after drug approval: selective COX-2 inhibitors (Vioxx and Celebrex), for example, were not withdrawn from the market until they had been given to millions of people (James et al. 2007).

Thus, we see that recording, reporting, assessing, and communicating adverse drug effects, as they occur during development and after approval, are essential. They guide the use of a drug during development and post-marketing administration. *Pharmacovigilance (PV)*, then, is the discipline that informs research on a drug and its use in the clinic, helping to ensure or at least maximize *safety*. Knowledge about potential benefits of a drug may evolve as well, though generally not as rapidly as safety information. The evolving safety profile is continually updated with ongoing evaluation of *risks* against anticipated or proven *benefits*—information that is included on the product label and used by medical practitioners. ▫ Figures 3, 4, and 5 show the results of recent PV studies in graphic form.

2.2 The Mandate and the Players

Clinical safety is of utmost importance as an element of clinical research. Individuals who volunteer as participants in a drug development trial need to be protected. Safety is addressed from the moment the drug first enters the pre-clinical (pre-human) phase of development. As the drug candidate goes through development, testing, and clinical studies, there will be a growing list of adverse reactions that may or may not be due to the drug. This list ultimately comes to be known by any of several names, one being the safety profile, which will inform those who administer the drug to humans in later studies and eventually in medical care, so they can maximize benefit and minimize toxicities. Because safety is so important, there are many activities devoted to it, and many players whose work on the safety profile overlaps, creating an intentional redundancy. Some of the phases and players are

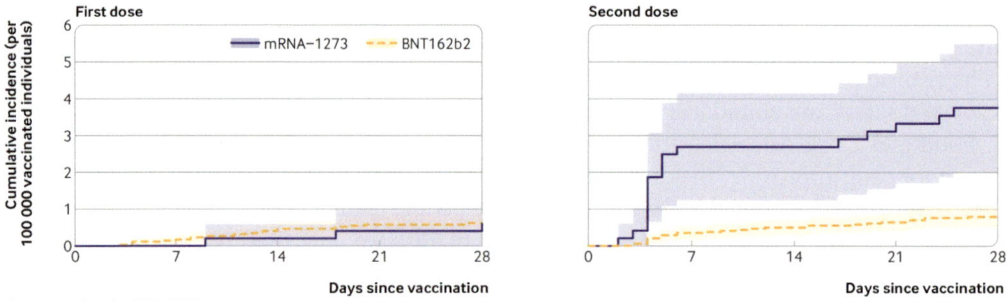

	First dose 0	7	14	21	28	Second dose 0	7	14	21	28
Cumulative No of mRNA-1273 events	0	0	<3	<3	3	0	13	13	16	18
Cumulative No of BNT162b2 events	0	6	16	20	21	0	12	17	22	27
No of individuals vaccinated with mRNA-1273	498 812	497 394	495 868	494 385	324 385	483 270	480 224	475 455	469 075	461 147
No of individuals vaccinated with BNT162b2	3 482 275	3 473 640	3 463 991	3 004 903	2 080 614	3 417 744	3 406 113	3 391 206	3 369 584	3 340 072

Fig. 3 Results of a pharmacovigilance study: cumulative incidence of myocarditis or myopericarditis events after COVID-19 mRNA vaccination, by vaccine type and dose number. (Husby et al. 2021)

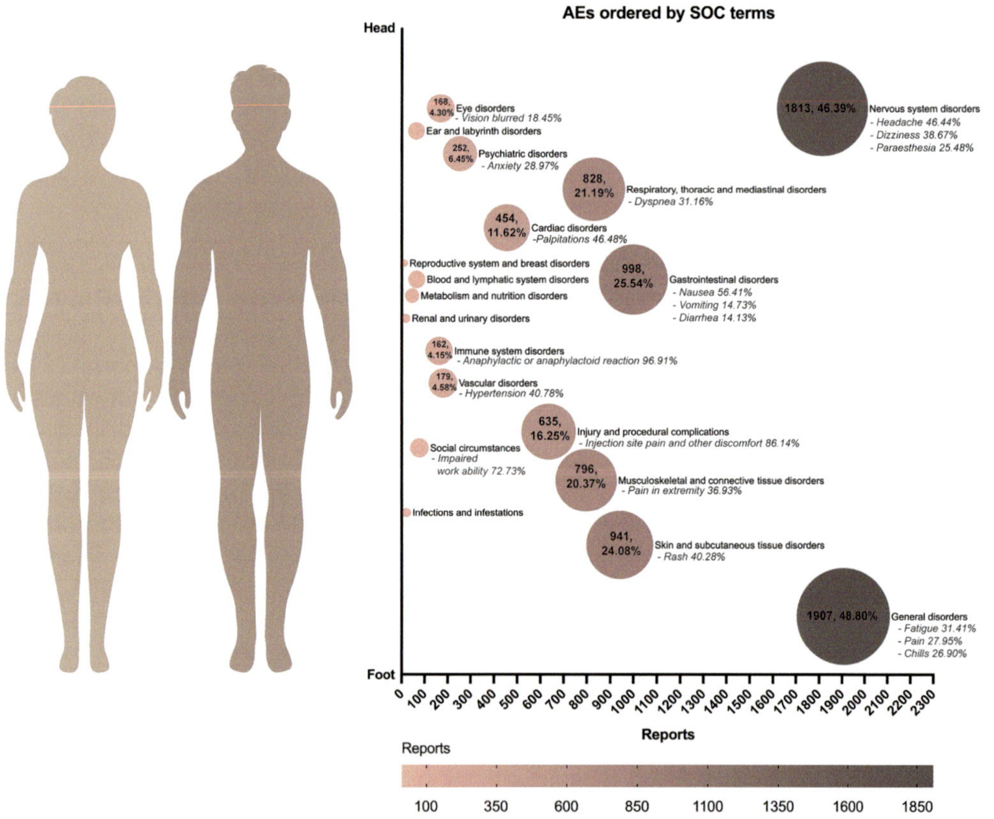

Fig. 4 A bubble plot displays the case numbers and percentages of AEs after COVID-19 mRNA vaccination. The size of the circles is determined by the number of patients with adverse events. (Chen et al. 2021; CC license to reprint with citation)

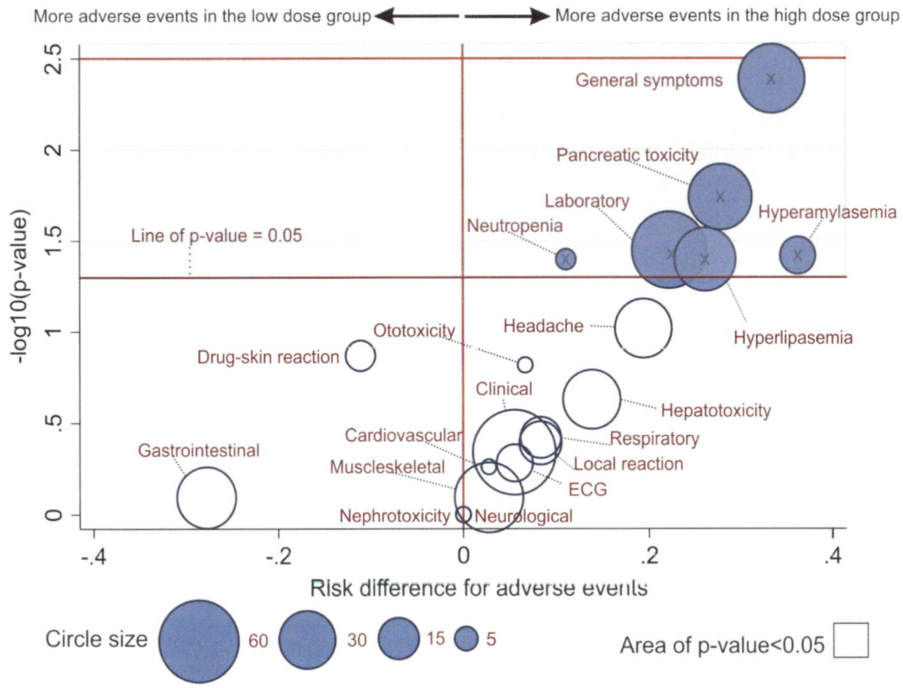

Fig. 5 A bubble plot displays the risk difference of AE in the high- vs. low-dose group in a clinical trial of antimony to treat leishmaniasis. The size of the circles is determined by the number of patients with adverse events. The blue circles indicate significantly more adverse events in the high-dose group. (Saheki et al. 2017; CC may be reused with attribution)

- *Preclinical scientists* do work that includes in silico (in silicon, or computer modeling) and in vitro (in glass, e.g., test tubes and flasks, often with specially developed cell lines) analysis to produce information on the chemical and biological properties of the compound, including target tissues, binding sites, and other parameters related to safety and efficacy.
- *Preclinical* work includes additional testing on how the compound behaves in a living creature, generally a small mammal for convenience, and often a larger mammal or nonhuman primate to better approximate behavior in a human. Reproductive toxicity work and vital organ changes, visible on histopathology after sacrifice, add to the safety profile.
- *First-in-human clinical investigators and safety teams* may then introduce the agent in Phase I trials that help define pharmacokinetics, pharmacodynamics, half-life, breakdown and elimination pathways, intermediate compounds, dosing and administration parameters, and the first list of observable human toxicities and laboratory findings. At this point, the major players on the safety stage are introduced and continue in the development program. They include.
  - *Regulatory agencies*: Governing bodies that implement national laws, regulations, and in many cases, internationally harmonized guidance and standards, for example, those of the International Conference on Harmonisation of Technical Requirements for Pharmaceuticals for Human Use (ICH 2023). These bodies set the boundaries for protection of humans and nonhuman animals when it comes to the development, testing, and marketed use of therapeutics. In the United States, this is primarily the FDA.
  - *Data safety monitoring boards and other safety monitoring and event adjudication and advisory teams*: These are panels of experts in clinical, scientific, pharma-

ceutical, statistical, data, and other fields. They are convened and empowered by drug development sponsors or by regulators to monitor and assess research data as it accumulates and upon completion of the research (▶ Chap. 23). Their mission is to identify signals of potential harm, or a clear lack of likely benefit or efficacy, or, conversely, a signal of such clear efficacy that the research needs to stop or be reconfigured to offer the drug to those who need it. Such panels are generally advisory, and although their determinations carry enormous weight, they normally act through a sponsoring or regulatory body.

- *The sponsor, sponsor medical monitor, and sponsor safety office*: This team, generally led by at least one physician or nurse specializing in the regulatory and clinical interface of drug development safety, also monitors and assesses incoming data from studies. Here, the focus is on a case-by-case and then cumulative view. Safety reports, particularly those indicating a serious event, are scrutinized, and queries are sent to the reporting physician or site to clarify details. The goal is multifold: ensure the quality of safety data (accuracy and completeness); assess reports individually and in clinically relevant groups (e.g., age, sex, comorbidities) to identify potential safety signals; act to help protect subjects in the study or those who may be using the same agent elsewhere; and report to regulators as required.
- *Research ethics committees (RECs) or institutional review boards (IRBs)*: Ethical review is mandated by drug regulators everywhere, although the RECs may differ in capacity and expertise. RECs usually include scientific, clinical, and ethical experts and nonscientists who represent the community. Members are trained in ethical principles and the practice of clinical research and are charged with acting not only to protect research volunteers from physiological harms, but to ensure that they are treated ethically, particularly when it comes to informing participants before they enroll in a study about the research and the risks they will face so they can provide their informed consent to participate. RECs have a great deal of input into and essentially veto power over the informed consent form (ICF) that research volunteers must agree to before they are enrolled in any study (▶ Chap. 33, In Practices 33.2, and 33.3).
- *Scientific and regulatory research reviewers and study monitors*: The sponsor is required to pick qualified individuals to assess the proposed research for scientific merit, safety and regulatory adherence, and subject protection, and to monitor the research to ensure that implementation is consistent with the research protocol. Monitoring informed consent is a major part of assessment once the trial has begun.
- *The principal investigator (PI) and site study team*: The sponsor is obligated to select investigators and teams who are qualified not only to conduct the research as outlined in the protocol, but monitor for, detect, and treat the most likely and most serious potential risks facing study participants. Failure here, aside from possible harm to volunteers, could lead to the entire study being halted because of safety concerns.
- *Pharmacists* plan the safe transport, storage, preparation, and administration of drugs with detailed standard operating procedures that cover everything from receipt through disposal, protecting not only subjects but the integrity of the trial and the well-being of those handling the drug (▶ Chap. 38).
- *Data and statistical specialists* design and test data collection forms, generally electronic, and design the summaries and reports that will go to other safety/PV-focused stakeholders to ensure they can identify single events and patterns that may indicate a problem (▶ Chap. 35) (◘ Fig. 6).

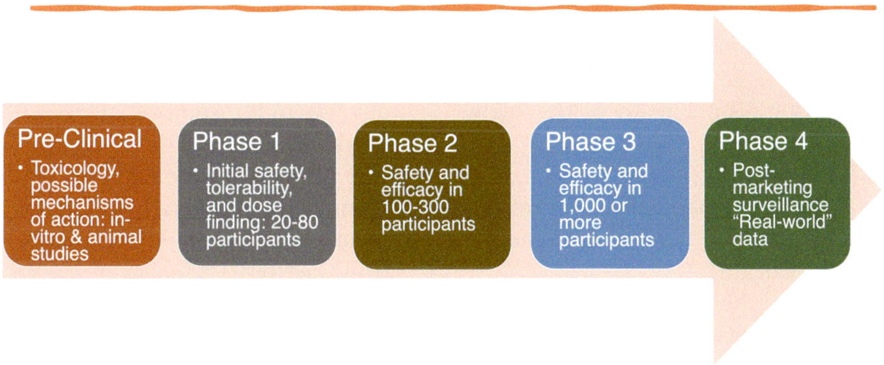

Fig. 6 Drug safety and pharmacovigilance activities during the life cycle of drug development. (Authors)

2.3 Methods

The methods of pharmacovigilance are, at their core, very simple, though the rules for what adverse events to collect and how they are reported and analyzed are quite complex:

- Early in the evaluation of a drug candidate, before human trials begin, preclinical research highlights areas of potential concern through a battery of tests and evaluations that help determine the route of administration, the initial dose, and the population best included in or excluded from clinical trials. These are addressed in an investigator's brochure, especially in sections on safety and guidance for the investigator, which are developed and maintained by the drug developer (FDA 1995).
- Each research protocol, illuminated by other, more detailed documents, such as the manual of operations (MOP), safety management plan (SMP), and clinical site monitoring plan (CSMP) for the study, lays out exclusion rules for research participants, safety management, monitoring, and other rules for human participants in the trial. A data and safety monitoring plan (DSMP) is also incorporated in each study. The DSMP, implemented by a data and safety monitoring board (DSMB) (▶ Chap. 23) "is a formalized process for reviewing accumulated outcome data from an ongoing research study to ensure the continuing safety and welfare of current research subjects and those yet to be enrolled, as well as the continuing validity and scientific merit of the study" (HHS 2018; NIH 2020). The purpose, again, is to minimize risks and keep the anticipated risk–benefit ratio acceptable, from initial enrollment through the duration of each subject's participation.
- Definitions and rules for identification, recording, assessment, and reporting of events are detailed in the protocol and the MOP. These include the criteria for the event's severity, or grade, based on a grading tool or table, as well as the event's seriousness, based on standard serious adverse event (SAE) definitions taken from regulatory and guidance documents. A selection of protocol templates with grading tools, definitions, and other guidelines may be accessed freely here (NIAID 2021).
- As research continues, adverse events affecting study participants are recorded in their records and entered into the study database. They are also assessed by the investigator and reported to the trial sponsor and the pharmacovigilance team through the safety database, in accordance with the protocol (▶ Chap. 35).
- The pharmacovigilance team reviews the incoming and accumulating safety data—essentially individual narratives of all serious safety reports, as well as a listing of all adverse events reported in the study—along with other safety-related information accumulating from the overall ongoing development program for the drug. This includes.

- *SAE:* Serious adverse events, or an adverse event or suspected adverse reaction that, in the view of the investigator or sponsor, results in any of the following outcomes:
  - Death
  - A life-threatening adverse event (one that places a person at immediate risk of death)
  - Inpatient hospitalization or prolongation of existing hospitalization
  - A persistent or significant incapacity or substantial disruption of the ability to conduct normal life functions or
  - A congenital anomaly/birth defect
  - Important medical events that may not result in death, be life-threatening, or require hospitalizations may be considered serious when, based upon appropriate medical judgment, they may jeopardize the patient or research participant and may require medical or surgical intervention to prevent one of the outcomes listed in this definition (CFR 2020)
- *SUSAR:* Suspected unanticipated serious adverse reactions, or SAEs that are suspected to have been caused by the study intervention or drug and are unexpected based on the safety information for the intervention being investigated. SUSARs call for analysis and if potential safety issues are identified, possible action.

- Safety-driven actions may be as mundane as updating details of the investigator's brochure or relatively minor updates to the likelihood of risks being disclosed to study participants in the informed consent process. They may be as significant as major modifications to study inclusion or exclusion criteria or major adjustments to safety monitoring activities, such as lab testing or medical imaging. They may in some cases require halting of enrollment or changing dosing of the drug. These safety actions may be limited to one study, or even one arm of a study, but they may also be serious enough to impact the use of the drug in any setting, including changes to the approved use of an already marketed drug.
- The pharmacovigilance team of the drug manufacturer generally maintains a complete database of safety events for the drug, performs analysis of similar events across multiple studies and usage globally, provides annual updates to the investigator's brochure, and provides notifications or submissions to collaborators and regulators as required. It is essential for any research with human subjects that the Safety/PV team communicate from the planning stages with their counterparts as all parties will have a keen interest in incoming safety information and related regulatory responsibilities. Such plans to share data are often worked out in detail, with contract-like agreements and detailed SOPs.
- Ultimately the drug may be approved for use based on the standard of having been judged *safe and efficacious.* A drug label is then prepared in a collaborative process including the developer, manufacturer, and applicable regulatory authority. The label explains the intended usage and includes a robust section on the relevant adverse events that have been observed. This information is updated as the drug is used by more people, further studied, used in different populations or for different purposes, or is combined in a product with a variety of other agents.

In this chapter, we will offer a functional definition of pharmacovigilance (PV) planning, implementation, and operations for a large-scale outbreak research program. Examples from the response to the global COVID-19 Pandemic, the 2014–2016 Ebola virus outbreak in West Africa, and the 2018–2020 Ebola outbreak in the northeastern Democratic Republic of the Congo (DRC) are based upon the authors' experience.

3 Pharmacovigilance in Action

3.1 Start with Trial Protocol Safety Section

Setting up a pharmacovigilance process always begins with the trial protocol. For emerging and re-emerging infectious disease (EID) emergencies, generic protocols that anticipate outbreaks and public health emergencies may have been drafted in advance to be adapted to specific circumstances when needed. Pre-outbreak protocols can save time and minimize problems and errors by allowing for review of as much as is possible without knowing the specific pathogen and circumstances. Once an EID outbreak occurs, the trial of an investigational new drug against the disease can be incorporated without re-inventing the wheel (Sigfrid et al. 2020).

The safety section of the trial protocol plays a key role as a rulebook. This is especially important in an EID emergency where morbidity and mortality are high. On the one hand, patients who are potential study participants must not be subjected to any risk that is not fully justified. On the other hand, in the absence of alternatives there may be demands from the population, politicians, and front-line medical practitioners to use experimental drugs more widely than is consistent with the protocol, or with rigorous determinations of safety and efficacy (Caluwaerts 2017; Schuklenk 2016; WHO 2014a, b).

While possibly starting from a generic draft, the pharmacovigilance professional will need to craft a more detailed, thoughtful safety section, focusing on the actual threat at hand, the population most at risk, the drug being tested, and the environment of the study. For example, during the COVID-19 pandemic it rapidly became evident that serious disease was highly correlated with both increased age and comorbidities that are more prevalent with age, for example, obesity and heart disease. Safety monitoring plans had to take these factors into account, requiring an accurate health history before a study drug was administered, both to correlate patient outcomes with factors predisposing them to severe disease and to prevent confusion between a pre-existing condition and a new safety signal.

Secondary documents such as SOPs, SMPs, MOPs, and diagrams showing how safety/PV activities flow from one stage to the next and from one team to another are of enormous help, and may well identify the gaps during the planning stage. The urgency of developing MCMs in a pandemic must be balanced with the need to comply with regulatory requirements, which may also be subject to adjustment in an EID emergency (▶ Chap. 6). Some flexibility is needed as any research program begins, as unpredicted events are expected. Nevertheless, practical adaptation must not contravene ethical or scientific principles. The clinical trial must incorporate two key roles of pharmacovigilance:

- Monitoring accumulating safety data in real time, facilitating the analysis, and sharing the data to help ensure that participants volunteering for the study are protected from unreasonable or unnecessary risks.
- Ensuring prompt review and systematic follow-up with medical care providers at the bedside and learning from their observations to help them gather high-quality data, so that the emerging safety profile of any study interventions develops into the most accurate, complete, and useful information possible.

These points apply whether the investigational interventions are licensed or are at the first-in-human stage of evaluation (Phase I) with limited information on human safety.

Box 1: Informed and Alert

It is essential that pharmacovigilance professionals in potential outbreak response roles remain alert and forward-thinking. "Peacetime" awareness is vital. A distant blip on the map, like a rat running down the cable of a merchant ship in Messina in 1347, or a mysterious respiratory outbreak in a city in China in late 2019, may all too quickly come to your neighborhood. One should not only be aware of the scientific and medical background of a situation but also strive to quickly understand the social, political, economic, and cultural factors that may shape the research response plan.

For response in an unfamiliar place, awareness of the local level of trust afforded outsiders is especially important for those following up with study participants in the community, since gaining trust can require subtlety, diligence, and time. Unfamiliar cultural mores must be understood and respected. Partnerships must be based on mutual respect and shared goals. Executing a pharmacovigilance program in a rapidly evolving epidemic is unsettling. A caring attitude and poise, as with a successful clinician, will serve safety/PV team members well. The time to focus on the background information and principles of PV in response research is *before* the call comes. The more best practices, regulations, and objectives have been ingrained in responders, the more they will be free to focus their response on the particular event. In an emergency, lines of demarcation are blurred, resources scarce, and people under stress. Any tension between patient-focused clinical care and rigorous, scientifically focused research may stand out in sharp relief.

It would be convenient for outbreaks to occur in well-resourced areas, but this does not appear to be the tendency (▶ Chap. 10), despite the counterexample of COVID-19. Those providing pharmacovigilance for investigational products are likely to be outsiders. No matter how well-intentioned and ready to help, they can easily put a foot wrong on unfamiliar terrain. Expressing exasperation over inefficient or nonexistent systems for pharmacovigilance will lead nowhere. Wide-ranging, mutual exchange of information can not only solve immediate problems but yield secondary benefits, as those working together to meet challenges become a cohesive pharmacovigilance team. Pharmacovigilance professionals, whose perspective and practice are rooted in rigorous compliance with regulatory requirements, will likely need to depart from their comfort zone. The often-overlooked "black box" statement at the top of many key FDA guidance documents is also worth noting:

> *This guidance represents … current thinking on this topic.…* ***You can use an alternative approach***.

3.2 Protocols for Emergency Response

Emergency response research protocols can differ considerably from those written for a more typical research setting. For those with experience in emergency clinical research, whether among vulnerable populations with life-threatening diseases, or in research-naïve and resource-poor settings, these challenges may be familiar. But as the old saying has it, "If you've seen one epidemic, you've seen one epidemic"—the challenges are never entirely predictable, and meeting them is never simple. For those accustomed to highly regulated, resource-rich, structured settings with established standard operating procedures, particularly for studies in healthy populations, expectations will be challenged from the outset.

It has been a century since we have seen a large-scale pandemic of an easily spread (airborne), frequently fatal disease. Sanitation and medical science have advanced to give us more tools to treat and prevent disease, but SARS-CoV 1 and 2 viewed together present the specter of a pathogen combining the virulence of the former with the asymptomatic transmission of the latter. When preparing for pharmacovigilance in EID response, one must envision what would be needed in that dire scenario.

Though the PV role would not change in principle, clearly the more dangerous the disease, the more acceptable adverse events become in pursuing MCMs. For example, Ebola virus disease (EVD) causes so many varied serious adverse events that investigators need to distinguish those most likely attributable to the disease from those that seem noteworthy, atypical, or the result of a potential drug toxicity.

In the DRC PALM therapeutics trial, sticking to the classical rules and definitions would have made the effort impossible and prevented the team from identifying two successful treatments (Mulangu et al. 2019). Additionally, the high likelihood of a poor outcome worked to the advantage of the PV team, which could monitor blinded aggregate data on deaths to see if numbers were at least no worse than the usual mortality for the disease under study. An experienced DSMB monitoring the unblinded data, comparing each investigational arm to the control arm, added a significant layer of protection. Finally, when deaths from EVD are frequent, it is easier to rapidly detect a change due to the intervention under study. Incidence impacts power, statistically speaking. This may mean the study will require fewer participants to identify a statistically significant benefit. Conversely, if a poor outcome is relatively rare and the disease relatively benign, the incidence of severe illness should be low, and any drug toxicity easily and rapidly detectable. These factors will play out in the statistical plan for the study but will also have an enormous impact on the clarity, confidence, and speed with which a PV team may identify the kinds of toxicity they are looking for.

What is known about the safety of a treatment candidate matters. If a licensed drug (e.g., dexamethasone) is being repurposed in an emergency, accumulated safety data will inform surveillance, in contrast to a drug candidate with little or no human data. Ultimately, regulators may be comfortable with relatively rapid emergency use authorization based on data from frequent past use. This may safely save time and resources from a safety and PV perspective.

In 2020, the healthcare systems of the richest nations, with the most highly developed and redundant clinical resources, were rapidly overwhelmed, to the point of potential or actual sharing of critical care measures (ventilators) meant for a single patient. In the 2014–2016 and 2018–2020 Ebola outbreaks, as in the COVID-19 pandemic, clinicians were pushed to the brink and beyond. In this situation, it is essential to distinguish between ethical and scientific requirements that must be upheld and the usual procedural requirements for ensuring standards are met, which can be streamlined, waived, or completed with a delay. To ignore such realities and impose unreasonable standards on research activities, which add to the demands on clinicians, is to invite failure.

While long-term safety assessment is indispensable, in 2020 the name of the game for many was to make it off the ventilator, out of the intensive care unit, and home. A punctilious adherence to procedure would not have helped. The FDA and other regulatory agencies, often derided as rigid and bureaucratic, were remarkably fleet-footed and flexible in response to COVID-19 (Kesselheim et al. 2021). We suggest that studies in this situation be designed to fit the most urgent scientific need and to answer the most pressing scientific questions by collecting the most essential data as a priority, in consultation with regulators and ethical and scientific reviewers. The rapid development, testing, emergency use approval, manufacturing, and deployment of MCMs in 2020–2021 exemplify reasonable adjustment to pandemic realities.

As in other spheres of action covered in this volume, this in no way suggests that the emergency is an excuse to dispense with any of the protections built into the pharmacovigilance system. Frequent consultation with regulators and reviewers is mandatory. At the same time, there is more room for discretion in implementing the regulations, and the systems and entities that enforce them, than may be obvious (FDA 2012). The response to the Ebola outbreaks in West Africa and the 2018–2020 northeastern DRC outbreak, where a four-arm randomized therapeutics trial was completed, demonstrate that scientifically rigorous and ethically sound research can be conducted in the most challenging conditions (Kennedy et al. 2017; Mulangu et al. 2019). The uneven global response to COVID-19, varying widely with popular opinion and political circumstances as well as response capacity, illustrates the key challenges.

What in normal times would be a routine and little noted halt in a trial in response to a potential safety signal can become headline news in a pandemic. COVID-19 has highlighted a large and apparently growing portion of the population in many if not most countries that does not trust scientific information and public health advice, especially when that advice is in flux. Those who stoke disinformation wait for opportunities to distort or fabricate news to buttress their narrative. This places a huge burden on those conducting pharmacovigilance. They must not only perform their duties soundly and diligently, but they must also consider how to convey information and cannot assume confidentiality is assured. Scientists and analysts need to be sensitive to how a malicious reader might misinterpret their reports. Their findings should be reported to the public by experienced communicators with a sense of how information may be received and distorted.

Many nations where COVID-19 vaccine is easily available have seen sharp drops in vaccination rates, with the oft-cited rationale, "I am not sure it is safe." Vaccine and drug skepticism has been around for as long as there have been vaccines and drugs, but 2021 brought this phenomenon into greater prominence, and it has done severe damage to the COVID-19 response (Dos Santos et al. 2023). The very concept of shared risk and responsibility, directly related to safety and pharmacovigilance, has in many quarters given way to distorted concepts of individual rights and freedom. Along with widespread skepticism about the safety and effectiveness of the vaccines, freedom has become a battle cry for those declining vaccination or evidence-based treatment, with safety concerns serving as the rationale for noncompliance with actions for the common good (AlShurman et al. 2021). The pharmacovigilance team must understand the reality not only at the research site level but how to convey it to the global village.

Professionals who routinely share information peer-to-peer, in blunt shorthand without fear of misinterpretation or misuse, *must* consider how information can be deliberately distorted, particularly if it is likely to get to the public via scientifically untrained, potentially biased messengers, such as bloggers, social media trendsetters, TV commentators, and factional opinion leaders. Safety messaging needs to be vetted to minimize misinterpretation.

4 Implementing Pharmacovigilance

4.1 Pharmacovigilance Capacity Assessment

The first step in building a pharmacovigilance process is to conduct a capacity assessment. Some documents useful for the assessment are listed below.

4.1.1 Pharmacovigilance Assessment Tools

Pharmacovigilance assessment tools include checklists, manuals, and guidebooks. *Pharmacovigilance Indicators: A Practical Manual for the Assessment of Pharmacovigilance Systems* (WHO 2015), based on prior experience in low-resource countries and reference guidelines, is (as of 2023) awaiting updates based on the COVID-19 experience. Answers to the checklist questions, which are aimed at elucidating existing pharmacovigilance capacity, are used to construct a pharmacovigilance response process that will work in a particular emergency.

4.1.2 Safety-Related SOPs

Safety-related SOPs are basic documents mapping the flow of adverse events and safety data, from the initial observation of the event through analysis and regulatory reporting. Key players need to be identified and will themselves provide additional valuable input, particularly those with prior experience and in-country knowledge. Following adaptation to meet the particulars of a specific outbreak research response, the SOPs should become very familiar to all study personnel, including those who will be carrying out pharmacovigilance.

4.1.3 A Safety Reporting Flow Chart

A safety reporting flow chart is a graphic representation of the SOP, protocol, and MOP content for safety data, critical to helping spot flaws, bottlenecks, and potentially dispensable steps that may consume precious time or resources (◘ Fig. 7). These will need to be customized for the specific safety team organization and requirements of the study at hand.

4.1.4 A Data and Safety Monitoring Board Charter

A data and safety monitoring board (DSMB) can be invaluable in a large-scale research project, particularly a randomly controlled, double-blinded trial, but whether it is required will be determined by sponsor policy and regulatory input. Should a DSMB or similar data monitoring committee be formed, a charter outlining the group's composition and mandate must be aligned with the statistical analysis plan for the study and the work plans of study statisticians and the pharmacovigilance team. An independent DSMB lends additional validity and scientific weight to study activities, including safety actions, through its expertise, independence, and access to unblinded data and statistics. Such an arrangement frees the pharmacovigilance team to perform blinded, unbiased analysis of incoming safety data, particularly serious events, and adds a major layer of real-time subject protection (▶ Chap. 23).

4.1.5 Transfer of Regulatory Obligation (TORO) Agreement

In major responses, there will be a need for a very rapid marshaling of resources, and this may require outsourcing some roles to trusted partners. TORO agreements make clear who is doing what to meet regulatory, ethical, and

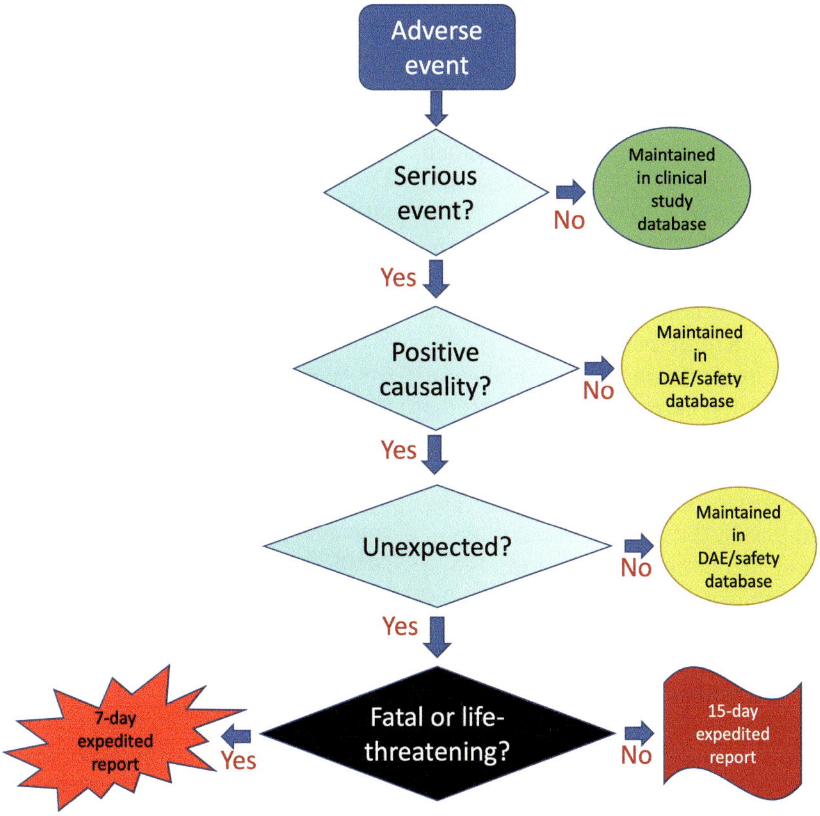

◘ **Fig. 7** A workflow chart for determining whether an adverse event must be reported to health authorities as an expedited safety report. (Adapted from NIA 2018; USG public domain)

operational requirements during the deployment of rapid response teams to establish necessary infrastructure and operations. TOROs may help clarify roles for in-country partners so a local expert can speed approvals and deployment of local resources. It is important that the sponsors remember that ultimately, from a regulatory, legal, ethical, and reputational perspective, they will still be held responsible for safety, so close oversight of activities undertaken under a TORO agreement is mandatory, along with an audit if necessary.

4.1.6 Publications Useful for Pharmacovigilance Planning and Implementation

Pharmacovigilance is a well-established, documented, and regulated element of the research enterprise in any moderately developed healthcare system. Information about regulatory requirements in most countries is publicly available in databases and documents regularly updated by the U.S. National Institute of Allergy and Infectious Diseases (NIAID), the U.S. Office of Human Research Protections, the European Clinical Research Information Network, and WHO (Baden et al. 2021; European Clinical Research Information Network 2023; NIAID 2023; OHRP 2020; WHO 2022). Country-specific safety reporting information included in these resources can be useful to quickly check on safety reporting requirements.

If detailed information is not available for a country, as in the case of DRC during the 2018–2020 Ebola outbreak, it can be developed during the response with in-country subject matter experts (SME). In the DRC case, foreign and local SMEs collaborated to compile accurate regulatory information. While the pharmacovigilance guidelines issued by the FDA, the European Medicines Agency, and WHO, along with a few others, remain the global standard, local publications may be available to help clarify local requirements for many pharmacovigilance activities. Likewise, partners may appreciate receiving documents that the sponsoring organization may take for granted. Examples include FDA requirements for investigational new drug safety reporting (FDA 2012), for institutional review board (research ethics committee) operations (FDA 2023), and widely accepted research guidance documents like those of the International Conference for Harmonisation of Technical Requirements for Pharmaceuticals for Human Use (ICH) (ICH 2016) or the Council for International Organizations of Medical Sciences (CIOMS 2016). Empty, formatted tables for adverse event and safety data (table shells) will help ensure that report contents match the data categories and formats needed by the pharmacovigilance team and DSMB. If the study does not have a DSMB, the pharmacovigilance team will find useful guidance in ICH guidelines on safety data management, which are also used as guidance by both the FDA and EMA (EMA 1995; FDA 1995; ICH 1994) (◘ Fig. 8).

In any case, for operations away from the home country of the sponsoring organization or pharmacovigilance team, identifying in-country partners—ideally including pharmacovigilance specialists—early in the project is essential to understand nuances that will need to be incorporated into an effective pharmacovigilance program. Some countries (e.g., DRC) already have established pharmacovigilance programs with knowledgeable staff (Nzolo et al. 2019), while others may have only a nascent pharmacovigilance program or none at all (e.g., countries most affected by the West Africa Ebola outbreak). Whether starting from scratch or with an established program, pharmacovigilance teams can gain experience and become familiar with global practices and standards, as well as how to adapt them to local circumstances, during emergency research. One goal of research partnerships is to demonstrate value, share knowledge, and establish practices customized to local requirements so that host nation programs are sustainable after the emergency research is completed.

Establishing a pharmacovigilance working group at the outset of a response and meeting as often as needed to establish a pharmacovigilance process should be a research response priority. Other working groups,

Table Display Shells

1. **AE Listing**

Site ID	Subject ID	First Dose Date	Preferred Term	Verbatim Term	Start Date/ Study Day	Stop Date/ Study Day	Days Since Last Dose	Outcome	Grade	Action Taken		Relationship	Infusion Reaction	AE of Special Interest	SAE
										Treatment	Other				

2. **SAE Listing**

Case Number	Site ID	Subject ID	First Dose Date	Preferred Term	Verbatim Term/ Case Number	Date AE Became Serious	Start Date/ Study Day	Stop Date/ Study Day	Days Since Last Dose	Outcome	Grade	Action Taken		Relationship	Infusion Reaction	AE of Special Interest	SAE
												Treatment	Other				

3. **Pregnancy Listing**

Case Number	Site ID	Subject ID	First Dose Date	Participant or Partner Pregnancy	Date of Last Menstrual Period/ Study Day	Days Since Prior Dose	Expected Delivery Date	Birth Date	Outcome	Birth Status	Description of Abnormalities

Fig. 8 Examples of table shells used to review safety events used at NIAID. (NIAID USG public domain)

including pharmacy, data management, social mobilization, and clinical operations, should participate where issues overlap. Lines of authority to make safety-related decisions should be clear. For example, deciding if a serious adverse event meets suspected unexpected serious adverse reaction (SUSAR) criteria and whether it triggers regulatory safety reporting requirements might be up to an individual study medical monitor or may be decided collaboratively by the pharmacovigilance working group. Beware of setting up overly sophisticated formal voting systems and criteria for determinations that speak for the group's thinking; team consensus building and trust are likely to be not only adequate but easier to achieve and more reassuring to those acting on pharmacovigilance team determinations.

Emergency research stakeholders often include pharmaceutical companies, nongovernmental organizations, multiple regulatory authorities, RECs/IRBs, Ministries of Health, WHO, the U.S. Centers for Disease Control and Prevention (CDC), U.S. National Institutes of Health (NIH), or equivalent institutions,[2] contractors and sub-contractors, safety oversight boards, and others. The flow of safety reporting in an emergency research response can be complex; mapping information flows to include all stakeholders is critical and should be accomplished early, subject to amendment as stakeholders or reporting requirements change. Pharmaceutical companies often have internal requirements for safety event reports, typically outlined in a clinical trials agreement (CTA). When collaborating with multiple pharmaceutical partners on a single study, it is imperative to incorporate the same safety reporting requirements in each CTA to avoid complex, duplicative reporting processes—something that requires flexibility from both pharmaceutical partners and other sponsors.

2 Such as Institut Pasteur (France), the Robert Koch Institute (Germany), or the National Biomedical Research Institute/*Institut National de Recherche Biomédicale* (DRC).

4.2 Procedure Development

In most cases, SOPs for pharmacovigilance need to cover, at a minimum, management and reporting of SAEs, unanticipated problems (UPs), pregnancy notification and outcomes, SUSARs, and protocol deviations. In emergent responses, research site staff may well have little or no research experience. As seen in 2020–21, healthcare capacity may be overwhelmed in areas affected by an EID emergency, even in resource-rich countries. Pharmacovigilance experts from each partner must provide input in the development of SOPs to meet the unique needs of research sites and maintain compliance with applicable laws, regulations, and guidelines of both the controlling jurisdiction and the sponsors. The pharmacovigilance team should be fully prepared to have regulators review SOPs and assess compliance in a regulatory inspection.

The FDA and many other oversight and regulatory entities exercised discretion and provided some degree of regulatory relief from the strains placed on local clinical and research resources during the height of the COVID-19 pandemic. However, the degree and form of any such latitude cannot be fully predicted, and the best policy is to plan for compliance with all regulations as they normally exist.

SOPs and many other critical documents may need translation into more than one language depending on the local linguistic landscape. If documents are translated by a commercial translation company, in-country pharmacovigilance experts or others with requisite medical and linguistic expertise should verify their accuracy. Translation of highly technical content can be a very specialized enterprise, and confusion and data shortfalls can result if it is not done properly (Hanrahan et al. 2015).

As time and resource consuming as all these steps may be in the face of a major outbreak, shortcuts pose a risk to the entire data collection endeavor and, thus, to the entire rationale for doing the research in the first place. Correcting inaccurate data once the study is underway—if it is possible at all—

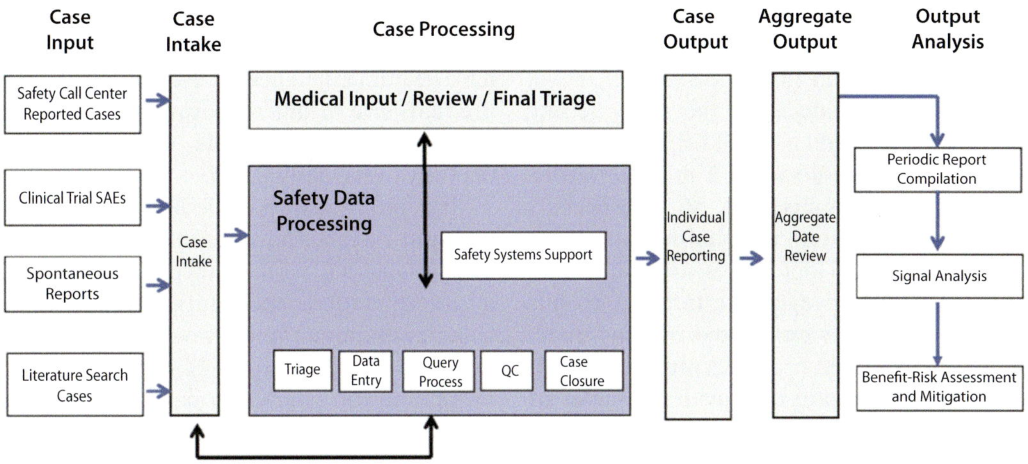

Fig. 9 Major pharmacovigilance activities. (Gagnon et al. 2012)

is likely to consume far more resources and time than it would have taken to set up and test solid procedures upfront. It is helpful to include concrete examples within SOPs, including likely issues and case studies of events similar to those that may occur. If a narrative section is required in a case report form (CRF), explain what is expected and provide an example. The pharmacovigilance working group should be in close contact with the training, monitoring, and site staff (▶ Chap. 42) to determine whether SOPs are clear and useful. A continuous feedback loop can help perfect SOPs. Well-translated fill-in-the-box templates, where appropriate, may reassure reporting personnel and help speed drafting of narrative portions of reports.

The reporting flow must ensure that all safety information is collected on the source medical record, that is, the clinical care record that would cover a patient not enrolled in a study. Study-specific information is then recorded on a CRF designed for the study, and reported and distributed per requirements of the sponsor, regulatory authorities, IRBs/RECs, safety oversight committees, and site investigators, and the principal investigator(s). Automation can ensure that information need not be entered twice (▶ Chap. 35). To avoid undue complexity, it is important that regulatory authorities, RECs/IRBs/ECs, and others agree on a single way of reporting SUSARs. There are several widely used options, such as MedWatch (FDA 2020) or the Council for International Organizations of Medical Sciences 1 Form (CIOMS 2019). If Internet access is sufficiently reliable, using an electronic form can be efficient, such as the UK MHRA gateway or a SUSAR report meeting the requirements of ICH and/or the European Medicines Agency (EMA 2021; ICH 2019; Medicines and Healthcare Products Regulatory Authority 2020). Along with a single form, it is useful to agree on a single reporting plan common to clinical trial and safety data exchange agreements. Automated alerts from the database are a good way to keep key players informed of safety-related issues in this complex structure (Fig. 9).

5 Training

Safety training for emergency research requires creativity, flexibility, and collaboration. Training material must meet the needs of overworked research and clinical care staff with widely varying degrees of experience. Training in-country pharmacovigilance staff who know the local language(s) is optimal as they are most aware of cultural factors, interpersonal interactions, and traditional attitudes about health, burial customs, etc., that may impact safety. Local experts are also best placed to address sensitive issues like pregnancy prevention when called for. Some of this information may be relevant and appropriate for inclusion in the protocol if it will help reviewers understand the study setting and constraints, and if it will help those carrying out the work do so in a more informed and sensitive manner. Site staff, especially expatriates and national capital-based personnel, rotate in and out of research sites, also requiring time for regular training. A mobile pharmacovigilance expert and training material with real-world examples are helpful. For example, it is helpful to provide examples of SAEs previously observed and reported during the study, followed by discussions about how to identify and report these and other potential SAEs.

Training programs should be planned for rapid expansion when needed. The clinical research team, including pharmacovigilance, must be prepared for a possible surge of resources and infrastructure, ranging from medical NGOs to official health response and even military assistance from various countries. Coordinators, investigators, clinicians, and others may need rapid training to meet the needs of an expanded research response. Training should be targeted bring medical personnel up to speed, cover likely problem areas and unique elements of the research, and address critical safety and data integrity issues. In an outbreak emergency, and even more so in a pandemic, must-have items come first, and nice-to-have knowledge may need to be provided in a document, video, or other format to be absorbed as time permits.

The mechanism for delivering training is also important: classroom methods should emphasize the Q and A session at the end of the material, as it may well be the most valuable, particularly with a novice team. Having a pharmacovigilance expert in the sessions, even remotely, is also valuable. It may be advisable for the expert to tread carefully and to avoid absolute statements where reasonable flexibility may be essential. As an example, work under the very harsh circumstances of the 2018–2020 DRC Ebola outbreak was subject to a protocol declaration that reporting deadlines would be respected but could not be absolutely guaranteed. This flexibility proved to be important, for despite enormous efforts teams could not meet all formal timelines. If hard deadlines had been presented as binding, it could have meant reallocation of precious resources from the bedside to the desk, particularly in the early going.

It is important to circle back to each site and staff member once the study is underway to assess actual performance and to correct misinterpretations and faulty processes early. Quality assurance/quality control of early safety data, focused queries, corrections, and re-training can pay off by halting errors that would otherwise continue. Expect training to be ongoing as staff changes occur. Documenting training and tracking these activities is required from a regulatory perspective (▸ Chap. 42).

6 PV Data Collection and Integrity

6.1 Safety Data Collection in an Emergency

It is important to remember that pharmacovigilance data, while primarily intended for the real-time protection of research study participants, will overlap with study data (endpoints) in many cases, and thus the data is collected in a single, ongoing stream and in a timely manner. Once collected, the single database can be drawn upon by researchers and study statisticians to fulfill the endpoint data need and serve the more immediate needs of the pharmacovigilance team in optimizing real-time safety assessment and action if needed.

Safety data collection during a high-risk public health emergency may be less comprehensive in a context of greater willingness to accept relatively minor risks in the face of widespread mortality and serious morbidity, coupled with resource constraints. This can mean a commensurate lessening of low-grade event reporting and collection and a focus on serious adverse events and unexpected events, as opposed to expected and low-grade events. Approval from oversight bodies is still required for such a shift.

The degree to which the pathophysiology and clinical course of the emerging condition are known also shape the safety data reporting process. In the case of Ebola, for example, the manifestations, course, and anticipated mortality of the disease may be known well enough to permit highly predictable symptoms to be collected as simply present or absent, without grading or severity assessment. In contrast, particularly early in the COVID 19 pandemic, relatively little was known about its clinical manifestations, and new ones seemed to appear with alarming frequency. In such cases, it is imperative to document events in greater detail, with precise grading of their severity, to establish a baseline against which any drug toxicity could be measured.

Data collection for safety should begin as soon as practicable, lest rapidly implemented public health measures (e.g., isolation, physical distancing, quarantine, etc.) and resource challenges make gathering data increasingly difficult over time. This difficulty may be compounded in areas of instability or conflict. In emergency settings, research participants may live or work in remote areas which are difficult to reach or have poor communications, making it more necessary to begin collecting accurate data in a timely manner. Such hurdles can make identifying safety signals difficult, and pharmacovigilance teams often rely on independent data and safety monitoring boards (▶ Chap. 23) to parse the data. Local teams and individuals were used in the DCR Ebola outbreak to follow up on participants and to collect data; they often visited participants' homes and were invaluable in collecting essential data for the research.

Purpose-hired data collectors can receive additional data from community health workers, often members of the community with limited to no formal medical education who provide patient-facing support and services for primary care (Hartzler et al. 2018; Miller et al. 2018). According to WHO, they should be members of the communities where they work, selected by the communities, answerable to them, and supported by the health system but not necessarily direct employees of the system. They typically have less training than professional health workers (Lehman and Sanders 2007). Community health workers are key personnel for pharmacovigilance and a useful link between the medical staff and the community, helping the populace to better understand medical recommendations while conveying community concerns and facilitating the reporting of AEs to medical staff.

6.2 Pharmacovigilance in Special Circumstances

6.2.1 Danger

In an environment where research staff and participants face personal risk, each focus area noted above needs to balance safety, data quality, and risk. Given the complexity, pace, staff rotations, and possible changes of sponsors or other stakeholders, quality management in such settings needs special attention. The northeastern DRC research response, for example, including the PALM study, took place against a background of armed civil conflict, mistrust of central authority among the populace, and hostility to Ebola response workers, who were identified with the authorities (Nguyen 2019). This meant that locally recruited data collectors, who could move with relative freedom in the area, collected most of the follow-up safety data required by the study protocol in homes and communities after study participant discharge. These data collectors were generally new to the task, requiring centralized quality control to ensure they collected quality data.

6.2.2 Unapproved Treatments

From a safety and research perspective, the collection and reporting of adverse events that may arise from alternative and traditional medicines are vital to keep the safety profile of authorized and investigational interventions clear and to help inform the public of adverse effects that can arise from alternative treatments. Self-medication, or medication prescribed by traditional practitioners or medical doctors operating outside medical consensus, became a major issue in all three of the outbreaks noted here. In the Ebola virus disease outbreaks, local healers and others encouraged the use of traditional healing practices and medicines. During the COVID-19 outbreak, misinformation led to many people dosing themselves with, and even being prescribed, ineffective medications with sometimes serious consequences (Farah et al. 2022). Having a reporting category for such exposures, with details of time, dose, and substance is essential. In research outside the researchers' home country, traditional medicines may be unfamiliar to the research team—one among the many reasons collaboration with local medical experts is necessary.

6.2.3 Investigational Product Quality Assurance

The transportation and storage of investigational medicinal products (IMPs) in resource-limited settings or under quarantine or conflict conditions is one of the major challenges of emergency research (▶ Chaps. 37–39). Quality problems associated with IMP(s) can have multiple safety implications that could put research participants at risk. Any reported problems require investigation, which is time-consuming for the pharmacovigilance and pharmacy teams, and may lead to a potentially life-saving IMP being set aside to sort out a quality concern. This is best avoided by meticulous quality management and documentation throughout production, transport, storage, and administration. In can be difficult to meet the requirement for the low temperatures (around −70 °C) required for transport and storage of many investigational products, as well as some of the COVID-19 vaccines. In the DRC PALM study, this was still more difficult since each of the four products under investigation required a different temperature range, despite limited and unreliable transport, power, and communications.

7 Conclusions

By definition, emergency research responds to a crisis, a situation that needs to be brought under control. Social, psychological, and political tensions are likely to increase and may have a profound impact on policies and funding for new studies, implementation, and social acceptance of study results, including medical countermeasures. Community outreach and consultation on clinical trials becomes more essential than ever (▶ Chap. 18). Be prepared for surprises in what the local community may find acceptable and unacceptable in research conduct: community consultation may lead to major changes in the safety monitoring and reporting plan, including events to emphasize and reports to local oversight bodies.

- *PV as part of preparedness and community acceptance*: Community response to vaccines, monoclonal agents, and other therapeutics can depend in large part on who provides information, how it is conveyed, and the prevalence of misinformation. Building a trustworthy drug safety and PV system and establishing a track record for transparency, public service, and reliability over time is necessary, though not sufficient, for public acceptance of messaging about research and the drugs and vaccines that may result. Adherence to rigorous ethical and scientific standards in conducting research and communicating results is essential and should reap rewards over time.
- *All timelines are shorter* (at least in concept) in an emergency response. Develop a good understanding of where major problems and risks tend to lie within your pharmacovigilance practice and focus your energy on addressing them proactively, with an emergency in mind. For example, you may have a robust expedited reporting pathway, but it may be highly dependent upon technology that may not work in a low-resource setting. Even in a developed setting, resources such as Internet bandwidth may be limited, and sometimes required adaptation during the COVID-19 pandemic. Technology, bandwidth, and access issues disproportionately affect remote and low-income areas, as well as underserved populations. There are many places where it is imprudent to assume an

adequate level of Internet availability, cellular or landline telephony, or even reliable electrical power (▶ Chaps. 37 and 39); by no means all of them are in lower-income countries. At some point, pen, paper, and couriers may become vital tools.

- *Focus on the key goals of pharmacovigilance*: Ensure that actionable safety information is gathered in raw form, recorded, and evaluated, with any safety signal identified appropriately and acted upon effectively. There is, for example, nothing magical about FDA's 15-day standard timeline for IMP safety reporting—it is simply the timeline that the agency has identified and set. There may be alarming event reports that warrant notification and widespread dissemination in far less time; in many, perhaps most cases, reports may not have any impact at all from a safety enhancement perspective.
- *Familiar definitions may need to be recalibrated* in the context of the emergency, available resources, the natural course of the condition under study, and other factors. Seriousness and expectedness can change, and it may not be possible to determine causality with the rigor desired. Events that would be dutifully reported as alarming in a study of healthy 20-year-olds may become resource-consuming clutter in a truly emergent research setting for a highly fatal disease or a global pandemic, even of a disease with modest fatality rates. Proper pharmacovigilance practices coupled with existing data will help ensure that signals are identified, verified, and acted upon in time to eliminate avoidable toxicities—but keep in mind that many adverse events may be acceptable in the absence of a less toxic alternative for a condition with high morbidity or mortality, just as the myriad toxicities of many chemotherapeutics are accepted for cancer therapy when the alternative is death.
- *The balance of risks can change dramatically*: If a disease has an established case fatality rate over 50% and several thousand people are infected or has a 2% CFR but has infected tens of millions worldwide, and pre-clinical or early clinical work suggests that the therapeutic interventions planned for the study are reasonably safe and unlikely to kill the patient, there is little point in devoting substantial resources to urgently reporting deaths typical of the disease within the anticipated numbers. Aggregate data remain essential, but immediate case-by-case reporting of expected and routine events is likely to be impractical in a real crisis. If subjects are likely to present with fulminant illness, there is little point, from a pharmacovigilance perspective, in reporting *any* SAEs until there has been a study intervention. Baseline signs and symptoms will be vital to making sense of safety data but reporting it "right now" is another matter.
- *Look critically at processes and flows in pharmacovigilance practice*: For your operating unit, do a stress test analogous to those used by financial oversight bodies to ensure banking liquidity in the event of a monetary crisis. How well would you handle a 50% increase in reporting volume, or the need to query sites frequently, or a major increase in required regulatory partner reporting? Consider whether your standards for timeliness are flexible enough to accommodate this; whether you could readily get added resources or staffing, or what other activities might need to be put on the back burner. Try to ensure that pharmacovigilance teams are included in table-top and larger-scale crisis exercises undertaken as part of pandemic preparedness planning and ensure incorporation of pharmacovigilance requirements into the resulting planning documents.
- *Distinguish between procedural and substantive requirements*: Thoroughly understand the applicable regulations for your likely sphere of action. This includes not only the hard requirements, but the key places in guidelines and regulations where "should" appears rather than "will" or "must." The word "should" will be your friend when you are at the end of your resources and you need to balance compliance against the needs of an unstructured crisis, especially if you find the time to

keep trial leadership and regulatory colleagues informed.

- *Establish the necessary flow of vital pharmacovigilance data* to ensure rapid, accurate safety signal detection, reporting, and action when required. The more serious the action contemplated, for example, dropping a trial arm or stopping a trial based on SUSARs, futility, or clearly shown efficacy, the more assurance of accuracy is required. Maintain a near-continuous and open line of two-way communication between the pharmacovigilance team and those at the bedside, making rapid queries and responses routine. In an unfamiliar environment, always include local partners on the team: this is not only essential for access and communications, but it also guards against the risk that data could suffer mistranslation or a "game of telephone" effect that renders the message received materially different from the one transmitted. Having PV/safety players in country and ideally on the scene to observe, adjust, and validate safety data process and collection methods was invaluable in the DRC effort in 2018, and is always best practice, as it converts events into the format and language of PV/Safety as close to the source as possible.

Pharmacovigilance is manageable in a dire emergency. Collaboration, adaptability, and adherence to principle are the watchwords.

Discussion Questions

1. What is pharmacovigilance? Discuss the key goals of a pharmacovigilance program.
2. Participants' safety is critical during clinical research; it must be addressed when a drug first enters pre-clinical (pre-human) development and through development, testing, and clinical studies.
   (a) Discuss the activities devoted to safety and players whose work on the safety profile overlaps to create intentional redundancy.
   (b) Discuss some methods of pharmacovigilance. (Remember that these methods are simple, but the rules for collecting, analyzing, and reporting adverse events are complex.)
3. Implementing a pharmacovigilance process begins with the trial protocol's safety section, which should be drafted before outbreaks occur. Pharmacovigilance professionals should then craft a more detailed, adaptable safety section focused on the threat, population at risk, drug being tested, and study environment.
4. What two key roles of pharmacovigilance must be incorporated into the safety section?
5. Discuss how emergency response research protocols differ considerably from the norm of a typical research setting.
6. The first step in building a pharmacovigilance process is to conduct a capacity assessment. What are some useful documents for this assessment?
7. Discuss the factors to consider when developing pharmacovigilance standard operating procedures in areas where the healthcare capacity is overwhelmed during an outbreak.
8. Safety training for emergency research requires creativity, flexibility, and collaboration. Discuss how training materials and methods can meet the needs of overworked research and clinical care staff with widely varying degrees of experience.
9. Since gathering data during a high-risk public health emergency becomes increasingly difficult, when should safety data collection begin? Discuss the factors that may affect data collection during an outbreak, especially in resource-constrained environments.
10. Emergency research responds to a crisis, a situation replete with tensions, surprises, and dangers that must be brought under control. Provide some practical, final recommendations for collaboration, adaptability, and adherence to principles to ensure that pharmacovigilance can be successfully managed in dire emergencies.

References

AlShurman BA, Khan AF, Mac C, Majeed M, Butt ZA. What demographic, social, and contextual factors influence the intention to use COVID-19 vaccines: a scoping review. Int J Environ Res Public Health. 2021;18(17):9342.

Baden LR, El Sahly HM, Essink B, Kotloff K, Frey S, Novak R, et al. Efficacy and safety of the mRNA-1273 SARS-CoV-2 vaccine. N Engl J Med. 2021;384(5):403–16. https://doi.org/10.1056/NEJMoa2035389.

BBC News. Johnson & Johnson vaccine paused over rare blood clots. 2021.

Caluwaerts S. Nubia's mother: being pregnant in the time of experimental vaccines and therapeutics for Ebola. Reprod Health. 2017;14(3):157. https://doi.org/10.1186/s12978-017-0429-8.

CFR. IND safety reporting, 21 CFR 312.32. 2020.

Chen G, Li X, Sun M, Zhou Y, Yin M, Zhao B, et al. COVID-19 mRNA vaccines are generally safe in the short term: a vaccine vigilance real-world study says. Front Immunol. 2021;12 https://doi.org/10.3389/fimmu.2021.669010.

CIOMS. International ethical guidelines for health-related research involving humans. Geneva: Council for International Organisations of Medical Sciences; 2016.

CIOMS. CIOMS 1 form. Geneva: Council for International Organizations of Medical Sciences; 2019. https://cioms.ch/cioms-i-form/. Accessed Jan 22 2020.

Cobert B, Gregory W, Thomas J-L. Cobert's manual of drug safety and pharmacovigilance. 3rd ed. Singapore: World Scientific Publishing Co.; 2019.

Dos Santos CVB, de Noronha TG, Werneck GL, Struchiner CJ, Villela DAM. Estimated COVID-19 severe cases and deaths averted in the first year of the vaccination campaign in Brazil: a retrospective observational study. Lancet Reg Health Am. 2023;17:100418. https://doi.org/10.1016/j.lana.2022.100418.

EMA. ICH E2A clinical safety data management: definitions and standards for expedited reporting. Amsterdam: European Medicines Agency; 1995.

EMA. EudraVigilance electronic reporting. In: Human regulatory. 2021. https://www.ema.europa.eu/en/human-regulatory/research-development/pharmacovigilance/eudravigilance/eudravigilance-electronic-reporting. Accessed 10 Oct 2021.

European Clinical Research Information Network. European Clinical Research Information. 2023. http://campus.ecrin.org. Accessed 27 Jan 2023.

Farah R, Kazzi Z, Brent J, Burkhart K, Wax P, Aldy K. Ivermectin associated adverse events in the treatment and prevention of COVID-19 reported to the FACT pharmacovigilance project. Clin Toxicol. 2022;60(8):942–6. https://doi.org/10.1080/15563650.2022.2070187.

FDA. In: Services USDoHaH, Administration FaD, (CDER) CfDEaR, (CBER) CfBEaR, editors. E2A clinical safety data management: definitions and standards for expedited reporting. Washington, DC: U.S. Department of Health and Human Services; 1995. p. 60.

FDA. Safety reporting requirements for INDs and BA/BE studies. Silver Spring, MD: U.S. Food and Drug Administration; 2012.

FDA. MedWatch: the FDA safety information and adverse event reporting program. Washington, DC: U.S. Food and Drug Administration; 2020. https://www.fda.gov/safety/medwatch-fda-safety-information-and-adverse-event-reporting-program. Accessed 22 Jan 2020.

FDA. Development and approval process—drugs. Silver Spring, MD: U.S. Food and Drug Administration; 2022. https://www.fda.gov/drugs/development-approval-process-drugs. Accessed 03 May 2023.

FDA. Institutional review boards (IRBs) and protection of human subjects in clinical trials. Silver Spring, MD: U.S. Food and Drug Administration; 2023. https://www.fda.gov/about-fda/center-drug-evaluation-and-research-cder/institutional-review-boards-irbs-and-protection-human-subjects-clinical-trials. Accessed 27 Jan 2023.

Fornasier G, Francescon S, Leone R, Baldo P. An historical overview over pharmacovigilance. Int J Clin Pharm. 2018;40(4):744–7. https://doi.org/10.1007/s11096-018-0657-1.

Gagnon S, Schueler P, Fan JD. Pharmacovigilance and risk management. In: Bairu M, Chin R, editors. Global clinical trials playbook: capacity and capability building. London: Elsevier; 2012.

Global Health Training Centre. Introduction to collecting and reporting adverse events. eLearning courses. 2021.

Hanrahan D, Sexton P, Hui K, Teitcher J, Sugarman J, London AJ, et al. Linguistic and cultural challenges in communication and translation in US-sponsored HIV prevention research in emerging economies. PLoS One. 2015;10(7):e0133394. https://doi.org/10.1371/journal.pone.0133394.

Hartzler AL, Tuzzio L, Hsu C, Wagner EH. Roles and functions of community health workers in primary care. Ann Fam Med. 2018;16(3):240–5. https://doi.org/10.1370/afm.2208.

HHS. Guidelines for developing a data and safety monitoring plan. Washington, DC: U.S. Department of Health and Human Services; 2018. https://www.hhs.gov/guidance/document/guidelines-developing-data-and-safety-monitoring-plan. Accessed 29 Sep 2021.

Husby A, Hansen JV, Fosbøl E, Thiesson EM, Madsen M, Thomsen RW, et al. SARS-CoV-2 vaccination and myocarditis or myopericarditis: population based cohort study. BMJ. 2021;375:e068665. https://doi.org/10.1136/bmj-2021-068665.

ICH. Clinical safety data management: definitions and standards for expedited reporting E2A. 1994.

ICH. Good clinical practice: ICH harmonised guideline. Integrated addendum to ICH E6(R1): guideline for good clinical practice ICH E6(R2) ICH consensus guideline. Geneva: International Council for Harmonisation of Technical Requirements for Pharmaceuticals for Human Use (ICH); 2016.

ICH. E2B(R3) individual case safety report (ICSR) specification and related files. Geneva: International Council for Harmonisation of Technical Requirements for Pharmaceuticals for Human Use; 2019. https://ich.org/page/e2br3-individual-case-safety-report-icsr-specification-and-related-files. Accessed 25 Jan 2020.

ICH. Quality guidelines. Geneva: International Council for Harmonisation; 2023. https://www.ich.org/page/quality-guidelines. Accessed 17 Apr 2023.

James MJ, Cook-Johnson RJ, Cleland LG. Selective COX-2 inhibitors, eicosanoid synthesis and clinical outcomes: a case study of system failure. Lipids. 2007;42(9):779–85. https://doi.org/10.1007/s11745-007-3069-x.

Kennedy SB, Bolay F, Kieh M, Grandits G, Badio M, Ballou R, et al. Phase 2 placebo-controlled trial of two vaccines to prevent Ebola in Liberia. N Engl J Med. 2017;377(15):1438–47. https://doi.org/10.1056/NEJMoa1614067.

Kesselheim AS, Darrow JJ, Kulldorff M, Brown BL, Mitra-Majumdar M, Lee CC, et al. An overview of vaccine development, approval, and regulation, with implications for COVID-19. Health Aff (Millwood). 2021;40(1):25–32. https://doi.org/10.1377/hlthaff.2020.01620.

Lehman U, Sanders D. Community health workers: what do we know about them? The state of the evidence on programmes, activities, costs and impact on health outcomes of using community health workers. Geneva: World Health Organization, Health DoHRf; 2007.

Medicines and Healthcare Products Regulatory Authority. Guidance on submitting clinical trial safety reports. In: Clinical trials and investigations. 2020. https://www.gov.uk/guidance/guidance-on-submitting-clinical-trial-safety-reports. Accessed 10 Oct 2021.

Miller NP, Milsom P, Johnson G, Bedford J, Kapeu AS, Diallo AO, et al. Community health workers during the Ebola outbreak in Guinea, Liberia, and Sierra Leone. J Glob Health. 2018;8(2):020601. https://doi.org/10.7189/jogh-08-020601.

Mulangu S, Dodd LE, Davey RT Jr, Tshiani Mbaya O, Proschan M, Mukadi D, et al. A randomized, controlled trial of Ebola virus disease therapeutics. N Engl J Med. 2019;381(24):2293–303. https://doi.org/10.1056/NEJMoa1910993.

Nguyen V-K. An epidemic of suspicion—Ebola and violence in the DRC. N Engl J Med. 2019;380:1298. https://doi.org/10.1056/NEJMp1902682.

NIA. NIA adverse event and serious adverse event guidelines. Bethesda, MD: National Institute on Aging; 2018.

NIAID. Rules and policies for clinical research. Bethesda, MD: National Institute for Allergy and Infectious Diseases; 2021. https://www.niaid.nih.gov/research/clinical-research. Accessed 29 Sep 2021.

NIAID. ClinRegs: aggregating clinical research regulations from around the globe. 2023. https://clinregs.niaid.nih.gov/. Accessed 27 Jan 2023.

NIH. Data and safety monitoring. Bethesda, MD: National Institutes of Health; 2020.

Nzolo D, Kuemmerle A, Lula Y, Ntamabyaliro N, Engo A, Mvete B, et al. Development of a pharmacovigilance system in a resource-limited country: the experience of the Democratic Republic of Congo. Ther Adv Drug Saf. 2019;10:2042098619864853. https://doi.org/10.1177/2042098619864853.

OHRP. International compilation of human research standards. Washington, DC: Office of Human Research Protection, U.S. Department of Health and Human Services; 2020.

Saheki MN, Lyra MR, Bedoya-Pacheco SJ, de Fátima Antônio L, Pimentel MIF, de Matos Salgueiro M, et al. Low versus high dose of antimony for American cutaneous leishmaniasis: a randomized controlled blind non-inferiority trial in Rio de Janeiro, Brazil. PLoS One. 2017;12(5):e0178592. https://doi.org/10.1371/journal.pone.0178592.

Schuklenk U. Future infectious disease outbreaks: ethics of emergency access to unregistered medical interventions and clinical trial designs. Dev World Bioeth. 2016;16(1):2–3. https://doi.org/10.1111/dewb.12102.

See I. Updates on thrombosis with thrombocytopenia syndrome (TTS). Atlanta: Centers for Disease Control and Prevention. Vaccine Safety Team CC-VTF; 2021.

Sigfrid L, Maskell K, Bannister PG, Ismail SA, Collinson S, Regmi S, et al. Addressing challenges for clinical research responses to emerging epidemics and pandemics: a scoping review. BMC Med. 2020;18(1):190. https://doi.org/10.1186/s12916-020-01624-8.

Waller P, Harrison-Woolrych M. An introduction to pharmacovigilance. 2nd ed. Wiley; 2017.

WHO. Pharmacovigilance: ensuring the safe use of medicines. Geneva: WHO; 2004.

WHO. Ethical considerations for use of unregistered interventions for Ebola viral disease. Geneva: World Health Organization; 2014a. Contract No.: WHO/HIS/KER/GHE/14.1.

WHO. Meeting summary of the WHO consultation on potential Ebola therapies and vaccines. Geneva: World Health Organization; 2014b.

WHO. Pharmacovigilance indicators: a practical manual for the assessment of pharmacovigilance systems. Geneva: World Health Organization; 2015.

WHO. REGTRAC: the WHO database of regulatory information, tracking of clinical trials registration & ethics committees. Geneva: World Health Organization; 2022. https://apps.who.int/trialsearch/Regtrac.aspx. Accessed 29 Sep 2021.

37 Supply and Logistics for Clinical Research in Low-Resource Settings

Beth Baseler, Calvin Proffitt, Jen Sandrus, Jonathan Marchand, and Eric Stavale

Contents

Learning Track Note: This chapter appears in Learning Tracks: Emergency Research Response, Research Operations

E. S. Higgs and R. A. Sorenson (eds.), *Principles and Practice of Emergency Research Response*,
https://doi.org/10.1007/978-3-031-48408-7_57

Learning Objectives

This chapter will help readers understand and describe the following:

- Logistics and inventory management for clinical research necessities during an outbreak in low-resource settings
- The role of the clinical research protocol team during an emergency clinical research response
- The roles of various agencies and organizations in getting equipment and supplies to where they are needed
- Paperwork requirements for shipping medical items
- Questions to be addressed for domestic transport
- Proactive steps to expedite procurement and transport of supplies
- Restrictions that may affect export of medical supplies
- Management of stocks and storage of adequate supplies
- Medical waste management
- Employment and training of local staff

1 Introduction

Implementing a research operation in an infectious disease emergency means resolving many urgent problems quickly, especially where infrastructure and resources are limited (▶ Chap. 32). And because infectious disease incidence often correlates with lower incomes and resources, clinical research managers will often have to cope with minimal healthcare infrastructure and unreliable communications, electrical power, water supply, and transportation—when these systems are functional at all. Add to that possible shortfalls in central and local government capacity, along with potential security threats, and you have supply and logistical challenges that will demand hard work and creative thinking to get equipment and supplies where they need to be for a functional clinical research program.

In this chapter, we explore logistics and inventory management (▶ Chap. 38) for clinical research during an outbreak in a low-resource setting. Roughly speaking, logistics lays out the steps for getting equipment and supplies to where they are needed when they are needed. Inventory management means ensuring that equipment functions properly and needed supplies are on hand to support the research but not in such oversupply as to be wasteful. The information presented here is based on the authors' experience establishing clinical research programs urgently in many parts of the world.

As we have seen in the COVID-19 pandemic, ideas may be about the only thing not in short supply during an emergency research response to an emerging or reemerging infectious disease. When promising therapeutic or vaccine candidates are identified, clinical trials to get them licensed are an arduous and often fruitless process. Many medical responders used to doubt the viability of setting up the many moving parts of a clinical trial and getting them to work in a least-developed country during an outbreak, especially at a site far from the capital. Such research is now widely recognized as a crucial element of response and preparedness, and though COVID-19 struck the whole world and not just places with few resources, it has, if anything, reinforced the idea that we need to be prepared to carry out such research anywhere (Carter et al. 2018; Devi 2020; GPMB 2020; Thompson 2021; WHO 2021).

Our aim here is to sketch out the basic logistical and supply management steps for setting up a clinical research response in a low-resource environment. A number of related topics are mentioned in this chapter, with references to where they are covered more fully elsewhere in this section of this book and in other literature. Infrastructure shortfalls may well include paved road networks reaching most areas, wireless and cabled communications, a reliable electric power supply, and clean, readily available water. Infrastructure systems also require a skilled workforce to keep them running; where there are few such systems, there are correspondingly few qualified personnel. Fragile, overburdened healthcare systems and scarce, overworked healthcare workers are very likely to be another of the difficulties the country faces. Moreover, we will surely not anticipate every problem that will come up, and there is no substitute for managers with expertise both in setting up a clinical research program and how to get things done in the country and locales where the research will take place—and a degree of problem-solving creativity.

2 First Steps: Assessment, Protocols, Partners, Presence, and Procurement

An urgent research response to an outbreak or epidemic must be an iterative process. Though neither scientific nor ethical standards can be relaxed in the name of the emergency, some of the procedures that assure the standards are met may be pursued in parallel rather than in sequence (▶ Chap. 31). Study design, site assessment, and logistical planning provide a good example of processes that need to happen urgently and simultaneously in an emergency. The assessment team traveling to the site of the outbreak needs to include experienced infectious disease investigators and experts in supply chain, administration, and logistics. As the research needs are defined, likely equipment and supply needs must be identified, along with study site and systems (power, water, etc.) requirements and transport needs that will likely include a cold chain (▶ Chap. 39). If research collaborators have not been identified, corresponding partnerships should be established. The sponsoring organization should maintain a local presence, beginning with a few staff members in a hotel if nothing else. Procurement of needed equipment and supplies, along with transport arrangements, should begin as the study protocol takes shape.

2.1 Research Protocol Team

The research protocol team defines the needs of an emergency clinical research response. Response may be hindered by local conditions; sometimes, the research will have to adapt, and sometimes conditions can be changed. In any case, establishing a team with well-integrated roles is critical to sharing developing information that will shape the research response. In response to the Ebola outbreak that began in the Democratic Republic of the Congo (DRC) in August 2018, for example, a research team was rapidly established with staff members from the study sponsor, operations management, and international and local collaborators (Mulangu et al. 2019). The team ensured cross-communication among participants and made rapid decisions to execute plans and meet emergency clinical research needs efficiently. This kind of collaborative effort is essential when protocols need frequent adjustment in light of developments that affect timelines for receiving equipment, supplies, and perishable items.

2.2 Partnerships

The necessity of partnerships for an emergency clinical research response is a theme throughout this book (▶ Chaps. 18, 29, and 30), but the need for strong partnerships is more acute the worse an emergency becomes. Civilian and military government agencies, international organizations, the diplomatic community, nongovernmental organizations (NGOs), regional and local governments, and informal community leadership bodies may all have roles in getting equipment and supplies to where they are needed.

2.2.1 National Partner

It is virtually always necessary to have a partner representing the national government of the country where the research will take place. This may be the ministry of health, national health research institute, or a national university. This leading partner should play a coequal role in management of the research. The imprimatur of the national government is essential for legitimacy, as is an effort to build up local research capacity in conjunction with the specific research program. For supply and logistics, the national partner should also provide the main channel to national authorities for transport questions and especially for import and export regulations and permissions. Entry and customs or tax requirements can be cumbersome and lengthy and sometimes further delayed by officials seeking to pocket extra "fees" (NASEM 2018). High-level pressure may be needed to enforce expeditious, duty-free entry of humanitarian goods.

Internal transport and security concerns, among others, can also be relayed through government channels. On the other hand, any consideration of close collaboration with national security forces, whether military or police, requires careful consideration of their effectiveness and how the populace views them, with the potential implications for the research program of such collaboration. In the eastern DRC during the 2018 Ebola outbreak, for example, much of the local population viewed the national government, and especially the military, with hostility, and a widespread perception that humanitarian medical response organizations were allied with the government was a factor in violence directed against their facilities and personnel (Wells et al. 2019).

2.2.2 NGOs

Emergency research programs can form valuable, mutually beneficial partnerships with NGOs, especially humanitarian medical response organizations like Médecins Sans Frontières (MSF), the Alliance for International Medical Action (ALIMA), and International Mercy Corps (IMC). NGOs can provide on-the-ground response support with medical supplies, doctors, nurses, and technical staff. Moreover, as in the DRC, their treatment centers can be the venue for critical research intended to mitigate morbidity and mortality, help end the epidemic, and lead to licensed treatments or vaccines (▶ In Practice 17.1 and In Focus 30.1).

Additionally, the WHO collaborates on a global scale during emergency responses and provides much needed diagnostics kits, equipment, medical/laboratory supplies, and staff. While working as an independent entity to provide logistical expertise, they have also collaborated with partners supporting randomized controlled trials (RCTs) and other clinical studies by supplying diagnostics kits, assays, and personal protective equipment (PPE). Major universities are frequent partners (e.g., the University of Massachusetts Amherst and its collaboration with the National Reference Laboratory in Liberia to support Lassa virus studies and the University of California Los Angeles and its collaboration in the DRC to support Ebola and other infectious disease response efforts).

2.2.3 International Organizations

Frequently, international organizations, like the United Nations (UN) System, may assist in building new permanent laboratory space, roads, and staff housing; connecting to electricity (via generators or solar panels) and water supplies; and providing critical training programs. These and national organizations may also provide expertise and information needed for nations to establish national public health systems subject matter experts, as they did in support of the National Public Health Institute of Liberia. The UN provided critical air support in transferring Ebola responders to North Kivu, DRC, accommodating equipment, supplies, and staff on weekly flights to the region. The WHO provided shipments of perishables, equipment, PPE, and investigational product on the weekly flights and also supported the transfer of clinical biological samples from field sites to biorepositories and national labs, maintaining cold chain (▶ Chap. 39) and safety for transporting Category A, B, and C biological samples (WHO 2012) (◘ Fig. 1).

2.2.4 Local Governments

Steps should always be taken to include local governments in planning and implementation. This is especially true when it comes to administering the supply chain and managing inventory. Local governments in resource-constrained areas are often ill-equipped to address the needs on their own but are almost always willing and able to understand that they have the most at stake in the response. Clinical research responders will find that local governments can provide significant guidance in identifying local resources and offices of national ministries that will need to be engaged. For example, in response to the

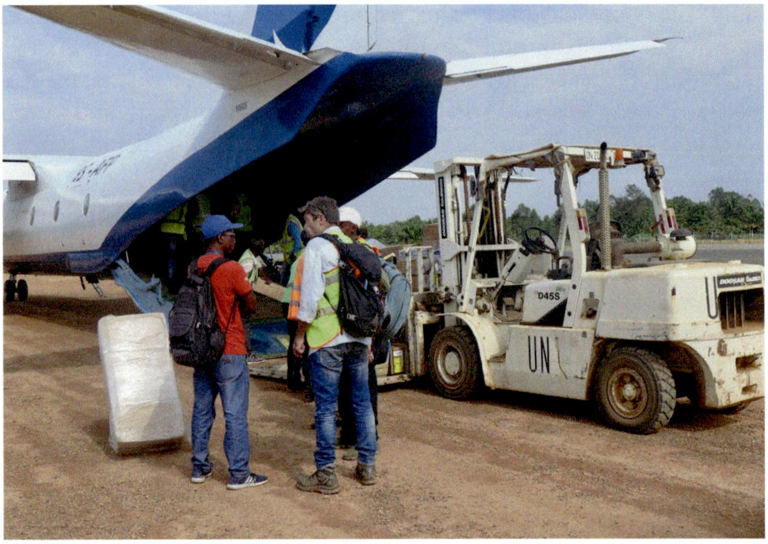

Fig. 1 MONUSCO, the UN Mission in the DRC, assists with delivery of medical supplies to Beni, North Kivu, DRC, during the 2018–2020 Ebola outbreak. (Photo: MONUSCO/Mamadou Alain Coulibaly)

2018–2019 Ebola outbreak in the DRC, responders faced daunting logistics challenges moving materials via air transport within the country. In addition, much of the international staff was not permitted to travel into the region where the studies were being conducted because of security considerations. During this time, the only way to move materials to the RCT sites was to utilize limited flight abilities available on domestic/national airlines and humanitarian flights. After engaging with the local airport authority in North Kivu, a mechanism was established to pay the local airport access tax to facilitate transport, removing one obstacle.

Adjacent countries could also be helpful, especially where a major airport or seaport in a neighboring country might be closer to the outbreak area than the primary national ports. This could be instrumental in meeting transportation needs, moving supplies or equipment across borders, or establishing staging locations that may be closer to remote areas affected by the outbreak.

2.2.5 Contractors and Vendors with a Local Presence

Using local contractors and vendors, including international firms with a local presence, is generally an advantage during an emergency clinical research response situation. Identifying resources that can be procured locally can expand supply chain capabilities and expedite urgent supply needs. Collaborating with entities that have a presence in and around the desired research area can save time on obtaining crucial resources for a quick emergency response. Neglecting the potential of local resources could result in unnecessary lead times, a lack of consumables, and/or insufficient resources.

2.2.6 Diplomatic Representations

If the study sponsor is a large, well-resourced country or a former colonial power, embassy staff may be able to overcome obstacles like customs and tax officials' reluctance to rapidly clear critical equipment and perishable items through ports of entry at local airports and facilitate prompt transportation to their intended destinations. This assistance may range from immediate clearance, in which supplies and equipment can be picked up as they are offloaded from commercial airlines, to clearance within a day or a few weeks. Diplomats may not have the capacity or connections to ensure such cooperation, however, depending on the countries involved.

2.2.7 Friends with Airplanes, Warehouses, and Trucks

When working with multiple partners providing supplies, organized and well-managed storage facilities are even more important. For a relatively large research program, multiple partners may provide supplies, each of them with its own inventory process. In this type of situation, coordination to establish which group will provide what is essential, and so is a central inventory management system to keep track of stock and ensure against interruptions. Partners that are better established in the country or region may have established supply chains into and within the country of operations, which can be invaluable when it comes to getting items to where they are needed when transport is tricky. Both formal and informal arrangements for cooperation among assistance actors can facilitate supply movements.

The UN can be very helpful in providing transport to humanitarian actors and supplies on its aircraft. In many cases, the World Food Programme, which leads the UN Logistics Cluster and operates most UN civilian aircraft, will provide support to non-UN humanitarian organizations (WFP 2020). In general, the importance of establishing good professional relations with other medical and non-medical humanitarian responders in the response area cannot be overstated (IASC 2020; Gralla and Goentzel 2018). Learning about each other's supply and logistics operations and sharing whenever possible help build up a robust, multifaceted response to infectious disease emergencies, including those that happen amidst a disaster with a different proximate cause, such as famine or war.

2.2.8 Military Assistance

Military organizations can also be mobilized for response. They often have well-defined supply chains and robust transport capacity operated by experienced personnel. In a number of fragile states, such as Liberia and the DRC, UN military missions are already present for peacekeeping operations (UN 2021). In other cases, foreign troops, often from a former colonial power, will have bases in such countries. Exceptionally, as during the 2014–2016 West Africa Ebola epidemic, foreign military units may arrive to help with response (Kamradt-Scott et al. 2016; Lu et al. 2016; Nevin and Anderson 2016). Additionally, multicountry, loosely formed coalitions aimed at the common goal may be established. Military forces may provide diagnostic equipment, PPE, and medical staff during an outbreak, either independently or in collaboration with other national and international organizations. However, not all military forces are as capable. For example, during the 2014–2016 Ebola outbreak in Sierra Leone, the Chinese military provided a humanitarian response, but, as they did not have an overseas logistics chain, critical supplies had to be shipped well in advance to meet the rapid response need (Lu et al. 2016).

2.3 Procurement

Whether through a formalized supply chain software system or an Excel sheet with pertinent data filters, a strong tracking system is needed for procurement success. Consider utilizing a SharePoint or cloud environment for remote file access by project staff. Categorizing functional areas for purchases (e.g., laboratory, pharmacy, clinic) can help create supply lists for historical reference and future orders. Vendors located near the emergency location should be considered first if availability and/or timelines are confirmed as shorter than vendors in other areas. However, it is important to verify that nearby vendors, especially those that may have less experience, can fulfill their promises and must always be prepared with a backup plan for critical supplies. Purchase and direct shipments from known and reliable manufacturers can be a solid solution to ensure the timely receipt of supplies and equipment. If at all possible, single purchases beyond a specified dollar amount (e.g., more than $5000) should include obtaining three quotations to properly review options, availability, timelines, and cost. Vendors providing high-value equipment (e.g., laboratory analyzers, low-temp freezers, etc.) should also commit to servicing the equipment when necessary. If in the event equipment warranties are not available, or invalid in the region of operation, alternative maintenance and upkeep mechanisms need to be implemented.

3 Export and Import Requirements

Proper research is necessary to ensure compliance with all domestic and international import and export requirements. In many developing countries, items being imported for medical response, including research, may be covered by special bilateral or multilateral agreements that exempt goods from the usual import taxes and fees. This is a complex area of international tax cooperation under continued discussion—yet another reason to bring in knowledgeable local partners (UN 2020).

3.1 Export Restrictions

Many countries instituted temporary export restrictions on medical supplies during the COVID-19 pandemic—a measure that may have been counterproductive to the goal of ending the pandemic and contrary to the spirit if not the letter of the binding International Health Regulations (2005), which are meant to deter unilateral actions by WHO member states that hinder worldwide infectious disease response (IMF 2020; WHO 2016). While the European Union (EU), for example, exempted products going to pandemic and humanitarian response from restrictions (EC 2020), such restrictions could still delay supplies needed for a research response until a waiver is granted.

Longer-standing export restrictions are based on controls designed to prevent exports of technology—both hardware and software—that could assist certain states or non-state actors in developing weapons, including biological weapons. These restrictions include UN and EU embargoes on certain countries, the U.S. export control system, and multilateral export control regimes including the Australia Group, the Missile Technology Control Regime, the Nuclear Suppliers Group, and the Wassenaar Arrangement (Bromley and Maletta 2018; U.S. Dept. of State 2011). Such restrictions would be most likely to affect computer hardware and software needed for program implementation, possibly including medical equipment and software. The freight forwarder is your first point of inquiry, and the manufacturer or supplier should also know of relevant export controls.

3.2 Documentation

Proper shipping paperwork must be prepared for each shipment. This is primarily the responsibility of the freight forwarder, but project managers will need to supply information and double-check documentation. Minimal requirements include an air waybill, a commercial invoice, and applicable customs declarations. A "pallet list" or spreadsheet identifying the contents of each container or pallet to facilitate inspection at the port of entry and inventory by the recipient is also a must. Shipping paperwork should be provided as soon as available to all interested parties, including the consignee and those handling the entry clearance and delivery of the shipment. The project team should determine country-specific import regulations and documentation in collaboration with the freight forwarder and in-country import experts and program staff. Shipments sent to and from multiple states will have to meet import-export requirements for all of them. It may be useful to include a statement on the invoice and container or packaging:

> No cost medical supplies disclaimer: Human Medical Welfare. No commercial value. Supplied free of charge. Not for sale or resale.

3.3 Customs, Duties, Inspections, Clearances, and Waivers

Customs brokers are generally available through the freight forwarder and are an option for paying customs fees and duties, clearing the shipment, and delivering it to the consignee. The clearing agent will advise whether to send the shipment door-to-door or door-to-airport. There should be an agreement in place with the host government that humanitarian response supplies will enter duty-free and not subject to national or local taxes or fees.

4 Transport

Successful shipment of goods, especially goods urgently needed where transport links are few, requires a dedicated and detail-oriented team ready to intervene day or night to find another flight, get a shipment cleared through customs, or find a truck to replace one that has broken down. Murphy's law applies—if it can go wrong, it will. Success depends on anticipating the unknown and openness to alternative solutions. The pallets sitting on the tarmac at airports across the world could be holding critical supplies, including investigational products and laboratory reagents that must be kept cold, that were desperately needed yesterday but are not moving. Even when one makes every effort to research, schedule, and plan the first shipment for an urgent project, one may find oneself in the situation of one of the authors, learning while preparing hors d'oeuvres for a Christmas Eve gathering that the special chartered airplane "guaranteed" to arrive by a critical deadline has been canceled. Finding a transportation solution may require many phone calls and other communications, even during holidays. Be sure to have a hands-free telephone option so as to continue your preparations—but be sure to answer the phone, no matter how inconvenient.

4.1 International Transport

4.1.1 Identifying a Freight Forwarder

A freight forwarder is a logistics company that handles much of the work of ensuring that shipments move to the right place on time. In the official definition of the international trade association FIATA (2017):

> Freight Forwarding and Logistic Services means services of any kind relating to the carriage … consolidation, storage, handling, packing or distribution of the Goods as well as ancillary and advisory services … including but not limited to customs and fiscal matters, declaring the Goods for official purposes, procuring insurance of the Goods and collecting or procuring payment or documents relating to the Goods.

Even with professional help, getting the specialized goods needed for a research program quickly to locations poorly served by commercial transportation is not simple, so identifying a reliable freight forwarder should begin early. Key criteria include a proven track record in international and domestic shipping, as well as experience with cold chains and established contacts and resources at all points of the shipping route. Initial discussions could start with estimated shipping weights, dimensions, and deadlines to seek comparative pricing and performance estimates. Perhaps more important is the reputation of the firm among its customers and competitors; medical NGOs and relief groups operating in remote areas might be able to provide useful recommendations.

Special items like heavy equipment, vaccines, and biological samples could require the expertise of more than one company. The freight forwarder should assist with identifying potential issues with aircraft reliability, expedited service for cold-chain shipments, entry permission issues (e.g., missing clearance documents, lack of donation letters), etc. Emergency response locations can present many challenges. You can never ask too many questions, but a good freight forwarder should be able to answer or find out the answer to most of them:

- Do they have experience with shipping biological samples?
- Do they have experience with −70 °C cold chain?
- What steps do they take to ensure cold-chain maintenance?
- What insurance do shipments have?
- What happens when a shipment is lost?
- What happens when there are delays during transit?

- Is the freight forwarder conversant with the documentation requirements of the receiving country? How would it learn if those requirements change?
- Is there adequate storage space or a staging area, including cold storage, in their facility to handle the shipments that need to be transported?
- Does the firm have an export requirements expert?

4.1.2 Identifying the Destination

The formal shipping consignee should be designated carefully. This will dictate, among other things, whether a shipment will be sent door-to-door or door-to-airport, which can have implications for who pays port clearance fees, duties, and/or taxes. If a shipment is going to an international capital, it may be beneficial to use the in-country embassy address of the sponsoring country, with the embassy's agreement if permissible under local and international law. Having a national government partner is essential to making this kind of arrangement, and embassy involvement may be important for seeing the agreement is fulfilled. With an official agreement, shipments can be sent door-to-door to a sponsor country embassy or assistance mission location customs and duty-free. It is important to check on this alternative when working from other countries as well.

4.1.3 Air Transport: Cargo Flights vs. Commercial Passenger

In an emergency clinical research response start-up, it is often necessary to handle air shipment pallets or containers that must hold the goods inside at specified internal temperatures until delivery. Cold-chain packaging calculations must be carried out by someone who knows the subject well, especially when scarce, costly investigational new products are at stake. Sufficient allowance in these calculations must be built in to allow for potential shipment delays. However, these additional allowances add to the bulk and expense that the extra insulation or active refrigeration would add to the shipment (▶ Chap. 39). Cargo-only flights are best for moving high volumes of supplies quickly and reliably, since cargo on passenger aircraft takes second priority to passengers and their baggage and can be bumped off one or more flights before it reaches the destination.

It may be possible or necessary to charter an aircraft, especially when there is a large volume of goods for initial delivery to set up a response operation. However, this is an expensive option. In an infectious disease or humanitarian emergency, there may be opportunities to charter aircraft jointly with other response organizations (IASC 2020). In some cases, there may even be military flights transporting supplies to the capital cities, such as those the German, UK, and U.S. militaries provided during the 2014–2016 Ebola epidemic in West Africa—although these may be less flexible than commercial alternatives and can engender public misunderstanding (De Waal 2014).

4.1.4 Surface Shipments

Air freight, whether by cargo or commercial passenger aircraft, is both faster and more expensive than surface options. There are also size and weight constraints on air shipments. Although all standard medical equipment and even vehicles can be accommodated on cargo aircraft, very large items and vehicles can be sent much more economically by ship, truck, or train if time, geography, and facilities allow. Special opportunities may arise during a large-scale, international response, as when the Royal Dutch Navy twice dispatched HNLMS *Karel Doorman*, a multifunction support vessel, to West Africa with supplies for the Ebola response in 2014 (EU ECHO 2014).

Scheduled maritime shipments are billed by shipping container units, so research program managers should take care to use container space efficiently and try to fill each container with items that will be useful to the project. For example, if the operation is shipping oversize equipment by sea, supplies currently being sent by air can be added to a container in order to fill it. International ground transportation by rail or truck is also less expensive than air but depends on geography and rail or road networks; trucks are particularly vulnerable in high-threat locations. Road shipment options need to be thoroughly reviewed, as road conditions, seasonal variations, security, driver skills, and availability of fuel must all be considered.

4.1.5 Passenger Baggage

Where shipping options are limited or timelines unworkable—especially in disasters or conflicts when transport links may be cut off—project team members may be asked to hand carry or check essential items in their passenger luggage. This will require confirmation that the items—which may require special packaging—are nonhazardous and permitted on passenger aircraft. The traveler should have sufficient documentation of the contents, purpose, and destination of the luggage and should be met at the port of arrival by team officials or leadership personnel to facilitate customs clearance. This is a great option when there is an urgent need to get supplies to sites quickly, as there are fewer hurdles than with cargo shipments and potential delays.

4.2 Domestic Transportation

4.2.1 Security

Although some shipments may be lost or stolen during international transit, the focus of security concerns will be domestic movement in the country of destination. Civil conflict, underlying discontent, banditry on the roads, and theft from storage sites are all possible. Transportation security needs may affect how items are shipped—for example, managers may decide to hire an armed escort or accept a government security escort for a convoy of trucks. Any decision about such matters should go to the principal investigator and the senior management team, since associating the research program with an armed force, especially a government one, may give rise to misperceptions among the local populace in many situations (Ilunga Kalenga et al. 2019). National government contacts must of course be consulted as well, whether or not government forces will be involved (▶ Chap. 41) (◘ Fig. 2).

4.2.2 Modes of Transport

Trucks (lorries) of various sizes and configurations and sport utility vehicles (four by fours) are commonly used to transport incom-

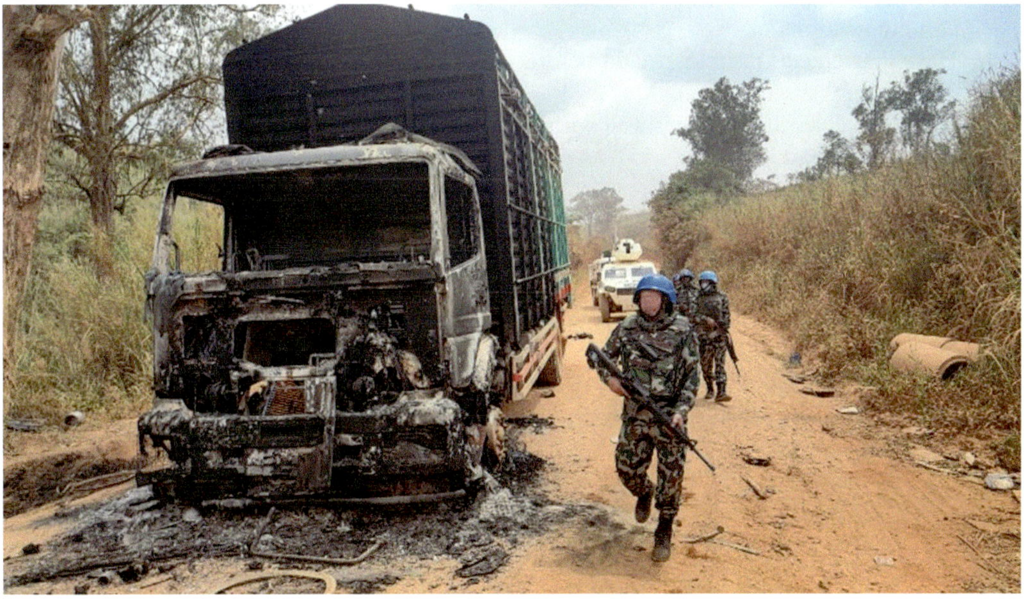

◘ **Fig. 2** Road transport can be dangerous, especially in areas of civil conflict. (Photo: MONUSCO-Force)

ing shipments from air or seaports. The type of vehicle generally used in country may be hired locally as long as the company providing service is favorably known to research partners. Experience has taught us to consult with the U.S. Embassy in selecting approved vendors for transporting shipments to remote locations. If shipments must leave major cities for remote locations, however, a number of additional questions should be considered. Not all of those listed below will be essential for relatively short trips.

- How far is it? How long should it take?
- What are the road conditions?
  - Are there up-to-date reports on the conditions of the route?
  - Paved, gravel, unimproved?
  - Passable during all seasons?
  - Accident frequency on road?
- What vehicles are proposed?
  - Can they handle the terrain?
  - Are the drivers experienced and qualified?
  - How many vehicles will be traveling together?
  - Is there enough redundancy to get the shipment through if one breaks down?
  - What assistance can the convoy provide, e.g., repairs, spare parts and tires, towing, winches, etc.?
  - Do the vehicles have reliable, tested communications?
  - Have the vehicles been inspected before departure?
  - Are all vehicles and cargoes well within their stated load limits?
- What assistance (mechanics, tires, fuel) is available en route?
- What is the security situation?
  - Are there checkpoints or other security challenges along the route that need to be considered?
- Are there biological or other potentially hazardous items on board?
  - Is there a mitigation plan in case of an accident or spill?
  - What laws govern hazardous spills?
- Has insurance coverage been carefully considered and decisions confirmed by the management team (▶ In Focus 32.2)?
- Are shipments packaged properly for the potential road conditions?
  - Is there a safety margin for cold-chain items (▶ Chap. 39)?
  - Is sensitive equipment well protected?

Roads can be unpredictable and sometimes impassible, particularly when it comes to remote and underserved areas of least developed countries. Alternative routes should be sought and mapped out if available. The likelihood of seasonal weather conditions leading to flooding, washouts, or wildfires must be considered—even earthquakes can prove a hazard, albeit one impossible to predict. Alternative means of transportation (water or air) should be considered if available. Skillful inventory management that takes predictable events like the rainy season into account will help obviate the need for extraordinary measures. Still, civil strife or rainy season washouts may mean that only rugged cargo aircraft, helicopters, or in a few cases watercraft remain as potential transport options. Air cargo is expensive, especially if chartered, and may be hard to hire. Helicopters are expensive and may not be a viable option outside extreme emergencies unless provided by the national government or military, the UN, or a military assistance operation. The UN Humanitarian Air Service, operated by the World Food Programme, provides access to humanitarian organizations in disaster situations (UN Logistics Cluster 2020; WFP 2021) and may be helpful. Water transport would be an unusual option in an infectious disease emergency but could be useful in some locations (◘ Fig. 3).

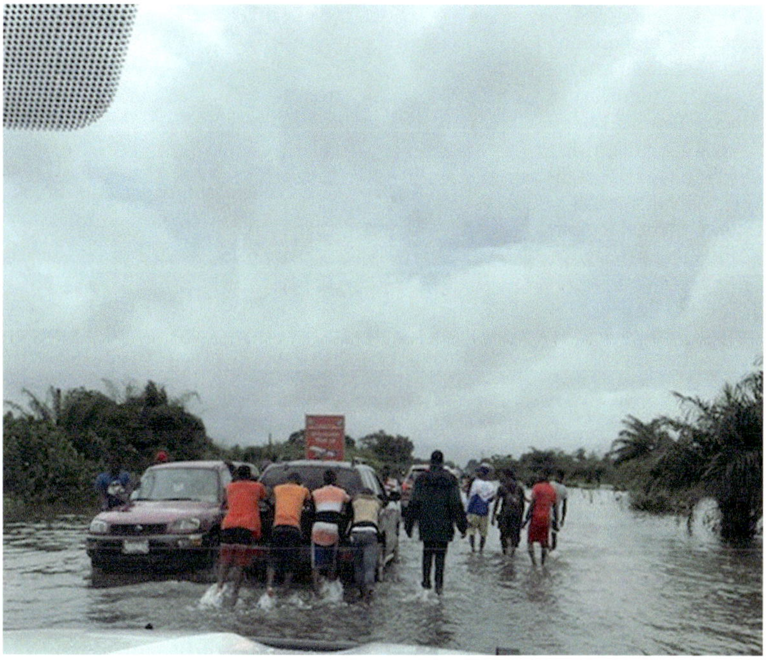

Fig. 3 It's not always easy getting around during the rainy season. (Photo: PREVAIL Research Team)

5 Supply and Equipment Management

5.1 Storage

Adequate supplies, stock confirmation, regular stock taking, and inventory management are all essential to a well-functioning research effort (▶ Chap. 38). A likely configuration is a centralized storage facility supporting multiple research sites; both central and peripheral sites will have dedicated areas and equipment for general medical supply, laboratory, and pharmacy storage. Establishing a central storage site facilitates consolidated supply requests and sharing similar research consumables. Study needs, space availability, and funding support will determine if a new facility must be built or if an existing structure can be used or renovated. Considerations should be made for space needed, truck or forklift access, refrigerator/freezer space, electrical requirements, and redundancy for cold storage (e.g., vaccine, reagents). With an adequate statement of work, local contractors can be used to do the work, though there should be close supervision to ensure work need not be redone. All contractors should have prior work referrals to ensure they have sufficient knowledge of the required construction/renovation elements (Figs. 4 and 5).

Attention to the storage requirements of all goods, especially temperature control and theft prevention, is essential. Investigational new drugs (IND), the lifeblood of a study, must often be stored at −70 °C; other medicines or vaccines may need to be refrigerated 2–8 °C but never frozen, while yet others may need to be at room temperature—which means an air-conditioned storage space. These requirements are covered in cold chain, but the supply manager and staff are one of the multiple layers of assurance that these items are put in the right place and kept in the right conditions. IND are of incalculable value as a scarce, potentially lifesaving commodity, which could be rendered useless simply by being left out on a shelf for a few minutes.

5.2 Inventory Management

At each site and facility, parallel practices and methods must be followed for supply management. Regular stock taking and calibration with current and projected "burn" or usage rates are fundamental to ensuring the study

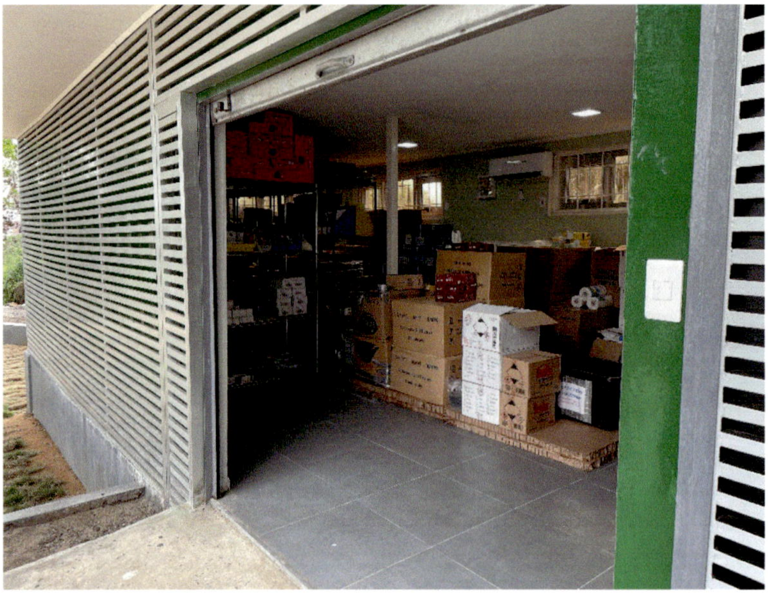

Fig. 4 Supply warehouse supporting multiple clinical research studies in Monrovia, Liberia. Photo taken in April 2022 at the AM Dogliotti Campus at the University of Liberia. (Photo: Clinical Research Team, Liberia)

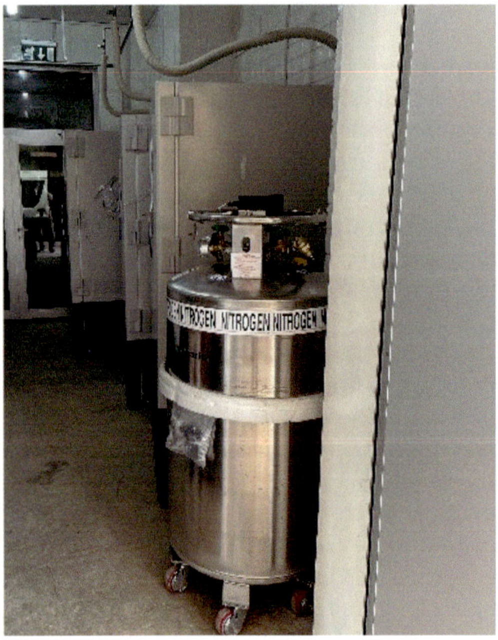

Fig. 5 A liquid nitrogen storage tank and three freezers at the Liberia Institute for Biomedical Research. Photo taken in April 2022. (Photo: Clinical Research team, Liberia/authors are members of the team)

has the supplies it needs. Burn rates continually change and should be frequently reevaluated in order to establish minimum quantities needed on hand in accordance with supply chain time requirements. Studying the protocol timelines, along with expected and actual study enrollment, will help determine the quantity of supplies that should always be available. The number of technicians and other workers at each site will help determine the amount of PPE needed. At each site, sufficient supplies must be available for daily activities, plus adequate stock to cover the site until new inventory arrives. The minimum amounts can change over time, so regular analysis may be necessary to meet changing demand.

Taking advantage of shipping opportunities—like extra space in a container—may justify ordering larger supply quantities than one would in other situations, since the savings on shipping costs can be considerable. A supply shortfall, even of seemingly minor items, can be very detrimental and even bring a clinical trial to a halt. An analogous example from the COVID-19 pandemic has been the shortage of long swabs bringing testing to a halt in some cases (Herper 2020).

In addition to usage rates, expiration dates must be taken into account to calculate supply needs. A good understanding of expiration dates and shelf life will help procurement managers get a supply order right: items with short shelf lives should be kept in smaller quantities so they do not expire before use, while items with longer shelf lives can be kept in larger quantities because there is less of a risk that they will not be used in time. Another impor-

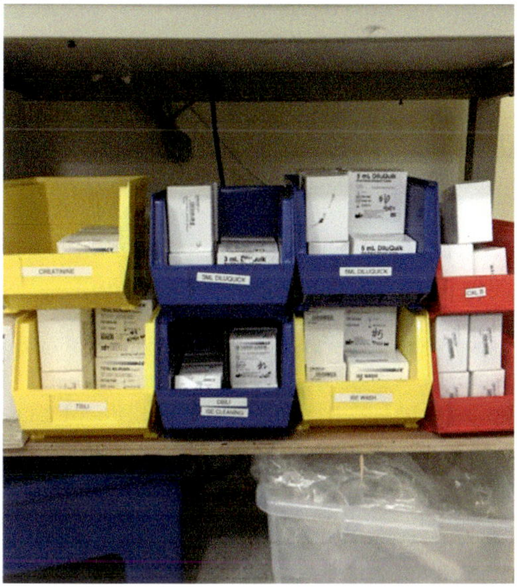

Fig. 6 Medical supplies organized and labeled for inventory at CH Rennie Hospital, Kakata, Liberia. Photo taken in April 2022. (Photo: Clinical Research team, Liberia)

tant aspect to consider is how long it takes for an item to be received at a storage site. If an item needs to be procured overseas, shipping, customs clearance, and transport to the site could take a few weeks to deliver it to the place of use. Managers will need to balance expiration dates with the need to have enough stock on hand and prolonged transportation timelines. It may be necessary to communicate with the supplier to ensure they are not shipping items that are close to their expiration dates. First-in, first-out policies and systems are a basic principle in many contexts and are essential to ensure reagents and other supplies with relatively short shelf lives do not expire before use. As items come into a site, they should be placed behind items that are already there, making it natural for staff to take out the supply that has been stored the longest (Fig. 6).

Even with essential risk mitigation policies in place, mistakes will happen, and there must be a way to correct them, for example, by asking traveling colleagues to hand carry critical reagents and supplies. Possibly there are medical NGOs or other missions in the field that could lend supplies until a shipment arrives. Be prepared to reciprocate. A note of caution is to ensure that the critical reagents and supplies that a colleague is carrying is approved by regulation and by the airline prior to boarding the airplane.

5.3 Requisition System

A standardized process for ordering, approvals, scheduling, tracking, and receiving all materials, supplies, and equipment purchased during an emergency clinical research response is essential for good management and for final reporting on the clinical research program. The requisition system must also ensure budget availability for all items and services ordered. Normally the project's chief financial officer or chief operating officer would approve all significant expenditures in advance. Although some decisions will have to be left to staff—emergency vehicle repair is one example—that expense should be incorporated into the accounting system as soon as possible. Common consumables and quantities should be harmonized to avoid over ordering and duplication. Timelines should be established to prioritize orders, considering long lead teams and evaluating possible alternatives. Location and sufficient space for shipment staging and storage should also be determined and may include direct shipments to the freight forwarder or site locations.

5.4 Equipment Maintenance

Regular maintenance is crucial to ensuring all equipment is performing at its best. Following maintenance schedules will help ensure that any issues are minimized. Skipping normal equipment maintenance can shorten the lifespan of the equipment, resulting in a need to purchase new equipment more often. A study can also be negatively affected if critical equipment malfunctions.

Maintenance and calibration are critical necessities when working with dangerous pathogens. Certification for biosafety cabinets must be obtained yearly, or whenever the biosafety cabinet is moved. Depending on the area where the biosafety cabinet is located, technicians who are trained on these types of certifications may not be available. In these

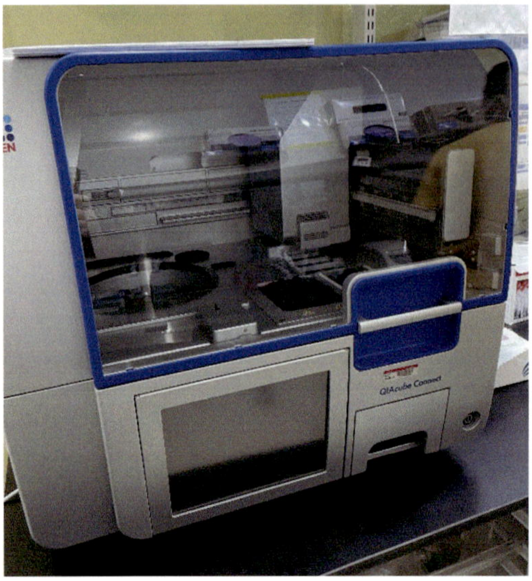

Fig. 7 An automated sample processor at the Liberia Institute for Biomedical Research requires regular maintenance. Photo taken in April 2022. (Photo: Clinical Research team, Liberia/authors are members of the team)

instances, outside companies can be brought in to decontaminate and provide certifications. Often the same companies can recertify biosafety cabinets that have malfunctioned if needed (Fig. 7).

When selecting equipment, choose items that are rated for the climate that they will be placed in. If available, select a tropical-rated freezer that has been built to withstand extreme heat and humidity over a freezer that is best suited for a more temperate environment. The procurement team should develop early plans and procedures for contacting local or international on-call vendors capable of quickly troubleshooting and repairing expensive, essential, and highly complex equipment. Ensure that the air conditioning units operating in the laboratory are routinely maintained.

5.5 Backup Requirements and Redundancies

In an ideal setting, all equipment would be placed in a facility with little risk of electrical surges or power outages. The environment would be clean and free of dust, maintenance would be performed regularly, and temperatures would be regulated and optimal for all equipment. In reality, studies take place in varied locations and environments, including those characterized by extreme heat, oppressive humidity, frequent electrical surges, and less than ideal maintenance standards. Extreme temperatures and humidity can wreak havoc on freezers, refrigerators, and other pieces of equipment. As mentioned previously, power surges can ruin electrical components. A backup plan and processes need to be established if a piece of equipment malfunctions or breaks down. Risk mitigation strategies for this scenario and others should always be built into planning and operations.

If a freezer storing study samples stops working, for example, what is the plan? Having a backup freezer in place that can be plugged in, brought to the correct temperature, and made available to transfer samples to is one option. Because it would take time to bring the new freezer to the proper temperature, perhaps it needs to be kept running. Protocols also need to be in place so staff members know what to do before and during such situations. The team needs to understand how long the malfunctioning freezer can hold its contents at the required temperature and the length of time it takes for the backup freezer to reach that temperature. Other questions to consider include the following: is there another freezer that is already plugged in and at the correct temperature, and could this freezer be used to store samples while the backup freezer is being plugged in and brought to the correct temperature? How are temperatures and freezer functions tracked outside of normal work hours, and what are the alert mechanisms to ensure human intervention for when there is an issue?

If a diagnostic instrument breaks down, malfunctions, or fails a calibration check, how quickly can it be repaired, or how quickly can a new instrument be brought in? If any downtime is detrimental to a study, adequate backup equipment is necessary. Prior to a study commencing, a list of required equipment and quantities should be prepared. A plan should also be developed to address equipment failure.

The amount of redundant (backup) equipment needed at a study site should be based on study activities, equipment availability, shipping arrival times, storage space, and study urgency. For example, if a PCR instrument stops working in the middle of an outbreak situation, it would be considered an urgent item, so immediate replacement would be necessary. However, if the item is used for downstream sample analysis that is not as urgent, immediate replacement would not be necessary.

5.6 Resupply Considerations

When establishing supply reordering points/stock alerts, it is critical to consider the time it takes to place an order, plus the time it takes to bring items into the country. Understanding this timeline will aid in establishing minimum supply amounts needed at sites in order to avoid study interruptions. For example, if it takes 1 week to order instrument controls and then takes 4–6 weeks for that item to be received at the site location, the supply reordering point/stock alert should be set to a minimum of a 7-week supply. This would allow adequate time for the material to be received in country without study interruption.

Various sociopolitical factors can cause disruptions and result in resupply issues. It is imperative to have a solid understanding of the sociopolitical landscape where a study is taking place. Elections, demonstrations, and holidays may shut down roads and facilities for days at a time. If you anticipate running out of supplies during an election, you might consider ordering a larger quantity beforehand to avoid any delays in getting extra supplies in country. Additionally, civil unrest in some regions may lead to damage or loss of equipment and supplies. Having a contingency plan if this occurs, such as having extra supplies stored in another location, will help ensure the study is not delayed.

5.7 Waste Management

When conducting emergency response clinical research, the waste generated must be managed appropriately. Local regulations for disposing of medical and chemical waste should be considered. It is essential to understand how waste needs to be treated and handled in order to protect workers in the facility and the community around the facility. These processes should be established and well understood before beginning any emergency response research. In the likely event that local regulations are inadequate or hard to comply with, treatment and disposal should follow appropriate waste management guidelines, for example, those published by WHO (2014) and the International Committee of the Red Cross (ICRC) (2011) (Fig. 8).

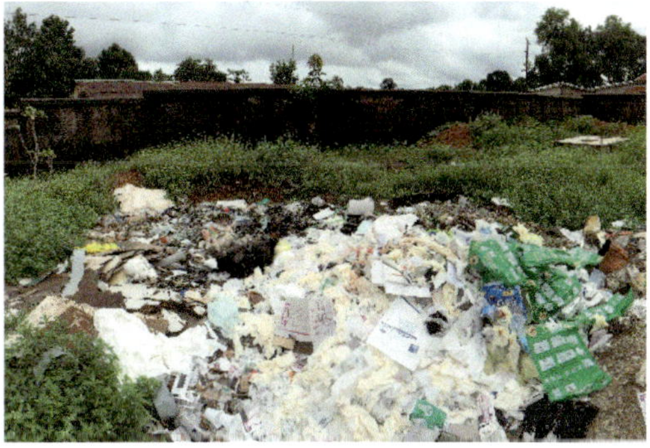

Fig. 8 Unmanaged waste. Photo taken in October 2015, Forécariah, Guinea. (Photo: Clinical Research team, Guinea/authors are members of the team)

Biohazardous and medical waste can be treated either chemically or thermally. If possible, all liquid waste potentially containing infectious agents should be chemically treated as soon as possible, following proper procedures and preparations of the chemical being used for treatment. For example, if sodium hypochlorite (bleach) is used to chemically disinfect, it needs to be at the proper concentration to be effective, and it needs to have appropriate contact time with the waste to ensure complete inactivation of any infectious agents. No matter the chemical disinfectant being used, proper procedures for preparations, storage, and use must be strictly followed.

If chemical disinfection is not a possibility or is not adequate for the waste, other techniques should be used to ensure waste is properly managed. Another technique is thermal treatment, such as incinerating or autoclaving

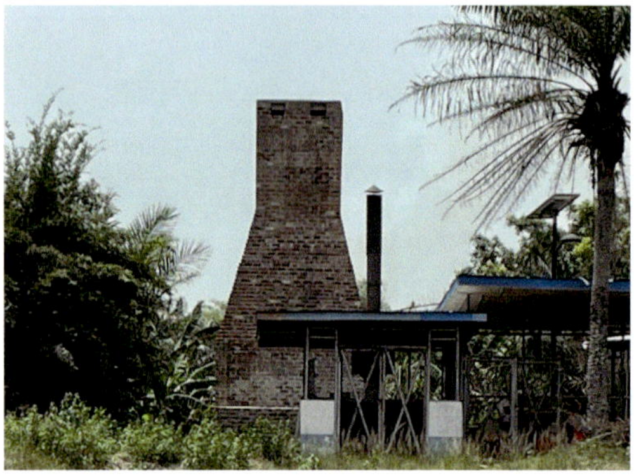

Fig. 9 An incinerator constructed at the Liberia Institute for Biomedical Research, Charlesville, Liberia. Photo taken in April 2022. (Photo: Clinical Research team, Liberia/authors are members of the team)

the waste. Chemical and thermal disinfection should be used in combination whenever possible. Staff members who are responsible for this process must be properly trained to handle the hazards and confirm that disinfection was successful. Training in these processes is essential, considering that the materials these staff members are handling could be grossly contaminated with an infectious agent. Additionally, if it is necessary to transport waste to the area where the thermal treatment will occur, the waste must be packaged appropriately to prevent accidental exposure and/or release. At a minimum, biohazardous waste should be sealed in biohazard waste bags (hard-sided boxes or cases are essential if there is potential for puncture) prior to transport (Fig. 9).

5.8 The Value of a Logistician

Logisticians analyze and coordinate supply chain and equipment management needs across an organization and projects. They manage the entire life cycle of a product, which includes how a product is sourced, acquired, delivered, set up, and maintained and its final disposition at the end of its life.

Supply chains are complex and sensitive as they depend on ever-changing customer and project/study demands. Implementing a research operation in an infectious disease emergency requires sophisticated logistics. The logistician uses a specialized set of knowledge, experience, professional management skills, and software systems designed specifically to manage logistical functions, to plan and coordinate the procurement, inventory management, and movement of products in a timely, safe, and effective manner. This management function facilitates the transport and delivery of supplies and investigational products to the right location at the needed time, decreasing (if not eliminating) waste of materials and time, thereby improving the quality and efficiency of clinical research projects.

Furthermore, the logistician has the necessary skills to ensure all aspects of supply management operations are coordinated. This involves planning, systems implementation, training, coordinating, and evaluating the actions required to support complex operations. Where resources and infrastructure are limited, this entails advising on the acquisition, shipment, tracking, storage, use, maintenance, and disposition of equipment and supplies, to support an evolving clinical research program.

6 Local Staff Requirements

The amount and sophistication of labor required when manipulating materials transfer is directly proportionate to the sensitivity of materials. In resource-constrained regions, there are specific opportunities to hire local staff that can assist in several ways (▶ Chap. 42). In some areas, there may be an oversupply of educated workers. In other, more remote regions of a country, the population may have had little access to education. In some areas, then, high numbers of unemployed workers with strong skills may be available; in others, such workers may have to be brought in from another part of the country or from outside.

Unskilled local temporary labor is rarely in short supply. When faced with a need to offload study supplies, such as PPE, gloves, beds, office supplies, and other nonspecialized equipment, this can be done relatively inexpensively and with little oversight. However, clinical research responders should take more care with more specialized equipment. For example, sensitive laboratory machinery that needs special handling and freezers that cannot be rotated more than a certain angle off of their vertical axis will require more supervision than a conference room table that simply requires many hands to move. If local labor is required to access more restricted facilities, such as embassies or government campuses, there may be more complex requirements, and alternative methods may need to be employed, such as using the local labor force to move materials to a gate and having individuals with access privileges move materials within the access-controlled areas.

As storage sites and plans are developed, training on these plans is also imperative. Determining who will be responsible for keeping inventory at the sites needs to be understood, and this person or group needs to be trained on the inventory processes. Ideally, this individual understands the processes well enough that he/she can train others to perform the same processes. Those responsible for performing stock takes and inventories need a full understanding of the importance of accurate stock takes and how errors can affect the study. Training plans, including refresher trainings, are important because they ensure staff members remain aware of the processes and this knowledge is not forgotten over time.

6.1 Implementation Checklists (▫ Fig. 10)

1. Reconnaissance and assessment
2. Establishment
3. Maintenance
4. Dissolution

6.2 Receiving Product

- Place in a secure area.
- Print off the packing slips from the pre-alert emails, and open the pallets, checking off that the supplies in the packing list match the description and quantity listed in the packing list.
- Once all the supplies have been confirmed as received, enter them into the inventory management system. Ensure that the quantities entered match the quantities in which the items will be removed.
- If using a barcoding application, print the barcodes and place them on the product.
- Once this is complete, the items can be moved to their final storage location.
- Ensure headquarters supply and shipping lead(s) are notified of receipt and any discrepancies.

▫ **Fig. 10** Sample inventory management checklist

	Pre-alert notification	**Notifies all involved parties of upcoming shipment**
	Commercial invoices	
	Packing lists	
	Carrier information	
	Clearance process	Steps taken to ensure shipment is cleared
	Airway bill	
	Commercial invoices	
	Packing lists	
	Payment(s) made	
	Reconcile packages	
	Receiving	Being ready for the supplies to arrive
	Review pre-alert	
	Perishables	
	Ambient	
	Local transport	
	Receipt at site	

- *If* items are damaged or missing, take photos of any damage and email the headquarters shipping lead to notify them of the discrepancy. Follow the above steps for all items correctly received in the remainder of the shipment.

6.3 Storing Product

- Storage areas should be kept clean and orderly at all times. Keep supplies in a cool or air-conditioned environment, away from the walls, off the floor, and away from sunlight exposure or risk of water damage.
- Where supplies are proprietary to one group (due to, e.g., budget restrictions), they need to be stored in a clearly labeled area that is distinct from other supplies (e.g., on their own racking or shelf in the fridge).
- For items that are shared by multiple entities, they should be grouped by usage, in the main body of the storeroom. For example, store reagents by equipment with which they are used, and place all apparel together, the same with site operations and clinical supplies.
- *Do not mix unopened inventory with opened stock* (this makes the unit of measure and quantities hard to track). Items should enter the facility *in the same unit of measure* in which they leave.
- Label stock supplies for ease of identification.
- If there are items with multiple expiration dates, place the items that are first to expire to the front of the shelf.

6.4 Performing a Stock Take

Stock takes are the physical verification of quantities of supplies held in inventory. This provides an audit of existing stock. It is also the source of stock discrepancy information.

- Choose a time when the site is quiet, and supplies are not likely to be removed as you are counting them. First thing in the morning or at the end of the day is usually best.
- Ensure the stock room is clean and tidy and inventory items are well laid out and labeled.
- If possible, use two people for the stock take—one person identifies the item held in inventory and calls out the physical count, while the other person finds that item in *the item description* column, checks the *unit of measure* column, and records the amount of stock in that unit of measure in the *stock take quantities* of the template.
- Only count unopened items. Opened packs are not considered part of inventory.
- Physically count every item in your inventory—do not estimate.
- Make a note of the expiration date of the items as you proceed. *The first item to expire should be at the front of the shelf and be the first to be removed and used.*
- Count in the same direction, for example, top to bottom for shelves starting on the far left and ending on the far right. This way you are less likely to miss an item.
- Your physical count should match the running total in final. Check any physical discrepancy between the two, and make a note of the item to report back to the accountable clinical research team members.

6.5 Key Terms

- *Lead time.* The time between when new stock is ordered and when it is received and available for use.
- *Maximum inventory.* The level of stock above which inventory levels should not rise under normal conditions. It is a set multiple of 1 month's usage.
- *Minimum inventory.* The lowest quantity of stock allowed in inventory *before an emergency order needs to be placed.* It is expressed in months of stock.
- *Recurring supplies.* Supplies the trial must never stock out of. They are the supplies that will form the bulk of regular subsequent scheduled resupply shipments.

- *Resupply.* Providing the sites with new inventory of supplies.
- *Stock on hand/quantity on hand.* Supplies available at the site at any given time. For inventory purposes, stock on hand is *all unopened stock*.
- *Stock take.* The physical verification of quantities of supplies held in inventory. This should be done every 2 weeks to provide an audit of existing stock. It is also the source of stock discrepancy information—a security measure ensuring proper inventory control to identify unauthorized use or theft of supplies, as well as an indispensable step to prevent stockouts.
- *Stockout.* This is where the existing supplies of an item at a site are exhausted—there is no more stock available of that product. The demand is greater than the supply. We want to *prevent* this at all costs, as it can halt the study.
- *Unit of measure.* A standard unit by which a quantity is accounted for and measured. It is very important that the units of measure are clear in any communication, and it is often one of the biggest challenges to understanding site needs and shipping the correct volumes.

6.6 Supply Staff Roles

- *Site supply manager.* This person has full accountability for stock entering and leaving the supply areas, ensuring the inventory management system is updated and performing stock takes every month.
- *In-country clinical laboratory supply lead* has full accountability of all clinical laboratory items, including supplies that are removed from the inventory management system as they are consumed, as well as performing monthly stock takes.
- *In-country research laboratory supply lead* has full accountability of all research laboratory items, including supplies that are removed from the inventory management system as they are consumed, as well as performing monthly stock takes.
- *Headquarters supply leads* review stock levels at headquarters and set the maximum and minimum stock levels in the inventory management system. They will have accountability for submitting reorder requests through the requisitioning system.
- *Headquarters supply and shipping team* receives order requests from the headquarters supply leads. They place orders and manage the shipping process to the site.

Discussion Questions

1. Define logistics and inventory management for clinical research during an outbreak in low-resource settings.
2. What is the role of the clinical research protocol team during an emergency clinical research response?
3. When an emergency worsens, the need for strong partnerships becomes more acute. In this context, discuss some roles of civilian government agencies, military, international organizations, diplomatic communities, nongovernmental organizations, regional and local governments, and informal community leadership bodies in getting equipment and supplies to where they are needed.
4. Procurement of needed equipment and supplies, along with transport arrangements, should begin as the study protocol takes shape. Furthermore, research is necessary to ensure compliance with all domestic and international import and export requirements.
   (a) Since these requirements are complex and under continued discussion, what could you do first to help ease the process?
   (b) Discuss some restrictions that may affect export of medical supplies during an outbreak emergency.
   (c) List some minimal paperwork requirements for shipping medical items.
5. Successful shipment of goods urgently needed where transport links are few requires a dedicated and detail-oriented team ready to facilitate the process day and night.

   (a) For international transport, discuss how to identify a freight forwarder and the destination. Further, what factors come into play when choosing between air transport, surface shipments, and passenger baggage transport?
6. For domestic transport, what questions must be answered to ensure shipments arrive safely at their destination despite unpredictable and insecure circumstances in underserved areas of least developed countries?
7. To ensure a well-functioning research effort, discuss the importance and management of adequate supplies, stock confirmation, regular stock taking, and inventory management at, most likely, a centralized storage facility supporting multiple research sites.
8. Appropriate waste management processes must be established and well understood before beginning the emergency response research. Discuss some important factors of waste management.
9. In resource-constrained regions, specific opportunities arise for hiring local staff to assist in several ways with research efforts. Describe factors related to employment and training of local staff.

References

Bromley M, Maletta G. The challenge of software and technology transfers to non-proliferation efforts: implementing and complying with export controls. Stockholm: Stockholm International Peace Research Institute; 2018.

Carter RJ, Idriss A, Widdowson M-A, Samai M, Schrag SJ, Legardy-Williams JK, et al. Implementing a multisite clinical trial in the midst of an Ebola outbreak: lessons learned from the Sierra Leone trial to introduce a vaccine against Ebola. J Infect Dis. 2018;217(Suppl_1):S16–23. https://doi.org/10.1093/infdis/jix657.

De Waal A. Militarizing global health. Boston Review; 2014.

Devi S. Travel restrictions hampering COVID-19 response. Lancet. 2020;395(10233):1331–2. https://doi.org/10.1016/S0140-6736(20)30967-3.

EC. Commission publishes guidance on export requirements for personal protective equipment. Brussels: European Commission; 2020.

EU ECHO. EU facilitates second rotation of Dutch vessel to Ebola affected region. 2014.

FIATA. Changing logistics: freight forwarders evolve with trade. Glattbrugg, CH: International Federation of Freight Forwarders Associations (FIATA); 2017.

GPMB. A world in disorder 2020. Global Preparedness Monitoring Board annual report 2020. Geneva: Global Preparedness Monitoring Board; 2020.

Gralla E, Goentzel J. Humanitarian transportation planning: evaluation of practice-based heuristics and recommendations for improvement. Eur J Oper Res. 2018;269(2):436–50. https://doi.org/10.1016/j.ejor.2018.02.012.

Herper M. To speed coronavirus testing. FDA greenlights a new type of nasal swab. STAT; 2020.

IASC. Step-by-step practical guide for humanitarian needs overviews, humanitarian response plans and updates. New York: Interagency Standing Committee. Cycle HP; 2020.

ICRC. Medical waste management. Geneva: International Committee of the Red Cross; 2011.

Ilunga Kalenga O, Moeti M, Sparrow A, Nguyen V-K, Lucey D, Ghebreyesus TA. The ongoing Ebola epidemic in the Democratic Republic of Congo, 2018–2019. N Engl J Med. 2019;381(4):373–83. https://doi.org/10.1056/nejmsr1904253.

IMF. WTO and IMF heads call for lifting trade restrictions on medical supplies and food. Washington, DC: International Monetary Fund; 2020.

Kamradt-Scott A, Harman S, Wenham C, Smith F. Civil–military cooperation in Ebola and beyond. Lancet. 2016;387(10014):104–5. https://doi.org/10.1016/s0140-6736(15)01128-9.

Lu Y, Rong G, Yu SP, Sun Z, Duan X, Dong Z, et al. Chinese military medical teams in the Ebola outbreak of Sierra Leone. J R Arm Med Corps. 2016;162(3):198–202. https://doi.org/10.1136/jramc-2015-000562.

Mulangu S, Dodd LE, Davey RT Jr, Tshiani Mbaya O, Proschan M, Mukadi D, et al. A randomized, controlled trial of Ebola virus disease therapeutics. N Engl J Med. 2019;381(24):2293–303. https://doi.org/10.1056/NEJMoa1910993.

NASEM. The critical health impacts of corruption. Crossing the global quality chasm: improving health care worldwide. The National Academies Collection: reports funded by National Institutes of Health. Washington, DC: National Academies Press; 2018.

Nevin RL, Anderson JN. The timeliness of the US military response to the 2014 Ebola disaster: a critical review. Med Conflict Surviv. 2016;32:1–30. https://doi.org/10.1080/13623699.2016.1212491.

Thompson DDP. Special issue: Preparing the humanitarian supply chain for epidemics and pandemic responses. J Humanit Logist Supply Chain Manag.

2021;11(2):157–75. https://doi.org/10.1108/JHLSCM-01-2021-0006. ISSN: 2042-6747
U.S. Dept. of State. Overview of U.S. export control system. Washington, DC: U.S. Dept. of State. 2011. https://2009-2017.state.gov/strategictrade/overview/index.htm. Accessed 27 Apr 2020.
UN. Discussion draft: guidelines on the tax treatment of government-to-government aid projects. New York: United Nations; 2020.
UN. Department of Peace Operations. New York: United Nations; 2021. https://peacekeeping.un.org/en/department-of-peace-operations. Accessed 19 May 2021.
UN Logistics Cluster. Logistics operational guide. Rome: UN Logistics Cluster; 2020. https://dlca.logcluster.org/display/LOG/Logistics+Operational+Guide+%28LOG%29+Home. Accessed 29 Apr 2020.
Wells CR, Pandey A, Ndeffo Mbah ML, Gauzere BA, Malvy D, Singer BH, et al. The exacerbation of Ebola outbreaks by conflict in the Democratic Republic of the Congo. Proc Natl Acad Sci USA. 2019;116(48):24366–72. https://doi.org/10.1073/pnas.1913980116.
WFP. Supply chain. Rome: World Food Programme; 2020. https://www.wfp.org/supply-chain. Accessed 29 Apr 2020.
WFP. UN Humanitarian Air Service. Rome: World Food Programme; 2021. https://www.wfp.org/unhas. Accessed 19 Oct 2021.
WHO. Guidance on regulations for the transport of infectious substances 2013–2014. Geneva: World Health Organization; 2012.
WHO. Safe management of wastes from health-care activities. Geneva: World Health Organizaion; 2014.
WHO. International Health Regulations (2005). 3rd ed. Geneva: World Health Organzation; 2016.
WHO. Building health systems resilience for universal health coverage and health security during the COVID-19 pandemic and beyond: WHO position paper. Geneva: World Health Organization; 2021. Contract No.: WHO/UHL/PHCSP/2021.01.

38 Pharmaceutical Management

Matthew Carl Kirchoff

Contents

Learning Track Note: This chapter appears in Learning Tracks: Clinical Research; Emergency Research Response, Research Operations

E. S. Higgs and R. A. Sorenson (eds.), *Principles and Practice of Emergency Research Response*,
https://doi.org/10.1007/978-3-031-48408-7_58

Learning Objectives

This chapter will help readers understand and describe

- Why investigational medicinal products (IMPs) require more careful management than approved products
- Methods for controlling the temperature, humidity, light exposure, physical agitation, and material compatibility of the IMP environment
- Considerations for labeling IMPs in a multilingual environment
- Questions to consider when analyzing possible shortfalls in essential requirements for clinical trial implementation
- Considerations for reviewing a new or existing pharmacy research facility during an outbreak in a resource-constrained area
- Equipment selection and procurement during an outbreak in a resource-constrained area
- Requirements for shipping IMP to a second trial site
- Donation or disposal of ancillary medicinal products

1 Introduction

The International Council for Harmonisation of Technical Requirements for Pharmaceuticals for Human Use (ICH) Efficacy Guidelines for Good Clinical Practice (GCP) define an investigational medicinal product (IMP) as

> A pharmaceutical form of an active ingredient or placebo being tested or used as a reference in a clinical trial, including a product with a marketing authorization when used or assembled (formulated or packaged) in a way different from the approved form, or when used for an unapproved indication, or when used to gain further information about an approved use (ICH 2016)

The management of investigational and approved drugs, biologics, and vaccines, as well as associated materials, equipment, and personnel for a clinical trial in the context of an infectious disease outbreak presents many challenges. These difficulties are compounded in low-resource and isolated settings, but even the best-resourced countries can be vulnerable, as evidenced by worldwide medical product shortages and supply-chain disruptions during the coronavirus disease 2019 (COVID-19) pandemic. The challenges clinical research programs encounter in low-resource and remote settings, particularly during an outbreak, are often more difficult versions of problems investigational pharmacy staff around the world face every day: varying regulatory considerations, shortages, facility shortcomings, storage issues, and logistical arrangements for moving products and associated supplies. In the context of an outbreak, these problems tend to come with greater frequency, urgency, and human consequences. It is a stressful juggling act to marshal both materiel and human resources quickly while aiming at a moving target as knowledge about the pathogen and disease course increases (▶ Chaps. 19 and 20). As we saw the healthcare resources of even the most developed countries overwhelmed by the COVID-19 pandemic, it became easier to appreciate the difficulties developing countries face in an infectious disease emergency.

The urgency and uncertainties of an outbreak response may leave research pharmacy staff dealing with more unknowns than is typical of clinical trials. It may be necessary, for example, to plan Phase II and III clinical trials while only limited knowledge from preclinical and Phase I studies are available. This is especially true for recently identified pathogens, rare pathogens, or pathogens endemic predominantly in less-developed countries with little clinical research infrastructure and few experienced local research personnel. If IMPs have already been developed to prevent or treat the outbreak's causative pathogen, they may be in an earlier stage of development when clinical trials begin than is typical during the usual course of drug development. In addition to efficacy, safety, and special population unknowns, only limited data and guidance may be available on the IMP's stability, material compatibility (e.g., with administration devices such as syringes, needles, and intravenous tubing), handling requirements, and hazards to staff. Products early in development or needed urgently worldwide are likely to be available in limited quantities initially, and resupply may take days, weeks, or be uncertain, so the loss of investigational medicinal products can be particularly devastating. A geographically and epidemiologically shifting epidemic compounds the complexities of planning ahead, building site infrastructure, and training research staff.

Many guidelines, manuals, and other resources are available on pharmacy operations and regulations as they relate to conducting clinical investigations (▶ Sect. 2). This chapter's primary focus is on considerations that may be overlooked while in the circumstances of a high-pressure, unfamiliar, and resource-constrained setting during an outbreak. The primary perspective is that of a pharmacist establishing and managing an investigational pharmacy on the ground, but the chapter includes additional research tasks which may naturally be delegated to or require input from a pharmacist.

The monumental task of storing and transporting investigational medicinal products and other products requiring a temperature-controlled environment (cold chain) is a significant challenge for pharmacy staff. This topic is covered in a dedicated chapter (▶ Chap. 39) due to its importance and multidisciplinary nature, often involving personnel from facilities, pharmacy, laboratory, other research team elements, and outside entities, such as consultants, equipment vendors, transport companies, and customs authorities.

2 Working with Investigational Medicinal Products in Early Development

During outbreaks, the challenges of working with IMPs are often amplified due to the urgency and unpredictability of the situation. For example, they may:

- Be in limited supply
- Require long lead times for resupply
- Require shipping between local sites during the study to manage scarce inventory
- Be shipped using a central vendor in different countries, with differing import and export requirements
- Have unusual storage requirements, such as below −60 °C
- Undergo revisions to storage and handling requirements, compatibility, administration, or dosing during a trial
- Require hazardous handling precaution
- Require more onerous blinding procedures
- Have complicated unblinding requirements
- Require frequent extensions to shelf life and relabeling
- Come with a limited, frequently updated pharmacy manual, or lack one completely
- Require regular revisions to associated processes, with tracking and documentation
- Have multiple investigational brochure updates and protocol amendments

Each of these challenges can significantly impact the conduct of clinical trials during outbreaks, requiring careful management and adaptability from research pharmacists and other clinical trial staff.

2.1 Stability of Investigational Medicinal Products

It is critical to develop an early understanding of storage and transport requirements, conduct thorough planning with detailed attention to circumstances in the study setting, and pay particularly close attention to operationalizing an acceptable environmental control plan that addresses temperature, humidity, light exposure, physical agitation, and material compatibility.

Departures, or excursions, from guideline-specified conditions for the IMP are protocol deviations or violations. These excursions require trial sponsor assessment, including consultations with the product manufacturer about product attributes and notifications of associated regulatory agencies and data safety monitoring boards. The pharmacy team must document these assessments, decisions, and follow up steps, which may include a corrective and preventive action plan to avoid repeated errors.

Limited stability data pose several issues. Products such as vaccines and monoclonal antibodies are often stored frozen or at ultra-cold temperatures with little allowance for temperature excursions until stability data at warmer temperatures can be established. In the event a low-temperature cooling device fails and the product must be moved to a warmer but acceptable storage location for a short period, the product rarely will be allowed to go back to the colder environment, often shortening the allowable stability time. Exacerbating these challenges, storage requirements may change during the trial as the sponsor continues to gather and analyze stability data.

Tip

Guidelines occasionally forget to specify a lower (coldest) temperature for product storage. Ensure this temperature is specified as storing at too low a temperature can result in container issues, such as vial stoppers becoming brittle.

Pharmaceutical management should make clear, in early and frequent consultations with the sponsor or manufacturer, the difficulties that may be involved in storing and transporting products at ultra-cold temperatures and push for guidance at the broadest range of temperatures that can be supported by data. Manufacturers are frequently inclined to specify temperature ranges more restrictive than necessary in order to provide a maximum safety margin. Worse yet, sponsors and manufacturers, or even different individuals within a company, may verbally provide similar but slightly different ranges, reflecting this ad hoc safety buffer. These inconsistencies may result in storage requirements that are difficult to maintain consistently at remote, austere research sites, risking the loss of scarce investigational medicinal products mid-outbreak. The research team may struggle to correct such problems, which could bring about a catastrophic pause or end to the trial.

The study sponsor should provide a certificate of analysis, certificate of suitability, certificate of compliance, or similar document which includes the current IMP stability date (which effectively functions as an expiration date), by lot number. This document is usually supplemented with information provided during shipments, in particular if the product is imported into a second country.

2.1.1 Temperature

Practical, effective temperature monitoring of product and storage locations is critical. Ideally, a continuous, real-time, electronic system with Internet connectivity can be implemented. If this setup is not available or will not be available at the study start, regular (i.e., twice daily or at staff changes) manual temperature recordings on a sheet of paper may be minimally acceptable, depending on a risk assessment of the cold-chain setup and the products being monitored (▶ Chap. 39). Although less critical, monitoring of “room temperature” surrounding a temperature-controlled storage space should also occur, even if the product is stored within a refrigerator or freezer, as this data may be critical in a manufacturer’s excursion assessment in the event of a prolonged malfunction of the cold-chain storage device.

Tip

A manufacturer may request an impractically narrow storage range, such as −20 to −25 °C, or − 65 to −75 °C. Given the normal temperature fluctuation within a freezer, any short-term loss of power, slightly longer than average door opening, or addition of thermal mass at a different temperature will almost certainly result in a temperature excursion and the quarantine of the investigational medicinal products. For sites with unreliable power, this is practically a certainty. While 2 to 8 °C is an acceptably narrow range for refrigerated products, as the temperature difference between the ambient environment and the required environment grows larger, so should the allowable temperature range.

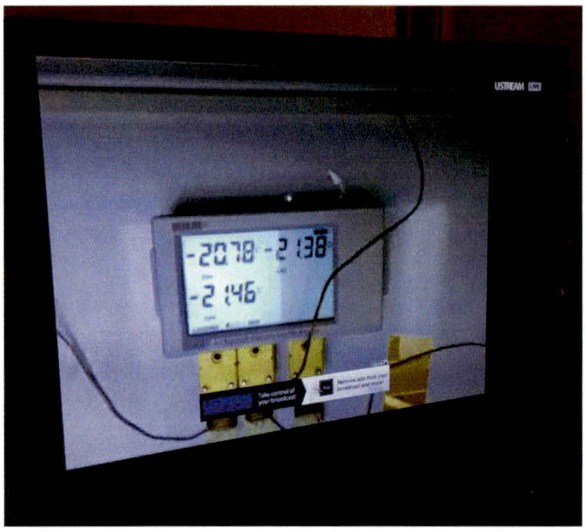

Fig. 1 Remote live stream of a temperature monitor for manual review and logging of temperatures. (Photo: Matthew Kirchoff)

In an outbreak or resource-constrained environment, creative solutions to operational problems are particularly important. Flexibility and ingenuity can help overcome unexpected challenges. For example, during one therapeutic trial for a monoclonal antibody to treat Ebola virus disease, a large amount of IMP was stored at frozen temperatures in a storage depot. Study staff were temporarily denied access to the site because of travel restrictions related to expected political unrest. In anticipation of the event, facility security staff were trained on emergency procedures related to equipment and power failure. As remote monitoring systems had not yet arrived, three extra computers and electronic tablets were positioned with remotely accessible cameras to view the local temperature readout of the freezer, enabling staff to regularly check freezer temperatures without traveling to the site during the travel moratorium (Fig. 1). At other times, a mobile phone hotspot function was used to set up remote temperature monitoring devices where land-based Internet coverage was unavailable but cellular Internet coverage was adequate.

2.1.2 Humidity

For pills, capsules, and powders, humidity can be a problem if they are not in a hermetically sealed container (i.e., completely airtight and impermeable to air and water vapor) or if they need to be stored for any length of time after opening. Exposure to high humidity can lead to product degradation and growth of microorganisms. The manufacturer should provide an acceptable relative humidity range along with storage temperature range. In practice, this is likely to entail air conditioning in tropical environments, as reducing air temperature also helps control relative humidity. In some cases, the use of desiccants (moisture-absorbing substances) within packaging can help control humidity levels for sensitive products. If relevant to the products being stored, humidity should be monitored and recorded along with the temperature. For liquid products in a sealed container such as a vial, humidity is generally not an issue and monitoring is not required but this should be verified in writing by the manufacturer.

2.1.3 Light

Light exposure can significantly affect the stability and efficacy of many medical products. Certain wavelengths of light, particularly ultraviolet (UV) light, can cause chemical reactions that degrade or alter the physical properties of medications. It is good practice to protect medical products from direct light exposure. The manufacturer may or may not provide information on light-related stability concerns, but in the absence of such data, light exposure should be minimized. Consider purchasing refrigerators with opaque doors rather than transparent windows. Room temperature medicines should be kept in closed cabinets, generally locked for security. Sterile drapes or similar materials can also be used to cover vials while thawing before preparation, and opaque bags may be used to cover prepared items, such as syringes with product drawn up, which have been removed from their original light-protecting containers. Record and justify the measures taken to protect products from light exposure. This documentation can be crucial for quality assurance and regulatory compliance.

2.1.4 Agitation

Agitating or shaking up an IMP may have adverse effects on stability such as protein denaturation, phase separation, or particle

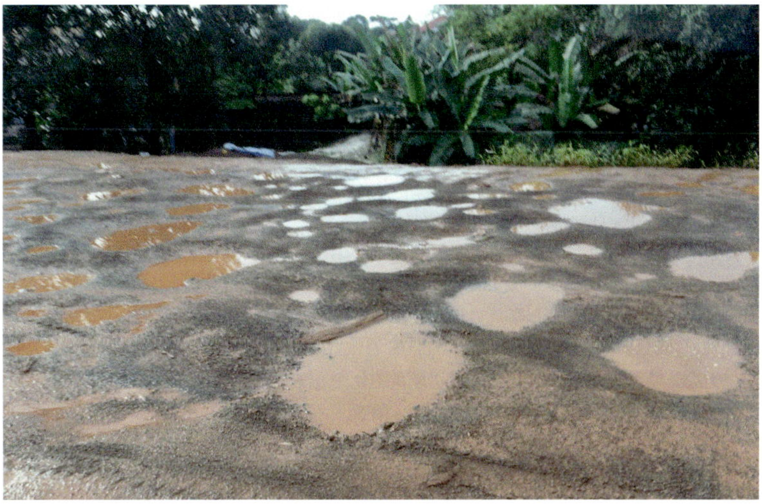

■ **Fig. 2** Potholes are common in dirt roads during and after the rainy season and can cause significant agitation. These potholes were present for the duration of a trip to a research lab in Monrovia, Liberia. (Photo: Matthew Kirchoff)

formation. Agitation is of particular concern in areas where roads may be poor, especially in rainy seasons. Investigators and pharmacists should make this a priority for discussion with the manufacturer as soon as an initial assessment finds that the product may need to be transported in difficult conditions (■ Fig. 2). Transport over any distance on bumpy roads should be authorized by the manufacturer based on thorough consideration, simulation if necessary, and cross-checking. This is a particular concern for liquid products, especially those that are protein-based such as monoclonal antibodies or certain vaccines.

2.1.5 Material Compatibility

Ensuring material compatibility is crucial for maintaining product stability, efficacy, and safety (Jenke 2009). Since investigational medicinal products are in an early stage of development, it may not be clear what materials could deleteriously affect them through contact. Examples of issues include leaching of plasticizers from IV bags, adsorption of protein-based drugs onto tubing or containers, degradation of light-sensitive compounds, and interactions with vial stoppers. This canpose significant challenges in remote locations or countries where a product manufacturer did not envision trials taking place, since procuring precisely specified compatible products may be difficult. Products in early development may only have one or two compatible materials listed, such as a single manufacturer's syringe or bag of intravenous fluids for product administration. Consider ordering compatible materials in advance along with the IMP. Sponsors may be willing to assist with procuring the required materials and will occasionally ship complete kits, which include the needed ancillary products for a single dose or single treatment course.

Tip

If multiple study products are used at a more research-naïve site, provision of kits for study products is particularly desirable to avoid inappropriate or accidental use of noncompatible products.

If the pharmacy manual details exact products for use with the IMP and those products are not available, notify the sponsor and ask whether a similar product is suitable. Request information on particular components of concern and details on what material components are known to be compatible or incompatible. Using this information, identify alternative products and provide their detailed component information to the sponsor for consideration. If a substitute is identified, obtain written agreement and file a copy in the study file.

2.2 Hazardous Material Precautions

Hazardous materials are substances that pose a potential risk to human health or the environment due to their physical, chemical, or biological properties. Perhaps the best-known guidance for the proper handling of hazardous drugs in healthcare settings, issued by the U.S. Pharmacopeial Convention, is referred to as USP 800 (USP 2020). Bernabeu-Martinez et al. (2018) note the availability of many sets of guidelines from around the world. Many investigational medicinal products are considered hazardous and require some level of precaution for handling and disposal. Pharmacy managers are responsible for ensuring that all staff are familiar with safe handling procedures, typically involving the use of personal protective equipment, containment systems during preparation, spill management procedures, and waste segregation. Many austere environments lack appropriate medical waste disposal systems, relying on incineration or dumping that allows access to scavengers seeking items for resale (Ali et al. 2017). Trial planning staff need to review site capabilities for product destruction before trial initiation so that alternative arrangements can be made if necessary, such as shipping selected products back to the sponsor or contracting with outside organizations. Regardless, a documented pharmacy IMP disposal plan with training provisions is required.

2.3 Labeling of Investigational Medicinal Products

2.3.1 Languages

The preferred language for labeling is the primary language where the product will be used, often the official or national language in a country with multiple languages. Professional staff anywhere are likely to know the official language well, but there may be environments in which other essential staff, for example, maintenance workers, drivers, etc., may not reliably understand that language. An official language may be widely spoken in the capital or major cities while other languages are more common in rural areas. An example of a complex labeling example arose in the Democratic Republic of Congo (DRC), where clinical trials of four experimental therapeutics for Ebola were conducted. With over 200 languages, the DRC is one of the more linguistically diverse countries in the world. While French is the official language and widely used in education and government, there are also four national languages: Kikongo (Kituba), Lingala, Swahili, and Tshiluba (Translators without Borders 2022).

In a multilingual environment, or when a product may go to sites with different primary languages, certified label translations in the most relevant languages should be available and provided with every IMP shipment. Deciding on the label language is essential in a multi-site study, as product loss at one site could necessitate temporary supply from another site with adequate inventory. Products labeled in one language may not be acceptable for import into another country. The labeling of IMP is regulated in many countries, and country-specific guidance should be sought. If labeling requirements are unavailable or unclear, regulatory bodies should be consulted prior to determining IMP labeling. This should be done as early as possible in a trial, as the labeling of IMP is often a process that must be scheduled in advance and integrated into a manufacturer's overall production schedule, often taking weeks or months of advance notice.

> **Tip**
>
> The manufacturer may be able to provide product packaging with multiple language translations on each package, accessed by peeling up the label to reveal an underside or additional folded labeling.

2.3.2 Stability Dates

Experience in the field suggests that for IMPs provided in unit-dose packaging or stored at frozen or ultra-low temperatures, the product

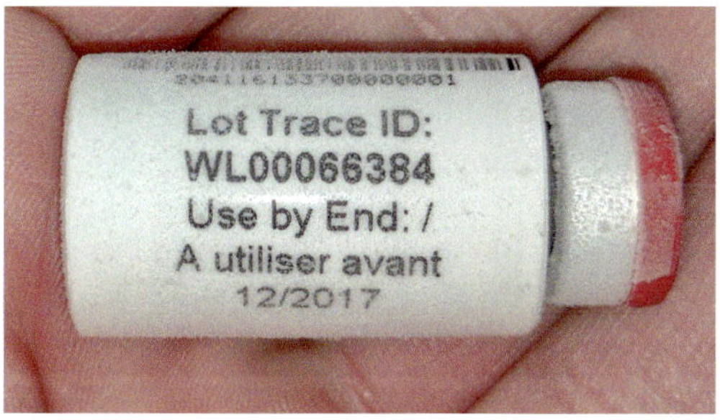

Fig. 3 A vial stored at less than −70 °C, which needs relabeling due to a pre-printed date. Writing or placing a new label is difficult due to the frozen temperature and layer of frost. (Photo: Matthew Kirchoff)

packaging should bear the printed lot number without a stability or use-by date, as the stability date is likely to be updated during the study, sometimes multiple times, necessitating relabeling if it were printed. Relabeling certain temperature-controlled products (Fig. 3) is time-consuming, complicated, and creates an additional risk of product loss, and relabeling products kept at ultra-low temperatures (less than −60 °C) is nearly impossible without materials specifically designed to function in the extreme cold. Relabeling products kept in a refrigerator or freezer may additionally cause degradation of the product when it is removed from the storage unit, and it may cause temperature excursions in the entire storage unit as a result of frequent door openings. At the same time, additional procedures must be put in place to ensure that products without printed stability dates are properly tracked and not inadvertently used past their stability date. A mix-up of products could be disastrous for a trial, resulting in participants receiving "expired" products of uncertain efficacy or the disposal of product due to uncertainty. Pharmacists may feel uncomfortable having vials without "use-by" dates, and risks and benefits should be evaluated for the particular trial and sites. An often-workable compromise is to label the cartons or boxes that contain products from the same lot. Prior to importing IMPs without printed dating on individually labeled units, consult country regulations to verify any related requirements specific to non-commercial investigational medicinal products.

2.3.3 Other Label Contents

In the United States, the Food and Drug Administration (FDA 2020) requires a label stating, "Caution: New Drug – Limited by Federal (or United States) law to investigational use." Requirements can differ for studies elsewhere: in principle, every sovereign country should have legislation and regulations covering such labeling issues, with some exceptions. The EU is moving away from national systems toward a unified European one (EMA 2022), and there are a number of gaps in the legislative and regulatory framework in some developing countries (Nuffield Council on Bioethics 2005). The U.S. National Institute of Allergy and Infectious Diseases (NIAID) is developing a compendium of clinical regulations from around the world, but its coverage is not universal (NIAID 2023). The World Health Organization (WHO) has an analogous Database of Regulatory Information Tracking of Clinical Trials Registration and Ethics Committees (REGTRAC), which provides links to many national regulatory authorities (WHO 2022). It is wise to make early contact on these and other regulatory issues with the Ministry of Health and the in-country partners cooperating on the research study.

3 Pre-response Planning

The quality of work performed during pre-response planning has a disproportionate influence on the launch and operational success of the trial. Elements deemed critical to trial initiation and success should be prioritized for careful consideration, broad consultation, and rigorous cross-checking.

3.1 Essential Elements

Actions or events that must occur for the project to begin or continue fall under the category of essential elements. An absence of or defect in any one of these factors may have a disproportionate effect on the success of trial operations, to the point of delaying or stopping the trial. Many tasks look essential at first glance. It is helpful to do a risk-based analysis of such elements during planning, considering the effect of each on trial readiness, scientific, and ethical standards, and staff and participant safety. Consider, for example, the following:

- Can the study start if element *x* is not complete, or can it wait until the trial is underway?
- If it can wait, what level of assurance is needed that it will happen?
- Will the element in question pose an unacceptable risk to participants, staff, or data quality?

Some examples:

- Inability to import and store the investigational medicinal product due to regulatory, political, or logistical constraints
- Inability to obtain required ancillary products for administration of the investigational medicinal product, for example, saline bags for infusion from a required manufacturer, infusion supplies, etc
- Inability to store or prepare the investigational medicinal product under the conditions required by the manufacturer because of shortfalls in power supply, facilities, trained personnel, or equipment
- Lack of personnel trained or licensed to execute required study procedures

Failure to maintain an adequate inventory of investigational medicinal product or associated medical supplies for administration is a trial-ending or pausing event. Other potential failure points relate to the inability to:

- Import the product while maintaining required temperatures due to customs and flight delays.
- Ensure 24/7/365 environmental conditions for product storage, including nights, weekends, and holidays.
- Secure the product from theft.
- Resupply the product as needed due to circumstances, including initial shortages, decisions to expand enrollment or add sites, or other changes in protocol.

There are other critical items that could be deferred to start a study expeditiously, but remain essential for the trial to proceed:

- Staff training. A core group may be able to begin implementing the study quickly and working out specific procedures, but additional trained staff will be needed as the study gets underway.
- Implementation of certain backup or secondary systems if they are not critical to protecting the health and well-being of participants. An example is uninterruptable power supply units if there is generator backup or secondary facilities with critical equipment.
- Dedicated and physically distinct investigational medicinal product quarantine space in a freezer, so long as there is room to quarantine the product and a way to physically separate and demarcate quarantined products with police tape or some other hard-to-miss visual indicator
- Acquisition of all study supplies necessary to support the study through complete enrollment and follow-up
- Implementation of electronic data capture and management systems when a paper system can be implemented
- Implementation of electronic temperature monitoring systems if regular temperature recordings on paper are acceptable.

3.2 Pharmacy Facilities and Infrastructure

In a traditional clinical trial, investigators can select research sites with capacity and support personnel ready to execute a study. During an outbreak in a resource-constrained area, sites may need to be developed *de novo,* or at least renovated, as proximity to the outbreak often becomes the most important selection criterion. Investigators and pharmacists may need to consider and recommend details such as selecting appropriate room surface finishes and developing power, water supply, plumbing, electrical wiring requirements, ventilation, cooling, etc., based on planned equipment (▶ Chap. 37). An example checklist of items to consider when developing or reviewing an existing facility follows.

1. Is the facility close enough to the product administration site to meet transport, temperature, and time standards for stability and sterility?
2. Does the facility have adequate space, and can this space be secured from unauthorized persons and accessed at all times by the pharmacy team?
3. Does the facility have sufficient power of the right type to support the cold-chain equipment, compounding hoods, or any other needs of the study? If not, can the power be rapidly augmented through generators, solar panels, or other means (▶ Chap. 39)?
4. Can the room temperature and humidity be maintained within the required parameters?
5. If needed for blinding, sterile product preparation, or counseling, can a portion of the space be made private?
6. Is there adequate space to prepare the investigational medicinal product, if needed?
7. Is there adequate space to securely store study records?
8. If phone or Internet connectivity is required for randomization or other critical tasks, is it available or can it be made available (▶ Chap. 34)?

3.3 Equipment Selection and Procurement

Pharmacy equipment is often specialized, heavy, sensitive, expensive, or all of these at once. Procurement time can be impressively long, with some equipment fabricated only once ordered, including many medical-grade refrigerators and freezers, and particularly ultra-low-temperature freezers. Consider the following questions during study startup:

- Where can equipment be procured, and how long will it take to purchase, receive, ship, clear customs, transport to the site, set up, qualify if needed, and train staff to use it? Is the equipment being sourced from Europe or another region of the world where companies may cease operations to give staff a month of vacation?
- Is there expertise at the site to:

- Assemble the equipment?
- Qualify the equipment for its intended use?
- Train other study staff on the equipment?

When choosing vendors, consider the availability of networks for service, spare parts, and repair, as well as whether the equipment can be serviced in the field by staff. A study could start without long-term maintenance plans in place, if necessary, but this presents an additional risk of having to rapidly procure replacement equipment or stop the study due to equipment malfunction.

3.3.1 Cold-Chain Equipment: Refrigerators and Freezers

An overview of cold-chain requirements follows (▶ Chap. 39), but a few cold-chain tips directly pertaining to the pharmacy are listed below. Refrigerators and freezers generally have a form factor of either upright (like a regular kitchen refrigerator), chest (approximately waist high), or portable (around the size of a drink cooler). ◘ Figure 4 compares several important form factor considerations when selecting a device, although individual devices vary in their capabilities.

When acquiring refrigerators and freezers, every possible attempt should be made to acquire a laboratory or pharmacy freezer (◘ Fig. 5) rather than a commercial freezer intended for food storage. Purpose-built units should have less variation in temperature ranges around the programmed set point, as well as a more uniform temperature throughout the storage space, which is essential when products must be stored within narrow ranges. Some manufacturers make specific models that are more robust for operation in adverse environments with unreliable power supply.

	Upright	Chest	Portable
Time to acquire	Slow: Often built to order. May incur shipping delays since usually must be shipped upright.	Medium: Unit is larger but can more easily fit in aircraft and truck beds for transport.	Medium-Fast: If in stock, can easily be shipped with other equipment and supplies.
Flexibility	Low: Large and difficult to move. Usually only capable of utilizing one power voltage, and has permanently attached plug.	Low: Large and difficult to move. Usually only capable of utilizing one power voltage, and has permanently attached plug.	Medium-High: Some models can run on 110-260 VAC and 12V DC (car outlet), with interchangeable plug types. Easily relocated by one or two people.
Internal storage space	High	High	Low
Temperature uniformity	OK	OK	Good
Contents organization and access	Excellent	Poor	OK-Poor
Needed room space	Medium	High	Low
Power requirement	Medium	Medium	Low
Service life	Medium	Medium	Low

Fig. 4 Refrigerator and freezer form factor comparison

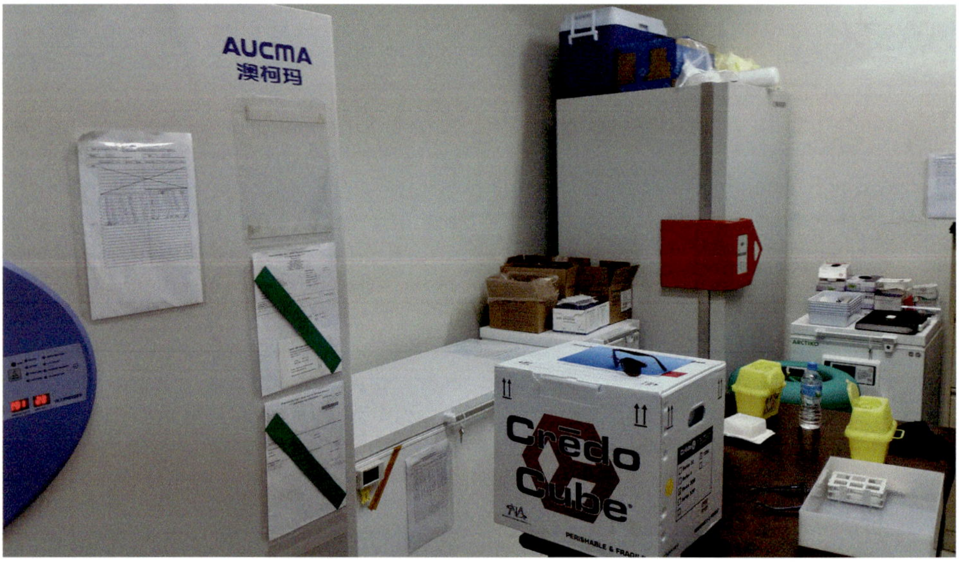

Fig. 5 A mixture of freezer types used at a study storage depot site in Freetown, Sierra Leone, including upright, chest, and passive transport containers. (Photo: Matthew Kirchoff)

A few other cold-chain tips useful to the pharmacy:

- Units filled with more mass are more stable in temperature and hold a temperature longer than a unit filled with mostly air. Consider filling up a portion of the empty space using bottles of water or other material with high specific heat, like phase change materials used in cold-chain shipping. It is critical that this mass is either added and allowed to stabilize at the correct temperature prior to the storage of temperature-sensitive products, or that the extra mass is brought to the same temperature as the unit before being placed inside. If done incorrectly, adding mass can cause a temperature excursion. Certain thermal phase change inserts for packaging can increase the temperature by tens of degrees Celsius and require days to stabilize.

- Ice packs or filled plastic water bottles can be used as thermal mass. Cool the thermal mass to the desired temperature in a storage unit not being used for product storage before transferring the thermal mass to a freezer with a temperature-sensitive product.
- Verify the definition of controlled room temperature for particular products.
- Temperatures in spaces that contain products labeled for storage at "Room Temperature" or "Controlled Room Temperature" need to be verified and recorded regularly.

The U.S. Pharmacopeial Convention revised its temperature and storage definitions in 2017 to meet the requirements of bodies like the FDA and ICH (► Sect. 6.2 includes a list of guidance). A useful note on current guidelines prepared by a commercial vendor has also been posted by USP, and WHO publishes a compendium of standards (USP 2017; Vaisala 2012; WHO 2003). Various standards and guidelines documents define controlled room temperature and other terms slightly differently, so it is important to be specific with temperatures rather than accepting terms like controlled room temperature without further specification.

Finally, if setting up a trial in a remote location, you may be required to rely on your partners to implement cold-chain and certain other systems. Be careful about ensuring that the partners agree in detail on a common standard for meeting regulatory expectations for controlled temperatures. It is critical to thoroughly assess each partner's storage for adequacy, including past performance, backup systems, procedures, and staff training. Regardless of the partner's reputation or assurances, pharmacists should meet in person to verify the setup and their common understanding of operating procedures, monitoring, etc. If the site is inaccessible, work through a copy of their standard operating procedures (SOPs) by videoconferencing, or at a minimum perform a step-by-step walk-through by telephone, covering critical procedures such as receipt, storage, and packaging of the product. Cold chain is a deceptively tricky process to implement effectively, and the quality tends to be variable. If the investigational medicinal product is highly temperature-sensitive, such as a messenger RNA (mRNA) vaccine or monoclonal antibody, there is no margin for misunderstanding.

3.3.2 Continuous, Real-Time Temperature Monitoring Systems

In our increasingly connected world, continuous, real-time temperature monitoring systems can be implemented almost anywhere, even in remote areas. Many monitoring devices run on batteries and can function two years or more before depletion, depending on the frequency of recordings and transmission. The final factor then becomes an Internet connection. Cellular data service is now available in most areas with sufficient population for an outbreak large enough to require a large-scale research response. Even with spotty connections, most remote monitors can store several days' worth of data, which are uploaded when the connection is restored. It is good practice to have a second Wi-Fi hotspot available but turned off, fully charged, topped up with account or subscriber identity module (SIM) card credit, and utilizing the same broadcast Service Set Identifier (SSID) and login credentials as the primary device (◘ Fig. 6). This allows for the second device to back up the first without reconfiguring site equipment.

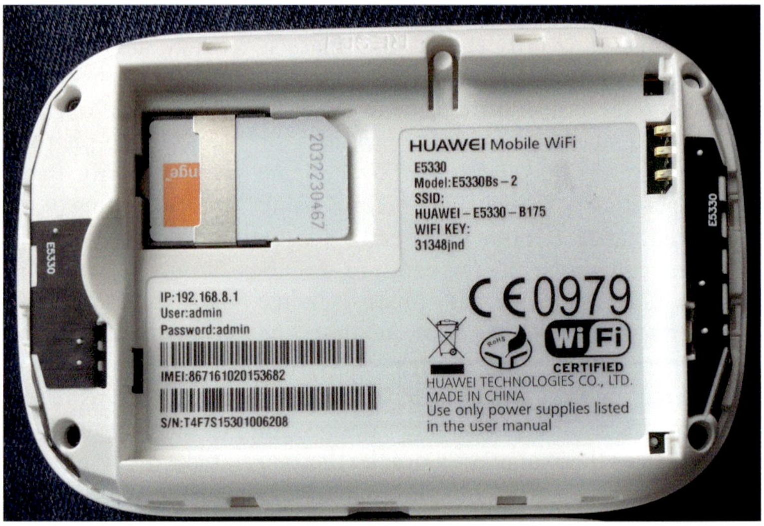

Fig. 6 A mobile hot spot device and SIM card used as an Internet backup device for real-time electronic temperature monitoring. (Photo: Matthew Kirchoff)

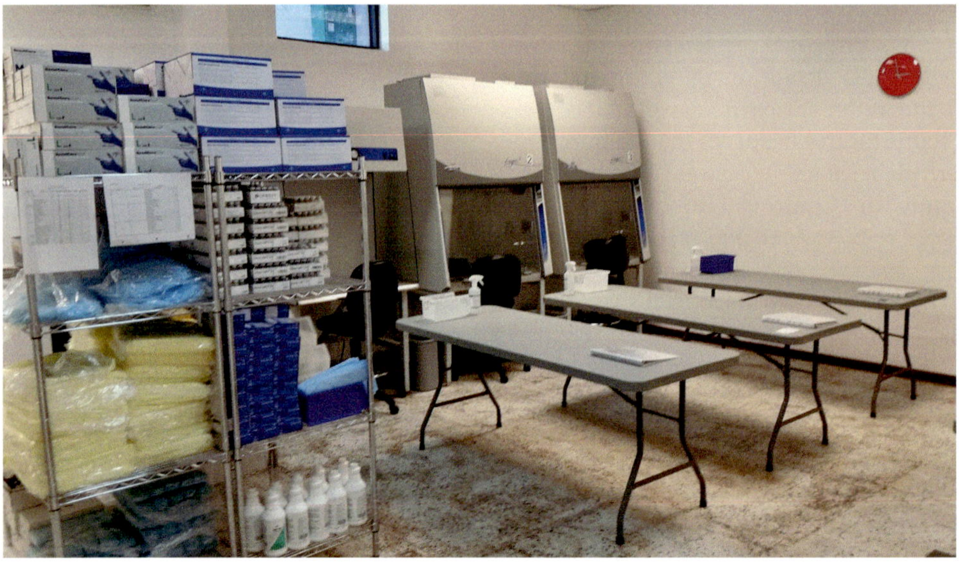

Fig. 7 Compounding space developed in West Africa from a storage facility. (Photo: Matthew Kirchoff)

3.3.3 Horizontal Flow Hoods and Biological Safety Cabinets

In an austere, remote environment, it may be impossible to locate or install a sterile compounding space (Fig. 7) for the preparation of sterile products. A pharmacist can, however, take measures to improve the conditions under which a sterile product is prepared. Simple precautions, when implemented correctly, can protect the product from significant contamination by the preparing staff and by the immediate environment. Such measures include wearing sterile gloves, sterile gowns, surgical/procedure masks, and bouffant caps. To mitigate contamination from the environment, a vertical or horizontal flow hood is called for, but if none is available the product may be prepared in a closed area sequestered from other activities, regularly cleaned with appropriate disinfectants, and with sterile drapes or other disposable sterile material

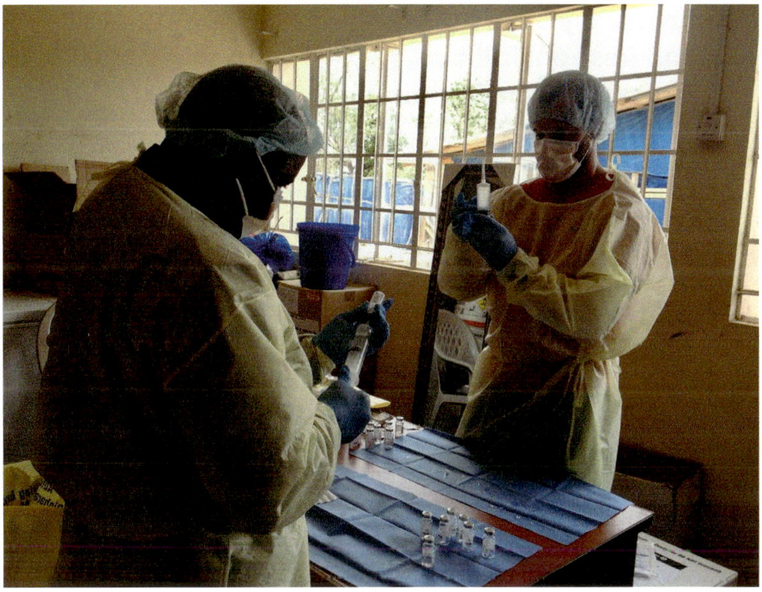

■ **Fig. 8** Compounding medications for administration to clinical trial participants. (Photo: Matthew Kirchoff)

used as a sterile field. If the space is a small, enclosed area, commercial high-efficiency particulate air (HEPA) filter devices can be added to the room. If light sockets are available and the area not continually occupied, an ultraviolet light bulb could be regularly run.

In an emergency, it is recommended that research pharmacists use their expertise in consultation with experts on the trial team or at the product manufacturer to determine if a basic solution, such as the one above, may be implemented until better equipment can be procured. The manufacturer may set the time for which the product can be held for use after final preparation based on advanced sterile compounding practices. Additional time and temperature restrictions may need to be placed on the compounded product to account for less-than-ideal sterility (■ Fig. 8).

3.4 Planning for Multiple Sites

In most multi-site trials, investigational medicinal products are shipped directly from the manufacturer to each research site, occasionally using a central shipping vendor that may ship to depots in different countries but seldom from one study site to another. Outbreaks can have several adverse effects on the supply chain, especially when countries cut transportation links in order to stop the spread of contagion or restrict exports to meet their own needs first. Add to that the overall difficulty of transport in underserved locations, and inter-site shipping may well become a more attractive logistics option than shipping from across the world.

When shipping an investigational medicinal product to a second site, consider the following steps:

- Obtain written permission from the sponsor and manufacturer.
- Obtain import and export permits, if needed.
- Notify regulatory authorities, if required.
- Ship product in thermal packaging, including a temperature monitor and copies of the temperature records for the product since receipt at the sending site (▶ Chap. 37).
- Include a product manifest.
- Write the allowable temperature range on the package or on a piece of paper inside.
- Provide clear written instructions to the receiving pharmacist. Instructions regarding whom to notify upon receipt of the product must be printed inside the package.

3.5 Pharmacy Staff Roles and Responsibilities, Education, and Training

According to the ICH E6 Efficacy Guidelines for Good Clinical Practice, "where allowed/required, the investigator/institution may/should assign some or all of the investigator's/institution's duties for IMP(s) accountability at the trial site(s) to an appropriate pharmacist or another appropriate individual who is under the supervision of the investigator/institution" (ICH 2016).

Clinical research pharmacists are critical members of the clinical study site team and must have the expertise to understand the special handling requirements of IMPs. Clinical research pharmacists assigned by the investigator or institute need to understand the management and documentation of IMP receipt, storage, dispensing, returns, and final disposition. They should possess an expert working knowledge of the clinical research study process, human subject protections, and national and local regulations governing drug research. They are responsible for providing information to the appropriate healthcare team members to enable correct dispensing of IMP (American Society of Health-System Pharmacists 2018).

It is critical to understand the educational and skill level of all partners and to arrange for additional training and assistance as needed. The practice of pharmacy across the world varies from pharmacists with doctorates, residencies, fellowships, and years of practicing bedside with physicians, to pharmacists with minimal specialized formal education (International Pharmaceutical Federation 1997). Some pharmacists lack the skills to administer vaccines, prepare intravenous admixtures, mix compounded medications, and ensure sterility where required. Some countries lack a legal and regulatory framework for pharmacists to practice at a level higher than product management and basic drug interaction checking. Pharmacists should not operate beyond their training or legal scope of practice. In an emergency, regulators may be willing to formally expand the scope of practice, in which case the pharmacists need to receive training on the new skills. The pharmaceutical manager in this scenario must document and sign off on the training received to ensure and be able to demonstrate that pharmacists do have the knowledge to fulfill their expanded duties. Regardless of the scope of practice, all research pharmacists should complete training and associated documentation on GCP, ICH guidelines, and ethical considerations, including aspects of patient safety and institutional procedures.

Visiting pharmacists not licensed in the country where research is conducted should seek clarity regarding their authorization to practice. Establishing a Memorandum of Understanding (MoU) with the host country allowing for recognition of foreign pharmacy licenses is an ideal scenario. Such an arrangement would generally be negotiated as part of a broader MoU covering healthcare personnel. In the absence of a formal agreement, ensure that all work requiring a licensed pharmacist is performed by or supervised by an appropriately licensed pharmacist. If a foreign pharmacist cannot practice pharmacy directly, they still may be able to advise and train the local pharmacists on study administration and procedures.

At a minimum, all staff should provide a current copy of their most recent pharmacy license, which should be maintained at the site and backed up at a second location. Expiration dates should be reviewed to ensure current licensure. A current *curriculum vitae* and any recent skill-specific training documentation should also be collected and kept with pharmacy licenses.

3.6 Concurrent Expanded Access Program Support

In an emergency, an investigational medicinal product may be made available for individual patients on a case-by-case basis, utilizing relevant programs or laws. A product may also be made more broadly available under an expanded access program, monitored emergency use of unregistered and experimental interventions (MEURI), or equivalent arrangements (FDA 2019; Lipsitch et al. 2016; WHO 2014). These programs do not have the scientific rigor of a controlled clinical trial and are a stopgap measure to provide some relief while trials can get underway, or for some patients who do not qualify for study enrollment. These programs may also be the unfortunate fallback if a trial is halted by extraneous circumstances (Rojek et al. 2020). Although it is preferable that an expanded access program not run concurrently at the same site as a trial using the same product, a site implementing an expanded access program could operate simultaneously with a clinical trial at nearby sites. Ring trial designs can also address the therapeutic misconception (the unwarranted belief that a candidate medical countermeasure is better for the recipient than alternatives or placebo), thus assuaging popular pressure for access to unproven medications. Pharmacists must be careful to ensure that the study product is not exchanged between the two programs. According to ICH (2016) E6(R2) 4.6.5, "The investigator should ensure that the investigational product(s) are used only in accordance with the approved protocol."

It is not appropriate for an expanded access site and a clinical trial site to exchange an investigational medicinal product, even during times of shortage. The primary risk falls on the trial site, as record-keeping at an expanded access site may not be adequate to verify the proper shipment and storage of the investigational medicinal product while it was held at the expanded access site.

4 Pharmacy Operations

4.1 Procuring Pharmacy Supplies

4.1.1 Importing Ancillary Pharmaceutical Products

A case can be made for procuring ancillary medications and supplies locally to take advantage of reduced export and import documentation, lower shipping costs, rapid availability, compliance with local regulations, and local staff familiarity with the products. Unfortunately, a number of factors may impede local procurement (Nebot Giralt et al. 2020):

- Specified products may not be available.
- Quality of generic products may not be assured.
- Products may not have been stored properly.
- Counterfeit products may be widespread.

For imports, follow general logistics guidelines (▶ Chap. 37), ensuring that any applicable export and import permits are in place and local procedures are followed. Include a copy of any permits with all shipments, placed in a location that will not require unpacking for access. A detailed inventory listing the products, identifier codes, lot number, and expiration dates should be included. Value of the products may also be needed for customs. Include information on whether the shipment contains products with specified temperature requirements on the outside of any packaging.

Be aware that many countries have laws and regulations governing the expiration dates of imported products. This is often a result of past experience with companies dumping short-dated or even expired products under the guise of assistance, often for tax advantages (Pinheiro 2008). Ideally, ensure that all products have an expiration date at least a year after import. Unless there is an MoU in place with a provision for duty-free import, be prepared to pay tax on imported medications. Finally, be aware that imported medications approved in another country, but not the host country, may be considered an unapproved, non-investigational medicinal product by the host country and require regulatory review or waiver. Ensure any waivers or determinations are documented in writing and readily available for inspection.

4.1.2 Management of Ancillary Products

It is strongly recommended that products critical to a trial be managed, segregated, and accounted for separately from identical or equivalent products used for general medical care. The separation of trial products serves two purposes. First, it creates barriers to accidental use of incorrect or incompatible supplies for preparation and administration. Second, it makes supply planning more predictable and accidental stockouts less probable. Keeping these products in the pharmacy near the investigational medicinal products helps ensure their careful management and prevents accidental use by a clinician at the site. Logs of these supplies and internal audits (stock takes) by staff should occur regularly, at least monthly. To explain one scenario, imagine a nurse selecting a 23-gauge needle and 3 mL syringe combination to administer a pharmaceutical. In general, clinical care needles of a given gauge, length, and associated syringes are interchangeable, so the nurse may or may not give a second thought as to which product is pulled, so long as it meets his or her requirement. In a clinical trial, limited compatibility data may require the use of one specified product, from a specific manufacturer, since it is possible that a syringe or needle containing different materials could interact chemically with the investigational medicinal product. It is critical, then, to ensure that the compatible product is available.

In scenarios where the preparation and/or administration of an investigational medicinal product requires a variety of ancillary products, consider creating "go bags" or "mobile kits" (Fig. 9). These can be particularly useful when conducting trials at multiple remote sites without dedicated clinical research staff, or if there is a significant chance of accidental use of trial supplies for regular care. This concept has been used with great success in several trials in West and Central Africa. Ideally, the investigational medicinal product owner, usually the manufacturer, will provide a quantity of prepackaged "kits" commensurate with the number of investigational medicinal product in each shipment, with some overage. Alternatively, a central coordinating site can create such kits and distribute them to sites. Kits should contain all necessary supplies to prepare and administer an investigational medicinal product. Overage should be included for critical items, such as sterile products that may accidentally become contaminated, or a certain number of backup kits should be provisioned with the full complement of required ancillary supplies. All kits should include an itemized contents log with expiration dates for perishable items and instructions for proper storage, and should be secured with serialized zip ties or other means to ensure the integrity of each kit. Contents of each kit must be regularly checked to ensure perishable items are replaced prior to their expiration.

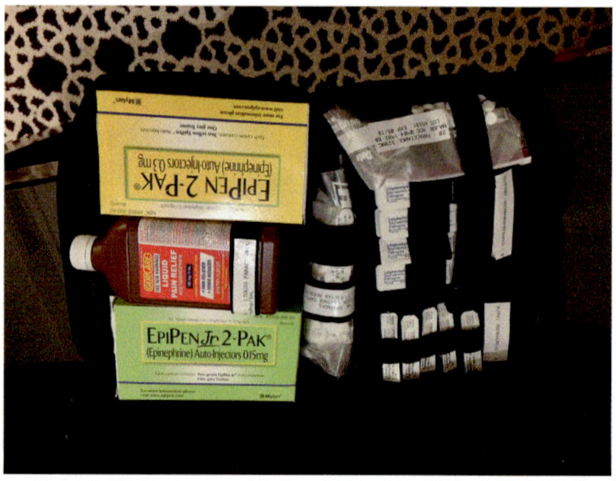

Fig. 9 An example of a "Go Bag" used in sites across West Africa to ensure basic supportive treatment for anaphylactic reactions. (Photo: Matthew Kirchoff)

5 Final Disposition

5.1 Final Disposition of Investigational Medicinal Products

Concurrence from the manufacturer should be documented in writing before any investigational medicinal products are destroyed. Guidance from the manufacturer should be followed, or if no guidance is provided, review local laws regarding destruction and follow them or exceed their requirements if they do not appear to ensure safety. Incineration is a common method and tends to be available in most locations. The standard for investigational medicinal product destruction in clinical research is to perform a witnessed destruction. A destruction form or memo placed in the study file should detail what products were destroyed, when, where, how, and by whom, with a second party witnessing the destruction and signing the form or memo.

5.2 Destruction or Donation of Ancillary Medical Products

Most countries will have a formalized process for the destruction of medical products. A local pharmacist should be well versed in those processes, including required notification to a regulatory authority or other documentation. For a variety of reasons such as accidental overstocking, order errors, or changes in protocol, pharmacists may find themselves with medical products which are not expired and no longer of use to the study. If it makes sense to donate these products locally, create a detailed list and obtain written concurrence from the principal investigator.

Under no circumstances should expired medications ever be donated (Pinheiro 2008). This has become a lively and sensitive political issue in many developing countries, and not without reason. Additionally, it may be illegal to donate medications that are not far from their expiration dates. Consult a local pharmacist or the regulatory authority for any requirements. If there are no prohibitions on short-dated approved medications, require assurance from recipients of any of these products that they will be used within the remaining unexpired time and that under no circumstances will these products be used after expiration. Your organization's reputation and possibly legal liability are on the line, and a well-intentioned but ill-judged donation could spell the end of your research. It is thus important to develop SOPs on the destruction and donation of medical products.

6 Foundational Guidance

Investigational pharmacy practice in an emergency has rarely been the focus of books, seminars, or training courses, but a few groups have produced articles or documents that provide a solid foundation when reviewed together. These materials should be shared with internal and partner pharmacy staff as reference and training materials. All documents and websites should be checked for updates; not only do laws and regulations change with developing technology, clinical practice, and new threats to human health, but organizations like ICH have established cycles of guideline revision. Pharmaceutical managers are critical during the investigational protocol because they ensure the integrity of IMP and ancillary therapy administration, compliance with the study protocol, GCP, and local and sponsor regulatory requirements. Investment in pharmaceutical management training is essential for current and future outbreak emergency responses since availability and management of clinical trial supplies typically become a bottleneck in the conduct of clinical studies.

6.1 Regulations

- National Institute of Allergy and Infectious Diseases (NIAID) ClinRegs, aggregating clinical research regulations from around the globe (NIAID 2023).
- Current ICH GCP and more than 50 additional clinical guideline documents are implemented by member regulatory agencies including the U.S. Food and Drug Administration (FDA), European Medicines Agency (EMA), and others (EMA 2021; FDA 2018; ICH 2016).
- FDA 21 CFR Part 11 or European Union Annex 11, and associated guidance documents (EC 2011; FDA 2003).

6.2 Operations

- American Society of Health-System Pharmacists (ASHP) Guidelines for the Management of Investigational Drug Products (American Society of Health-System Pharmacists 2018).
- Hematology/Oncology Pharmacy Association (HOPA) Investigational Drug Service Best Practice Standards (HOPA 2014).
- NIAID Division of Microbiology and Infectious Diseases (DMID) Guidelines for Clinical Study Product Management (NIAID 2015).
- Pharmacist-Prepared Dispensing Guidelines for Drugs Used in Clinical Research (Siden et al. 2012).
- Pharmacy Guidelines & Instructions for DAIT-Sponsored Clinical Trials & Networks (NIAID 2016).
- Practice Guidance on Pharmacy Services for Clinical Trials (Royal Pharmaceutical Society of Great Britain 2019).
- Requirements for Pharmacy Activities at [Division of AIDS] DAIDS-Supported Clinical Research Sites Conducting Clinical Trials Outside of the HIV/AIDS Clinical Trials Networks (NIAID 2014).

Discussion Questions

1. How is working with investigational medicinal products (IMPs) generally more challenging than working with approved pharmaceutical products?
2. Regarding IMP stability, it is critical to develop an early understanding of storage and transport requirements, conduct thorough planning with detailed attention to circumstances in the study setting, and pay close attention to an environmental control plan. Discuss methods for controlling the temperature, humidity, light exposure, physical agitation, and material compatibility of the IMP environment.
3. Describe some considerations for labeling IMPs in a multilingual environment.
4. An absence of or defect in any essential element for project initiation and continuation may have a disproportionate effect on the success of trial operations, to the point of delaying or stopping the trial. Considering the effect of each element on trial conduct, what questions should you consider first when performing a risk-based analysis of such elements during planning?
5. Discuss critical items to consider when developing or reviewing an existing pharmacy research facility during an outbreak in a resource-constrained area.
6. Pharmacy equipment is often specialized, heavy, sensitive, and expensive. Procurement time can be long, with some equipment fabricated only once ordered, including many medical-grade refrigerators and freezers, particularly ultra-low-temperature freezers. List important considerations of equipment selection and procurement during an outbreak in a resource-constrained area.
7. What are some important steps to consider when shipping an investigational medicinal product from one study site to a second site?
8. Why is it strongly recommended that ancillary products critical to a trial be managed, segregated, and accounted for separately from identical or equivalent products used for general medical care? Discuss the donation or disposal of ancillary medical products.

References

Ali M, Wang W, Chaudhry N, Geng Y. Hospital waste management in developing countries: a mini review. Waste Manag Res. 2017;35(6):581–92. https://doi.org/10.1177/0734242x17691344.

American Society of Health-System Pharmacists. ASHP guidelines for the management of investigational drug products. Am J Health Syst Pharm. 2018;75:561–73.

Bernabeu-Martinez MA, Ramos Merino M, Santos Gago JM, Alvarez Sabucedo LM, Wanden-Berghe C, Sanz-Valero J. Guidelines for safe handling of hazardous drugs: a systematic review. PLoS One.

2018;13(5):e0197172. https://doi.org/10.1371/journal.pone.0197172.
EC. EudraLex: the rules governing medicinal products in the European Union, Good manufacturing practice: medicinal products for human and veterinary use, annex 11: computerised systems, vol. 4. Brussels: European Commission, Health and Consumers Directorate-General; 2011.
EMA. Good clinical practice. Amsterdam: European Medicines Agency; 2021. https://www.ema.europa.eu/en/human-regulatory/research-development/compliance/good-clinical-practice. Accessed 27 May 2021.
EMA. COVID-19 vaccines: development, evaluation, approval and monitoring. Brussels: European Medicines Agency; 2022. https://www.ema.europa.eu/en/human-regulatory/overview/public-health-threats/coronavirus-disease-covid-19/treatments-vaccines/vaccines-covid-19/covid-19-vaccines-development-evaluation-approval-monitoring. Accessed 7 Feb 2022.
FDA. Part 11: electronic-records—electronic-signatures—scope-and-application. Washington, DC: U.S. Department of Health and Human Services, Food and Drug Administration; 2003.
FDA. E6(R2) good clinical practice: integrated addendum to ICH E6(R1) guidance for industry. In: Services USDoHaH, Administration FaD, (CDER) CfDEaR, (CBER) CfBEaR, editors. Washington, DC: U.S. Department of Health and Human Services; 2018. p. 60.
FDA. Expanded access: information for physicians. Washington, DC: U.S. Food and Drug Administration; 2019. https://www.fda.gov/news-events/expanded-access/expanded-access-information-physicians#ExpandedAccess. Accessed 3 Aug 2020.
FDA. Investigational new drug application. 2020.
HOPA. HOPA investigational drug service best practice standards. Chicago: Hematology/Oncology Pharmacy Association; 2014.
ICH. Good clinical practice: ICH harmonised guideline. Integrated addendum to ICH E6(R1): guideline for good clinical practice ICH E6(R2) ICH consensus guideline. Geneva: International Council for Harmonisation of Technical Requirements for Pharmaceuticals for Human Use (ICH); 2016.
International Pharmaceutical Federation. Standards for quality of pharmacy services: good pharmacy practice. The Hague: International Pharmaceutical Federation; 1997.
Jenke D. In compatibility of pharmaceutical products and contact materials. John Wiley & Sons, Ltd; 2009. https://onlinelibrary.wiley.com/doi/abs/10.1002/9780470459416.
Lipsitch M, Jha A, Simonsen L. Observational studies and the difficult quest for causality: lessons from vaccine effectiveness and impact studies. Int J Epidemiol. 2016;45(6):2060–74. https://doi.org/10.1093/ije/dyw124.
Nebot Giralt A, Bourasseau A, White G, Pouget C, Tabernero P, Van Assche K, et al. Quality assurance systems of pharmaceutical distributors in low-income and middle-income countries: weaknesses and ways forward. BMJ Glob Health. 2020;5(10) https://doi.org/10.1136/bmjgh-2020-003147.
NIAID. Requirements for pharmacy activities at DAIDS supported clinical research sites conducting clinical trials outside of the HIV/AIDS clinical trials networks. Bethesda, MD: National Institute of Allergy and Infectious Diseases, Division of Acquired Immunodeficiency Syndrome; 2014.
NIAID. DMID guidelines for clinical study product management. Bethesda, MD: National Institute of Allergy and Infectious Diseases, Division of Microbiology and Infectious Diseases; 2015.
NIAID. Pharmacy guidelines & instructions for DAIT-sponsored clinical trials & networks. Bethesda, MD: National Institute for Allergy and Infectious Diseases, Division of Allergy, Immunology, and Transplantation; 2016.
NIAID. ClinRegs: aggregating clinical research regulations from around the globe. 2023. https://clinregs.niaid.nih.gov/. Accessed 27 Jan 2023.
Nuffield Council on Bioethics. The ethics of research related to healthcare in developing countries: a follow-up discussion paper based on the workshop held in Cape Town, South Africa 12–14th February 2004. London: Nuffield Council on Bioethics; 2005.
Pinheiro CP. Drug donations: what lies beneath. Bull World Health Organ. 2008;86(8):580.
Rojek AM, Martin GE, Horby PW. Compassionate drug (mis)use during pandemics: lessons for COVID-19 from 2009. BMC Med. 2020;18(1):265. https://doi.org/10.1186/s12916-020-01732-5.
Royal Pharmaceutical Society of Great Britain. Practice guidance on pharmacy services for clinical trials. London: Royal Pharmaceutical Society of Great Britain; 2019.
Siden R, Tamer HR, Skyles AJ, Weadock S, Redic K. Pharmacist-prepared dispensing guidelines for drugs used in clinical research. Am J Health Syst Pharm. 2012;69(12):1021–6. https://doi.org/10.2146/ajhp110082.
Translators without Borders. Language data for the Democratic Republic of Congo. Garden City, ID: Translators without Borders; 2022. https://translatorswithoutborders.org/language-data-for-the-democratic-republic-of-congo-drc. Accessed 17 Dec 2022.
USP. Packaging and storage requirements. Rockville, MD: The United States Pharmacopeial Convention; 2017.
USP. (800) Hazardous drugs: handling in healthcare settings. Rockville, MD: The United States Pharmacopeial Convention; 2020.
Vaisala. FDA & ICH: regulations and standards for temperature-controlled supply chains. Vantaa, FI: Vaisala; 2012.

WHO. WHO Expert Committee on Specifications for Pharmaceutical Preparations—WHO technical report series, no. 908—thirty-seventh report. Geneva: World Health Organization; 2003.

WHO. Ethical considerations for use of unregistered interventions for Ebola viral disease. Geneva: World Health Organization; 2014. Contract No.: WHO/HIS/KER/GHE/14.1.

WHO. REGTRAC: the WHO database of regulatory information, tracking of clinical trials registration & ethics committees. Geneva: World Health Organization; 2022. https://apps.who.int/trialsearch/Regtrac.aspx. Accessed 29 Sep 2021.

39 Cold Chain and Electrical Power for Emergency Research Response

Daniel J. Littlefield

Contents

Learning Track Note: This chapter appears in Learning Tracks: Emergency Research Response, Research Operations

E. S. Higgs and R. A. Sorenson (eds.), *Principles and Practice of Emergency Research Response*,
https://doi.org/10.1007/978-3-031-48408-7_59

Owen Glendower: I can summon spirits from the vasty deeps.
Harry Hotspur: Why, so can I, or so can any man;
But will they come when you do call for them?
—Shakespeare, Henry IV, Part 1

Learning Objectives

This chapter will help readers understand and describe the following:

- The many requirements and backup measures needed to ensure that investigational medicinal products stay at specified temperatures during manufacturing, shipment, and storage (cold chain)
- Mitigation strategies for identified risks
- Steps to ensure a reliable electrical power supply and backup measures
- How to generate an impact and effort matrix for prioritizing mitigation strategies

1 Introduction

The system for keeping a product at a specified temperature from the point of production to final delivery is called a cold chain—a term used for food and some other commercial deliveries as well as in science and medicine. At each stage of production, storage, transport, and delivery, the product must be kept at the specified temperature. Many routinely administered vaccines and many advanced treatments, as well as investigational medicinal products (IMPs)—both vaccines and therapeutics—are highly sensitive to temperature excursions, that is, failure to maintain the prescribed temperature at all times. Some products must be kept at very low temperature (under −60 °C), where a nominal −80 °C freezer or dry ice might be used; others must be kept cold (2–8 °C) but protected from freezing (Wirkas et al. 2007); still others must be kept at controlled room temperature (15–25 °C) (ECA Academy 2017).

IMPs require particular attention because they are generally in short supply and have not been fully tested for tolerance of temperature variations. Biological samples from patients that must be analyzed must also be kept at specified temperatures (Gordy et al. 2019). It is not unusual to have temperature specifications that differ during the stages of shipment, storage, and use of the product (e.g., store frozen product at less than −60 °C; store at 2–8 °C after reconstitution). If that is not complex enough, clinical trials and laboratories can use multiple products with different temperature specifications. A temperature excursion, as a significant departure from the required temperature is known, can have dire consequences, such as rendering a pharmaceutical product or biological sample useless. Any temperature excursion will require that the affected product be quarantined, pending an assessment of whether it can still be used. An unrecorded excursion could lead to loss of product potency and failure of a trial and even endanger the lives of trial participants.

Such temperature specifications require attention to detail but are routine in developed countries with a reliable power supply, established distribution networks, readily available laboratory-grade freezers,[1] skilled maintenance personnel, and specialized packaging for transport. When a research program must be set up urgently in a low-resource environment, setting especially in a remote location like, say, the eastern Democratic Republic of the Congo (DRC), all of these requirements may be absent. While ▶ Chap. 37 discusses supply and logistics challenges more generally, this guidance is intended to help the reader cope with the specific challenges of the cold chain—something essential to virtually every clinical trial. It can be done wherever it must be done, but it requires careful planning and execution at every step.

This chapter starts with an overview of the distribution process, followed by good distribution practice and risk assessments and then preparedness and mitigation. We also outline how to ensure a reliable electrical power supply. Finally, we lay out some standard operat-

1 "Freezers" is used throughout the text to refer to various units ranging from ultracold or −80 °C units to 2–8 °C refrigerators. Likewise, while the text generally refers to INDs (investigational new drugs), the same considerations apply to other temperature-sensitive medications and supplies coming in and biological samples going out.

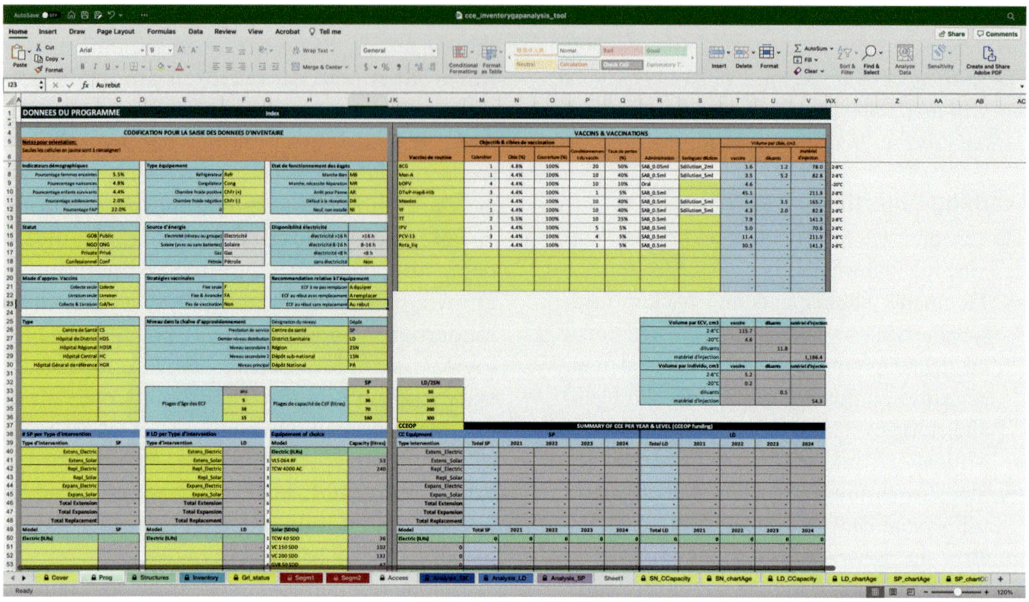

Fig. 1 Worksheet from a WHO cold chain inventory and gap analysis for an immunization program. (WHO 2021; Courtesy WHO)

ing procedures to help ensure success and prevent problems from turning into failures. We have cited more detailed guidance on specific aspects of cold chain management below. The World Health Organization (WHO) has produced a more detailed overview (WHO 2015); however, it is oriented to distribution of standard vaccines, which generally do not require the very low temperatures needed for many experimental products. Finally, just to make it abundantly clear that this short chapter cannot fully cover the subject, Fig. 1 is a screenshot of one worksheet of a WHO workbook produced to assist with practical cold chain inventory.

2 Process Overview

"Distribution of pharmaceutical products" (Fig. 2) covers the process by which products move from the manufacturer to the point of use, in conformity with temperature and other guidelines for their shipping and storage. While distribution focuses on storage locations or depots, products must also be kept at the specified temperatures during transport and at point of use.

2.1 Storage Locations or Depots

A storage site or depot that stores temperature-sensitive products for a clinical trial will require freezers (Fig. 3) and refrigerators to handle the specified temperature ranges of all the products and supplies needed for the trial.

Each type of unit should have at least one backup unit in case of malfunction. The freezers will generally need to be in air-conditioned rooms: freezers produce heat during operation, and most will not operate effectively if the ambient temperature is above 30 °C. Tropical-rated freezers can operate at up to 43 °C, but ambient room temperature is still important for efficiency and to minimize the chance of a temperature excursion during put-away, picking, or packing and for storage of room-temperature items. Ambient air-conditioning in the depot should be monitored, controlled, and operated with the same level of monitoring and safeguards applied to freezers. All of this equipment will need a reliable power supply, as explained below.

Freezers and refrigerators used for storage of investigational new drugs (INDs) should be designed for this purpose. Commercial, nonpharmaceutical-grade freezers and refrig-

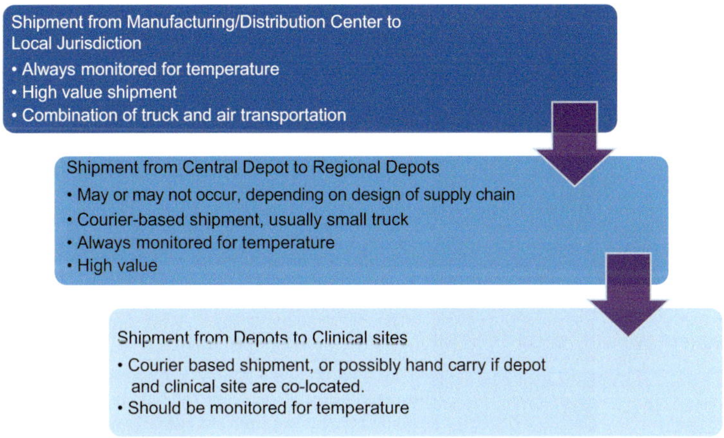

Fig. 2 Distribution of pharmaceutical products: basic elements of a cold chain system. (Author)

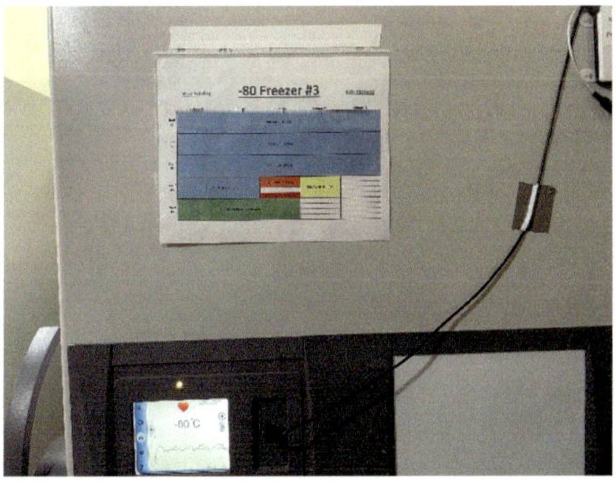

Fig. 3 −80 °C storage freezer at the Liberian Institute for Biomedical Research (LIBR). (Photo: Dan Littlefield)

erators are fine for storage of phase change materials but are not as consistent with their temperature control as pharmaceutical-grade freezers and refrigerators.

All depots have a standard set of steps that apply to the distribution process: receive, put away, store, pick, pack, and ship. The six steps shown in Fig. 4 are the framework for assessment and operation of the depot.

2.2 Transport and Packaging

Success in packing and shipping temperature-sensitive INDs requires qualified thermal packaging, good standard operating procedures (SOPs) for packing and shipping, and properly trained staff to implement SOPs. Transport disruptions can occur anywhere and anytime but are especially likely in poorly served, remote areas during emergencies. Less developed transportation networks may be subject to additional delays during rainy seasons or because of other factors. Shipments into and out of a country may also be held up by customs, port clearance, and other administrative and entry-exit requirements.

Thermal packaging is broadly separated into two categories: active and passive. Some characteristics of active and passive cooling are outlined in Fig. 5. Active shipping solutions are defined as those that provide cooling rather than just insulation and therefore require electrical power. Batteries are used to power active packaging while they are in transit and unplugged. Active "shippers" (shipping units) also have power cords that can be plugged into electrical outlets at storage locations and in a vehicle if so designed. Most active shippers use a compressor and refrigeration system and heating system to maintain temperature in the payload area. Active packaging is heavy and expensive but provides good temperature control. Passive thermal packaging uses the thermodynamic properties of a phase change material (frequently water-based for refrigerated products and dry ice for deep frozen) to counteract the heat that is transferred from the environment into the product packaging. Passive thermal packaging is much more economical and lighter than active packaging but has limited duration and is not as forgiving of extreme environmental conditions or delays.

Depot Process Step	Considerations
Receive	Products should be received and inspected immediately upon delivery. This includes recording temperature of product as received and inspection of the temperature monitor and packaging.
Put away	IND should be put away in the correct storage location promptly to prevent temperature excursions. The newly received product should be placed in a separate location and identified as "quarantine" until released by quality control. Temperature data from the shipment's temperature monitor should be reviewed and sent promptly to the appropriate quality reviewer, usually the trial sponsor.
Store	Storage equipment should be qualified, temperature mapped (ISPE 2016; WHO 2019), continuously monitored, and manually inspected at least once a day by local staff. All of this should be appropriately documented.
Pick	When a request for a product is received by the depot, the local staff must be certain they are selecting the right product for the request. The product should be removed from storage only when thermal packaging is ready for use.
Pack	The time between when the product is removed from storage and properly packed should be minimized. Packing should be done promptly and correctly, consistent with standard operating procedures (SOP).
Ship	Shipping arrangements must be consistent with the qualification of the thermal packaging used. That is, the packaging should be rated to hold the internal temperature within the specified range for the duration and ambient temperature exposure expected, plus a safety margin.

Fig. 4 Process steps in depot operation. (Author)

	Active Cooling	Passive Cooling
Equipment examples	Air conditioning units, refrigerators, freezersand active shippers	Ice chests(including dry ice), thermal shippers with phase-change materials (PCM)
Electricity requirements	Required: grid / mains power; battery for shippers	PCM and gel pack inserts need conditioning in a refrigerator or freezer prior to use
Ability to regulate temperature	Yes, usually able to set and vary temperature throughout a range	Only moves toward the gradient of the ambient
		environmental temperature, usually colder to warmer
Ruggedness	Has moving parts that can break, susceptible to electrical damage	Usually high, with no moving parts or possibility for electrical damage
Ease of use	After setup, typically requires little maintenance other than an air filter and battery change, occasional defrost	Requires processes to ensure duration and proper conditioning of PCM prior to each use
Cost	Higher ($2,000 - $15,000)	Lower ($100 - $1,000)
Mobility	Conventional units may weigh several hundred kilos; portable units which can be carried by one to two people are becoming more available	High, shipment packages can usually be carried by one to two people
Duration of hold	Indefinite if supplied with power	Commonly up to 96 hours, some capable of around a month
Temperature monitoring	Preferably internet-connected continuous monitoring	Battery-operated data logger
Other requirements	Back-up power supply (UPS), voltage regulator	None

Fig. 5 Features of active vs. passive cooling. (Author)

Thermal packaging is qualified for a product temperature range, duration of shipment, and expected ambient conditions. First, the product temperature specification *must* match the temperature range for the thermal packaging. Second, the planned shipping route should take no longer than the qualified duration of the thermal packaging. Finally, the shipment should be protected from unusual ambient temperature extremes. Keep in mind that one cannot rely on transportation companies or customs agents to follow instructions on packages or shipping documents rigorously.

Qualification is often done by the supplier of thermal packaging and can be generally relied on, especially for reputable suppliers of thermal packaging. If this documentation is not readily available, a field expedient qualification can be done. The qualification should have a protocol that describes how the qualification will be done. Temperature monitors are used to confirm that temperature is maintained appropriately within the thermal packaging. The packaging should be exposed to the expected worst-case temperature environment as far as is practical for the expected shipment duration. Data from the temperature monitors should confirm that the payload area of the thermal packaging maintained adequate temperature control through the qualification. The results should be documented in a report.

Phase change material (PCM) packaging and gel packs used for passive thermal packaging must be brought to the needed temperature, or preconditioned, in a freezer or refrigerator before they are used. *The preconditioning cannot be done in a freezer where IND is being stored:* the phase change (liquid to solid) is an energetic process and can cause a temperature excursion inside the freezer as it occurs. Once the PCM/gel pack is preconditioned to the proper temperature, it will be ready to use for transport or can be moved to a freezer that is storing IND—where it will provide the benefit of additional time to act in the event of a power loss.

Data loggers that record time and temperature inside the package during shipping should always be used, if at all possible, because they can confirm that the product has stayed within temperature specifications. Quality cannot be inspected into a flawed process, so monitoring is not a substitute for qualified thermal packaging, effective SOPs, and training. Many passive thermal packaging systems will provide 72 hours or more of controlled temperature storage for an IND, and, as noted, the packing materials, once they are cold, can help safeguard against the consequences of a power loss.

The transportation process can be broadly separated into two parts: shipment of IND from manufacturing/distribution center to the local jurisdiction and shipment of IND within the local jurisdiction from cold chain storage depots to clinical sites. The movement of IND into the local jurisdiction is normally via international shipments that are a combination of truck and air shipping modes. Challenges in this part of the supply chain include long routes, delays in customs, and restrictions based on flight availability. Best practices for these shipments are use of high-quality thermal packaging and reputable logistics companies that have the capability to intervene in a shipment in the event of delays (i.e., addition of dry ice to a shipment that is running low or even repackaging of a shipment as needed with fresh phase change materials).

Within the local jurisdiction, the transport process is likely to be via courier and small vehicles (trucks, autos, even motorcycles). The emphasis should be on determining the worst-case duration for each mode, which is commonly much longer than is typical. For example, a truck shipment from depot to clinical site on an unpaved road during rainy season may normally take 2 hours but up to 16 hours if the road is flooded. These issues are captured during the risk assessment discussed in ▶ Sect. 3 below.

3 Assessment

The two cold chain assessment methodologies we recommend are good distribution practice (GDP) assessment and risk assessment. By performing the GDP assessment, you ensure that the distribution process is consistent with regulatory guidelines and industry best practices. The risk assessment ensures that you have investigated failure modes of the process and completed risk identification, analysis, and evaluation. Both analyses are critical to success in distribution of temperature-sensitive IMPs in challenging circumstances. The initial step of any assessment is to create a good process map of the cold chain process, one which identifies each distribution step, describes the storage and transportation conditions for the products, and outlines the activities at each location.

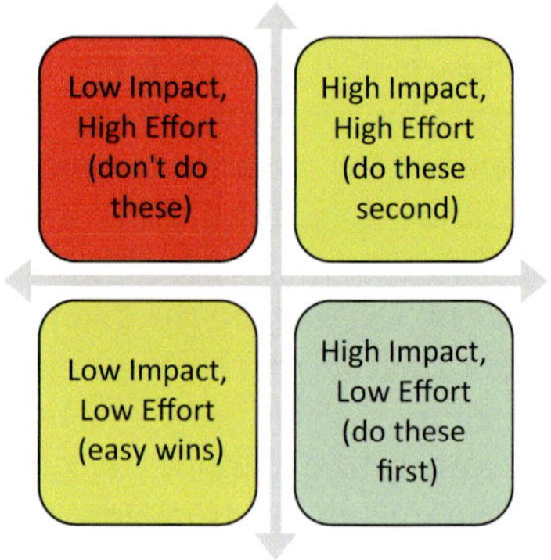

Fig. 6 Impact/effort matrix. (Author)

3.1 Good Distribution Practice (GDP) Assessment

The objective of the GDP assessment is to identify any gaps between current practice at a depot and industry guidance. This can be in the form of a questionnaire based on appropriate industry guidance. We recommend the U.S. Food and Drug Administration (FDA) Good Manufacturing Practices, European Medicines Agency (EMA) Guidelines for Good Distribution Practices, and Health Canada Guidelines for Temperature Control of Drug Products during Storage and Transportation (CFR 1999; EMA 2020; Health Canada 2011). WHO Annex 9 can also be used as a basis for a GDP assessment (WHO 2011). FDA guidance for good distribution practices has little detail. EMA and Health Canada guidance is more thorough but more prescriptive. WHO Annex 9 is a long, detailed, and prescriptive document, almost impossible to follow exactly in most emergency response clinical trials, but the WHO has also issued a user-friendly pamphlet version (John Snow Inc. and WHO 2003). Our recommendation is to use these documents as they pertain to local needs.

If a depot location has not been finalized or there are options to choose from, GDP assessment can help determine their relative suitability. The technique we recommend is an impact/effort matrix to map out the resources needed to bring each of the options into acceptable compliance. The impact/effort matrix (Fig. 6) is a commonly used Six Sigma tool that can be used to map mitigation tasks into one of four quadrants: high impact and low effort, high impact and high effort, low impact and low effort, and low impact and high effort. The object is to prioritize work to do the easiest, most useful tasks first.

3.2 Risk Assessment

Risks to the cold chain must be assessed to improve the robustness of the distribution process during trial operation. There are a number of methodologies used in the industry, and any are suitable. The International Conference on Harmonization of Technical Requirements for Pharmaceuticals for Human Use (ICH) Q9 Quality Risk Management covers all the common techniques (ICH 2005). Failure mode effect analysis (FMEA) is commonly used in the industry; another good method is a hazard and operability study (HAZOP). Both methods are described in versions of ICH Q9 promulgated by the FDA (FDA and ICH 2006) and EMA (EMA and ICH 2015).

There are two key points to risk assessment in emergency response clinical trials:

1. Murphy's law: if it can go wrong, it will.
2. A redundant layer of protection is needed for all quality critical processes.

In a real-world example we experienced, one research program had a cold chain depot powered by the national electrical grid and

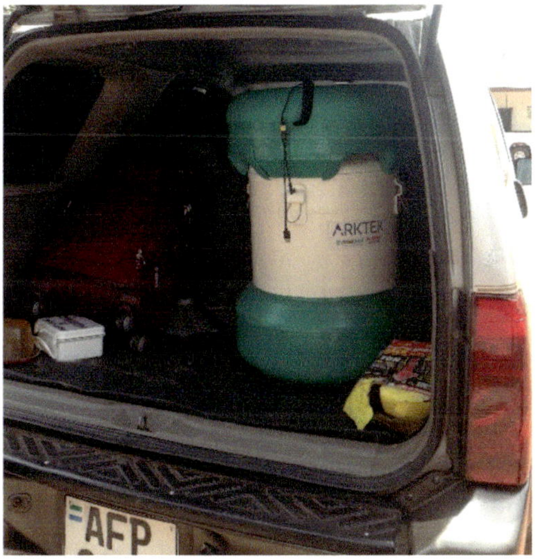

Fig. 7 Transporting passive storage containers (ARKTEK®) for last-ditch emergency response. (Photo: Dan Littlefield)

three backup generators operated by a global social welfare organization. A last-ditch emergency response plan using passive storage containers (Fig. 7) was also in place.

Electrical grid power was cut during road maintenance, and the first backup generator was started up; ran out of oil thanks to leaks; and burned up after about 12 h of operation. The second and third generators suffered similar fates in 12-h increments, leaving the site without power in under 36 h. We were never advised of the issues until all the generators had failed. We implemented our emergency response plan (good for 96 h) and arranged to have a generator installed and operated by our organization. No product was lost in the incident, but it illustrates that even what seems to be a triply redundant system may not be as strong as it seems, especially if all the backup units can fail for the same reason.

4 Electrical Power

Electrical power can be unreliable in many places and yet is essential for successful research operations. Brief and practical information for managers is below, but note well that electricity is complicated and can be dangerous. An appropriately trained and licensed individual should review critical decisions involving electrical supply and equipment selection. Expertise in both the particular features of local electricity supply and the power requirements of scientific equipment may be needed—another instance where full partnership between local and foreign experts may be essential. In any case, untrained individuals should not attempt to wire, modify, or test electrical connections, as this can result in serious injury or death.

4.1 The Basics

Some basic concepts include supply current (amperage, amps, or A), number of phases (single or three phase), voltage (volts, or V), hertz (Hz), plug type, grounding, power supply type, and backup electricity. Electricity is supplied via direct current (DC) and alternating current (AC). DC electricity is most commonly supplied from batteries, such as from a car's electrical system. AC is used in building electrical systems and some solar refrigeration or freezing systems and is typically used in more powerful motors and fans. Note that DC electricity may be converted to AC if needed, and vice versa, using a device called an inverter.

Electrical current, or the amount of electricity flowing, is measured in amps (A). Voltage, or volts (V), is a measure of electromotive force. AC power also has a frequency represented by hertz (Hz), which is the rate at which current changes direction per second and is discussed in ▶ Sect. 4.3 below. Pharmacy equipment and building electrical supply are usually either 50 or 60 Hz.

Power, measured in Watts (W), is calculated for DC and AC electricity as follows:

$$\text{Watts}\left(\text{DC Power}\right) = \text{Amps} * \text{Volts}$$

$$W = A * V$$

$$\text{Watts}\left(\text{AC Power}\right) = \text{Amps} * \text{Volts} * \text{Power Factor}$$

$$W = A * V * \text{PF}$$

This calculation is useful to estimate the size of a generator to provide backup power to an equipment set. The easiest way to estimate a generator's size is to use the rated watts for all the equipment it will supply. Once the total wattage is known, a generator should be selected where the total wattage needed is 85% of the rated generator power.

4.2 Connectors (Receptacles and Plugs)

Different regions of the world also use different AC plugs and receptacles. In nations relying on substantial international donor support for facilities and equipment, a room or building may use an unexpected electrical plug. Adaptors may be obtained to convert between one adaptor plug type to another, but care must be taken to ensure that the adaptor is rated to handle the maximum current of the equipment being plugged in. Underrated plugs may catch fire or otherwise fail. Plugging equipment into a receptacle with the wrong power supply could immediately destroy the equipment or, possibly worse, result in the equipment initially appearing to function but causing insidious malfunctions and eventual failure over time. *Always test electrical outlets before use.* The handheld-sized devices used to test a receptacle are called "multimeters" and are available at hardware and online stores. Electrical receptacles in a building use unique plug types intended to prevent their accidental use, giving a clue as to the power supply at the receptacle (assuming correct wiring).

4.3 Power (Amps, Volts, Hertz)

The installed receptacle in a facility should indicate the amperage rating of the receptacle. However, critical equipment such as ultralow temperature freezers should be plugged into outlets which are on their own wiring circuit so that the full amount of rated current is available to the equipment. Multiple pieces of equipment wired on the same circuit could deplete the available current.

Electrical motors often have a much higher power draw on startup than would otherwise be calculated using $W = V * A$. This consideration is critical when selecting equipment such as an uninterruptible power supply (UPS) (◘ Fig. 8), which may stop supplying power to the attached equipment if overloaded. A single power outage could also cause a large spike in energy demand if multiple motor-driven pieces of equipment are attached to the same electrical supply and simultaneously pull a large electrical load to start backup.

4.3.1 Voltage and Cycle

The voltage of a building's electrical outlets will likely be 100–120 or 230–240 V. Outlets may have a higher voltage if wired to support specific equipment. AC electrical outlets in

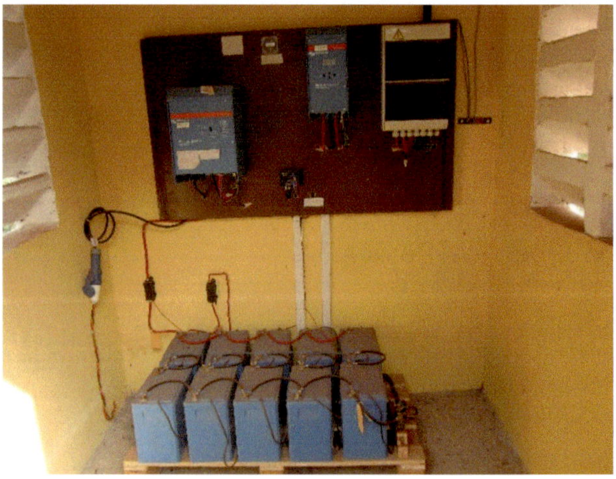

◘ **Fig. 8** Uninterruptable power supply, Sierra Leone. (Photo: Dan Littlefield)

buildings will be either 50 or 60 Hz, and selected equipment should be built to run on the available electrical supply frequency or risk abnormal operation. A motor designed to run at one frequency, or hertz, will run proportionally slower at a lower hertz and faster at a higher hertz.

4.3.2 Grounding (Earthing)

Countries with strict enforcement of building codes are likely to be grounded (earthed) as required per appropriate guidelines. Facilities which are older or in a country with less strict code enforcement may be grounded inappropriately, inadequately, or not at all, despite the presence of a ground pin receptacle on an electrical receptacle. Improper grounding is particularly concerning as it could result in electrocution to an equipment user or more frequently the insidious malfunction and eventually complete failure of equipment. Ground wires are often grounded by running and burying the ground in the earth. This is often not found in older buildings in countries without strict code enforcement.

4.3.3 Power Supply Type: Grid, Generator, Solar

There are three primary types of power supply to a cold chain facility. Each has its own advantages and disadvantages. In all cases, multiple different sources (primary and backup) are recommended to reduce the chance of common failure modes.

Grid or "national" power is provided from dispersed sites by generating stations. It has the advantages of low cost and minimal support required from the research program team. The disadvantages include more or less frequent outages, and often relatively poor quality of power, e.g., fluctuations in voltage that can burn out unprotected equipment.

Generator power has the advantage of reasonably high reliability and ease of operation. Generators are commonly used in developing countries, and high-quality generators are readily available, as is maintenance assistance. Operating costs—chiefly fuel—can be very high, and proper maintenance is essential for good operation.

Solar power has become more popular as it comes down in cost but has significant limitations. Solar power generation itself is zero cost, but a solar power system requires not only solar panels but batteries to store power, along with inverters and transfer switches to supply power to end use locations. At least until recently, solar power has been useful primarily for low-current services and is of course rendered less useful when sunshine is reduced or when dust covers the panels.

The standard mix in low-resource situations, as long as a grid connection is available, is primary use of national (grid) power with generator backups.

4.3.4 Backup Electrical Power Source

When the primary source of electrical power goes down, there are several backup options. A good rule is to have two alternatives to the primary source of electrical power. Use of a UPS is an effective means to ensure continuous supply of power in the event of a limited outage from the primary power source. A UPS should be sized to support critical equipment, and noncritical equipment should not be connected to it. The sizing should match the expected duration of most power outages. The other advantage of a UPS is that it also provides protection from voltage fluctuations, eliminating the need for separate voltage regulators.

Ahead of the UPS, backup power should generally be provided by one or more generators sized to support critical equipment. Generators can be installed with automatic startup and automatic transfer switches (ATS) to eliminate the need for someone to intervene and start the backup generator (Fig. 9) when it is needed. Care should be taken to be sure the ATS is properly installed, as they can be damaged, especially in areas with poor grounding.

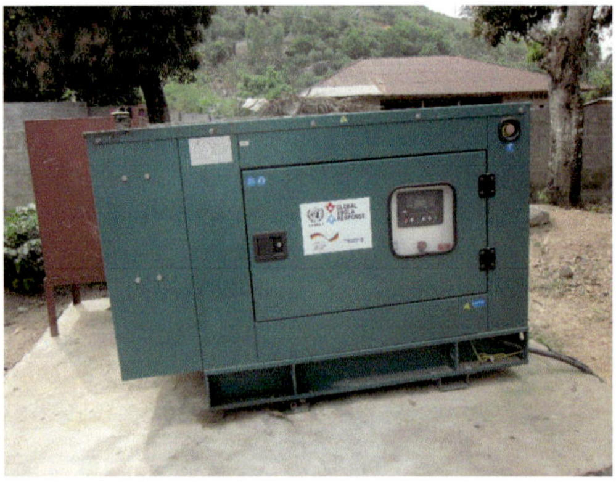

Fig. 9 Backup generator, Sierra Leone. (Photo: Dan Littlefield)

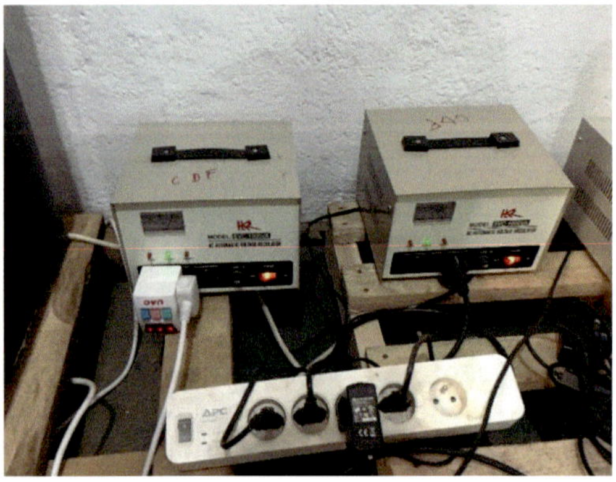

Fig. 10 Voltage regulators mounted on pallets in case of standing water in the building. (Photo: Dan Littlefield)

4.3.5 Surge Protectors and Voltage Regulators

Surge protectors guard against damage to sensitive equipment from voltage spikes. In other words, they can protect equipment from high voltage conditions, but not if voltages drop. For this reason, they are best used only in low power services. Voltage regulators (Fig. 10) have the advantage of protecting from high and low voltage conditions. This makes them optimal for sensitive equipment that could be affected by low voltage as well. Voltage regulators are sized for a maximum wattage and should be selected to ensure they are adequate for the maximum power required by the equipment.

Electrical power is often very unstable in developing countries. Daily outages and voltage swings large enough to damage equipment are commonplace. All sensitive equipment should be provided with a voltage regulator to protect it from damage from voltage swings. In addition, most countries use alternating current (AC) electricity at 50 Hz, rather than the 60 Hz used in the United States. Before procurement of any electrical equipment, specifications must be reviewed to ensure it can be used where intended.

5 Preparedness and Problem-Solving (Mitigation)

The logical follow-on to good distribution practice (GDP) and risk assessment is to develop and practice implementation of a mitigation strategy. GDP gaps and hazards that have a moderate to high likelihood of affecting patient safety or the success of a trial must be addressed. In emergency response clinical trials, the most important mitigations will ensure successful operation during power outages, robust packing and shipping processes, regular preventative maintenance (PM), and effective response to emergencies. Implementation of the mitigation measures that follow will significantly improve IND storage and distribution.

5.1 Redundancy

The most common strategy to mitigate equipment failure is redundancy. Two freezers are better than one, as the second can be used as a spare in the event of failure of the first freezer. However, the two freezers also have a common failure mode—loss of power—just as multiple generators can have a common failure mode, such as loss of lubricating oil. Using a strategy that accounts for common failure modes will thus help reduce the likelihood of failure. One might, for example, want to install both a gasoline-powered and a diesel-powered generator made by different manufacturers in order to guard against fuel supply interruptions and any weaknesses common to a single manufacturer's products. It is also important to have a passive (non-powered) storage alternative based on thermal packaging materials for INDs; we have experienced failures of triply and even quadruply redundant power systems.

5.2 Qualification

Freezers must be qualified to confirm that they are suitable for storage of INDs. There are three primary steps to qualification: installation qualification (IQ), operational qualification (OQ), and performance qualification (PQ). Once user requirements are defined, the correct freezer can be selected. Freezers/refrigerators fall into three broad temperature categories: −80, −30, and 2–8 °C. Residential/commercial nonpharma equipment is not recommended for the storage of INDs, because they cannot be successfully qualified. The installation qualification for a freezer is focused on ensuring that the equipment is designed and built to meet the user requirements (primarily temperature range and storage volume). The operational and performance qualifications are commonly combined for freezers and refrigerators. The objectives of the OQ/PQ are to map the interior of the freezer and find the hottest and coldest locations, demonstrate adequate temperature performance after installation, and demonstrate adequate performance during upset conditions (open door and loss of power).

5.3 Monitoring

Remote continuous monitoring is very useful for process documentation and oversight. The challenge may be Internet availability. A sophisticated process is needed to install a Wi-Fi hotspot and ensure it is maintained, regularly refilled with credit, and connected. Access to the hotspot should be restricted to prevent inappropriate use of the limited bandwidth (▶ Chap. 34). When selecting a continuous temperature monitoring system, consider battery backup with a data storage and push system that can overcome temporary losses of Internet connection.

5.4 Preventing Shipment Failures

Storage equipment and power failure are of greatest concern because the result can mean catastrophic loss of all IND, but the most *likely* failure to occur is loss of temperature control during shipment because of errors in packing and shipping. The most egregious shipping error we have experienced was shipping a frozen product in only corrugated cardboard with no insulation. A key part of SOPs for thermal packaging is proper preconditioning of gel packs/PCMs (phase change materials). Failure to follow these procedures will result in temperature excursions in passive thermal packaging. It pays to think through all the risks: the most common problem in shipping many vaccines for routine immunizations is that they are damaged by freezing when packed with materials cooled to too low a temperature (PATH 2003).

5.5 Standard Operating Procedures for Mitigation

SOPs should be easy to follow, written in a language the expected users can read, and readily available in the work area. We have encountered organizations that assured us they had SOPs, but they were locked up and the person with the key was not available. We interpret that as "we do not have SOPs." The users should be trained and drilled on the SOPs regularly. This means more than reading the procedures; hands-on training and performance of critical functions such as starting up and checking generators must be practiced and assessed, along with implementing passive backup using thermal packaging materials.

Training in basic concepts of heat transfer and thermodynamics can also be valuable. Most staff working in depots and pharmacies have no engineering background, but training in the basics will help them think problems through rather than follow SOPs by rote. Some of the more important concepts include the following:

Equipment Type	Recommended Inspections
Temperature Monitors	Check battery life, check and/or replace calibrated probes.
Freezers	Listen for unusual sounds, check for liquids under equipment, check for frost buildup around seals, check air filters, check alarm conditions.
Air conditioning (HVAC)	Check for proper drainage, check air filters and replace on schedule.
Electrical outlets	Check all outlets for discoloration or warping from high temperature, inspect all plugs and cords for same.
Voltage Regulators	Check alarm conditions, inspect all plugs and cords for discoloration or warping from high temperature.

Fig. 11 Preventive maintenance inspections by equipment type

- Mass of material directly affects the rate of temperature change; greater mass means lower rate of change.
- Thickness of insulation affects rate of heat transfer.
- Temperature difference (ambient vs. packaged material) affects rate of heat transfer.
- Most of the heat sink in passive thermal packaging is in the phase change of the gel packs/PCM.
- For any given rate of heat transfer (q), the rate of change of the temperature of the contents of a freezer is q/mc_p, where "m" is the mass of the contents and c_p is the specific heat of the contents.

For example, a −80 °C freezer with 100 2 mL vials of IND and insulation that allows about 2 kcal/h of heat transfer will reach −60 °C in just about 1 h. If 10 kg of already frozen gel packs are added into the same freezer (note: gel packs must be frozen *before* placing them in a freezer with product because the phase change of the gel packs requires a lot of energy and can cause a temperature excursion in the freezer), the time to reach −60 °C is closer to 50 h. The additional gel packs, because of their much larger mass (10 kg vs. 0.2 kg IND), will require much more heat to raise their temperature.

5.6 Preventive Maintenance

Equipment and facilities need systematic inspection and maintenance as specified by the manufacturer. Ideally, incipient failures will be detected and corrected before they occur or at least before they turn into major defects requiring expensive and hard to arrange repairs. Figure 11 provides a useful list of equipment and recommended basic inspections.

5.7 Emergency Response

In spite of best efforts by all involved, failures will occur (see Murphy's law). Timely, effective response will protect your IND. Assuming your SOPs are in place, the first important step to emergency response is to recognize there is an emergency. Remote monitoring and alarming of freezer temperatures and electrical power help with this. If that is not possible, 24-h staffing of the facility can meet the same need. Emergency phone call/SMS lists should be prominently posted within the site and outside the storage facility. Provision should be made for the emergency contacts to travel quickly to the facility if needed. Many local staff members may not have vehicles, and response cannot be left to rely on public transport during off hours. Role-play scenarios should be created and exercised to give staff the opportunity to troubleshoot and anticipate problems. Such scenarios can help uncover problems with emergency response SOPs, allow staff to talk through troubleshooting strategies for various equipment failures, and provide real-life illustrations for training on concepts of heat transfer and thermodynamics.

6 Case Study

Storage of Ebola vaccine at central depot in Freetown, Sierra Leone. Frozen vaccine is stored at <−60 °C. The freezer is a four-shelf unit kept at −86 °C. Onset® Hobo® brand temperature monitors are used to continuously monitor the product temperature. Two additional −80 °C freezers are maintained in the depot to store phase change materials for use in shipping and passive storage. In addition, the two spare freezers are fully qualified to store product in the event the main freezer fails. All the freezers share the same electrical source, which creates a potential common failure mode (identified in the risk assessment). Because of the common failure mode, additional emergency response plans were developed to protect the product.

First, passive storage containers capable of maintaining <−60 °C for 4 days were put in service and kept as emergency storage in the event of loss of power. These were specialized passive thermal packaging, and two were always available. Because of the unreliability of power from the site generators, an additional generator dedicated to the cold chain depot was installed. The quality of power from the national power supply was not good, and automatic transfer switches failed multiple times. Therefore, manual switching of power to the backup generator was required. Since security guards were available around the clock, they were trained to respond to a power outage by switching the transfer switch and turning on the generator. Because the security guards were motivated and competent, they were also trained on basic preventive maintenance and operation of the generator. They were responsible for checking water, oil, and diesel levels in the generator; they ran the generator under load every week to confirm it functioned and were responsible for emergency response and notification in the event of a power outage. Their work resulted in three successful interventions to prevent possible temperature excursions, and they maintained critical preventive maintenance documentation. In addition to product storage, vaccine syringes were prepared in the depot. The vials were thawed so the product could be diluted and placed in syringes. The syringes were then stored in passive thermal packaging at 2–8 °C, where they were good for 12 h. The packaging available in Sierra Leone was a good returnable package, but the pack-out procedures had not been designed or qualified. The initial pack-out, with three frozen gel packs and one refrigerated gel pack, resulted in temperatures that were too low. The pack-out was optimized to two frozen gel packs and two refrigerated gel packs, and the thermal packaging was then highly successful. During an 8-month period where more than 12,000 vaccine syringes were prepared, there were 4 deviations, but no product loss from temperature excursions. The deviations were all electrical power related.

7 Conclusion

Consistent temperature control remains a challenge even for routine vaccine delivery in many countries (Kristensen et al. 2016), but with the right expertise, sufficient funding, and attention to training and operations, it can be achieved even in the most difficult environments. Given the indications that the world is seeing novel pathogens at an increasing rate (Frutos et al. 2020), and the reality that many of these will emerge in low-resource environments (Di Marco et al. 2020), it is essential to maintain and improve cold chain expertise and methodology so that the necessary research to counter EID threats to humankind, as well as distribution of the resulting vaccines and therapies, can continue as universally and equitably as possible.

Case Study and Discussion Questions

Observations During Site Assessment

Storage of Ebola vaccine at central depot in Freetown, Sierra Leone. Frozen vaccine is stored at <−60 °C. The freezer is a four-shelf unit kept at −86 °C. Onset® Hobo® brand temperature monitors are used to continuously monitor the product temperature. Two additional −80 °C freezers are maintained in the depot to store phase change materials for use in shipping and passive storage. In addition, the two spare freezers are fully qualified to store product in the event the main freezer fails. All the freezers share the same electrical source. Site staff tell you that the quality of power from the national supply as well as the power from site generators is unreliable. The automatic transfer switch has failed multiple times. Security is available around the clock. In addition to product storage, vaccine syringes were prepared in the depot. The vials were thawed so the product could be diluted and placed in syringes. The syringes were then stored in passive thermal packaging at 2–8 °C, where they were good for 12 h. The packaging available in Sierra Leone was a good returnable package, but the pack-out procedures had not been designed or qualified. The initial pack-out, with three frozen gel packs and one refrigerated gel pack, resulted in temperatures that were too low.

1. *Identify and list potential risks based on the observations in the site assessment. Several examples follow*:
   - The shared electrical source between the freezers is a potential common failure mode.
   - No backup storage option is available to maintain the vaccine temperature <−60 °C if power is lost.
   - There are no pack-out procedures for the passive thermal packaging, and the packaging is not qualified.

2. *Generate and discuss possible mitigation strategies for identified risks. Several examples follow*:
   - Because of the electrical common failure mode, additional emergency response plans should be developed to protect the product. Consider how new procedures can be implemented at the site.
   - Obtain and use passive storage containers capable of maintaining <−60 °C for 4 days as emergency storage in the event of loss of power. How many passive thermal packages are needed? How long must they be qualified for?
   - Because of the unreliability of power from the site generators, an additional generator dedicated to the cold chain depot should be installed. Consider the preventative maintenance that is required for a generator and who will be expected to perform it.
   - Due to failure of the automatic transfer switch, manual switching of power to the backup generator will be required. The 24/7 security guards can be trained to respond to a power outage by switching the transfer switch and turning on the generator.
   - Review and optimize the passive thermal packaging pack-out, and perform shipments with temperature monitors included to monitor the internal temperature. Consider the number and temperature of the phase change material.

3. *Create an impact and effort matrix for the mitigation strategies such that they can be prioritized.*

   The risk ranking scale used is as follows:
   - High impact—failure to mitigate could result in adverse impact to operations
   - Low impact—would be helpful to have

   The effort score represents the amount of effort required to implement the mitigation strategy:
   - Low effort
   - High effort

   The prioritization can then be done focusing on high impact, low effort items first (refer to the impact and effort matrix).

   Fill in the table below and discuss.

Identifier	Description	Mitigation Strategy	Responsible party	Impact	Effort
A	–	–	–	–	–
B	–	–	–	–	–
C	–	–	–	–	–
–	–	–	–	–	–
–	–	–	–	–	–
–	–	–	–	–	–
–	–	–	–	–	–
–	–	–	–	–	–
–	–	–	–	–	–
–	–	–	–	–	–
–	–	–	–	–	–

Foundational Guidelines

- International Society of Pharmaceutical Engineers Good Practice Guide: Controlled Temperature Chamber Mapping and Monitoring, 2016 (ISPE 2016).
- U.S. Code of Federal Regulations, Current Good Manufacturing Practices for Finished Pharmaceuticals (CFR 2022).
- European Commission, Guidelines of 5 November 2013 on Good Distribution Practice of medicinal products for human use (EC 2013).
- WHO, Model guidance for the storage and transport of time- and temperature-sensitive pharmaceutical products (Annex 9) (WHO 2011).
- ICH, Q9 Quality Risk Management (ICH 2005).
- Parenteral Drug Association, Technical Report No. 52 Guidance for Good Distribution Practices (GDPs) for the Pharmaceutical Supply Chain (Parenteral Drug Association 2011).

References

CFR. Minimum requirements for the storage and handling of prescription drugs and for the establishment and maintenance of prescription drug distribution records. Sect. Chapter I, Sub-Chapter C, Part 205, 205.50. 1999.

CFR. Current good manufacturing practices for finished pharmaceuticals, Title 21, Chapter I, Subchapter C, Part 211. 2022.

Di Marco M, Baker ML, Daszak P, De Barro P, Eskew EA, Godde CM, et al. Opinion: sustainable development must account for pandemic risk. Proc Natl Acad Sci USA. 2020;117(8):3888–92. https://doi.org/10.1073/pnas.2001655117.

EC. Guidelines of 5 November 2013 on good distribution practice of medicinal products for human use. 2013.

ECA Academy. What are the regulatory definitions for "ambient", "room temperature" and "cold chain"? Mannhein, DE: ECA Foundation; 2017. https://www.gmp-compliance.org/gmp-news/what-are-the-regulatory-definitions-for-ambient-room-temperature-and-cold-chain. Accessed 2 Apr 2020.

EMA. Good distribution practice. Amsterdam: European Medicines Agency; 2020. https://www.ema.europa.eu/en/human-regulatory/post-authorisation/compliance/good-distribution-practice. Accessed 2 Apr 2020.

EMA, ICH. Guideline Q9 on quality risk management. London: European Medicines Agency; 2015.

FDA, ICH. Guidance for industry: Q9 quality risk management. Washington, DC: U.S. Department of Health and Human Services; 2006.

Frutos R, Lopez Roig M, Serra-Cobo J, Devaux CA. COVID-19: the conjunction of events leading to the coronavirus pandemic and lessons to learn for

future threats. Front Med. 2020:7. https://doi.org/10.3389/fmed.2020.00223.
Gordy D, Tashjian RS, Lee H, Movassaghi M, Yong WH. Domestic and international shipping of biospecimens. Methods Mol Biol. 2019;1897:433–43. https://doi.org/10.1007/978-1-4939-8935-5_35.
Health Canada. Guidelines for temperature control of drug products during storage and transportation. Ottowa: Health Canada; 2011.
ICH. Quality risk management Q9. Geneva: International Conference on Harmonisation of Technical Requirements for Registration of Pharmaceuticals for Human Use; 2005.
ISPE. Good practice guide: controlled temperature chamber mapping & monitoring. Bethesda, MD: International Society for Pharmaceutical Engineering; 2016.
John Snow Inc., WHO. Guidelines for the storage of essential medicines and other health commodities. Arlington, VA. John Snow, Inc./DELIVER, for the U.S. Agency for International Development; 2003.
Kristensen DD, Lorenson T, Bartholomew K, Villadiego S. Can thermostable vaccines help address cold-chain challenges? Results from stakeholder interviews in six low- and middle-income countries. Vaccine. 2016;34(7):899–904. https://doi.org/10.1016/j.vaccine.2016.01.001.
Parenteral Drug Association. Technical report no. 52: guidance for good distribution practices (GDPs) for the pharmaceutical supply chain. Bethesda, MD: Force PGfGDPftPSCT; 2011.
PATH. Protocol for evaluating freezing in the vaccine cold chain. Seattle: Program for Appropriate Technology in Health; 2003.
WHO. Model guidance for the storage and transport of time- and temperature-sensitive pharmaceutical products (Annex 9). Geneva: World Health Organization; 2011. Contract No.: 961.
WHO. The vaccine cold chain. Immunization in practice: a practical guide for health staff—2015 update. Geneva: World Health Organization; 2015.
WHO. Cold chain equipment inventory and gap analysis tool. Geneva: World Health Organization; 2021.
Wirkas T, Toikilik S, Miller N, Morgan C, Clements CJ. A vaccine cold chain freezing study in PNG highlights technology needs for hot climate countries. Vaccine. 2007;25(4):691–7. https://doi.org/10.1016/j.vaccine.2006.08.028.

40 Selecting and Opening a Clinical Research Site in a Low-Resource Setting

Olivier Tshiani Mbaya, Wissedi Njoh, Kevin Barrett, Mary Smolskis, Alejandra Miranda, and Nikki Gettinger

Contents

Learning Track Note: This chapter appears in Learning Tracks: Clinical Research; Emergency Research Response, Research Operations; Research Ethics; Social Science Response Research

E. S. Higgs and R. A. Sorenson (eds.), *Principles and Practice of Emergency Research Response*,
https://doi.org/10.1007/978-3-031-48408-7_60

Learning Objectives

This chapter will help readers understand and describe the following:

- Essential requirements for a clinical research site
- How a "roadmap" and flowcharts can help ensure proper implementation of clinical protocols
- What is required for conducting clinical research in an infectious disease emergency in a remote area with limited resources
- The roles of different agencies and institutions in providing clinical care and conducting quality clinical research
- Contingency planning to safeguard the successful implementation of a research study
- Examples of creative problem-solving in previous emergency clinical research response

1 Introduction

This chapter covers principles and practicalities for selecting research sites during an infectious disease emergency and getting them into operation. While the coronavirus disease 2019 (COVID-19) pandemic has demonstrated that emergency research response even in the most developed countries needs improvement, it is very likely that the next outbreak with pandemic potential will occur in more challenging circumstances in a developing country (Jones et al. 2008; Morens and Fauci 2020). We thus focus on resource-constrained locations with limited infrastructure, where various obstacles can impede rapid implementation of a research agenda, even setting aside possible civil or military strife. It is important to understand the tribal, ethnic, religious, political, and economic circumstances in the research area (▶ Chap. 18)—one of many reasons it is essential to have in-country partners (▶ Chap. 30). The disease outbreak itself may have caused or intensified societal conflict, while compromised health status prevalent in a population may have exacerbated the outbreak, especially if the outbreak affects refugee or displaced populations (Braveman 2011). The baseline assumption for this chapter is that the emergency response research program is conducted in a challenging, resource-limited location and requires detailed planning and tireless attention to ensure that site selection and preparations satisfy research needs.

The better developed and more stable the research location is, the less likely all the steps outlined here will be necessary. A lower security risk level, sound infrastructure, and a population with secure livelihoods are all important: the disease burden may be lessened by effective community education, the local medical system may be better able to cope, power and water may be more readily available, etc. However, the considerations, precautions, checklists, actions, and processes presented here can still serve as a fundamental baseline of structural needs relevant to any research program, regardless of external circumstances.

As we hope this book makes clear, scientifically rigorous, ethically sound clinical research during outbreaks is possible even where there are few resources and considerable dangers (Mulangu et al. 2019; NASEM 2017). Other chapters cover many other requirements, but on the most basic level, one cannot conduct research without a sound structure. In some of the examples we describe from the 2014–2016 West Africa and 2018–2020 Democratic Republic of the Congo (DRC) Ebola outbreaks, there was no such place, or there were bare walls and a roof but little else (Kennedy et al. 2016; Mulangu et al. 2019). We hope our experiences in setting up research sites will prove useful to anyone who needs to establish one, whether they are starting with an empty field or a well-equipped medical facility.

2 Primary Considerations

Before initiating any research project, the protocol team should identify a group of people within the team who will oversee identifying and securing the research site. These team members, referenced as "planners" in this chapter, will need to consider these important questions:

- What must be done?
- Where can it be done?
- When does it need to be done?
- Who will do it?

Thinking through these basic questions in advance will inform protocol development, site assessment and selection, and study implementation (Brett-Major and Lawler 2018). Throughout the project, these concepts should be continually evaluated to determine whether changes or adaptations are needed.

2.1 What Must Be Done?

The research question to be answered is always the primary determinant of the "what" (Sigfrid et al. 2019). Prevention and treatment studies (vaccines as opposed to therapeutic agents) may have quite different requirements, especially when considering the disease epidemiology, geography, infrastructure, and resource needs—perhaps the primary consideration for site planning being whether the study participants will be hospitalized patients, people coming from the community for appointments, or people in the community contacted by mobile research staff.

2.2 Where Will It Be Done?

A disease outbreak can occur over a wide geographic area, and the choice of where to locate research sites within that area will be influenced by multiple factors, some of which the people planning the research project have little control over. These include political circumstances, operational security, disease incidence and other epidemiologic factors, population density, and infrastructure. As these factors become understood, planners will make and refine their decisions about where to locate both central and satellite research sites—bearing in mind that location choices might be revisited as the epidemic develops.

2.3 When Does It Need to Be Done?

In an outbreak or other infectious disease emergency, the answer to "when" is usually "as soon as possible." When the goal of the research is not only to assess the safety and efficacy of medical countermeasures (MCMs) but to mitigate and control an outbreak, lives are at stake, and successful protocol implementation has a corresponding urgency. Nonetheless, planners also need to consider the entire life cycle of the study, from recruitment through follow-up and making conclusions available. The outbreak itself could be viewed as a "stakeholder" in the planning since it could change the protocol at any moment through a decrease or increase in disease incidence or a change in pathogen phenotype.

The initial protocol implementation schedule guides staff members in the preparation and hiring of staff, procurement and delivery of equipment and supplies, and infrastructure requirements like power and water. At the same time, understanding the potential trajectory of external factors which could impact the protocol allows the operations team to anticipate how quickly implementation can occur and how a changing situation could affect the study timeline. While planning a research response to an epidemic, though, the primary consideration will be urgency. In the case of Ebola in West Africa, most research studies did not get well underway before the outbreak started to wane, leaving too few Ebola cases for statistically significant results (Kennedy et al. 2016). Site selection is among the first things that must be done, since just about every other necessary step—equipment, staff, power, and water installation—requires that the research site be identified and modifications planned, scheduled, and accomplished.

2.4 Who Will Do It?

Protocol research teams comprising principal investigators, clinicians, pharmacists, laboratory technicians, psychosocial and social mobilization experts, data managers, statisticians, community engagement staff, participant trackers, trainers, project managers, etc. are generally the "who" (▶ Chap. 42). Additionally, for the overall success of the project, research collaborators and partners, including the local community, need to be informed and engaged (▶ Chap. 18). These groups may include the following:

- Governments, national and foreign
  - Health ministries
  - Government-supported research institutions
  - National healthcare system
  - Universities
  - Official development assistance agencies, disaster assistance if warranted
  - Military and security personnel (may complicate community acceptance)
- Private sector healthcare and educational institutions
- International organizations and diplomatic representatives, e.g., the World Health Organization (WHO), the United Nations (UN), bilateral embassies
- Nongovernmental organizations (NGOs) including medical response, e.g., Doctors Without Borders (MSF) and the International Medical Corps (IMC)
- Stakeholders affected by the outbreak, e.g., community leaders and advocacy groups
- International and local contractors
  - Supply vendors
  - Staffing agencies
  - Pharmacies
  - Clinical and research laboratories
  - Local storage facilities
- Transportation and logistics companies

3 Site Selection Criteria

Identifying and qualifying a research site for use in a protocol is a multifaceted process that requires extensive consultations with operational group leads, research collaborators, local partners, and often contractors. It requires considerable expertise to translate the objectives of the protocol, which are stated on paper in relatively abstract terms, into physical and resource requirements needed to accomplish the objectives and then into actual walls, roofs, beds, sphygmomanometers, and freezers. It also requires expertise to be flexible: if brand Y isn't available, is brand Z acceptable? If there is no running water available at a site, but the site looks good otherwise, how can we get enough clean water?

While the specific requirements for a research site will change depending on the protocol and/or the country involved, the process employed to reach either final activation or disqualification of a site can be standardized. In general, any research site will have to meet the following criteria:

- Local community acceptance
- Governmental approval, be it local, regional, or national
- Access to a sufficient population that meets criteria for inclusion in the study
- Access to qualified staff members: ability to hire them from the community or provide housing for staff
- For outpatient and in-patient studies alike, facilities that can accommodate
  - Secure offices
  - Labs
  - Pharmacy
  - Staff areas
  - Waiting rooms
  - Patient care facilities for in-patient research
- Reliable electricity and clean water (present or to be installed)
- Communications infrastructure, including Internet, mobile phones, and/or landlines (present or to be installed)
- Security, especially in areas beset by armed conflict or substantial unrest
- Waste management

4 Types of Research Sites

4.1 Sites Within an Existing Health Facility

Having fixed research sites established in existing institutions, as during the 2014–2016 Ebola outbreak in Liberia, provided a central location that proved invaluable for a large vaccine study and a continuing research program. The PREVAIL[1] site, in the John F. Kennedy Hospital in Monrovia, Liberia's major tertiary referral hospital, provided facilities (after renovation) and access to the capital's population, the largest in the country, whose demographics ran the full gamut of the socioeconomic, educational, and age spectrum.

The Duport Road site in a Monrovia suburb was selected to accommodate additional participants closer to their place of residence. The CH Rennie Hospital site was selected for its essentially rural population within reasonable proximity, under an hour's drive to Monrovia. This improved the demographic diversity of the study population. The Redemption Hospital site (◘ Fig. 1), located at one of the epicenters of the Ebola outbreak, a community hospital in the borough of New Kru Town, added another dimension of diversity. Although the population was considered urban, it was among the most socially and economically disadvantaged communities in Liberia. Areas of the hospital needed to be reconfigured and renovated for informed consent procedures, phlebotomy, processing and testing of protocol-defined lab specimens, and vaccination and observation rooms.

4.2 Research Site Within an Ebola Treatment Center

Bringing investigational agents to sick patients can often best be accomplished where the patients are being treated. The PALM (short for "Pamoja Tulinde Maisha," a Kiswahili phrase that translates to "together save lives") randomized controlled trial, conducted in the Democratic Republic of the Congo (DRC), tested four investigational agents against Ebola at four locations (► In Practice 17.1 and 23.1) in Ebola treatment

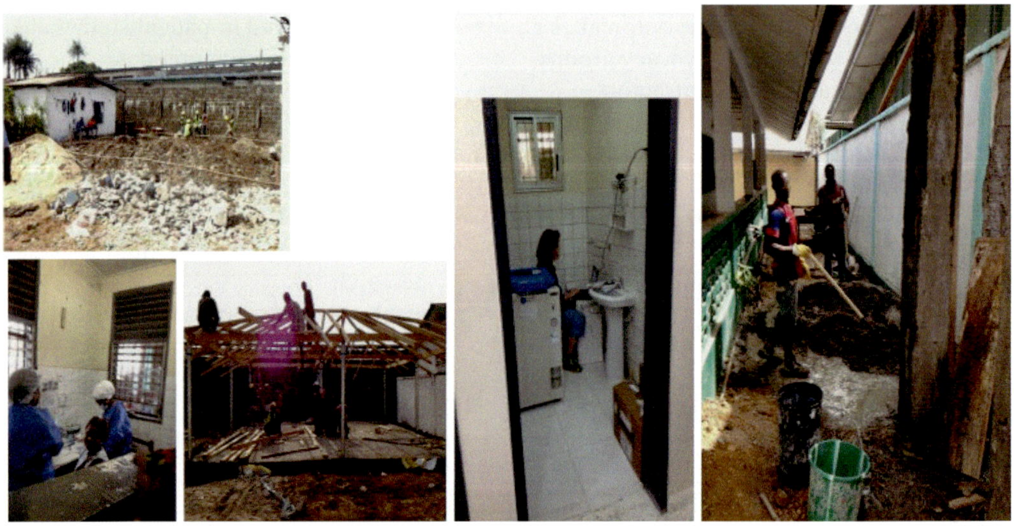

◘ **Fig. 1** Before and after photos of renovations at Redemption Hospital, site of a large, randomized Ebola vaccine study. (Photos: Leidos Biomedical Research, Inc.)

1 Partnership for Research on Ebola Virus in Liberia.

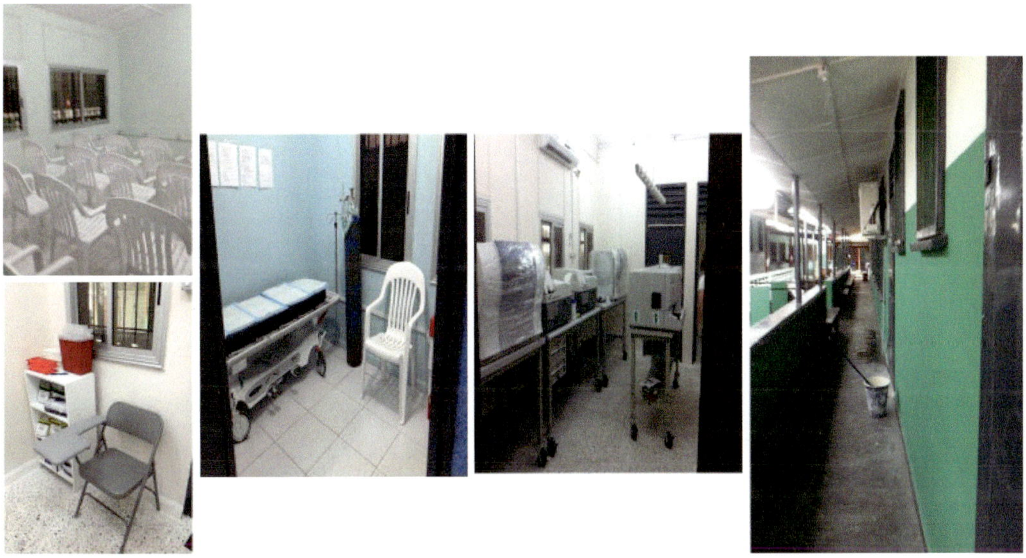

Fig. 1 (continued)

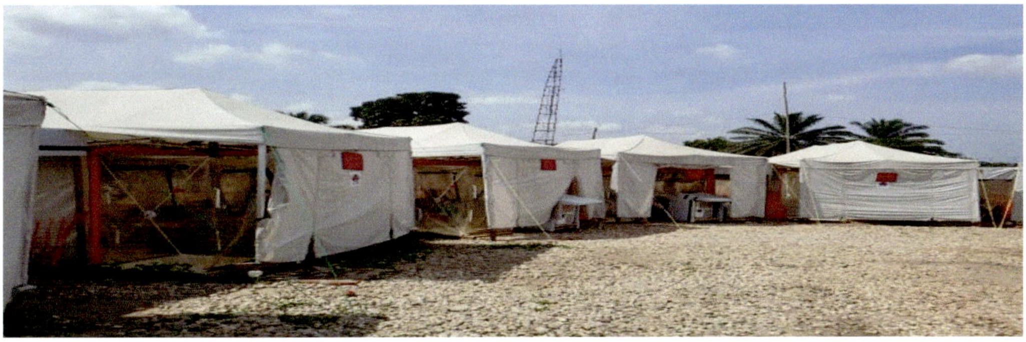

Fig. 2 Ebola treatment center in Beni. (Leidos Biomedical Research, Inc.)

centers set up for the 2018–2020 outbreak (Mulangu et al. 2019). The clinical and research teams needed to be well-coordinated, with their duties and expectations clearly delineated. For example, as in the PALM study, a protocol enrolling participants who have tested positive for disease in an outbreak may rely on NGOs to assist with infrastructure and clinical care at the research sites; as the epidemiological curve begins to flatten and cases decrease, the NGO may close down well in advance of scheduled participant follow-up appointments, potentially affecting the continuation of the research study activities.

4.3 Mobile Site

A cluster vaccine study of the investigational rVSV-ZEBOV vaccine was part of the November 2015 response to a small Ebola virus disease (EVD) outbreak in Cow Field, Liberia (Figs. 2 and 3). Because of Liberia's earlier experience in conducting vaccine research during an outbreak, procedures and practices needed to open a mobile site were already in place, and the site was quickly established. Trained staff were deployed to the area, and a protocol was implemented just 4 days after the first new EVD case was confirmed. Only three cases occurred during the outbreak, and none after research response had

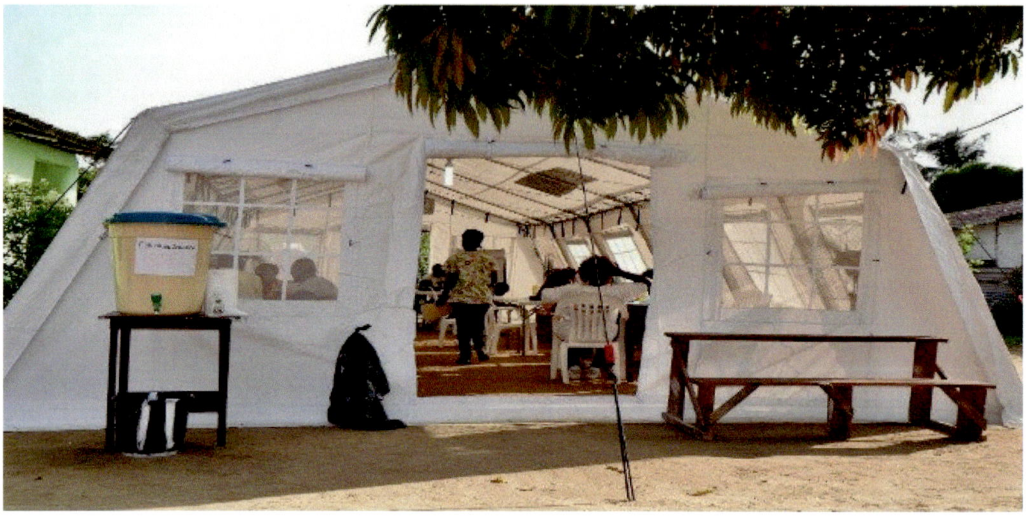

Fig. 3 Mobile vaccination study site in Cow Field, Liberia. (Photo: Leidos Biomedical Research, Inc.)

Fig. 4 Mobile clinical research site in Cow Field, Liberia. (Credit: Leidos Biomedical Research, Inc.)

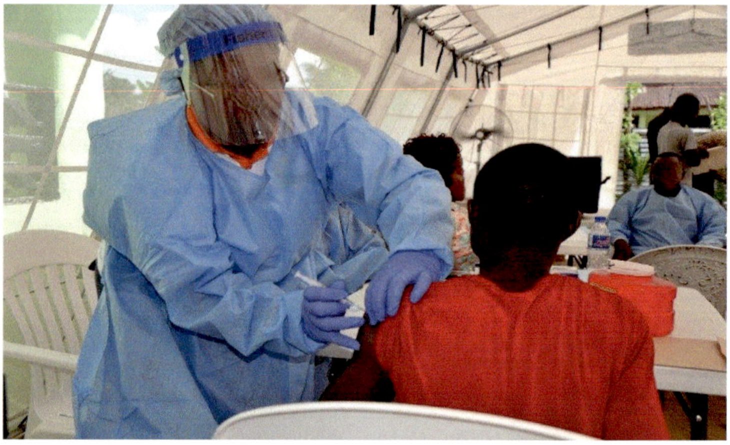

begun (Bolay et al. 2019). The Ebola Ça Suffit! (Ebola that's enough!) ring vaccination (cluster-randomized) trial in Guinea was also structured in such a way that it required mobile vaccination and follow-up teams (Henao-Restrepo et al. 2015, 2017) (Fig. 4).

5 Activating a Site

5.1 Minimum Requirements

In a resource-restricted environment, steps to operationalize a protocol in an emergency are at first guided by the essential minimum requirements to start a research program. Many of these topics are covered by other chapters in this volume; in many cases, specialized expertise—preferably combined with personal experience operating in remote areas with little infrastructure — will be essential to get some of the needed elements in place. Some early acquisition decisions may also depend on the short-term or long-term level of commitment from the sponsoring organization as well as the level of expenditure the sponsoring organizations have available.

The following are key questions to determine minimal requirements to start a research program:

1. Is there an adaptable facility available with power, water, communications, staff, equipment, etc.? Is the current infrastructure sufficient for the demands of the study? If not, will the infrastructure installed for the study remain and contribute to the longer-term needs of the host country?
2. Are the equipment and supplies being provided specifically for the clinical research study? Patient beds, monitoring equipment, etc. primarily intended for patient care may be difficult for the clinical research team to justify.
3. Is the long-term sustainability of the project part of the planning? Can the clinical, laboratory, and information technology (IT) infrastructure be locally operated and maintained? Will doing so require additional training?

Most sponsoring organizations will accept a degree of over-procurement in the initial stages of an emergency—it is better to have some excess than to lack items essential to getting the research program started. The longer-term prospects of the project and the distinction between essential and nonessential (but justifiable) items should be a planning factor at all stages, especially once the site has been activated and the study is underway.

5.2 Tools for Site Activation

Developing standardized toolkits for use when preparing to implement a protocol can speed site activation and provide a common platform for communicating with the protocol team and other stakeholders. The most frequently used tools are flowcharts and checklists. While task-based checklists are commonly used in the implementation of research studies, the site operations unit of the research team is responsible for determining and assessing the protocol requirements and maintaining primary checklists to guide the site activation process.

5.2.1 Flowcharts and Lists

A flowchart is a diagram that outlines a process in a way that is easy to follow, often using shapes and/or graphics to visually represent a sequence of events from start to finish. Flowcharts can allow for easier visualization of study participant activities, physical space and layout requirements, and staffing needs and roles. They provide a visual of how the study schedule can be implemented, identifying problem areas before activation of a study site. For protocols involving multiple therapeutic drug arms, this is also an excellent way to determine if multiple drug administrations will occur concurrently, which could impact staffing, space, and supply needs. Other operational groups will often benefit from their process flowcharts; for example, data management may map out the process for capturing source documentation, and the laboratory team may map how samples move from the clinical area to the lab and how results are communicated back to the clinical team.

5.2.2 The Clinical Flowchart

The clinical flowchart outlines participant flow and organization of assessment, procedure, and discharge. This chart helps to identify which staff are needed for each procedure, how best to distribute supplies, and potential issues with participant flow or space constraints. For example, if an observation area for participants after they receive a vaccine injection is needed, a flowchart in conjunction with a schematic of the research site layout can identify where this area should be or identify a need for more space. A flowchart prepared for PREVAIL (◘ Fig. 5) later served as a template for other trials based on different protocols.

5.2.3 Data Management Flowchart

This chart is focused on data collection (case report forms and source documents) and transmission of data from the site. Source documents are the *original* records of clinical findings, observations, or other activities in a clinical trial necessary for the reconstruction and evaluation of the trial; they provide source data used to reconstruct the trial as it

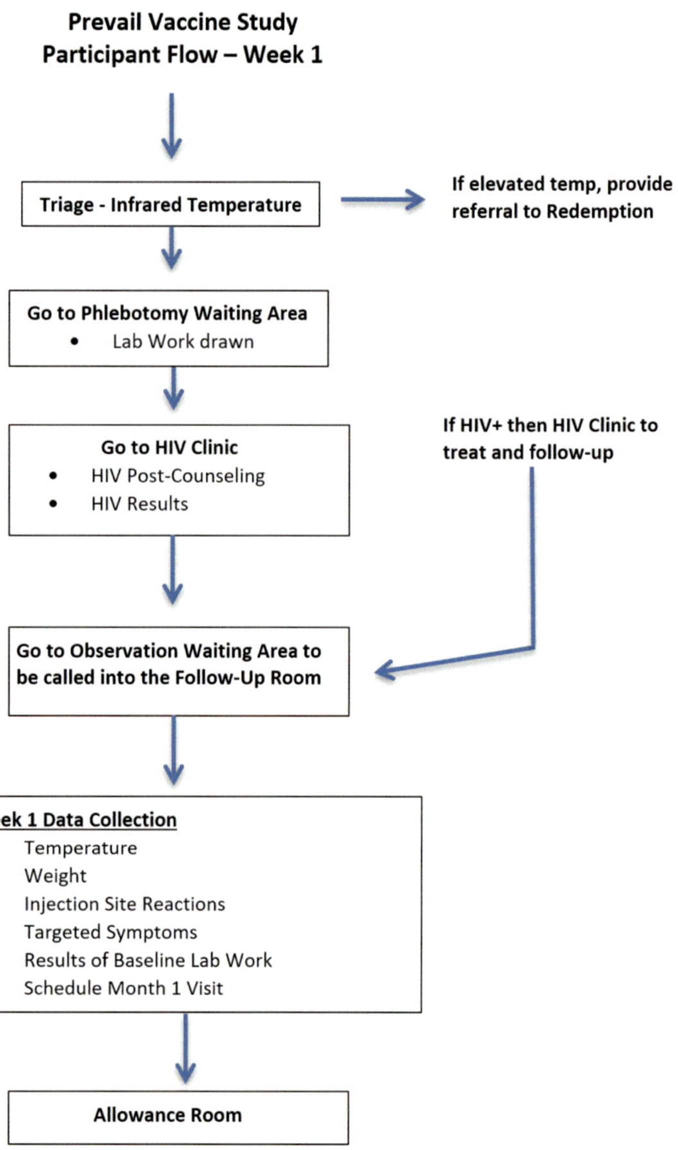

Fig. 5 A clinical flowchart used by PREVAIL researchers. (Courtesy PREVAIL)

happened. This is particularly vital for protocols involving participants exposed to a high-consequence pathogen where data collection may occur in the restricted "hot zone," preventing immediate transfer of documents to the area where data entry is done (▶ Chap. 35).

5.2.4 Site Assessment Checklist

A site assessment checklist is a tool for understanding the current capabilities, capacity, and available resources of the potential research site. While it will need to be adapted to the needs of each particular protocol (observational study or randomized controlled trial), it will generally cover most of the same operational areas, though some headings may not be needed:

- Principal investigator requirements
- Site staffing (including role identification)
- Data management
- Laboratory
- Pharmacy
- Site operations
- Cold chain
- Psychosocial/social mobilization team
- Safety/pharmacovigilance
- Monitoring or quality assurance/control

5.2.5 Site Activation Checklist

A tracking document maintained by the site operations team, it reflects both the information received from the initial site assessment checklist and updated entries based on feedback from operational groups and the research site team. Once every item identified on the activation checklist (◘ Fig. 6) has been confirmed, the site can be considered ready for activation.

The site activation checklist and the site assessment checklist have much in common but

BENI		
Training	**Status:**	**Comments:**
* RCT v3.0 Training Logs	🟢	Initial v2.0 completed 11/14/18-11/19/18; v3.0 completed 1/22/19
* Pharmacy Training Logs		
* Laboratory Training Logs	🟢	Completed 11/20/18-11/21/19
Laboratory	**Status:**	**Comments:**
* GeneXpert (minimum: 2; optimal: 4)	🟢	Current: 5 (3/22/2019)
* GeneXpert Cartridges	🟢	Current: 6361 (3/22/2019)
* Picolo (minimum: 2; optimal: 4)	🟢	Current: 2 (3/22/2019)
* AmLyte13 Discs for Picolo	🟢	Current: 290 (3/22/2019)
* Lithium Tubes for Picolo		
* Training	🟢	Refresher training for Mrs. Doe 2/6/19
Pharmacy	**Status:**	**Comments:**
* ZMapp Treatment Courses (TCs)	🟢	TCs: ~10.7 available (1072 vials) 6/20/19 (RCT)
* ZMapp IV Set (0.2 μ low-protein binding PES in-line filter)		
* ZMapp Compounding (250, 500, 1000mL D5W and/or Normal Saline)		
* mAb114 Treatment Courses (TCs)	🟢	TCs: ~22.3 available (156 vials) 6/20/19 (RCT)
* mAb114 IV Set (1.2 μ PES filter membrane; DEHP-free; Latex-free)	🔴	
* mAb114 Compounding (Sterile Water for injection; 250mL Normal Saline)	🔴	
* REGN-EB3 Treatment Courses (TCs)	🟢	TCs: ~8.4 available (109 vials) 6/20/19 (RCT)
* REGN-EB3 IV Set (0.2μ in-line filter)		
* REGN-EB3 Compounding (100, 250, 500, 1000mL Normal Saline, D5W or Lactated Ringer's)	🔴	
* Remdesivir Treatment Courses (TCs)	🟢	TCs: ~27 available (383 vials) 6/20/19 (RCT)
Cold-Chain Supply	**Status:**	**Comments:**
* Temperature-control containers for investigational drug transport	🟢	Onsite: 1 (Portable)
* Refrigerators +2°C to +8°C (minimum of 2 for investigational drug storage)	🟢	Vestfrost: 1 for IDP Back-up: Need top select from multiple VestFrost AKG 377 Upright Refrigerators (not tropical rated), 2 × VF 400A arrived in Kinshasa 10APR19 (Tropical rated)
* Continuous temperature monitoring with alarms (72 hours of data monitoring is required)	🟢	All monitored and all TempTales replaced every 9 months (no audible alarms)
* Freezers -15°C to -25°C (for ZMapp storage only)	🟢	Freezer: 2 chest for IDP & 1 portable for quarantine and gel-pack conditioning Back-up: Need to select from 1 VestFrost MF 314 (Tropical) and 2 Revco DXF Ultra-Low -40 Uprights
* Continuous temperature monitoring with alarms (72 hours of data monitoring is required)	🟢	All monitored and all TempTales replaced every 9 months (no audible alarms)

◘ **Fig. 6** An excerpted site activation checklist. (Courtesy PALM)

are used in different ways. While the site *assessment* checklist is a static document intended to provide a snapshot of a site's initial feasibility and resource availability, the *activation* checklist is a living document tracking completion of the tasks required before an activation letter can be issued by the controlling regulatory body or study sponsor. The site activation checklist also provides a much more detailed outline of what is needed. For example, the site assessment checklist will list general printer requirements and whether printers need to be procured. The site activation checklist will specify types of printers and necessary supply orders like paper, ink, connectivity cables, etc. Color coding of the status of each item is a simple way to quickly communicate how much work remains before the site can be activated.

5.3 The Site Activation Process in Outline

5.3.1 Organize the Operations Team

- Identify points of contact for the following:
  - Clinical team and research study team if separate, e.g., where study takes place in an existing ETU
  - Operational areas: data management, logistics, laboratory, etc.
  - In-country partners and operational liaisons
  - Pharmaceutical companies as necessary
  - Others as needed
- Determine procurement responsibility delegation
  - Will each operational area order their own supplies, or will clinical operations consolidate supply ordering from all sites (see ◘ Fig. 7)?

5.3.2 Map the Protocol

- Review schedule of events and create a flowchart of activities (see site assessment, ▸ Sects. 5.3.3 and 5.3.4)
- Identify post-discharge needs for participants (if in-patient)
- Prepare additional flowcharts or process documents for the following:
  - Data management
  - Pharmacy

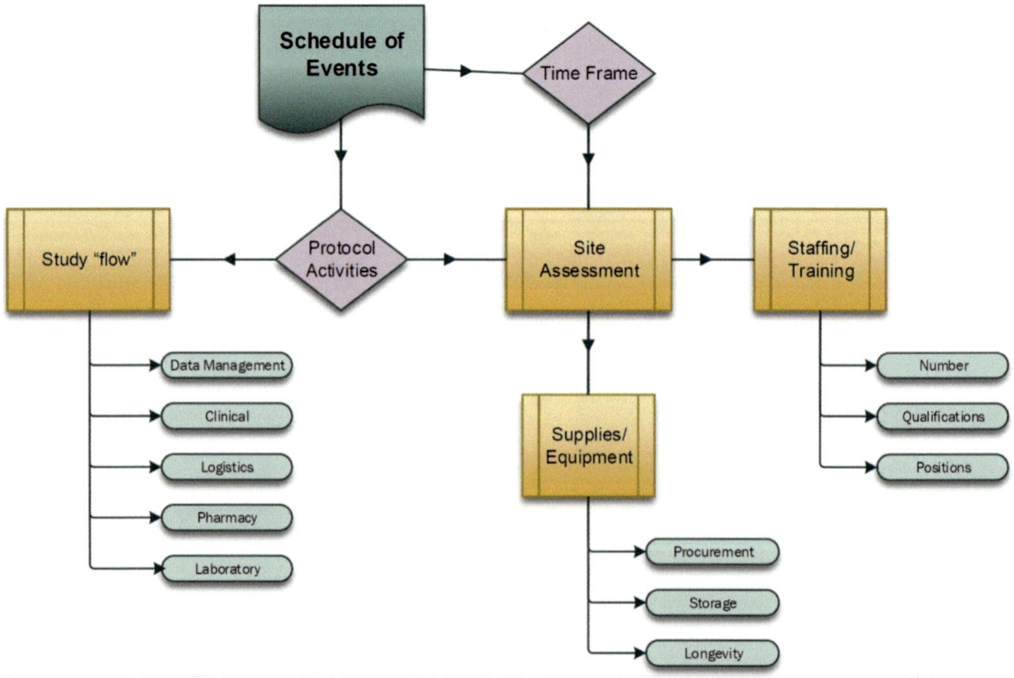

◘ **Fig. 7** Flowchart showing sequence of events essential to opening a research site. (Kevin Barrett, NIAID/NIH)

  - Laboratory
  - Logistics
  - Planning process for equipment maintenance, replacement of faulty or broken equipment, and disposition (donation or disposal)
  - Lead times for new order delivery
- Update site assessment checklist using the schedule of events and flowchart as guides (see ▶ Sect. 5.2.4). To ensure it captures all information relevant to the study, ask all operational areas to review and include additional items as needed. Some areas where detail is essential are as follows:
  - Supplies (▶ Chap. 37)
    - Are protocol-specific supplies available?
    - Special lab collection devices, including consumables
    - Drug-specific intravenous (IV) infusion kits and/or anaphylaxis kits
  - Staffing (▶ Chap. 42)
    - Qualifications (curricula vitae, medical licenses, etc.)
    - Number of staff, required level of effort, and availability
    - Positions and responsibilities
    - Personal protective equipment (PPE) stock needed
    - Cross-training and training supplies
  - Data management (▶ Chap. 35)
    - Documentation: how will we document it (electronic or paper)?
    - Assess current documentation systems and if they can be utilized
    - Consider consolidated worksheets as the source document if CRF are cumbersome
    - Availability of secure, environmentally stable storage for CRFs and/or source documents
    - Plan for long-term storage of protocol documents
  - Infrastructure
    - Operating hours
      - Are protocol activities scheduled on weekends or local holidays?
    - Physical layout, available space at the site
    - Cold chain equipment (▶ Chap. 39)
    - Electricity (▶ Chap. 39)
    - Communications (Internet, telephony, etc.) (▶ Chap. 34)

5.3.3 Assess the Site

Once the site assessment checklist has been completed, it must be reviewed to determine the initial viability of the site. The assessment should be reviewed by representatives from each operational area, as well as those who perform specialized assessments in response to requests from the research team.

- Site assessment checklist review: possible outcomes.
  - The individual who performed the assessment may provide additional relevant information that was not anticipated on the original form.
  - Operational areas may realize they neglected to add certain assessment criteria to the original form.
  - An additional site visit may be found necessary to collect or confirm information not initially identified as important.
  - Operational groups may need to commit to providing specific solutions for areas where the site does not meet activation criteria.
  - If "deal-breaker" issues are identified—problems at the site for which there is no reasonable solution and which would prohibit the start of the protocol regardless of other criteria—alert the principal investigator (PI) and other stakeholders. Finding a solution may require a high-level decision to either modify the protocol or invest significant funding.
- Conduct additional site assessments as needed.
- Proceed with necessary procurement, and set up activities as identified on the assessment checklist.

5.3.4 Run the Site Assessment Checklist

- Transfer the site activation checklist items to a new document (such as a spreadsheet).
  - For each operational area, ask the lead for that area to populate the section with line items detailing the specific

equipment or resources that must be available on site to activate.

- Track site activation status.
  - An assigned project manager will schedule regular status update meetings with all operational leads and relevant stakeholders to ensure that each line item is up to date. Often, there will be overlap among operational areas, so that a problem solved by pharmacy staff may solve a problem for the site operations team as well. The project manager will ensure version control and will manage the document through site activation.
- Submit request for activation once all items on the activation checklist have been confirmed.

6 Triage and Infection Control

Triage and infection control practices are integral to healthcare and clinical research, especially in an outbreak of an infectious disease with few or no approved MCMs. Implementation of triage and infection control depend on the layout and on the sequence, duration, and physical proximity of interactions between patients and healthcare workers and so must be a factor in choosing a site that can accommodate the required facilities. A clean water supply is a requirement as well.

Human nature being what it is, there is a tendency to become complacent and less attentive than at first to established standards and practices. The two large Ebola outbreaks in West Africa and in the northeastern DRC and the COVID-19 pandemic compelled healthcare workers and the public to start paying attention and implement practices to prevent or minimize the spread of infection. With its demonstrated high mortality and initial lack of MCMs, EVD may have been more compelling than COVID-19 in this respect, but of course the Ebola virus was much less transmissible than severe acute respiratory system coronavirus 2 (SARS-CoV-2). Be that as it may, it is essential to provide for infection control with strategically located, hard-to-ignore cleanliness stations, among other measures like PPE and careful waste disposal.

Emergency transport and medical admission processes, such as triage, are high-risk areas for disease transmission during an outbreak. Identification and isolation of potentially infectious patients may be delayed because of a high work burden, lack of specific training and skills, and unavailability of adequate isolation measures. This poses a special risk for nosocomial transmission unless adequate triage and infection control procedures are in place and observed.

6.1 Study Participant Triage

Since research sites during the West Africa Ebola response were embedded in clinical care facilities, triaging procedures for the host facility, based on national triage procedures, had to be followed. PREVAIL's research sites implemented additional screening procedures for all participants entering the research facilities. Triage forms were developed specifically to screen individuals who came as potential research participants. All individuals first had to go through the screening procedures and then were subject to the PREVAIL-specific triage.

6.2 Universal Precautions

Universal precautions should be practiced and implemented continuously. As specified in regulations from, e.g., the U.S Occupational Safety and Health Administration, universal precautions are an approach to infection control that treats all human blood and certain human body fluids as if they were known to be infectious for human immunodeficiency virus (HIV), hepatitis B virus (HBV), and other bloodborne pathogens (OSHA 2019). During the Ebola outbreak, the importance of this precaution was reemphasized and imbedded in all study-specific training. The Ministry of Health of Liberia, PREVAIL's primary partner in the research response, developed a standard training program which was provided to all Ministry of Health facilities. This training was also extended to all research staff to ensure they had the most updated information on infection control and universal precautions. With a respiratory pathogen like (SARS-CoV-2), different precautionary measures apply (WHO 2021).

6.3 Environmental Considerations

It is necessary to ensure adequate biohazard containers (burn boxes/sharps containers) are available for the safe disposal of used syringes, unused or compromised experimental product, and other research supplies. Additionally, it needs to be established upfront how these contaminated items will be disposed of. Planners must ensure the availability of functional incinerators with capacity and fuel, locations for safe burial, or other means for proper disposal.

7 Some Lessons Learned and Conclusion

7.1 Every Emergency Is Different from the Previous One

Experience with implementing emergency research responses over the last decade—in Liberia, the DRC, and worldwide for COVID-19—has repeatedly demonstrated the pitfalls of conventional wisdom. The synthesis of preliminary assumptions, standard operating procedures, existing literature on the disease or family of diseases, cultural presuppositions, and previous emergency response may suggest solutions but cannot serve as an accurate guide to implementing a research response. Creative thinking to fight the current outbreak and a real understanding of and commitment to scientific and ethical standards are essential to a successful study (Larson et al. 2017). Solutions that worked in a previous outbreak may not apply to current situations. Some examples include the following:

- *Security guards or soldiers?* It is important to ensure that research staff, participants, and research facilities are protected. In situations where there is public distrust of the government or military, it may be advisable to consider hiring civilian security personnel who are less threatening than official security personnel and will follow research team instructions on admission of potential research participants and patients to the site (▶ Chap. 41).
- *Branding.* Some collaborations have successfully "branded" the research initiatives to allow the branding to be recognizable to those outside of the research while maintaining equity for all partners and stakeholders. It can be useful for communities to learn to recognize logos or a memorable name to spread the word about the study. In other cases, the need for neutrality and a low profile may take precedence. Fear of the disease itself, suspicion of authorities or researchers, or misunderstanding of the goals of clinical research could make discretion the best course. This is a question where the advice of local partners is indispensable.
- *Fixed or rotational staffing?* Conventional wisdom has it that each site should be staffed by a fixed, trained contingent which understands the site and the research catchment area. This also makes for straightforward accountability and known personnel for data and safety queries (FDA 2019). In some instances, however, especially in remote sites, personnel must travel great distances, be away from family, and stay in temporary lodging during their work on the research program. This can mean a large portion of the staff rotates every few weeks or months, in which case careful records, or an accountability matrix, should be kept to record when staff members were on site, what responsibilities they had at a given time, and documented transitions to incoming staff.
- *Supplies.* Clinical and research supplies common in one setting may not be usable in another. Established medical facilities have had time to work any incompatibili-

ties between frequently used items out of the system, e.g., that they have the right tubing for the saline bags on hand. All of this must be rapidly established during an emergency research response (▶ Chap. 37).

7.2 Conclusion

The concepts presented in here are a basic framework to quickly initiate and implement infectious disease clinical research. All topics can be adapted as needed and should be continually evaluated to make for a more proactive rather than reactive approach. It is essential to act quickly to ensure important research can be conducted and the research questions can be answered during the height of a disease outbreak, so no opportunities are missed to demonstrate a vaccine or treatment safely and significantly improves outcomes.

As Jeremy Farrar (2018) has noted, "It's time to stop reacting to these outbreaks as discrete episodes and instead work together with a coordinated, nationally led, and internationally supported approach that learns from each outbreak so we can better prepare for the next."

Discussion Questions

1. Why is contingency planning essential to ensure the success of a research study?
2. There is an urgent infectious disease outbreak in a remote Asian village.
   (a) What key questions determine the minimal requirements to start a research program?
   (b) What questions must be answered by the planners before the research project begins?
   (c) What criteria must the research site meet?
   (d) What other steps should the research team consider?
3. How can response agencies divide clinical research responsibilities while maintaining research and patient care quality?
4. What is the role of flowcharts and checklists in site activation and facilitating communications between the protocol team and other stakeholders?
5. Briefly outline site activation.
6. Why must triage and infection control practices be integral components of healthcare and clinical research, especially during infectious disease outbreaks with few or no approved MCMs?

References

Bolay FK, Grandits G, Lane HC, Kennedy SB, Johnson MP, Fallah MP, et al. PREVAIL I cluster vaccination study with rVSVΔG-ZEBOV-GP as part of a public health response in Liberia. J Infect Dis. 2019;219(10):1634–41. https://doi.org/10.1093/infdis/jiy698.

Braveman P. Accumulating knowledge on the social determinants of health and infectious disease. Public Health Rep. 2011;126(Suppl 3) https://doi.org/10.1177/00333549111260S306.

Brett-Major D, Lawler J. Catching chances: the movement to be on the ground and research ready before an outbreak. Viruses. 2018;10(8) https://doi.org/10.3390/v10080439.

Farrar J. It isn't crazy to conduct an Ebola clinical trial in a war zone—it's necessary. Stat; 2018.

FDA. Statement of investigator (form 1572). Washington, DC: Food and Drug Administration, U.S. Department of Health and Human Services; 2019.

Henao-Restrepo AM, Longini IM, Egger M, Dean NE, Edmunds WJ, Camacho A, et al. Efficacy and effectiveness of an rVSV-vectored vaccine expressing Ebola surface glycoprotein: interim results from the Guinea ring vaccination cluster-randomised trial. Lancet. 2015;386(9996):857–66. https://doi.org/10.1016/s0140-6736(15)61117-5.

Henao-Restrepo AM, Camacho A, Longini IM, Watson CH, Edmunds WJ, Egger M, et al. Efficacy and effectiveness of an rVSV-vectored vaccine in preventing Ebola virus disease: final results from the Guinea ring vaccination, open-label, cluster-randomised trial (Ebola Ca Suffit!). Lancet. 2017;389(10068):505–18. https://doi.org/10.1016/S0140-6736(16)32621-6.

Jones KE, Patel NG, Levy MA, Storeygard A, Balk D, Gittleman JL, et al. Global trends in emerging infectious diseases. Nature. 2008;451(7181):990–3. https://doi.org/10.1038/nature06536.

Kennedy SB, Neaton JD, Lane HC, Kieh MWS, Massaquoi MBF, Touchette NA, et al. Implementation of an Ebola virus disease vaccine clinical trial during the Ebola epidemic in Liberia: design, procedures, and challenges. Clin Trials (London, England). 2016;13(1):49–56. https://doi.org/10.1177/1740774515621037.

Larson GS, Baseler BR, Hoover ML, Pierson JF, Tegli JK, Johnson MP, et al. Conventional wisdom versus actual outcomes: challenges in the conduct of an Ebola vaccine trial in Liberia during the international public health emergency. Am J Trop Med Hyg. 2017;97(1):10–5. https://doi.org/10.4269/ajtmh.16-1015.

Morens DM, Fauci AS. Emerging pandemic diseases: how we got to COVID-19. Cell. 2020;182(5):1077–92. https://doi.org/10.1016/j.cell.2020.08.021.

Mulangu S, Dodd LE, Davey RT Jr, Tshiani Mbaya O, Proschan M, Mukadi D, et al. A randomized, controlled trial of Ebola virus disease therapeutics. N Engl J Med. 2019;381(24):2293–303. https://doi.org/10.1056/NEJMoa1910993.

NASEM. Integrating clinical research into epidemic response: the Ebola experience. Washington, DC: National Academies of Sciences Engineering and Medicine Publications, The National Academies Press; 2017.

OSHA. Bloodborne pathogens. In: Occupational safety and health standards. Washington, DC: Occupational Safety and Health Administration, U.S. Department of Labor; 2019. https://www.osha.gov/laws-regs/regulations/standardnumber/1910/1910.1030. Accessed 30 Mar 2022 2022.

Sigfrid L, Moore C, Salam AP, Maayan N, Hamel C, Garritty C, et al. A rapid research needs appraisal methodology to identify evidence gaps to inform clinical research priorities in response to outbreaks-results from the Lassa fever pilot. BMC Med. 2019;17(1):107. https://doi.org/10.1186/s12916-019-1338-1.

WHO. Infection prevention and control during health care when coronavirus disease (COVID-19) is suspected or confirmed. Geneva: World Health Organization; 2021. Contract No.: WHO/2019-nCoV/IPC/2021.1.

40.1 In Practice: Improving Patient Care in the Field: The CUBE Isolation Unit

Richard Kojan

Contents

Learning Track Note: This chapter appears in Learning Tracks: Emergency Research Response, Research Operations; Research Ethics; Social Science Response Research

E. S. Higgs and R. A. Sorenson (eds.), *Principles and Practice of Emergency Research Response*, https://doi.org/10.1007/978-3-031-48408-7_61

Learning Objectives

This chapter will help readers understand and describe

- The advantages and disadvantages of the traditional Ebola treatment unit (ETU) design with the Emergency biosecurity chamber for epidemics (CUBE)
- How maintaining family and community relationships affects patient morale and recovery
- How an ETU layout can take advantage of CUBE
- Steps that can enhance adherence to strict infection and prevention control measures

1 Ebola: Isolation and Treatment

The CUBE (◘ Fig. 1) is an innovative, field-deployable shelter and isolation system for treating patients with dangerous infectious diseases. The development of the CUBE unit dates to the experience of caring for patients in Conakry, Guinea, during the 2014–2016 West Africa Ebola epidemic, by the Alliance for International Medical Action (ALIMA). Ebola Treatment Units (ETUs) that ALIMA and others built and managed during that outbreak were based on a model of care developed 40 years earlier. Their purpose was to provide patient care while protecting caregivers and the community from infection. The units were housed in large tents, with separate sections for people with suspected and confirmed infection. Entry into the patient areas was restricted to healthcare providers in full personal protective equipment (PPE).

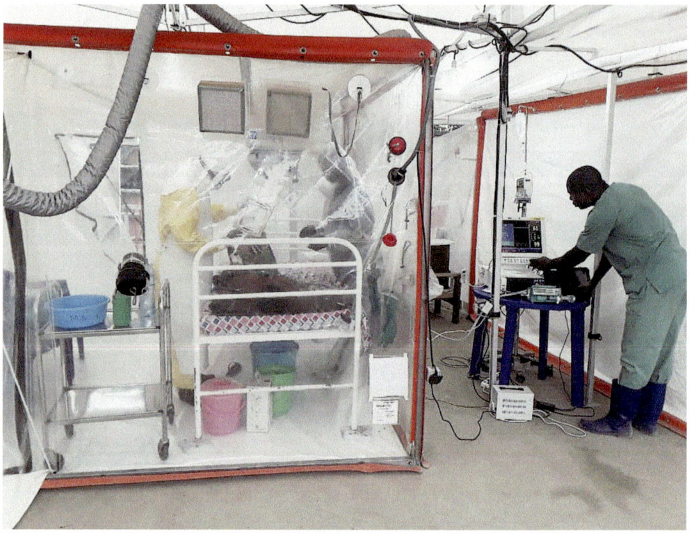

◘ **Fig. 1** CUBE in operation. (Fischer et al. 2019)

2 The Old ETU Design

The old ETU design had serious disadvantages for patients, caregivers, and families. Patients were isolated, cut off from contact with family, friends, and relatives. They could hardly see even the faces of their caregivers through the personal protective equipment (PPE) (◘ Fig. 2). Facing death from Ebola virus disease (EVD) alone, while separated from loved ones, multiplied patients' fear and suffering. At the time, caregivers had limited knowledge about the most effective supportive care and interventions; moreover, the inside temperature meant caregivers could only remain in the hot tents in full PPE for a short time before risking severe dehydration, heat illness, and heat stroke (Sprecher et al. 2015).

For ALIMA, a medical organization dedicated to providing both medical and compassionate care to the sick, the experience was beyond frustrating. The entire care team soon expressed a deep need for psychological support themselves. Patients and their loved ones began to see enforced isolation for the sake of minimal, often fruitless, medical care as a kind of physical and mental aggression, rather than their best hope of survival. This perception, especially natural to the impoverished and disadvantaged, soon began to discourage newly infected people from seeking care that could contribute to their own survival and stem the spread of the disease.

After this harsh experience, we were determined to improve the quality and humanity of patient care in similar circumstances. ALIMA designated a small working group to lead a design process. As members of the group, medical caregivers, psychologists, and logisticians reflected on how to improve the

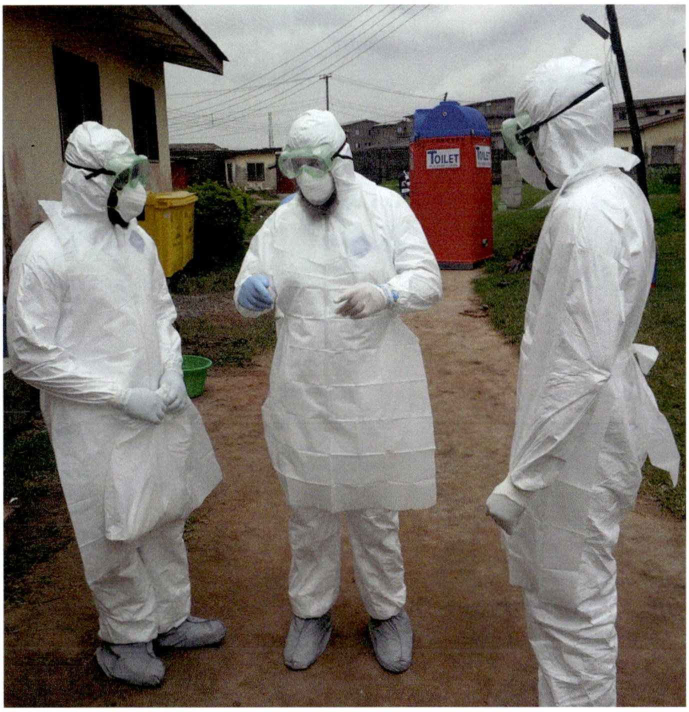

◘ **Fig. 2** Nigerian physicians being trained by the World Health Organization (WHO) on how to put on and remove PPE to treat Ebola patients. All this equipment must be donned and doffed for each foray into an old-standard Ebola treatment unit (ETU). (CDC Global, CC 2.0; ▶ https://commons.wikimedia.org/w/index.php?search=ebola+ppe&title=Special:MediaSearch&go=Go&type=image)

design and standards of optimized care facilities for the next epidemic. After several national consultations in Guinea, regional consultations in West and Central Africa, and further discussions in developed countries—an approach that brought in public, private, humanitarian, scientific, academic, military, and civilian nuclear specialists—the CUBE took shape.

3 The CUBE Is Born

The conceptual shift was to stop trying to isolate an entire patient ward, and instead build a smaller containment structure for each patient. The CUBEs have transparent plastic walls (◘ Fig. 3a), with built-in ports resembling full-body gloves and airlock door and window portals. The CUBE can be placed under negative pressure, and it can be decontaminated with hydrogen peroxide gas between patients or before unit closure. The CUBE was deployed to the field for the first time in response to a 2018 Lassa fever outbreak in Nigeria (◘ Fig. 3b), and has since been used extensively for EVD response in the DRC (Fischer et al. 2019).

The advantages are many. At under 300 kg, each unit can be moved far more easily than a large temporary structure, even by small vehicles over rough roads. Patients can be continually monitored from outside the CUBE by health providers unencumbered by full PPE; most procedures can be carried out through the access portals without the caregiver entering the CUBE. The CUBEs do not get nearly as hot as the old isolation units, a tremendous advantage in equatorial Africa. And last but certainly not least, patients and their loved ones can communicate with one another frequently and face to face.

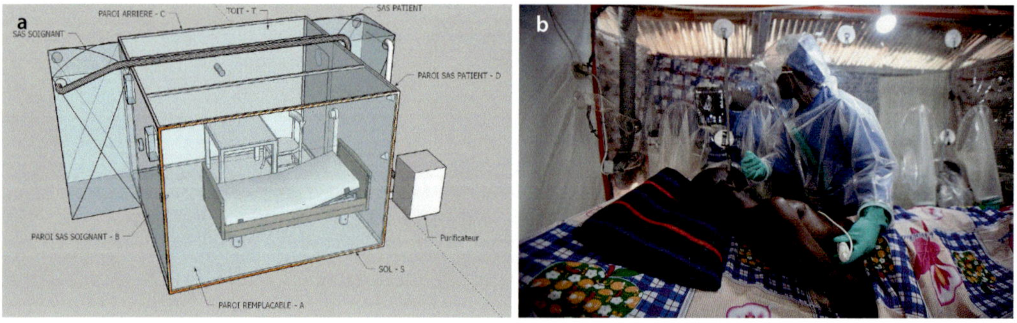

◘ **Fig. 3** **a** Cube diagram showing ports for access to patient and ventilation and doorways for entry. (ALIMA). **b** Ultrasound assessment: note doctor is in direct contact with patient through portals in CUBE. (ALIMA)

4 Better Patient Care

The development of the CUBE has allowed us to improve the standard of care for EVD patients in a low-resource setting. This also makes clinical trials, which require at least a minimal standard of care, more feasible on an emergency basis. The CUBE can be installed within or just outside existing medical facilities, closer to patients' homes, preventing the spread of infection but preserving their interactions with family and community. The value to patient morale and ultimate recovery of maintaining these irreplaceable relationships would be hard to overstate. Knowing that family members can see the patient also reduces fear in the community that seeking treatment for EVD means going off to a lonely death. Among the many advantages of the CUBE we have seen are

- Much simpler access to the patient for most purposes
- Continuous observation as needed
- Lack of convection heat enables staff to provide hands-on care for longer periods
- Broader range of care providers can interact with patients without spending time donning and doffing PPE
- Easier coordination of care and research, for example, mutual decisions on some medical procedures and level of critical care
- Cross-control of case report forms (CRF)
- CRFs can be filed rather than transcribed and incinerated because of possible contamination
- Better monitoring facilitates multidisciplinary consultation (mental health care, clinicians, lab, researchers, members of family)
- Group therapy for mental health with family participation
- Easier and better consent process, with family support and advice

This approach of integrating EVD care into existing health facilities in affected communities (Fig. 4) also facilitates the training of healthcare workers and builds on and builds up existing resources—even if they are at first minimal—in a way appropriate to the existing health systems we find in our interventions in Africa.

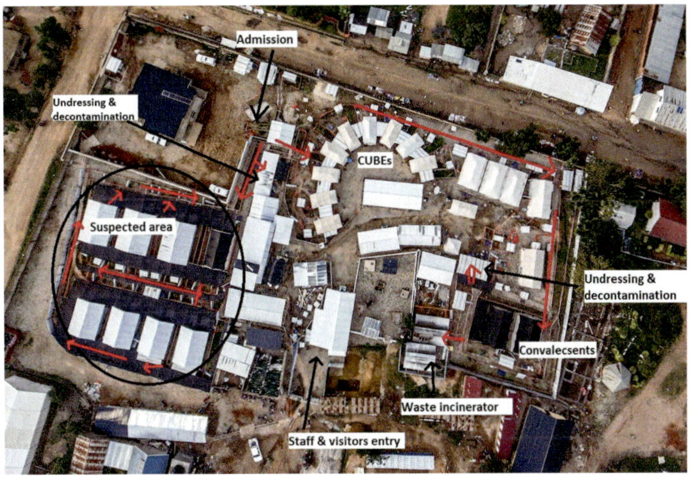

Fig. 4 New ETU layout with CUBEs. (ALIMA)

5 New Layout for ETUs

We have adapted the layout of the treatment sites to take full advantage of the CUBEs:

- The *triage area*, which receives patients awaiting diagnosis and testing, is in a building with one patient per room; the rooms have a glass window so the patient and caregivers can still see one another.
- The *intensive care* section receives unstable cases, whether confirmed or still suspect, as well as stable patients enrolling in a clinical trial; this section is housed entirely in CUBEs and is monitored by an ICU specialist.
- The *transition* section receives stabilized patients who are no longer critical, housed in space similar to the triage area.
- The *convalescent* section houses completely stable patients, who are out of danger from EVD and only waiting to be discharged; patients are generally in group wards but can be isolated if needed.

6 Infection Prevention and Control (IPC)

Patient care, procuring bodily fluid samples for diagnosis and research, and interactions connected with the research program all require strict control of the environment to minimize the risk of infection. Sufficient resources, mastery of IPC practices, and effective decontamination techniques must be integrated from design through implementation. In low-resource countries, and by no means only low-resource countries, adherence to strict IPC measures may often be spotty, resulting in exposure of both patients and medical staff to infection; for example, many healthcare workers (HCW) succumbed to EVD, in countries that could ill afford to lose them, during the West African outbreak (Evans et al. 2015). As the required expertise for care and research is often unavailable in remote regions, supervision and ongoing training becomes a fundamental element for both patient care and research. One of the major contributions of the CUBE system is to make IPC easier by greatly reducing the need for donning and doffing cumbersome PPE. When procedures are simpler and less troublesome, adherence is more likely.

7 Conclusions

Clinical research that meets internationally required ethical and scientific standards (► Chap. 33, In Practice 33.2, and 33.3) becomes feasible in low-resource areas through innovative, not necessarily high-tech problem solving. We believe the CUBE is just such an innovation, but of course good patient care and clinical research require a host of other inputs, starting with HCW familiar with and capable of implementing good patient care, clinical research practices, and participatory practices. By facilitating the standard of optimized care for patients, the CUBE also facilitates not only the implementation of research; it provides a better, less isolated treatment experience for patients and improves the morale of patients, their families, and their communities—the veil of mystery that was fertile ground for many rumors has been lifted from the closed Ebola ward.

? Discussion Questions

1. Contrast and compare the advantages and disadvantages of the traditional ETU design with the CUBE for treating patients with dangerous infectious diseases.
2. How does maintaining family and community relationships affect patient morale and ultimate recovery?
3. Discuss how the new layout for ETUs takes full advantage of CUBE.
4. Adherence to strict IPC measures is often inconsistent. What steps can enhance adherence? What difference does the CUBE make?

References

Evans D, Goldstein MP, Popova A. The next wave of deaths from Ebola? The impact of health care worker mortality. Washington, DC: World Bank Group; 2015. Contract No.: WPS 7344.

Fischer WA, Crozier I, Bausch DG, Muyembe J-J, Mulangu S, Diaz JV, et al. Shifting the paradigm—applying universal standards of care to Ebola virus disease. N Engl J Med. 2019;380(15):1389–91. https://doi.org/10.1056/NEJMp1817070.

Sprecher AG, Caluwaerts A, Draper M, Feldmann H, Frey CP, Funk RH, et al. Personal protective equipment for filovirus epidemics: a call for better evidence. J Infect Dis. 2015;212(Suppl 2):S98–S100. https://doi.org/10.1093/infdis/jiv153.

41 Management of Security for Clinical Trials During Emergencies

Billy Sivahera Muyisa, Eric Barte de Sainte Fare, and Jamila Aboulhab

Contents

Learning Track Note: This chapter appears in Learning Tracks: Emergency Research Response, Research Operations; Research Ethics

E. S. Higgs and R. A. Sorenson (eds.), *Principles and Practice of Emergency Research Response*,
https://doi.org/10.1007/978-3-031-48408-7_62

Learning Objectives

This chapter will help readers understand and describe the following:

- The terms risk, threat, and vulnerability
- The issue of sponsor institutions and countries prohibiting illicit payments in environments where such payments are widely accepted
- How security measures to protect a research site in a hostile environment might affect the quality of the research
- How adhering to the Golden Rule contributes to the security of a research site
- Ways of securing the pharmacy, laboratory, and cold chain
- Vital communication rules that ensure security and facilitate response actions in case of an incident
- Social communication strategies that enhance transparency and dispel conspiracy theories and scurrilous rumors
- The process of ethically selecting research participants and avoiding security
- Problems or threats from aggrieved community members not selected for trial participation
- Some useful precepts for cash withdrawals at the bank

1 Introduction

Conducting clinical research in emergency situations requires a prior analysis of the country and locality and potential risks which could jeopardize the research, research staff, participants, and their communities. Because research projects involve all these stakeholders within a surrounding environment, there are always potential safety concerns during a clinical trial, many of them specific to the time and place. Since infectious disease outbreaks are especially likely to appear and spread where poverty, malnutrition, and insecurity are already prevalent, participants and communities may have been at risk even before the trial. For example, in the northeastern Democratic Republic of the Congo (DRC) from 2018 to 2020, an Ebola outbreak coincided with a tense election in provinces far from the capital where several armed groups were already operating and violence was directed against Ebola responders (UN 2019). Especially in places where there is deep disaffection from central authorities, the arrival of treatment and research teams whose intentions are not clear to the populace, who promote unwelcome public health measures, and whose relative material wealth is apparent, can engender additional risks. Since medical responders seem to appear along with the disease itself, the idea that the newcomers are bringing the disease, rather than responding to it, can gain a foothold (Muzembo et al. 2020).

Given such potential dangers, it is essential to assess the threat environment where the response and research team will be operating, what additional risks the conduct of the trial could engender, and how to mitigate risks through community outreach to explain the relevance and the potential immediate and long-term benefits of the project for local communities.

A great many of the standard precepts of any medical or development project's security management apply to emergency clinical research, just as many of the standards applying to any sort of biomedical research will apply in the emergency context.

This chapter will focus on the environment analysis, potential risks, and management of security issues, as well as measures to mitigate risk.

Three principles apply:

- *No research begins without considering security.*
- *Security of staff and participants is paramount and shall never be neglected.*
- *Adherence to high standards of ethics and courtesy helps guard against anger and resentment.*

2 Evaluation and Analysis of Security Issues

2.1 Contextual Analysis of the Environment

As complete an analysis of the political, social, and environmental context as possible, including a threat assessment, must be conducted before clinical trials and other research projects begin. Such analyses will primarily use qualitative rather than quantitative techniques. Information may be gathered from a variety of sources: observation, informed sources, local and international media, government organizations, and documents from reliable sources. Environmental analysis will provide a clear understanding of infrastructure, sanitation, climate, and pollution hazards. Health system performance and health risk analysis will be based on quantitative as well as qualitative information. ▶ Box 1 shows elements to be considered for each of three components.

Box 1: Context Analysis

Political: Key elements of the country's history; political actors and their respective roles and influence; civil society; type of governance; elections; democracy, freedoms, and human rights advocacy groups; causes of political and social tensions; information about parties in conflict; etc.

Environment: Weather forecasts; flooding risk; road practicability; hygiene and sanitation status; air pollution; etc.

Health: Health indicators; health system organization and performance; referral system; epidemic and endemic diseases; bacterial and viral infection risks; etc.

2.2 Risk and Threat

Security professionals define risk and threat in a particular way. The United Nations (UN) Security Policy Manual (2017), for example, stipulates that a threat is "a potential cause of harm initiated by deliberate actions," while risk is "the likelihood of a harmful event occurring and the impact of the event if it were to occur (Risk = Likelihood × Impact)." Put another way, a threat is a possible cause of harm; a risk is a calculation of the probability of the threat and the amount of harm it would cause. Another useful term, vulnerability, refers to things that program managers may be able to correct to reduce risk: "a weakness that can allow a threat or hazard to cause harm." To state a simple example, there is always a *threat* of theft where valuable equipment, drugs, and money are concerned. The *risk* of a theft could be determined by estimating its prevalence in the research locale and the effect it would have on the program: if all the investigational new drugs are stolen, the program would have to stop. The possible *vulnerabilities* the managers would want to consider include whether the facility is guarded at all times, the vetting of the guards, and whether the storage space is secured (◘ Fig. 1).

2.3 Security Assessment and Analysis

Security analysis should produce what the UN calls a structured threat assessment, which evaluates five categories: armed conflict, terrorism, crime, civil unrest, and hazards (UN 2017). Each category is evaluated using a point system, and the combination of these separate scores determines a security level. Many security assessment tools are available to download or use online (Open Briefing 2020). ▶ Box 2 describes the five threat categories used by the UN and how they could affect a clinical trial. Each category is analyzed based on three variables: the intent/mindset (i.e., the intention or disposition to cause harm), the capability (i.e., the ability to cause harm), and the inhibiting context (i.e., existing deterrents to the threat). A threat level is then identified on a scale of 1 (minimal threat) to 5 (maximum threat, incidents already occurring).

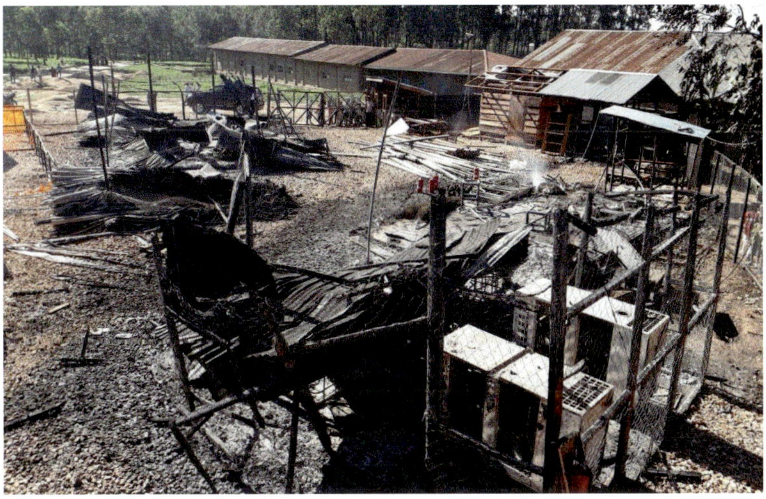

Fig. 1 Unidentified attackers set fire to a 70-bed Ebola treatment center in Katwa, North Kivu, DRC, in early 2019. (Laurie Bonnaud/MSF)

Box 2: Threats Defined

Armed conflict: Organized violence by groups fighting each other. Noninvolved parties would most likely be indirectly affected by this threat, although Ebola treatment centers (ETCs) in DRC were attacked directly by armed groups in 2018 and 2019.

Terrorism: Violence by individuals or groups against civilians or other noncombatant targets. Clinical trial staff, participants, and assets could be directly or indirectly affected by this threat.

Crime: Illegal activities undertaken for economic or personal gain, with or without violence. Trial staff, operating funds, equipment, and infrastructure are a potential target even when the project is welcomed by the community.

Civil unrest: Organized demonstrations or unauthorized disturbances to public order (e.g., rioting, looting). It may or may not involve violence. The trial could be directly or indirectly affected by this threat.

Hazards: Natural events (such as earthquakes or extreme weather) or human-caused incidents (such as fires, road accidents, industrial disasters) can lead to destruction, injury, or death.

Figure 2 shows the threat assessment and the scale of threat for an armed conflict.

Such a systematic approach will identify existing and potential threats and the risks they pose to the conduct of the trial. Security analyses should be updated regularly and after any significant change in the security context. Comparing your risk and threat assessment with that of other partners present in the field helps ensure your own analysis is complete and realistic. Security information may also be collected through the UN Department of Safety and Security, UNDSS, which has a mandate to cooperate with "relevant NGOs" under the Saving Lives Together framework (UN 2017). Researchers sponsored by national government institutions may also be able to work with security professionals at their embassy or at their headquarters to conduct security assessments and take necessary steps to reduce risk. For example, the US. Embassy in Liberia conducted a security review of the first Ebola clinical trial vaccination site in Monrovia. As a matter of principle, differences over the existing threat level should be resolved in favor of greater protection.

Threat level	Intent or mind-set	Capability	Inhibiting context
1	No intention to use armed or military force	No presence of or very limited hostile military type capability, weapons, and training; small numbers of disorganized groups/factions	Strong deterrents against initiating conflict
2	Indications that military force is an option or statements threatening attack, but political solution still possible.	Small arms and automatic weapons, but limited/minimal military type training and experience; loosely organized	Pressure and other incentives or agreements against hostilities occurring
3	Clear statements of imminent attack, peaceful options exhausted, and/or limited military operations	Organized and structured forces but without a deployed heavy weapons (HW) capability	Peace talks or unstable peace/ cease-fire agreement
4	Limited armed conflict	Organized and structured forces with HW deployed, and/or large numbers of forces and intensified military style operations.	No political or other restraints or pressure to prevent the outbreak of conflict
5	Widespread armed conflict	Organized structured forces with HW capability deployed or large number of disorganized forces fully engaged	Armed conflict already occurring in the area

Fig. 2 Threat assessment for an armed conflict. (Billy Sivahera Muyisa)

3 Management of Security Issues

3.1 Security Organization

A clear organizational chart defining security roles and responsibilities must be prepared with project managers and made known to all staff, who are responsible for complying with guidelines and fulfilling their security roles. A security grid defines the measures or actions corresponding to a particular security situation. To protect the staff and the assets of the research project, security rules need to be respected and enforced by the persons in charge. Planning should cover foreseeable contingencies and include evacuation plans and shelter-in-place procedures known to all staff. Based on the criteria defined above, a security level is defined by the designated person or group, often a committee comprising top management and the person(s) responsible for security. When a given security level is adopted, all staff working in the clinical trial must comply with the corresponding security guidance. Normally any substantial violation would result in the violator being removed from the team.

Specific actions taken in response to rising threat levels may include adjustment of working hours, closure of sites or offices, restrictions on movement, stricter site access control, a decision to shelter in place at the organization base, or even a partial or full evacuation of staff from the project site.

3.2 Communications

A few simple rules for communications are vital to ensure security and coordinate actions in case of an incident or worsening situation. Since wired landline telephones are the least secure, calls should be made via either mobile telephony provided by local operators or satellite phones (e.g., Thuraya, Inmarsat), which should be available to the project as an emergency backup; high cost per minute is the main obstacle to routine use of satellite phones. Internet connection may be made via GPRS (General Packet Radio Services) and Wi-Fi mobile modems (mobile hotspots) at remote sites. An updated research response telephone directory must be available to all staff involved in the research project but should not be kept within the project and "need-to-know" contacts like headquarters or security resources.

Vehicle radios can serve as an additional communications backup in some cases, but their primary purpose is for personnel out of range of other networks and for vehicles to do a regular communications check with their departure and destination points when traveling between sites. Communications procedures for security operations need to be tightly controlled: only authorized security personnel, the security chief, or the project lead is authorized to communicate security instructions.

3.3 Behavior

Adherence to high ethical standards (▶ Chaps. 33, 33.2, and 33.3) helps guard against resentment and anger on the part of the local population and even other staff members. Just as important is personal commitment by staff members to help patients, trial participants, and their community. The attitude and behavior of research team members must express these values; this is a moral imperative but also a practical necessity. Failure to respect other persons not only violates a key ethical norm, but it could also undermine the research program's security and credibility. While several ethical codes related to clinical research and infectious disease response are covered in earlier chapters (▶ Chap. 5), the WHO Code of Conduct (2017) is a more general practical guide that expresses the principles of a humanitarian project in day-to-day behavior. It includes the following key points:

- A respectful attitude toward research participants and a friendly demeanor toward the partners and the populations involved
- Good communication between team members to coordinate effectively and promote harmony in the workplace
- Maintaining a calm demeanor in stressful and demanding situations
- Understanding the customs of the locality and population without condemning them

3.4 Corruption

No matter how widespread or customary they might be, corrupt practices are not tolerated by international organizations, government agencies, or academic institutions. The definition used by the leading anti-corruption NGO, Transparency International (2014), is widely accepted: "the abuse of entrusted power for private gain." Whether it takes the form of paying inflated prices for contracts or procurement, preferential hiring for the relatives of local power brokers, or paying unauthorized "tolls" for transport, corrupt practices not only violate the policies of sponsoring organizations and governments—they detract from the reputation of a research project, feed the perception that it is just another group of people feathering their own nests, and can lead to ever-increasing demands for payoffs.

3.5 Human Resource Management

Personnel recruitment can be sensitive in certain contexts and even generate security problems. Especially in remote areas where relations with central authorities are troubled, rumors that expatriates and experts from the national capital are there for personal gain can poison relations with the community. But research requires experienced staff members with specific skills. It may be necessary to explain carefully why specialists from elsewhere are needed to implement the research project (▶ Chap. 18).

Once again, this a matter of ethics and equity that also has practical implications for security. To the extent possible, the research project should endeavor to build capacity for and transfer skills to the national and local communities. It is good policy to focus on local recruitment for positions that do not have specific requirements. Transparent human resource procedures and policies and an open recruitment process are a must for limiting resentment, suspicion, and protest by local communities—and therefore for limiting security threats. In some contexts, all individuals who have submitted their application files must be "selected" and interviews conducted orally and in public to satisfy the community that the hiring process is honest. Multiethnic conflict can further complicate personnel considerations; recruiting staff from all significant communities in the research area is another principle based on moral values that can help minimize suspicions and resentment in the surrounding population.

3.6 Selection of Research Participants

Recruitment of study participants is crucial and must be transparent. All ethnicities, tribes, social strata, and other significant groups should be included, taking into account eligibility criteria for the trial, Good Participatory Practice (GPP) (▶ Chap. 18) and Good Clinical Practice (GCP) (ICH 2016; UNAIDS and AVAC 2011). The sensitivities of the population should also be considered, more so because existing poverty is likely to have been aggravated, in many cases, by the outbreak or epidemic. Benefits received—better medical care, meals, transport costs, per diem—can loom large, in some cases becoming the only income of the trial participants. Since the number of participants in clinical trials is usually limited and based on strict eligibility criteria, some would-be participants are likely to feel aggrieved. Transparency in recruitment and the involvement of local communities in all stages of the project's implementation can minimize any potential increased threat on this basis. A means of identifying research participants will also be needed. Depending on the environment, this could be simple ID cards or biometric security arrangements. A database to track scheduled and unscheduled visits by research participants is also useful.

3.7 Visibility and External Communication

Some organizations and their logos can be a target from the outset of an emergency. This is yet another instance where local cultural and political knowledge is essential to gauge the extent of threats that may arise from hostility to a particular organization or country. Threat analysis should determine whether one of the research sponsors or implementing organizations is likely to be attacked. Since emergency research is a multidisciplinary effort with several actors, it might be best to use a neutral logo that has no previous history and brings together all research actors. That does not prevent organizations from pursuing logos for their own assets if that is deemed safe. Both as a security matter and for consistency of messages, all oral, written, or visual external communications must be made in consultation with the principal investigators in charge of the research.

3.8 Photography

In general, photography should take place only with sufficient knowledge of local culture and norms. Never photograph or interview people without their express consent. If there is any chance the photograph or interview will be published, there should be written informed consent in the form of a signed document. The consent document should be translated into a language the person signing knows. When photos are taken, their purpose must be compatible with the mandate of the research sponsors and partners. Photos of vulnerable people at sensitive moments, such as when they are ill, can easily cross the invisible line into exploitation or be seen to do so. We recommend staff never take pictures of soldiers, police officers, government officials, military installations, or other sites that may be deemed sensitive by authorities.

4 Social Mobilization, Communications, and Community Engagement

4.1 Social Science Surveys

Anthropological research and surveys of community sentiment before and during a clinical research study can also help mitigate risks and anticipate security issues. A community engagement strategy is essential for such research projects for many reasons, and ongoing surveys must be carried out on all operational issues in order to adapt the appropriate strategies to the field. It is important to be aware that "community" is not a simple concept but can refer to multiple overlapping categories people belong to, for example, their village, tribe or clan, religion, occupation, social class, and, of course, gender (Wilkinson et al. 2017).

4.2 Social Communications

Maximum transparency is a sacrosanct principle for research project implementation. Effective explanation of the methods and objectives of the project helps build the support of surrounding communities for the project and its staff. People need to understand the added value of the research project in the short, medium, and long term. The better they understand the project, the more they will defend it with their communities, families, and peers (▶ Chap. 18). Such alliances with local stakeholders must be based on achieving the objectives of the project and providing any promised benefits and should not be based on cash payment as the primary incentive. The subject is one of continued disagreement and controversy (Largent and Fernandez 2017), but the ongoing involvement of legitimate leaders and their participation in outreach activities for community ownership of the messages are important, as are community-based chats, meetings, and advocacy activities. The organization of guided tours of research sites with community members and leaders reduces rumors and promotes acceptance of the project.

Beyond medical management of serious adverse events (SAEs), such as anaphylactic shock, a participant's death must be handled according to the protocol procedures in place, which should have been developed with local partners. Community-based plans for group insurance services need to take local socio-anthropological norms into account for effective management of serious events and communications with family, communities, and local authorities. Clumsy or inappropriate handling of deaths or severe injuries could lead to violent reactions against the research site or personnel, which family or community members blame for the deaths or injuries. If disease mortality rates are high, as with Ebola, or if the interventions under investigation prove not to be efficacious or even cause harm, the risk to staff and research sites increases. The pharmacovigilance team and local staff members who know the community should report regularly on community attitudes toward the research project.

Conspiracy theories and scurrilous rumors about research projects, especially those testing experimental products, are all too common. The idea that the project's real purpose is human experimentation, sterilization, or even extermination can find fertile ground. While the principle of transparency remains paramount in clinical research, in some contexts, the impact of large-scale communication of research objectives with poorly formulated messages may be misunderstood, and excessive public messaging may be counterproductive. A lower public profile, limiting full communications to trial participants, implementers, and officials who need to know, may be preferable. Such a decision would only be made with the advice of knowledgeable local partners.

4.3 Disaffected Communities

There are times and places where national and local governments have lost their popular legitimacy—where people's needs, safety, and protection have been neglected by authorities or where epidemic response has been inadequate. Since research projects need government authorities for authorization and implementation, the national government is nearly always an official partner in an emergency research endeavor. While remaining in partnership with the country's authorities, research stakeholders may need to differentiate themselves through professional and neutral implementation of the research and equal respect for members of all social groups. Research actors may need to negotiate with rebellious or criminal armed groups opposed to the government.

5 Securing Research Assets

5.1 Research Sites

Research facilities—both physical facilities and electronic systems for data and communications—must always be secured against unauthorized entry in order to protect people, property, confidentiality, and scientific value of data, biological samples, experimental products, etc.

Physical security of a research project begins with site selection (▶ Chap. 40). A participatory process with the surrounding community in choosing and setting up the site is essential. It is often preferable for research sites to be integrated with existing structures such as hospitals or health facilities, which may facilitate acceptance of the research by populations who know them as medical locations. Such sites often have existing physical security measures (walls, access-controlled entries, etc.) conducive to good security management. The establishment of isolated sites may fuel rumors about secrecy for hidden purposes. Unless infection prevention and control or biosafety considerations require an isolated location, it is good practice to locate in populated areas.

This chapter will not go into great detail about specific security procedures, especially since they depend so heavily on local conditions. There are many practical security manuals and guidelines for humanitarian operations in difficult environments (Davis et al. 2017; Overseas Development Institute 2010; Oxfam. 2014; Stoddard et al. 2019). Even more useful is consultation with health emergency responders and other assistance groups already operating in the area to take advantage of their experience. A complex research program is unlikely to be the first organization to set up in an emergency.

5.2 Securing Energy, Information and Communications Technology, and Inventory

Monitoring of electrical installations must be continuous, and regular tests and preventive maintenance must be carried out. Local staff may be trained on the basics of energy security and the standard operating procedures (SOPs) defining the rules to be developed (see ▶ Chap. 35).

Security for information and communications technology is a field of its own (▶ Chap. 34). Many of the operational principles and practices will be the same as they are anywhere in the world; most of the differences in a low-resource research setting will be related to the fragility and inadequacy of existing infrastructure.

5.3 Pharmacy, Laboratory, and Cold Chain Security

Pharmacy operations include importation, safekeeping, inventory management, and transport (▶ Chap. 38). The premises housing the pharmacy and investigational product preparation must meet well-defined security criteria in accordance with the research protocol. Laboratories must also be built or renovated in accordance with the research to be done there (▶ Chap. 9). Detailed specifications must be put in place before tenders for laboratory construction or renovation are issued. The space(s) housing the pharmacy and laboratory must have an additional level of physical protection and access control over and above that of the research site as a whole, and entry should be strictly limited to personnel authorized by the principal investigator or site manager.

Most clinical research projects will require a cold chain to transport investigational products, reagents, and other needed supplies to the site, sometimes with special requirements for maintaining a very cold temperature (−80 °C) (▶ Chap. 39). The transfer of biological samples can also have specific biosafety requirements to ensure they do not leak into the environment even in extreme events like a plane crash. Specific procedures for the safety of the cold chain are to be developed according to the requirements of the project.

5.4 Money

Research projects in low-resource, emergency contexts will often have to do much of their business in cash, sometimes quite a lot of it. Because research projects usually require that some compensation be paid to participants to cover their expenses and inconvenience, cash payments may regularly coincide with participant visits. Goods and services like motor vehicle and generator fuel, food supplies, payment of personnel, etc. will sometimes have to be in cash. Specific security rules will limit financial and human risks. The project finance coordinator manages cash as well as accounts. The specific rules governing security of funds should not be shared beyond senior staff and those who must actually implement them, since dissemination of this sensitive information could compromise the security of fund transport, storage, and disbursement (Gordon 2015). When possible, payments should be made by bank transfer only, rather than by check or cash. Crisis conditions are often associated with banditry, and research programs may be seen as easy and lucrative targets. Security risks associated with cash are important, and liquidity management requires attention.

Project accounts must operate with a dual signature to ensure no one person has unchecked control of funds. The signers are often the project manager and the financial administrator, who approve the operations according to the internal administrative and financial procedures of the organization. Finally, note that risks increase at the end of the month, with the payment of staff salaries; before important holidays (Eid al-Fitr, Easter, New Year) because these may require seasonal expenditures among the local communities; when the local economy is depressed by the emergency; and if soldiers or civilian officials have not been paid.

6 Conclusion

As with so many aspects of an emergency clinical research response, ensuring security for sites and personnel requires upholding the fundamental standards that pertain to a nonemergency situation, by applying both professional expertise and sufficient flexibility to cope with the emergency circumstances. Not all threats can be averted, but good security practices will prevent the vast majority of potential incidents that can harm the research program, its personnel and participants, and the communities in which it is implemented.

Box 3: An Example of Specific Security Procedures

Cash withdrawals are made at the bank under the following rules:

- Avoid as much as possible withdrawals between the 25th and 5th of the month, since salaries, rents, etc. are often due at the end or beginning of the month.
- The day of withdrawal should vary with each withdrawal.
- The administrator making the withdrawal is accompanied only by a driver, who must remain on standby.
- The travel destination is not communicated to the guards or on motor pool movement tables; it should be replaced with an innocuous destination like the market.
- The destination is communicated orally to other senior staff present at the office.
- The destination is communicated to the driver only en route.
- Routes are varied if possible and safe.
- During the return, the windows of the vehicle must be closed, and the doors locked.
- No other stops can be considered while traveling to and from the bank.
- The frequency and timing of cash transfers, whether from the bank or between project locations, must appear random.
- At the bank, cash withdrawals must be done in a private room.
- The return path must vary with each withdrawal if at all possible. The administrator should tell the driver which route to take as they are returning.

Discussion Questions

1. Define the terms risk, threat, and vulnerability.
2. The United States and other industrialized nations have strict laws forbidding kickbacks, bribes, or other illicit payments, especially when government funds are involved. In many countries, such illicit payments are tacitly accepted. If you were involved in contracting or other business affairs for a research site, how would you reconcile this conflict?
3. If a research site had to be protected at all times from a hostile local population, how would this affect the quality of the research?
4. The Golden Rule–treat others as you wish to be treated, or another of its varying formulations–is an accepted ethical principle in many if not most religions and cultures. How can adhering to the Golden Rule contribute to the security of your research site?
5. Research facilities must be secured against unauthorized entry. Discuss ways to secure the pharmacy, laboratory, and cold chain.
6. Discuss a few simple but vital communication rules to ensure security and coordinate actions in case of an incident or worsening situation.
7. Maximum transparency is critical when implementing a research project. Transparency demands effectively explaining the methods and objectives of the project to help build the support of surrounding communities for the project and its staff. Discuss social communication strategies that enhance transparency, and dispel conspiracy theories and scurrilous rumors.
8. Discuss the process of ethically selecting research participants and avoiding security problems or threats from aggrieved community members unable to meet inclusion criteria for trial participation.
9. Discuss some cash withdrawal rules to be followed at the bank.

References

Davis J, Reilly L, Vazquez Llorente R, Williamson C, Fairbanks A. Security to go: a risk-management toolkit for humanitarian aid-agencies. London: European Interagency Security Forum; 2017.

Gordon L. Risk and humanitarian cash transfer programming. London: Overseas Development Institute; 2015.

ICH. Good clinical practice: ICH harmonised guideline. Integrated addendum to ICH E6(R1): guideline for good clinical practice ICH E6(R2) ICH consensus guideline. Geneva: International Council for Harmonisation of Technical Requirements for Pharmaceuticals for Human Use (ICH); 2016.

Largent EA, Fernandez Lynch H. Paying research participants: regulatory uncertainty, conceptual confusion, and a path forward. Yale J Health Policy Law Ethics. 2017;17(1):61–141.

Muzembo BA, Ntontolo NP, Ngatu NR, Khatiwada J, Ngombe KL, Numbi OL, et al. Local perspectives on Ebola during its tenth outbreak in DR Congo: a nationwide qualitative study. PLoS One. 2020;15(10):e0241120. https://doi.org/10.1371/journal.pone.0241120.

Open Briefing. Security risk assessment tool. Penzance: Open Briefing Ltd.; 2020. https://www.openbriefing.org/resources/security-risk-assessment-tool/. Accessed 16 Mar 2020.

Overseas Development Institute. Good practice review: operational security management in violent environments. London: Overseas Development Institute; 2010.

Oxfam. Oxfam security policy. Nairobi: Oxfam; 2014. p. 21.

Stoddard A, Czwarno M, Hamsik L. NGOs & risk: managing uncertainty in local-international partnerships: interaction. 2019.

Transparency International. Preventing corruption in humanitarian operations. Berlin: Transparency International; 2014.

UN. Security policy manual. New York: United Nations; 2017.

UN. Armed groups kill Ebola health workers in eastern DR Congo. UN News; 2019.

UNAIDS, AVAC. Good participatory practice: guidelines for biomedical HIV prevention trials. Geneva: UNAIDS (Joint United Nations Programme on HIV/AIDS); 2011.

WHO. Code of conduct for responsible research. Geneva: World Health Organization; 2017. p. 26.

Wilkinson A, Parker M, Martineau F, Leach M. Engaging 'communities': anthropological insights from the West African Ebola epidemic. Philos Trans R Soc Lond B Biol Sci. 2017;372(1721) https://doi.org/10.1098/rstb.2016.0305.

42 Locally Hired Staff for Clinical Research Sites in Low-Resource Settings

Beth Baseler, Mary Smolskis, Jestina Doe-Anderson, Melvin Johnson, Wissedi Njoh, Sara Albert, and Chris Worthington

Contents

Learning Track Note: This chapter appears in Learning Tracks: Emergency Research Response, Research Operations; Research Ethics

E. S. Higgs and R. A. Sorenson (eds.), *Principles and Practice of Emergency Research Response*,
https://doi.org/10.1007/978-3-031-48408-7_63

Learning Objectives

This chapter will help readers understand and describe the following:

- The main requirements for a human resource plan
- The importance of team communication and partnership when hiring and managing staff
- The roles of various staff positions in a research program, using the PREVAIL Ebola vaccine study as an example
- The adaptive approach to clinical research conduct in a setting with little experience of research and shortcomings in basic staffing and infrastructure
- The value of social mobilization, communications, and community outreach (SMC) throughout a research study
- Some ethical and pragmatic dilemmas in recruiting scarce skilled personnel during an emergency outbreak
- Training staff members during an emergency response
- Workarounds if more experienced personnel are prohibited from traveling to sites where the research protocol is being implemented because of security concerns

1 Background

Human resources must meet the requirements of regulatory and ethics compliance and scientific rigor even during time-sensitive, high-risk scenarios. The examples below are drawn from multiple studies and the authors' experience, primarily in the response to Ebola virus disease (EVD) in Liberia during the 2014–2016 outbreak in West Africa and to a lesser degree in the 2018–2020 outbreak in the eastern Democratic Republic of the Congo (DRC). All three of the countries most affected in 2014–2016, as well as the DRC, are classified as low income by the World Bank and least developed by the United Nations (OECD 2021). For this reason and because of past or present civil conflict, infrastructure was lacking, the health system was overtaxed, and qualified personnel—especially medical personnel—were in short supply. Operations in the eastern DRC outbreak were further complicated by current civil unrest and multiple armed groups moving amid a population mistrustful of central government authority (Nguyen 2019).

Most of the potential challenges to establishing a research program will be encountered in low-resource settings like these; similar difficulties will occur even in high-income countries during a public health emergency. Clinical trial partners must work together to design and conduct scientifically rigorous, ethical, and culturally appropriate clinical studies that meet international standards for clinical research, with the goal of (a) mitigating and helping to end the outbreak and (b) gathering regulatory-level data on investigational products, while active human-to-human transmission of the pathogen in question continues.

Human resource planning and identification should commence when a protocol concept is defined in parallel with other activities required for planning, initiating, and conducting clinical studies. It is critical to initiate this process as early as possible, with the expectation that the planning will be refined based on new information and experience.

2 Emergency Response Clinical Trials

Examples from two separate Ebola outbreaks illustrate lessons learned in collaborative efforts to engage locally hired staff to carry out essential functions in the research responses.

The first example comes from the U.S. National Institute of Allergy and Infectious Diseases' (NIAID) experience with the inaugural trial of the Partnership for Research on Ebola Vaccines in Liberia (PREVAIL)[1] during the 2014–2016 West Africa outbreak (Kennedy et al. 2016; Larson et al. 2017).

1 As the PREVAIL program expanded, the full name is changed to Partnership for Research on Vaccines and Infectious Diseases in Liberia to include other types of infectious disease research, but the PREVAIL acronym remains.

PREVAIL I was a Phase II placebo-controlled randomized clinical trial designed to evaluate the safety and efficacy of two candidate Ebola vaccines. It was initially planned as a Phase III trial that would enroll up to 28,000 participants, but with a decline in new cases of Ebola virus infection as the outbreak waned, the Phase III design was no longer deemed to be feasible. Following safety, ethical, and U.S. Food and Drug Administration (FDA) approval/concurrence, the study was amended to a more robust 1500-person Phase II design. PREVAIL nevertheless proved to be a pivotal example for increased acceptance of clinical research as an integral part of an infectious disease emergency response (NASEM 2017; Thielman et al. 2016). For a study of this magnitude, effective human resource management was vital to identifying, recruiting, training, motivating, and retaining staff for an effective and productive workforce aligned with the strategic priorities of the program. Most of this chapter is based on the PREVAIL experience.

Lessons from PREVAIL also informed the planning and implementation of the DRC PALM trial (*Pamoja Tulinde Maisha*, meaning "Together Save Lives" in Swahili), and elements of PREVAIL adapted to PALM will be described in the training section of this chapter. This was a NIAID collaboration with the DRC *Institut National de Recherche Biomédicale* (INRB) during the 2018–2020 EVD outbreak in the North Kivu and Ituri provinces (Mulangu et al. 2019; WHO 2020a). The DRC Ebola PALM therapeutics trial provided most of the data that led to FDA approval of two Ebola treatments (FDA 2020a, b). Planning for both studies moved as expeditiously as possible. The PREVAIL I study in Liberia took 3 months from initial planning to enrollment of the first study participant in a naïve clinical research setting.

2.1 PREVAIL

PREVAIL serves in several chapters of this volume (▶ Chaps. 17, and 40, In Practice 32.1) as a paradigmatic example of how to overcome barriers and carry out a research program under demanding circumstances. The 2014–2016 Ebola outbreak in West Africa, in which Liberia was one of three countries hit hardest, was a test case for quickly implementing clinical research programs on new Ebola vaccine candidates to mitigate a major outbreak while it was occurring.

2.1.1 PREVAIL Background

PREVAIL was the outcome of an overture from the Liberian Minister of Health to the U.S. Secretary of Health and Human Services for a suggested research collaboration. The objective was to conduct research on promising therapeutics and vaccines for EVD, which had been identified in West Africa for the first time (Doe-Anderson et al. 2016). A panel of researchers and scientists from the U.S. National Institutes of Health (NIH), NIAID, and the Ebola Incident Management Team designated by the Liberian Ministry of Health (MoH) discussed how to mitigate the outbreak and decided to conduct clinical trials on existing investigational vaccines (Lane et al. 2016). Fundamental aspects of ensuring a successful clinical research partnership included quickly defining roles and responsibilities to establish a partnership agreement and governance and organizational structures.

Liberia had hosted little clinical research before 2014, and the necessary infrastructure and human resource capabilities for clinical research were limited at best. While much has been written on how to conduct clinical research, there are few written resources on infrastructure and staffing in research-naïve, resource-limited settings (Koita et al. 2016; NASEM 2017).

Liberian infrastructure and healthcare still suffered the lingering consequences of years of civil war between 1989 and 2003. Conflict effectively destroyed most of the medical clinics and hospitals in the nation and severely depleted the medical workforce. By 2008, only 51 physicians were practicing in a country of 3.9 million people—1.4 physicians per 100,000 citizens. Although this number had grown to 90 doctors in 2010 (WHO 2020b), it was still a tiny fraction of the needed proportion of physicians to population. The country's only medical school had few faculty members

(Challoner and Forget 2011) and shut down with the onset of the EVD outbreak in 2014. Most Liberian medical students and residents left their training to work in Ebola treatment units (ETUs) or in other positions with international agencies. Most non-Ebola health facilities had closed by the fall of 2014. The weaknesses in Liberia's healthcare system were exacerbated by the epidemic; 8% of healthcare workers died from the disease, including 5 doctors and 78 nurses (Evans et al. 2015).

Even in places where infrastructure and trained research support specialists are available, it usually takes many months to start a clinical research study. Rising death tolls during an infectious disease emergency such as the global COVID-19 pandemic or the West African EVD outbreak make this timeline unacceptable. Efforts in Liberia prefigured global efforts in 2020 to mount an all-fronts response to the outbreak, with expedited clinical research at the core of the response. An urgent yet well-planned process for hiring and training local staff is an essential element of setting up an emergency research program. Along with developing and refining the trial protocol, the PREVAIL team had to determine the level of staffing required to prepare and operate the clinical research facility and secondary trial sites and reconcile the requirements with the available labor force and the number of staff members who could be brought in from outside the country.

Box 1: Initial Short-Term Employment for In-Country and International Staff

The urgency of the Ebola response in West Africa meant that the host countries and their foreign partners had to quickly identify staff, whether through recruitment or reassignment, willing to support rapid-response operations in Liberia and other West African countries. In the case of PREVAIL, the U.S. government and contract staff volunteered to partner with Liberian colleagues to establish the program in Liberia, which got underway in early February 2015. Many other medical personnel from other countries volunteered to work in the West Africa emergency response, despite the risks of working amidst an Ebola epidemic. This led to a widespread short-term employment model comprising a mix of foreign and in-country staff, including many with rotating deployments in and out of West Africa.

Factors leading to the initial success of the collaborations were constant communications between the partners, many of which were face-to-face engagements, mutual knowledge sharing, and identifying and relying on subject matter experts to solve daily challenges and obstacles.

Although this chapter focuses on local hiring, it is worth noting that those who travel from other countries should develop a list of considerations for deployment during an infectious disease outbreak (e.g., risk factors, provision for medical evacuation insurance, international health insurance, medical clearance and required vaccinations, identification of health facilities in the host country where foreign staff can be evaluated and receive medical care, UN or embassy briefings, in-country logistics, visa requirements, and security requirements, among others).

As the PREVAIL partnership got under way, the collaborating U.S.-Liberia team of experts appointed the first three positions by consensus, a Director of Operations and two Assistant Directors, who made up the PREVAIL Operations Team. Once in place, the Operations Team reviewed the protocol concept to identify staff positions, recruit and hire staff, and adapt or establish infrastructure to meet the logistical requirements of the trial.

Moving swiftly required the negotiation and execution of contracts needed to recruit and hire in-country staff to support the human resource management plan. Staffing contracts were legally mandated in Liberia, and though employment law was often skirted, the NIAID-MoH partnership was obligated to comply with them.

The outbreak response required international and in-country experts from the scientific, technical, public health, security, and medical communities to work in concert with the Liberian Ministry of Health and Ministry of Labor to develop mechanisms to hire in-country staff. Rotating clinical research operations staff from the United States, including volunteers from institutions including the NIH, FDA, Centers for Disease Control and Prevention (CDC), U.S. Public Health Service, and others, was also essential to the launch and continuation of the study.

3 Hiring Amid an Emergency

3.1 Human Resource Management

> Establish hiring mechanisms quickly by negotiating and executing contracts that meet the needs of all parties.

Human resource management is vital to identifying, recruiting, retaining, training, and motivating staff members for an effective and productive workforce aligned with the strategic priorities of a program. A human resource management plan guides leadership's human resource actions throughout the study/program. At a minimum, the human resource management plan must include the following:

- Foundational framework for personnel needs
- Planned roles and responsibilities
- Project organization and governance chart(s)
- Staffing management plan(s)
- Recruitment plan and mechanism(s)
- Onboarding plan/employee handbook
- Performance monitoring and evaluation plan
- Fair and reasonable salary scale
- Initial and ongoing training to include leadership and management training as well as scientific and clinical training
- Termination or transition plan for the end of the program and/or transition from emergency response to a sustainable clinical research program
- Inherent flexibility to adjust for rotation of international-local support staff and for modifications to effectively meet evolving resource needs and strategic priorities

While the items listed above are all part of initiating and implementing a robust human resource management plan, not all can realistically be fully developed before the study begins. With PREVAIL, aspects of the essential elements listed above were initially established, while others were enhanced as the Partnership expanded from one vaccine trial in early 2015 to ten interventional and observational studies, including malaria and HIV as well as EVD and involving thousands of participants by the end of 2019.

An emergency research response project in a developing country must include building research capacity in the host country so that the infrastructure, equipment, and personnel can transition to a sustained national research program that addresses an expanded portfolio of diseases (NASEM 2017).

One cannot overemphasize the importance of team communication, collaboration, partnership, and mutual respect in enabling the successful conduct of clinical research during an outbreak, especially when it comes to hiring and managing staff. Full engagement among team members to understand both cultural nuances and standard global requirements is paramount.

Sharing knowledge within the clinical research partnership and capitalizing on the innate strengths of partners involved are also invaluable in emergency response. In PREVAIL, Liberian partners understood and shared specific local factors, such as the Liberian healthcare system and its human resource structure; the cultural norms and practices of potential study participants; and in-country connections, capabilities, and motivations of in-country staff. Communication was crucial to understanding cultural and business-custom nuances related to employing and training physicians, nurses, phlebotomists, pharmacists, and other key staff.

3.2 Key Staff Positions

Personnel who have specific training and competencies are needed to achieve a high standard of design, management, and operational execution of a clinical study (Gobat et al. 2018). Not all the positions listed here are found in standard staffing charts for clinical trials. They represent the adaptive approach used to conduct research in a clinical research-naïve setting with shortcomings in basic infrastructure like power, water, sanitation systems, and communications. Adaptability is fundamental—clinical trial circumstances for emerging or reemerging infectious diseases will vary depending on the nature and burden of the disease, the location, the medical countermeasures available (investigational or licensed), and many other factors. Investigators and operational staff will not find an "off-the-shelf" procedural template in such circumstances, though with proper preparedness they can have one ready to adapt. The task is to apply the principles of clinical research and trial operations in diverse and challenging conditions.

The Operations Team determined that the following positions needed to be staffed for PREVAIL's Ebola vaccine study. The list is indicative and may vary depending on the nature and circumstances of an emergency response and what is required for the study. Therefore, when considering key staff positions, one must be cognizant of the staffing needs of the study while avoiding competition with the national public health emergency response.

3.2.1 The Principal Investigator (PI)

The principal investigator (PI) is the overall chief and manager of a clinical trial and must have the appropriate education (generally MD, PhD, or both), further post-degree training, and considerable trial experience. The PI takes overall responsibility for all aspects of the trial.

3.2.2 Site Physicians and Physician Assistants

Site physicians and physician assistants were on site daily and were responsible for conducting physical exams, reviewing laboratory results, and monitoring the medical condition of participants during their participation. In Liberia, they were often referred to as "medical monitors," although in the clinical research context elsewhere the term usually means "medically qualified individuals … involved in safety oversight and pharmacovigilance" (NIH 2014). It took a little time to straighten out mutual understanding of the term—a case in point of the necessity for agreed terminology among all parties working together.

3.2.3 Subject Matter Experts (SMEs)

Subject matter experts (SMEs) may be needed depending on circumstances in fields such as clinical trial operations, clinical research science, project management, clinical and research laboratory, regulatory, logistics, biostatisticians, pharmacy, data management, quality control, and information and communications technology.

3.2.4 Site Managers

Site managers are responsible for day-to-day operations at the individual sites. The site manager oversees the site, communicates effectively with all stakeholders, and is the primary liaison between the site and the management operations center. They must be capable of implementing and amending site standard operating procedures.

3.2.5 Clinical Site Coordinators

Clinical site coordinators are responsible for monitoring operational activities at all research sites and serving as a liaison with partners and stakeholders. This position might include ensuring appropriate equipment is ordered and delivered, site infrastructure is maintained, staffing is appropriate, etc.

3.2.6 Nurses

- *Research nurses* educate participants about the study, obtain informed consent, perform study-related procedures (such as vital signs assessments and pregnancy testing), record study data, and administer study vaccines.

- *Follow-up nurses* keep track of participants between study visits to monitor potential adverse events and encourage participants to return for subsequent visits. Though follow-up nurses often worked closely with participant trackers, their roles and scopes differed. The participant trackers were members of the local communities who worked in the field, while follow-up nurses were medically trained staff who worked in the clinic and were not necessarily members of the local community.

3.2.7 Case Managers

Case managers work with participants referred for medical issues unrelated to the study to ensure they receive appropriate medical care. They coordinate with the site manager, physicians, and referral centers. They also serve as patient advocates and collaborate to maximize the participant's and family's ability to make informed decisions.

- *Participant trackers*. This position was created by PREVAIL based on a need to follow the vaccine trial participants for the duration of the study to ensure their return for scheduled visits and minimize loss to follow-up. These were known and trusted individuals from the local communities near the study site who talked with the study participants about their concerns, whether medical symptoms, social or personal issues, or community perceptions of the study. The trackers reported relevant information from the participants and the community to the site manager, medical monitor, case manager, and social mobilization team. They helped to minimize community fears and suspicions by conveying accurate information and updates about the research program. The trackers were a key factor in achieving high compliance with follow-up schedules.
- *Psychosocial counselors*, usually social workers or mental health practitioners, provide psychological and social support to participants. Since the Ebola vaccine protocol included HIV/AIDS testing, related counseling was provided in accordance with Liberian MoH mandates for HIV testing.

3.2.8 Study Coordinators

Study coordinators complete case report forms and ensure that all aspects of the protocol have been implemented. They also ensure compliance with international standards such as good clinical practice (GCP) and good participatory practice (GPP) (EMA 2016; FDA 1995; ICH 2016; UNAIDS/AVAC 2011; WHO 2016). The study coordinators ensure quality control and participate in trial procedures on an ongoing basis with research staff to ensure clinical support for the trial is in accordance with the protocol. Although this position was not in the original PREVAIL staffing plan, the study coordinator role was identified later as having been immensely valuable in the EVD and other emerging and reemerging infectious disease (EID) responses. During the COVID-19 pandemic, study coordinators were recruited through domestic and international staffing agencies to supplement clinical site staff who did not have the time to manage all the research aspects of the study due to their patient care responsibilities.

3.2.9 The Laboratory Manager

The laboratory manager ensures that on-site and central laboratory requirements are fulfilled, supervises laboratory technicians and assistants, and implements day-to-day laboratory testing schedules. The laboratory manager may devise and test improved laboratory methods and procedures, represent the clinical laboratory working group as the functional lead, train new technicians on all laboratory standard operating procedures, and evaluate the performance of all laboratory staff. In addition to having the required competencies and skills, the laboratory manager must be flexible and available at all hours to participate in after-hours emergency response when required.

- *Laboratory technicians and lab assistants* collect, process, analyze, and often transport research and clinical samples between clinical research sites and the central clinical lab or the research lab. They are involved in the collection and processing of research samples (blood, urine, breast milk, semen, cord blood, cerebral spinal fluid) and perform chemistry, bacteriology, urine, and hematology analyses.

3.2.10 Pharmacists and Pharmacy Technicians

Pharmacists and pharmacy technicians receive and ensure proper storage, handling, and shipment of investigational products and other pharmaceutical agents (▶ Chap. 38). They prepare products for dispensing in accordance with study protocols and are responsible for ancillary supplies ranging from alcohol swabs to syringes. PREVAIL pharmacists ensured that cold chain requirements were understood, complied with, and documented throughout the study—a mission-critical requirement for sound data (▶ Chap. 39).

3.2.11 Data Management Staff

Data management staff work with the clinical staff to confirm that data collection on study participants is in accordance with the study protocol and that the number of errors and missing data is minimized. They ensure that the data are complete, accurate, and suitable for statistical analysis and fulfill relevant regulatory standards for data quality and integrity. They also support the development of case report forms. These individuals are required to have basic computer proficiency, data entry and presentation skills, and ability to pay close attention to detail in organizing and entering study data, reporting on data entry status, and identifying and communicating data entry queries and complications.

- *Quality control staff* ensure that all data collected fulfill the integrity standards required for future regulatory approval of the investigational product. Quality control staff collaborate extensively with the physicians, site managers, study coordinators, data management, and other research staff to ensure the quality and completeness of study records and documentation.

3.2.12 Information and Communications Technology (ICT)

ICT is the backbone for all operations and can demand improvisational skills that may be hard to find when communications infrastructure is unreliable or lacking (▶ Chap. 34). ICT staff perform setup and troubleshooting on all ICT issues including computers, Internet connectivity, telephones, and radio for communications with drivers; between study sites, staff, and participants; and with national and international sponsors and stakeholders.

3.2.13 Administrative Staff

Administrative staff include administrative assistants, receptionists, office assistants, logistics, and finance clerks. They are essential for the operations of any organization, but the special circumstances of an emergency response clinical research program in a low-resource setting require a special combination of local knowledge and adaptability. The PREVAIL management team identified individuals who not only had administrative skills but also had flexibility and mastery of the local terrain to function and navigate successfully under emergency conditions.

3.2.14 Facilities Management Staff

Facilities management staff includes janitors ("hygienists" in Liberia), security guards, drivers, and maintenance technicians. The many tasks they perform ensure that the physical infrastructure is kept clean, secure, and functional to support the conduct of the research and the safety and well-being of the study participants and staff and that staff and supplies are where they need to be. Maintaining power supply where grid supplies are unreliable is a matter of special importance (▶ Chap. 39).

3.2.15 Communications and Social Mobilization Coordinator

Communications and social mobilization coordinator roles were created in response to the EVD outbreak based on a requirement from the Liberian Ministry of Health because of the positive impact they would have on the outbreak response and mitigating spread.

Social mobilization (▶ Case Study 32.1) ensures that community members and potential study participants are well informed about the purpose and details of the clinical trial and receive ongoing information on new findings and other relevant updates.

- *The communications manager* educated PREVAIL scientists on how to effectively communicate scientific concepts in lay language; trained local journalists on science and health-sensitive reporting; interacted closely with the local and international media to proactively facilitate media coverage of PREVAIL activities, events, and dissemination of research findings; and worked with the SMC team and the MoH to develop appropriate messages for the Liberian public (▶ In Practice 32.1).
- *Social mobilization, communications, and community engagement teams* ensured good participatory practice (GPP) (MacQueen et al. 2015; UNAIDS/AVAC 2011; WHO 2016, 2017) and were also a key factor for the success of Liberia's national effort to reduce EVD transmission, not only through clinical trials but also through broader measures of public health and medical treatment. The Liberian Minister of Health rightly insisted on incorporating social mobilization strategies for outreach to communities as well as for recruitment and retention of study participants, which would have been difficult without a background of community support.
- *Social mobilization coordinators* facilitated entry and acceptance into targeted communities by engaging influential, trusted local community and national stakeholders. In the absence of a formal stakeholder advisory mechanism, such as a community advisory board, the social mobilization coordinators were the primary liaison between the PREVAIL research team and the community. Through high-level advocacy meetings with stakeholders and community engagement events, the social mobilization coordinators ensured that community members and potential study participants were well informed about the purpose and details of the clinical trial and received ongoing information on new findings and other relevant updates. They also provided the PREVAIL researchers and leadership team with feedback and concerns about the research from the community members and study participants. They must be excellent communicators and well-received by community members.

In the DRC, the overall human resources strategy included operational management staff as well as a plan for recruiting and hiring dedicated on-the-ground clinical research site, laboratory, pharmacy, and other protocol-associated staff. The staff performed activities such as the safe and efficient preparation and administration of therapeutics, sample collection and transport, data entry and quality control activities, safety reporting, and regulatory support. In addition, the subcontractor hired a management team that included clinical, data management, logistical, operations, administrative, and financial expertise.

The human resources requirements for the PALM trial in the DRC included the following:

- Executive committee
  - Chair
  - Deputy chair
  - Members (4)
- Program operations
  - Operations manager
  - Clinical coordinator
  - Training coordinator
  - Finance
  - Supply logistician
  - Human resources (HR)/regulatory support
  - Administrative assistants (2)
  - Driver
- Laboratory
  - Lab coordinator
  - Lab supervisor
  - Research lab support (2)
  - Research lab data
- Data and information
  - Data manager
  - Data manager assistant/data entry supervisor
  - Data assistants (2)
  - Information technology (IT) manager
  - IT assistant

- Pharmacy and pharmacovigilance (PV)
  - Pharmacy/PV coordinator
  - Safety physicians (4)
  - Pharmacists (2)
  - Assistant pharmacy supervisors (2)
- Social mobilization and communication
  - Communications officers (3)
  - Psychosocial counselors (2)
  - Participant trackers (6)
- Site development and management
  - Site PIs (2)
  - Assistant clinical research associates (3)
  - Pediatrician (1)
  - Clinicians (7)
  - Study nurses (4)
- Subcontractor field office
  - Country operations manager
  - Chief accountant
  - Accountants (2)
  - Payroll assistant
  - Human resource manager
  - Administrative assistant
  - Procurement/inventory control officer
  - Travel counselor
  - IT specialist
  - Logistician/fleet officer
  - Project coordinator assistant
  - Finance clerk
  - HR clerk
  - Facilities manager
  - Site administration assistant
- The Mitchell Group (TMG) home office staff
  - Project director
  - Clinical project manager
  - Program manager
  - Program associate/travel counselor
  - Financial management specialist

The position descriptions were similar to those described for the Liberian team.

3.3 Recruitment, Interview, and Selection

In responding to an emergency outbreak situation, one must consider the source(s) for staff, as well as recruiting and hiring. In a government-to-government relationship, both governments will generally provide and help to recruit human resources. Contract support is also a source to supplement existing staffing. Early determination of requirements and recruitment methods is advised since there may be other outbreak response and clinical research organizations vying for a very limited pool of skilled personnel. Terms of reference for both clinical and nonclinical positions should also be quickly developed to illustrate the scope of work needed for the effort. Advertising should be considered and processes for interviewing and hiring should begin early. A graphic for this process (◘ Fig. 1) is shown below. Establishing terms

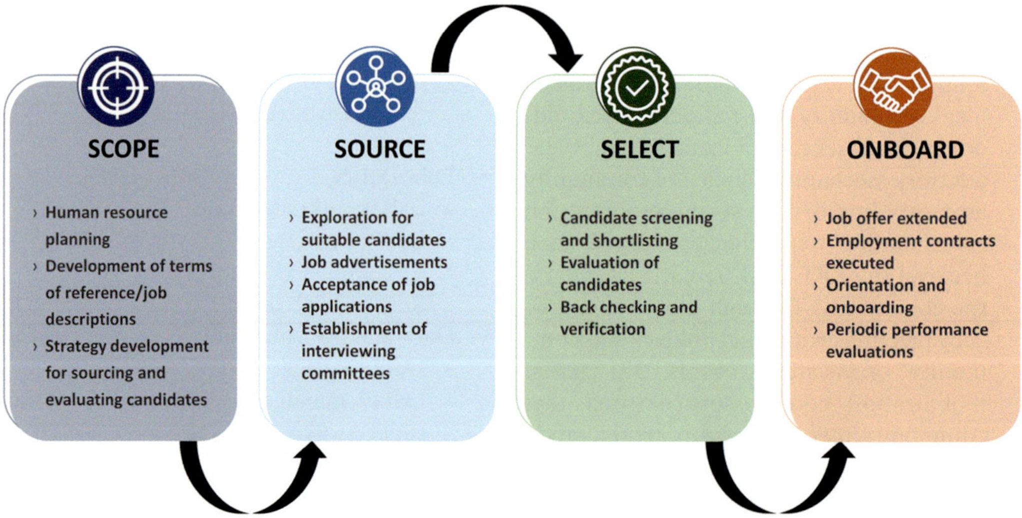

◘ **Fig. 1** Hiring process: planning, employee sourcing, recruiting, hiring, and onboarding. (Beth Baseler, author)

within the contract for participation in the interview and selection process is an important consideration.

3.4 Human Resources Contracting

Staffing in Liberia was handled by a subcontractor, hired by a prime contractor to the U.S. government to assist with local staff hiring and payroll management. This worked well because the subcontractor had both a U.S. and host country presence and was familiar with both federal acquisition regulations and host country labor laws.

In the DRC, there was an initial 2-month period during which the team relied on an existing subcontract for IT, logistics, operations, and clinical support. During that period, a higher-tier subcontract was executed for similar support, after which the original contractor's staff shifted to Ebola treatment unit support in the field rather than central support in Kinshasa. The new subcontractor performed a staffing needs assessment and implemented a strategy that included operational management as well as a plan for recruiting and hiring dedicated on-the-ground clinical research site, laboratory, pharmacy, and other protocol-associated staff.

3.4.1 Using an Established Legal Entity for Employment of Local Staff

In many low-income nations, the bulk of economic activity takes place in a "gray," unregistered zone, but it is prudent—and usually a legal requirement—for foreign partners to have an authorized way of operating. In Liberia, Most businesses are not formal legal entities but working with an established entity licensed to do business, such as a clinical-research organization (CRO), non-governmental organization (NGO), temporary manpower agency, or academic institution facilitates compliance with the local rules. In this arrangement, the licensed business in the host country is the employer of record; is licensed, registered, and insured to employ and pay staff; and administers all local employment procedures, including contracts, payroll, tax withholdings, and other requirements. Direct employment of local staff requires a thorough understanding of business, regulatory, and legal requirements, and most often it makes sense to delegate it to an entity registered and permitted to conduct business in the country where the study is implemented. The benefits of engaging a local subcontractor include the following:

- Quick and effective deployment/engagement of staff
- Established salary scales
- Legal responsibility for complying with all U.S. and host country local laws and relevant national regulations as well as donor/sponsor policies
- Historical knowledge and relationships that facilitate rapid implementation of requirements
- Existing knowledge of cultural sensitivities, business operations, and logistics
- Established trust and good will
- Existing partnerships with stakeholders and institutions
- Established communication channels

It may take 3–6 weeks to contract with an entity licensed to do business within the host country. It is helpful to identify reputable organizations that conduct business in areas with high potential for infectious disease outbreaks. Ascertaining options for contract and acquisitions processes for specific combinations of funding, operating, and local partners and awarding contracts beforehand insofar as possible can accelerate response once an emergency starts. Firms with "peacetime" experience in a particular operating environment will cope much better in an emergency than newcomers.

3.4.2 Contracts

Developing and executing staff contracts during an infectious disease outbreak must be flexible, time sensitive, and fair. Without appropriate preparation and due attention, contracting can seriously delay clinical trials. Templates for terms of reference, job specifications, contracts, checklists, onboarding tools, etc. should be developed beforehand (Lang 2015; Lang and Siribaddana 2012).

Developing and sharing these tools and templates is a vital preparedness measure. Time spent explaining contracts and adjusting to local needs is not time wasted, though: "The basis for a good collaboration should be trust and openness. A well-negotiated contract will ensure that all partners achieve a fair share of both the benefits and the costs. It is worth spending time on, and will help to ensure minimization of problems in project execution further on" (Edwards et al. 2014).

With donor-funded activities, the operations leaders in the partnership must also have or obtain a thorough understanding of donor regulations and comply with both local and donor-country laws and regulations. For projects funded by the U.S. government, directly or indirectly, there are detailed rules on cost principles, administration, and audit standards. Other countries, NGOs, foundations, and academia have similar guidance for internationally funded clinical research projects.

An alternative to contracting with an authorized legal entity in the host country is to employ a staffing agency to directly employ personnel and manage human resource functions. Hiring firms, such as CROs, labor brokers, or staffing agencies, can be helpful in identifying and hiring local staff. A drawback to utilizing a staffing agency is the cost (an agency's fee can be upward of 50% of the employee's annual salary). Due diligence is required prior to using staffing agencies as there are many different methods of negotiating and charging fees. How much and on what basis an employment agency may charge can depend on a variety of factors, such as the difficulty of the placement, the industry, the position, and market conditions. The need for early planning once again is paramount.

If the partnership is expected to continue over a longer term, a potential option is to establish a legal business entity in the host country. However, this may take too long to meet immediate needs during a rapid response and may require substantial initial outlays.

4 Clinical Trial Training During Emergency Response

The time is urgent, the stakes are high, and the atmosphere is tense, but fundamental decisions on resources and the way ahead to implement a safe, high-quality clinical trial remain. After the research team has identified the study staff, it is imperative that they ensure the protocol is carried out punctiliously, that participants are safe, and that data are of high quality and acceptable to data safety and monitoring reviewers and regulators.

Clinical protocol training (Fig. 2) is vital (Lescano et al. 2019; Sam-Agudu et al. 2016). There are multiple levels and methodologies of training. Before assigning staff members to training, it is essential to assess

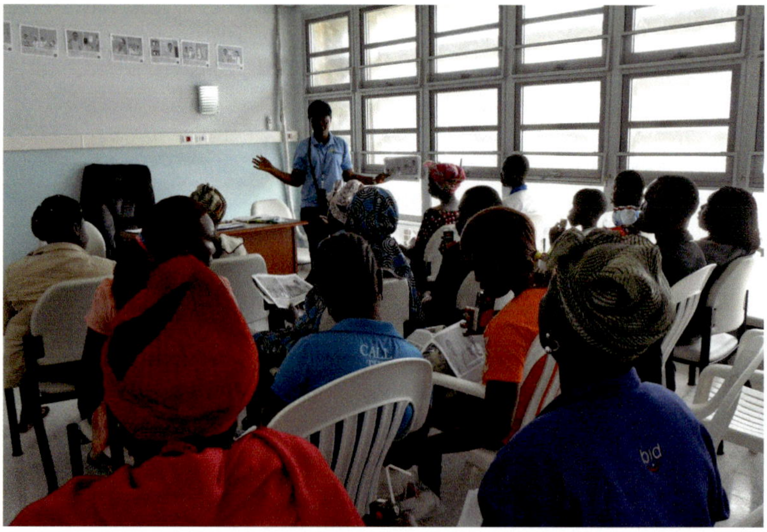

Fig. 2 Classroom training for the PREVAIL study in Liberia. (Photo: Beth Baseler)

them, including their clinical background, experience, skills, and motivation. The time available to make these observations is limited, so one starts by specifying training goals and tailoring the training to the individuals involved, setting up a feedback loop to learn what works best for individuals with varying levels of education and experience. Training takes the cultural background and the individual learner into account; flexibility and mutual exchange allow for growth and change and help build productive, respectful interactions. As the trainee learns about clinical research, the trainer learns about the physical and cultural environment in which the clinical trials will take place. Training practices should thus align with the ethical principle of respect for persons, and the GPP principle of mutual understanding, where partners, respectively, build competencies in sociocultural issues and research processes (UNAIDS/AVAC 2011).

4.1 Timing

It is important not to conduct training too far in advance of when it will be applied, or the recipient will not be able to properly connect what is learned in the classroom to what happens in practice. Working backward from an anticipated, realistic start date is a good way to determine the training date, generally to begin no more than 2 weeks before the start of the study. This timeframe is reasonable for retaining material (memory) and allows for reading of pertinent material and practice of procedures before the study is to begin. Another important planning point is to ensure that study staff who will attend training have completed the appropriate contract and onboarding steps before training if possible. If staff agree to attend the training but have not formally been hired, it may be difficult or impossible to pay them for their time retroactively.

4.2 Fundamentals

All study staff need to understand the fundamental rationale of a study during an emergency—the requirement for expeditious

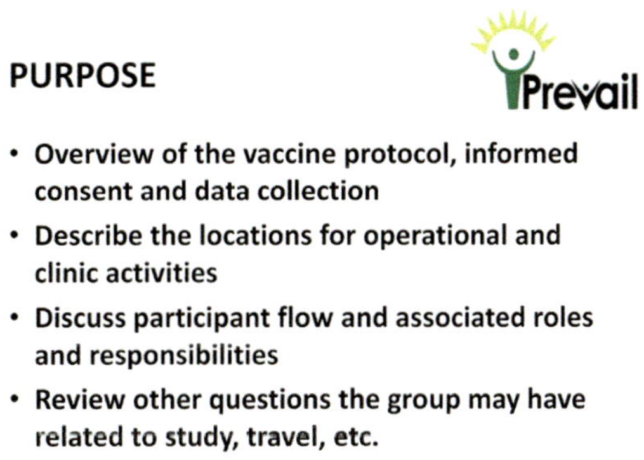

Fig. 3 Introductory training slide. (Courtesy PREVAIL)

implementation, the importance of participant and staff safety, and the indispensability of high-quality data. The urgency of an outbreak requires concentrated and immediate didactic training, yet training is an ongoing, interactive process, with multiple clinical research SMEs assisting the study staff through the duration of the program. It is also important for trainers to be flexible in adapting training to different environments. The opening slide for a PREVAIL training (Fig. 3) is captured below.

4.3 Training Methods

The level and type of training needed was different for various staff positions and research settings, yet all the training relied to a great extent on four basic concepts of medical training:

1. *Didactic teaching* using traditional lecture methods to provide information to students.
2. *Buddy system*, in which two students work together to advance their understanding under the guidance of a trainer.
3. *Train-the-trainer*: training focused not only on subject matter but teaching the trainee to train others.
4. *Simulation*, interactive exercise, and eventually carrying out actual tasks under guidance.

Didactic learning methods (Fig. 4) build on students' existing baseline knowledge while

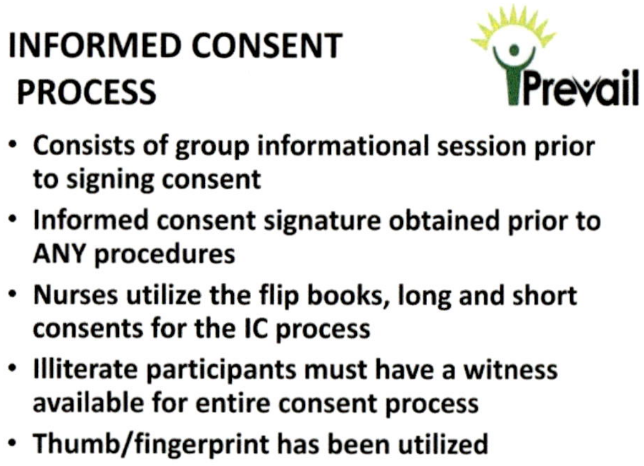

Fig. 4 Informed consent training slide. (Courtesy PREVAIL)

conveying new information. Baseline knowledge is the starting point in a lesson plan, where a student needs to attain a certain minimal level of knowledge before engaging in more interactive forms of learning. A teacher or educator functions in this role as an authoritative figure but also as a guide and resource for students (Austin 2013).

Didactic training will not serve its purpose without more robust dialectical training. Didactic training should lead to interactive training, allowing for dialog. With open dialog, it can be more difficult to maintain a schedule, but it develops trust and mutual understanding. In diverse research settings, advice and feedback from locally based SMEs and program leadership are essential.

4.4 Training Topics

> Identify knowledge gaps in key areas and address them.

In cases where collaborating partners have little or no experience with the terminology and regulatory requirements of clinical research, the following topics are essential training topics:

1. Overview of the study
2. Purpose of conducting this study in this setting
3. Study design
4. Primary study objective
5. Enrollment criteria
6. Sample size
7. International Conference on Harmonisation (ICH), good clinical practice guidelines
8. Informed consent process
9. Laboratory procedures, including clinical and research procedures, good laboratory practice guidelines
10. Data management methods
11. Adverse/serious adverse event reporting
12. Quality assurance/quality control procedures
13. Study monitoring—safety and site monitoring

4.5 Dry Runs or Simulations

After leaving the classroom, it is hardly reasonable to go straight to implementing the protocol, enrolling study participants, and collecting data. The next training phase, an interactive exercise conducted according to how the study was to be performed at each site, came to be termed "dry runs" in Liberia and "simulations" in the DRC (Fig. 5).

Simulations are designed so each staff member becomes well-versed in the duties of a particular study station with a certain study procedure, allowing inexperienced staff to become proficient in one task to start with, thus decreasing the risk of jeopardizing the safety of the participant or the quality of the data collected at that point in the process. They serve as study procedure practice; iden-

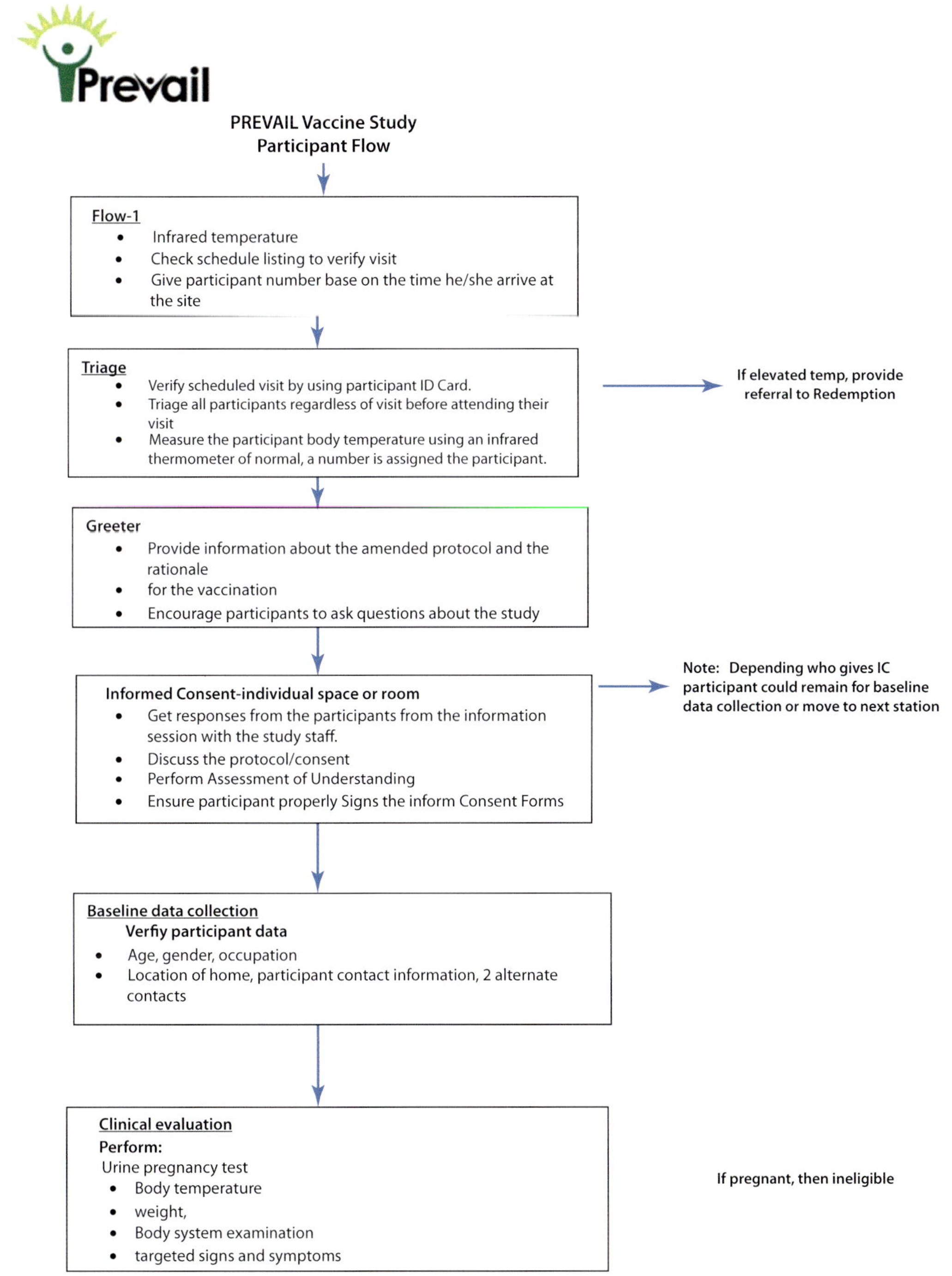

Fig. 5 Flowchart for a practice run. (Courtesy PREVAIL)

tify unclear protocol areas, inefficiencies, or missteps in the procedures; provide a realistic estimate of the time it would take a participant to go through a study; and inculcate attention to detail in quality control/quality assurance (QA/QC) of the data collected. The time that staff members spent in-country was dependent on the available resources and the study needs. Some people stayed more than 3 weeks, depending on their roles.

4.6 Train-the-Trainer

The train-the-trainer model is widespread in both development assistance and medical response (Atindehou et al. 2019; Tobin et al. 2020). In PREVAIL, this method was used when both the Liberian and U.S. staff agreed it was time for training to progress to a new level, with more in-country trainers rather than foreign staff. This was not an abrupt or complete transition but one that occurred as development of local skills allowed.

In the DRC, by contrast, the train-the-trainer model was needed at program outset in October 2018 because of U.S. government restrictions on employees traveling to the outbreak area where the research protocol was being implemented, since it was designated a conflict zone (▶ In Practice 17.1 and 23.1). The northeastern region's longstanding disaffection from the DRC government in the capital city of Kinshasa was evident not only in popular mistrust but in the presence of armed rebel groups. It had been exacerbated by the EVD outbreak, rumors EVD was imported as a moneymaking scheme, and then postponement of national elections in the northeast region (Kraemer et al. 2020; Nguyen 2019). Initial train-the-trainer sessions had to be conducted in Kinshasa. The primary participants in the training were staff from the leading DRC collaborating organization: members of the *Institut National de Recherche Biomédicale* (INRB), the national medical research institute of the DRC. The in-country trainers were provided comprehensive information in the form of PowerPoint presentations and standard operating procedures.

The train-the-trainer model in these settings is practical and effective. The key trainers in this case were the staff administering the medications, pharmacy, laboratory and data management personnel, and social mobilization and community engagement (SMC) staff and psychosocial counselors. The training sessions were documented in the form of standard sign-in sheets and logs, to provide evidence of compliance with training requirements for regulators. The training team also became proficient in responding to questions they could not answer immediately by obtaining responses from SMEs and relaying them to the study team members. This allowed for recordings of important supplementary information for future use.

As mobile telephony and Internet service become readily available, virtual meetings are becoming an option in even very remote locations, and videoconferencing has taken a key role in research development, implementation, training, and closeouts.

5 Conclusions

Skillful human resource management, though not a prominent topic in the clinical research literature, was critical to the successful clinical research response to the public health emergencies created by the Ebola outbreaks in West Africa and the DRC. The human resource management challenges faced by the NIAID Division of Clinical Research in emergency clinical research response were not always easy to resolve, but they became opportunities to devise and implement solutions that worked in those settings. It is very likely that emergency research responders will face similar challenges, even in quite distinct situations. The authors hope that lessons learned from the Ebola experience can help establish an adaptable framework for future emergency response. A number of general precepts are globally applicable and especially worth remembering: (1) be committed and fair to all partners, (2) listen to input from all partners and staff members, (3) maintain openness to new approaches, (4) move quickly to implement solutions, and (5) quickly reject or adapt approaches that do not work.

? Discussion Questions

1. Initiating and implementing a robust human resource management plan is vital to identifying, recruiting, retaining, training, and motivating staff members for an effective and productive workforce aligned with the strategic priorities of a program.
   (a) List and discuss minimum requirements for a human resource management plan.

   (b) Discuss the importance of team communication, collaboration, partnership, and mutual respect when hiring and managing staff.
2. Please review ▶ Sect. 3.2, which emphasizes that personnel who have specific training and competencies are needed to achieve a high standard of design, management, and operational execution of a clinical study in diverse and challenging conditions.
   (a) Discuss the roles of several staff positions for PREVAIL's Ebola vaccine study, emphasizing the adaptive approach used to conduct research in a clinical research-naïve setting with shortcomings in basic staffing infrastructure.
   (b) Discuss the value of the communications and social mobilization team across the spectrum of a research study, including the research team, members of the media, and community members and potential study participants.
   (c) Given that naming conventions for staff positions with the same roles and responsibilities are not always uniform, discuss how you would come to agreement on staff titles.
3. Discuss staff recruitment, interview, and selection when vying for a limited pool of skilled personnel during an emergency outbreak situation. What are some benefits of engaging a local subcontractor?
4. Discuss the fundamental principles or major factors (e.g., adaptability, flexibility, creativity) to consider when conducting clinical trials in response to emerging infectious disease outbreaks, particularly in challenging and resource-limited settings.
5. To ensure that the protocol is carried out punctiliously, participants are safe, and data are of high quality and acceptable to data safety and monitoring reviewers and regulators, clinical protocol training is vital for study staff.
   (a) Discuss some fundamental aspects and methods of this training during an emergency response.
   (b) When collaborating partners have little or no experience with the terminology and regulatory requirements of clinical research, what training topics are essential?
   (c) Describe how a practice run may proceed so that each staff member becomes well-versed in the duties of a particular study station.
   (d) How can you continue training staff if the U.S. government places restrictions on employees traveling to an outbreak area where the research protocol is being implemented in a conflict zone?

References

Atindehou M, Adéoti K, Estelle L, Loko Y, Beulé T, Paradis E, et al. MooSciTIC: training of trainers in West African research and higher education. PLoS Biol. 2019;17(6) https://doi.org/10.1371/journal.pbio.3000312.

Austin S. Didactic approaches. In: Volkmar FR, editor. Encyclopedia of autism spectrum disorders. New York: Springer; 2013. p. 947–8.

Challoner KR, Forget N. Effect of civil war on medical education in Liberia. Int J Emerg Med. 2011;4(1):6. https://doi.org/10.1186/1865-1380-4-6.

Doe-Anderson J, Baseler B, Driscoll P, Johnson M, Lysander J, McNay L, et al. Beating the odds: successful establishment of a phase II/III clinical research trial in resource-poor Liberia during the largest-ever Ebola outbreak. Contemp Clin Trials Commun. 2016;4:68–73. https://doi.org/10.1016/j.conctc.2016.06.008.

Edwards D, Toohey J, IJsselmuiden C. Negotiating research contracts: creating opportunities for stronger research and innovation systems. Geneva: Council on Health Research for Development; 2014.

EMA. Good clinical practice: ICH harmonised guideline. Integrated addendum to ICH E6(R1): guideline for good clinical practice ICH E6(R2) ICH consensus guideline. European Medicines Agency; 2016.

Evans D, Goldstein MP, Popova A. The next wave of deaths from Ebola? The impact of health care worker mortality. Washington, DC: World Bank Group; 2015. Contract No.: WPS 7344.

FDA. E2A clinical safety data management: definitions and standards for expedited reporting. In: Services USDoHaH, Administration FaD, (CDER) CfDEaR, (CBER) CfBEaR, editors. Washington, DC: U.S. Department of Health and Human Services; 1995. p. 60.

FDA. FDA approves first treatment for Ebola virus. Washington, DC: U.S. Food and Drug Administration; 2020a.

FDA. FDA approves treatment for Ebola virus. Washington, DC: U.S. Food and Drug Administration; 2020b.

Gobat NH, Gal M, Butler CC, Webb SAR, Francis NA, Stanton H, et al. Talking to the people that really matter about their participation in pandemic clinical research: a qualitative study in four European countries. Health Expect. 2018;21(1):387–95. https://doi.org/10.1111/hex.12634.

ICH. ICH harmonised guideline: integrated addendum to ICH E6(R1): guideline for good clinical practice E6(R2). Geneva: International Council for Harmonisation of Technical Requirements for Pharmaceuticals for Human Use (ICH); 2016.

Kennedy SB, Neaton JD, Lane HC, Kieh MWS, Massaquoi MBF, Touchette NA, et al. Implementation of an Ebola virus disease vaccine clinical trial during the Ebola epidemic in Liberia: design, procedures, and challenges. Clin Trials (London, England). 2016;13(1):49–56. https://doi.org/10.1177/1740774515621037.

Koita OA, Murphy RL, Fongoro S, Diallo B, Doumbia SO, Traore M, et al. Clinical research and the training of host country investigators: essential health priorities for disease-endemic regions. Am J Trop Med Hyg. 2016;94(2):253–7. https://doi.org/10.4269/ajtmh.15-0366.

Kraemer MUG, Pigott DM, Hill SC, Vanderslott S, Reiner RC Jr, Stasse S, et al. Dynamics of conflict during the Ebola outbreak in the Democratic Republic of the Congo 2018–2019. BMC Med. 2020;18(1):113. https://doi.org/10.1186/s12916-020-01574-1.

Lane HC, Marston HD, Fauci AS. Conducting clinical trials in outbreak settings: points to consider. Clin Trials (London, England). 2016;13(1):92–5. https://doi.org/10.1177/1740774515618198.

Lang T. Ebola: embed research in outbreak response. Nature. 2015;524(7563):29–31. https://doi.org/10.1038/524029a.

Lang T, Siribaddana S. Clinical trials have gone global: is this a good thing? PLoS Med. 2012;9(6):e1001228. https://doi.org/10.1371/journal.pmed.1001228.

Larson GS, Baseler BR, Hoover ML, Pierson JF, Tegli JK, Johnson MP, et al. Conventional wisdom versus actual outcomes: challenges in the conduct of an Ebola vaccine trial in Liberia during the international public health emergency. Am J Trop Med Hyg. 2017;97(1):10–5. https://doi.org/10.4269/ajtmh.16-1015.

Lescano AG, Cohen CR, Raj T, Rispel L, Garcia PJ, Zunt JR, et al. Strengthening mentoring in low- and middle-income countries to advance global health research: an overview. Am J Trop Med Hyg. 2019;100(1_Suppl):3–8. Published online 14 Nov 2018. https://doi.org/10.4269/ajtmh.18-0556.

MacQueen KM, Bhan A, Frohlich J, Holzer J, Sugarman J, Ethics Working Group of the HIVPTN. Evaluating community engagement in global health research: the need for metrics. BMC Med Ethics. 2015;16:44. https://doi.org/10.1186/s12910-015-0033-9.

Mulangu S, Dodd LE, Davey RT Jr, Tshiani Mbaya O, Proschan M, Mukadi D, et al. A randomized, controlled trial of Ebola virus disease therapeutics. N Engl J Med. 2019;381(24):2293–303. https://doi.org/10.1056/NEJMoa1910993.

NASEM. Integrating clinical research into epidemic response: the Ebola experience. Washington, DC: National Academies of Sciences Engineering and Medicine Publications, The National Academies Press; 2017.

Nguyen V-K. An epidemic of suspicion—Ebola and violence in the DRC. N Engl J Med. 2019; https://doi.org/10.1056/NEJMp1902682.

NIH. The role of DMID medical monitors in safety oversight. In: Service USHaH, Health NIo, Diseaes NIoAaI, Diseases DoMaI, editors. Bethesda, MD: NIH; 2014. p. 3.

OECD. DAC list of ODA recipients. In: Financing for sustainable development. Paris: Organisation for Economic Co-operation and Development; 2021. https://www.oecd.org/dac/financing-sustainable-development/development-finance-standards/daclist.htm. Accessed 23 Sep 2021.

Sam-Agudu NA, Paintsil E, Aliyu MH, Kwara A, Ogunsola F, Afrane YA, et al. Building sustainable local capacity for global health research in West Africa. Ann Glob Health. 2016;82(6):1010–25. https://doi.org/10.1016/j.aogh.2016.10.011.

Thielman NM, Cunningham CK, Woods C, Petzold E, Sprenz M, Russell J. Ebola clinical trials: five lessons learned and a way forward. Clin Trials (London, England). 2016;13(1):83–6. https://doi.org/10.1177/1740774515619897.

Tobin CD, Alfred M, Wilson DA, MenkinSmith L, Lehman-Huskamp KL, Schaefer JJ, et al. Train-the-trainer: pilot trial for Ebola virus disease simulation training. Educ Health (Abingdon). 2020;33(2):37–45. https://doi.org/10.4103/efh.EfH_262_19.

UNAIDS/AVAC. Good participatory practice: guidelines for biomedical HIV prevention trials. Geneva: UNAIDS (Joint United Nations Programme on HIV/AIDS); 2011.

WHO. Good participatory practice guidelines for trials of emerging (and re-emerging) pathogens that are likely to cause severe outbreaks in the near future and for which few or no medical countermeasures exist (GPP-EP). Geneva: World Health Organization; 2016. p. 53.

WHO. Community engagement framework for quality, people-centred and resilient health services. Geneva: WHO; 2017.

WHO. 10th Ebola outbreak in the Democratic Republic of the Congo declared over; vigilance against flare-ups and support for survivors must continue. Geneva: World Health Organization; 2020a.

WHO. Global Health Observatory data repository: medical doctors. Geneva: World Health Organization; 2020b. https://apps.who.int/gho/data/node.main.HWFGRP_0020?lang=en. Accessed 30 Jan 2021.

Supplementary Information

E. S. Higgs and R. A. Sorenson (eds.), *Principles and Practice of Emergency Research Response*,
https://doi.org/10.1007/978-3-031-48408-7

Index

D

E

L

M

N

O

P

Y

Z